THE WASHINGTON MANUAL™
OF SURGERY
Fifth Edition

THE WASHINGTON MANUAL™ OF SURGERY

Fifth Edition

Department of Surgery
Washington University
School of Medicine
St. Louis, Missouri

Mary E. Klingensmith, MD
Li Ern Chen, MD
Sean C. Glasgow, MD
Trudie A. Goers, MD
Spencer J. Melby, MD

Foreword by
Timothy J. Eberlein, MD
Bixby Professor and
Chair of Surgery
Director, Siteman Cancer Center
Washington University
School of Medicine
St. Louis, Missouri

Wolters Kluwer | Lippincott Williams & Wilkins
Health

Philadelphia · Baltimore · New York · London
Buenos Aires · Hong Kong · Sydney · Tokyo

Acquisitions Editor: Brian Brown
Managing Editor: Julia Seto
Project Manager: Nicole Walz
Manufacturing Coordinator: Kathleen Brown
Marketing Manager: Lisa Parry
Design Coordinator: Terry Mallon
Cover Designer: Becky Baxendell
Compositor: Aptara, Inc.

Library of Congress Cataloging-in-Publication Data

The Washington manual of surgery / Department of Surgery, Washington University School of Medicine, St. Louis, Missouri; Mary E. Klingensmith . . . [et al.]; foreword by Timothy J. Eberlein. – 5th ed.
    p. ; cm.
Includes bibliographical references and index.
ISBN-13: 978-0-7817-7447-5 (alk. paper)
ISBN-10: 0-7817-7447-0 (alk. paper)
    1. Surgery, Operative–Handbooks, manuals, etc.   I. Klingensmith, Mary E.
II. Washington University (Saint Louis, Mo.). Dept. of Surgery.
III. Title: Manual of surgery.
    [DNLM: 1. Surgical Procedures, Operative–methods. WO 500 W317 2008]
    RD37.W37 2008
    617′.91–dc22
                                                              2007042869

The Washington Manual™ is an intent-to-use mark belonging to Washington University in St. Louis to which international legal protection applies. The mark is used in this publication by LWW under license from Washington University.

Care has been taken to confirm the accuracy of the information presented and to describe generally accepted practices. However, the authors, editors, and publisher are not responsible for errors or omissions or for any consequences from application of the information in this book and make no warranty, expressed or implied, with respect to the currency, completeness, or accuracy of the contents of the publication. Application of the information in a particular situation remains the professional responsibility of the practitioner.

The authors, editors, and publisher have exerted every effort to ensure that drug selection and dosage set forth in this text are in accordance with current recommendations and practice at the time of publication. However, in view of ongoing research, changes in government regulations, and the constant flow of information relating to drug therapy and drug reactions, the reader is urged to check the package insert for each drug for any change in indications and dosage and for added warnings and precautions. This is particularly important when the recommended agent is a new or infrequently employed drug.

Some drugs and medical devices presented in the publication have Food and Drug Administration (FDA) clearance for limited use in restricted research settings. It is the responsibility of the health care provider to ascertain the FDA status of each drug or device planned for use in their clinical practice.

To purchase additional copies of this book, call our customer service department at (800) 638-3030 or fax orders to (301) 223-2320. International customers should call (301) 223-2300.

Visit Lippincott Williams & Wilkins on the Internet: at LWW.com. Lippincott Williams & Wilkins customer service representatives are available from 8:30 am to 6 pm, EST.

2 3 4 5 6 7 8 9 10

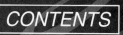

CONTENTS

*W*elcome to the fifth edition of *The Washington Manual* ™ *of Surgery.* The most important focus of our Department of Surgery is medical education of students, residents, fellows, and practicing surgeons. This commitment is no more evident than in the current edition of *The Washington Manual* ™ *of Surgery.*

The educational focus of our Department of Surgery has a rich tradition. The first full-time Head of the Department of Surgery at Washington University was Dr. Evarts A. Graham (1919–1951). Dr. Graham was a superb educator. Not only was he an outstanding technical surgeon, but his insightful comments at conferences and ward rounds were well known and appreciated by a generation of surgeons who learned at his elbow. Dr. Graham was a founding member of the American Board of Surgery and made many seminal contributions to the management of surgical patients. His work in the development of oral cholecystography actually helped establish the Mallinckrodt Institute of Radiology at Washington University. Dr. Graham was among the first to identify the epidemiological link of cigarette smoking to lung cancer and was instrumental in raising public health consciousness about the deleterious effect on health from cigarette smoke.

Dr. Carl Moyer (1951–1965) succeeded Dr. Graham. Dr. Moyer is still regarded as a legendary educator at Washington University. He was particularly known for his bedside teaching techniques as well as for linking pathophysiology to patient care outcomes. Dr. Walter Ballinger (1967–1978) came from Johns Hopkins University and incorporated the Halsted traditions of resident education. Dr. Ballinger introduced the importance of laboratory investigation and began to foster development of the surgeon/scientist in our department. Dr. Samuel A. Wells (1978–1997) is credited with establishing one of the most accomplished academic Departments of Surgery in the United States. Not only did he recruit world-class faculty, but he increased the focus on research and patient care. Dr. Wells also placed a great emphasis on educating the future academic leaders of surgery.

As in previous editions, this fifth edition of *The Washington Manual* ™ *of Surgery* combines authorship of residents ably assisted by faculty coauthors and our senior editor, Dr. Mary Klingensmith. This combination of resident and faculty participation has helped to focus the chapters on issues that will be particularly helpful to the trainee in surgery. This new edition of the manual provides a complete list of references that will serve medical students, residents, and practicing surgeons who wish to delve more deeply into a particular topic. This manual does not attempt to extensively cover pathophysiology or history, but it presents brief and logical approaches to the management of patients with comprehensive surgical problems. In each of the chapters, the authors have attempted to provide the most up-to-date and important diagnostic and management information for a given topic. We have attempted to standardize each of the chapters so that the reader will be able to most easily obtain information regardless of subject matter.

The fifth edition has undergone a major reorganization of chapters with an emphasis on clarity and consistency. There are several new sections and there has been expansion of other sections. Most importantly, there has been incorporation of a significant amount of evidence-based medicine into each of the chapters. This is so readers can better understand the reasoning behind all of the information presented. Finally, all of the sections have been updated and rewritten to reflect the most current standards of practice in each topic. These updates have been carefully edited and integrated so that the volume of pages remains approximately the same. The goal is to keep this volume concise, portable, and the most user-friendly edition that we have published.

I am truly indebted to Dr. Klingensmith for her passion for education and her specific devotion to this project. Additionally, I am proud of the residents in the Department of Surgery at Washington University who have done such an outstanding job with their faculty members in this fifth edition. I hope that you will find *The Washington Manual*™ *of Surgery* a reference you commonly utilize in the care of your patient with surgical disease.

Timothy J. Eberlein, MD
St. Louis, Missouri

*A*s with the previous four editions, this fifth edition of *The Washington Manual* ™ *of Surgery* is designed to complement *The Washington Manual* ™ *of Medical Therapeutics.* Written by resident and faculty members of the Department of Surgery, it presents a brief, rational approach to the management of patients with surgical problems. The text is directed to the reader at the level of the second- or third-year surgical resident, although surgical and nonsurgical attendings, medical students, physician assistants, and others who provide care for patients with surgical problems will find it of interest and assistance. The book provides a succinct discussion of surgical diseases, with algorithms for addressing problems based on the opinions of the physician authors. Although multiple approaches may be reasonable for some clinical situations, this manual attempts to present a single, effective approach for each. We have limited coverage of diagnosis and therapy; this is not an exhaustive surgical reference. Coverage of pathophysiology, the history of surgery, and extensive reference lists have been excluded from most areas. This is the fifth edition of the manual; the first edition was published in 1996, followed by editions in 1999, 2002, and 2005. New to this volume is the incorporation of evidence-based medicine into each chapter. As with previous editions, this fifth edition includes updates on each topic as well as substantial new material.

This is a resident-prepared manual. Each chapter was updated and revised by a resident with assistance from a faculty coauthor. Editorial oversight for the manual was shared by four senior resident coeditors (Li Ern Chen, MD, Chapters 1–7, 12, and 16; Sean C. Glasgow, MD, Chapters 8–11, 13–15, and 17–19; Trudie A. Goers, MD, Chapters 20–27 and 30; and Spencer J. Melby, MD, Chapters 28–29 and 31–37). The tremendous effort of all involved—residents and faculty members and particularly the senior resident coeditors—is reflected in the quality and consistency of the chapters.

I am indebted to the former senior editor of this work, Gerard M. Doherty, MD, who developed and oversaw the first three editions, then handed over to me an exceptionally well-organized project. I am grateful for the continued tremendous support from Lippincott Williams & Wilkins, who have been supportive of the effort and have supplied dedicated assistance. Brian Brown has been tremendously helpful, and Julia Seto has been a terrific developmental editor, keeping me in line and on schedule.

Finally, I am grateful to have an outstanding mentor and friend in my department chair, Timothy J. Eberlein, MD. Dr. Eberlein has a very full professional life, overseeing both a productive department and cancer center. Despite this, he continues to appreciate the individuals with whom he interacts. He is an inspiration for his friendship, leadership, and dedication.

M.E.K.

Rebecca L. Aft, MD, PhD
Associate Professor of Surgery
Washington University School of Medicine
St. Louis, Missouri

Richard J. Battafarano, MD, PhD
Associate Professor of Surgery
University of Maryland School of Medicine
Baltimore, Maryland

Daniel C. Brennan, MD
Professor of Medicine
Washington University School of Medicine
St. Louis, Missouri

Rebecca A. Brooks, MD
Resident in Obstetrics and Gynecology
Washington University School of Medicine
St. Louis, Missouri

L. Michael Brunt, MD
Professor of Surgery
Washington University School of Medicine
St. Louis, Missouri

Timothy G. Buchman, PhD, MD
Professor of Surgery
Washington University School of Medicine
St. Louis, Missouri

Arnold D. Bullock, MD
Associate Professor of Urologic Surgery
Washington University School of Medicine
St. Louis, Missouri

Christopher Chambers, MD, PhD
Resident in Surgery
Washington University School of Medicine
St. Louis, Missouri

William C. Chapman, MD
Professor of Surgery
Washington University School of Medicine
St. Louis, Missouri

Li Ern Chen, MD
Resident in Surgery
Washington University School of Medicine
St. Louis, Missouri

Michael R. Chicoine, MD
Associate Professor of Neurosurgery
Washington University School of Medicine
St. Louis, Missouri

Tyler L. Christensen, MD
Resident in Urologic Surgery
Washington University School of Medicine
St. Louis, Missouri

J. Perren Cobb, MD
Professor of Surgery and Genetics
Washington University School of Medicine
St. Louis, Missouri

Craig M. Coopersmith, MD
Associate Professor of Surgery
Washington University School of Medicine
St. Louis, Missouri

Ralph J. Damiano, Jr., MD
Professor of Surgery
Washington University School of Medicine
St. Louis, Missouri

Sekhar Dharmarajan, MD
Resident in Surgery
Washington University School of Medicine
St. Louis, Missouri

David W. Dietz, MD
Assistant Professor of Surgery
Washington University School of Medicine
St. Louis, Missouri

xiii

Patrick A. Dillon, MD
Assistant Professor of Surgery and
  Pediatrics
Washington University School of Medicine
St. Louis, Missouri

J. Chris Eagon, MD
Assistant Professor of Surgery
Washington University School of Medicine
St. Louis, Missouri

Felix G. Fernandez, MD
Resident in Surgery
Washington University School of Medicine
St. Louis, Missouri

Elizabeth A. Fialkowski, MD
Resident in Surgery
Washington University School of Medicine
St. Louis, Missouri

Ryan C. Fields, MD
Resident in Surgery
Washington University School of Medicine
St. Louis, Missouri

Steven E. Finkelstein, MD
Resident in Surgery
Washington University School of Medicine
St. Louis, Missouri

James W. Fleshman, MD
Professor of Surgery
Washington University School of Medicine
St. Louis, Missouri

Amy Fox, MD
Resident in Surgery
Washington University School of Medicine
St. Louis, Missouri

Bradley D. Freeman, MD
Associate Professor of Surgery
Washington University School of Medicine
St. Louis, Missouri

Patrick J. Geraghty, MD
Assistant Professor of Surgery
Washington University School of Medicine
St. Louis, Missouri

Sean C. Glasgow, MD
Resident in Surgery
Washington University School of Medicine
St. Louis, Missouri

Jennifer L. Gnerlich, MD
Resident in Surgery
Washington University School of Medicine
St. Louis, Missouri

Trudie A. Goers, MD
Resident in Surgery
Washington University School of Medicine
St. Louis, Missouri

Bruce L. Hall, MD, PhD
Associate Professor of Surgery
Washington University School of Medicine
St. Louis, Missouri

Valerie J. Halpin, MD
Assistant Professor of Surgery
Washington University School of Medicine
St. Louis, Missouri

Bruce H. Haughey, MD
Professor of Otolaryngology
Washington University School of Medicine
St. Louis, Missouri

William G. Hawkins, MD
Assistant Professor of Surgery
Washington University School of Medicine
St. Louis, Missouri

Richard S. Hotchkiss, MD, PhD
Professor of Anesthesiology
Washington University School of Medicine
St. Louis, Missouri

Kareem D. Husain, MD
Resident in Surgery
Washington University School of Medicine
St. Louis, Missouri

James Johnston, MD
Resident in Neurosurgery
Washington University School of Medicine
St. Louis, Missouri

John P. Kirby, MD
Assistant Professor of Surgery
Washington University School of Medicine
St. Louis, Missouri

Mary E. Klingensmith, MD
Associate Professor of Surgery
Washington University School of Medicine
St. Louis, Missouri

Elbert Y. Kuo, MD
Resident in Surgery
Washington University School of Medicine
St. Louis, Missouri

David C. Linehan, MD
Associate Professor of Surgery
Washington University School of Medicine
St. Louis, Missouri

Jeffrey A. Lowell, MD
Professor of Surgery and Pediatrics
Washington University School of Medicine
St. Louis, Missouri

Susan E. Mackinnon, MD
Professor of Plastic and Reconstructive
 Surgery
Washington University School of Medicine
St. Louis, Missouri

Brent D. Matthews, MD
Associate Professor of Surgery
Washington University School of Medicine
St. Louis, Missouri

John E. Mazuski, MD
Associate Professor of Surgery
Washington University School of Medicine
St. Louis, Missouri

Kevin McConnell, MD
Resident in Surgery
Washington University School of Medicine
St. Louis, Missouri

Spencer J. Melby, MD
Resident in Surgery
Washington University School of Medicine
St. Louis, Missouri

Bryan F. Meyers, MD, MPH
Associate Professor of Surgery
Washington University School of Medicine
St. Louis, Missouri

Nader Moazami, MD
Assistant Professor of Surgery
Washington University School of Medicine
St. Louis, Missouri

Jeffrey F. Moley, MD
Professor of Surgery
Washington University School of Medicine
St. Louis, Missouri

Tricia A. Moo-Young, MD
Resident in Surgery
Washington University School of Medicine
St. Louis, Missouri

Robert G. Neumann, MD
Resident in Surgery
Washington University School of Medicine
St. Louis, Missouri

Jack R. Oak, MD
Resident in Surgery
Washington University School of Medicine
St. Louis, Missouri

Giao Q. Phan, MD
Resident in Surgery
Washington University School of Medicine
St. Louis, Missouri

Richard A. Pierce, MD, PhD
Resident in Surgery
Washington University School of Medicine
St. Louis, Missouri

Frank J. Quayle, MD
Resident in Surgery
Washington University School of Medicine
St. Louis, Missouri

Rishindra M. Reddy, MD
Resident in Surgery
Washington University School of Medicine
St. Louis, Missouri

Daniel Refai, MD
Resident in Neurosurgery
Washington University School of Medicine
St. Louis, Missouri

William M. Ricci, MD
Associate Professor of Orthopedics
Washington University School of Medicine
St. Louis, Missouri

Jason T. Rich, MD
Resident in Otolaryngology
Washington University School of Medicine
St. Louis, Missouri

Emily B. Rivet, MD
Resident in Surgery
Washington University School of Medicine
St. Louis, Missouri

Charles Robertson, MD
Resident in Surgery
Washington University School of Medicine
St. Louis, Missouri

T. Elizabeth Robertson, MD
Resident in Surgery
Washington University School of Medicine
St. Louis, Missouri

Jason Robison, MD
Resident in Orthopedic Surgery
Washington University School of Medicine
St. Louis, Missouri

Jason M. Rovak, MD
Resident in Plastic Surgery
Washington University School of Medicine
St. Louis, Missouri

Brian Rubin, MD
Professor of Surgery and Radiology
Washington University School of Medicine
St. Louis, Missouri

Luis A. Sanchez, MD
Professor of Surgery
Washington University School of Medicine
St. Louis, Missouri

Douglas J.E. Schuerer, MD
Assistant Professor of Surgery
Washington University School of Medicine
St. Louis, Missouri

Steven J. Schwulst, MD
Resident in Surgery
Washington University School of Medicine
St. Louis, Missouri

Gregorio A. Sicard, MD
Professor of Surgery
Washington University School of Medicine
St. Louis, Missouri

Peter O. Simon, Jr., MD
Resident in Surgery
Washington University School of Medicine
St. Louis, Missouri

Steven M. Strasberg, MD
Professor of Surgery
Washington University School of Medicine
St. Louis, Missouri

Marcus Tan, MD
Resident in Surgery
Washington University School of Medicine
St. Louis, Missouri

Marissa J. Tenenbaum, MD
Resident in Plastic Surgery
Washington University School of Medicine
St. Louis, Missouri

Premal H. Thaker, MD
Assistant Professor of Obstetrics and
Gynecology, Washington University School
of Medicine
St. Louis, Missouri

Thomas H. Tung, MD
Assistant Professor of Surgery
Washington University School of Medicine
St. Louis, Missouri

Aislinn Vaughan, MD
Instructor in Surgery
Washington University School of Medicine
St. Louis, Missouri

Rochus K. Voeller, MD
Resident in Surgery
Washington University School of Medicine
St. Louis, Missouri

Scott J. Ziporin, MD
Resident in Surgery
Washington University School of Medicine
St. Louis, Missouri

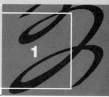

GENERAL AND PERIOPERATIVE CARE OF THE SURGICAL PATIENT
Elbert Y. Kuo and Mary E. Klingensmith

I. PREOPERATIVE EVALUATION AND MANAGEMENT

A. General evaluation of the surgical patient. The goals of preoperative evaluation are to (1) identify the patient's medical problems, (2) determine if further information is needed to characterize the patient's medical status, (3) establish if the patient is medically optimized, and (4) confirm the appropriateness of the planned procedure.

1. **History and physical examination.** A thorough history and physical are essential in evaluating surgical patients. Key elements of the history should include preexisting medical conditions known to increase operative risk, such as ischemic heart disease, congestive heart failure (CHF), renal insufficiency, prior cerebrovascular accident (CVA), and diabetes mellitus. Prior operations, operative complications, and the patient's use of tobacco, alcohol, and/or drugs should also be noted.

2. **Routine diagnostic testing.** Minor surgical procedures and procedures on young, healthy patients often require minimal or no diagnostic testing. Table 1-1 lists routine preoperative diagnostic tests and reasons for their use. Inclusion or exclusion of these tests should be selected on a case-by-case basis with consideration of the probability that results will alter management.

3. **Preoperative medications.** In general, patients should continue their medications in the immediate preoperative period. Exceptions to this rule include diabetic medications (see Section I.B.6), anticoagulants (see Section I.B.8.a), and antiplatelet agents. The use of some medications such as statins and angiotensin-converting-enzyme inhibitors should be individualized. It is important to query patients regarding their use of over-the-counter and herbal medications.

B. Specific considerations in preoperative management

1. **Cerebrovascular disease.** Perioperative stroke is an uncommon surgical complication, occurring in less than 1% of general patients and in 2% to 5% of cardiac surgical patients. The majority (>80%) of these events are postoperative, and they most often are caused by hypotension or cardiogenic emboli during atrial fibrillation. Acute surgical stress might cause focal signs from a previous stroke to recur, mimicking acute ischemia.

a. **Risk factors** for perioperative stroke include previous CVA, age, hypertension, coronary artery disease (CAD), diabetes, and tobacco use. Known or suspected cerebrovascular disease requires special consideration.

(1) **The asymptomatic carotid bruit** is relatively common, occurring in approximately 14% of surgical patients older than 55 years. However, fewer than 50% of bruits reflect hemodynamically significant disease. No increase in risk of stroke has been demonstrated during noncardiac surgery in the presence of an asymptomatic bruit.

(2) **Patients with recent transient ischemic attacks** are at increased risk for perioperative stroke and should have preoperative neurologic evaluation [e.g., computed tomography (CT) of the head, echocardiography, carotid Doppler]. Patients with symptomatic carotid artery stenosis should have an endarterectomy or carotid stenting before elective surgery.

(3) **Elective surgery for patients with recent cerebrovascular accident** should be delayed for a minimum of 2 weeks, ideally for 6 weeks.

TABLE 1-1	Routine Preoperative Testing
Test	**Comment**
Complete blood cell count	Possibility of substantial blood loss, patients with chronic illnesses or symptoms of anemia
Urinalysis	Urologic symptoms, instrumentation of the urinary tract, possibility of surgical placement of prosthetic materials
Serum electrolytes, creatinine, and blood urea nitrogen	Age >50, chronic diarrhea, renal disease, liver disease, diabetes, CHF or other cardiac disease, HTN, major procedure, diuretic use, digoxin use, ACE inhibitor use
Coagulation studies	Family history of bleeding disorder, patient history of abnormal bleeding, anticoagulant usage, liver disease, malnutrition, chronic antibiotics
Biochemical and profiles (including liver enzymes)	History of liver or biliary disease (albumin is a strong predictor of perioperative morbidity and mortality and should be considered for major procedures)
Pregnancy testing	Any woman of childbearing age (except posthysterectomy patients)
Chest x-ray	Acute cardiac or pulmonary symptoms
Electrocardiogram	Men >40, women >50, history of cardiovascular disease or arrhythmia, diabetes, HTN
Type and cross/type and screen	None if very low risk of blood loss; type and screen if risk of substantial blood loss is low to moderate; type and cross if moderate to high risk of substantial blood loss

ACE, angiotensin converting enzyme; CHF, congestive heart failure; HTN, hypertension.

2. **Cardiovascular disease.** Cardiovascular disease is one of the leading causes of death after noncardiac surgery. Patients who experience a myocardial infarction (MI) after noncardiac surgery have a hospital mortality rate of 15% to 25% (*CMAJ* 2005;173:627). A study of 4,315 patients older than 50 years between 1989 and 1994 undergoing nonemergent, noncardiac surgery with expected postoperative stays greater than 48 hours found that major perioperative cardiac events occur in 1.4% of the patients (*Circulation* 1999;100:1043). More than 100 million adults worldwide undergo noncardiac surgery annually. Therefore, each year it is likely that 500,000 to 900,000 patients worldwide experience perioperative cardiac death, a nonfatal MI, or nonfatal cardiac arrest postoperatively. Risk stratification by the operating surgeon, anesthesiologist, and consulting internist is important.
   a. **Risk factors.** The following risk factors have been associated with perioperative cardiac morbidity:
      (1) **The patient's age** (>70 years) has been identified as an independent multivariate risk factor for cardiac morbidity.
      (2) **Unstable angina** is defined as chest pain that does not correlate with the level of physical activity and, therefore, occurs at rest or with minimal physical exertion. Elective operation in patients with unstable angina is contraindicated and should be postponed pending further evaluation.
      (3) **Recent myocardial infarction (MI)** is a well-defined risk factor for cardiac morbidity. The risk of reinfarction is significant if an operation is performed within 6 months of an MI (11% to 16% at 3 to 6 months). This risk is still increased substantially after 6 months, in contrast to patients without a history of MI (4% to 5% vs. 0.13%).
      (4) **Untreated congestive heart failure (CHF)** is a predictor of perioperative cardiac morbidity. Consequently, these patients should be optimized before any operative procedures are performed.

TABLE 1-2	Antibiotic Prophylaxis of Bacterial Endocarditis for Adult Patients	
Procedure	**Situation**	**Regimen**
Dental, oral, respiratory, esophageal	Standard	**Amoxicillin** 2 g PO 1 hr before procedure
	Unable to take PO	**Ampicillin** 2 g IM or IV 30 min before procedure
	Penicillin-allergic	**Clindamycin** 600 mg PO 1 hr before procedure; or **cephalexin**[a] or **cefadroxil**[a] 2 g PO 1 hr before procedure; or **clarithromycin** or **azithromycin** 500 mg PO 1 hr before procedure
	Penicillin-allergic and unable to take PO	**Clindamycin** 600 mg IV within 30 min before procedure or **cefazolin**[a] 1 g IV within 30 min before procedure
Gastrointestinal and genitourinary	High-risk patients	**Ampicillin** 2 g IM or IV, plus **gentamicin** 1.5 mg/kg (max 120 mg) within 30 min before procedure; 6 hr later, **ampicillin** 1 g IV/IM or **amoxicillin** 1 g PO
	High-risk, penicillin-allergic patients	**Vancomycin** 1 g IV plus **gentamicin** 1.5 mg/kg (max 120 mg) timed to finish within 30 min of starting procedure
	Moderate-risk patients	**Amoxicillin** 2 g PO 1 hr before procedure or **ampicillin** 2 g IM or IV 30 min before procedure
	Moderate-risk, penicillin allergic patients	**Vancomycin** 1 g IV timed to finish within 30 min of starting procedure

IM, intravascular; IV, intravenous; PO, by mouth.
[a]Cephalosporins should not be used in patients with anaphylactic or urticarial reactions to penicillin.

(5) **Diabetes mellitus,** especially in those requiring insulin, is thought to confer additional independent risk for an adverse cardiac outcome.

(6) **Valvular heart disease.** Aortic stenosis is a significant risk factor and may confer a 14-fold increase in relative risk independent of the manifestations of CHF. Patients with unexplained symptoms of dyspnea on exertion, shortness of breath, chest pain, or syncope or an uncharacterized systolic ejection murmur should undergo further diagnostic evaluation before elective operation. All patients with valvular heart disease, even hemodynamically insignificant disease (excluding patients with mitral valve prolapse alone without a murmur), should receive prophylactic antibiotics before any operation that can introduce bacteria into the bloodstream or any dental procedure to reduce the risk of infectious endocarditis (Table 1-2).

(7) **Arrhythmias and conduction defects.** Both supraventricular and ventricular arrhythmias have been identified as independent risk factors for perioperative coronary events. The existence of a preoperative arrhythmia should prompt a search for underlying cardiac or pulmonary disease.

(8) **Peripheral vascular disease.** Because of the high coexistence of CAD with peripheral vascular disease, a lower threshold for obtaining diagnostic testing is warranted.

(9) **Type of procedure.** Patients who are undergoing thoracic surgery, vascular surgery, or upper abdominal surgery are at a higher risk of adverse cardiac outcome. Other procedures considered high risk include emergent

TABLE 1-3	Revised Cardiac Risk Index[a]
Risk factor	**Comment**
High-risk type of surgery	Intrathoracic, intraperitoneal, major vascular
Ischemic heart disease	History of myocardial infarction, positive exercise test, angina, nitrate therapy, electrocardiogram with abnormal Q waves
History of CHF	History of CHF, pulmonary edema, or paroxysmal nocturnal dyspnea, bilateral rales, S_3 gallop, chest x-ray showing pulmonary vascular redistribution
History of cerebrovascular disease	History of transient ischemic attack or stroke
Preoperative insulin therapy for diabetes	—
Preoperative serum creatinine >2 mg/dL	

CHF, congestive heart failure.
[a]Rates of major cardiac complication with 0, 1, 2, or 3 of these factors were 0.4%, 0.9%, 7.0%, and 11.0%, respectively.
Adapted with permission from Lee TH, Marcantonio ER, Mangione CM, et al. Derivation and prospective validation of a simple index for prediction of cardiac risk of major noncardiac surgery. *Circulation* 1999;100:1043.

major operations, especially in the elderly, and prolonged procedures associated with large fluid shifts or significant blood loss.

(10) Functional impairment. Patients with a poor functional capacity have a significantly higher risk of experiencing a postoperative cardiac event. Poor function is an indication for more aggressive preoperative evaluation, whereas patients who exercise regularly generally have sufficient cardiac reserve to withstand stressful operations.

b. **Revised cardiac risk index.** See Table 1-3.

c. **Preoperative testing.** Patients at intermediate risk for a perioperative myocardial event may require additional studies to determine if further therapy is needed to optimize their status.

(1) A preoperative electrocardiogram (ECG) is warranted in intermediate- or high-risk patients with a history of recent chest pain scheduled for an intermediate- or high-risk procedure. In addition, our policy is to obtain an ECG on any patients with a cardiac history, concerning symptoms, or significant risk factors, especially diabetes and renal failure. A screening ECG is obtained on any patients over the age of 50 years.

(2) Noninvasive testing. Patients who are identified to be at risk of a perioperative cardiovascular event by the revised cardiac risk index or who have other risk factors (e.g., peripheral vascular disease, unexplained chest pain, diabetes, ECG abnormalities) should undergo further evaluation.

(a) Exercise stress testing provides useful information for risk stratification. An inability to achieve even modest levels of exercise or the presence of ECG changes with exercise identifies patients at significant risk of adverse outcome.

(b) Dipyridamole thallium imaging has a very high negative predictive value of approximately 99% but a moderate positive predictive value ranging from 4% to 20%.

(c) Dobutamine stress echocardiography is believed to provide similar adrenergic stimulus to perioperative stress. A meta-analysis of eight studies and 1,877 patients suggested a trend toward superior prognostic accuracy with dobutamine stress echocardiography compared to other tests, with a sensitivity of 85% and a specificity of 70% for predicting perioperative cardiac death or nonfatal MI in patients undergoing vascular surgery (*Heart* 2003;89:1327).

(3) **Invasive testing.** Patients identified as high risk on noninvasive testing can be further evaluated with angiography. Patients with significant cardiac lesions should have definitive treatment (angioplasty or coronary artery bypass grafting) prior to an elective surgical procedure.

d. Preoperative management

(1) **Patients with pacemakers** should have their pacemakers turned to the uninhibited mode (e.g., DOO) before surgery. In addition, a bipolar cautery should be used when possible in these patients. If a unipolar cautery is necessary, the grounding pad should be placed away from the heart.

(2) **Patients with internal defibrillators** should have these devices turned off during surgery.

(3) **Perioperative beta-blockade** can be used for intermediate-risk patients with good functional status. A randomized, multicenter trial of 112 patients with positive dobutamine echocardiography undergoing major vascular surgery demonstrated that patients who received perioperative blockade of beta-adrenergic receptors had a significantly lower death rate from cardiac causes (3.4% vs. 17%) and rate of nonfatal myocardial infarctions (0% vs. 17%) than those who did not (*N Engl J Med* 1999;341:1789). However, a recent study from Canada of 496 patients undergoing major vascular surgery randomized to either perioperative metoprolol or placebo failed to demonstrate a reduction in 30-day or 6-month postoperative cardiac events rate (*Am Heart J* 2006;152:983). Major differences between the two studies included the following: (1) Patients in the Canadian study received beta-blockade 2 hours preoperatively and 5 days postoperatively, compared to an average of 37 days preoperatively and 30 days postoperatively in the first study; and (2) of 1,351 patients screened, only 112 patients who had positive dobutamine echocardiography were randomized to beta-blockade versus placebo in the first study. The Canadian study did not include positive dobutamine echocardiography as a criterion for its patients. In conclusion, perioperative beta-blockade appears to have a role in preventing perioperative cardiac complications in selected patients.

(4) **Patients with recent angioplasty or stenting.** Over the last few years, use of coronary angioplasty and stenting has increased dramatically. Several studies have shown a high incidence of cardiovascular complications when noncardiac surgery is performed shortly after coronary angioplasty or stenting. A study of 216 consecutive patients who underwent noncardiac surgery within 3 months of percutaneous coronary intervention demonstrated that significantly more adverse clinical events (acute myocardial infarction, major bleeding, and death) occurred when noncardiac surgery was performed within 2 weeks of percutaneous coronary intervention (*Am J Cardiol* 2006;97:1188). Current guidelines are to delay noncardiac surgery at least 6 weeks after coronary angioplasty or stenting.

3. Pulmonary disease. Preexisting lung disease confers a dramatically increased risk of perioperative pulmonary complications.

a. Preoperative evaluation and screening

(1) **Risk factors**

(a) **Chronic obstructive pulmonary disease (COPD)** is by far the most important risk factor, increasing pulmonary complications three- to fourfold.

(b) **Smoking** is also a significant risk factor. Operative risk reduction has only been documented after 8 weeks of smoking cessation; however, there are physiologic benefits to stopping as little as 48 hours before surgery.

(c) **Advanced age,** older than 60 years.

(d) **Obesity.** Body mass index (BMI) greater than 27 kg/m^2, in some studies.

      (e) **Type of surgery.** Pulmonary complications occur at a much higher rate for thoracic and upper abdominal procedures.

      (f) **Acute respiratory infections.** Postoperative pulmonary complications occur at a much higher rate for patients with acute respiratory infections; therefore, elective operations should be postponed in these individuals.

      (g) **Functional status.** In the patient with pulmonary disease or a history of smoking, a detailed evaluation of the patient's ability to climb stairs, walk, and perform daily duties is vital to stratify risk. Clinical judgment has been shown to be of value equal to or greater than pulmonary function testing for most patients.

    (2) **Physical examination** should be performed carefully, with attention paid to signs of lung disease (e.g., wheezing, prolonged expiratory–inspiratory ratio, clubbing, or use of accessory muscles of respiration).

    (3) **Diagnostic evaluation**

      (a) **Chest x-ray (CXR)** should be done for acute symptoms related to pulmonary disease.

      (b) An **arterial blood gas (ABG)** should be considered in patients with a history of lung disease or smoking to provide a baseline for comparison with postoperative studies.

      (c) **Preoperative pulmonary function testing** is controversial and probably unnecessary in stable patients with previously characterized pulmonary disease undergoing nonthoracic procedures.

  b. **Preoperative prophylaxis and management**

    (1) **Pulmonary toilet.** Increasing lung volume by the use of preoperative incentive spirometry is potentially effective in reducing pulmonary complications.

    (2) **Antibiotics** do not reduce pulmonary infectious complications in the absence of preoperative infection. Elective operations should be postponed in patients with respiratory infections. If emergent surgery is required, patients with acute pulmonary infections should receive intravenous antibiotic therapy.

    (3) **Cessation of smoking.** All patients should be encouraged and assisted to stop smoking before surgery.

    (4) **Bronchodilators.** In the patient with obstructive airway disease and evidence of a significant reactive component, bronchodilators may be required in the perioperative period. When possible, elective operation should be postponed in the patient who is actively wheezing.

4. **Renal disease**

  a. **Preoperative evaluation of patients with existing renal insufficiency**

    (1) **Risk factors**

      (a) **Underlying medical disease.** A substantial percentage of patients who require chronic hemodialysis for chronic renal insufficiency (CRI) have diabetes or hypertension. The incidence of CAD is substantially higher in these patients. Much of the perioperative morbidity and mortality arises from these coexisting illnesses.

      (b) **Metabolic and physiologic derangements of chronic renal insufficiency.** A variety of abnormalities in normal physiology that occur as a result of CRI can affect operative outcome adversely; these include alterations in electrolytes, acid-base balance, platelet function, the cardiovascular system, and the immune system. Specifically, the most common abnormalities in the perioperative period include hyperkalemia, intravascular volume overload, and infectious complications.

      (c) **Type of operative procedure.** Minor procedures under local or regional anesthesia are usually well tolerated in patients with CRI; however, major procedures are associated with increased morbidity and mortality.

(2) Evaluation

   (a) History. It is important to ascertain the specific etiology of CRI because patients with hypertension or diabetes and CRI are at a substantially increased risk of perioperative morbidity and mortality. The timing of last dialysis, the amount of fluid removed, and the preoperative weight provide important information about the patient's expected volume status.

   (b) Physical examination should be performed carefully to assess the volume status. Elevated jugular venous pulsations or crackles on lung examination can indicate intravascular volume overload.

   (c) Diagnostic testing

   (i) Laboratory data. Serum sodium, potassium, calcium, phosphorus, magnesium, and bicarbonate levels should be measured, as well as blood urea nitrogen (BUN) and creatinine levels. A complete blood cell (CBC) count should be obtained to evaluate for significant anemia or a low platelet level. Normal platelet numbers can mask platelet dysfunction in patients with chronic uremia.

   (ii) Supplemental tests such as noninvasive cardiac evaluation may be warranted in patients with CRI and other risk factors.

(3) Management

   (a) Timing of dialysis. Dialysis should be performed within 24 hours of the planned operative procedure.

   (b) Intravascular volume status. CAD is the most common cause of death in patients with CRI. Consequently, because of the high incidence of coexisting CAD, patients with CRI undergoing major operations may require invasive monitoring in the intraoperative and postoperative periods. Hypovolemia and volume overload are both poorly tolerated.

b. Patients at risk for perioperative renal dysfunction. The reported incidence of acute renal failure (ARF) after operations in patients without preexisting CRI ranges from 1.5% to 2.5% for cardiac surgical procedures to more than 10% for patients undergoing repair of supraceliac abdominal aortic aneurysm.

   (1) Risk factors for the development of ARF include elevated preoperative BUN or creatinine, CHF, advanced age, intraoperative hypotension, sepsis, aortic cross-clamping, and intravascular volume contraction. Additional risk factors include administration of nephrotoxic drugs, such as aminoglycosides, and the administration of radiocontrast agents.

   (2) Prevention

   (a) Intravascular volume expansion. Adequate hydration is the most important preventive measure for reducing the incidence of ARF because all mechanisms of renal failure are exacerbated by renal hypoperfusion caused by intravascular volume contraction.

   (b) Radiocontrast dye administration. Patients undergoing radiocontrast dye studies have an increased incidence of postoperative renal failure. Fluid administration (1 to 2 L of isotonic saline) alone appears to confer protection against ARF. Additional measures for reducing the incidence of contrast dye–mediated ARF include the use of low-osmolality contrast agents, a bicarbonate drip, and oral N-acetylcysteine (600 mg orally two times a day on the day of and day after contrast agent administration). A prospective, single-center, randomized trial conducted from 2002 to 2003 of 119 patients with stable serum creatinine levels of at least 1.1 mg/dL demonstrated that patients randomized to receive an infusion of sodium bicarbonate before and after intravenous (IV) contrast administration had a significantly lower rate of contrast-induced nephropathy than patients randomized to receive sodium chloride (13.5% vs. 1.7%) (*JAMA* 2004;291:2376).

A meta-analysis of 7 studies and 805 patients found that compared with preprocedural hydration alone, the administration of acetylcysteine and hydration significantly reduced the relative risk of contrast nephropathy by 56% in patients with chronic renal insufficiency (*Lancet* 2003;362:598). However, a follow-up meta-analysis of 13 randomized trials including 1,892 patients did not find conclusive evidence that N-acetylcysteine administration before coronary angiography in patients with impaired renal function reduced the incidence of contrast nephropathy (*Am J Heart* 2006;151:140). N-acetylcysteine has minimal toxicity, and further studies are needed to define its exact role.

- (c) **Other nephrotoxins,** including aminoglycoside antibiotics, nonsteroidal antiinflammatory drugs, and various anesthetic drugs, can predispose to renal failure and should be used judiciously in patients with other risk factors for the development of ARF.

5. **Infectious complications.** Infectious complications may arise in the surgical wound itself or in other organ systems. They may be initiated by changes in the physiologic state of the respiratory, genitourinary, or immune systems associated with surgery. It is impossible to overemphasize the importance of frequent hand washing or antiseptic foam use by all health care workers to prevent the spread of infection.

   a. **Assessment of risk.** Risk factors for infectious complications after surgery can be grouped into risk factors arising from the type of procedure and patient-specific risk factors.

      (1) **Surgical risk factors** include the type of procedure and degree of wound contamination (Table 1-4) and the duration and urgency of the operation.

TABLE 1-4   **Classification of Surgical Wounds**

Wound class	Definition	Examples of typical procedures	Wound infection rate (%)	Usual organisms
Clean	Nontraumatic, elective surgery; no entry of GI, biliary, tracheo bronchial, respiratory, or GU tracts	Wide local excision of breast mass	2	*Staphylococcus aureus*
Clean-contaminated	Respiratory, genitourinary, GI tract entered but minimal contamination	Gastrectomy, hysterectomy	<10	Related to the viscus entered
Contaminated	Open, fresh, traumatic wounds; uncontrolled spillage from an unprepared hollow viscus; minor break in sterile technique	Ruptured appendix; resection of unprepared bowel	20	Depends on underlying disease
Dirty	Open, traumatic, dirty wounds; traumatic perforated viscus; pus in the operative field	Intestinal fistula resection	28–70	Depends on underlying disease

GI, gastrointestinal.

(2) Patient-specific risk factors include age, diabetes, obesity, immunosuppression, malnutrition, preexisting infection, and chronic illness.

b. Prophylaxis

(1) Nonantimicrobial strategies documented to decrease the risk of postoperative infection include strict sterile technique, maintaining normal body temperature, maintaining normal blood glucose levels, and hyperoxygenation.

(2) Surgical wound infection. Antibiotic prophylaxis has contributed to a reduction in superficial wound infection rates (see Table 1-5 for specific recommendations). Coverage should be initiated not more than 2 hours (oral administration) or 1/2 hour (intramuscularly or intravenously) before the skin incision is made and, in the absence of gross contamination or overt infection, should not be administered beyond 24 to 48 hours after surgery. A prospective study of 2,847 patients undergoing elective clean or clean-contaminated surgical procedures in a community hospital demonstrated that prophylactic administration of antibiotics 2 hours before surgery significantly reduced the risk of postoperative wound infection to 1.4% compared to 3.3% and 3.8%, respectively, in patients who received antibiotics postoperatively and prior to 2 hours before surgery (*N Engl J Med* 1992;325:281). Repeat doses should be administered according to the usual dosing protocol during prolonged procedures.

(3) Respiratory infections. Risk factors and measures for preventing pulmonary complications are discussed in Section I.B.3.

(4) Genitourinary infections may be caused by instrumentation of the urinary tract or an indwelling urinary catheter. Preventive measures include sterile insertion of the catheter and removal of the catheter as soon as possible postoperatively. A prophylactic dose of antibiotics should be given after a difficult catheter insertion or excessive manipulation of the urinary tract.

6. Diabetes mellitus. Diabetic patients experience significant stress during the perioperative period and are at an estimated 50% increased risk of morbidity and mortality over nondiabetic patients. Diabetic patients experience more infectious complications and have impaired wound healing. Most important, vascular disease is common in diabetics, and silent CAD must always be considered. MI, often with an atypical presentation, is the leading cause of perioperative death among diabetic patients.

a. Preoperative evaluation. All diabetic patients should have their blood glucose checked on call to the operating room and during general anesthesia to prevent unrecognized hyperglycemia or hypoglycemia.

(1) Patients with **diet-controlled diabetes mellitus** can be maintained safely without food or glucose infusion before surgery.

(2) Patients who are taking oral hypoglycemic agents should discontinue these medications the evening before scheduled surgery. Patients who take such long-acting agents as chlorpropamide or glyburide should discontinue these medications 2 to 3 days before surgery.

(3) Patients who normally take insulin require insulin and glucose preoperatively to prevent ketosis and catabolism. Patients undergoing major surgery should receive one half of their morning insulin dose and 5% dextrose intravenously at 100 to 125 mL/hour. Subsequent insulin administration by either subcutaneous sliding-scale or insulin infusion is guided by frequent (every 4 to 6 hours) blood glucose determinations. Subcutaneous insulin pumps should be inactivated the morning of surgery.

7. Adrenal insufficiency and steroid dependence

a. Exogenous steroids are used to treat a variety of diseases that are encountered in surgical patients. Perioperative management of these individuals requires knowledge of the dose and type of steroid (long acting vs. short acting), schedule, and length of treatment with exogenous steroids.

TABLE 1-5   Recommendations for Antibiotic Prophylaxis

Nature of operation	Likely pathogens	Recommended antibiotics	Adult dose before surgery[a]
Cardiac: prosthetic valve and other procedures	Staphylococci, corynebacteria, enteric Gram-negative bacilli	Cefazolin Vancomycin Cefuroxime	1–2 g IV 1 g IV 1.5 g IV
Vascular: peripheral bypass or aortic surgery with prosthetic graft	Staphylococci, streptococci, enteric Gram-negative bacilli, clostridia	Cefazolin Vancomycin Cefoxitin	1–2 g IV 1–2 g IV 1–2 g IV
Orthopedic: total joint replacement or internal fixation of fractures	Staphylococci	Cefazolin Vancomycin	1–2 g IV 1 g IV
Ophthalmic	Staphylococci, streptococci, enteric Gram-negative bacilli, *Pseudomonas* spp.	Gentamicin Tobramycin Ciprofloxacin Ofloxacin Neomycin-gramicidin-polymyxin B	Multiple drops topically over 2–24 hr
Head and neck, entering oral cavity or pharynx	Oral anaerobes, enteric Gram-negative bacilli, staphylococci	Cefazolin Ampicillin-sulbactam Clindamycin Gentamicin	1–2 g IV 1.5–3 g IV 600–900 mg IV 1.5 mg/kg IV
Gastroduodenal (high-risk patient)	Enteric Gram-negative bacilli, Gram-positive cocci	Cefazolin	1–2 g IV
Biliary	Enteric Gram-negative bacilli, enterococci, clostridia	Cefazolin Cefoxitin Cefotetan	1–2 g IV 1–2 g IV 1–2 g IV

Procedure	Likely pathogens	Recommended antibiotic	Dose
Colorectal	Enteric Gram-negative bacilli, anaerobes, enterococci	Oral: neomycin + erythromycin base	1 g of each at 1 PM, 2 PM, and 11 PM the day before an 8 AM operation
		IV:	
		Cefoxitin	1–2 g IV
		Cefotetan	1–2 g IV
		Cefazolin plus flagyl	1–2 g IV; 500 mg IV
		Parenteral: cefoxitin	1 g IV
Appendectomy (no perforation)	Enteric Gram-negative bacilli, anaerobes, enterococci	Cefoxitin	1–2 g IV
		Cefotetan	1–2 g IV
Vaginal or abdominal hysterectomy	Enteric Gram-negative bacilli, anaerobes, group B streptococci, enterococci	Cefazolin	1–2 g IV
		Cefoxitin	1–2 g IV
		Cefotetan	1–2 g IV
Cesarean section (high-risk patient)	Same as for hysterectomy	Cefazolin	1 g IV after cord clamped
Traumatic wound	Staphylococci, group A streptococci, clostridia	Cefazolin or	1 g IV q8h
		Ampicillin-sulbactam	1.5–3 g IV q6h

IV, intravenous.

[a]Parenteral antibiotics for clean and clean-contaminated surgery can be given as a single intravenous dose completed 30 min before incision. For prolonged procedures, additional doses should be administered at usual dosing intervals. In general, antibiotics should not be continued postoperatively except in dirty wounds.

TABLE 1-6	Recommendations for Preoperative and Postoperative Anticoagulation in Patients Taking Oral Anticoagulants[a]	
Indication	**Preoperative**	**Postoperative**
Acute venous thromboembolism		
Within 1 mo of surgery	IV heparin[b]	IV heparin[b]
Within 3 mo of surgery	No therapy[d]	IV heparin
Recurrent venous thromboembolism[c]	No therapy[d]	SC heparin
Acute arterial embolism (within 30 days)	IV heparin	IV heparin[e]
Mechanical heart valve	No therapy[d]	SC heparin
Nonvalvular atrial fibrillation	No therapy[d]	SC heparin

[a]*IV heparin* denotes intravenous heparin at therapeutic doses, and *SC heparin* denotes subcutaneous unfractionated and low-molecular-weight heparin at doses recommended for prophylaxis against venous thromboembolism.
[b]A vena caval filter should be considered if acute venous thromboembolism has occurred within 2 wk or if the risk of bleeding during IV heparin therapy is high.
[c]*Recurrent venous thromboembolism* refers to patients whose last episode of venous thromboembolism occurred more than 3 mo before evaluation but who require long-term anticoagulation because of a high risk of recurrence.
[d]If patients are hospitalized, SC heparin can be administered, but hospitalization is not necessary solely for this purpose.
[e]IV heparin should be used after surgery only if the risk of bleeding is low.
Adapted with permission from Kearon C, Hirsh J. Management of anticoagulation before and after elective surgery. *N Engl J Med* 1997;336:1506. Copyright ⓒ1997, Massachusetts Medical Society. All rights reserved.

    b. Perioperative stress-dose steroids are indicated for patients undergoing major surgery who have received chronic steroid replacement or immunosuppressive steroid therapy within the last year.

    c. Dosage recommendations for perioperative steroids reflect estimates of normal adrenal responses to major surgical stress. The normal adrenal gland produces 250 to 300 mg cortisol per day under maximal stress, peaking at 6 hours after surgery and returning to baseline after 24 hours unless stress continues. A regimen of hydrocortisone sodium succinate, 100 mg intravenously, on the evening before major surgery, at the beginning of surgery, and every 8 hours on the day of surgery approximates the normal adrenal stress response. Tapering is not necessary in uncomplicated cases. Patients who are undergoing minor surgery or diagnostic procedures usually do not require stress-dose steroids.

8. Anticoagulation. The most common indications for warfarin therapy are atrial fibrillation, venous thromboembolism, and mechanical heart valves. Mitigation of warfarin's anticoagulant effect occurs only after several days of cessation from the drug, and it requires several days to reestablish the effect after warfarin is resumed. Recommendations for the management of anticoagulation (summarized in Table 1-6) in the perioperative period require weighing the risk of subtherapeutic anticoagulation (thromboembolic events) against the benefits (reduced incidence of perioperative bleeding).

    a. Preoperative anticoagulation. It is generally considered safe to perform surgery when the international normalized ratio (INR) value is below 1.5. Patients whose INR is maintained between 2.0 and 3.0 normally require withholding of the medication for 4 days preoperatively. For patients whose INR is maintained at a value greater than 3.0, withholding medication for a longer period of time is necessary. The INR should be measured the day before surgery, if possible, to confirm that the anticoagulation is reversed. Alternate prophylaxis should be considered for the preoperative period when the INR is less than 2.0.

TABLE 1-7	Prophylaxis for Deep Venous Thrombosis and Pulmonary Embolus	
Patient group[a]	**Surgery type**	**Prophylaxis**
Low risk	Minor	None
Low or moderate risk	Major	GCS, SQH-12, or IPC
High risk	Major	SQH-8 or LMWH[b]
Highest risk	Major	SQH-8/12 or LMWH + IPC

GCS, graded compression stockings; IPC, intermittent pneumatic compression; LMWH, low-molecular-weight heparin; SQH-8, subcutaneous heparin every 8 hr; SQH-12, subcutaneous heparin every 12 hr.
[a]Low risk, age less than 40 yr, no risk factors; moderate risk, major surgery and age less than 40 yr or minor procedure with risk factors or between 40 and 60 yr of age; high risk, major procedure over age 40 yr with risk factors, or minor procedure over age 60 yr or with risk factors; highest risk, age greater than 40 yr, multiple risk factors present, major procedure.
[b]Can use IPC if risk of hematoma or infection is high.

   b. Postoperative anticoagulation. The anticoagulant effects of warfarin require several doses before therapeutic levels are reached. For this reason, in patients who can tolerate oral or nasogastric medications, warfarin therapy can be resumed on postoperative days 1 or 2. If indicated (Table 1-6), intravenous heparin should generally not be restarted until 12 hours after surgery and should be delayed even longer if there is any evidence of bleeding.
   c. Emergent procedures. In an urgent or emergent situation in which there is no time to reverse anticoagulation before surgery, plasma products must be administered. In addition, Factor VII can have immediate effects, whereas vitamin K will have observable effects within 8 hours.
II. POSTOPERATIVE CARE OF THE PATIENT. This section summarizes general considerations in all postoperative patients.
  A. Routine postoperative care
   1. Intravenous fluids. The intravascular volume of surgical patients is depleted by both insensible fluid losses and redistribution into the third space. As a general rule, patients should be maintained on intravenous fluids until they are tolerating oral intake. Extensive abdominal procedures require aggressive fluid resuscitation (see Chapter 4). Insensible fluid losses associated with an open abdomen can reach 500 to 1,000 mL/hour.
   2. Deep venous thrombosis prophylaxis. Many postoperative patients are not immediately ambulatory. In these individuals, it is important to provide prophylactic therapy to reduce the risk of deep venous thrombosis (DVT) and pulmonary embolism (PE) (see Table 1-7). Prophylaxis should be started preoperatively in patients undergoing major procedures because venous stasis and relative hypercoagulability occur during the operation. The American College of Chest Physicians recommends the use of pharmacologic methods combined with the use of intermittent pneumatic compression devices in high-risk general surgery patients with multiple risk factors. Prophylaxis and management of patients with a history of DVT or PE is discussed in Chapter 20.
   3. Pulmonary toilet. Pain and immobilization in the postoperative patient decrease the clearance of pulmonary secretions and alveolar recruitment. Patients with inadequate pulmonary toilet can develop fevers, hypoxemia, and pneumonia. Early mobilization, incentive spirometry, and cough and deep breathing exercises are indispensable to avoid these complications.
   4. Medications
    a. Antiemetics. Postoperative nausea is common in patients after general anesthesia and in patients receiving narcotics.
    b. Ulcer prophylaxis. Patients with a history of peptic ulcer disease should have some form of ulcer prophylaxis in the perioperative period with either acid-reducing agents or cytoprotective agents, such as sucralfate. Routine ulcer

prophylaxis in patients without a history of peptic ulcer disease has only been of proven benefit in those with a coagulopathy or prolonged ventilator dependence.

c. Pain control. Inadequate pain control can slow recovery or contribute to complications in postoperative patients. Individuals whose pain is poorly controlled are less likely to ambulate and take deep breaths and are more likely to be tachycardic.

d. Antibiotics. Surgeon preferences often dictate the use of postoperative antibiotics in particular cases. Recommendations for specific procedures are given in Table 1-5. Antibiotic therapy for specific infectious etiologies is discussed in Section III.E.2.

5. Laboratory tests. Postoperative laboratory tests should be individualized; however, the following considerations are important when planning laboratory evaluations:

    a. A **complete blood count** should be obtained in the immediate postoperative period and on subsequent postoperative days in any procedure in which significant blood loss occurred. If there is a concern for ongoing blood loss, serial hematocrits should be followed.

    b. Serum electrolytes, blood urea nitrogen, and creatinine are important postoperatively in patients on nothing-by-mouth (NPO) status or who are receiving large volumes of intravenous fluids, total parenteral nutrition, or transfusions. In patients with large transfusion requirements, it is important to keep track of calcium and magnesium levels.

    c. Coagulation studies are important in patients who have had insults to the liver or large transfusion requirements.

    d. Daily **ECGs** and a series of three **troponin I** levels 12 hours apart are appropriate ways to monitor for myocardial ischemia in patients with significant cardiac risk factors.

    e. Chest x-rays are a necessity after any procedure in which the thoracic cavity is entered or when central venous access is attempted. CXRs on subsequent postoperative days should be considered on an individual basis if significant pulmonary or cardiovascular disease is present.

III. COMPLICATIONS

A. Neurologic complications

1. Perioperative stroke

    a. Presentation. Patients usually describe a rapid onset of focal loss of neurologic function (unilateral weakness or clumsiness, sensory loss, speech disorder, diplopia, or vertigo). Massive strokes can present with altered mental status.

    b. Examination. A thorough neurologic examination, in addition to vital signs, finger-stick glucose, and pulse oximetry, should be assessed.

    c. Evaluation

       (1) Laboratory evaluation should include a CBC, electrolytes, BUN, creatinine, and coagulation studies. An ECG should be done to rule out cardiac arrhythmia.

       (2) A **CT scan of the head** should be obtained urgently to rule out a hemorrhagic stroke.

       (3) Further studies, including echocardiography, carotid and transcranial ultrasound, and magnetic resonance imaging (MRI), may be ordered in consultation with a neurologist.

    d. Treatment

       (1) General supportive measures include supplemental oxygen and intravenous fluid.

       (2) Aspirin (325 mg orally) should be given immediately in ischemic stroke.

       (3) Thrombolysis has been proven effective in improving outcomes from ischemic strokes; however, it is usually contraindicated in postoperative patients and should only be initiated in close consultation with a neurologist.

2. Seizures. Evaluation and treatment of postoperative seizures involve the same principles as those encountered in other settings. Most seizures in surgical patients without a history of seizure can be attributed to metabolic derangements, including electrolyte abnormalities (e.g., hyponatremia, hypocalcemia), hypoglycemia, sepsis, fever, and drugs (e.g., imipenem).

a. Determine from patient history whether a true seizure was witnessed; if so, note its type, characteristics (i.e., general versus focal onset), and similarity to any previous seizures. New-onset seizures are worrisome, and iatrogenic causes (e.g., medications) and cerebrovascular accident must be considered. A history of preoperative alcohol use may indicate withdrawal.

b. Complete physical and neurologic examination should focus on airway, oxygenation, and hemodynamics and then on any sequelae of seizure, including trauma, aspiration, or rhabdomyolysis. A focally abnormal neurologic examination, especially in the setting of a new-onset focal seizure, suggests a possible cerebrovascular event.

c. Laboratory and diagnostic studies. The immediate evaluation of a patient should consist of vital signs, a blood glucose determination, CBC, and serum chemistries, including calcium and magnesium. Serum levels of anticonvulsants should be measured in patients receiving these medications. Patients with new-onset seizures who do not have identifiable metabolic or systemic causes warrant further evaluation with a head CT scan followed by a lumbar puncture.

d. Treatment of new-onset, single, nonrecurring seizures or recurrent generalized seizures with identifiable metabolic or systemic causes usually requires only correction of the underlying abnormality.

(1) Recurrent generalized tonic–clonic seizures require anticonvulsant therapy. A 15- to 20-mg/kg load of phenytoin, given parenterally in three divided doses followed by maintenance dosing of 5 mg/kg/day in three divided doses, controls most seizures. Therapeutic serum levels are 10 to 20 mg/mL.

(2) Status epilepticus is a medical emergency.

(a) Monitor cardiopulmonary parameters and stabilize the patient's airway with a soft oral or nasal airway. Endotracheal intubation might be required to protect the airway. Phenobarbital and benzodiazepines in combination severely depress the respiratory drive. Intravenous access should be established immediately.

(b) Administer parenteral anticonvulsants promptly.

(i) Diazepam (5 to 10 mg intravenously every 5 to 10 minutes) or **lorazepam** (1 to 2 mg intravenously every 5 to 10 minutes) should be administered to patients with generalized convulsions lasting longer than 5 minutes. Results are usually seen within 10 minutes. These agents are relatively short acting, and a second parenteral anticonvulsant should be started concurrently.

(ii) Phenytoin administered parenterally is the first choice to supplement the benzodiazepines in this setting.

(iii) Phenobarbital is a second-line agent and should be used when phenytoin is contraindicated (e.g., heart block) or ineffective. A loading dose of 10 mg/kg can be given at 100 mg/minute. Maintenance doses of 1 to 5 mg/kg/day intravenously or orally are required to achieve therapeutic plasma levels. Institution of a phenobarbital coma should be considered if status epilepticus continues.

3. Delirium. Delirium is fairly common in patients (especially the elderly) who undergo the stress of operation. An underlying cause usually can be identified, and in most cases it involves medications or infection. Other causes include hypoxemia, electrolyte abnormalities, cardiac arrhythmias, MI, and stroke. Alcohol withdrawal, discussed in Section III.A.4, is another common cause of postoperative delirium.

a. Symptoms include impaired memory, altered perception, and paranoia. Altered sleep patterns result in drowsiness during the day and wakefulness and agitation at night (sundowning). Disorientation and combativeness are common.

   b. **Management** begins with eliminating the possibility of an underlying physiologic or metabolic derangement. Pulse, blood pressure (BP), temperature, and pulse oximetry should be assessed and a thorough physical exam performed with attention to the possibility of infection. CBC and electrolytes should be obtained. Other testing, including ECG, ABG, urinalysis (UA), and CXR, is dictated by clinical suspicion. Medications should be reviewed carefully, with consideration directed toward anticholinergic agents, opiate analgesics, and antihistamines. If no underlying organic cause is identified, alteration in sleep patterns or sensory deprivation can be invoked, and haloperidol (1 to 5 mg orally or intramuscularly) can be prescribed. Often, family reassurance or transfer to a naturally lighted room is curative. Physical restraints might be necessary to prevent self-harm.

4. **Alcohol withdrawal.** Alcohol withdrawal carries a significant risk of morbidity and mortality and requires a high level of vigilance.

   a. **Symptoms.** Minor withdrawal can begin 6 to 8 hours after cessation of alcohol intake and is characterized by anxiety, tremulousness, anorexia, and nausea. Signs include tachycardia, hypertension, and hyperreflexia. These signs and symptoms generally resolve within 24 to 48 hours. **Delirium tremens** typically occurs 72 to 96 hours or longer after cessation of alcohol intake and is characterized by disorientation, hallucinations, and autonomic lability that includes tachycardia, hypertension, fever, and profuse diaphoresis.

   b. **Treatment**

      (1) **Benzodiazepines**—such as chlordiazepoxide, 25 to 100 mg orally every 6 hours; oxazepam, 5 to 15 mg orally every 6 hours; or diazepam, 5 to 20 mg orally or intravenously every 6 hours—can be used as prophylaxis in alcoholics who have a history of withdrawal or to alleviate symptoms of minor withdrawal. Patients with delirium tremens should be given diazepam, 5 to 10 mg intravenously every 10 to 15 minutes, to control symptoms. Oversedation must be avoided through close monitoring. The dose of benzodiazepines should be reduced in patients with liver impairment. Moderate alcohol intake with meals can be a simple way to prevent and treat alcohol withdrawal.

      (2) **Clonidine,** 0.1 mg orally four times a day, or atenolol, 50 to 100 mg orally, every day, can be used to treat tachycardia or hypertension resulting from autonomic hyperactivity. Close hemodynamic monitoring is required during therapy.

      (3) **General medical care.** Fluid and electrolyte abnormalities should be corrected, and fever should be treated with acetaminophen or cooling blankets as needed. Thiamine, 100 mg intramuscularly for 3 days, followed by 100 mg orally every day, should be given to all suspected alcoholic patients to prevent development of Wernicke encephalopathy. Many chronic alcoholics have hypomagnesemia; if it is present, magnesium sulfate should be administered to patients with normal renal function. Folate should be given 1 mg intramuscularly or orally every day.

      (4) **Restraints** should be used only when necessary to protect the patient from self-harm.

      (5) **Alcohol withdrawal seizures** occur 12 to 48 hours after cessation of alcohol and are most often generalized tonic–clonic. They are usually brief and self-limited, although status epilepticus occurs in approximately 3% of cases. Benzodiazepines are most helpful in preventing recurrent seizures.

B. **Cardiovascular complications**

   1. **Myocardial ischemia and infarction**

      a. The **presentation** of myocardial ischemia in the postoperative patient is often subtle. Frequently, perioperative MI is silent or presents with dyspnea, hypotension, or atypical pain.

b. In postoperative patients who present with chest pain, the **differential diagnosis** includes myocardial ischemia or infarction, PE, pneumonia, pericarditis, aortic dissection, and pneumothorax.
c. Evaluation
  (1) Physical examination should be performed carefully to assess BP, heart rate, and organ and tissue perfusion. The lungs should be auscultated for signs of pulmonary edema and diminished or absent breath sounds unilaterally (pneumothorax). Auscultation of the heart can reveal a new murmur suggestive of ischemic mitral regurgitation or a pericardial friction rub suggestive of pericarditis.
  (2) Diagnostic testing
    (a) An **electrocardiogram** is warranted in virtually all cases of postoperative chest pain, with comparison to prior tracings. Sinus tachycardia is one of the most common rhythms associated with myocardial ischemia.
    (b) Laboratory data
      (i) Cardiac enzymes. An elevated troponin I level is diagnostic of MI. A series of three samplings of troponin I 12 hours apart has a sensitivity and specificity of greater than 90% for detecting myocardial injury.
      (ii) Routine serum chemistries and hemoglobin.
      (iii) Oxygen saturation should be determined via pulse oximetry, and supplemental oxygen should be administered. Significant hypoxia can be seen with MI, CHF, pneumonia, and PE.
    (c) Chest x-rays should be obtained to evaluate for pneumothorax, infiltrate, or evidence of pulmonary edema.
    (d) Further diagnostic evaluation [e.g., echocardiography, coronary catheterization, ventilation-perfusion (V/Q) scintigraphy, or CT scan] should be pursued as indicated by the diagnostic workup.
  (3) Treatment
    (a) Telemetry should be used in all patients with suspected myocardial ischemia.
    (b) Oxygen therapy. The arterial oxygen saturation should be kept greater than 90% with supplemental oxygen. Endotracheal intubation and mechanical ventilation are indicated for patients with hypoxia that is refractory to supplemental oxygen therapy, progressive hypercapnia, or respiratory fatigue.
    (c) Pharmacologic therapy
      (i) Nitrates. In the absence of hypotension (systemic BP <90 mm Hg), initial management of patients with chest pain of presumed cardiac origin includes the use of sublingual nitroglycerin (0.4 mg), which can be repeated every 5 minutes. Additionally, topical nitrate therapy (0.5 to 2 in. every 6 hours) can be instituted. Ongoing myocardial ischemia or infarction should be treated with intravenous nitroglycerin, starting with an infusion rate of 5 μg/minute and increased at 5-μg/minute increments until the chest pain is relieved or significant hypotension develops (systemic BP <90 mm Hg).
      (ii) Beta-adrenergic receptor antagonists. In the absence of significant contraindications (e.g., heart failure, bradycardia, heart block, or significant COPD), patients should be treated with intravenous beta-adrenergic receptor antagonists (e.g., metoprolol, 15 mg intravenously, in 5-mg doses every 5 minutes, followed by a 50- to 100-mg oral dose every 12 hours).
      (iii) Intravenous morphine sulfate (1 to 4 mg intravenously every hour) is also useful in the acute management of chest pain to decrease the sympathetic drive of an anxious patient.
      (iv) Antiplatelet therapy in the form of a non–enteric-coated aspirin (325 mg) can also be given if the patient is at low risk of perioperative bleeding.

(d) Other therapeutic measures. Thrombolytic therapy, anticoagulation, or coronary catheterization should be considered on an individual basis in consultation with a cardiologist.

2. Congestive heart failure

   a. Differential diagnosis of shortness of breath or hypoxia in the perioperative period includes CHF, pneumonia, atelectasis, PE, reactive airway disease (asthma, COPD exacerbation), and pneumothorax. These pulmonary conditions are discussed in Section III.C.

   b. Evaluation

   (1) History. CHF can occur immediately postoperatively as a result of excessive intraoperative administration of fluids or 24 to 48 hours postoperatively related to mobilization of fluids that are sequestered in the extracellular space. Myocardial ischemia or infarct can also result in CHF. Net fluid balance and weight for the preceding days should be assessed.

   (2) Physical examination should be directed toward signs and symptoms of fluid overload and myocardial ischemia.

   (3) Diagnostic testing

   (a) Laboratory data. Troponin I, B-type natriuretic peptide (BNP), ABG, CBC, electrolytes, and renal function tests should be obtained.

   (b) Pulse oximetry.

   (c) Electrocardiogram.

   (d) Chest x-ray.

   (e) An **echocardiogram** is frequently indicated in patients with new CHF to evaluate valves, assess the contractility and dimensions of each cardiac chamber, and rule out tamponade.

   (f) Invasive measurement of cardiac output with a **pulmonary artery catheter** may be of use in assessing volume status.

   c. Management of congestive heart failure

   (1) Supplemental oxygen should be administered. Mechanical ventilation is indicated in patients with refractory hypoxemia.

   (2) Diuretics. Treatment should be initiated with furosemide (20 to 40 mg intravenous push), with doses up to 200 mg every 6 hours as necessary to achieve adequate diuresis. Furosemide drips can be effective in promoting diuresis. Fluid intake should be limited, and serum potassium should be monitored closely.

   (3) Morphine (1 to 4 mg intravenous push every hour)

   (4) Arterial vasodilators. To reduce afterload and help the failing heart in the acute setting, sodium nitroprusside or angiotensin-converting-enzyme inhibitors can be used to lower the systolic BP to 90 to 100 mm Hg.

   (5) Inotropic agents. Digoxin increases myocardial contractility and can be used to treat patients with mild failure. Patients with florid failure may need invasive monitoring and titration of drips if they do not respond to these measures. If there is a low cardiac index (<2.5 L/minute/m^2) with elevated filling pressures, inotropic agents are indicated. Therapy can be initiated with dobutamine (3 to 20 μg/kg/minute) to increase the cardiac index to a value near 3 L/minute/m^2. Milrinone is also a useful agent for refractory CHF. (A loading dose of 50 μg/kg is administered over 10 minutes, followed by a continuous infusion of 0.375 to 0.750 μg/kg/minute titrated for clinical response.) If hypotension is accompanied by low systemic vascular resistance, vasopressors may be useful (Table 1-8).

C. Pulmonary complications

   1. The **differential diagnosis** of dyspnea includes atelectasis, lobar collapse, pneumonia, CHF, COPD, asthma exacerbation, pneumothorax, PE, and aspiration.

   2. Evaluation

   a. History. Additional factors that help to differentiate disease entities include the presence of a fever, chest pain, and the time since surgery.

   b. Physical examination with attention to jugular venous distention, breath sounds (wheezing, crackles), symmetry, and respiratory effort.

| TABLE 1-8 | Doses of Commonly Used Vasopressors | | |

Vasopressor	Preparation	Infusion	Comments
Dobutamine	250 mg/250 mL NS or D5W	Start at 3 μg/kg/min and titrate up to 20 μg/kg/min based on clinical response	Beta agonist
Dopamine	800 mg in 500 mL NS or D5W	Start at 3 μg/kg/min and titrate to systolic BP	Beta-adrenergic effects dominate at lower infusion rates
Epinephrine	5 mg/500 mL NS or D5W	1–4 μg/min, titrate to effect	Alpha and beta
Norepinephrine	8 mg in 500 mL D5W	Start at 2 μg/min and titrate to systolic BP	Strong alpha-adrenergic agonist
Phenylephrine (NeoSynephrine)	10 mg in 250 mL D5W or NS	Start at 10 μg/min and titrate to systolic BP	May be ineffective in severe distributive shock

BP, blood pressure; D5W, 5% dextrose in water; NS, normal saline.

- c. **Diagnostic testing**
  - (1) **Laboratory.** CBC, chemistry profile, and pulse oximetry or ABG.
  - (2) **Electrocardiograms** should be obtained for any patient older than 30 years with significant dyspnea or tachypnea to exclude myocardial ischemia and in any patient who is dyspneic in the setting of tachycardia.
  - (3) **Chest x-rays** are mandatory in all dyspneic patients.
  - (4) **V/Q scan, pulmonary embolism protocol chest computed tomography scan,** or pulmonary angiogram may be helpful.
- 3. **Management** of specific diagnoses
  - a. **Atelectasis** commonly occurs in the first 36 hours after operation and typically presents with dyspnea and hypoxia. Therapy is aimed at reexpanding the collapsed alveoli. For most patients, deep breathing and coughing along with the use of incentive spirometry are adequate. Postoperative pain should be sufficiently controlled so that pulmonary mechanics are not significantly impaired. In patients with significant atelectasis or lobar collapse, chest physical therapy and nasotracheal suctioning might be required. In rare cases, bronchoscopy can aid in clearing mucus plugs that cannot be cleared using less invasive measures.
  - b. **Pneumonia** is discussed in Section III.E.2.b.
  - c. **Pulmonary embolism** is discussed in Section III.F.
  - d. **Gastric aspiration** usually presents with acute dyspnea and fever. CXR might be normal initially but subsequently demonstrate a pattern of diffuse interstitial infiltrates. Therapy is supportive, and antibiotics are typically not given empirically.
  - e. **Pneumothorax** is treated with tube thoracostomy. If tension pneumothorax is suspected, immediate needle decompression through the second intercostal space in the midclavicular line using a 14-gauge needle should precede controlled placement of a thoracostomy tube.
  - f. **Chronic obstructive pulmonary disease and asthma exacerbations** present with dyspnea or tachypnea, wheezing, hypoxemia, and possibly hypercapnia. Acute therapy includes administration of supplemental oxygen and inhaled beta-adrenergic agonists [albuterol, 3.0 mL (2.5 mg) in 2 mL normal saline every 4 to 6 hours of nebulization]. Beta-adrenergic agonists are indicated primarily for acute exacerbations rather than for long-term use. Anticholinergics such as ipratropium bromide metered-dose inhaler (Atrovent, 2

TABLE 1-9	Laboratory Evaluation of Oliguria and Acute Renal Failure				
Category	FE_{Na}	U_{Osm}	RFI	U_{Cr}/P_{Cr}	U_{Na}
Prerenal	<1	>500	<1	>40	<20
Renal (acute tubular necrosis)	>1	<350	>1	<20	>40
Postrenal	>1	<50	>1	<20	>40

FE_{Na}, fractional excretion of sodium; RFI, renal failure index; U_{Cr}/P_{Cr}, urine–plasma creatinine ratio; U_{Na}, urine sodium; U_{Osm}, urine osmolality.

puffs every 4 to 6 hours) can also be used in the perioperative period, especially if the patient has significant pulmonary secretions. Patients with severe asthma or COPD may benefit from parenteral steroid therapy (methylprednisolone, 50 to 250 mg intravenously every 4 to 6 hours) as well as inhaled steroids (beclomethasone metered-dose inhaler, 2 puffs four times a day), but steroids require 6 to 12 hours to take effect.

D. Renal complications

1. Acute renal failure

  a. Causes. The etiologies of postoperative renal insufficiency can be divided into prerenal, intrinsic renal, and postrenal classes (Table 1-9).

    (1) Prerenal azotemia results from decreased renal perfusion that might be secondary to hypotension, intravascular volume contraction, or decreased effective renal perfusion.

    (2) Renal. Intrinsic renal causes of ARF include drug-induced acute tubular necrosis, pigment-induced renal injury, radiocontrast dye administration, acute interstitial nephritis, and prolonged ischemia from suprarenal aortic cross-clamping.

    (3) Postrenal causes of ARF can result from obstruction of the ureters or bladder. Operations that involve dissection near the ureters, such as colectomy, colostomy closure, or total abdominal hysterectomy, have a higher incidence of ureteral injuries. In addition to ureteral injuries or obstruction, obstruction of the bladder from an enlarged prostate, postoperative pain and medication administration, or obstructed urinary catheter can occur.

  b. General evaluation

    (1) History and physical examination.

    (2) Laboratory evaluation

      (a) Urinalysis can help to differentiate between etiologies of renal failure.

      (b) Serum chemistries.

      (c) Urinary indices help to classify ARF into prerenal, postrenal, or intrinsic renal categories (Table 1-9). Fractional excretion of sodium (FE_{Na}) can be calculated from

$$FE_{Na} = (U_{Na}/P_{Na})/(U_{Cr}/P_{Cr}),$$

where U_{Na} is urine sodium, P_{Na} is plasma sodium, and U_{Cr}/P_{Cr} is urine–plasma creatinine ratio. The renal failure index (RFI) is $(U_{Na})(P_{Cr})/U_{Cr}$. These measurements must be obtained before diuretic administration.

    (3) Other diagnostic testing

      (a) Renal ultrasonography can be used to exclude the diagnosis of obstructive uropathy, evaluate the chronicity of renal disease, and evaluate the renal vasculature with Doppler.

      (b) Radiologic studies using intravenous contrast are contraindicated in patients with suspected ARF due to the potential to exacerbate renal injury.

  c. Management of specific problems

    (1) Oliguria (<500 mL/day) in the postoperative period

      (a) Evaluation. The goal of this evaluation is to determine the patient's intravascular volume status and to differentiate the causes of oliguria.

Cardiac echocardiography, central venous pressures, and pulmonary artery pressures can assist with the evaluation of volume status.

(b) Management

(i) Prerenal. In most surgical patients, oliguria is caused by hypovolemia. Initial management includes fluid challenges (normal saline, 500 mL). Patients with adequate fluid resuscitation and CHF may benefit from invasive monitoring and optimization of cardiac function.

(ii) Intrinsic renal. Treat the underlying cause, if possible, and manage volume status.

(iii) Postrenal. Ureteral injuries or obstruction can be treated with percutaneous nephrostomy tubes and generally are managed in consultation with a urologist. Urinary retention and urethral obstruction can be managed by placement of a Foley catheter or, if necessary, a suprapubic catheter.

(2) Elevated creatinine and acute renal failure

(a) Evaluation. The laboratory and diagnostic evaluation for patients with a rising creatinine is similar to the evaluation for patients with oliguria.

(b) Management includes careful attention to the intravascular volume status. The patient should be weighed daily, and intakes and outputs should be recorded carefully. Serum electrolytes should be monitored closely. The patient should be maintained in a euvolemic state. Hyperkalemia, metabolic acidosis, and hyperphosphatemia are common problems in patients with ARF and should be managed as discussed in Chapter 4. Medication doses should be adjusted appropriately and potassium removed from maintenance intravenous fluids (IVF).

(i) Dialysis. Indications for dialysis include intravascular volume overload, hyperkalemia, severe metabolic acidosis, and complications of uremia (encephalopathy, pericarditis).

E. Infectious complications

1. Management of infection and fever

a. Evaluation of fever should take into context the time after operation in which the fever occurs.

(1) Intraoperative fever may be secondary to malignant hyperthermia, a transfusion reaction, or a preexisting infection.

(a) Diagnosis and management of a transfusion reaction are discussed in Chapter 5.

(b) Malignant hyperthermia is discussed in Chapter 3.

(c) Preexisting infections should be treated with empiric intravenous antibiotics.

(2) High fever (>39°C) in the first 24 hours is commonly the result of a streptococcal or clostridial wound infection, aspiration pneumonitis, or a preexisting infection.

(a) Streptococcal wound infections present with severe local erythema and incisional pain. Penicillin G (2 million units intravenously every 6 hours) or ampicillin (1 to 2 g intravenously every 6 hours) is effective therapy. Patients with a **severe necrotizing clostridial infection** present with systemic toxemia, pain, and crepitus near the incision. Treatment includes emergent operative débridement and metronidazole (500 mg intravenously every 6 hours) or clindamycin (600 to 900 mg intravenously every 8 hours).

(3) Fever that occurs more than 72 hours after surgery has a broad differential diagnosis, including pneumonia, urinary tract infection, thrombophlebitis, wound infection, intraabdominal abscess, and drug allergy.

b. Diagnostic evaluation. The new onset of fever or leukocytosis without an obvious source of infection requires a thorough history and physical examination (including inspection of all wounds, tubes, and catheter sites) and selected laboratory tests.

   c. Specific laboratory tests
   (1) Complete blood count.
   (2) Urinalysis.
   (3) Chest x-ray.
   (4) Gram stain/culture. Cultures of the blood, sputum, urine, or wound should be dictated by the clinical situation.
   d. Antibiotics. Empiric antibiotics can be initiated, with therapy directed by clinical suspicion.
   e. Imaging studies such as ultrasound or CT should be chosen based on clinical context.
2. **Management of specific infectious etiologies**
   a. Wound infection is diagnosed by local erythema, swelling, pain, tenderness, and wound drainage. Fever and leukocytosis are usually present but may be absent in superficial wound infections. The primary treatment is to open the wound to allow drainage. The wound should be cultured. If the infection is contained in the superficial tissue layers, antibiotics are not required. In the case of a clean procedure that did not enter the bowel, the usual pathogens are staphylococcal and streptococcal species. If surrounding erythema is extensive, parenteral antibiotics should be initiated. Wound infections in the perineum or after bowel surgery are more likely to be caused by enteric pathogens and anaerobes. More-aggressive infections with involvement of underlying fascia require emergent operative débridement and broad-spectrum intravenous antibiotics.
   b. Respiratory infections. Pneumonia is diagnosed by the presence of fever, leukocytosis, purulent sputum production, and an infiltrate on CXR. After Gram stain and culture of the sputum and blood is performed, empiric antibiotics can be started. Pneumonias that occur in postoperative patients should be treated as nosocomial infections. Patients requiring mechanical ventilation for longer than 48 hours are at risk for ventilator-associated pneumonia (VAP), which may require bronchoscopy for diagnosis.
   c. Gastrointestinal infections may present with fever, leukocytosis, and diarrhea. *Clostridium difficile* is a common cause of diarrhea in hospitalized patients, and assay for the C. *difficile* organism or toxin should be performed. Initial therapy includes fluid resuscitation and metronidazole (500 mg orally every 6 to 8 hours) or vancomycin (250 to 500 mg orally every 6 hours).
   d. Intraabdominal abscess or peritonitis presents with fever, leukocytosis, abdominal pain, and tenderness. If the patient has generalized peritonitis, emergency laparotomy is indicated. If the inflammation appears to be localized, a CT scan of the patient's abdomen and pelvis should be obtained. The primary management of an intraabdominal abscess is drainage. In some circumstances, this can be performed percutaneously with radiologic guidance. In other situations, operative débridement and drainage are required. Empiric antibiotic therapy should cover enteric pathogens and anaerobes.
   e. Genitourinary infections. After the urine is cultured, simple lower-tract infections can be managed with oral antibiotics. Ill patients or those with pyelonephritis require more aggressive therapy.
   f. Prosthetic device–related infections may present with fever, leukocytosis, and systemic bacteremia. Infection of prosthetic valves may present with a new murmur. Management may require removal of the infected device and the use of long-term antibiotics.
   g. Catheter-related infections also are diagnosed by the presence of fever, leukocytosis, and systemic bacteremia. Local erythema and purulence may be present around central venous catheter insertion sites. Erythema, purulence, a tender thrombosed vein, or lymphangitis may be present near an infected peripheral intravenous line. Management includes removal of the catheter and intravenous antibiotic coverage.
   h. Fascial or muscle infections may result from gross contamination of a surgical wound or from a previously infected wound. Fasciitis and deep-muscle

infections present with hemorrhagic bullae over the infected area, rapidly progressive edema, erythema, pain, and crepitus. Fever, tachycardia, and ultimately cardiovascular collapse occur in rapid succession. Therapy includes emergent operative débridement, management of shock, and broad-spectrum antibiotics (including anaerobic coverage). Necrotizing fasciitis is a surgical emergency; death may result within a few hours of the development of symptoms.

  i. **Viral infections** complicating operations are uncommon in immunocompetent patients.

  j. **Fungal infections** (primarily with *Candida* species) occur most commonly after long-term antibiotic administration. In these patients, evaluation of persistent fever without an identified bacterial source should include several sets of routine and fungal blood cultures, removal of all intravenous catheters, and examination of the retina for *Candida endophthalmitis*. Therapy includes either amphotericin B or fluconazole.

F. Deep venous thrombosis and pulmonary embolism

  1. Diagnosis and treatment of deep venous thrombosis

   a. Diagnosis

   (1) Symptoms of DVT vary greatly, although classically they include pain and swelling of the affected extremity distal to the site of venous obstruction. Signs of DVT on physical examination may include edema, erythema, warmth, a palpable cord, or calf pain with dorsiflexion of the foot (Homans' sign). Physical examination alone is notoriously inaccurate (<50%) in the diagnosis of DVT.

   (2) Noninvasive studies of the venous system, most notably B-mode ultrasonography plus color Doppler (duplex scanning), have revolutionized the diagnosis and management of suspected DVT. Reported sensitivity and specificity of this test for the detection of proximal DVT are greater than 90%, with nearly 100% positive predictive value. This modality is less reliable in the detection of infrapopliteal thrombi, and a negative study in symptomatic patients should be followed by repeat examination in 48 to 72 hours to evaluate for propagation of clot proximally. Patients in whom a negative study contrasts with a strong clinical suspicion may require contrast venography, the gold standard for diagnosis of DVT.

   b. Treatment. See Chapter 5.

  2. Diagnosis and treatment of pulmonary embolism

   a. Diagnosis

   (1) Symptoms of PE are neither sensitive nor specific. Mental status changes, dyspnea, pleuritic chest pain, and cough can occur, and hemoptysis is encountered occasionally. Signs of PE most commonly include tachypnea and tachycardia. Patients with massive PE may experience syncope or cardiovascular collapse. PE should be considered in any postoperative patient with unexplained dyspnea, hypoxia, tachycardia, or dysrhythmia.

   (2) Laboratory studies. Initial evaluation of patients with suspected PE must include noninvasive arterial oxygen saturation, ECG, and CXR. Findings that are suggestive of PE include arterial oxygen desaturation, nonspecific ST-wave or T-wave changes on ECG, and atelectasis, parenchymal abnormalities, or pleural effusion on CXR. Such classic signs as $S_1Q_3T_3$ on ECG or a prominent central pulmonary artery with decreased pulmonary vascularity (Westermark's sign) on CXR are uncommon. ABG determination is a helpful adjunctive test; a decreased arterial oxygen tension (Pao_2) (<80 mm Hg), an elevated alveolar–arterial oxygen gradient, or a respiratory alkalosis may support clinical suspicion. Data that are obtained from these initial studies collectively may corroborate clinical suspicion but alone are neither sensitive nor specific for PE. **D-Dimer** assays have a high negative predictive value; however, positive values, particularly in the setting of recent surgery, are less helpful because the postoperative period is one of many conditions that can cause an elevation of this test.

(3) Imaging studies

(a) Spiral computed tomography scan is becoming the primary diagnostic modality for PE. The advantages of CT scans for PE include increased sensitivity, the ability simultaneously to evaluate other pulmonary and mediastinal abnormalities, greater after-hours availability, and the ability to obtain a CT venogram with the same dye load. This study subjects the patient to a contrast dye load and requires a large (18 g) IV in the antecubital vein, but it is not invasive. There are still wide variations in technology and institutional expertise with this modality, with reported sensitivities ranging from 57% to 100% and specificity ranging from 78% to 100%.

(b) A **V/Q scan** that demonstrates one or more perfusion defects in the absence of matched ventilation defects is abnormal and may be interpreted as high, intermediate, or low probability for PE, depending on the type and degree of abnormality. V/Q scans alone are neither sensitive nor specific for PE, and their interpretation may be difficult in patients with preexisting lung disease, especially COPD. Nevertheless, high-probability scans are 90% predictive and suffice for diagnosis of PE. In the appropriate clinical setting, a high-probability V/Q scan should prompt treatment. Likewise, a normal scan virtually excludes PE (96%). Scans of intermediate probability require additional confirmatory tests.

(c) Pulmonary angiography is the reference standard for the diagnosis of PE, but it is an invasive test with some element of risk. This test is rapidly being supplanted by spiral CT for most circumstances. Its use should be reserved for (1) resolution of conflicting or inconclusive clinical and noninvasive data; (2) patients with high clinical suspicion for PE and extensive preexisting pulmonary disease in whom interpretation of V/Q scans is difficult without access to spiral CT; and (3) confirmation of clinical and noninvasive data in patients who are at high risk for anticoagulation or in unstable patients being considered for thrombolytic therapy, pulmonary embolectomy, or vena caval interruption.

b. Treatment

(1) Supportive measures include administration of oxygen to correct hypoxemia and use of intravenous fluids to maintain BP. Hypotensive patients with high clinical suspicion of PE (i.e., high-risk patients, patients with acute right heart failure or right ventricular ischemia on ECG) require immediate transfer to an intensive care unit, where hemodynamic monitoring and vasoactive medications may be required.

(2) Anticoagulation with intravenous heparin should be started immediately with a target activated partial thromboplastin time (PTT) of 50 to 80 seconds. Oral warfarin can be started concurrently while heparin is continued until a therapeutic prothrombin time is achieved. Anticoagulation should continue for 6 months unless risk factors persist or DVT recurs. Some studies have shown that low-molecular-weight heparin administered subcutaneously (1 mg/kg every 12 hours) may be as effective as intravenous heparin.

(3) Thrombolytic therapy is not indicated in the routine treatment of PE in surgical patients because the risk of hemorrhage in individuals with recent (<10 days) surgery outweighs the uncertain long-term benefits of this therapy. Surgical patients with shock secondary to angiographically proven massive PE that is refractory to anticoagulation should be considered for either transvenous embolectomy or open pulmonary embolectomy. These aggressive measures are rarely successful.

(4) Inferior vena caval filter placement is indicated when a contraindication to anticoagulation exists, a bleeding complication occurs while receiving anticoagulation, or a DVT or PE recurs during anticoagulation therapy.

G. Complications of diabetes

1. **Tight blood glucose control.** A recent prospective study of 1,548 patients who were admitted to a surgical intensive care unit on mechanical ventilation randomly assigned patients to tight control with intensive insulin therapy (sugar between 80 and 110 mg/dL) versus conventional control (blood glucose between 180 and 200 mg/dL and treatment only for levels >215 mg/dL). This study showed nearly a twofold decrease in mortality in the tight-glucose-control group. Intensive insulin therapy also reduced overall in-hospital mortality, bloodstream infections, acute renal failure, the median number of red cell transfusions, and critical illness polyneuropathy (*N Engl J Med* 2001;345:1359).

2. **Diabetic ketoacidosis (DKA)** may occur in any diabetic patient who is sufficiently stressed by illness or surgery. DKA patients who require an operation should be provided every attempt at correction of metabolic abnormalities before surgery, although in cases such as gangrene, surgery may be essential for treatment of the underlying cause of DKA. DKA may occur without excessive elevation of the blood glucose. Management of this disorder should emphasize volume repletion, correction of acidosis and electrolyte abnormalities, and regulation of blood glucose with insulin infusion.

   a. **Laboratory evaluation**

      (1) **Blood glucose.**

      (2) **Complete blood count.**

      (3) **Serum electrolytes.**

      (4) **Serum osmolarity.**

      (5) **Arterial blood gas.**

   b. **Restoration of intravascular volume** should be initiated with isotonic (0.9%) saline or lactated Ringer's solution without glucose. Patients without cardiac disease should receive 1 L or more of fluid per hour until objective evidence of normalization of intravascular volume is demonstrated by a urine output greater than 30 mL/hour and stabilization of hemodynamics. Invasive hemodynamic monitoring may be required to guide fluid replacement in some circumstances (i.e., CHF, MI, and renal failure). Maintenance fluids of 0.45% NaCl with potassium (20 to 40 mEq/L) can be instituted when intravascular volume has been restored. Dextrose can be added to fluids when the blood glucose is less than 400 mg/dL.

   c. **Correction of acidosis** with bicarbonate therapy is controversial but should be considered if the blood pH is less than 7.1 or shock is present. Two ampules (88 mEq $NaHCO_3$) of bicarbonate can be added to 0.45% NaCl and given during the initial resuscitation.

   d. **Potassium replacement** should be instituted immediately unless hyperkalemia with ECG changes exists. In nonoliguric patients, replacement should begin with 30 to 40 mEq/hour of KCl for serum potassium of less than 3; 20 to 30 mEq/hour of KCl for serum potassium of 3 to 4; and 10 to 20 mEq/hour of KCl for potassium of greater than 4 mEq/L.

   e. **Blood glucose** can be controlled with 10 units of insulin as an intravenous bolus followed by insulin infusion at 2 to 10 units per hour to a target range of 200 to 300 mg/dL. When the blood glucose falls below 400 mg/dL, 5% dextrose must be added to the intravenous fluids. Therapy is guided by hourly blood glucose determinations.

3. **Nonketotic hyperosmolar syndrome** is characterized by severe hyperglycemia and dehydration without ketoacidosis. This occurs most often in elderly non–insulin-dependent diabetes mellitus patients with renal impairment and may be precipitated by surgical illness or stress. Laboratory findings include blood glucose that exceeds 600 mg/dL and serum osmolarity of greater than 350 mOsm/L. Therapy is similar to that for DKA but with two notable exceptions: (1) Fluid requirements are often higher, and replacement should be with 0.45% saline, and (2) total insulin requirements are less.

H. Hypertension

1. **Definition.** Postoperative hypertension should be defined by the patient's preoperative blood pressure. Patients with chronic hypertension have a shift in

their cerebral autoregulatory system that may not allow for adequate cerebral perfusion at normotensive blood pressures. A reasonable goal of therapy for acute postoperative hypertension is within 10% of the patient's normal blood pressure.

2. **Treatment.** Before using antihypertensive drugs in the treatment of postoperative hypertension, it is essential to diagnose and treat underlying causes, such as pain, hypoxemia, hypothermia, and acidosis. Acute hypertension can be managed with clonidine (0.1 mg orally every 6 hours), hydralazine (10 to 20 mg intravenously every 6 hours), labetalol (10 to 20 mg intravenously every 10 minutes, to a total dose of 300 mg), or a nitroprusside drip (0.25 to 8 μg/kg/minute intravenously). In situations in which the patient is unable to take oral medications and intravenous medications are not appropriate, nitroglycerin paste (0.5 to 2 in. every 6 hours) can be used.

IV. DOCUMENTATION

Optimal patient care requires not only appropriate management, but also effective communication and documentation. Documentation is essential for communication among members of the health care team, risk management, and reimbursement. All documentation should include a date, time, legible signature, and contact information (such as phone or pager number) in case clarification is necessary.

A. **Hospital orders**

1. **Admission orders** should detail every aspect of a patient's care. **ADCVAANDIML** is a simple mnemonic to help in organizing admission, postoperative, and transfer orders:

   a. **Admit.** Include nursing division, surgical service, attending physician, and admission status (in-patient versus 23-hour observation).

   b. **Diagnosis.** The principal diagnosis and, if relevant, care path. Include the operation or procedure performed.

   c. **Condition.** Distinguish among good, satisfactory, serious, and critical.

   d. **Vitals.** Include the frequency that vital signs should be obtained and special instructions such as pulse oximetry and neurologic and vascular checks.

   e. **Allergies.** Include specific reactions if known.

   f. **Activity.** Include necessary supervision and weight-bearing status, if applicable. If mobilizing the patient, include specific instructions for ambulation. Patients on bedrest should be considered for DVT prophylaxis.

   g. **Nursing orders.** These may include dressing care, drain care, urine output monitoring, antiembolic stockings, and sequential compression devices. Include specific parameters for physician notification for abnormal results (such as low urine output or low blood pressure). Daily weights, intake and output, pulmonary toilet (such as incentive spirometry), and regimens for turning patients should be addressed here. So should **ventilator settings,** if applicable. Include mode, rate, tidal volume or pressure support, positive end-expiratory pressure, and oxygen percentage (FiO_2).

   h. **Diet.** Include diet type (regular, American Diabetes Association, renal, etc.) and consistency (clear liquids, full liquids, pureed, etc.) as well as supervision instructions, if applicable. Patients are NPO after midnight if a procedure requiring sedation is planned for the following day.

   i. **Intravenous fluids.** Include fluid type, rate, and time interval.

   j. **Medications.** Include home medicines if appropriate. Reference to patient-controlled anesthesia forms should be made here. Indications for new medications should be provided. Include the dose, route, and frequency of each medication ordered.

   k. **Laboratories.** All necessary laboratory and radiographic investigations should be listed here, as well as electrocardiograms, cardiac diagnostic laboratory testing, pulmonary function tests, and other special procedures.

2. **Review orders with nursing staff.** All orders should be reviewed with the nursing staff, particularly any unusual orders or orders that must be expedited.

3. **STAT (immediately) orders** should be designated as such on the order form and brought to the attention of the nursing staff. This is especially true for orders for

new medicines because the pharmacy must be notified and the medicine brought to the floor.

4. Discharge orders
   a. Discharge should include location and condition. If a transfer to another institution is planned, copies of all medical records and a copy of current orders should be included.
   b. Activity limitations, if applicable, should be included. Workplace or school documentation may also be necessary.
   c. Medicines. Prescriptions for new medicines as well as detailed instructions are required.
   d. Follow-up. Follow-up plans with the appropriate physicians should be clearly indicated, with contact information for their offices.
   e. Special. Wound care, catheter care, physical therapy, home health care needs, or special studies should be described before discharge.

B. Hospital notes
   1. History and physical examination. The admission history and physical examination should be a complete record of the patient's history. Include past medical and surgical history, social history and family history, allergies, and home medicines with dose and schedule. A complete review of systems should be documented. Outpatient records are often helpful and should be obtained if possible.
   2. Preoperative notes summarize the results of pertinent laboratory tests and other investigations before one proceeds to the operating room (Table 1-10).
   3. Operative notes. A brief operative note should be placed in the written medical record immediately following the operation, including the operative findings and the patient's condition at the conclusion of the procedure (Table 1-11). The surgeon should also complete a dictated operative note immediately after the operation. In addition, a dictated note should include specific operative indications, preparation and drape position, sponge and instrument count, and copy distribution.
   4. Postoperative check. Several hours after an operation, a patient should be examined and vital signs and urine output reviewed. Documentation in the medical record in the form of a SOAP (subjective-objective-assessment-plan) note should be included.
   5. Discharge summary. A detailed account of a patient's hospitalization should be dictated at the time of discharge (Table 1-12). If a dictation confirmation number is provided, it should be recorded in the written medical record as the final note of the hospitalization. A discharge summary must accompany any patient who is being transferred to another institution.

V. INFORMED CONSENT
   A. Obtaining informed consent. Recognition of patient autonomy dictates that physicians provide adequate information so that patients can make informed decisions regarding their medical care. Patients should understand the disease process, the

TABLE 1-10	Preoperative Note

Preoperative diagnosis
Procedure planned
Attending physician
Laboratory investigations
Electrocardiogram (if applicable)
Chest x-ray and other radiology (if applicable)
Informed consent
NPO (nothing by mouth) past midnight
Type and screen/cross (if applicable)

TABLE 1-11	Brief Operative Note

Preoperative diagnosis
Postoperative diagnosis
Procedure performed
Attending surgeon
Assistant/resident surgeons
Type of anesthesia
Operative findings and complications
Specimens removed
Packs, drains, and catheters
Estimated blood loss
Urine output
Fluids administered
   Blood products administered
   Antibiotics administered
Documentation that "time-out" to verify correct patient, procedure, and site was performed
Patient disposition and condition

natural course of the disease, the risks and benefits of the procedure under consideration, and potential alternative therapies. The most common and serious risks of the procedure and the patient's condition that might affect the outcome of a planned procedure or might place the patient at increased risk should be discussed. Recovery time, including amount and expected duration of postoperative pain, hospitalization, and future functional status, should also be reviewed. The use of invasive monitoring devices, including arterial and pulmonary artery catheters, should be explained. These discussions should use terms that are readily understood by the patient. This is also an important opportunity for a physician to learn about the patient's wishes for aggressive treatment and acceptance of limitations to functional status.

B. Documentation of informed consent. An informed consent form is completed and signed by the patient before any elective operative procedure. In addition to the generic consent form, informed consent discussions should be documented in the progress notes section of the medical record. These notes should document the salient features of the informed consent discussion and specifically document that the potential complications and outcomes were explained to the patient. The patient's refusal to undergo a procedure that has been recommended by the physician should

TABLE 1-12	Discharge Summary (Dictated)

Your name, date, and time of dictation
Patient name
Patient registration number
Attending physician
Date of admission
Date of discharge
Principal diagnosis
Secondary diagnosis
Brief history and physical examination
Laboratory/radiographic findings
Hospital course
List of procedures performed with dates
Discharge instructions
Discharge condition
Copy distribution

be documented clearly in the chart. In certain situations, such as a medical emergency, it is impossible to obtain informed consent. Inability to obtain consent should be documented carefully in the medical record. Local medical bylaws generally have provisions for these types of situations and should be consulted on a case-by-case basis.

VI. ADVANCE DIRECTIVES. These are legal documents that allow patients to provide specific instructions for health care treatment in the event that the patient is unable to make or communicate these decisions personally. Advance directives commonly include standard living wills and durable powers of attorney for health care. With the growing realization that medical technology can prolong life considerably and sometimes even indefinitely beyond the point of significant or meaningful recovery, the importance of these issues is clear. Patients should be offered the opportunity to execute an advance directive on admission to the hospital.

  A. Living wills provide specific instructions for the withdrawal of medical treatment in the event that a patient is unable to make treatment decisions and is terminally ill. Living wills do not include withdrawal or withholding of any procedure to provide nutrition or hydration.

  B. Durable powers of attorney for health care. These directives allow a patient to legally designate a surrogate or proxy to make health care decisions if the patient is unable to do so. Because of the difficulty of predicting the complexities of aggressive medical management, powers of attorney are often more helpful than living wills in making difficult treatment decisions.

  C. Implementation. Advance directives are personal documents and therefore differ from patient to patient. These documents should be reviewed carefully before implementation. Advanced directives are legal documents, and they should be displayed prominently in the medical record. To be legally binding, the documents must be executed properly. If there is any question of validity, the risk management or legal staff of the hospital should be consulted. The most effective advance directives include specific instructions for health care decisions. Important issues to be addressed include the following:

   1. Intravenous fluids.
   2. Enteral and parenteral nutrition.
   3. Medicines.
   4. Inotropic support.
   5. Renal dialysis.
   6. Mechanical ventilation.
   7. Cardiopulmonary resuscitation.

  D. Conflicts. Although advance directives can be helpful in the management of critically ill patients, their implementation often is difficult. Advance directives, by their nature, cannot provide for every medical situation. For this reason, it is important to communicate with the patient and family before the execution of an advance directive and with the family in the event that a patient becomes incapacitated. If no advance directive is available, the physician and family must consider carefully when life-prolonging medical treatments are no longer beneficial to the patient. In such a case, the state's interest in preserving life might conflict with the desires of the family and physician. If the family and physician do not agree, the hospital ethics committee or risk management staff should be consulted.

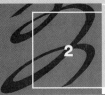

NUTRITION

Elizabeth A. Fialkowski and J. Chris Eagon

Nutrition plays a vital and often overlooked role in the care of patients on a surgical service. Between 30% and 50% of hospitalized patients are malnourished, and malnutrition is clearly associated with increased morbidity and mortality in select general surgical patients. Although most healthy patients can tolerate 7 days of starvation (with adequate glucose and fluid replacement), those who have been subject to major trauma, a prolonged operative course, sepsis, cancer-related cachexia, or other physiologic stressors require earlier nutritional intervention. However, the prudent use of nutritional support is important because not only is misuse cost-inefficient, but it also can adversely affect patient recovery. The only patient populations that have been identified as clearly benefiting from perioperative nutrition support are severely malnourished patients (*J Parenter Enteral Nutr* 2002;26:1SA).

METABOLISM

I. METABOLISM OF PROTEINS, CARBOHYDRATES, AND FATS

A. Proteins are important for the biosynthesis of enzymes, structural molecules, and immunoglobulins; the balance between protein synthesis and degradation is critical.

1. **Digestion of proteins** yields dipeptides and single amino acids, which are actively absorbed. Gastric pepsin initiates the process of digestion. Pancreatic proteases, activated on exposure to enterokinase found throughout the duodenal mucosa, are the principal effectors of protein degradation. Once digested, almost 50% of protein absorption occurs in the duodenum, and complete protein absorption is achieved by the midjejunum. Protein absorption can effectively occur at every level of the small intestine; therefore, clinically significant protein malabsorption is relatively infrequent, even after extensive intestinal resection. The 20 amino acids are divided into essential and nonessential groups, depending on whether they can be synthesized *de novo* in the body. Only the L isotype is utilized in human protein.

2. **Major roles of amino acids** include the following:
   a. **Synthesis and recycling** of proteins.
   b. **Catabolic reactions,** resulting in energy generation and CO_2 production.
   c. **Incorporation of nitrogen** into nonessential amino acids and nucleotides.
   d. **Transport and storage** of small molecules and ions.

3. **Metabolism of absorbed amino acids,** primarily by the liver, regulates accumulation of plasma amino acids. Parenteral nutrition initially bypasses the liver by delivering amino acids directly into the systemic circulation. A baseline nitrogen loss of 10 to 15 g/day occurs through urinary excretion.

4. **Total body protein** in a 70-kg person is approximately 10 to 11 kg, concentrated mostly in skeletal muscle. Daily protein turnover is 250 to 300 g, or approximately 3% of total body protein. The primary site of turnover is the gastrointestinal (GI) tract, where shed enterocytes and secreted digestive enzymes are regularly lost. Excessive GI tract losses from a fistula, ileostomy, or draining gastrostomy and losses from partial- or full-thickness skin burns or seeping wounds provide other potential sources of significant protein loss in surgical patients. Protein turnover decreases with age, from 25 g/kg per day in the neonate to 3 g/kg per day in the adult.

5. **Protein requirements** in the average healthy adult without excessive losses are approximately 0.8 g/kg body weight. In the United States, the typical daily intake averages twice this amount. Requirements for patients with acute illness increase to 1.2 g/kg/day and up to 2.5 g/kg/day in severely physiologically stressed patients in the intensive care unit (ICU). Generally, protein intake of 6.25 g is equivalent to 1 g of nitrogen. Amino acids contribute only 15% of the normal energy expenditure, with the remainder supplied by carbohydrates and fat. Each gram of protein can be converted into **4 kcal** of energy.

B. **Carbohydrates** are the body's primary energy source, providing 30% to 40% of calories in a typical diet.

1. **Carbohydrate digestion** is initiated by the action of salivary amylase, and absorption is generally completed within the first 1 to 1.5 m of small intestine. Salivary and pancreatic amylases cleave starches into oligosaccharides. Surface oligosaccharidases then hydrolyze and transport these molecules across the GI tract mucosa. Deficiencies in carbohydrate digestion and absorption are rare in surgical patients. Because pancreatic amylase is abundant, even in patients with limited pancreatic function, maldigestion of starch does not usually occur. Diseases that result in generalized mucosal flattening (e.g., celiac sprue, Whipple disease, and hypogammaglobulinemia) may cause diminished uptake of carbohydrates because of resultant deficiencies in oligosaccharidases.

2. **Glucose stores.** More than 75% of ingested carbohydrate is broken down and absorbed as glucose. Hyperglycemia leads to insulin secretion, which in turn influences protein synthesis. A minimum intake of 400 calories of carbohydrate per day minimizes protein breakdown, particularly after adaptation to starvation. Cellular uptake of glucose (stimulated by insulin) also inhibits lipolysis and promotes glycogen formation. Conversely, glucagon is released in response to starvation or stress; it promotes proteolysis, glycogenolysis, lipolysis, and increased serum glucose. Glucose is essential for wound repair, but excessive amounts can have adverse effects, including hepatic steatosis and neutrophil dysfunction. Each gram of enteral carbohydrate provides **4 kcal** of energy. Parenteral carbohydrate (e.g., dextrose) provides **3.4 kcal/g.**

C. **Lipids** comprise the remaining 25% to 45% of calories in the typical diet. During starvation, lipids provide the majority of energy in the form of ketone bodies converted by the liver from long-chain fatty acids (see Section II.A).

1. **Digestion and absorption of lipids** is complex and requires coordination between **biliary and pancreatic secretions**, as well as a functional jejunum and ileum. The introduction of fat to the duodenum produces secretion of cholecystokinin and secretin, which lead to gallbladder contraction and pancreatic enzyme release, respectively. **Pancreatic secretions** contain a combination of lipase, cholesterol esterase, and phospholipase A_2. In the alkaline environment of the duodenum, lipase hydrolyzes triglycerides to one monoglyceride and two fatty acids. Bile salts lead to emulsification. **Micelle formation** is the most important step in lipid absorption, facilitating absorption of fats across the mucosal barrier. Reabsorption of bile salts is necessary to maintain the bile salt pool (i.e., the enterohepatic circulation). The liver is able to compensate for moderate intestinal bile salt losses by increased synthesis from cholesterol. Major ileal resection may lead to depletion of the bile salt pool and subsequent fat malabsorption. Lipolysis is stimulated by steroids, catecholamines, and glucagon but is inhibited by insulin. **Stress causes dramatic lipolysis.** Each gram of lipid provides **9 kcal** of energy.

2. The **essential fatty acids** linoleic acid and linolenic acid are required for cell membrane integrity. Dietary fats are the sole precursors to eicosanoid production and as such are potent immunomodulators. Arachidonic acid, a vital component in prostaglandin synthesis, can be manufactured from linoleic acid. Clinical deficiency results in a generalized scaling rash, poor wound healing, hepatic steatosis, and bone changes. This condition is usually a consequence of long-term fat-free parenteral nutrition, in which high glucose levels stimulate relative hyperinsulinemia, thus inhibiting lipolysis and preventing peripheral essential fatty acid liberation. This can be avoided by providing at least 3% of caloric intake as parenteral lipid.

II. STRESS METABOLISM

A. Starvation. After an overnight fast, liver glycogen is rapidly depleted due to decreased plasma insulin and a rise in glucagon levels. Carbohydrate stores are exhausted after a 24-hour fast. Liver glycogen is used first, followed by muscle glycogen. In the first few days of starvation, caloric needs are supplied by fat and protein degradation. Most of the available protein is from breakdown of skeletal and visceral muscle. Protein is converted to glucose via hepatic gluconeogenesis. The brain preferentially uses this endogenously produced glucose, with the remainder consumed by red blood cells and leukocytes. Within approximately 10 days of starvation, the brain adapts to use fat as its fuel source. Because the brain cannot use free fatty acids in the same manner as other tissues do, it relies on ketoacids produced by the liver. This adaptation to ketone usage has a protein-sparing effect. In summary, the adaptive changes to starvation are a decrease in basal energy expenditure (up to 30%), a change in the type of fuel consumed (which maximizes the caloric potential), and relative preservation of protein.

B. Physiologic stress. The interaction of metabolic and endocrine responses that result from major operation, trauma, or sepsis can be divided into three phases.

1. Catabolic phase. After major injury, the metabolic demand is dramatically increased, as reflected in a significant rise in the urinary excretion of nitrogen (beyond that seen in simple starvation). Following a major surgical procedure, protein depletion inevitably occurs because patients are commonly prevented from eating in addition to having an elevated basal metabolic rate. The hormonal response of physiologic stress includes elevation in the serum levels of glucagon, glucocorticoids, and catecholamines and reduction in insulin.

2. The **early anabolic phase** is also called the *corticoid-withdrawal phase* as the body shifts from catabolism to anabolism. The timing of this event is variable, depending on the severity of stress, and ranges from several days to several weeks. The period of anabolism can last from a few weeks to a few months, depending on many factors, including the ability of the patient to obtain and use nutrients and the extent to which protein stores have been depleted. This phase is marked by a positive nitrogen balance, and there is a rapid and progressive gain in weight and muscular strength. The total amount of nitrogen gained is equivalent to the amount lost in the catabolic phase; however, the rate of repletion is much slower than the rapid rate of protein depletion after the original insult.

3. The **late anabolic phase** is the final period of recovery and may last from several weeks to months. Adipose stores are replenished gradually, and nitrogen balance equilibrates. Weight gain is much slower during this period than in the early anabolic phase due to the higher caloric content of fat—the primary energy stores deposited during the early anabolic phase—as compared to protein.

NUTRITIONAL ASSESSMENT AND ADMINISTRATION

I. NUTRITIONAL ASSESSMENT is essential for identifying patients who are at risk of developing complications related to significant malnutrition. Preoperative nutritional support can significantly reduce perioperative morbidity and mortality in patients with severe malnutrition (*N Engl J Med* 1991;325:52). In addition, the incidence of postoperative morbidities, such as intra-abdominal abscess, anastomotic leakage, and ileus, may be decreased by the use of preoperative enteral or parenteral hyperalimentation in malnourished patients. Preoperative nutritional support for patients with only mild or moderate malnutrition is not routinely indicated. Table 2-1 presents nutritional and biologic indices developed to predict the risk of perioperative morbidity and mortality.

A. Types of malnutrition. Originally identified in children, two forms of malnutrition can be generalized to adults.

1. Marasmus is characterized by inadequate protein *and* caloric intake, typically caused by illness-induced anorexia. It is a chronic nutritional deficiency marked by losses in weight, body fat, and skeletal muscle mass (as identified by

TABLE 2-1	Nutritional Indices

Body mass index (BMI)
BMI = weight (kg)/[height (m)]^2 = 703 × weight (lb)/[height (in.)]^2
BMI: normal 18.5–24.9, overweight 25–29.9, obese 30–40, morbid obesity >40

Prognostic nutritional index (PNI)
PNI = 158 − 16.6 (Alb) − 0.78 (TSF) − 0.2 (TFN) − 5.8 (DH)
DH: >5 mm induration = 2; 1–5 mm induration = 1; anergy = 0
PNI: >50% = high risk for complications; 40%–49% = intermediate risk; <40% = low risk

Nutrition risk index
NRI = 15.19 (Alb) + 41.7 [weight (kg)/ideal weight (kg)]
NRI: <100 = malnourished

Catabolic index (CI)
CI = UUN − [0.5 (dietary nitrogen intake in g)]
CI: 0 = no significant stress; 0–5 = mild stress; >5 = moderate to severe stress

Alb, albumin (g/dL); DH, delayed cutaneous hypersensitivity; TFN, transferrin (mg/dL); TSF, triceps skinfold thickness (mm); UUN, 24-hr urine urea nitrogen excretion (g).
Adapted from Charney PJ. Nutrition screening and assessment. In: Skipper A, ed. *Dietitian's Handbook of Enteral and Parenteral Nutrition*, 2nd ed. Gaithersburg, MD: Aspen Publishers; 1998:324.

anthropometric measurements). Visceral protein stores remain normal, as do most lab indices. Patients with marasmus may lose substantial body weight but are able to resist infection and respond appropriately to minor or moderate stress.

2. **Kwashiorkor** is characterized by catabolic protein loss, resulting in **hypoalbuminemia** and generalized **edema**. This form of malnutrition develops with prolonged starvation or severe stress. Even in a well-nourished patient, a severe stress (e.g., major burn or prolonged sepsis) may rapidly lead to depletion of visceral protein stores and impairment in immune function. Conventional anthropometric measurements may not identify these patients as being significantly malnourished.

B. **Evaluation of preexisting deficits.** A dietary history, physical examination (including anthropometric measurements), and relevant labs are the appropriate tools needed for an accurate evaluation of a patient's preoperative nutritional status. The Subjective Global Assessment (*J Parenter Enteral Nutr* 1987;11:8), based on key history and physical exam findings, is the only method that has been validated as reliably stratifying patients according to nutritional status (*J Parenter Enteral Nutr* 2002;26:1SA).

1. A **history** of weight fluctuation or a change in dietary habits is particularly relevant. In most cases, the possibility of malnutrition is suggested by the underlying disease or by a history of recent weight loss. Anorexia, nausea, vomiting, dysphagia, odynophagia, gastroesophageal reflux, or a history of generalized muscle weakness should prompt further evaluation. Recent weight loss (5% in the last month or 10% over 6 months) or a current body weight of 80% to 85% (or less) of ideal body weight suggests significant malnutrition. A complete history of current medications is essential to alert caretakers to potential underlying deficiencies as well as drug–nutrient interactions.

2. **Physical examination** may identify muscle wasting (especially thenar and temporal muscles), loose or flabby skin (indicating loss of subcutaneous fat), and peripheral edema and/or ascites (as a result of hypoproteinemia). Subtler findings of nutritional deficiency include skin rash, pallor, glossitis, gingival lesions, hair changes, hepatomegaly, neuropathy, and dementia (*A.S.P.E.N. Nutrition Support Practice Manual*, 2nd ed. Gaithersburg, MD: Aspen; 1998).

3. **Anthropometric measurements** such as triceps skinfold thickness and midarm muscle circumference reflect body-fat stores and skeletal muscle mass, respectively. These values are standardized for gender and height and should be reported as a percentage of the predicted value. Along with body mass index, these values allow the clinician to assess the patient's visceral and somatic protein mass and fat reserve.

4. **Laboratory tests** associated with nutrition have been shown to predict perioperative morbidity (*N Engl J Med* 1991;325:525) and mortality (*Arch Surg* 1999;134:36). As negative acute-phase proteins, albumin, prealbumin, and transferrin are indicators of the *degree of illness* rather than strictly nutritional status, their levels vary with the hepatic metabolic response (decreased synthesis) and capillary leak response (diluted serum levels) to inflammation (*J Am Diet Assoc* 2004;104:1258). Given their increased morbidity, patients with altered levels are more likely to need nutritional support. Levels associated with illness are as follows:

   a. **Serum albumin** of less than 3.5 g/dL (35 g/L) in a stable, hydrated patient; half-life is 14 to 20 days.

   b. **Serum prealbumin** may be a more useful indicator of acute changes: 10 to 17 mg/dL corresponds to mild depletion, 5 to 10 mg/dL to moderate depletion, and less than 5 mg/dL to severe depletion; half-life is 2 to 3 days.

   c. **Serum transferrin** of less than 200 mg/dL; half-life is 8 to 10 days.

5. **Immune function** is frequently altered by malnutrition. The degree of derangement can be determined by assessing the following:

   a. **Delayed-type hypersensitivity** (anergy to common skin antigens).

   b. **Total lymphocyte count (TLC),** as calculated by the formula

$$\mathrm{TLC} = \frac{\%\ \mathrm{lymphocytes} \times \mathrm{WBC}}{100},$$

where WBC is the white blood cell count. TLC of 1,500 to 1,800/mm^3 corresponds to mild depletion, 900 to 1,500/mm^3 to moderate depletion, and less than 900/mm^3 to severe depletion.

C. **Estimation of caloric requirements** is necessary to provide adequate substrates for healing and tissue repair. Failure to provide sufficient calories and protein leads to further depletion of lean body mass.

   1. **Basal energy expenditure (BEE)** can be predicted by using the Harris-Benedict equation:

      a. BEE in kilocalories per day for men equals 66.4 + [13.7 × weight (kg)] + [5 × height (cm)] – [6.8 × age (years)].

      b. BEE in kilocalories per day for women equals 655 + [9.6 × weight (kg)] + [1.7 × height (cm)] – [4.7 × age (years)].

   2. These equations provide a reliable estimate of the energy requirements in approximately 80% of hospitalized patients. The actual caloric need is obtained by multiplying BEE by specific stress factors (Table 2-2). Most stressed patients require 25 to 35 kcal/kg/day. In obese patients, these equations tend to overestimate caloric needs.

D. **Estimates of protein requirements.** The appropriate calorie:nitrogen ratio is approximately 150:1 (calorie:protein ratio of 24:1), which increases to 300:1 to 400:1 in uremia. In the absence of severe renal or hepatic dysfunction, approximately 1.5 g protein per kilogram body weight should be provided daily (Table 2-3).

   1. **Twenty-four–hour nitrogen balance** is calculated by subtracting nitrogen loss from nitrogen intake. Nitrogen intake is the sum of nitrogen delivered from enteral and parenteral feedings. Nitrogen is lost through urine, fistula drainage, diarrhea, and so on. The usual approach is to measure the urine urea nitrogen (UUN) concentration of a 24-hour urine collection and multiply by urine volume to estimate 24-hour urinary loss. Nitrogen loss equals 1.2 × [24-hour UUN (g per day)] + 2 g per day as a correction factor to account for nitrogen losses in stool and skin exfoliation.

| TABLE 2-2 | Disease Stress Factors Used in Calculation of Total Energy Expenditure |

Clinical condition	Stress factor
Starvation	0.80–1.00
Elective operation	1.00–1.10
Peritonitis or other infections	1.05–1.25
Adult respiratory distress syndrome or sepsis	1.30–1.35
Bone marrow transplant	1.20–1.30
Cardiopulmonary disease (noncomplicated)	0.80–1.00
Cardiopulmonary disease with dialysis or sepsis	1.20–1.30
Cardiopulmonary disease with major surgery	1.30–1.55
Acute renal failure	1.30
Liver failure	1.30–1.55
Liver transplant	1.20–1.50
Pancreatitis	1.30–1.80

Adapted from Shoppell JM, Hopkins B, Shronts EP. Nutrition screening and assessment. In: Gottschlich M, ed. *The Science and Practice of Nutrition Support: A Case Based Core Curriculum*. Dubuque, IA: Kendall/Hunt; 2001:107–140.

2. **Creatinine-height index (CHI)** can be used to determine the degree of malnutrition. A 24-hour urinary creatinine excretion is measured and compared to normal standards. The creatinine height index is calculated using the following equation:

$$CHI = \frac{\text{actual 24-hour creatinine excretion}}{\text{predicted creatinine excretion}}.$$

Greater than 80% represents no to mild protein depletion, 60% to 80% represents moderate depletion, and less than 60% represents severe depletion.

| TABLE 2-3 | Estimated Protein Requirements in Various Disease States |

Clinical condition	Protein requirements (g/kg ideal body weight per day)
Healthy, nonstressed	0.80
Bone marrow transplant	1.40–1.50
Liver disease without encephalopathy	1.00–1.50
Liver disease with encephalopathy	0.50–0.75 (advance as tolerated)
Renal failure without dialysis	0.60–1.00
Renal failure with dialysis	1.00–1.30
Pregnancy	1.30–1.50
Simplified estimates	
Mild metabolic stress (elective hospitalization)	1.00–1.10
Moderate metabolic stress (complicated postoperative care, infection)	1.20–1.40
Severe metabolic stress (major trauma, pancreatitis, sepsis)	1.50–2.50

Adapted from Nagel M. Nutrition screening: identifying patients at risk for malnutrition. *Nutr Clin Pract* 1998;8:171–175.

II. ADMINISTRATION OF NUTRITION

A. Indications. The need for nutritional support should be assessed continually in patients preoperatively and postoperatively. The majority of surgical patients do not require nutritional supplementation; perioperative dietary supplements provide no clinical benefit to well-nourished patients (*Nutrition* 2000;16:723). Most patients have adequate fuel reserves to withstand common catabolic stresses and partial starvation for at least 1 week. For these patients, intravenous fluids with appropriate electrolytes and a minimum of 100 g glucose daily (to minimize protein catabolism) is adequate. However, even patients who were well nourished before a major operation or trauma but subsequently enter a prolonged hypermetabolic or severely catabolic period may require nutritional support (*Curr Probl Surg* 1995;32:833). Without nutritional intervention, these patients may have complications related to impaired immune function and poor wound healing from depletion of visceral protein stores (see Chapter 6). Patients with a significant degree of preoperative malnutrition have less reserve, tolerate catabolic stress and starvation poorly, and are at higher risk for postoperative complications.

B. Enteral nutrition. In general, the enteral route is preferred over the parenteral route. Enteral feeding is simple, physiologic, relatively inexpensive, and well tolerated by most patients. Enteral feeding maintains the GI tract cytoarchitecture and mucosal integrity (via trophic effects), absorptive function, and normal microbial flora. This results in less bacterial translocation and endotoxin release from the intestinal lumen into the bloodstream (*Nutrition* 2000;16:606). **Enteral feedings are indicated** for patients who have a functional GI tract but are unable to sustain an adequate oral diet. **Enteral feedings may be contraindicated** in patients with an intestinal obstruction, ileus, GI bleeding, severe diarrhea, vomiting, enterocolitis, or a high-output enterocutaneous fistula. Choice of appropriate feeding site, administration technique, formula, and equipment may circumvent these problems.

1. Feeding tubes. Nasogastric, nasojejunal (e.g., Dobhoff), gastrostomy, and jejunal tubes are available for the administration of enteral feeds. Percutaneous gastrostomy tubes can be placed endoscopically or under fluoroscopy. The techniques for tube placement and the common complications associated with their use are discussed in Chapters 9 and 10.

2. Enteral feeding products. A variety of commercially available enteral formulas are available. Standard solutions provide 1 kcal/mL; calorically concentrated solutions (>1 kcal/mL) are available for patients who require volume restriction. The available dietary formulations for enteral feedings can be divided into polymeric (blenderized and nutritionally complete commercial formulas), chemically defined formulas (elemental diets), and modular formulas (Table 2-4).

a. Blenderized tube feedings can contain any food that can be blenderized. Caloric distribution of these formulas should parallel that of a normal diet.

b. Nutritionally complete formulas (standard enteral diets) vary in protein, carbohydrate, and fat composition. Several formulas use sucrose or glucose as carbohydrates and are suitable for lactose-deficient patients. Commercial formulas are convenient, sterile, and inexpensive. They are recommended for patients with minimal metabolic stress and normal gut function.

c. Chemically defined formulas (*elemental diets*). The nutrients are provided in predigested and readily absorbed form. They contain protein in the form of free amino acids or polypeptides. They are hyperosmolar, which may cause cramping and diarrhea. Elemental diets are efficiently absorbed in the presence of compromised gut function. However, they are costlier.

d. Modular formulations are designed for use in specific clinical situations (e.g., pulmonary, renal, or hepatic failure or immune dysfunction).

3. Enteral feeding protocols. It is recommended to start with a full-strength formula at a slow rate, which is steadily advanced. This reduces the risk of microbial contamination and achieves goal intake earlier. This approach can also be used with high-osmolarity or elemental feeds. Conservative initiation and advancement are recommended for patients who are critically ill, those who have not been fed for some time, and those receiving a high-osmolarity or calorie-dense formula.

TABLE 2-4 Enteral Formulas

Product	Description	kcal/mL	mOsm	Protein [g (% kcal)]	Carbo-hydrates [g (% kcal)]	Fat [g (% kcal)]	H₂O (mL)	Na (mEq)	K (mEq)	Ca (mg)	PO₄ (mg)	Vitamin K (mg)
Standard												
Ensure	Lactose-free, low residue	1.06	470	37.2 (14)	145 (54.5)	37.2 (31.5)	845	36.8	40	530	530	43
Osmolite	Isotonic, lactose-free, low residue	1.06	300	37.2 (14)	145 (54.6)	38.5 (31.4)	841	27.6	25.9	530	530	43
Jevity	Isotonic, lactose-free, high dietary fiber (14.4 g/L), high nitrogen content	1.06	310	44.4 (16.7)	151.7 (53.3)	36.8 (30)	833	40.4	40	909	756	61
Glucerna	Lactose-free, low carbohydrates, high fiber (14.4 g/L)	1	375	41.8 (16.7)	93.7 (33.3)	55.7 (50)	873	40.3	40	703	703	57
Low volume												
Ensure Plus	Lactose-free, low residue	1.5	690	54.9 (14.7)	200 (53.3)	53.3 (32)	769	45.9	49.7	704	704	57
Magnacal	Lactose-free, low residue	2	590	70 (14)	250 (50)	80 (34)	690	43.5	32	1,000	1,000	300
Low volume, high nitrogen												
Ensure Plus HN	Lactose-free, low residue	1.5	650	62.6 (16.7)	199.9 (53.3)	50 (30)	769	51.5	46.5	1,056	1,056	85

(continued)

TABLE 2-4 Enteral Formulas (Continued)

Product	Description	kcal/mL	mOsm	Protein [g (% kcal)]	Carbohydrates [g (% kcal)]	Fat [g (% kcal)]	H$_2$O (mL)	Na (mEq)	K (mEq)	Ca (mg)	PO$_4$ (mg)	Vitamin K (mg)
						Per 1,000 mL						
Perative	Lactose-free, low residue	1.3	425	66.6 (20.5)	177 (54.5)	37.3 (25)	789	45.2	44.3	867	867	70
Very high nitrogen												
Replete with Fiber	Lactose-free, high fiber (14 g/L)	1	300	62.5 (25)	113 (45)	34 (30)	840	21.7	40	1,000	1,000	80
Sustacal	Lactose-free, low residue	1.01	650	61 (24)	140 (55)	23 (21)	840	40	54	1,010	930	240
Elemental												
Vivonex TEN	Elemental, low fat, low residue	1	630	38.2 (15.3)	205.6 (82.2)	2.77 (2.5)	845	20	20	500	500	22.3
Pudding (per 5-oz serving)												
Ensure Pudding	Contains lactose	250		6.8	34.0	9.7		10.4	8.5	200	200	12
Modulars (analysis per tablespoon)												
Polycose Liquid	Glucose polymer	30			7.5							
ProMod	Protein supplement	17		3	0.4	0.4		0	1			
Microlipid	Fat supplement	67.5				7.5				15.6	15.6	
MCT Oil	MCT supplement	115.5				14						

MCT, medium-chain triglycerides.

a. **Bolus feedings** are reserved for patients with nasogastric or gastrostomy feeding tubes. Feedings are administered by gravity, begin at 50 to 100 mL every 4 hours, and are increased in 50-mL increments until goal intake is reached (usually 240 to 360 mL every 4 hours). Tracheobronchial aspiration is a potentially serious complication because feedings are prepyloric. To reduce the risk of aspiration, the patient's head and body should be elevated to 30 to 45 degrees during feeding and for 1 to 2 hours after each feeding. The gastric residual volume should be measured before administration of the feeding bolus. If this volume is greater than 50% of the previous bolus, the next feeding should be held. The feeding tube should be flushed with approximately 30 mL of water after each use. Free water volume can be adjusted as needed to treat hypo- or hypernatremia.

b. **Continuous infusion** administered by a pump is generally required for nasojejunal, gastrojejunal, or jejunal tubes. Feedings are initiated at 20 mL/hour and increased in 10- to 20-mL/hour increments every 4 to 6 hours until the desired goal is reached. The feeding tube should be flushed with approximately 30 mL of water every 4 hours. Feedings should be held or advancement should be slowed if abdominal distension or pain develops. For some patients, the entire day's feeding can be infused over 8 to 12 hours at night to allow the patient mobility free from the infusion pump during the day.

c. **Conversion to oral feeding.** When indicated, an oral diet is resumed gradually. In an effort to stimulate appetite, enteral feeding can be modified by the following measures:

   (1) **Providing fewer feedings.**

   (2) **Holding daytime feedings.**

   (3) **Decreasing the volume of feedings.** When oral intake provides approximately 75% of the required calories, tube feedings can be stopped.

d. **Administration of medications.** Many oral medications can be administered through feeding tubes. The elixir form is preferred but is not always available. Medications that are not suitable for administration through a feeding tube include the following:

   (1) Enteric-coated medications.

   (2) Drugs in gelatinous capsules.

   (3) Medications that are designed for sublingual use.

   (4) Most sustained-release medications.

4. **Complications**

   a. **Metabolic complications.** Abnormalities in serum electrolytes, calcium, magnesium, and phosphorus can be minimized through vigilant monitoring. **Hyperosmolarity** (hypernatremia) may lead to the development of mental lethargy or obtundation. This is treated with the administration of free water by giving either dextrose 5% in water (D_5W) intravenously or additional water in the tube feedings. Volume overload and subsequent congestive heart failure may occur as a result of **excess sodium administration**, observed especially in patients with impaired ventricular function or valvular heart disease. **Hyperglycemia** may occur in any patient but is particularly common in individuals with pre-existing diabetes or sepsis. Insulin should be used to control serum glucose level.

   b. **Clogging** can usually be prevented by careful routine flushing of the feeding tube. Wire stylets should not be used to unclog a feeding tube because of the risk of tube perforation and injury to the GI tract. Instillation of carbonated soda, cranberry juice, pancreatic enzyme replacement, or meat tenderizer (1 teaspoon papain in 30 mL of water) is sometimes useful for unclogging feeding tubes. Tubes that are refractory to these remedies, as well as those with cracks, leaks, or defective connectors, should be replaced.

   c. **Tracheobronchial aspiration** of tube feeds may occur with patients who are fed into the stomach or proximal small intestine and may lead to the development of pneumonia. Patients at particular risk are those with central nervous system abnormalities and those who are sedated. Testing tracheal aspirates with glucose strips or adding methylene blue (1 mL/L) to the tube feeds aids in assessing for aspiration. Historically, jejunal feeding has been the preferred route for patients who are at risk for aspiration. Two recent meta-analyses compared prepyloric to postpyloric feeds (*J Parenter Enteral Nutr* 2003;27:355; *Crit Care* 2003;7:R46). One found a significant reduction in aspiration with postpyloric feeds when aggregate data from ten trials were analyzed (*J Parenter Enteral Nutr* 2003.) The second demonstrated no significant difference in aspiration but did see a trend toward lower rates of aspiration with postpyloric feeds (*Crit Care* 2003.)

d. High gastric residuals as a result of outlet obstruction, dysmotility, intestinal ileus, or bowel obstruction may limit the usefulness of nasogastric or gastrostomy feeding tubes. Treatment of this problem should be directed at the underlying cause. Gastroparesis frequently occurs in diabetic or head-injured patients. Promotility agents such as metoclopramide or erythromycin may aid in gastric emptying. If gastric retention prevents the administration of sufficient calories and intestinal ileus or obstruction can be excluded, a nasojejunal or jejunostomy feeding tube may be necessary.

e. Diarrhea occurs in 10% to 20% of patients; however, other causes of diarrhea (e.g., *Clostridium difficile* colitis) should be considered. Diarrhea may result from an overly rapid increase in the volume of hyperosmolar tube feedings, medications (e.g., metoclopramide), a high-fat diet, or the presence of components not tolerated by the patient (e.g., lactose). If other causes of diarrhea can be excluded, the volume or concentration of tube feedings should be decreased. If no improvement occurs, a different formula should be used. Antidiarrheal agents such as loperamide should be reserved for patients with severe diarrhea. In surgical patients, *C. difficile* is a frequent cause of diarrhea due to the common use of perioperative antibiotics. Diagnosis can be confirmed with a *C. difficile* toxin assay or colonoscopy. Treatment includes stopping unnecessary antibiotics, followed by either oral or intravenous metronidazole or vancomycin orally or as a retention enema.

C. Parenteral nutrition is indicated for patients who require nutritional support but cannot meet their needs through oral intake and for whom enteral feeding is contraindicated or not tolerated.

1. Peripheral parenteral nutrition (PPN) is administered through a peripheral intravenous catheter. The osmolarity of PPN solutions generally is limited to 1,000 mOsm (approximately 12% dextrose solution) to avoid phlebitis. Consequently, unacceptably large volumes (>2,500 mL) are necessary to meet the typical patient's nutritional requirements. Temporary nutritional supplementation with PPN may be useful in selected patients but is not typically indicated.

2. Total parenteral nutrition (TPN) provides complete nutritional support (*Surgery* 1968;64:134). The solution, volume of administration, and additives are individualized based on an assessment of the nutritional requirements.

a. Access. TPN solutions must be administered through a central venous catheter. A dedicated single-lumen catheter or a multilumen catheter can be used. Catheters should be replaced for unexplained fever or bacteremia.

b. TPN solutions. TPN solutions generally are administered as a 3-in-1 admixture of protein, as amino acids (10%; 4 kcal/g); carbohydrate, as dextrose (70%; 3.4 kcal/g); and fat, as a lipid emulsion of soybean or safflower oil (20%; 9 kcal/g). Alternatively, the lipid emulsion can be administered as a separate intravenous "piggyback" infusion. Standard preparations are used for most patients (Table 2-5). Special solutions that contain low, intermediate, or high nitrogen concentrations as well as varying amounts of fat and carbohydrate are available for patients with diabetes, renal or pulmonary failure, or hepatic dysfunction.

c. Additives. Other elements can be added to the basic TPN solutions.

(1) Electrolytes (i.e., sodium, potassium, chloride, acetate, calcium, magnesium, phosphate) should be adjusted daily. A suggested formulation is often listed on a prewritten order sheet, with concentrations designed for patients

TABLE 2-5	Barnes-Jewish Hospital Parenteral Nutrition Form

Date Due _____   Bag No. _____
Calories to the nearest 100 kcal/24 hr _____

Check one	Standard solutions	% Total kcal provided as AA/Dex/fat	Grams/1,000 kcal of AA/Dex/fat	mL/1,000 kcal
	a) Intermediate nitrogen	16/60/24	40/176/27	786
	b) High nitrogen	20/55/25	50/162/28	843
	c) Very high nitrogen	24/56/20	60/165/22	946
	d) Low nitrogen	12/65/23	30/191/26	680
	e) Peripheral	16/32/52	40/94/58	1,429
	f) Amino acid/dextrose	10% Amino acid _____ mL		
		70% Dextrose _____ mL		
	Lipids (as separate infusion)	Circle one: 100 mL, 250 mL, 500 mL, 20% intralipid _____ mL/hr		

Electrolytes	Suggested amount	Amount ordered	Other additives	Suggested amount	Amount ordered
Na	60–120 mEq		MVI-12	10 mL/day	
K	30–80 mEq		Trace element-5	1 mL/day	
Cl	80–140 mEq		Vitamin K	10 mg/wk	
Acetate	a	Balance	Regular insulin		units
Ca	4.6–9.2 mEq		Pepcid		mg
Mg	8.1–24.3 mEq				
PO$_4$	12–24 mmol				

AA, amino acids; Dex, dextrose; MVI, multivitamin.
[a]Cations (sodium and potassium) must be balanced by anions (chloride and acetate). In patients with normal electrolytes, the acetate:chloride ratio should be approximately 1:2.

with normal serum electrolytes and renal function. The number of cations and anions must balance; this is achieved by altering the concentrations of chloride and acetate. If the serum bicarbonate is low, the solution should contain more acetate. The calcium:phosphate ratio must be monitored to prevent salt precipitation.

(2) Medications such as albumin, H$_2$-receptor antagonists, heparin, iron, dextran, insulin, and metoclopramide can be administered in TPN solutions. However, not all medications are compatible with 3-in-1 admixtures. Regular insulin should initially be administered subcutaneously according to a sliding scale, based on a determination of the blood glucose level. After a stable insulin requirement has been established, insulin can be administered in the TPN solution, generally at two thirds of the daily subcutaneous insulin dose.

(3) Other additives. Trace elements are added daily using a commercially prepared mixture (e.g., 1 mL trace element-5: 1 mg copper, 12 μg chromium, 0.3 μg manganese, 60 μg selenium, 5 mg zinc). Multivitamins generally are added daily using a commercially prepared mixture (e.g., 10 mL MVI-12). Vitamin K is not included in most multivitamin mixtures and must be added separately (10 mg once a week). Vitamins A and C and zinc are essential for proper wound healing.

d. Routine physiologic and laboratory monitoring should occur on a scheduled basis. This can be performed less frequently for patients whose postoperative course has stabilized and who are receiving a consistent TPN regimen.

The initial frequency of monitoring includes vital signs and serum glucose every 6 hours; weight, serum electrolytes, and blood urea nitrogen daily; and triglycerides, complete blood cell count, prothrombin time, liver enzymes, and bilirubin weekly.

- **e. Administration of TPN.** Orders, written daily, should reflect the patient's dynamic nutritional status and biochemical profile (Table 2-5).
  - **(1) Introduction of TPN** should be gradual. For example, approximately 1,000 kcal is provided the first day. If there is metabolic stability (i.e., normoglycemia), this is increased to the caloric goal over 1 to 2 days.
  - **(2) TPN solutions** are delivered most commonly as a continuous infusion. A new 3-in-1 admixture bag of TPN is administered daily at a constant infusion rate over 24 hours. Additional maintenance intravenous fluids are unnecessary, and total infused volume should be kept constant while nutritional content is increased.
  - **(3) Cyclic administration of TPN** solutions may be useful for selected patients, including (1) those who will be discharged from the hospital and subsequently receive home TPN, (2) those with limited intravenous access who require administration of other medications, and (3) those who are metabolically stable and desire a period during the day when they can be free of an infusion pump. Cyclic TPN is administered for 8 to 16 hours, most commonly at night. This should not be done until metabolic stability has been demonstrated for patients on standard, continuous TPN infusions.
  - **(4) Discontinuation of TPN** should take place when the patient can satisfy 75% of his or her caloric and protein needs with oral intake or enteral feeding. The calories provided by TPN can be decreased in proportion to calories from the patient's increasing enteral intake. To discontinue TPN, the infusion rate should be halved for 1 hour, halved again the next hour, and then discontinued. Tapering in this manner prevents rebound hypoglycemia from hyperinsulinemia. It is not necessary to taper the rate if the patient demonstrates glycemic stability when TPN is abruptly discontinued (i.e., cycled TPN) or receives less than 1,000 kcal/day.
- **f. Complications associated with TPN**
  - **(1) Catheter-related complications** can be minimized by strict aseptic technique and routine catheter care (*Surg Clin North Am* 1985;65:835).
  - **(2) Metabolic complications.** A large parenteral sodium load in a severely malnourished patient may precipitate congestive heart failure. Without daily monitoring and correction, electrolyte abnormalities can occur rapidly; the consequences of various imbalances are discussed in Chapter 4. Hyperglycemia and hyperosmolarity may lead to coma or death. In addition, hyperglycemia may be the first indication of occult infection. As noted in Section II.C.2.d, the serum glucose level should be monitored frequently. Strict maintenance of serum glucose level below 110 mg/dL improves mortality and reduces infectious complications in surgical ICU patients (*New Engl J Med* 2001;345:1359). Table 2-6 depicts the standard insulin regimen used in the ICU at Barnes-Jewish Hospital.
  - **(3) Refeeding syndrome** occurs when TPN is administered to a severely malnourished patient, resulting in anabolism, a dramatic shift of extracellular ions into the intracellular space, and rapid depletion of ATP stores. Refeeding syndrome can present insidiously as respiratory failure. For this reason, frequent monitoring and additional supplementation of potassium, manganese, and phosphate are required in severely malnourished patients.
  - **(4) Hepatic dysfunction** is a common manifestation of long-term TPN support. Steatosis is associated with mild elevations of the transaminases, alkaline phosphate, and bilirubin. Cirrhosis is the end result.
  - **(5) Cholecystitis,** particularly the acalculous type, may occur in patients who receive TPN for extended periods. Cholecystostomy or cholecystectomy is indicated for symptomatic patients. To avoid cholestasis, gallbladder

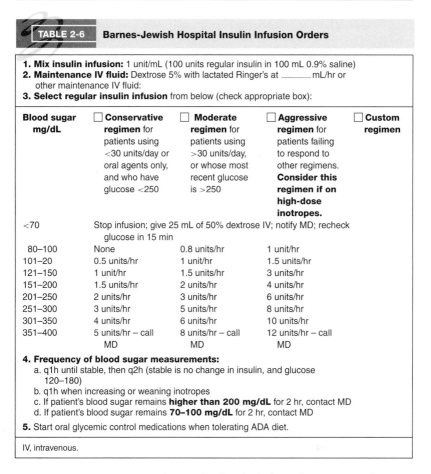

| TABLE 2-6 | Barnes-Jewish Hospital Insulin Infusion Orders |

1. Mix insulin infusion: 1 unit/mL (100 units regular insulin in 100 mL 0.9% saline)
2. Maintenance IV fluid: Dextrose 5% with lactated Ringer's at _____mL/hr or
other maintenance IV fluid:
3. Select regular insulin infusion from below (check appropriate box):

Blood sugar mg/dL	☐ Conservative regimen for patients using <30 units/day or oral agents only, and who have glucose <250	☐ Moderate regimen for patients using >30 units/day, or whose most recent glucose is >250	☐ Aggressive regimen for patients failing to respond to other regimens. **Consider this regimen if on high-dose inotropes.**	☐ Custom regimen
<70	Stop infusion; give 25 mL of 50% dextrose IV; notify MD; recheck glucose in 15 min			
80–100	None	0.8 units/hr	1 unit/hr	
101–20	0.5 units/hr	1 unit/hr	1.5 units/hr	
121–150	1 unit/hr	1.5 units/hr	3 units/hr	
151–200	1.5 units/hr	2 units/hr	4 units/hr	
201–250	2 units/hr	3 units/hr	6 units/hr	
251–300	3 units/hr	5 units/hr	8 units/hr	
301–350	4 units/hr	6 units/hr	10 units/hr	
351–400	5 units/hr – call MD	8 units/hr – call MD	12 units/hr – call MD	

4. Frequency of blood sugar measurements:
   a. q1h until stable, then q2h (stable is no change in insulin, and glucose 120–180)
   b. q1h when increasing or weaning inotropes
   c. If patient's blood sugar remains **higher than 200 mg/dL** for 2 hr, contact MD
   d. If patient's blood sugar remains **70–100 mg/dL** for 2 hr, contact MD
5. Start oral glycemic control medications when tolerating ADA diet.

IV, intravenous.

contraction can be stimulated with cholecystokinin (0.02 μg/kg intravenously per day).
  D. Specialized substrates. Promise has been shown for "nutritional pharmacology," in which interventions with cytokines, hormones, and substrates can augment basic nutritional repletion.
    1. Cytokines such as interleukin-1 (IL-1), IL-6, and tumor necrosis factor-α (TNF-α) contribute to the acute-phase response of inflammation, loss of skeletal muscle protein, and use of exogenous nutrients. Pharmacologic manipulation of these agents may reverse their deleterious effects (*Cancer* 1997;79:1828). For example, recent studies have shown that the TNF-α–blocking agent infliximab (monoclonal antibody) can induce remission in Crohn disease and ulcerative colitis (*Cochrane Database Syst Rev.* 2004;1:CD003574; *Cochrane Database Syst Rev* 2006;19;3:CD005112.)
    2. Exogenous **growth hormone** has been shown to increase amino acid uptake, decrease nitrogen loss, and hasten weaning from mechanical ventilation (*Am J Surg* 1996;171:576). Ongoing trials are exploring its use in critical illness.
    3. Immunonutrition is the use of nutrition to modulate a patient's immune response. Arginine and glutamine stimulate immune response and may improve gut integrity, thereby preventing bacterial translocation. Synthetic nucleotides can also enhance host defenses. Omega-3 fatty acids attenuate the inflammatory response by

shifting fatty acid metabolism toward anti-inflammatory mediators and may be beneficial in patients with acute respiratory distress syndrome. Recent meta-analyses of studies using combination immunonutrition demonstrated reductions in infectious complications and length of hospital stay but failed to show any improvement in mortality among complex surgical and critical care patients (*Ann Surg* 1999;229:467; *JAMA* 2001;286:944).

E. Disease-specific nutrition

1. **Thermal injury** has a tremendous impact on metabolism because of prolonged, intense neuroendocrine stimulation. The increase in metabolic demands following thermal injury correlates with the extent of ungrafted body surface area. Decreasing the intensity of neuroendocrine stimulation by providing analgesia and thermoneutral environments lowers the accelerated metabolic rate in many of these patients and helps to decrease catabolic protein loss until the burned surface can be grafted (*Compr Ther* 1991;17:47).

2. **Diabetes** often complicates nutritional management. Complications associated with TPN administration (e.g., catheter-related sepsis) are more common with prolonged hyperglycemia. Unopposed glycosuria may cause osmotic diuresis, loss of electrolytes in urine, and nonketotic coma. The goal in glucose-intolerant patients is to maintain the serum glucose within the normal range. Hypoglycemia can result in shock, seizures, or vascular instability. This can be avoided by adjusting the insulin dosing, with the understanding that insulin requirements will decrease as the patient recovers from the initial stress.

3. **Difficulty weaning** a patient from mechanical ventilation can be caused by excessive carbohydrate administration. Patients with marginal pulmonary reserve who are ventilator dependent may be particularly difficult to wean (*JAMA* 1980;243:1444). The respiratory quotient (**RQ**) represents the balance between CO_2 production and O_2 consumption and is a general indicator of metabolism. It is calculated from

$$RQ = \frac{\dot{V}_{CO_2}}{\dot{V}_{O_2}},$$

where $\dot{V}_{CO_2}$ is carbon dioxide output rate and $\dot{V}_{O_2}$ is oxygen uptake rate. RQ can be measured by indirect calorimetry. Patients given only lipids will have an RQ of 0.67, whereas the RQ equals 1 in those receiving only carbohydrates. It is important to note that patients with excess caloric intake will begin producing fat and have an RQ greater than 1. A higher RQ reflects increased CO_2 production, which can impair weaning from the ventilator.

4. **Renal failure** may be associated with glucose intolerance, negative nitrogen balance from increased losses through dialysis, loss of protein with decreased protein synthesis, hyperkalemia, and diminished excretion of phosphorus. Dialysis should be adjusted accordingly, and these patients should be nutritionally replenished according to their calculated needs. Patients who receive peritoneal dialysis absorb approximately 80% of the dextrose in the dialysate fluid (assuming a normal serum glucose level). These factors must be considered when designing a nutritional support strategy.

5. **Hepatic failure** may result in wasting of lean body mass, fluid retention, vitamin and trace metal deficiencies, anemia, and encephalopathy. It may be difficult or impossible to limit the amount of nitrogen that a patient receives each day yet still provide adequate nutritional support. Branched-chain amino acids (BCAA) are metabolized by skeletal muscle and serve as an energy source during periods of stress. These amino acids are available enterally or parenterally to decrease the levels of aromatic amino acids and, therefore, the severity of encephalopathy (*J Nutr* 2006;136(1 Suppl):295S). The largest randomized, controlled trial evaluating BCAA-enriched therapy included 646 cirrhotic patients (*Clin Gastroenterol Hepatol* 2005;3:705) and showed a significant decrease in complication rates (progression of liver failure, development of liver cancer, rupture of esophageal varices)

in patients receiving oral supplementation with BCAA. Further studies are needed to define the role of BCAA.

6. **Cancer-related cachexia** is a syndrome of lean muscle wasting, peripheral insulin resistance, and increased lipolysis. More than two thirds of cancer patients experience significant weight loss (*J Parenter Enteral Nutr* 2002;26:S63). Antineoplastic therapies, such as chemotherapy, radiation, or operative extirpation, can worsen preexisting malnutrition. Although adding TPN to these modalities in clinical trials has shown improvement in weight, nitrogen balance, and biochemical markers, there is little evidence to suggest improved survival. Megestrol acetate (Megace) improves food intake, fat gain, and patient mood but does not alter outcome.

7. **Short-bowel syndrome** occurs in patients with less than 180 cm of functional small bowel. It may result from mesenteric ischemia, Crohn disease, or necrotizing enterocolitis. The estimated length of small bowel that is required for adult patients to become independent of TPN is greater than 120 cm without colon or greater than 60 cm with some colonic continuity. Salvage of the ileocecal valve improves outcome. Dietary management includes consuming frequent small meals, avoiding hyperosmolar foods, restricting fat intake, and limiting consumption of foods high in oxalate (precipitates nephrolithiasis). Intestinal adaptation may occur in some patients. In addition to glutamine, recombinant human growth hormone (r-HGH) assists these patients in weaning from parenteral nutrition (*J Clin Gastroenterol* 2006;40(5 Suppl 2):S99). Recently, the Food and Drug Administration approved r-HGH (Somatropin) for use in this patient population.

8. **Patients with AIDS** develop protein-calorie malnutrition and lose weight. Malnourished AIDS patients require 35 to 40 kcal and 2 to 2.5 g protein/kg/day. In addition to the required electrolytes, vitamins, and minerals, they should receive glutamine, arginine, nucleotides, omega-3 polyunsaturated fats, branched-chain amino acids, and trace metal supplements. Those with normal gut function should be given a high-protein, high-calorie, low-fat, lactose-free oral diet. Patients with compromised gut function require an enteral (amino acid–enriched, polypeptide-enriched, or immunoenhancing) diet or TPN.

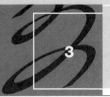

LIFE SUPPORT AND ANESTHESIA

Kareem D. Husain, John E. Mazuski, and Richard S. Hotchkiss

LIFE SUPPORT

The **time** from cardiopulmonary arrest to the initiation of **basic life support (BLS)** and **advanced cardiac life support (ACLS)** is critical to outcome. According to recent American Heart Association (AHA) guidelines, survival from out-of-hospital cardiac arrest in the United States remains about 6%, yet survival rates can be greater than 50% for victims when immediate and effective cardiopulmonary resuscitation (CPR) is combined with prompt use of an automated external defibrillator. The following guidelines were developed by the AHA to standardize treatment for adults (*Circulation* 2005;112(Suppl I):IV-1).

Life Support and Cardiopulmonary Arrest Algorithms

- **I. BLS.** The ABCDs of BLS are *a*irway, *b*reathing, *c*irculation, and early *d*efibrillation.
  - ■ **Determine unresponsiveness** by gently tapping or shaking the victim and asking, "Are you okay?" **Do not shake the victim's head or neck** unless trauma to these areas has been excluded.
  - ■ **Call for help if there is no response.** In the field, activate the emergency medical service system (e.g., 911). Call for a defibrillator/AED (automated external defibrillator).
  - ■ The most recent **AHA guidelines for BLS and CPR** are summarized in Table 3-1 and Figure 3-1.
- **II. ACLS.** Properly performed BLS is critical to the successful performance of ACLS, which is a team effort that depends on effective supervision by a team leader. The leader should ensure that the ABCDs of ACLS are expediently executed by the team.
  - **A. Airway**
    1. **Proper airway management** is essential to the resuscitative effort. Endotracheal intubation remains the procedure of choice for the unconscious and/or apneic patient. When intubation is not possible, several alternative airway ventilation methods, such as the **Laryngeal Mask Airway** or the **Esophageal-Tracheal Combitube**, may provide more effective ventilation than a bag-mask apparatus. Emphasis should be placed on minimizing the interruption of chest compressions.
  - **B. Breathing**
    1. For endotracheal intubation, tube placement should be directly assessed by visualization of the tube passing through the vocal cords, auscultation of bilateral breath sounds, and the absence of gastric insufflation by epigastric auscultation. Additional confirmation should be determined by an **end-tidal carbon dioxide detector** or an **esophageal detector device.** Once appropriate position is confirmed, the endotracheal tube should be secured to prevent dislodgment.
  - **C. Circulation**
    1. Adequate **intravenous access** should be obtained expediently. The antecubital vein should be the first target for access. If central venous catheterization is required to obtain access, the femoral vein usually provides the easiest and fastest access.
    2. **Normal saline** is the recommended intravenous fluid vehicle. A bolus of intravenous fluid should follow administration of medications because this enhances delivery to the central circulation.

| **TABLE 3-1** | **Basic Life Support ABCD Maneuvers for Laypersons and Health Care Providers for Infants, Children, and Adults (Newborn Information Not Included)**[a] |

Maneuver	**Adult** Lay rescuer: ≥ 8 yr HCP: adolescent and older	**Child** Lay rescuer: 1–8 yr HCP: 1 yr to adolescent	Infant <1 yr of age
Airway	Assess responsiveness, then perform head tilt–chin lift (HCP: suspected trauma, use jaw thrust)		
Breathing: Initial	2 breaths at 1 s/breath	2 effective breaths at 1 s/breath	
HCP: Rescue breathing without chest compressions	10–12 breaths/min (approximate)	12–20 breaths/min (approximate)	
HCP: Rescue breaths for CPR with advanced airway		8–10 breaths/min (approximately)	
Foreign-body airway obstruction		Abdominal thrusts	Back slaps and chest thrusts
Circulation: HCP, pulse check (≤10 s)		Carotid	Brachial or femoral
Compression landmarks	Lower half of sternum, between nipples		Just below nipple line (lower half of sternum)
Compression method: push hard and fast, allow complete recoil	Heel of one hand, other hand on top	Heel of one hand or as for adults	2 or 3 fingers HCP (2 rescuers): 2 thumb–encircling hands
Compression depth	1½–2 in.	Approximately one-third to one-half the depth of the chest	
Compression rate		Approximately 100/min	
Compression–ventilation ratio	30:2 (one or two rescuers)	30:2 (single rescuer), HCP: 15:2 (2 rescuers)	
Defibrillation: AED	Use adult pads, do not use child pads	Use AED after 5 cycles of CPR (out of hospital)	No recommendation for infants <1 yr of age
	Use pediatric system for child 1–8 yr if available		
		HCP: For sudden collapse (out of hospital) or in-hospital arrest, use AED as soon as available	

AED, automated external defibrillator; CPR, cardiopulmonary resuscitation.
[a]Maneuvers used by only health care providers are indicated by HCP. With permission from *Circulation* 2005;112(Suppl I):IV-15.

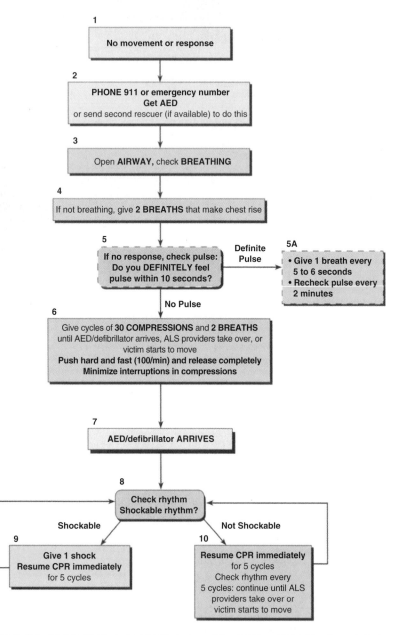

Figure 3-1. Adult basic life support health care provider algorithm. Dashed-line boxes indicate health care provider maneuvers not provided by the lay rescuer. AED, automated external defibrillator; ALS, advanced life support; CPR, cardiopulmonary resuscitation. (With permission from *Circulation* 2005:112(Suppl I):IV-22.)

3. Appropriate monitor leads should be attached and rhythms and rates identified. A noninvasive measurement of blood pressure should be obtained. If intravenous access cannot be established, **epinephrine, lidocaine,** and **atropine** can be administered via the endotracheal tube.

D. Differential diagnosis

1. One must attempt to determine the etiology of the arrest to search for, identify, and treat reversible causes of cardiopulmonary arrest with specific therapy. The differential diagnosis of cardiopulmonary arrest can be generally divided into three broad categories of shock—**hypovolemic, cardiogenic,** and **distributive**— the etiologies and therapies of which are discussed in Chapter 7.

III. UNIVERSAL ALGORITHM OF ADULT EMERGENCY CARDIAC CARE (Fig. 3-1 and Table 3-1)

A. Institute BLS protocols.

1. Assess responsiveness, breathing, and circulation.

2. Defibrillate early for ventricular fibrillation (VF) or pulseless ventricular tachycardia (VT).

B. Institute ACLS and arrhythmia-specific algorithm.

1. VF or pulseless VT (Fig. 3-2)

a. There are **two phases in the algorithm** for this dysrhythmia: The first involves electrocardioversion, and the second involves pharmacologic cardioversion and electrocardioversion. In the first phase, defibrillate **one** time at 200 J with a manual biphasic device or 360 J with a monophasic device for refractory VF or VT. Do *not* pause for a pulse check if the monitor clearly displays persistent VF or VT—resume CPR immediately.

b. There are **four guidelines for the second phase:** Follow a **drug–shock, drug–shock** sequence, shock within 30 to 60 seconds of drug administration, do not assess for a pulse after each shock, and maximize one antiarrhythmic before administering another to limit proarrhythmic drug–drug interactions.

c. First-line antiarrhythmic medications are either **epinephrine**, 1 mg intravenously every 3 to 5 minutes, or **vasopressin**, 40 units intravenously once. After the administration of vasopressin, 10 to 20 minutes should elapse before epinephrine can be given. **Epinephrine** increases myocardial and cerebral blood flow during cardiopulmonary resuscitation, principally because of its α-adrenergic receptor–stimulating properties. There is no evidence to support the use of high-dose or escalating doses of epinephrine in VF or/pulseless VT. **Vasopressin (arginine vasopressin)** has vasoconstrictive properties at pharmacologic doses and may have a more favorable side effect profile than epinephrine. Vasopressin has not been found to be superior to epinephrine for resuscitation from VF or pulseless VT in recent randomized, controlled trials, although there is evidence that vasopressin followed by epinephrine may be more effective than epinephrine alone in the treatment of refractory cardiac arrest (*Lancet* 2001;358:105, *N Engl J Med* 2004;350:105). There also exist conflicting data in more recent studies suggesting that the vasopressin/epinephrine combination or vasopressin alone may or may not improve outcomes in out-of-hospital cardiac arrest (*Am J Cardiol* 2006;98:1316, *Crit Care* 2006;10:R13).

d. Antiarrhythmic drugs are used as second-line medications for the treatment of persistent or refractory VF or/pulseless VT. **Amiodarone** has been shown in recent trials to be the drug of choice in shock-refractory VF or/pulseless VT and is also used for the management of atrial fibrillation and hemodynamically stable ventricular tachycardia (*N Engl J Med* 1999;341:871, *N Engl J Med* 2002;346:884, *Pharmacotherapy* 2006;26:1703). Amiodarone affects the sodium, potassium, and calcium channels and is an α- and β-adrenergic antagonist. Amiodarone is initially administered as an intravenous bolus of 300 mg in 20 to 30 mL of dextrose 5% in water (D5W), and a second dose of 150 mg can be used in case of recurrence. With return of a spontaneous perfusing rhythm, an amiodarone drip is administered, consisting of 150 mg

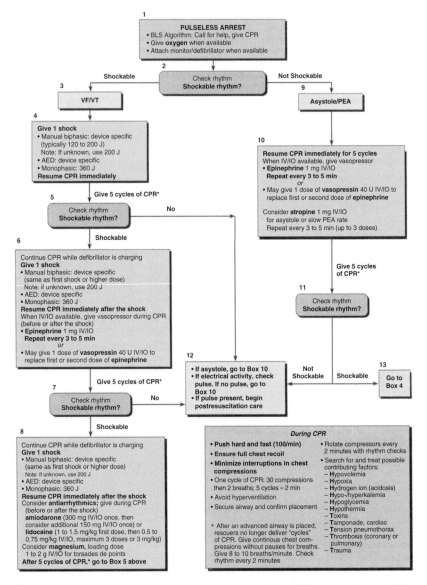

Figure 3-2. Advanced cardiac life support pulseless arrest algorithm. AED, automated external defibrillator; BLS, basic life support; CPR, cardiopulmonary resuscitation; IO, intraosseous; IV, intravenous; PEA, pulseless electrical activity; VF, ventricular fibrillation; VT, ventricular tachycardia. (With permission from *Circulation* 2005;112(Suppl I):IV-59.)

over the first 10 minutes, followed by 1 mg/minute over the next 6 hours, and finally a maintenance infusion of 0.5 mg/minute over the next 18 hours.

  e. Other antiarrhythmics that may be of benefit in refractory or persistent cases include **lidocaine** and **procainamide.** The initial dose of **lidocaine** for VF is 0.50 to 0.75 mg/kg intravenously every 5 to 10 minutes, with electrocardioversion attempts after the medication. The maximal dose is 3 mg/kg. With return of a spontaneous perfusing rhythm, a lidocaine drip can begin with a loading dose of 1 to 1.5 mg/kg followed by a continuous infusion of 1 to 4 mg/minute. **Central nervous system symptoms,** especially seizure, are an early manifestation of lidocaine toxicity. **Procainamide** is loaded at 30 mg/minute up to a total of 17 mg/kg (1.2 g for a 70-kg patient), followed by a maintenance infusion of 1 to 4 mg/minute. Procainamide may induce hypotension, heart block, or even cardiac arrest.

  f. Magnesium sulfate is the treatment of choice in patients with **torsades de pointes** (polymorphic VT). For torsades de pointes, higher doses (up to 5 to 10 g) may be used. Rapid administration of magnesium can cause flushing, sweating, mild bradycardia, and hypotension. Depressed reflexes, flaccid paralysis, circulatory collapse, respiratory paralysis, and diarrhea may occur with hypermagnesemia.

  g. A solitary precordial thump can convert pulseless VT (and, less often, VF) to sinus rhythm, but it should only be used for witnessed arrests when a defibrillator is not available and the patient is pulseless.

2. Pulseless electrical activity (PEA) (Fig. 3-2)

  a. PEA is almost uniformly fatal unless an underlying cause can be identified and treated, usually because it represents a preterminal rhythm. Resuscitation rates from PEA are only 20%, with only 4% to 5% of patients surviving to hospital discharge. Potentially reversible causes follow the acronym 6H 5T:

  (1) Hypovolemia, especially resulting from hemorrhage, is the most common cause of pulseless electrical activity.

  (2) Hypoxia.

  (3) Hypothermia.

  (4) Hydrogen ions (severe acidosis).

  (5) Hyperkalemia or hypokalemia.

  (6) Hypoglycemia.

  (7) Tablets/toxins.

  (8) Tension pneumothorax, evidenced by tracheal deviation and decreased ipsilateral breath sounds, should be treated by insertion of a large-bore angiocatheter (14-gauge) into the pleural space through the second intercostal space in the midclavicular line, followed by a thoracostomy tube.

  (9) Tamponade (pericardial) is treated by pericardiocentesis.

  (10) Thrombosis of coronary vessels (acute coronary syndromes).

  (11) Thrombosis of pulmonary vessels (pulmonary embolism).

  b. Sodium bicarbonate may be beneficial in patients with preexisting metabolic acidosis, hyperkalemia, or tricyclic or phenobarbital overdose. When bicarbonate is used, 1 mEq/kg should be given as the initial dose, with 0.5 mEq/kg administered every 10 minutes thereafter. One ampule of sodium bicarbonate contains 8.4% bicarbonate (50 mEq/50 mL).

  c. Calcium is indicated for the treatment of myocardial instability secondary to hypocalcemia or hyperkalemia. A 10% calcium chloride solution may be given as an intravenous bolus of 2 to 4 mg/kg.

3. Asystole (Fig. 3-2)

  a. Survival rates from **asystole** are only 1% to 2%. Asystole should be confirmed in two leads because fine VF may be difficult to distinguish from asystole. If the rhythm is unclear, the presence of fine VF should be assumed. **Transcutaneous pacing** may be useful if the asystolic period is brief. **Epinephrine, vasopressin,** and **atropine** are the mainstays of pharmacologic therapy. A recent clinical trial indicates that vasopressin is superior to epinephrine in the resuscitation of patients from asystolic cardiac arrest (*N Engl J Med* 2004;350:105), and current guidelines state that one dose of vasopressin may replace the first or second dose of epinephrine in the treatment algorithm for asystole or PEA.

(1) Atropine may have some benefit in the treatment of asystole (1 mg every 3 to 5 minutes intravenously). A total dose of 3 mg may result in full vagal blockade and should not be exceeded. The denervated transplanted heart does not respond to atropine and requires pacing, catecholamine infusion, or both. Anticholinergic syndrome comprising delirium, tachycardia, coma, flushed and hot skin, ataxia, and blurred vision can occur with excessive doses of atropine.

b. Asystole most often represents a confirmation of death rather than a rhythm to be treated. With the exception of cardiac arrests in special situations such as hypothermia, electrocution, and drug overdose, team leaders may terminate resuscitation efforts under the following circumstances:

(1) Asystole persists for at least 10 minutes after CPR has been performed.

(2) VF, if present, has been eliminated.

(3) Successful endotracheal intubation has been accomplished and confirmed.

(4) Adequate ventilation has been provided as determined by oxygen saturation and, if possible, end-tidal CO_2 monitoring.

(5) A successful intravenous line has been established, and rhythm-appropriate medications have been administered.

4. Bradycardia (Fig. 3-3)

a. The indications for treatment of bradycardia include associated signs and symptoms (e.g., chest pain, shortness of breath, decreased level of consciousness, hypotension, or congestive heart failure). It should be remembered that some athletes and patients on beta-blockers might have a resting heart rate of less than 60 beats/minute. The sequential intervention sequence is as follows:

(1) Atropine, 0.5 to 1 mg intravenously every 3 to 5 minutes, up to a 3-mg total dose, may be used. Use with caution in patients with acute coronary ischemia or myocardial infarction.

(2) Transcutaneous pacing is indicated in patients with hemodynamically unstable bradycardia unresponsive to pharmacologic treatments (e.g., atropine, dopamine) and is first-line therapy for type II second-degree and third-degree atrioventricular (AV) block. Transcutaneous cardiac pacing is the initial method of choice because of the speed with which it can be initiated and because it is widely available. **Transvenous pacing** is best instituted in the postresuscitation period.

(3) Dopamine infusion, 5 to 20 μg/kg intravenously per minute, may be used for symptomatic bradycardia not responding to atropine if transcutaneous pacing is not immediately available. At lower doses of dopamine, the α_1- and β-adrenergic effects cause increased myocardial contractility, cardiac output, heart rate, and blood pressure. The infusion may be increased to 20 μg/kg/minute for a predominant α-adrenergic effect if hypotension is associated with the bradycardia.

(4) Epinephrine, 2 to 10 mg intravenously per minute, may be used.

(5) Glucagon, 3 mg intravenously followed by a 3-mg/hour infusion, has been shown to improve signs and symptoms of drug-induced symptomatic bradycardia refractory to atropine (*Chest* 1998;114:323).

5. Tachycardia (Fig. 3-4)

a. Tachyarrhythmias can be classified based on the appearance of the QRS complex:

(1) Narrow-complex (supraventricular) tachycardia (QRS <0.12 seconds)
- Sinus tachycardia
- Atrial fibrillation
- Atrial flutter
- AV nodal re-entry

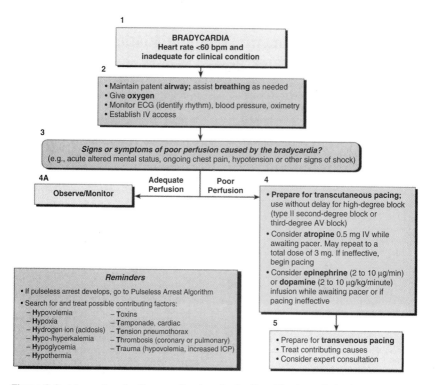

Figure 3-3. Advanced cardiac life support bradycardia algorithm. AV, atrioventricular; bpm, beats per minute; ECG, electrocardiogram; ICP, intracranial pressure; IV, intravenous; WPW, Wolff-Parkinson-White syndrome. (With permission from *Circulation* 2005;112(Suppl I):IV-68.)

    ○ Ectopic atrial tachycardia
    ○ Multifocal atrial tachycardia
    ○ Junctional tachycardia
  (2) Wide-complex (ventricular) tachycardia (QRS ≥ 0.12 seconds)
    ○ Ventricular tachycardia
    ○ SVT with aberrancy
    ○ Pre-excited tachycardia

IV. POSTRESUSCITATION MANAGEMENT depends on the underlying disease process and the continued maintenance of hemodynamic and electrical stability. All patients should be transferred to an intensive care unit for continued care.

  A. The ultimate goal of resuscitation is not merely to restore spontaneous circulation, but also to achieve long-term neurologically intact survival. Two recent clinical trials suggest that treatment of patients successfully resuscitated from cardiac arrest with **mild to moderate therapeutic hypothermia** improves outcomes, increases the rate of a favorable neurologic outcome, and reduces mortality (*N Engl J Med* 2002;346:549, *N Engl J Med* 2002;346:557). The routine use of hypothermia in the management of postarrest patients awaits additional confirmatory studies.

V. Long-term survival among persons who have undergone successful early defibrillation after cardiac arrest is similar to that for matched patients who did not suffer cardiac arrest. The quality of life of survivors is similar to that of the general population (*N Engl J Med* 2003;348:2626).

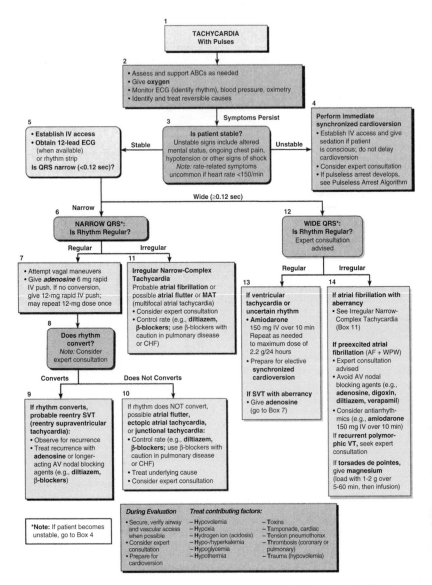

Figure 3-4. Advanced cardiac life support tachycardia algorithm. AF, atrial fibrillation; AV, atrioventricular; CHF, congestive heart failure; ECG, electrocardiogram; IV, intravenous; VT, ventricular tachycardia. (With permission from *Circulation* 2005;112(Suppl I):IV-70.)

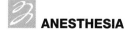

ANESTHESIA

Preparing the Patient

I. PATIENT PREPARATION FOR OPERATION

A. Preoperative evaluation

1. A **comprehensive preoperative evaluation** is critical to the safe administration of anesthetic care.

   a. A **complete history,** including medication usage and prior anesthetic usage, should be obtained.

   b. An **examination of airway,** vascular access, and other pertinent anatomy tailored to the anticipated operation should be undertaken.

2. In **patients without preexisting disease,** preoperative screening and testing are determined primarily by age.

   a. **Hemoglobin or hematocrit** may be the only test required in healthy patients younger than 40 years.

   b. A **serum pregnancy test** should be obtained for female patients of childbearing age.

   c. A **screening chest x-ray and electrocardiogram (ECG)** are obtained for patients who are 50 years or older, unless an indication is found from the history or physical examination, or both.

3. **Additional testing** may be required when clinically indicated.

   a. **Serum electrolytes** must be evaluated in patients with diabetes or renal insufficiency and in patients who are taking diuretics.

   b. **Coagulation studies** (prothrombin time, partial thromboplastin time, bleeding time) must be evaluated in patients who are receiving anticoagulation therapy or have a personal or family history that is suggestive of abnormal bleeding.

   c. **Additional testing or consultation** may be required in patients with evidence of severe coexisting disease, especially those with cardiac, pulmonary, or renal compromise.

4. Unstable or uncontrolled medical conditions, upper respiratory infections, and solid food ingestion within 6 hours of surgery are **indications to cancel or postpone elective surgery.**

5. **American Society of Anesthesiologists (ASA) criteria** (see Table 3-2)

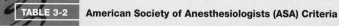

TABLE 3-2	American Society of Anesthesiologists (ASA) Criteria

ASA Grade	Description
I	There is no organic, physiologic, biochemical, or psychiatric disturbance; the pathologic process for which the operation is to be performed is localized and is not a systemic disturbance.
II	Mild to moderate systemic disturbance caused either by the condition to be treated or by other pathophysiologic processes
III	Severe systemic disturbance or disease for whatever cause, even though it may not be possible to define the degree of disability
IV	Indicative of the patient with severe systemic disorder that is already life-threatening and not always correctable by the operative procedure
V	The moribund patient who has little chance of survival but is submitted to operation in desperation

An E is added after a grade to indicate emergency surgery (e.g., IVE).

B. Nothing by mouth (NPO) status

1. For all patients, it is customary to abstain from any oral intake except for medications with sips of water for 8 hours before elective surgery. However, for adult patients who are not considered to be at increased risk for aspiration of gastric contents, the following **aspiration prophylaxis regimens** can be used.

   a. Solid food is permitted until 6 hours before surgery.

   b. Clear liquids (which do not include milk or juices containing pulp) are permitted until 2 hours before surgery (*Anesthesiology* 1999;90:896).

2. **Patients with slowed or incomplete gastric emptying** (e.g., those who are morbidly obese, diabetic, or on narcotic therapy) **may require longer fasting periods and additional pretreatment with metoclopramide, histamine H_2-receptor antagonists, or sodium citrate.** Rapid-sequence induction can be considered in these patients. Maintenance intravenous fluids should be started in NPO inpatients.

C. Medications

1. Patients can receive **benzodiazepines or narcotics** to alleviate preoperative anxiety.

2. **Cardiovascular or other pertinent medications** usually are administered on the morning of surgery with small sips of water. Inpatients who normally receive scheduled insulin doses should instead be placed on sliding-scale insulin, with blood sugars checked frequently every 2 to 6 hours while NPO, depending on difficulty of their diabetic control. Outpatients should be instructed to take one half to one third of their regular insulin dose the morning of surgery and to check blood sugars frequently. **It is essential to avoid hypoglycemia.**

3. In general, antiplatelet medications such as **aspirin** or **clopidogrel** should be held 5 days prior to surgery unless otherwise specified.

D. Obstructive sleep apnea (OSA)

1. **Over the last few years,** OSA has been recognized as a significant source of perioperative morbidity and mortality in the United States. The American Society of Anesthesiology guidelines for the perioperative management of OSA are shown in Tables 3-3 and 3-4 (*Anesthesiology* 2006,104:1081).

Types of Anesthesia

I. LOCAL ANESTHETICS are categorized into two groups. **Esters** include tetracaine, procaine, cocaine, and chloroprocaine. **Amides** include lidocaine, mepivacaine, bupivacaine, and etidocaine. Characteristics of commonly used local anesthetic agents are summarized in Table 3-5.

A. Mechanism of action

1. **Local anesthetics** work by diffusing through the nerve plasma membrane and causing blockade of sodium channels. The nerve cell is unable to depolarize, and axonal conduction is inhibited.

2. **Local tissue acidosis** (e.g., from infection) slows the onset and decreases the intensity of analgesia by causing local anesthetic molecules to become positively charged and less able to diffuse into the neuron.

B. Toxicity (dose dependent, except for allergic reactions)

1. **Central nervous system (CNS) toxicity**

   a. Signs and symptoms include mental status changes, dizziness, perioral numbness, a metallic taste, tinnitus, visual disturbances, and seizures. Seizures resulting from inadvertent intravascular injection usually last only minutes. Continuous infusion of local anesthetics may result in high plasma levels and prolonged seizures.

   b. Treatment involves airway support and ventilation with 100% oxygen, which should always be available. Prolonged seizures may require administration of benzodiazepines (midazolam, 1 to 5 mg intravenously; diazepam, 5 to 15 mg intravenously; or lorazepam, 1 to 4 mg intravenously). Intubation may be required to ensure adequate ventilation.

2. **Cardiovascular toxicity**

   a. Signs and symptoms range from decreased cardiac output to hypotension and cardiovascular collapse. Most local anesthetics cause CNS toxicity

TABLE 3-3	Identification and Assessment of Obstructive Sleep Apnea[a]

A. Clinical signs and symptoms suggesting the possibility of OSA
  1. Predisposing physical characteristics
    a. BMI 55 kg/m^2 [95th percentile for age and gender]
    b. Neck circumference 17 in. (men) or 16 in. (women)
    c. Craniofacial abnormalities affecting the airway
    d. Anatomic nasal obstruction
    e. Tonsils nearly touching or touching in the midline
  2. History of apparent airway obstruction during sleep (two or more of the following are present; if patient lives alone or sleep is not observed by another person, then only one of the following needs to be present)
    a. Snoring (loud enough to be heard through closed door)
    b. Frequent snoring
    c. Observed pauses in breathing during sleep
    d. Awakens from sleep with choking sensation
    e. Frequent arousals from sleep
    f. Intermittent vocalization during sleep
    g. Parental report of restless sleep, difficulty breathing, or struggling respiratory efforts during sleep
  3. Somnolence [one or more of the following is present]
    a. Frequent somnolence or fatigue despite adequate "sleep"
    b. Falls asleep easily in a nonstimulating environment [e.g., watching TV, reading, riding in or driving a car, despite adequate "sleep"]
    c. Parent or teacher comments that child appears sleepy during the day, is easily distracted, is overly aggressive, or has difficulty concentrating
    d. Child often difficult to arouse at usual awakening time
  If a patient has signs or symptoms in two or more of the foregoing categories, there is a significant probability that he or she has OSA. The severity of OSA may be determined by sleep study (see following tabulation). If a sleep study is not available, such patients should be treated as though they have moderate sleep apnea unless one or more of the foregoing signs or symptoms is severely abnormal (e.g., markedly increased BMI or neck circumference, respiratory pauses that are frightening to the observer, patient regularly falls asleep within minutes after being left unstimulated). In these cases patients should be treated as though they have severe sleep apnea.
B. If a sleep study has been done, the results should be used to determine the perioperative anesthetic management of a patient. However, because sleep laboratories differ in their criteria for detecting episodes of apnea and hypopnea, the Task Force believes that the sleep laboratory's assessment (none, mild, moderate, or severe) should take precedence over the actual AHI (the number of episodes of sleep-disordered breathing per hour). If the overall severity is not indicated, it may be determined by using the following table.

Severity of OSA	Adult AHI	Pediatric AHI
None	0–5	0
Mild OSA	6–20	1–5
Moderate OSA	21–40	6–10
Severe OSA	>40	>10

AHI, apnea-hypopnea index; BMI, body mass index; OSA, obstructive sleep apnea; TV, television.
[a] Items in brackets refer to pediatric patients.
With permission from *Anesthesiology* 2006;104:1081–1093.

TABLE 3-4	Obstructive Sleep Apnea Scoring System

	Points
A. Severity of sleep apnea based on sleep study (or clinical indicators if sleep study not available). Point score (0–3)[a,b] Severity of OSA (Table 3-3)	
None	0
Mild	1
Moderate	2
Severe	3
B. Invasiveness of surgery and anesthesia. Point score– (0–3) Type of surgery and anesthesia	
Superficial surgery under local or peripheral nerve block anesthesia without sedation	0
Superficial surgery with moderate sedation or general anesthesia	1
Peripheral surgery with spinal or epidural anesthesia (with no more than moderate sedation)	1
Peripheral surgery with general anesthesia	2
Airway surgery with moderate sedation	2
Major surgery, general anesthesia	3
Airway surgery, general anesthesia	3
C. Requirement for postoperative opiolds. Point score– (0–3) Opioid requirement	
None	0
Low-dose oral opioids	1
High-dose oral opioids, parenteral or neuraxial opioids	3
D. Estimation of perioperative risk. Overall score = score for A plus the greater of the score for either B or C. Point score– (0–6)[c]	

A scoring system similar to this table can be used to estimate whether a patient is at increased perioperative risk of complications from obstructive sleep apnea (OSA). This example, which has not been clinically validated, is meant only as a guide, and clinical judgment should be used to assess the risk of an individual patient.

[a] One point may be subtracted if a patient has been on continuous positive airway pressure (CPAP) or noninvasive positive-pressure ventilation (NIPPV) before surgery and will be using his or her appliance consistently during the postoperative period.

[b] One point should be added if a patient with mild or moderate OSA also has a resting arterial carbon dioxide tension ($Paco_2$) >60 mm Hg.

[c] Patients with score of 4 may be at increased perioperative risk from OSA; patients with a score of 5 or 6 may be at significantly increased perioperative risk from OSA.

With permission from *Anesthesiology* 2006;104:1081–1093.

before cardiovascular toxicity. Bupivacaine is an exception, and its intravascular injection can result in severe cardiac compromise.

    b. Treatment includes fluid resuscitation, administration of vasopressors, and cardiopulmonary resuscitation, if necessary.

  3. Hypersensitivity reactions, although rare, have been described with **ester**-based local anesthetics and are attributed to the metabolite *p*-aminobenzoic acid. True amide-based local anesthetic anaphylactic reactions are questionable.

    a. Signs and symptoms can range from urticaria to bronchospasm, hypotension, and anaphylactic shock.

    b. Treatment is similar to that for hypersensitivity reactions from other etiologies. Urticaria responds to diphenhydramine, 25 to 50 mg intravenously. Bronchospasm is treated with inhaled bronchodilators (e.g., albuterol) and oxygen.

TABLE 3-5 Local Anesthetics for Infiltration

Agent	Maximum dose (mg/kg)		Length of action (hr)	
	Plain	With epinephrine[a]	Plain	With epinephrine[a]
Procaine	—	8	0.25–1	0.5–1.5
Lidocaine	5	7	0.5–1	2–6
Mepivacaine	5	7	0.75–1.5	2–6
Bupivacaine	2.5	3	2–4	3–7
Tetracaine	1.5		24	

[a] 1:200,000.

Hypotension is treated with fluid resuscitation and vasopressors [e.g., phenylephrine hydrochloride (Neo-Synephrine)] as required. Anaphylactic cardiovascular collapse can be treated with epinephrine, 0.5 to 1 mg, administered as an intravenous bolus.

C. Epinephrine (1:200,000, 5 μg/mL) is mixed with local anesthetic solutions to prolong the duration of neural blockade and reduce systemic drug absorption. Its use is **contraindicated** in areas where arterial spasm would lead to tissue necrosis (e.g., nose, ears, fingers, toes, penis).

II. REGIONAL ANESTHESIA

A. In the operating room

1. **General considerations**

   a. The **importance of preoperative communication between anesthesiologist and surgeon** cannot be overemphasized. The extent and duration of the procedure must be appreciated by the anesthesiologist so that the appropriate area and duration of analgesia can be achieved. If the possibility of a prolonged or involved operative procedure is likely, a general anesthetic may be more appropriate. Certain surgical positions are poorly tolerated by awake patients (e.g., steep Trendelenburg may cause respiratory compromise); in these instances, a general anesthetic is appropriate.

   b. **Supplements to regional anesthesia.** No regional anesthetic technique is foolproof, and local infiltration by the surgeon may be required if there is an incomplete block. Intravenous sedation using short-acting benzodiazepines, narcotics, barbiturates, or propofol can also be helpful. General anesthesia may be required when a regional technique provides inadequate analgesia.

   c. **NPO status.** Because any regional anesthetic may progress to a general anesthetic, NPO requirements for regional and general anesthetics are identical.

   d. **Monitoring requirements** are no different from those for general anesthesia. Heart rhythm, blood pressure (BP), and arterial oxygen saturation should be monitored regularly during regional or general anesthesia. Other monitoring may be indicated, depending on coexisting disease states.

2. **Types of regional anesthesia**

   a. **Spinal anesthesia** involves the injection of small volumes of local anesthetic solution into the subarachnoid space at the level of the lumbar spine.

   (1) Anatomy and placement (Fig. 3-5)

   (a) With the use of sterile technique and after local anesthetic infiltration of the skin and subcutaneous tissues, a small (22- to 27-gauge) **spinal needle is passed between two adjacent lumbar spinous processes.** The needle is passed through the following structures: supraspinous ligament, interspinous ligament, ligamentum flavum, dura mater, and arachnoid mater. Cerebrospinal fluid (CSF) is aspirated, and the appropriate local anesthetic solution is injected.

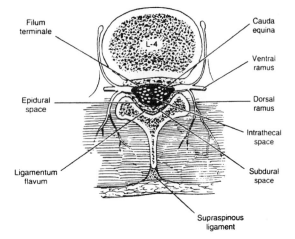

Figure 3-5. Anatomy for spinal and epidural anesthesia.

   (b) The needle can be removed (single-shot method), or a catheter can be placed to allow repeated dosing for potentially longer procedures (continuous spinal).

  (2) Level of analgesia

   (a) Multiple variables affect the spread of analgesia. The **baricity** of the agent (solution density compared to that of CSF) and the position of the patient immediately after injection are major determinants of level. The **total dose injected** (increased dose results in higher spread) and the **total volume injected** (increased volume results in higher spread) are also important determinants of anesthetic level.

   (b) Older patients tend to have greater spread of anesthesia by a few dermatomes, but clinical significance is variable.

  (3) Onset and duration of analgesia

   (a) The **specific characteristics of the local anesthetic** used and the **total dose injected** are the primary determinants of onset and duration of action. Epinephrine added to the solution increases the duration of analgesia.

   (b) The variability in length of analgesia is significant, ranging from as little as 30 minutes (lidocaine) to up to 6 hours (tetracaine with epinephrine).

  (4) Complications

   (a) Hypotension may occur as a result of sympatholytic-induced vasodilation and bradycardia. It may be more severe in hypovolemic patients or in those with preexisting cardiac dysfunction. Treatment includes volume resuscitation with crystalloid, vasopressors (epinephrine, 5 to 10 μg intravenously or phenylephrine hydrochloride, 50 to 100 μg intravenously), and positive chronotropic drugs. It is advisable to administer 500 to 1,000 mL of crystalloid prior to spinal block to avoid hypotension due to spinal anesthesia.

   (b) High spinal blockade. Inadvertently high levels of spinal blockade may result in hypotension, dyspnea (loss of chest proprioception or intercostal muscle function), or apnea (decreased medullary perfusion secondary to hypotension). Respiratory dysfunction may necessitate intubation and ventilatory support.

   (c) Headache after spinal anesthesia or diagnostic lumbar puncture is encountered with higher frequency in young or female patients. This is usually the result of leakage of CSF from the puncture site. A postural component is always present (i.e., symptoms worsened by sitting up or standing). The recent use of smaller-gauge spinal needles has reduced the frequency of this complication. Treatment includes oral or intravenous fluids, oral analgesics, and caffeinated beverages. Severe refractory headache may require placement of an epidural blood patch to prevent ongoing leakage of CSF.

- **(d) CNS infection** after spinal anesthesia, although extremely rare, may result in meningitis, epidural abscess, or arachnoiditis.
- **(e) Permanent nerve injury** is exceedingly rare and is seen with the same frequency as in general anesthesia.
- **(f) Urinary retention with bladder distention** occurs in patients with spinal anesthesia whose bladders are not drained by urethral catheters, which should remain in place until after the spinal anesthesia has been stopped and full sensation has returned.

(5) Contraindications
- **(a) Absolute contraindications** to spinal anesthesia are localized infection at the planned puncture site, increased intracranial pressure, generalized sepsis, coagulopathy, and lack of consent.
- **(b) Relative contraindications** include hypovolemia, preexisting CNS disease, chronic low back pain, platelet dysfunction, and aortic stenosis.

b. Epidural anesthesia

(1) Anatomy and placement (Fig. 3-5)
- **(a)** Inserting an epidural needle is similar to placing a spinal needle except that the **epidural needle is not advanced through the dura**. No CSF is obtained. The tip of the epidural needle lies in the epidural space between the ligamentum flavum posteriorly and the dura mater anteriorly. Local anesthetic solution can then be injected.
- **(b)** Either the **needle is removed** (single-shot method) or, more commonly, **a flexible catheter is passed through the needle** into the space and the needle is withdrawn over the catheter (continuous catheter technique). Local anesthetics or opiates can be infused as needed.

(2) Level of analgesia
- **(a)** Once injected into the epidural space, the local anesthetic solution diffuses through the dura and into the spinal nerve roots, resulting in a **bilateral dermatomal distribution of analgesia.**
- **(b)** The spread of nerve root blockade is primarily determined by the **volume** of injection and, to a lesser degree, by patient **position and age** and **area of placement.**

(3) Onset and duration of analgesia
- **(a) Epidural anesthesia develops more slowly than does spinal anesthesia** because the local anesthetic solution must diffuse farther. The rate of onset of sympathetic blockade and hypotension also is slowed, enabling more precise titration of hemodynamic therapy compared with spinal anesthesia.
- **(b)** The **dosing interval** depends on the agent used.

(4) Complications are similar to those encountered with spinal anesthesia.
- **(a) Spinal headache** may result from inadvertent perforation of the dura.
- **(b) Epidural hematoma** is rare and usually occurs with coexisting coagulopathy. Emergent laminectomy may be required to decompress the spinal cord and avoid permanent neurologic injury.
- **(c)** If a patient with an epidural catheter in place becomes **hypotensive,** stopping the infusion of anesthetic will often correct the blood pressure.

c. Combined spinal and epidural anesthesia

(1) Anatomy and placement
- **(a)** A **small-gauge spinal needle** is placed through an epidural needle once the epidural space has been located. The dura is punctured only by the

spinal needle, and placement is verified by CSF withdrawal. Subarachnoid local anesthetics or narcotics can then be administered via the spinal needle.

   (b) The **spinal needle** is withdrawn after the initial dosing, and an epidural catheter is threaded into the epidural space through the existing epidural needle.

   (2) Onset and duration. This procedure combines the quick onset of spinal analgesia with the continuous dosing advantages of epidural analgesia.

   (3) Complications are similar to those seen in spinal and epidural anesthesia.

d. Comparison of spinal or epidural anesthesia with general anesthesia. Although the incidence of thromboembolic complications and total blood loss is reduced in certain surgical procedures with spinal or epidural anesthesia, there is no evidence that long-term mortality is reduced compared with general anesthesia (*Br J Anaesth* 1986;58:284).

e. Brachial plexus blockade. Injection of local anesthetic solution into the sheath surrounding the brachial plexus results in varying degrees of upper extremity blockade. This technique is indicated for any procedure involving the patient's shoulders, arms, or hands. The approach taken depends on the distribution of blockade desired.

   (1) Axillary block. The needle is placed into the brachial plexus sheath from the axilla. Blockade above the patient's elbow is unreliable.

   (2) Supraclavicular blockade. The needle is directed caudally from behind the posterior border of the inner one third of the clavicle. This technique reliably blocks the entire upper extremity, sparing the patient's shoulder. The risk of pneumothorax is low.

   (3) Interscalene blockade involves the cervical as well as brachial plexus and reliably blocks the patient's shoulder. There is a high incidence of phrenic nerve block, which increases the risk of pulmonary complications in patients with chronic obstructive pulmonary disease. This also serves as a contraindication to bilateral blockade.

f. Cervical plexus blockade blocks the anterior divisions of C1 to C4 and is the anesthetic method of choice for carotid endarterectomy at many institutions. Inadvertent blockade of neighboring structures does occur.

   (1) Phrenic nerve blockade may result in transient diaphragmatic paralysis. Simultaneous bilateral cervical plexus blockade is therefore contraindicated.

   (2) Ipsilateral cervical sympathetic plexus blockade may result in Horner syndrome, producing transient ptosis, miosis, and facial anhidrosis.

B. Outside the operating room

1. Intercostal nerve block is indicated after thoracotomy or before chest tube placement.

a. Anatomy and placement (Fig. 3-6)

   (1) The **posterior axillary line is identified,** and with the use of sterile technique, a 23-gauge needle is placed perpendicular to the patient's skin until contact is made with his or her rib. The needle is then walked caudad off the patient's rib and advanced several millimeters. After negative aspiration, 5 mL of bupivacaine 0.25% to 0.50% with epinephrine (1:200,000) is injected.

   (2) Usually, **five interspaces** (including two above and two below the interspace of interest) are injected.

b. Complications include pneumothorax and intravascular injection causing arrhythmias. Injection into the nerve sheath with retrograde spread back to the spinal cord can produce a high spinal or epidural block.

2. Digital block is indicated for minor procedures of the fingers.

a. Anatomy and placement

   (1) From the **dorsal surface of the hand,** a 23-gauge needle is placed on either side of the metatarsal head and inserted until the increased resistance of the palmar connective tissue is felt. An injection of 1 to 2 mL of lidocaine 1% to 2% is made as the needle is withdrawn.

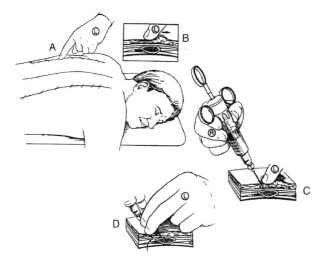

Figure 3-6. Anatomy and placement for intercostal nerve block. **A:** The administerer's hand closest to the patient's head (cephalic) first locates the target interspace and then **(B)** retracts the skin over the rib above. **C:** The hand closest to the patient's feet (caudad) places the needle and attached syringe containing local anesthetic through the skin onto the rib at approximately a 30-degree angle, with the needle bevel directed cephalad. **D:** The cephalic hand then grasps the needle while maintaining contact with the patient and allows the tension of the retracted skin to walk the needle off the inferior edge of the rib and advance 2 to 3 mm.

   (2) Supplemental injection of 0.5 to 1 mL of lidocaine 1% to 2% in the interdigital web on either side may be required.
   b. Epinephrine is contraindicated.
C. Local infiltration
   1. In the operating room, the area of incision can be infiltrated before incision or at the conclusion of the operation. Some evidence suggests that infiltration before incision is associated with less postoperative discomfort and reduced analgesic use (*Anesth Analg* 1992;74:495). Bupivacaine is frequently used.
   2. Outside the operating room, local anesthetic infiltration may also be useful during wound débridement, central venous catheter placement, or repair of minor lacerations. The agent of choice is lidocaine 1% to 2% due to its quick onset and low toxicity. The area of interest should be injected liberally. Frequent aspiration helps to avoid intravascular injection. Injection should be repeated as necessary.
   3. Local anesthetics containing **epinephrine** are **contraindicated** in areas where arterial spasm would lead to tissue necrosis (e.g., nose, ears, fingers, toes, penis).
III. GENERAL ANESTHESIA PROVIDES HYPNOSIS (UNCONSCIOUSNESS), ANALGESIA, AMNESIA, AND SKELETAL MUSCLE RELAXATION.
   A. All patients who are undergoing general anesthesia require an appropriate **preoperative evaluation** and optimization of any coexisting medical problems (see "Preparing the Patient," Sections I.A.1 and I.A.2).
   B. Monitoring. Basic monitoring requirements for general anesthesia are similar to those for regional anesthesia.
   C. Induction of general anesthesia. Intravenous agents are most widely used owing to rapid onset and ease of administration.
      1. Thiopental, a barbiturate (3 to 5 mg/kg intravenously), has a rapid onset and redistribution. However, there is often an associated decrease in cardiac output, BP, and cerebral blood flow. It should be used with caution in patients with hypotension or active coronary ischemia.

2. **Propofol,** a phenol derivative (1 to 3 mg/kg intravenously), is used for both induction and maintenance of anesthesia. Onset of action is immediate. It has hemodynamic properties that are similar to those of thiopental but is associated with a low incidence of postoperative nausea and vomiting. The pharmacokinetics is not changed by chronic hepatic or renal failure.

3. **Etomidate,** an imidazole derivative (0.3 mg/kg intravenously), has an onset of 30 to 60 seconds and only mild direct hemodynamic depressant effects.

4. **Ketamine,** a phencyclidine derivative (1 to 4 mg/kg intravenously), increases cardiac output and BP in patients who are not catecholamine depleted and provides dissociative anesthesia. Ketamine raises intracranial pressure and **is not** used in patients with head trauma. The **use of ketamine is limited** owing to emergence delirium and nightmares and is often reserved for use in the pediatric population.

D. **Airway management.** Ventilation during general anesthesia may be spontaneous, assisted, or controlled.

1. **Mask ventilation** with spontaneous respiratory effort can be used during limited (usually peripheral) procedures that do not require neuromuscular relaxation. Because the airway is unprotected, this technique is contraindicated in patients at risk for aspiration.

2. **Endotracheal intubation** secures the airway, allows control of ventilation, and protects against aspiration. Although frequently performed orally with the laryngoscope, intubation can also be accomplished nasally and, in anatomically challenging patients, can be performed with the aid of a fiberoptic bronchoscope via oral or nasal routes.

3. The **Laryngeal Mask Airway (LMA)** is an alternative airway device used for anesthesia and airway support consisting of an inflatable silicone mask and rubber connecting tube. It is inserted blindly into the pharynx, forming a low-pressure seal around the laryngeal inlet and permitting gentle positive pressure ventilation. It is an appropriate airway choice when mask ventilation can be used but endotracheal intubation is not necessary. The use of LMA is contraindicated in nonfasted patients, morbidly obese patients, and patients with obstructive or abnormal lesions of the oropharynx.

E. **Neuromuscular blockade** facilitates tracheal intubation and is required for many surgical procedures. It provides the surgeon with improved working conditions and optimizes ventilatory support. Agents that produce neuromuscular blockade act on postsynaptic receptors in the neuromuscular junction to antagonize the effects of acetylcholine competitively. Agents are categorized as either depolarizing or nondepolarizing (Table 3-6).

1. **Succinylcholine** is a rapidly acting (60 seconds), rapidly metabolized (by plasma cholinesterase) depolarizing agent that allows return of neuromuscular function in 5 to 10 minutes. This agent causes a transient mild hyperkalemia that may be exaggerated in patients with severe burns, trauma, or paralysis or patients with other neuromuscular disorders. In addition, it can cause increases in intraocular, intracranial, and gastric pressures. **Malignant hyperthermia** is a rare but deadly complication (see Section H.1.).

2. **Nondepolarizing muscle relaxants** can be divided into short-, intermediate-, and long-acting agents. Associated hemodynamic effects and elimination pathways vary.

a. **These agents are often used in an intensive care setting** when paralysis is necessary for adequate ventilation of an intubated patient. Such patients must have adequate sedation and analgesia before and during paralysis. Dosage should be monitored by train-of-four stimulus every 4 hours, with the goal being one out of four twitches. Corticosteroids, aminoglycosides, and long-term use of neuromuscular blockers potentiate the risk of a critical level of neuromyopathy.

b. **Reversal of neuromuscular blockade** for patients who are receiving nondepolarizing muscle relaxants usually is performed before extubation to ensure full return of respiratory muscle function and protective airway reflexes. The

TABLE 3-6	Agents Producing Neuromuscular Blockade			
Agent	**Initial dose (mg/kg)**	**Duration (min)**	**Elimination**	**Associated effects**
Depolarizing				
Succinylcholine	1–1.5	3–5	Plasma cholinesterase	Fasciculations, increase or decrease in heart rate, transient hyperkalemia, known malignant hyperthermia trigger agent
Nondepolarizing				
Mivacurium	0.15	8–10	Plasma cholinesterase	Flushing, decrease in BP
Atracurium	0.2–0.4	20–35	Ester hydrolysis	Histamine release
Cisatracurium	0.1–0.2	20–35	Ester hydrolysis	—
Vecuronium	0.1–0.2	25–40	Primarily hepatic	—
Rocuronium	0.6–1.2	30	Primarily hepatic	—
d-Tubocurare	0.5–0.6	75–100	Primarily renal	Histamine release, decrease in BP
Pancuronium	0.04–0.1	45–90	Primarily renal	Increase in heart rate, mean arterial BP, and caredic output
Doxacurium	0.05–0.08	90–180	Primarily renal	Decrease in BP

BP, blood pressure.

diaphragm is less sensitive to muscle relaxants than are the muscles of the head and neck. A spontaneously ventilating patient **may be unable to protect the airway.** The definitive test for assessing the degree of remaining paralysis is to have the patient raise the head from the bed for 5 seconds or more. **Anticholinesterases** (neostigmine, 0.06 to 0.07 mg/kg, and edrophonium, 0.1 mg/kg) act to increase the availability of acetylcholine at the neuromuscular junction. They reverse the blockade by reducing the binding frequency of the nondepolarizing muscle relaxant (a competitive acetylcholine antagonist).

F. **Maintenance of anesthesia**
1. The **goal of anesthesia** is to provide unconsciousness, amnesia, analgesia, and, usually, muscle relaxation. Balanced anesthesia involves the combined use of inhalational agents, narcotics, and muscle relaxants to attain this goal.
2. **Inhalational agents**
   a. All inhalational agents provide varying degrees of unconsciousness, amnesia, analgesia, and muscle relaxation.
   b. **Isoflurane** is the most commonly used inhalational agent due to its low rate of metabolism. It causes less cardiovascular depression than other agents. Enflurane, halothane, sevoflurane, and desflurane are also used.
   c. **Halothane** has a rapid onset of action. Its use is excellent for asthmatics because of its bronchial smooth muscle–relaxing properties. However, it does sensitize the myocardium to catecholamines, increasing the rate of ventricular arrhythmias. Halothane should also be used with caution in patients with brain lesions because it is a potent vasodilator and can increase cerebral perfusion and intracranial pressure. It is used extensively as an induction agent for pediatric patients because of the decreased irritating effects of halothane on the airway. Sevoflurane is also used in children for the same reason.

  d. Nitrous oxide by itself cannot provide surgical anesthesia. When combined with other inhalational agents, it reduces the required dose and subsequent side effects of the other agents. Nitrous oxide is extremely soluble and readily diffuses into any closed gas space, increasing its pressure. As a result, this agent should not be administered to patients with intestinal obstruction or suspected pneumothorax.

 3. Intravenous agents

  a. Narcotics can be administered continuously or intermittently. These agents provide superior analgesia but unreliable amnesia. Commonly used narcotics include fentanyl, sufentanil, alfentanil, remifentanil, morphine, and meperidine.

  b. Hypnotics, benzodiazepines, and propofol. Propofol infusion provides excellent hypnosis (unconsciousness) but insignificant analgesia and unreliable amnesia. The rapid dissipation of its effects and the low incidence of postoperative nausea have contributed to its widespread use in outpatient surgery. The maintenance dose is 0.1 to 0.2 mg/kg/minute.

  c. Ketamine by itself can provide total anesthesia. The associated emergence of delirium and nightmares limits its use.

G. Recovery from general anesthesia. The goal at the conclusion of surgery is to provide a smooth, rapid return to consciousness, with stable hemodynamics and pulmonary function, protective airway reflexes, and continued analgesia.

 1. Preparation for emergence from anesthesia usually begins before surgical closure, and communication between the surgeon and anesthesiologist facilitates prompt emergence of the patient at the procedure's termination.

 2. Patients recover from the effects of sedation or general or regional anesthesia in the **postanesthesia care unit.** Once they are oriented, comfortable, hemodynamically stable, ventilating adequately, and without signs of anesthetic or surgical complications, they are discharged to the appropriate ward or to home.

H. Complications of general anesthesia

 1. Malignant hyperthermia is a hypermetabolic disorder of skeletal muscle that is characterized by intracellular hypercalcemia and rapid adenosine triphosphate consumption. This condition is initiated by exposure to one or more anesthetic-triggering agents, including desflurane, enflurane, halothane, isoflurane, sevoflurane, and succinylcholine. Its incidence is approximately 1 in 50,000 in adults and 1 in 15,000 in children.

  a. Signs and symptoms may occur in the operating room or more than 24 hours postoperatively and include tachycardia, tachypnea, hypertension, hypercapnia, hyperthermia, acidosis, and skeletal muscle rigidity.

  b. Treatment involves immediate administration of dantrolene (1 mg/kg intravenously up to a cumulative dose of 10 mg/kg). This attenuates the rise in intracellular calcium. Repeat doses are given as needed if symptoms persist. Each vial commonly contains 20 mg of dantrolene and 3 g of mannitol and must be mixed with 50 mL of sterile water. Acidosis and hyperkalemia should be monitored and treated appropriately. Intensive care monitoring for 48 to 72 hours is indicated after an acute episode of malignant hyperthermia to evaluate for recurrence, acute tubular necrosis, pulmonary edema, and disseminated intravascular coagulation.

 2. Laryngospasm

  a. During emergence from anesthesia, noxious stimulation of the vocal cords can occur at light phases of anesthesia. In addition, blood or other oral secretions can irritate the larynx. As a result, the vocal cords may be brought into forceful apposition, and the flow of gas through the larynx may then be restricted or prevented completely. This alone may cause airway compromise or may lead to **negative-pressure pulmonary edema.**

  b. Treatment involves the use of positive-pressure ventilation by mask to break the spasm. Such therapy usually is sufficient. Succinylcholine may be required in refractory cases to allow successful ventilation.

3. **Nausea and vomiting**
   a. **Cortical** (pain, hypotension, hypoxia), **visceral** (gastric distention, visceral traction), **vestibular,** and **chemoreceptor trigger zone** (narcotics) afferent stimuli all can play a role in postoperative nausea and vomiting. The overall incidence is approximately 30%. It is more common in preadolescents 11 to 14 years old, women, and obese patients. Narcotics, etomidate, and isoflurane have been implicated.
   b. **Treatment** includes avoiding gastric distention during ventilation as well as administering prochlorperazine (Compazine), an antidopaminergic agent, 10 mg intravenously or orally every 4 to 6 hours as needed. For severe cases of postoperative nausea and vomiting, ondansetron (Zofran), 4 mg intravenously, can be given. The dosing can be repeated every 6 to 8 hours if symptoms persist.
4. **Urinary retention**
   a. Although very common with spinal anesthesia [see Section II.A.2.a(4)(f)], **urinary retention occurs in only 1% to 3% of cases involving general anesthesia.** It most commonly occurs after pelvic operations and in conjunction with benign prostatic hypertrophy.
   b. **Treatment** ranges from conservative (early ambulation, having patient sit or stand while attempting to micturate) to aggressive (bladder catheterization).
5. **Hypothermia**
   a. General anesthesia induction causes **peripheral vasodilation,** which leads to internal redistribution of heat, resulting in an increase in peripheral temperature at the expense of the core temperature. The core temperature then decreases in a linear manner until a plateau is reached. Such hypothermia is more pronounced in the elderly. Hypothermia may provoke cardiac arrhythmias.
   b. **Treatment** includes passive warming during an operation by insulation of all exposed surfaces. In addition, active warming with forced-air convective warmers is effective, but care should be taken in using warmers with patients with vascular insufficiency (warmers should not be used on ischemic extremities).
6. **Nerve injury**
   a. **Nerve palsies** can occur secondary to improper positioning of the patient on the operating table or insufficient padding of dependent regions. Such palsies can be long lasting and debilitating.
   b. **Prophylactic padding** of sensitive regions and attention to **proper positioning** remain the most effective therapies.
7. **Postanesthesia shaking**
   a. **Meperidine** or **butorphanol tartrate** may relieve postanesthesia shaking, which spontaneously and unpredictably occurs in up to two thirds of patients emerging from anesthesia.

Intubation and Sedation

I. EMERGENT INTUBATION BY RAPID-SEQUENCE INDUCTION

A. **Patients in respiratory distress** outside the operating room may require intubation to ensure adequate oxygenation and ventilatory support. Whenever possible, an anesthesiologist should be alerted and present at the time of intubation to assist if necessary; however, intubation should not be unduly delayed while waiting for an anesthesiologist to arrive.

B. **Airway support with 100% oxygen mask ventilation should be initiated before intubation.** In the emergent setting or with the hemodynamically unstable patient, rapid-sequence induction of anesthesia with etomidate followed by succinylcholine may be preferred. Succinylcholine should be avoided in patients with severe burns, intracranial bleeds, and eye trauma. Intubation can then be performed via laryngoscopy using an endotracheal tube of appropriate size—in general, a size 8 tube for men and a size 7 tube for women. After inflation of the cuff, bilateral and equal breath sounds should be auscultated, end-tidal CO_2 and pulse oximetry measured, and a portable chest x-ray ordered to ensure proper placement. The patient should be continued on 100% oxygen until transfer to an intensive care setting.

II. SEDATION FOR PROCEDURES

A. Monitored anesthesia care

1. In monitored anesthesia care or local standby cases, **an anesthesiologist is present** to monitor and sedate the patient during the procedure. The surgeon is responsible for analgesia, which is accomplished with local infiltration or peripheral nerve blockade. Sedating or hypnotic medications (e.g., propofol) provide sedation only, and when given in conjunction with inadequate analgesia, they may result in a disinhibited, uncooperative patient.

2. **Monitoring is identical to that required for general or regional anesthesia.** Supplemental oxygen is provided by facemask or nasal cannula.

3. **NPO criteria** are identical to those for general or regional anesthesia.

4. **Considerable variation exists** regarding the response of patients to sedating medications, and protective airway reflexes may be diminished with even small doses.

B. Local procedures in the operating room

1. *Local* implies that **an anesthesiologist is not required** to monitor the patient or provide sedation. It still is advisable for the physician performing the procedure to monitor the ECG, arterial oxygen saturation, and BP even if sedation is not given.

2. **Painful stimuli** can increase vagal tone, resulting in bradycardia, hypotension, and hypoventilation.

C. Sedation outside the operating room

1. **Indications** are to relieve patient anxiety and avoid potentially detrimental hemodynamic sequelae during invasive procedures or diagnostic tests.

2. **Oxygen** should be supplied by nasal cannula or facemask when sedation is given. When benzodiazepines and narcotics are combined, even healthy patients breathing room air may become hypoxic.

3. **Monitoring** should include pulse oximetry, continuous ECG, and BP.

4. The end result should be a calm, easily arousable, cooperative patient. Oversedation may result in hypoventilation, airway obstruction, or disinhibition. Doses of commonly used sedatives are summarized in Table 3-7.

5. **Side effects** that result from benzodiazepine administration include oversedation, respiratory depression, and depressed airway reflexes. Flumazenil (Romazicon), a benzodiazepine antagonist, can be used to reverse such effects. A dose of 0.2 mg intravenously should be administered and repeated every 60 seconds as required to a total dose of 1 mg. It can produce seizures and cardiac arrhythmias. Sedation can recur after 30 to 60 minutes, requiring repeated dosing.

TABLE 3-7	**Medications for Short-Term Sedation and Analgesia During Procedures**		
Agent	**Route**	**Dose (as needed)**	**Comments**
Midazolam (Versed)	IV	1–2 mg q5min	Benzodiazepines provide sedation only
Meperidine (Demerol)	IV	25–50 mg q10–15min	Narcotics provide analgesia with unpredictable sedative effects
Fentanyl	IV	25–50 μg q5–10min	Narcotics provide analgesia with unpredictable sedative effects
Propofol (Diprivan)	IV	10–20 mg over 3–5 min q10min	May cause hypotension, especially with boluses
IV, intravenous; q, every.			

Postoperative Medication and Complications

I. POSTOPERATIVE ANALGESIA is provided to minimize patient discomfort and anxiety, attenuate the physiologic stress response to pain, enable optimal pulmonary toilet, and enable early ambulation. Analgesics can be administered by the oral, intravenous, or epidural route.

A. Intravenous route. Many patients are unable to tolerate oral medications in the immediate postoperative period. For these patients, narcotics can be administered intravenously by several mechanisms.

1. As needed (PRN)

a. Narcotics

(1) The **intermittent administration of intravenous or intramuscular narcotics by nursing staff** has the disadvantage that the narcotics may be given too infrequently, too late, and in insufficient amounts to provide adequate pain control. This may be the only choice in patients who are functionally unable to operate a patient-controlled analgesia device.

(2) Morphine, 2 to 4 mg intravenously every 30 to 60 minutes, or **meperidine,** 50 to 100 mg intravenously every 30 to 60 minutes, should provide adequate analgesia for most patients. Orders should be written to withhold further injections for a respiratory rate of less than 12 breaths/minute or in cases of oversedation.

b. Nonsteroidal anti-inflammatory drugs (NSAIDs)

(1) Ketorolac is an NSAID that is available in oral and in injectable forms and is an effective adjunct to opioid therapy. The usual adult dose is 30 mg intramuscularly, followed by 15 to 30 mg every 6 hours for no longer than 48 hours.

(2) Ketorolac shares the potential side effects of other NSAIDs and should be used cautiously in the elderly and in patients with a history of peptic ulcer disease, renal insufficiency, steroid use, or volume depletion.

2. Patient-controlled analgesia (PCA)

a. With PCA, the patient has the ability to self-deliver analgesics within **preset safety parameters.** It is imperative to stress to family and friends that only the patient should administer the analgesic.

b. Patients initially receive **morphine** (100 mg in 100 mL, with each dose delivering 1 mg), **hydromorphone** (50 mg in 100 mL, with each dose delivering 0.25 mg), or **meperidine** (1,000 mg in 100 mL, with each dose delivering 20 mg), with a maximum of one dose every 10 minutes. If this treatment provides inadequate pain control, the concentration of the drug can be increased and/or the lockout time period can be reduced.

3. Continuous "basal" narcotic infusions are rarely used in the surgical population. Respiratory arrest can occur with the "buildup" of narcotic levels.

B. Epidural infusions are useful for treating postoperative pain caused by thoracotomy, extensive abdominal incisions, or orthopedic lower-extremity procedures. Narcotics, local anesthetics, or a mixture of the two can be infused continuously through catheters placed in the patient's lumbar or thoracic epidural space.

C. Oral agents. There are multiple oral agents and combination analgesics.

D. Side effects and complications

1. Oversedation and respiratory depression

a. Arousable, spontaneously breathing patients should be given supplemental oxygen and be monitored closely for signs of respiratory depression until mental status improves. Medications for pain or sedation should be decreased accordingly.

b. Unarousable but spontaneously breathing patients should be treated with oxygen and naloxone (Narcan). One vial of naloxone (0.4 mg) should be diluted in a 10-mL syringe, and 1 mL (0.04 mg) should be administered every 30 to 60 seconds until the patient is arousable. Adequate ventilation should be confirmed by arterial blood gas measurement. Current opioid administration should be stopped and the regimen decreased. In addition to continuous-pulse oximetry, the patient should be monitored closely for potential recurrence of sedation as the effects of naloxone dissipate.

2. **Apnea**
   a. **Treatment** involves immediate intubation and ventilation.
   b. **Naloxone,** 0.2 to 0.4 mg intravenously, should be given immediately.

3. **Hypotension and bradycardia**
   a. **Local anesthetics administered via lumbar epidurals** decrease sympathetic tone to the abdominal viscera and lower extremities and greatly increase venous capacitance. Thoracic epidurals can additionally block the cardioaccelerator fibers, resulting in bradycardia.
   b. The **treatment** of choice for any of these situations (excluding bradycardia) is cessation of epidural infusion followed by volume resuscitation. Epinephrine can be used to raise BP acutely; 10 mg is diluted in 100 mL and given intravenously 1 mL at a time. If needed, this mixture can be infused intravenously starting at 15 mL/hour (25 μg/minute). Bradycardia can be treated with atropine, 0.4 to 1 mg intravenously, or glycopyrrolate given intravenously in 0.2-mg increments every 3 to 5 minutes as needed.

4. **Nausea and vomiting**
   a. **Naloxone** in small doses (0.04 to 0.1 mg intravenously as needed).
   b. **Metoclopramide** (10 mg intravenously every 6 hours).
   c. **Zofran** (4 mg intravenously every 6 to 8 hours).
   d. **Compazine** (10 mg intravenously or orally every 4 to 6 hours).

5. **Pruritus**
   a. **Naloxone,** 0.04 to 0.1 mg intravenously, is effective.
   b. **Diphenhydramine,** 25 to 50 mg intravenously as needed, may provide symptomatic relief.

6. **Monoamine oxidase inhibitors** (e.g., isocarboxazid, phenelzine) may **interact adversely with narcotics,** resulting in severe hemodynamic swings, respiratory depression, seizures, diaphoresis, hyperthermia, and coma. Meperidine has been most frequently implicated and should be avoided. Although morphine and fentanyl are believed to be safe, narcotics should be avoided whenever possible.

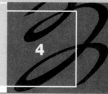

FLUID, ELECTROLYTE, AND ACID-BASE DISORDERS

Jennifer L. Gnerlich and Timothy G. Buchman

4

DIAGNOSIS AND TREATMENT OF FLUID, ELECTROLYTE, AND ACID-BASE DISORDERS

I. **DEFINITION OF BODY FLUID COMPARTMENTS.** Water constitutes 50% to 70% of lean body weight. Total body water content is slightly higher in men, is most concentrated in skeletal muscle, and declines steadily with age. Total body water is divided into an intracellular fluid compartment, comprising 40% of total body weight, and an extracellular fluid compartment, comprising 20%. The extracellular fluid compartment consists of a plasma or intravascular compartment, comprising 5% of total body weight, and an interstitial compartment, comprising 15%. The extracellular and intracellular compartments have distinct electrolyte compositions. The principal extracellular cation is Na^+, and the principal extracellular anions are Cl^- and HCO_3^-. In contrast, the principal intracellular cations are K^+ and Mg^{2+}, and the principal intracellular anions are phosphates and negatively charged proteins.

II. **OSMOLALITY AND TONICITY.** *Osmolality* refers to the number of osmoles of solute particles per kilogram of water. Total osmolality is composed of both effective and ineffective components. Effective osmoles cannot freely permeate cell membranes and are restricted to either the intracellular or extracellular fluid compartments. The asymmetric accumulation of effective osmoles in either extracellular fluid (e.g., Na^+, glucose, mannitol, glycine) or intracellular fluid (e.g., K^+, amino acids, organic acids) causes transcompartmental movement of water. Because the cell membrane is freely permeable to water, the osmolalities of the extracellular and intracellular compartments are equal. The effective osmolality of a solution is equivalent to its tonicity. Ineffective osmoles, in contrast, freely cross cell membranes and therefore are unable to affect shifts in water between fluid compartments. Such ineffective solutes (e.g., urea, ethanol, and methanol) contribute to total osmolality but not to tonicity. *Tonicity*, not osmolality, is the physiologic parameter that the body attempts to regulate.

III. **COMMON ELECTROLYTE DISORDERS**
   A. **Sodium**
      1. **Physiology.** The normal individual consumes 3 to 5 g of NaCl (130 to 217 mmol Na^+)/day. Balance is maintained primarily by the kidneys. Normal Na^+ concentration is 135 to 145 mmol/L (310 to 333 mg/dL). Potential sources of significant Na^+ loss include sweat, urine, and gastrointestinal (GI) secretions (Table 4-1). The Na^+ concentration largely determines the plasma osmolality (P_{osm}), which can be approximated by the following equation:

$$P_{osm}(mOsm/L) = 2 \times serum[Na^+ (mmol/L) + K^+ (mmol/L)] + \frac{glucose\ (mg/dL)}{18} + \frac{BUN\ (mg/DL)}{2.8},$$

where BUN is blood urea nitrogen. Normal P_{osm} is 290 to 310 mOsm/L. In general, hypotonicity and hypertonicity coincide with hyponatremia and hypernatremia, respectively. However, Na^+ concentration and total body water are controlled by independent mechanisms. As a consequence, hyponatremia or

TABLE 4-1 Composition of Gastrointestinal Secretions

Source	Volume (mL/24 hr)[a]	Na^+ (mmol/L)[b]	K^+ (mmol/L)[b]	Cl^- (mmol/L)[b]	HCO_3^- (mmol/L)[b]
Salivary	1,500 (500–2,000)	10 (2–10)	26 (20–30)	10 (8–18)	30
Stomach	1,500 (100–4,000)	60 (9–116)	10 (0–32)	130 (8–154)	0
Duodenum	(100–2,000)	140	5	80	0
Ileum	3,000	140 (80–150)	5 (2–8)	104 (43–137)	30
Colon	(100–9,000)	60	30	40	0
Pancreas	(100–800)	140 (113–185)	5 (3–7)	75 (54–95)	115
Bile	(50–800)	145 (131–164)	5 (312)	100 (89–180)	35

[a]Average volume (range).
[b]Average concentration (range).
Reprinted with permission from Faber MD, Schmidt RJ, Bear RA, et al. Management of fluid, electrolyte, and acid-base disorders in surgical patients. In: Narins RG, ed. *Clinical Disorders of Fluid and Electrolyte Metabolism*. New York: McGraw-Hill; 1994:1424.

hypernatremia may occur in conjunction with hypovolemia, hypervolemia, or euvolemia.

2. Hyponatremia

a. Causes and diagnosis. The diagnostic approach to hyponatremia is illustrated in Figure 4-1. Hyponatremia may occur in conjunction with hypertonicity, isotonicity, or hypotonicity. Consequently, it is necessary to measure the serum osmolality to evaluate patients with hyponatremia.

(1) Isotonic hyponatremia. Hyperlipidemic and hyperproteinemic states result in an isotonic expansion of the circulating plasma volume and cause a decrease in serum Na^+ concentration, although total body Na^+ remains the same. The reduction in serum sodium (mmol/L) can be estimated by multiplying the measured plasma lipid concentration (mg/dL) by 0.002 or the increment in serum protein concentration above 8 g/dL by 0.25. Isotonic, sodium-free solutions of glucose, mannitol, and glycine are restricted initially to the extracellular fluid and may similarly result in transient hyponatremia [see Section III.A.2.c(5)].

(2) Hypertonic hyponatremia. Hyperglycemia may result in transient fluid shift from the intracellular to the extracellular compartment, thus diluting the serum Na^+ concentration. The expected decrease in serum Na^+ is approximately 1.3 to 1.6 mmol/L (2.99 to 3.68 mg/dL) for each 100-mg/dL increase in blood glucose above 200 mg/dL. Rapid infusion of hypertonic solutions of glucose, mannitol, or glycine may have a similar effect on Na^+ concentration [see Section III.A.2.c(5)].

(3) Hypotonic hyponatremia is classified on the basis of extracellular fluid volume. Hypotonic hyponatremia generally develops as a consequence of the administration and retention of hypotonic fluids [e.g., dextrose 5% in water (D5W), 0.45% NaCl] and rarely from the loss of salt-containing fluids alone.

(a) Hypovolemic hypotonic hyponatremia in the surgical patient most commonly results from replacement of sodium-rich fluid losses (e.g., from the GI tract, skin, or lungs) with an insufficient volume of hypotonic fluid (e.g., D5W, 0.45% NaCl).

(b) Hypervolemic hypotonic hyponatremia. The edematous states of congestive heart failure, liver disease, and nephrosis occur in conjunction with inadequate circulating blood volume. This serves as a stimulus for the renal retention of sodium and of water. Disproportionate accumulation of water results in hyponatremia.

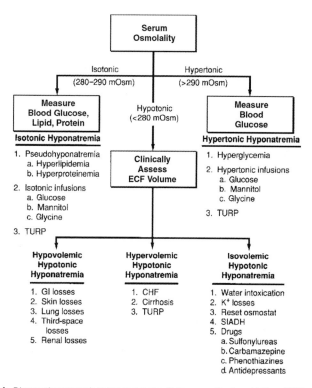

Figure 4-1. Diagnostic approach to hyponatremia. CHF, congestive heart failure; ECF, extracellular fluid; GI, gastrointestinal; SIADH, syndrome of inappropriate antidiuretic hormone secretion; TURP, transurethral resection of the prostate. (Adapted with permission from Narins RG, Jones ER, Stom MC, et al. Diagnostic strategies in disorders of fluid, electrolyte, and acid-base homeostasis. *Am J Med* 1982;72:496–520.)

(c) Isovolemic hypotonic hyponatremia

(i) Water intoxication typically occurs in the patient who consumes large quantities of water and has mildly impaired renal function (primary polydipsia). Alternatively, it may be the result of the administration of large quantities of hypotonic fluid in the patient with generalized renal failure.

(ii) K$^+$ loss, either from GI fluid loss or secondary to diuretics, may result in isovolemic hyponatremia due to cellular exchange of these cations.

(iii) Reset osmostat. Normally, the serum "osmostat" is set at 285 mOsm/L. In some individuals, the osmostat is "reset" downward, thus maintaining a lower serum osmolality. Several chronic diseases (e.g., tuberculosis and cirrhosis) predispose to this condition. Patients thus affected respond normally to water loads with suppression of antidiuretic hormone (ADH) secretion and excretion of free water.

(iv) SIADH (syndrome of inappropriate ADH) is characterized by low plasma osmolality (<280 mOsm/L), hyponatremia (<135 mmol/L), low urine output with concentrated urine (>100 mOsm/kg), elevated urine sodium (>20 mEq/L), and clinical euvolemia. The major causes of SIADH include pulmonary disorders (e.g., atelectasis, empyema, pneumothorax, respiratory failure), central nervous system disorders (e.g., trauma, meningitis, tumors, subarachnoid hemorrhage), drugs (e.g., cyclophosphamide, cisplatin, nonsteroidal anti-inflammatory drugs), and ectopic ADH production (e.g., small-cell lung carcinoma).

(4) Transurethral resection syndrome refers to hyponatremia in conjunction with cardiovascular and neurologic manifestations, which infrequently follow transurethral resection of the prostate. This syndrome results from intraoperative absorption of significant amounts of irrigation fluid (e.g., glycine, sorbitol, or mannitol). Isotonic, hypotonic, or hypertonic hyponatremia may occur. Management of these patients may be complicated.

b. Clinical manifestations. Symptoms associated with hyponatremia are predominantly neurologic and result from hypoosmolality. A decrease in P_{osm} causes intracellular water influx, increased intracellular volume, and cerebral edema. Symptoms include lethargy, confusion, nausea, vomiting, seizures, and coma. The likelihood that symptoms will occur is related to the degree of hyponatremia and to the rapidity with which it develops. Chronic hyponatremia is often asymptomatic until the serum Na^+ concentration falls below 110 to 120 mEq/L (253 to 276 mg/dL). An acute drop in the serum Na^+ concentration to 120 to 130 mEq/L (276 to 299 mg/dL), conversely, may produce symptoms.

c. Treatment
(1) Isotonic and hypertonic hyponatremia correct with resolution of the underlying disorder.
(2) Hypovolemic hyponatremia can be managed with administration of 0.9% NaCl to correct volume deficits and replace ongoing losses.
(3) Water intoxication responds to fluid restriction (1,000 mL/day).
(4) For **SIADH,** water restriction (1,000 mL/day) should be attempted initially. The addition of a loop diuretic (furosemide) or an osmotic diuretic (mannitol) may be necessary in refractory cases.
(5) Hypervolemic hyponatremia may respond to water restriction (1,000 mL/day) to return Na^+ to greater than 130 mmol/L (299 mg/dL). In cases of severe congestive heart failure, optimizing cardiac performance may assist in Na^+ correction. If the edematous hyponatremic patient becomes symptomatic, plasma Na^+ can be increased to a safe level by the use of a loop diuretic (furosemide, 20 to 200 mg intravenously every 6 hours) while replacing urinary Na^+ losses with 3% NaCl. A reasonable approach is to replace approximately 25% of the hourly urine output with 3% NaCl. Hypertonic saline should not be administered to these patients without concomitant diuretic therapy. Administration of synthetic brain natriuretic peptide (BNP) is also useful therapeutically in the setting of acute heart failure because it inhibits Na^+ reabsorption at the cortical collecting duct and inhibits the action of vasopressin on water permeability at the inner medullary collecting duct.
(6) In the presence of symptoms or extreme hyponatremia [Na^+ <110 mmol/L (253 mg/dL)] hypertonic saline (3% NaCl) is indicated. Serum Na^+ should be corrected to approximately 120 mmol/L (276 mg/dL). The quantity of 3% NaCl that is required to increase serum Na^+ to 120 mmol/L (276 mg/dL) can be estimated by calculating the Na^+ deficit:

$$Na^+ \text{deficit (mmol)} = 0.60 \times \text{lean body weight (kg)}$$
$$\times [120 - \text{measured serum } Na^+ \text{ (mmol/L)}].$$

(Each liter of 3% NaCl provides 513 mmol Na^+.) The use of a loop diuretic (furosemide, 20 to 200 mg intravenously every 6 hours) may increase the effectiveness of 3% NaCl administration. Central pontine demyelination occurs in the setting of correction of hyponatremia. The risk factors for

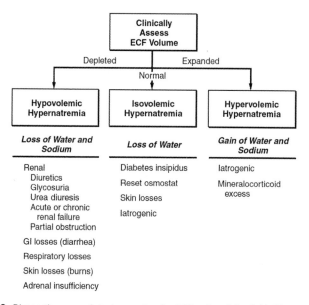

Figure 4-2. Diagnostic approach to hypernatremia. ECF, extracellular fluid; GI, gastrointestinal. (Adapted from Narins RG, Jones ER, Stom MC, et al. Diagnostic strategies in disorders of fluid, electrolyte, and acid-base homeostasis. *Am J Med* 1982;72:496–520.)

demyelination are controversial but appear to be related to the chronicity of hyponatremia (>48 hours) and the rate of correction. The serum Na^+ should be increased by no more than 12 mmol/L (27.6 mg/dL) in 24 hours of treatment [i.e., Na^+ <0.5 mmol (1.15 mg/dL)/hour]. For acute hyponatremia (<48 hours), the serum Na^+ may be corrected more rapidly [i.e., Na^+ = 1 to 2 mmol (2.3 to 4.6 mg/dL)/hour]. The patient's volume status should be carefully monitored over this time, and the serum Na^+ should be determined frequently (every 1 to 2 hours). Once the serum Na^+ concentration reaches 120 mmol/L (276 mg/dL) and symptoms have resolved, administration of hypertonic saline can be discontinued.

3. Hypernatremia

    a. Diagnosis. Hypernatremia is uniformly hypertonic and typically the result of water loss in excess of solute. Patients are categorized on the basis of their extracellular fluid volume status. The diagnostic approach to hypernatremia is illustrated in Figure 4-2.

        (1) Hypovolemic hypernatremia. Any net loss of hypotonic body fluid results in extracellular volume depletion and hypernatremia. Common causes in the surgical patient include diuresis as well as GI, respiratory, and cutaneous (e.g., burns) fluid losses. Chronic renal failure and partial urinary tract obstruction also may cause hypovolemic hypernatremia.

        (2) Hypervolemic hypernatremia in the surgical patient is most commonly iatrogenic and results from the parenteral administration of hypertonic solutions (e.g., $NaHCO_3$, saline, medications, and nutrition).

        (3) Isovolemic hypernatremia

            (a) Hypotonic losses. Constant evaporative losses from the skin and respiratory tract, in addition to ongoing urinary free water losses, require the administration of approximately 750 mL of electrolyte-free water (e.g., D5W) daily to parenterally maintained afebrile patients. Inappropriate replacement of these hypotonic losses with isotonic fluids is the most common cause of isovolemic hypernatremia in the hospitalized surgical patient.

(b) Diabetes insipidus is characterized by polyuria and polydipsia in association with hypotonic urine (urine osmolality <200 mOsm/kg or a specific gravity of <1.005) and a high plasma osmolality (>287 mOsm/kg). *Central diabetes insipidus* (CDI) describes a defect in the hypothalamic secretion of ADH and is commonly seen after head trauma or hypophysectomy. CDI may also occur as a result of intracranial tumors, infections, vascular disorders (aneurysms), hypoxia, or medications (e.g., clonidine, phencyclidine). *Nephrogenic diabetes insipidus* (NDI) describes renal insensitivity to normally secreted ADH. NDI may be familial or drug induced (e.g., lithium, demeclocycline, methoxyflurane, glyburide) or may occur as a result of hypokalemia, hypercalcemia, or intrinsic renal disease. If CDI and NDI are not distinguishable clinically, they can be differentiated by dehydration testing.

(c) Therapeutic. Hypertonic saline may be administered for deliberate hypernatremia to control elevated intracranial pressure and cerebral edema after head injury. Apart from osmotic properties, hypertonic saline also has hemodynamic, vasoregulatory, and immunomodulatory effects after traumatic brain injury. Two prospective, randomized studies demonstrated the efficacy of using hypertonic saline to reduce intracranial pressure (ICP). One study of adult patients with brain injury in an intensive care unit (ICU) comparing a 7.5% saline/6% dextran solution (HSD) and a 20% mannitol solution showed that HSD lowered ICP more effectively and for a longer duration than did mannitol (*Crit Care Med* 2005;33:196). Another study in children with severe head injury comparing hypertonic saline (Na$^+$ 268 mmol/L) with lactated Ringer's solution (Na$^+$ 131 mmol/L) demonstrated that an increase in serum sodium concentration was correlated with a reduction in ICP and an elevation in cerebral perfusion pressure. The children receiving hypertonic saline had fewer complications and a shorter ICU stay than the children receiving lactated Ringer's solution (*Crit Care Med* 1998;26:1265).

b. Clinical manifestations. Symptoms of hypernatremia that are related to the hyperosmolar state are primarily neurologic. These initially include lethargy, weakness, and irritability and may progress to fasciculations, seizures, coma, and irreversible neurologic damage.

c. Treatment

(1) Water deficit associated with hypernatremia can be estimated using the following equation:

$$\text{Water deficit (L)} = 0.60 \times \text{total body weight (kg)}$$
$$\times \; [(\text{serum Na}^+ \text{ in mmol/L}/140) = 1].$$

Rapid correction of hypernatremia can result in cerebral edema and permanent neurologic damage. Consequently, only one half of the water deficit should be corrected over the first 24 hours, with the remainder being corrected over the following 2 to 3 days. Serial Na$^+$ determinations are necessary to ensure that the rate of correction is adequate but not excessive. Oral fluid intake is acceptable for replacing water deficits. If oral intake is not possible, D5W or D5/0.45% NaCl can be substituted. In addition to the actual water deficit, insensible losses and urinary output must be replaced.

(2) Diabetes insipidus

(a) Central diabetes insipidus can be treated with desmopressin acetate administered intranasally [0.1 to 0.4 mL (10 to 40 μg) daily] or subcutaneously or intravenously [0.5 to 1 mL (2 to 4 μg) daily].

(b) **Nephrogenic diabetes insipidus** treatment requires removal of any potentially offending drug and correction of electrolyte abnormalities. If these measures are ineffective, dietary sodium restriction in conjunction with a thiazide diuretic may be useful (hydrochlorothiazide, 50 to 100 mg/day orally).

B. Potassium

1. Physiology. K^+ is the major intracellular cation, with only 2% of total body K^+ located in the extracellular space. The normal serum concentration is 3.3 to 4.9 mmol/L (12.9 to 19.1 mg/dL). Approximately 50 to 100 mmol (195 to 390 mg/dL) K^+ is ingested and absorbed daily. Ninety percent of K^+ is renally excreted, with the remainder eliminated in stools.

2. Hypokalemia

  a. Causes. K^+ depletion from inadequate intake alone is rare. Common causes of K^+ depletion in the surgical patient include GI losses (e.g., diarrhea, persistent vomiting, nasogastric suctioning), renal losses (e.g., diuretics, fluid mobilization, amphotericin B), and cutaneous losses (e.g., burns). Other causes of hypokalemia include acute intracellular K^+ uptake (associated with insulin excess, metabolic alkalosis, myocardial infarction, delirium tremens, hypothermia, and theophylline toxicity). Hypokalemia may also occur in the malnourished patient after initiation of total parenteral nutrition (refeeding syndrome), caused by the incorporation of K^+ into rapidly dividing cells.

  b. Clinical manifestations. Mild hypokalemia [K^+ >3 mmol/L (11.7 mg/ dL)] is generally asymptomatic. The symptoms present with severe K^+ deficiency [K^+ <3 mmol/L (11.7 mg/dL)] and are primarily cardiovascular. Early electroencephalogram (ECG) manifestations include ectopy, T-wave depression, and prominent U waves. Severe depletion increases susceptibility to reentrant arrhythmias.

  c. Treatment. In mild hypokalemia, oral replacement is suitable. Typical daily therapy for the treatment of mild hypokalemia in the patient with intact renal function is 40 to 100 mmol (156 to 390 mg) KCl orally in single or divided doses. Parenteral therapy is indicated in the presence of severe depletion, significant symptoms, or oral intolerance. K^+ concentrations (administered as chloride, acetate, or phosphate) in peripherally administered intravenous fluids should not exceed 40 mmol/L (156 mg/dL), and the rate of administration should not exceed 20 mmol (78 mg)/hour. However, higher K^+ concentrations [60 to 80 mmol/L (234 to 312 mg/dL)] administered more rapidly (with cardiac monitoring) are indicated in cases of severe hypokalemia, for cardiac arrhythmias, and in the management of diabetic ketoacidosis. Administration of high K^+ concentrations via subclavian, jugular, or right atrial catheters should be avoided because local K^+ concentrations may be cardiotoxic. Hypomagnesemia frequently accompanies hypokalemia and generally must be corrected to successfully replenish K^+.

3. Hyperkalemia

  a. Causes and diagnosis. Hyperkalemia may occur with normal or elevated stores of total body K^+. Pseudohyperkalemia is a laboratory abnormality that reflects K^+ release from leukocytes and platelets during coagulation. Spurious elevation in K^+ may result from hemolysis or phlebotomy from a strangulated arm. Abnormal redistribution of K^+ from the intracellular to the extracellular compartment may occur as a result of insulin deficiency, β-adrenergic receptor blockade, acute acidemia, rhabdomyolysis, cell lysis (after chemotherapy), digitalis intoxication, reperfusion of ischemic limbs, and succinylcholine administration.

  b. Clinical manifestations. Mild hyperkalemia [K^+ = 5 to 6 mmol/L (19.5 to 23.4 mg/dL)] is generally asymptomatic. Signs of significant hyperkalemia [K^+ >6.5 mmol/L (25.4 mg/dL)] are, most notably, ECG abnormalities: symmetric peaking of T waves, reduced P-wave voltage, and widening of the QRS complex. If untreated, severe hyperkalemia ultimately may cause a sinusoidal ECG pattern.

c. Treatment

(1) Mild hyperkalemia [$K^+ = 5$ to 6 mmol/L (19.5 to 23.4 mg/dL)] can be treated conservatively by the reduction of daily K^+ intake and the possible addition of a loop diuretic (e.g., furosemide) to promote renal elimination. Any medication that is capable of impairing K^+ homeostasis (e.g., nonselective β-adrenergic antagonists, angiotensin-converting enzyme inhibitors, K^+-sparing diuretics, nonsteroidal anti-inflammatory drugs) should be discontinued, if possible.

(2) Severe hyperkalemia [$K^+ >6.5$ mmol/L (25.4 mg/dL)]

(a) Temporizing measures produce shifts of potassium from the extracellular to the intracellular space.

(i) NaHCO$_3$ [1 mmol/kg or 1 to 2 ampules (50 mL each) of 8.4% NaHCO$_3$] can be infused intravenously over a 3- to 5-minute period. This dose can be repeated after 10 to 15 minutes if ECG abnormalities persist.

(ii) Dextrose (0.5 g/kg body weight) **infused with insulin** (0.3 unit of regular insulin/g of dextrose) transiently lowers serum K^+ (the usual dose is 25 g dextrose, with 6 to 10 units of regular insulin given simultaneously as an intravenous bolus).

(iii) Inhaled β-agonists [e.g., albuterol sulfate, 2 to 4 mL of 0.5% solution (10 to 20 mg) delivered via nebulizer] have been shown to lower plasma K^+, with a duration of action of up to 2 hours. Although only modest increases in heart rate and blood pressure have been reported when the nebulized form of this drug is used, caution is warranted in patients with known or suspected cardiovascular disease.

(iv) Calcium gluconate 10% (5 to 10 mL intravenously over 2 minutes) should be administered to patients with profound ECG changes who are not receiving digitalis preparations. Calcium functions to stabilize the myocardium.

(b) Therapeutic measures to definitively decrease total body potassium by increasing potassium excretion.

(i) Sodium polystyrene sulfonate (Kayexalate), a Na^+-K^+ exchange resin, can be administered orally (20 to 50 g of the resin in 100 to 200 mL of 20% sorbitol every 4 hours) or rectally (as a retention enema, 50 g of the resin in 50 mL of 70% sorbitol added to 100 to 200 mL of water every 1 to 2 hours initially, followed by administration every 6 hours) to promote K^+ elimination. A decrease in serum K^+ level typically occurs 2 to 4 hours after administration.

(ii) Hydration with 0.9% NaCl in combination with a **loop diuretic** (e.g., furosemide, 20 to 100 mg intravenously) should be administered to patients with adequate renal function to promote renal K^+ excretion.

(iii) Dialysis is definitive therapy in severe, refractory, or life-threatening hyperkalemia.

C. Calcium

1. Physiology. Serum calcium (8.9 to 10.3 mg/dL or 2.23 to 2.57 mmol/L) exists in three forms: ionized (45%), protein bound (40%), and complexed to freely diffusible compounds (15%). Only free ionized Ca^{2+} (4.6 to 5.1 mg/dL or 1.15 to 1.27 mmol/L) is physiologically active. Daily calcium intake ranges from 500 to 1,000 mg, with absorption varying considerably. Normal calcium metabolism is under the influence of parathyroid hormone (PTH) and vitamin D. PTH promotes calcium resorption from bone and reclamation of calcium from the glomerular filtrate. Vitamin D increases calcium absorption from the intestinal tract.

2. Hypocalcemia

a. Causes and diagnosis. Hypocalcemia most commonly occurs as a consequence of calcium sequestration or vitamin D deficiency. Calcium sequestration may occur in the setting of acute pancreatitis, rhabdomyolysis, or rapid administration of blood (citrate acting as a calcium chelator). Transient hypocalcemia may occur after total thyroidectomy, secondary to vascular compromise of the parathyroid glands, and after parathyroidectomy. In the latter case, serum Ca^{2+} reaches its lowest level within 48 to 72 hours after operation, returning to normal in 2 to 3 days. Hypocalcemia may occur in conjunction with Mg^{2+} depletion, which simultaneously impairs PTH secretion and function. Acute alkalemia (e.g., from rapid administration of parenteral bicarbonate or hyperventilation) may produce clinical hypocalcemia with a normal serum calcium concentration due to an abrupt decrease in the ionized fraction. Because 40% of serum calcium is bound to albumin, hypoalbuminemia may decrease total serum calcium significantly. A fall in serum albumin of 1 g/dL decreases serum calcium by approximately 0.8 mg/dL (0.2 mmol/L). Ionized Ca^{2+} is unaffected by albumin. As a consequence, the diagnosis of hypocalcemia should be based on ionized, not total serum, calcium.

b. Clinical manifestations. Tetany is the major clinical finding and may be demonstrated by Chvostek's sign (facial muscle spasm elicited by tapping over the branches of the facial nerve). The patient may also complain of perioral numbness and tingling. In addition, hypocalcemia can be associated with QT-interval prolongation and ventricular arrhythmias.

c. Treatment

(1) Parenteral therapy. Asymptomatic patients, even those with moderate hypocalcemia (calcium 6 to 7 mg/dL or 1.5 to 1.75 mmol/L), do not require parenteral therapy. Symptoms such as overt tetany, laryngeal spasm, or seizures are indications for parenteral calcium. Approximately 200 mg of elemental calcium is needed to abort an attack of tetany. Initial therapy consists in the administration of a calcium bolus (10 to 20 mL of 10% calcium gluconate over 10 minutes) followed by a maintenance infusion of 1 to 2 mg/kg elemental calcium/hour. Calcium chloride contains three times more elemental calcium than calcium gluconate; one 10-mL ampule of 10% calcium chloride contains 272 mg (13.6 mEq) elemental calcium, whereas one 10-mL ampule of 10% calcium gluconate contains only 90 mg (4.6 mEq) elemental calcium. The serum calcium level typically normalizes in 6 to 12 hours with this regimen, at which time the maintenance rate can be decreased to 0.3 to 0.5 mg/kg/hour. In addition to monitoring calcium levels frequently during therapy, one should check Mg^{2+}, phosphorus, and K^+ levels and supplement as necessary. Calcium should be administered cautiously to patients who are receiving digitalis preparations because digitalis toxicity may be potentiated. Once the serum calcium level is normal, patients can be switched to oral therapy.

(2) Oral therapy. Calcium salts are available for oral administration (calcium carbonate, calcium gluconate). Each 1,250-mg tablet of calcium carbonate provides 500 mg of elemental calcium (25.4 mEq), and a 1,000-mg tablet of calcium gluconate has 90 mg (4.6 mEq) of elemental calcium. In chronic hypocalcemia, with serum calcium levels of 7.6 mg/dL (1.9 mmol/L) or higher, the daily administration of 1,000 to 2,000 mg of elemental calcium alone may suffice. When hypocalcemia is more severe, calcium salts should be supplemented with a vitamin D preparation. Daily therapy can be initiated with 50,000 IU of calciferol, 0.4 mg of dihydrotachysterol, or 0.25 to 0.50 μg of 1,25-dihydroxyvitamin D_3 orally. Subsequent therapy should be adjusted as necessary.

3. Hypercalcemia

a. Causes and diagnosis. Causes of hypercalcemia include malignancy, hyperparathyroidism, hyperthyroidism, vitamin D intoxication, immobilization, long-term total parenteral nutrition, thiazide diuretics, and granulomatous disease. The finding of an elevated PTH level in the face of hypercalcemia supports the diagnosis of hyperparathyroidism. If the PTH level is normal or low, further evaluation is necessary to identify one of the previously cited diagnoses.

b. Clinical manifestations. Mild hypercalcemia (calcium <12 mg/dL or <3 mmol/L) is generally asymptomatic. The hypercalcemia of hyperparathyroidism is associated infrequently with classic parathyroid bone disease and nephrolithiasis. Manifestations of severe hypercalcemia include altered mental status, diffuse weakness, dehydration, adynamic ileus, nausea, vomiting, and severe constipation. The cardiac effects of hypercalcemia include QT-interval shortening and arrhythmias.

c. Treatment of hypercalcemia depends on the severity of the symptoms. Mild hypercalcemia (calcium <12 mg/dL or <3 mmol/L) can be managed conservatively by restricting calcium intake and treating the underlying disorder. Volume depletion should be corrected if present, and vitamin D, calcium supplements, and thiazide diuretics should be discontinued. The treatment of more severe hypercalcemia may require the following measures:

(1) NaCl 0.9% and loop diuretics may rapidly correct hypercalcemia. In the patient with normal cardiovascular and renal function, 0.9% NaCl (250 to 500 mL/hour) with furosemide (20 mg intravenously every 4 to 6 hours) can be administered initially. The rate of 0.9% NaCl infusion and the dose of furosemide should subsequently be adjusted to maintain a urine output of 200 to 300 mL/hour. Serum Mg^{2+}, phosphorus, and K^+ levels should be monitored and replaced as necessary. The inclusion of KCl (20 mmol) and $MgSO_4$ (8 to 16 mEq or 1 to 2 g) in each liter of fluid may prevent hypokalemia and hypomagnesemia. This treatment may promote the loss of as much as 2 g of calcium over 24 hours.

(2) Salmon calcitonin, in conjunction with adequate hydration, is useful for the treatment of hypercalcemia associated with malignancy and with primary hyperparathyroidism. Salmon calcitonin can be administered either subcutaneously or intramuscularly. Skin testing by subcutaneous injection of 1 IU is recommended before progressing to the initial dose of 4 IU/kg intravenously or subcutaneously every 12 hours. A hypocalcemic effect may be seen as early as 6 to 10 hours after administration. The dose may be doubled if unsuccessful after 48 hours of treatment. The maximum recommended dose is 8 IU/kg every 6 hours.

(3) Pamidronate disodium, in conjunction with adequate hydration, is useful for the treatment of hypercalcemia associated with malignancy. For moderate hypercalcemia (calcium 12 to 13.5 mg/dL or 3 to 3.38 mmol/L), 60 mg of pamidronate diluted in 1 L of 0.45% NaCl, 0.9% NaCl, or D5W should be infused over 24 hours. For severe hypercalcemia, the dose of pamidronate is 90 mg. If hypercalcemia recurs, a repeat dose of pamidronate can be given after 7 days. The safety of pamidronate for use in patients with significant renal impairment is not established.

(4) Plicamycin (25 μg/kg, diluted in 1 L of 0.9% NaCl or D5W, infused over 4 to 6 hours each day for 3 to 4 days) is useful for treatment of hypercalcemia associated with malignancy. The onset of action is between 1 and 2 days, with a duration of action of up to 1 week.

D. Phosphorus

1. Physiology. Extracellular fluid contains less than 1% of total body stores at a concentration of 2.5 to 4.5 mg/dL (0.81 to 1.45 mmol/L). Phosphorus balance is regulated by a number of hormones that also control calcium metabolism. As a consequence, derangements in concentrations of phosphorus and calcium frequently coexist. The average adult consumes 800 to 1,000 mg of phosphorus daily, which is predominantly renally excreted.

2. Hypophosphatemia

a. Causes

(1) Decreased intestinal phosphate absorption results from vitamin D deficiency, malabsorption, and the use of phosphate binders (e.g., aluminum-, magnesium-, calcium-, or iron-containing compounds).

TABLE 4-2	Phosphorus Repletion Protocol		

Phosphorus level	Weight 40–60 kg	Weight 61–80 kg	Weight 81–120 kg
<1 mg/dL	30 mmol Phos IV	40 mmol Phos IV	50 mmol Phos IV
1–1.7 mg/dL	20 mmol Phos IV	30 mmol Phos IV	40 mmol Phos IV
1.8–2.2 mg/dL	10 mmol Phos IV	15 mmol Phos IV	20 mmol Phos IV
If the patient's potassium is <4, use potassium phosphorus			
If the patient's potassium is >4, use sodium phosphorus			

IV, intravenous; Phos, phosphorus.
Adapted with permission from Taylor BE, Huey WY, Buchman TG, et al. Effectiveness of a protocol based on patient weight and serum phosphorus levels in repleting hypophosphatemia in a surgical ICU. *J Am Coll Surg* 2004;198:198–204.

(2) **Renal phosphate loss** may occur with acidosis, alkalosis, diuretic therapy (particularly acetazolamide), during recovery from acute tubular necrosis, and during hyperglycemia as a result of osmotic diuresis.

(3) **Phosphorus redistribution** from the extracellular to the intracellular compartment occurs principally with respiratory alkalosis and administration of nutrients such as glucose (particularly in the malnourished patient). This transient decrease in serum phosphorus is of no clinical significance unless there is a significant total body deficit. Significant hypophosphatemia may also occur in malnourished patients after the initiation of total parenteral nutrition (refeeding syndrome) as a result of the incorporation of phosphorus into rapidly dividing cells.

(4) Hypophosphatemia may develop in **burn patients** as a result of excessive phosphaturia during fluid mobilization and incorporation of phosphorus into new tissues during wound healing.

b. **Clinical manifestations.** Moderate hypophosphatemia (phosphorus 1 to 2.5 mg/dL or 0.32 to 0.81 mmol/L) is usually asymptomatic. Severe hypophosphatemia (phosphorus <1 mg/dL or 0.32 mmol/L) may result in respiratory muscle dysfunction, diffuse weakness, and flaccid paralysis.

c. **Treatment.** A recent study of patients at Barnes-Jewish Hospital's surgical intensive care unit (Saint Louis, MO) demonstrated that the use of an aggressive phosphorus repletion protocol based on a patient's admission weight (kg) and most recent phosphorus level (mg/dL) leads to more successful treatment of hypophosphatemia than physician-directed therapy (see Table 4-2). Adequate repletion of phosphorus is especially important in critically ill patients, who are more likely to experience adverse physiologic consequences from hypophosphatemia, including the inability to be weaned from the ventilator, organ dysfunction, and death. Phosphorus replacement should begin with intravenous therapy, especially for moderate (1 to 1.7 mg/dL) or severe (<1 mg/dL) hypophosphatemia (*J Am Coll Surg* 2004;198:198). Risks of intravenous therapy include hyperphosphatemia, hypocalcemia, hypotension, hyperkalemia (with potassium phosphate), hypomagnesemia, hyperosmolality, metastatic calcification, and renal failure. Five to 7 days of intravenous repletion may be required before intracellular stores are replenished. Once the serum phosphorus level exceeds 2 mg/dL (0.65 mmol/L), the patient can be switched to oral therapy. Oral therapy can be initiated with a sodium-potassium phosphate salt [e.g., Neutra-Phos, 250 to 500 mg (8 to 16 mmol phosphorus) orally four times a day; each 250-mg tablet of Neutra-Phos contains 7 mmol each of K^+ and Na^+].

3. **Hyperphosphatemia**

a. **Causes** include impaired renal excretion and transcellular shifts of phosphorus from the intracellular to the extracellular compartment (e.g., tissue trauma, tumor lysis, insulin deficiency, or acidosis). Hyperphosphatemia is also a common feature of postoperative hypoparathyroidism.

b. Clinical manifestations, in the short term, include hypocalcemia and tetany. In contrast, soft tissue calcification and secondary hyperparathyroidism occur with chronicity.

c. Treatment of hyperphosphatemia, in general, should eliminate the phosphorus source, remove phosphorus from the circulation, and correct any coexisting hypocalcemia. Dietary phosphorus should be restricted. Urinary phosphorus excretion can be increased by hydration (0.9% NaCl at 250 to 500 mL/hour) and diuresis (acetazolamide, 500 mg every 6 hours orally or intravenously). Phosphate binders (aluminum hydroxide, 30 to 120 mL orally every 6 hours) minimize intestinal phosphate absorption and can induce a negative balance of greater than 250 mg of phosphorus daily, even in the absence of dietary phosphorus. Hyperphosphatemia secondary to conditions that cause phosphorus redistribution (e.g., diabetic ketoacidosis) resolves with the treatment of the underlying condition and requires no specific therapy. Dialysis can be used to correct hyperphosphatemia in extreme conditions.

E. Magnesium

1. Physiology. Mg^{2+} (1.3 to 2.2 mEq/L or 0.65 to 1.10 mmol/L) is predominantly an intracellular cation. Renal excretion and retention play the major physiologic role in regulating body stores. Mg^{2+} is not under direct hormonal regulation.

2. Hypomagnesemia

a. Causes. Hypomagnesemia on the basis of dietary insufficiency is rare. Common etiologies include excessive GI or renal Mg^{2+} loss. GI loss may result from diarrhea, malabsorption, vomiting, or biliary fistulas. Urinary loss occurs with marked diuresis, primary hyperaldosteronism, renal tubular dysfunction (e.g., renal tubular acidosis), or chronic alcoholism or as a drug side effect (e.g., loop diuretics, cyclosporine, amphotericin B, aminoglycosides, cisplatin). Hypomagnesemia may also result from shifts of Mg^{2+} from the extracellular to the intracellular space, particularly in conjunction with acute myocardial infarction, alcohol withdrawal, or after receiving glucose-containing solutions. After parathyroidectomy for hyperparathyroidism, the redeposition of calcium and Mg^{2+} in bone may cause dramatic hypocalcemia and hypomagnesemia. Hypomagnesemia is usually accompanied by hypokalemia and hypophosphatemia and is frequently encountered in the trauma patient.

b. Clinical manifestations. Symptoms of hypomagnesemia are predominantly neuromuscular and cardiovascular. With severe depletion, altered mental status, tremors, hyperreflexia, and tetany may be present. The cardiovascular effects of hypomagnesemia are similar to those of hypokalemia and include T-wave and QRS-complex broadening as well as prolongation of the PR and QT intervals. Ventricular arrhythmias most commonly occur in patients who receive digitalis preparations.

c. Treatment

(1) Parenteral therapy is preferred for the treatment of severe hypomagnesemia (Mg^{2+} <1 mEq/L or 0.5 mmol/L) or in symptomatic patients. In cases of life-threatening arrhythmias, 1 to 2 g (8 to 16 mEq) of $MgSO_4$ can be administered over 5 minutes, followed by a continuous infusion of 1 to 2 g/hour for the next several hours. The infusion subsequently can be reduced to 0.5 to 1 g/hour for maintenance. The normal range of Mg^{2+} (1.3 to 2.2 mEq/L or 0.65 to 1.10 mmol/L) is probably below its physiologic optimum. Thus, except in cases of renal failure, vigorous correction of either severe or symptomatic hypomagnesemia is warranted. In less urgent situations, $MgSO_4$ infusion may begin at 1 to 2 g/hour for 3 to 6 hours, with the rate subsequently adjusted to 0.5 to 1 g/hour for maintenance. Mild hypomagnesemia (1.1 to 1.4 mEq/L or 0.5 to 0.7 mmol/L) in an asymptomatic patient can be treated initially with the parenteral administration of 50 to 100 mEq (6 to 12 g) of $MgSO_4$ daily until body stores are replenished. Treatment should be continued for 3 to 5 days, at which time the patient can be switched to an oral maintenance dose. Intravenous $MgSO_4$ remains the initial therapy of choice for torsades de pointes (polymorphologic ventricular tachycardia). Furthermore, it is used to achieve hypermagnesemia that is therapeutic for eclampsia and pre-eclampsia.

(2) Oral therapy. Magnesium oxide is the preferred oral agent. Each 400-mg tablet provides 241 mg (20 mEq) of Mg^{2+}. Other formulations include magnesium gluconate [each 500-mg tablet provides 27 mg (2.3 mEq) of Mg^{2+}] and magnesium chloride [each 535-mg tablet provides 64 mg (5.5 mEq) of Mg^{2+}]. Depending on the level of depletion, oral therapy should provide 20 to 80 mEq of Mg^{2+}/day in divided doses.

(3) Prevention of hypomagnesemia in the hospitalized patient who is receiving prolonged parenteral nutritional therapy can be accomplished by providing 0.35 to 0.45 mEq/kg of Mg^{2+}/day [i.e., by adding 8 to 16 mEq (1 to 2 g) of $MgSO_4$ to each liter of intravenous fluids].

3. Serum Mg^{2+} levels should be monitored during therapy. Reduce the dose of Mg^{2+} in patients with renal insufficiency.

4. Hypermagnesemia

a. Causes. Hypermagnesemia occurs infrequently, is usually iatrogenic, and is seen most commonly in the setting of renal failure.

b. Clinical manifestations. Mild hypermagnesemia (Mg^{2+} 5 to 6 mEq/L or 2.5 to 3 mmol/L) is generally asymptomatic. Severe hypermagnesemia (Mg^{2+} >8 mEq/L or 4 mmol/L) is associated with depression of deep tendon reflexes, paralysis of voluntary muscles, hypotension, sinus bradycardia, and prolongation of PR, QRS, and QT intervals.

c. Treatment. Cessation of exogenous Mg^{2+} is necessary. Calcium gluconate 10% (10 to 20 mL over 5 to 10 minutes intravenously) is indicated in the presence of life-threatening symptoms (e.g., hyporeflexia, respiratory depression, or cardiac conduction disturbances) to antagonize the effects of Mg^{2+}. A 0.9% NaCl (250 to 500 mL/hour) infusion with loop diuretic (furosemide, 20 mg intravenously every 4 to 6 hours) in the patient with intact renal function promotes renal elimination. Dialysis is the definitive therapy in the presence of intractable symptomatic hypermagnesemia.

IV. PARENTERAL FLUID THERAPY. The composition of commonly used parenteral fluids is presented in Table 4-3.

A. Crystalloids, in general, are solutions that contain sodium as the major osmotically active particle. Crystalloids are relatively inexpensive and are useful for volume expansion, maintenance infusion, and correction of electrolyte disturbances.

1. Isotonic crystalloids (e.g., lactated Ringer's solution, 0.9% NaCl) distribute uniformly throughout the extracellular fluid compartment so that after 1 hour, only 25% of the total volume infused remains in the intravascular space. Lactated Ringer's solution is designed to mimic extracellular fluid and is considered a balanced salt solution. This solution provides a HCO_3^- precursor and is useful for replacing GI losses and extracellular fluid volume deficits. In general, lactated Ringer's solution and 0.9% NaCl can be used interchangeably. However, 0.9% NaCl is preferred in the presence of hyperkalemia, hypercalcemia, hyponatremia, hypochloremia, or metabolic alkalosis.

2. Hypertonic saline solutions alone and in combination with colloids, such as dextran, have generated interest as a resuscitation fluid for patients with shock or burns. These fluids are appealing because, relative to isotonic crystalloids, smaller quantities are required initially for resuscitation. A randomized, double-blinded study of a 250-mL dose of hypertonic saline (7.5% NaCl, 6% dextran-70) compared to placebo (0.9% NaCl) given to patients in hemorrhagic shock after sustaining blunt trauma showed that the patients receiving the hypertonic saline bolus had significant blunting of neutrophil activation and alteration of the pattern of monocyte activation and cytokine secretion with a only a transient increase in serum sodium that normalized within 24 hours. This immunomodulatory effect of hypertonic saline plus dextran may help to prevent widespread tissue damage and multiorgan dysfunction seen after traumatic injury (*Ann Surg* 2006;243:47).

TABLE 4-3 Composition of Common Parenteral Fluids[a]

Solution	Volume[b]	Na+	K+	Ca2+	Mg2+	Cl−	HCO3 (as lactate)	Dextrose (g/L)	mOsm/L
Extracellular fluid	—	142	4	5	3	103	27	—	280–310
Lactated Ringer's	—	130	4	3	—	109	28	—	273
0.9% NaCl	—	154	—	—	—	154	—	—	308
0.45% NaCl	—	77	—	—	—	77	—	—	154
D5W	—	—	—	—	—	—	—	50	252
D5/0.45% NaCl	—	77	—	—	—	77	—	50	406
D5LR	—	130	4	3	—	109	28	50	525
3% NaCl	—	513	—	—	—	513	—	—	1,026
7.5% NaCl	—	1,283	—	—	—	1,283	—	—	2,567
6% hetastarch	500	154	—	—	—	154	—	—	310
10% dextran-40	500	0/154[c]	—	—	—	0/154[c]	—	—	300
6% dextran-70	500	0/154[c]	—	—	—	0/154[c]	—	—	300
5% albumin	250, 500	130–160	<2.5	—	—	130–160	—	—	330
25% albumin	20, 50, 100	130–160	<2.5	—	—	130–160	—	—	330
Plasma protein fraction	250, 500	145	—	—	—	145	—	—	300

D5LR, 5% dextrose in lactated Ringer's solution; D5/0.45% NaCl, 5% dextrose per 0.45% NaCl; D5W, 5% dextrose in water.
[a]Electrolyte concentrations in mmol/L.
[b]Available volumes (mL) of colloid solutions.
[c]Dextran solutions available in 5% dextrose (0 Na+, 0 Cl) or 0.9% NaCl (154 mmol Na+, 154 mmol Cl).

The possible side effects of hypertonic solutions include hypernatremia, hyperosmolality, hyperchloremia, hypokalemia, and central pontine demyelination with rapid infusion and should be administered with caution until more research becomes available.

B. Hypotonic solutions (D5W, 0.45% NaCl) distribute throughout the total body water compartment, expanding the intravascular compartment by as little as 10% of the volume infused. For this reason, hypotonic solutions should not be used for volume expansion. They are used to replace free water deficits.

C. Colloid solutions contain high-molecular-weight substances that remain in the intravascular space. Early use of colloids in the resuscitation regimen may result in more prompt restoration of tissue perfusion and may lessen the total volume of fluid required for resuscitation. However, there are no situations in which colloids have unequivocally been shown to be superior to crystalloids for volume expansion. In fact, the SAFE (Saline versus Albumin Fluid Evaluation) study, which randomized 6,997 patients in the ICU to receive either 4% albumin or normal saline for fluid resuscitation, found no significant difference in outcomes, including mortality and organ failure, between the two groups (*N Engl J Med* 2004;350:2247). Because colloid solutions are substantially more expensive than crystalloids, their routine use in hypovolemic shock is controversial. The use of colloids is indicated when crystalloids fail to sustain plasma volume because of low colloid osmotic pressure (e.g., increased protein loss from the vascular space, as in burns and peritonitis).

1. **Albumin preparations** ultimately distribute throughout the extracellular space, although the initial location of distribution is the vascular compartment. Preparations of 25% albumin (100 mL) and 5% albumin (500 mL) expand the intravascular volume by an equivalent amount (450 to 500 mL). Albumin 25% is indicated in the edematous patient to mobilize interstitial fluid into the intravascular space. The cost per liter of albumin is more than that of other colloid solutions and 30 times the cost of the intravascular volume–equivalent amount of crystalloid solutions; albumin preparations should be used judiciously. They are not indicated in the patient with adequate colloid oncotic pressure (serum albumin >2.5 mg/dL, total protein >5 mg/dL), for augmenting serum albumin in chronic illness (cirrhosis or nephrotic syndrome), or as a nutritional source.

2. **Dextran** is a synthetic glucose polymer that undergoes predominantly renal elimination. In addition to its indications for volume expansion, dextran also is used for thromboembolism prophylaxis and promotion of peripheral perfusion. Dextran solutions expand the intravascular volume by an amount equal to the volume infused. Side effects include renal failure, osmotic diuresis, coagulopathy, and laboratory abnormalities (i.e., elevations in blood glucose and protein, interference with blood cross-matching). Preparations of 40- and 70-kD dextran are available (dextran-40 and dextran-70, respectively).

3. **Hydroxyethyl starch (hetastarch)** is a synthetic molecule resembling glycogen that is available as a 6% solution in 0.9% NaCl. Hetastarch, like 5% albumin, increases the intravascular volume by an amount equal to or greater than the volume infused. Hetastarch is less expensive than albumin and has a more favorable side effect profile than dextran formulations, making it an appealing colloid preparation. Hextend is a recently Food and Drug Administration–approved colloid that contains 6% hetastarch, balanced electrolytes, a lactate buffer, and physiologic levels of glucose. Relative to hetastarch in saline, Hextend seems to have a more beneficial coagulation profile, less antigenicity, and antioxidant properties.

   a. **Indications** include use as a plasma volume–expanding agent in shock from hemorrhage, trauma, sepsis, and burns. Urine output typically increases acutely secondary to osmotic diuresis and must not be misinterpreted as a sign of adequate peripheral perfusion in this setting.

   b. **Elimination** is hepatic and renal. Patients with renal impairment are particularly subject to initial volume overload and tissue accumulation of hetastarch with repeated administration. In these patients, initial volume resuscitation accomplished with hetastarch should be maintained with another plasma volume expander, such as albumin or crystalloid.

      c. Laboratory abnormalities include elevations in serum amylase to approximately twice normal without alteration in pancreatic function.

      d. Dosing of hetastarch 6% solution is 30 to 60 g (500 to 1,000 mL), with the total daily dose not exceeding 1.2 g/kg (20 mL/kg) or 90 g (1,500 mL). In hemorrhagic shock, hetastarch solution can be administered at a rate of 1.2 g/kg/hour (20 mL/kg/hour). Slower rates of administration generally are used in patients with burns or septic shock. In individuals with severe renal impairment (creatinine clearance <10 mL/minute), the usual dose of hetastarch can be administered initially, but subsequent dose should be reduced 50% to 75%.

D. Principles of fluid management. A normal individual consumes an average of 2,000 to 2,500 mL of water daily. Daily water losses include approximately 1,000 to 1,500 mL in urine and 250 mL in stool. The minimum amount of urinary output that is required to excrete the catabolic end products of metabolism is approximately 800 mL. An additional 750 mL of insensible water loss occurs daily via the skin and respiratory tract. Insensible losses increase with hypermetabolism, fever, and hyperventilation.

    1. Maintenance. Maintenance fluids should be administered at a rate that is sufficient to maintain a urine output of 0.5 to 1 mL/kg/hour. Maintenance fluid requirements can be approximated on the basis of body weight as follows: 100 mL/kg/day for the first 10 kg, 50 mL/kg/day for the second 10 kg, and 20 mL/kg/day for each subsequent 10 kg. Maintenance fluids in general should contain Na^+ (1 to 2 mmol/kg/day) and K^+ [0.5 to 1 mmol/kg/day (e.g., D5/0.45% NaCl + 20 to 30 mmol K^+/L)].

    2. Preoperative management. Pre-existing volume and electrolyte abnormalities should be corrected before operation whenever possible. Consideration of duration and route of loss provides important information regarding the extent of fluid and electrolyte abnormalities.

    3. Intraoperative fluid management requires replacement of preoperative deficit as well as ongoing losses (Table 4-4). Intraoperative losses include maintenance fluids for the duration of the case, hemorrhage, and "third-space losses." The maintenance fluid requirement is calculated as detailed previously (see Section IV.D.1). Acute blood loss can be replaced with a volume of crystalloid that is three to four times the blood loss or with an equal volume of colloid or blood. Intraoperative insensible and third-space fluid losses depend on the size of the incision and the extent of tissue trauma and dissection and can be replaced with an appropriate volume of lactated Ringer's solution. Small incisions with minor tissue trauma (e.g., inguinal hernia repair) result in third-space losses of approximately 1 to 3 mL/kg/hour. Medium-sized incisions with moderate tissue trauma (e.g., uncomplicated sigmoidectomy) result in third-space losses of approximately

---

TABLE 4-4   **Estimation of Intraoperative Fluid Loss and Guide for Replacement**

Preoperative deficit	Maintenance IVF × hr NPO, plus preexisting deficit related to disease state
Maintenance fluids	Maintenance IVF × duration of case
Third-space and insensible losses	1–3 mL/kg/hr for minor procedure (small incision) 3–7 mL/kg/hr for moderate procedure (medium incision) 9–11 mL/kg/hr for extensive procedure (large incision)
Blood loss	1 mL blood or colloid per 1 mL blood loss, or 3 mL crystalloid per 1 mL blood loss

IVF, intravenous fluids; NPO, nothing by mouth.

3 to 7 mL/kg/hour. Larger incisions and operations with extensive tissue trauma and dissection (e.g., pancreaticoduodenectomy) can result in third-space losses of approximately 9 to 11 mL/kg/hour or greater.

4. **Postoperative fluid management** requires careful evaluation of the patient. Sequestration of extracellular fluid into the sites of injury or operative trauma can continue for 12 or more hours after operation. Urine output should be monitored closely and intravascular volume repleted to maintain a urine output of 0.5 to 1 mL/kg/hour. GI losses that exceed 250 mL/day from nasogastric or gastrostomy tube suction should be replaced with an equal volume of crystalloid. Mobilization of perioperative third-space fluid losses typically begins 2 to 3 days after operation. Anticipation of postoperative fluid shifts should prompt careful evaluation of the patient's volume status and, if needed, consideration of diuresis before the development of symptomatic hypervolemia.

V. ACID-BASE DISORDERS
A. Diagnostic approach
1. General concepts
   a. **Acid-base homeostasis** represents equilibrium among the concentration of H^+, partial pressure of CO_2 (Pco_2), and HCO_3^-. Clinically, H^+ concentration is expressed as pH.

   b. **Normal pH** is 7.35 to 7.45. **Acidemia** refers to pH of less than 7.35, and **alkalemia** refers to pH of greater than 7.45.

   c. **Acidosis and alkalosis** describe processes that cause the accumulation of acid or alkali, respectively. The terms *acidosis* and *acidemia* and the terms *alkalosis* and *alkalemia* are often used interchangeably, but such usage is inaccurate. A patient, for example, may be acidemic while alkalosis is occurring.

   d. **Laboratory studies** that are necessary for the initial evaluation of acid-base disturbances include arterial pH, arterial Pco_2 ($Paco_2$) (normal is 35 to 45 mm Hg), and serum electrolytes [HCO_3^- (normal is 22 to 31 mmol/L)]. Although base-excess or base-deficit calculations can be made, this information does not add substantially to the evaluation.

2. Compensatory response to primary disorders.
Disorders that initially alter $Paco_2$ are termed *respiratory acidosis* or *alkalosis*. Alternatively, disorders that initially affect plasma HCO_3^- concentration are termed *metabolic acidosis* or *alkalosis*. Primary metabolic disorders stimulate respiratory responses that act to return the ratio of Pco_2 to HCO_3^- (and therefore the pH) toward normal. Similarly, primary respiratory disturbances elicit countervailing metabolic responses that also act to normalize pH. As a general rule, these compensatory responses do not normalize pH because to do so would remove the stimulus for compensation. By convention, these compensating changes are termed *secondary*, *respiratory*, or *metabolic* compensation for the primary disturbance. The amount of compensation to be expected from either a primary respiratory or metabolic disorder is presented in Table 4-5. Significant deviations from these expected values suggest the presence of a mixed acid-base disturbance.

B. Primary metabolic disorders
1. Metabolic acidosis
results from the accumulation of nonvolatile acids, reduction of renal acid excretion, or loss of alkali. The most common causes of metabolic acidosis are listed in Table 4-6. Metabolic acidosis has few specific signs. The appropriate diagnosis depends on the clinical setting and laboratory tests.

   a. **The anion gap** (AG; normal = 12 ± 2 mmol/L) represents the anions, other than Cl^- and HCO_3^-, that are necessary to counterbalance Na^+ electrically:

$$AG \text{ (mmol/L)} = Na^+ \text{ (mmol/L)} + [Cl \text{ (mmol/L)} + HCO_3^- \text{ (mmol/L)}]$$

   It is useful diagnostically to classify metabolic acidosis into increased or normal AG metabolic acidosis.

   (1) Increased AG metabolic acidosis (Table 4-6).

   (2) Normal AG (hyperchloremic) metabolic acidosis (Table 4-6).

| TABLE 4-5 | Expected Compensation for Simple Acid-base Disorders | | |

Primary disorder	Initial change	Compensatory response	Expected compensation
Metabolic acidosis	HCO_3^- decrease	Pco_2 decrease	Pco_2 decrease = 1.2 × ΔHCO_3^-
Metabolic alkalosis	HCO_3^- increase	Pco_2 increase	Pco_2 increase = 0.7 × ΔHCO_3^-
Respiratory acidosis	Pco_2 increase	HCO_3^- increase	Acute: HCO_3^- increase = 0.1 × ΔPco_2 Chronic: HCO_3^- increase = 0.35 × ΔPco_2
Respiratory alkalosis	Pco_2 decrease	HCO_3^- decrease	Acute: HCO_3^- decrease = 0.2 × ΔPco_2 Chronic: HCO_3^- decrease = 0.5 × ΔPco_2

b. Treatment of metabolic acidosis must be directed primarily at the underlying cause of the acid-base disturbance. Bicarbonate therapy should be considered in patients with moderate to severe metabolic acidosis only after the primary cause has been addressed. The HCO_3^- deficit (mmol/L) can be estimated using the following equation:

$$HCO_3^- \text{ deficit (mmol/L)} = \text{body weight (kg)} \times 0.4$$
$$\times [(\text{desired } HCO_3^- \text{ [mmol/L]}) - (\text{measured } HCO_3^- \text{ [mmol/L]})]$$

This equation serves to provide only a rough estimate of the deficit because the volume of HCO_3^- distribution and the rate of ongoing H^+ production are variable.

| TABLE 4-6 | Causes of Metabolic Acidosis |

Increased anion gap
  Increased acid production
    Ketoacidosis
      Diabetic
      Alcoholic
      Starvation
    Lactic acidosis
    Toxic ingestion (salicylates, ethylene glycol, methanol)
  Renal failure

Normal anion gap (hyperchloremic)
  Renal tubular dysfunction
    Renal tubular acidosis
    Hypoaldosteronism
    Potassium-sparing diuretics
  Loss of alkali
    Diarrhea
    Ureterosigmoidostomy
    Carbonic anhydrase inhibitors
  Administration of HCl (ammonium chloride, cationic amino acids)

TABLE 4-7	Causes of Metabolic Alkalosis

Associated with extracellular fluid volume (chloride) depletion
  Vomiting or gastric drainage
  Diuretic therapy
  Posthypercapnic alkalosis
Associated with mineralocorticoid excess
  Cushing syndrome
  Primary aldosteronism
  Bartter syndrome
Severe K^+ depletion
Excessive alkali intake

(1) **Rate of HCO3$_3^-$ replacement.** In nonurgent situations, the estimated HCO_3^- deficit can be repaired by administering a continuous intravenous infusion over 4 to 8 hours [a 50-mL ampule of 8.4% $NaHCO_3$ solution (provides 50 mmol HCO_3^-) can be added to 1 L of D5W or 0.45% of NaCl]. In urgent situations, the entire deficit can be repaired by administering a bolus over several minutes. The goal of HCO_3^- therapy should be to raise the arterial blood pH to 7.20 or the HCO_3^- concentration to 10 mmol/L. One should not attempt to normalize pH with bicarbonate administration because the risks of bicarbonate therapy (e.g., hypernatremia, hypercapnia, cerebrospinal fluid acidosis, or overshoot alkalosis) are likely to be increased. Serial arterial blood gases and serum electrolytes should be obtained to assess the response to HCO_3^- therapy.

(2) **Lactic acidosis.** Correction of the underlying disorder is the primary therapy for lactic acidosis. Reversal of circulatory failure, hypoxemia, or sepsis reduces the rate of lactate production and enhances its removal. Because the use of $NaHCO_3$ in lactic acidosis is controversial, no definite recommendations can be made.

2. **Metabolic alkalosis** (Table 4-7)

  a. **Causes**

  (1) **Chloride-responsive metabolic alkalosis** in the surgical patient is typically associated with extracellular fluid volume deficits. The most common causes of metabolic alkalosis in the surgical patient include inadequate fluid resuscitation or diuretic therapy (e.g., contraction alkalosis), acid loss through GI secretions (e.g.. nasogastric suctioning, vomiting), and the exogenous administration of HCO_3^- or HCO_3^- precursors (e.g.. citrate in blood). Posthypercapnic metabolic alkalosis occurs after the rapid correction of chronic respiratory acidosis. Under normal circumstances, the excess in bicarbonate that is generated by any of these processes is excreted rapidly in the urine. Consequently, maintenance of metabolic alkalosis requires impairment of renal HCO_3^- excretion, most commonly due to volume and chloride depletion. Because replenishment of Cl^- corrects the metabolic alkalosis in these conditions, each is classified as Cl^--responsive metabolic alkalosis.

  (2) **Chloride-unresponsive metabolic alkalosis** is encountered less frequently in surgical patients and usually results from mineralocorticoid excess. Hyperaldosteronism, marked hypokalemia, renal failure, renal tubular Cl^- wasting (Bartter syndrome), and chronic edematous states are associated with chloride-unresponsive metabolic alkalosis.

  b. **Diagnosis.** Although the cause of metabolic alkalosis is usually apparent in the surgical patient, measurement of the urinary chloride concentration may be useful for differentiating these disorders. A urine Cl^- concentration of less than 15 mmol/L suggests inadequate fluid resuscitation, ongoing GI loss from emesis or nasogastric suctioning, diuretic administration, or posthypercapnia as the cause of the metabolic alkalosis. A urine Cl^- concentration of greater than 20 mmol/L suggests mineralocorticoid excess, alkali loading, concurrent diuretic administration, or the presence of severe hypokalemia.

   c. **Treatment principles** in metabolic alkalosis include identifying and removing underlying causes, discontinuing exogenous alkali, and repairing Cl^-, K^+, and volume deficits. Because metabolic alkalosis generally is well tolerated, rapid correction of this disorder usually is not necessary.

   (1) **Initial therapy** should include the correction of volume deficits (with 0.9% NaCl) and hypokalemia. Patients with vomiting or nasogastric suctioning also may benefit from H_2-receptor antagonists or other acid-suppressing medications.

   (2) **Edematous patients.** Chloride administration does not enhance HCO_3^- excretion because it does not correct the reduced effective arterial blood volume. Acetazolamide (5 mg/kg/day intravenously or orally) facilitates fluid mobilization while decreasing renal HCO_3^- reabsorption. However, tolerance to this diuretic may develop after 2 to 3 days.

   (3) **Severe alkalemia** (HCO_3^- >40 mmol/L), especially in the presence of symptoms, may require more aggressive correction. The infusion of acidic solutions is occasionally indicated in the patient with severe refractory metabolic alkalosis and chloride loss, typically due to massive nasogastric drainage or complete prepyloric obstruction. Ammonium chloride (NH_4Cl) is hepatically converted to urea and HCl. The amount of NH_4Cl that is required can be estimated using the following equation:

$$NH_4Cl \ (mmol) = 0.2 \times weight \ (kg) \times [103 - serum \ Cl^- \ (mmol)].$$

   NH_4Cl is prepared by adding 100 or 200 mmol (20 to 40 mL of the 26.75% NH_4Cl concentrate) to 500 to 1,000 mL of 0.9% NaCl. This solution should be administered at a rate that does not exceed 5 mL/minute. Approximately one half of the calculated volume of NH_4Cl should be administered, at which time the acid-base status and Cl^- concentration should be repeated to determine the necessity for further therapy. NH_4Cl is contraindicated in hepatic failure.

   (4) **HCl** [0.1 N (normal), administered intravenously] corrects metabolic alkalosis more rapidly. The amount of H^+ to administer can be estimated using the following equation:

$$H^+ \ (mmol) = 0.5 \times weight \ (kg) \times [103 - serum \ Cl^- \ (mmol/L)].$$

   To prepare 0.1 N HCl, mix 100 mmol of HCl in 1 L of sterile water. The calculated amount of 0.1 N HCl must be administered via a central venous catheter over 24 hours. The HCO_3^- concentration can be safely reduced by 8 to 12 mmol/L over 12 to 24 hours.

   (5) **Dialysis** can be considered in the volume-overloaded patient with renal failure and intractable metabolic alkalosis.

C. Primary respiratory disorders

   1. **Respiratory acidosis** occurs when alveolar ventilation is insufficient to excrete metabolically produced CO_2. Common causes in the surgical patient include respiratory center depression (e.g., drugs, organic disease), neuromuscular disorders, and cardiopulmonary arrest. Chronic respiratory acidosis may occur in pulmonary diseases, such as chronic emphysema and bronchitis. Chronic hypercapnia may also result from primary alveolar hypoventilation or alveolar hypoventilation related to extreme obesity (e.g., pickwickian syndrome) or from thoracic skeletal abnormalities. The diagnosis of acute respiratory acidosis usually is evident from the clinical situation, especially if respiration is obviously depressed. Appropriate therapy is correction of the underlying disorder. In cases of acute respiratory acidosis, there is no indication for $NaHCO_3$ administration.

TABLE 4-8	Common Causes of Mixed Acid-base Disorders

Metabolic acidosis and respiratory acidosis
  Cardiopulmonary arrest
  Severe pulmonary edema
  Salicylate and sedative overdose
  Pulmonary disease with superimposed renal failure or sepsis

Metabolic acidosis and respiratory alkalosis
  Salicylate overdose
  Sepsis
  Combined hepatic and renal insufficiency

Metabolic alkalosis and respiratory acidosis
  Chronic pulmonary disease, with superimposed:
    Diuretic therapy
    Steroid therapy
    Vomiting
    Reduction of hypercapnia by mechanical ventilation

Metabolic alkalosis and respiratory alkalosis
  Pregnancy with vomiting
  Chronic liver disease treated with diuretic therapy
  Cardiopulmonary arrest treated with bicarbonate therapy and mechanical ventilation

Metabolic acidosis and alkalosis
  Vomiting superimposed on
    Renal failure
    Diabetic ketoacidosis
  Alcoholic ketoacidosis

2. **Respiratory alkalosis** is the result of acute or chronic hyperventilation. The causes of respiratory alkalosis include acute hypoxia (e.g., pneumonia, pneumothorax, pulmonary edema, bronchospasm), chronic hypoxia (e.g., cyanotic heart disease, anemia), and respiratory center stimulation (e.g., anxiety, fever, Gram-negative sepsis, salicylate intoxication, central nervous system disease, cirrhosis, pregnancy). Excessive ventilation may also cause respiratory alkalosis in the mechanically ventilated patient. Depending on its severity and acuteness, hyperventilation may or may not be clinically apparent. Clinical findings are nonspecific. As in respiratory acidosis, the only effective treatment is correction of the underlying disorder.

D. **Mixed acid-base disorders.** When two or three primary acid-base disturbances occur simultaneously, a patient is said to have a mixed acid-base disorder. As summarized in Table 4-5, the respiratory or metabolic compensation for a simple primary disorder follows a predictable pattern. Significant deviation from these patterns suggests the presence of a mixed disorder. Table 4-8 lists some common causes of mixed acid-base disturbances. The diagnosis of mixed acid-base disorders depends principally on evaluation of the clinical setting and on interpretation of acid-base patterns. However, even normal acid-base patterns may conceal mixed disorders.

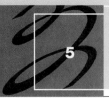

HEMOSTASIS AND TRANSFUSION THERAPY
Amy Fox and Craig M. Coopersmith

I. HEMOSTASIS
A. Mechanisms of hemostasis.
Coagulation is a complex equilibrium among thrombotic, anticoagulant, and fibrinolytic processes. Disruption of these processes can lead to severe hemorrhagic or thrombotic complications.

1. **Platelets** serve a primary role in hemostasis by filling defects in the vessel wall and by releasing thrombotic mediators. Endothelial injury exposes platelets to underlying collagen, which activates them. Von Willebrand factor (vWF) binds to platelet glycoprotein Ib/IX, allowing platelet adhesion. Bridges between activated platelets are formed through fibrinogen interaction with glycoprotein IIb/IIIa. Activated platelets release vasoactive agents and express binding sites for coagulation factors, causing platelet aggregation and thrombus formation.

2. **The coagulation cascade** is a series of reactions involving the activation of serine proteases (factors), which eventually leads to the formation of a cross-linked fibrin and platelet thrombus. Activation of two different pathways can initiate the coagulation cascade (Fig. 5-1). The **extrinsic pathway** begins when activated factor VIIa interacts with tissue factor, a lipoprotein released by injured cells. The **intrinsic pathway** is initiated by activation of factor XI to XIa by contact with activated factor XII, plasma prekallikrein, and high-molecular-weight kininogen (HMWK). Although the extrinsic pathway appears to be more important in initiating coagulation, both pathways are required for normal hemostasis. Both pathways merge in the production of factor Xa, the first enzyme of the common pathway. In the final step of the cascade, fibrin is produced by the action of thrombin on fibrinogen. Insoluble fibrin is then cross-linked by activated factor XIII. In addition to the enzymatic clotting factors, cofactors (e.g., factors V and VIII) and calcium are required for normal coagulation to occur on platelet phospholipid surfaces. Deficiencies of any of the coagulation factors, except for factor XII, HMWK, and prekallikrein, can lead to abnormal bleeding.

B. Endogenous anticoagulants
are important to restrict coagulation to the specific area of vascular injury. Deficiencies in these anticoagulants can lead to thrombosis.

1. **Antithrombin (AT, previously known as antithrombin III)** inhibits coagulation by binding several clotting factors (e.g., thrombin, factor Xa) and producing complexes that are cleared from the circulation. Heparin markedly accelerates AT-induced factor inhibition, increasing factor clearance and leading to anticoagulation.

2. **The thrombomodulin–protein C–protein S system** is also important in the regulation of hemostasis. Thrombomodulin binds with thrombin to accelerate the activation of protein C, a vitamin K–dependent proenzyme. Activated protein C inactivates factors Va and VIIIa in the presence of protein S.

C. Fibrinolytic system.
Once formed, fibrin can be degraded by plasmin, which allows for natural dissolution or remodeling of a clot. Exogenous streptokinase or endogenous tissue plasminogen activator and urokinase help to activate fibrin-bound plasminogen into plasmin.

D. Evaluation.
A detailed history and physical examination constitute the most important screening tools for hemostasis disorders in surgical patients. A family history of bleeding or bleeding disorders should be elicited. Laboratory studies can further

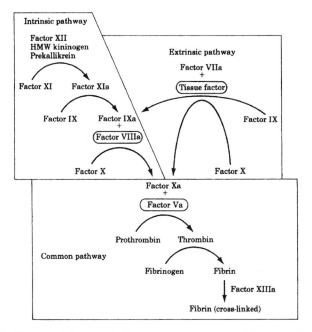

Figure 5-1. Blood coagulation cascade. Plasma zymogens are sequentially converted to active proteases (*arrows*). Nonenzymatic protein cofactors (*ovals*) are required at several stages of the cascade. Factors IX and X and prothrombin are activated on phospholipid surfaces. Thrombin cleaves fibrinogen, yielding fibrin monomers that polymerize to form a clot. HMW, high molecular weight. (Reprinted with permission from Ewald GS, McKenzie CR, eds. *Manual of Medical Therapeutics*, 28th ed. Boston: Little, Brown; 1995.)

characterize or identify clinical suspicion. Although surgical patients can have hereditary disorders of hemostasis, acquired defects and medications affecting hemostasis are most common in this patient population. In cases of hereditary hemostasis disorders, it is often helpful to work with the patient's hematologist in perioperative management.

II. EVALUATION OF PLATELETS

A. History and physical examination. Patients with a platelet disorder may complain of frequent bruising, epistaxis, or prolonged bleeding after minor injuries or surgical and dental procedures. A medication list should be reviewed to determine if any affect platelet function, such as aspirin, clopidogrel, and nonsteroidal anti-inflammatory drugs. Physical examination may reveal mucosal bleeding, petechiae, or purpura.

B. Laboratory evaluation

1. **Platelet count** (140,000 to 400,000/μL) is often determined as part of an automated blood count. If thrombocytopenia is noted, a peripheral smear must be obtained to confirm low platelet count because platelet clumping may lead to artifactually low platelet counts. The smear may also show evidence of abnormalities in white and red blood cells, which may help to elucidate an etiology.

2. **Platelet function** can be evaluated by multiple tests, but none is adequate for screening platelet dysfunction due to limited sensitivity. The risk or severity of surgical bleeding cannot be reliably assessed. **Bleeding time** (2.5 to 9 minutes) measures the duration of bleeding to stop after a standardized superficial cut. Qualitative platelet disorders, von Willebrand disease (vWD), vasculitides, and connective tissue disorders prolong bleeding time. **The platelet function analyzer**

TABLE 5-1	Commonly Used Drugs Affecting Platelet Number and Function

Drugs causing decreased platelet production
Thiazide diuretics
Amrinone
Ethanol
Estrogens
Trimethoprim-sulfamethoxazole
Chemotherapeutic agents

Drugs causing increased platelet destruction
Heparin
Quinidine
Quinine
Gold salts
Rifampin
Sulfonamides
Penicillins
Valproic acid

Drugs affecting platelet function
Nonsteroidal anti-inflammatory drugs
Aspirin
Dipyridamole

(PFA-100) measures the time for platelet aggregation and is useful for measuring global platelet function or assessing the efficacy of antiplatelet therapy.
C. **Platelet disorders**
   1. **Thrombocytopenia** is defined as a platelet count of less than 140,000/μL. If platelet function is normal, thrombocytopenia is usually not the cause of bleeding unless counts are less than 50,000/μL. Severe spontaneous bleeding may occur with platelet counts less than 10,000/μL. Intramuscular injections and rectal examinations, suppositories, or enemas should be limited in patients with severe thrombocytopenia (<10,000/μL).
      a. **Drug-induced thrombocytopenia.** Many drugs can affect platelet production or cause increased platelet destruction (Table 5-1) and are associated with bleeding. Increased destruction of platelets is most commonly the result of an immune mechanism in which platelets are destroyed by complement activation by drug–antibody complexes. **All nonessential drugs should be discontinued until the cause of the thrombocytopenia is identified.** Drug-induced thrombocytopenia typically resolves within 7 to 10 days after cessation and clearance of the offending agent. Prednisone (1 mg/kg/day orally) may facilitate recovery of platelet counts.
      b. **Heparin-induced thrombocytopenia (HIT)** is a unique form of drug-induced thrombocytopenia in which two different forms have been recognized.
         (1) **HIT type I** is a nonimmune, heparin-associated thrombocytopenia that typically begins within 4 days of initiation of heparin therapy. Platelet counts typically range between 100,000 and 140,000/μL. The incidence ranges from 5% to 30%. This form of HIT may not require cessation of heparin.
         (2) **HIT type II** is a severe immune-mediated syndrome caused by heparin-dependent antiplatelet antibodies occurring 5 to 10 days after initial exposure to heparin but within hours after re-exposure. Platelet counts are often less than 100,000/μL or drop by more than 50%. In 20% to 50% of cases, thrombotic events ensue, including extensive arterial and venous thrombosis (*N Engl J Med* 2006;355:809). Although diagnosis is clinical, the serotonin release assay or the enzyme-linked immunosorbent assay

may confirm the diagnosis. The serotonin release assay is the gold standard due to its high sensitivity and specificity, although it is expensive and not widely available. HIT is not type, dose, or route dependent, so care must be taken to discontinue and remove all sources of heparin, including flushes and heparin-coated catheters. If HIT is suspected, heparin should be stopped immediately prior to laboratory confirmation. Because thrombotic complications can continue even after the cessation of heparin, anticoagulation with a direct thrombin inhibitor (lepirudin or argatroban; see Section III.D.3) is recommended if there are no contraindications to anticoagulation. **If HIT is present, warfarin administration can potentiate a hypercoagulable state and has been associated with the development of venous limb gangrene.** Therefore, warfarin therapy should not be initiated until adequate alternative anticoagulant control has been achieved.

   c. **Dilutional thrombocytopenia** can occur with rapid blood product replacement for massive hemorrhage. No formula predicts accurate platelet requirements in this setting. Therefore, frequent platelet counts should be used to guide platelet transfusion therapy. In the setting of ongoing hemorrhage, empiric platelet transfusion may be appropriate.

   d. **Other causes of thrombocytopenia** include disseminated intravascular coagulation (DIC), sepsis, immune thrombycytopenic purpura (ITP), thrombotic thrombocytopenic purpura (TTP), hemolytic uremic syndrome (HUS), dialysis, and hematopoietic disorders. Therapy should be directed at the underlying disorder.

2. **Thrombocytosis** is defined as a platelet count greater than $600,000/\mu L$. Essential thrombocytosis is caused by myeloproliferative disease. Secondary thrombocytosis occurs with splenectomy, iron deficiency, malignancy, or chronic inflammatory disease. Aspirin therapy (81 mg/day orally) is useful in the treatment of thrombotic events in patients with myeloproliferative disorders and in decreasing fetal loss in pregnant women. Secondary thrombocytosis is generally not associated with an increased thrombotic risk and usually requires no specific therapy.

3. **Qualitative platelet dysfunction**

   a. **Medications** causing acquired defects of platelets account for most qualitative platelet disorders. Treatment is aimed at identifying the medication and ceasing usage if clinically appropriate. In cases of severe bleeding, platelet transfusions may be necessary.

      (1) **Aspirin** irreversibly acetylates cyclo-oxygenase, inhibiting platelet synthesis of thromboxane A2 and causing decreased platelet function. It is often used in the prevention and treatment of acute transient ischemic attacks, stroke, myocardial infarction, and coronary and vascular graft occlusion. Patients who are receiving anticoagulation therapy in addition to aspirin are at increased risk for bleeding complications and should be monitored closely. Aspirin should be discontinued about 1 week before elective nonvascular operations to allow new, functional platelets to form.

      (2) **Clopidogrel** is a thienopyridine that irreversibly inhibits platelet function by binding to the adenosine diphosphate (ADP) receptor that promotes aggregation and secretion. It is used to decrease thrombotic events in percutaneous stenting and patients with unstable angina. Although the half-life of clopidogrel is 8 hours, the bleeding time remains prolonged over 3 to 7 days, reflecting the fact that complete recovery of platelet function takes 5 days. Therefore, patients should discontinue clopidogrel therapy 7 days prior to elective operations to decrease the risk of bleeding complications.

      (3) **Glycoprotein IIb/IIIa inhibitors** (abciximab, tirofiban, eptifibatide) bind to the fibrinogen receptor, blocking platelet adhesion to fibrin. These agents are used in preventing coronary artery thrombosis after coronary angioplasty or in unstable angina. Although they have relatively short half-lives (0.5 to 2.5 hours), the bleeding time may remain elevated for longer periods. It is recommended that surgery be delayed 12 hours after discontinuing abciximab and 4 hours after discontinuing tirofiban or eptifibatide.

Zero-balance ultrafiltration may be beneficial in patients who need immediate surgical interventions (*Perfusion* 2002;17:33).

(4) Other medications. Dextran is used to reduce perioperative thrombotic events such as bypass graft occlusion because of its ability to decrease platelet aggregation and adhesion. **Nonsteroidal anti-inflammatory drugs (NSAIDS)** such as ketorolac (Toradol) inhibit cyclo-oxygenase, reversibly inhibiting platelet aggregation. **Hetastarch** can cause a transient decrease in platelet counts.

b. Other acquired defects of platelets are caused by uremia, liver disease, or cardiopulmonary bypass. Treatment is aimed at the underlying cause. Desmopressin acetate (DDAVP, 0.3 μg/kg intravenously 1 hour before operation) may limit bleeding from platelet dysfunction, particularly in uremic patients. Conjugated estrogens (0.6 mg/kg/day intravenously for 5 days) also can improve hemostatic function.

c. Hereditary defects of platelet dysfunction (e.g., von Willebrand disease, Bernard-Soulier syndrome, Glanzmann thrombasthenia, storage pool defects) are less common and usually warrant consultation with a hematologist.

D. Platelet transfusions

1. Indications. Platelet transfusions are used to control bleeding that is caused by thrombocytopenia or platelet dysfunction and to prevent spontaneous bleeding in situations of severe thrombocytopenia. Platelet transfusions should be considered for a platelet count of less than 10,000/μL to prevent spontaneous bleeding. In cases of bleeding or for minor surgical procedures, the transfusion threshold is often increased to a platelet count of less than 50,000/μL. For severe ongoing hemorrhage and before major operations, platelet counts greater than 100,000/μL should be the goal.

2. Complications associated with platelet transfusions

a. Alloimmunization occurs in 50% to 75% of patients receiving repeated platelet transfusions and presents as a failure of the platelet count to increase significantly after a transfusion. In patients who need long-term platelet therapy, human leukocyte antigen–matched single-donor platelets slow the onset of alloimmunization.

b. Posttransfusion purpura is a rare complication of platelet transfusions seen in previously transfused individuals and multiparous women. It is usually caused by antibodies that develop in response to a specific platelet antigen Pl^{A1} from the donor platelets. This condition presents with severe thrombocytopenia, purpura, and bleeding occurring 7 to 10 days after platelet transfusion. Although fatal bleeding can occur, the disease is typically self-limiting. Plasmapheresis or an infusion of intravenous immunoglobulin may be helpful.

III. EVALUATION OF COAGULATION

A. History and physical examination. Patients with a coagulopathy may typically show delayed development of soft-tissue hematomas and hemarthroses. Warfarin and heparin are common medications that affect coagulation. A patient's nutritional status such as vitamin K deficiency can also affect coagulation.

B. Laboratory evaluation

1. Prothrombin time (PT) (11 to 14 seconds) is the clotting time measured after the addition of thromboplastin, phospholipids, and calcium to citrated plasma. This test assesses the factors of the extrinsic and common pathways and is most sensitive to factor VII deficiency. Test reagents vary in their responsiveness to warfarin-induced anticoagulation; therefore, the **international normalized ratio (INR)** is used to standardize PT reporting between laboratories. The INR is the ratio of the measured PT to a mean laboratory control PT corrected for the sensitivity of testing reagents.

2. Partial thromboplastin time (PTT) (26 to 36 seconds) is the clotting time for plasma that is preincubated in particulate material (causing contact activation) followed by the addition of phospholipid and calcium. Inhibitors or deficiencies of factors in the intrinsic or common pathways cause prolongation of the PTT. A prolonged PTT should be evaluated by a 50:50 mixture with normal plasma.

Factor deficiencies are corrected by the addition of normal plasma, whereas prolongation due to inhibitors is not.

3. **Activated clotting time (ACT)** assesses the clotting time of whole blood. A blood sample is added to a diatomate-containing tube, leading to activation of the intrinsic pathway. The ACT is used to follow coagulation in patients requiring heparin during vascular procedures, percutaneous coronary interventions, or cardiopulmonary bypass. Automated systems are available for bedside use, allowing accurate and rapid determinations of the state of anticoagulation. Normal ACT is 150 to 180 seconds, with therapeutic target values ranging from 300 to 500 seconds for cardiac bypass procedures and 250 to 350 seconds for noncardiac vascular procedures (*Ann Pharm* 1995;29:1015).

4. **Thrombin time (TT)** (11 to 18 seconds) is the clotting time for plasma after the addition of thrombin. Patients with a fibrinogen level of less than 100 mg/dL or with abnormal fibrinogen will have a prolonged TT. The presence of fibrin degradation products (FDPs) or heparin can also elevate the TT. Prolongation of the TT by heparin can be confirmed by the addition of protamine sulfate to the assay, resulting in normalization of the test.

5. **Factor assays.** A fibrinogen level (150 to 360 mg/dL) can be measured directly by functional or immunologic quantitative assays. This level can be underestimated by the TT. FDP elevations (>8 μg/mL) occur in many disease states with increased fibrinogen turnover, including DIC, thromboembolic events, and during administration of fibrinolytic therapy. D-dimer levels reflect fibrinolysis and are useful in outpatient evaluations for pulmonary embolism. The utility in surgical patients is less clear due to its nonspecific elevation in response to inflammation.

C. **Disorders of coagulation**

1. **Acquired factor deficiencies** in surgical patients commonly result from a nutritional deficiency (e.g., vitamin K) or from medical conditions such as liver failure and DIC.

   a. **Vitamin K deficiency** leads to the production of inactive, noncarboxylated forms of prothrombin, factors VII, IX, and X, and proteins C and S. The diagnosis should be considered in a patient with a prolonged PTT that corrects with a 50:50 mixture of normal plasma. Vitamin K deficiency can occur in patients without oral intake within 1 week, with biliary obstruction, with malabsorption, and in those receiving antibiotics or warfarin.

   b. **Sepsis** stimulates the coagulation cascade, whereas levels of anticoagulant factors such as protein C, protein S, and antithrombin III are decreased. This represents an imbalance in hemostasis, causing microvascular thrombi to form. These thrombi further amplify injury and cause distal tissue ischemia and hypoxia. Therapy with activated protein C has been reported to decrease mortality in patients with severe sepsis as defined by an Acute Physiology and Chronic Health Evaluation (APACHE) II score greater than or equal to 25. Higher rates of bleeding have been noted in patients receiving activated protein C compared to placebo (*N Engl J Med* 2001;344:699).

   c. **Liver dysfunction** leads to complex alterations in coagulation through decreased synthesis of all clotting factors and inhibitors except vWF. The coagulopathy can be worsened by thrombocytopenia from associated hypersplenism. Spontaneous bleeding is infrequent, but coagulation defects should be corrected prior to invasive procedures. Fresh-frozen plasma (FFP) administration often improves the coagulopathy transiently (*Semin Liver Dis* 2002; 22:83).

   d. **Disseminated intravascular coagulation** has many inciting causes, including sepsis, extensive trauma or burns, necrotic tissue, intravascular antibody–antigen immune reactions, malignancies, liver failure, obstetric complications, and intravascular prosthetic devices. The pathogenesis of DIC is due to the inappropriate generation of thrombin within the vasculature, leading to the formation of fibrin thrombi, platelet activation, and fibrinolytic activity. DIC often presents with complications from microvascular thrombi that involve the vascular beds of the kidney, brain, lung, and skin. In some patients, the consumption of coagulation factors, particularly fibrinogen, and the activation of the fibrinolytic pathway can lead to bleeding. Laboratory findings in DIC include thrombocytopenia, hypofibrinogenemia, increased FDPs, and prolonged TT and PTT. Therapy begins with treatment of the underlying cause. Management of hemodynamics and oxygenation is critical. Correction of coagulopathy with platelet transfusions, FFP, and cryoprecipitate should be undertaken for bleeding complications but should not be given empirically. Although not well defined, prophylactic anticoagulation with heparin (500 to 1,000 units/hour intravenously) should be considered in patients with DIC.

2. **Hemophilia** is an inherited factor deficiency of either factor VIII (hemophilia A) or factor IX (hemophilia B, Christmas disease). The severity of the disease depends on the factor activity level. The diagnosis is suggested by patient history and an elevated PTT, normal PT, and normal bleeding time. Factor activity assays confirm the diagnosis. Minor bleeding can often be controlled locally without the need for factor replacement therapy. DDAVP stimulates the release of vWF into the circulation, which increases factor VIII levels two- to sixfold. This may control minor bleeding in patients with mild disease (*Semin Thromb Hemost* 2003;29:101). Major bleeding (e.g., during a surgical procedure) requires factor VIII replacement. Cryoprecipitate contains factor VIII, vWF, and fibrinogen and can be used to treat patients with hemophilia A for control of bleeding. Purified factor IX is the treatment of choice for hemophilia B.

3. **Other inherited factor deficiencies** account for fewer than 10% of severe factor deficiencies. Deficiencies of factor XII, HMWK, or prekallikrein do not cause bleeding and require no treatment.

4. **Inherited hypercoagulable disorders** place patients at risk for thrombosis and include deficiencies in body anticoagulants (antithrombin, protein C, and protein S deficiencies), hyperhomocystinemia, and prothrombin gene mutations. Indications for anticoagulation depend on type, severity, and clinical situation of the disorder.

    a. **Antithrombin deficiency** is an autosomal dominant disorder that presents with recurrent venous thromboembolism, usually in the second decade of life. Assays for AT levels are typically decreased in the setting of acute thrombosis and also if the patient is receiving heparin. Patients with acute thromboembolism or previous history of thrombosis are typically anticoagulated. AT-deficient patients should have the AT level restored to more than 80% of normal activity with AT concentrate prior to operation or childbirth.

    b. **Protein C deficiency and protein S deficiency** are risk factors for venous thrombosis. In a state of protein C or S deficiency, factors Va and VIIIa are not adequately inactivated, thereby allowing unchecked coagulation. Besides the inherited type, protein C deficiency is encountered in patients with liver failure and in those who are receiving warfarin therapy. Symptomatic patients are treated with heparin [or low-molecular-weight heparin (LMWH)] anticoagulation followed by warfarin therapy. In individuals with diminished protein C activity, effective heparin anticoagulation must be confirmed before warfarin initiation because warfarin transiently lowers protein C levels further and potentially worsens the hypercoagulable state. Patients with protein C or S deficiency but with no history of thrombosis typically do not require prophylactic anticoagulation.

    c. **Activated protein C resistance (factor V Leiden)** is a genetic mutation in factor V that renders it resistant to breakdown by activated protein C, placing patients at increased risk for thromboembolism. Routine preoperative screening in asymptomatic patients is unnecessary. Therapy for venous thrombosis consists of anticoagulation with heparin followed by warfarin therapy. The role of long-term warfarin anticoagulation for patients with a single thrombotic event is undefined.

5. **Acquired hypercoagulable disorders**

    a. **Antiphospholipid antibodies** are immunoglobulins that are targeted against antigens composed in part of platelet and endothelial cell phospholipids.

TABLE 5-2	Relative Contraindications to Anticoagulation Therapy

Ongoing bleeding
Recent surgical or invasive procedure
Recent severe trauma
Bleeding tendency (e.g., hemophilia, thrombocytopenia)
Intracranial hemorrhage
Malignant hypertension
Patients prone to falling
Pericarditis or pericardial effusion
Inadequate laboratory facilities
Noncompliant patient

Antiphospholipid antibody disorders may be detected by **lupus anticoagulant, anticardiolipin, or other antiphospholipid antibodies.** Patients with these antibodies are at risk for arterial and venous thrombosis, recurrent miscarriages, and thrombocytopenia.

  b. Other acquired hypercoagulable states include malignancies, pregnancy or the use of estrogen therapy, intravascular hemolysis (e.g., hemolytic anemia or after cardiopulmonary bypass), and the localized propensity for thrombosis in arteries that have recently undergone endarterectomy, angioplasty, or placement of prosthetic vascular grafts. Along with effective anticoagulation therapy, treatment should be directed at any identified underlying risk factor.

D. Anticoagulation medications

  1. Principles and indications. Anticoagulation is used to prevent and treat thrombosis and thromboembolic events. Before therapy is instituted, careful consideration must be given to the risk of thromboembolism and to anticoagulation-induced bleeding complications. Specific indications for anticoagulation therapy are discussed in detail in other chapters; they include atrial fibrillation, mechanical prosthetic heart valves, venous thromboembolism, stroke prevention, and acute arterial or graft occlusion. Table 5-2 shows relative contraindications to anticoagulation therapy.

  2. Heparin

  a. Unfractionated heparin (MW 10,000 to 20,000) acts by potentiating the action of AT, leading to accelerated inhibition of thrombin, factor Xa, and other coagulation proteases.

  (1) Administration. Heparin is administered parenterally, either subcutaneously or intravenously. PTT should be measured before initiation of heparin, 6 hours after the initial bolus, and 6 hours after each change in dosing. A therapeutic PTT of 1.5 to 2.5 times the control (approximately 50 to 80 seconds) should be maintained. Platelet counts should be measured daily until a maintenance dose of heparin is achieved and periodically thereafter.

  (2) Complications that occur with heparin therapy include bleeding and HIT. If bleeding occurs, heparin should be discontinued, and immediate assessment of the PT, PTT, and complete blood count (CBC) should be undertaken. Gastrointestinal (GI) bleeding that occurs while a patient is therapeutically anticoagulated suggests an occult source and warrants further evaluation. HIT is an uncommon but potentially devastating complication of heparin therapy and must be recognized early (see Section II.C.1.b).

  (3) Heparin clearance is rapid, occurring with a half-life of about 90 minutes. Reversal can be achieved more quickly with intravenous protamine sulfate. Each milligram of protamine sulfate reverses 100 units of heparin. The PTT or ACT can be used to assess the adequacy of the reversal. Protamine should be used with caution because it can induce anaphylactic reactions, especially in diabetic patients who have received protamine-insulin [neutral protamine Hagedorn (NPH)] preparations.

   b. LMWH preparations (enoxaparin, dalteparin, and tinzaparin) are depolymerized, yielding fragments of 3,000 to 7,000 daltons. The anticoagulant effect of LMWH is predominantly due to factor Xa inhibition, and LMWH results in less thrombin inhibition than unfractionated heparin. The advantages of LMWH include a more predictable anticoagulant effect, less platelet interaction, and a longer half-life. Dosing is based on weight, and laboratory monitoring is not typically needed. LMWH may be used for longer-term therapy in patients with a contraindication to oral anticoagulant treatment (e.g., pregnant patients who cannot take warfarin). Because LMWH has a longer half-life and no effective antidote, it must be used with caution in surgical patients and in those in whom a bleeding risk has been substantiated.

 3. **Direct thrombin inhibitors** are a class of compounds that bind to free and fibrin-bound thrombin. These agents inhibit thrombin activation of clotting factors, fibrin formation, and platelet aggregation.

   a. **Hirudin,** an anticoagulant originally derived from leeches, has been formulated as lepirudin and bivalirudin. Lepirudin, recombinant hirudin, binds irreversibly to thrombin, providing effective anticoagulation. The drug is approved in patients with HIT but may be considered in other severe clotting disorders. Lepirudin is cleared unmodified by the kidney, so dosing is adjusted in patients with renal insufficiency. Monitoring of anticoagulation is by the PTT, similar to heparin. Bivalirudin is a truncated form of recombinant hirudin that targets only the active site of thrombin. Bivalirudin is Food and Drug Administration approved for use during percutaneous coronary angioplasty and stenting.

   b. **Argatroban** is a synthetic thrombin inhibitor that is also approved for treatment of HIT. Therapy is monitored by the PTT. Elimination is primarily through the liver and should be used with caution in patients with hepatic insufficiency.

 4. **Warfarin** is a vitamin K antagonist that causes anticoagulation by inhibiting vitamin K–mediated carboxylation of factors II, VII, IX, and X as well as proteins C and S. The vitamin K–dependent factors decay with varying half-lives, so the full warfarin anticoagulant effect is not apparent for 5 to 7 days. When immediate anticoagulation is necessary, heparin or another agent must be used initially.

   a. **Administration.** Warfarin usually is initiated with a loading dose of 5 to 10 mg/day for 2 days, followed by dose adjustment based on daily INR results. The smaller dose is more likely to produce an INR of 2 to 3 with less excess anticoagulation and decreases the risk of a hypercoagulable state caused by precipitous drops in protein C levels during initiation of warfarin therapy (*Arch Int Med* 1999;159:46). Use of the INR provides a standard for the assessment of anticoagulation by warfarin and should be used in place of the PT or a PT ratio. Elderly patients, those with hepatic insufficiency, and those who are receiving parenteral nutrition or broad-spectrum antibiotics should be given lower initial doses of warfarin. A daily dose of warfarin needed to achieve therapeutic anticoagulation usually ranges from 2 to 15 mg/day. An INR of 2 to 3 is therapeutic for most indications, but patients with prosthetic heart valves should be maintained with an INR of 2.5 to 3.5. Once a stable INR is obtained on a stable warfarin dose, it can be monitored biweekly or monthly.

   b. **Complications.** The bleeding risk in patients who are treated with warfarin is estimated to be approximately 10% per year. The risk of bleeding correlates directly with the INR. Warfarin-induced skin necrosis, caused by dermal venous thrombosis, occurs rarely when warfarin therapy is initiated in patients who are not already anticoagulated and is often associated with hypercoagulability caused by protein C deficiency. Warfarin can produce significant birth defects and fetal death and should not be used during pregnancy. Changes in medications and diet that affect warfarin or vitamin K levels (Table 5-3) require more vigilant INR monitoring and dose adjustment.

TABLE 5-3	Commonly Used Drugs That Affect the International Normalized Ratio (INR) in Patients Receiving Oral Anticoagulation

Prolong INR
Anabolic steroids
Cimetidine
Clofibrate
Dipyridamole
Disulfiram
Erythromycin
Fluconazole
Metronidazole
Oral hypoglycemic agents
Quinidine
Second- and third-generation cephalosporins
Trimethoprim-sulfamethoxazole

Shorten INR
Antihistamines
Cholestyramine
Haloperidol
Oral contraceptives
Penicillins
Phenobarbital
Rifampin
Spironolactone
Vitamin K

    c. Reversal of warfarin-induced anticoagulation requires up to 1 week after discontinuation of therapy. Vitamin K administration can be used to reverse warfarin anticoagulation within 1 to 2 days, but the effect can last for up to 1 week longer. The appropriate vitamin K dose depends on the INR and the urgency with which correction must be accomplished. For patients with bleeding or extremely high INR levels (>10), 10 mg of vitamin K should be administered intravenously. Serial INR levels should be followed every 6 hours. In addition, FFP can be administered to patients with ongoing hemorrhage. Recombinant human factor VIIa has also been used (100 μg/kg) in cases of life-threatening bleeding.

  5. Indirect factor Xa inhibitors (Fondaparinux) are small, synthetic, heparin-like molecules that enhance AT-mediated inhibition of factor Xa. Fondaparinux has been shown to be as effective in preventing DVT after hip and knee replacement. Monitoring of coagulation parameters is usually not necessary. If bleeding complications occur, the drug should be stopped. FFP should be given, depending on the clinical situation. No specific antidote is available.

E. Fibrinolytic therapy

  1. Indications and contraindications. Thrombolytic therapy is most often used for iliofemoral deep venous thrombosis (DVT), superior vena caval thrombosis, pulmonary embolism (PE) resulting in a hemodynamically unstable patient, acute thrombosis of peripheral, mesenteric, and coronary arteries, acute vascular graft occlusion, thrombosis of hemodialysis access grafts, and occlusion of venous catheters. Contraindications to fibrinolytic therapy are listed in Table 5-4.

  2. Dosage depends on the agent and the indication. Tissue plasminogen activator (alteplase) or a recombinant analog (reteplase), as well as urokinase (Abbokinase), are used for lysis of catheter, venous, and peripheral arterial thrombi.

F. Transfusion products for coagulopathy

  1. FFP contains all the coagulation factors. However, factors V and VIII may not be stable through the thawing process and are not reliably recovered from FFP.

TABLE 5-4	Contraindications to Fibrinolytic Therapy

Absolute contraindications
Intolerable ischemia (for arterial thrombosis)
Active bleeding (not including menses)
Recent (<2 mo) stroke or neurosurgical procedure
Intracranial pathology such as neoplasm

Relative contraindications
Recent (<10 d) major surgery, major trauma, parturition, or organ biopsy
Active peptic ulcer or recent gastrointestinal bleeding (within 2 wk)
Uncontrolled hypertension (blood pressure >180/110 mm Hg)
Recent cardiopulmonary resuscitation
Presence or high likelihood of left heart thrombus
Bacterial endocarditis
Coagulopathy or current use of warfarin
Pregnancy
Hemorrhagic diabetic retinopathy

Therefore, it can be used to correct coagulopathies that are due to deficiencies of any other coagulation factor and is particularly useful when multiple factor deficiencies exist (e.g., liver disease or massive transfusion). FFP effects are immediate and typically last about 6 hours. Factor VIII and IX deficiencies are best treated using specific factor concentrates.

2. **Cryoprecipitate** is the cold-insoluble precipitate of fresh plasma and is rich in factor VIII and vWF as well as fibrinogen, fibronectin, and factor XIII. Cryoprecipitate may be used as second-line therapy in vWD or hemophilia but is most often used to correct fibrinogen deficiency in DIC or during massive transfusion.

3. **Recombinant human factor VIIa (rhFVIIa)** is used primarily in the treatment of patients with hemophilia or factor VIII inhibitors. However, it may be considered for patients with difficult bleeding problems for which therapy is inadequate or not available. The recommended dose is 100 μg/kg, which can be repeated at 1- to 2-hour intervals if needed. The PT is used to monitor drug effect. Use of rhFVIIa in blunt trauma patients requiring massive transfusions has been shown to reduce the overall blood transfusion requirements. There was also a trend in reduction of the incidence of multiple system organ failure and acute respiratory distress syndrome with its use (*Crit Care* 2006;10:R178, *J Trauma* 2006;60:242).

IV. **ANEMIA**
   A. **Evaluation.** Anemia is a decreased circulating red blood cell (RBC) mass and is defined as a hemoglobin level of less than 12 g/dL in women and less than 14 g/dL in men. A history and physical examination may determine the cause of anemia or indicate the acuity of the problem. Initial laboratory evaluation is usually a complete blood count, but a peripheral blood smear, reticulocyte count, and mean cellular volume may further help to evaluate and identify the cause of the anemia. The blood smear is used to identify abnormalities in RBCs, white blood cells (WBCs), and platelets. The reticulocyte count assesses the bone marrow response to anemia. A normal or low reticulocyte count in the presence of anemia suggests an inadequate bone marrow response. The mean cellular volume differentiates different types of anemia. Causes of anemia are summarized in Table 5-5.
   B. **Anemias associated with RBC loss or increased RBC destruction**
   1. **Bleeding** is the most frequently encountered cause of RBC destruction. Most postoperative patients have an obvious etiology for blood loss; however, sources of occult bleeding include the GI tract, uterus, urinary tract, and retroperitoneum. The hematocrit is not a reliable method to determine blood loss after an acute hemorrhage because the patient loses plasma in addition to RBCs.

TABLE 5-5	Classification of Anemia Based on Red Blood Cell (RBC) Kinetics

Anemias associated with impaired RBC production
Aplastic anemia
Iron-deficiency anemia
Thalassemia
Myelodysplastic syndromes and sideroblastic anemia
Megaloblastic anemia
Anemia of chronic renal insufficiency
Anemia of chronic disease
Zidovudine- and cancer chemotherapy–induced anemia
Anemias associated with increased RBC loss or destruction
Bleeding
Hereditary hemolytic anemias
    Hemoglobinopathies (e.g., sickle cell disease)
    Primary disorders of RBC membrane
    RBC enzymopathies (e.g., glucose 6-phosphate dehydrogenase)
Acquired hemolytic anemias
    Autoimmune hemolytic anemia
    Drug-induced hemolytic anemia
    Microangiopathic hemolytic anemia
    Traumatic hemolytic anemia
Paroxysmal nocturnal hemoglobinuria

2. **Sepsis.** Anemia is common is sepsis and is partially due to a decreased expression of the erythropoietin gene, but treatment with recombinant human erythropoietin has failed to demonstrate an increase in survival. Transfusions for hematocrits lower than 30% earlier in the stages of sepsis is associated with a decreased risk of mortality (*N Engl J Med* 2001;345:1368).

3. **Hemolytic anemias**
   a. **Acquired hemolytic anemias** are caused by autoimmune disorders, medications, or trauma. The direct Coombs test usually identifies autoimmune hemolytic anemia. Idiosyncratic drug-induced hemolytic anemia rarely occurs with a range of medications, but cefotetan-induced hemolysis is noteworthy because of its frequency and severity. Traumatic hemolytic anemias are often induced by malfunctioning prosthetic heart valves or vascular grafts.
   b. **Hereditary hemolytic anemias** include the hemoglobinopathy of sickle cell disease, which is caused by abnormal hemoglobin that polymerizes under decreased oxygen tension. Dehydration and hypoxia must be avoided to prevent sickling, which is critical in patients who undergo general anesthesia. Other hereditary hemolytic anemias include RBC membrane abnormalities (e.g., hereditary spherocytosis) and RBC enzymopathies (e.g., glucose 6-phosphate dehydrogenase deficiency).

C. **Anemias associated with decreased RBC production**
   1. **Iron-deficiency anemia** is most commonly caused by menstrual bleeding or occult GI blood loss. Sources of GI blood loss include gastritis, peptic ulcer disease, angiodysplasia, hemorrhoids, and colon adenocarcinoma. In men and postmenopausal women with iron-deficiency anemia, a complete GI evaluation for a potential source of blood loss is strongly recommended. Iron requirements for women increase during pregnancy owing to the transfer of iron to the fetus. Patients with a gastrectomy, achlorhydria, chronic diarrhea, or intestinal malabsorption may have diminished intestinal absorption of iron. The diagnosis is suggested by a hypochromic microcytic anemia, low serum iron levels (<60 μg/dL), increased total iron-binding capacity (>360 μg/dL), and low serum ferritin levels

(<14 ng/L). A trial of iron therapy typically establishes the diagnosis. Oral iron replacement (ferrous sulfate 325 mg orally three times a day) is usually sufficient treatment. It is generally administered with a stool softener, such as docusate sodium, to prevent constipation. Iron dextran also can be administered intramuscularly (100 mg/day) or as a single-dose intravenous preparation (1 to 2 g over 3 to 6 hours) in patients with malabsorption, poor compliance, or intolerance of oral preparations.

2. **Megaloblastic anemias** are associated with a deficiency of cobalamin (vitamin B_{12}) or folic acid. These deficiencies cause decreased DNA synthesis in all cells but primarily manifest in the hematopoietic tissue. Cobalamin, derived in the diet from meat and dairy products, is dependent on intrinsic factor (IF) for absorption. IF is produced by gastric parietal cells, and the IF-cobalamin complex is absorbed in the terminal ileum. Pernicious anemia in which anti-IF antibodies occur places patients at risk. In addition, patients with gastrectomy, ileal resection or ileitis, intestinal parasites, or bacterial overgrowth can develop vitamin B_{12} deficiency. However, because only a small portion of the body's stores is used each day, vitamin B_{12} deficiency takes several years to manifest. In addition to anemia, vitamin B_{12} deficiency often causes a neuropathy (extremity paresthesias), weakness, ataxia, and poor coordination. In contrast to vitamin B_{12} deficiency, folic acid deficiency can develop within weeks from decreased intake (e.g., alcohol abuse), malabsorption, or increased use (e.g., pregnancy or hemolysis). Clinical suspicion and serum vitamin B_{12} or folate levels establish the diagnosis. Therapy for vitamin B_{12} deficiency involves replacement with cyanocobalamin (1 mg/day intramuscularly for 7 days, then weekly for 2 months, then monthly). Folic acid is replenished (1 mg/day orally) until the deficiency is corrected. An incomplete response to therapy might indicate a coexisting iron deficiency, which occurs in one third of patients with megaloblastic anemia.

3. **Other anemias** associated with decreased RBC production include anemia due to renal insufficiency, chronic disease, chemotherapy, and the thalassemias. Aplastic anemia is an acquired defect of bone marrow stem cells and is associated with pancytopenia. The majority of cases are idiopathic or autoimmune, but approximately 20% are drug related (e.g., gold, benzene, chemotherapeutics, anticonvulsants, sulfonamides, chloramphenicol). Some are associated with an antecedent viral infection. A bone marrow biopsy helps to establish the diagnosis.

V. **TRANSFUSION THERAPY.** The risks and benefits of transfusion therapy must be considered carefully in each situation. Informed consent should be obtained before blood products are administered. The indications for transfusion should be noted in the medical record. Before elective procedures that are likely to require blood transfusion, the options of autologous or directed blood donation should be discussed with the patient in time to allow for the collection process.

A. **Indications.** RBC transfusions are used to treat anemia to improve the oxygen-carrying capacity of the blood. A hemoglobin level of 7 to 8 g/dL is adequate for tissue oxygenation in most normovolemic patients. However, therapy must be individualized based on the clinical situation rather than a hemoglobin level. The patient's age, cardiovascular and pulmonary status, volume status, the type of transfusion (i.e., homologous vs. autologous), and the expectation of further blood loss should guide transfusion decisions.

B. **Transfusions in critically ill patients.** Critically ill patients may be at increased risk for the immunosuppressive complications of transfusions and may benefit from a more restrictive transfusion protocol. A randomized, controlled clinical trial examined 838 critically ill patients with hemoglobin concentrations of less than 9 g/dL admitted to an intensive care unit. A restrictive transfusion strategy (transfusion for hemoglobin concentration <7 g/dL; maintain hemoglobin between 7 and 9 g/dL) was compared to a liberal transfusion strategy (transfusion for hemoglobin concentration <10 g/dL; maintain hemoglobin between 10 and 12 g/dL). Mortality rates were significantly lower with the restrictive transfusion strategy among patients who were less acutely ill or less than 55 years of age. A restrictive transfusion strategy was not as effective in patients with acute cardiac disease such as myocardial infarction or acute ischemia (*N Engl J Med* 1999;340:409).

C. Preparation. RBCs are most commonly administered as packed RBCs. When available, whole blood can be used for blood volume replacement associated with recent hemorrhage (i.e., in GI bleeding, major surgery, or trauma). Before administration, both donor blood and recipient blood are tested to decrease transfusion reactions. Blood typing tests the recipient's RBCs for antigens (A, B, and Rh) and screens the recipient's serum for the presence of antibodies to a panel of known RBC antigens. Each unit to be transfused is then cross-matched against the recipient's serum to check for preformed antibodies against antigens on the donor's RBCs. In an emergency situation, type O/Rh-negative blood that has been prescreened for reactive antibodies may be administered prior to blood typing and cross-matching. After blood typing, type-specific blood can be given.

D. Administration. Proper identification of the blood and patient is necessary to prevent transfusion errors. Packed RBCs should be administered through a standard filter (170 to 260 μm) and an 18-gauge or larger intravenous catheter. One unit of packed RBCs raises the hemoglobin approximately 1 g/dL and the hematocrit approximately 3%. The rate of transfusion is determined by the clinical situation; typically, however, each unit of blood must be administered within 4 hours. Patients are monitored for adverse reactions during the first 5 to 10 minutes of the transfusion and frequently thereafter. Those who need chronic transfusion therapy and organ transplant patients should be administered leukocyte-depleted blood. Immunocompromised patients and those receiving blood from first-degree relatives should be given irradiated blood to prevent graft versus host disease.

E. Alternatives to homologous transfusion exist and may provide advantages in safety and cost when used in elective procedures with a high likelihood of significant blood loss.

1. Autologous predonation is the preferred alternative for elective transfusions. Up to 20% of patients still require allogeneic transfusion, however, and transfusion reactions may still result from clerical errors in storage. Despite its intrinsic advantages, predonation is not cost-effective when the risk of transfusion is moderate or low.

2. Isovolemic hemodilution is a technique in which whole fresh blood is removed and crystalloid is simultaneously infused in the immediate preoperative period. The blood is stored at room temperature and reinfused after acute blood loss has ceased. Moderate hemodilution (hematocrit 32% to 33%) is as effective as autologous predonation in reducing the need for allogeneic transfusion and is much less costly.

3. Intraoperative autotransfusion, in which blood from the operative field is returned to the patient, can decrease allogeneic transfusion requirements. Equipment to separate and wash recovered RBCs is required. Contraindications include neoplasm and enteric or purulent contamination.

4. Erythropoietin may be effective in decreasing allogeneic transfusion requirements when given preoperatively. Appropriate dose can be calculated based on anticipated transfusion requirements and is administered weekly over 2 to 4 weeks. Adjunctive use with autologous predonation has not consistently been shown to be effective. Chronic anemia, particularly anemia due to renal disease, is usually treated with erythropoietin (50 to 100 U/kg subcutaneously three times a week) rather than with transfusions.

F. Complications of Transfusions

1. Infections. Despite aggressive testing of the blood supply, the spread of transmissible agents is still a concern with homologous blood. However, the use of polymerase chain reaction (PCR)–based testing of blood products has greatly reduced transmission rates of viral diseases. Hepatitis B transmission is in the range of 1 in 205,000 units transfused. The risk of HIV or hepatitis C transmission is in the range of 1 in 2 million units transfused. Blood is tested for human T-cell lymphoma viruses and syphilis. In 2003, PCR testing for West Nile virus was also initiated. Cytomegalovirus (CMV) transmission is a risk in CMV-negative immunocompromised patients and can be lowered by using either leukocyte-depleted or CMV-negative blood products. Bacteria and endotoxins can be infused with blood products, particularly in platelets that are stored at room temperature. Parasitic infections also can be transmitted, although rarely, with blood products.

2. **Transfusion reactions**

   a. **Allergic reactions** are the most common type of transfusion reactions and occur when the patient reacts to donated plasma proteins in the blood. Symptoms include itching or hives and can often be treated with antihistamines such as diphenhydramine (25 to 50 mg orally or intravenously). Prophylactic administration of benadryl and prednisone prior to a transfusion may be considered in patients with a previous history of allergic reaction. Rarely, severe reactions may involve bronchospasm or laryngospasm, which should prompt discontinuation of the infusion. Steroids and subcutaneous epinephrine may also be required.

   b. **Febrile nonhemolytic reactions** involve the development of a high fever during or within 24 hours of a transfusion. This reaction is mediated by the body's response to white blood cells in donated blood. General malaise, chills, nausea, or headaches may accompany the fever. Because fever can be the first manifestation of a more serious transfusion reaction, the situation must be promptly evaluated. Patients with a previous history of a febrile reaction should receive leukoreduced blood products.

   c. **Acute immune hemolytic reactions** are the most serious transfusion reactions, in which patient antibodies react to transfused RBC antigens causing intravascular hemolysis. This typically occurs with ABO or Rh incompatibility. Symptoms include nausea, chills, anxiety, flushing, and chest or back pain. Anesthetized or comatose patients may show signs of excessive incisional bleeding or oozing from mucous membranes. The reaction may progress to shock or renal failure with hemoglobinuria. If a transfusion reaction is suspected, the infusion should be stopped immediately. Identities of the donor unit and recipient should be rechecked because clerical error is the most common cause. A repeat cross-match should be performed in addition to a complete blood count, coagulation studies, and serum bilirubin. Treatment includes maintenance of intravascular volume, hemodynamic support as needed, and preservation of renal function. Urine output should be maintained at greater than 100 mL/hour using volume resuscitation and possibly diuretics if resuscitation is attained. Alkalinization of the urine to a pH of greater than 7.5 by adding sodium bicarbonate to the intravenous fluids (two to three ampules of 7.5% sodium bicarbonate in 1,000 mL of D5W) helps to prevent precipitation of hemoglobin in the renal tubules.

   d. **Delayed hemolytic reactions** result from an anamnestic antibody response to antigens other than the ABO antigens to which the recipient has been previously exposed. Transfused blood cells may take days or weeks to hemolyze after transfusion. Typically there are few signs or symptoms other than a falling red blood cell count or elevated bilirubin. Specific treatment is rarely necessary, but severe cases should be treated like acute hemolytic reactions, with volume support and maintenance of urine output.

   e. **Transfusion-related acute lung injury (TRALI)** is a serious reaction that typically occurs within 1 to 2 hours of transfusion but can occur any time up to 6 hours later. Patients complain of shortness of breath and may have a fever. Support can vary from supplemental oxygen to intubation and ventilation. Although most cases resolve on their own, severe cases can be fatal.

   f. **Graft versus host disease (GVHD)** can occur after transfusion of immunocompetent T cells into immunocompromised recipients or human leukocyte antigen–identical family members. GVHD presents with a rash, elevated liver function tests, and pancytopenia and has an associated mortality of greater than 80%. Irradiation of donor blood from first-degree relatives of immunocompetent patients and all blood for immunocompromised patients prevents this complication.

3. **Volume overload after blood transfusion** can occur in patients with poor cardiac or renal function. Careful monitoring of the volume status and judicious use of diuretic therapy can reduce the risk of this complication.

4. **Massive transfusion,** usually defined as the transfusion of blood products that are greater in volume than a patient's normal blood volume in less than 24 hours, creates several risks not encountered with a lesser volume or rate of transfusion. **Coagulopathy** might arise as a result of platelet or coagulation factor depletion. Transfusion of platelets, FFP, or cryoprecipitate should be based on the clinical situation and laboratory values rather than empirically based. **Hypothermia** can result from massive volume resuscitation with chilled blood products but can be prevented by using blood warmers. Hypothermia can lead to cardiac dysrhythmias and coagulopathy. **Citrate toxicity** can develop after massive transfusion in patients with hepatic dysfunction. Hypocalcemia can be treated with intravenous administration of 10% calcium gluconate. **Electrolyte abnormalities,** including acidosis and hyperkalemia, occur rarely after massive transfusions, especially in patients with preexisting hyperkalemia.

VI. **LOCAL HEMOSTATIC AGENTS** can aid in the intraoperative control of bleeding from needle punctures, vascular suture lines, or areas of extensive tissue dissection. Anastomotic bleeding usually is best controlled with local pressure or a simple suture. Local hemostatic agents promote hemostasis by providing a matrix for thrombus formation.

A. **Gelatin sponge** (e.g., Gelfoam) can absorb many times its weight of whole blood by capillary action and provides a platform for coagulation. Gelfoam itself is not intrinsically hemostatic. It resorbs in 4 to 6 weeks without a significant inflammatory reaction.

B. **Oxidized cellulose** (e.g., Surgicel) is a knitted fabric of cellulose that allows clotting by absorbing blood and swelling into a scaffold. Its slow resorption can create a foreign body reaction.

C. **Collagen sponge** (e.g., Helistat) is produced from bovine tendon collagen and promotes platelet adhesion. It is slowly resorbed and creates a foreign body reaction similar to that of cellulose.

D. **Microfibrillar collagen** (e.g., Avitene, Hemotene) can be sprayed onto wounds and anastomoses for hemostasis, particularly in areas that are difficult to reach. It stimulates platelet adhesion and promotes thrombus formation. Because microfibrillar collagen can pass through autotransfusion device filters, it should be avoided during procedures that utilize the cell-saver.

E. **Topical thrombin** can be applied to the various hemostatic agents or to dressings and placed onto bleeding sites to achieve a fibrin-rich hemostatic plug. Topical thrombin, usually of bovine origin, is supplied as a lyophilized powder and can be applied directly to dressings or dissolved in saline and sprayed onto the wound. Repeated use of bovine thrombin may result in formation of inhibitors to thrombin or factor V, which is not usually associated with a clinical bleeding disorder, although there may be dramatic alterations in the coagulation testing. Topical thrombin can be used effectively in anticoagulated patients.

F. **Gelatin matrices** (e.g., FloSeal) are often used in combination with topical thrombin intraoperatively. Typically, bovine thrombin (5,000 units) is sprayed onto the matrix, which is then applied to the site of bleeding.

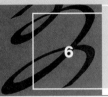

WOUND HEALING AND CARE
Robert G. Neumann, Thomas H. Tung, and John P. Kirby

6

*W*ound healing is the normal body response to injury. The goal of modern wound care is to promote the timely restoration of the body to a previous state of normal form and function. Wound healing is often divided into acute wound healing and chronic wound healing. *Acute wound healing* is the normal orderly process that occurs after a typical injury and requires minimal practitioner intervention. *Chronic wound healing* often necessitates a variety of interventions to correct and shift the healing process toward a more normal state of wound healing. An understanding of the basic processes found in normal wound healing allows for better insight into how alterations lead to abnormal wound healing and how interventions can result in restoration of normal healing.

ACUTE WOUND HEALING

I. **PHYSIOLOGY OF THE ACUTE WOUND.** The disruption of the integrity of tissues, whether surgical or traumatic, stimulates a series of events that attempts to restore the injured tissue to a normal state. The process of wound healing occurs in an orderly fashion and strikes a fine balance between repair and regeneration of tissue. Normal wound healing is affected by the extent of injury, tissue type, and existence of comorbid conditions in the patient. The steps of wound healing can be grouped into early, intermediate, and late stages.

A. **Early wound healing**
1. This stage involves the **establishment of hemostasis** (day of wounding) and the onset of inflammation (days 1 to 4 postwounding). With the onset of injury, blood vessels are disrupted, with subsequent hemorrhage. Severed blood vessels with any smooth muscles in their walls immediately constrict, and within minutes, the coagulation cascade is initiated and produces the end-product fibrin, which plays an important role in the formation of clot and in wound healing. Fibrin forms the initial matrix for early wound healing. In later phases of wound healing, the fibrin-formed matrix facilitates cell attachment and migration. It also serves as a reservoir for cytokines. With the production of fibrin, platelets are activated, and they bind to and aggregate on the fibrin lattice to form the clot that is necessary to achieve hemostasis.
2. The **inflammatory phase** (days 1 to 4 postwounding) is the initial response of the body to injury. It is recognized at the skin level by the cardinal signs of inflammation—*rubor* (redness), *calor* (heat), *tumor* (swelling), and *dolor* (pain), which result from changes in the microcirculation. As hemostasis is established, leukocytes begin to migrate out of the intravascular space through gaps between endothelial cells and bind to the provisional wound matrix. Polymorphonuclear leukocytes (PMNs) are the dominant inflammatory cells in the wound for the first 24 to 48 hours, and they phagocytize bacteria, foreign material, and damaged tissue. They also release cytokines that stimulate fibroblasts and keratinocytes.
   a. The inflammatory phase progresses with the infiltration of circulating **monocytes** into the wound. Monocytes migrate into the extravascular space through capillaries and differentiate into **macrophages** under the influence of cytokines and fibronectin. Macrophages are activated by several cytokines and are essential for normal healing because of their important role in the coordination of the

healing process. They function to phagocytize bacteria and damaged tissue, secrete enzymes for the degradation of tissue and extracellular matrix, and release cytokines for inflammatory cell recruitment and fibroblast proliferation.

    b. The inflammatory phase lasts a well-defined period of time in primarily closed wounds (approximately 4 days), but it continues indefinitely to the endpoint of complete epithelialization in wounds that close by secondary or tertiary intention. Foreign material or bacteria can change a normal healing wound into one with chronic inflammation.

B. Intermediate wound-healing events involve mesenchymal cell migration and proliferation, angiogenesis, and epithelialization.

    1. Two to 4 days after wounding, chemotactic cytokines influence fibroblasts to migrate into the wound from undamaged tissue. Movement of cells occurs on the extracellular matrix, consisting of fibrin, fibronectin, and vitronectin.

    2. While the wound is infiltrated by mesenchymal cells, **angiogenesis** takes place to restore the vasculature that has been disrupted by the wound.

    3. Epithelialization is the third critical aspect of intermediate wound-healing events. It restores the barrier between the wound and the external environment. Epithelialization of wounds occurs via the migration of epithelial cells from the edges of the wound and from remaining epidermal skin appendages. Migration of epithelial cells occurs at the rate of 1 mm/day in clean, open wounds. Primarily closed wounds have a contiguous epithelial layer at 24 to 48 hours.

C. Late wound-healing events involve the deposition of collagen and other matrix proteins and wound contraction. After being present in the wound, the primary function of the fibroblast becomes protein synthesis. Fibroblasts produce several proteins that are components of the extracellular matrix, including collagen, fibronectin, and proteoglycans. Glucocorticoids inhibit protein production by fibroblasts.

    1. Collagen is the main protein secreted by fibroblasts. It provides strength and structure and facilitates cell motility in the wound. Collagen is synthesized at an accelerated rate for 2 to 4 weeks, greatly contributing to the tensile strength of the wound. Oxygen, vitamin C, α-ketoglutarate, and iron are important cofactors for the cross-linkage of collagen fibers. If these are not present, wound healing may be poor.

    2. Wound contraction, another aspect of late wound healing, is a decrease in the size of the wound without an increase in the number of tissue elements that are present. It involves movement of the wound edge toward the center of the wound through the action of myofibroblasts. It is differentiated from contracture, which is the pathologic and movement-limiting result of prolonged wound contraction across a joint primarily from scar formation. Wound contraction begins 4 to 5 days after wounding and continues for 12 to 15 days or longer if the wound remains open.

D. The final wound-healing event is **scar formation and remodeling**. It begins at approximately 21 days after wounding. At the outset of scar remodeling, collagen synthesis is downregulated, and the cellularity of the wound decreases. During scar remodeling, collagen is broken down and replaced by new collagen that is denser and organized along the lines of stress. By 6 months, the wound reaches 80% of the bursting strength of unwounded tissue. It is important to note that a well-healed wound never achieves the strength of unwounded tissue. This process reaches a plateau at 12 to 18 months, but it may last indefinitely.

CHRONIC WOUND HEALING

I. PHYSIOLOGY OF THE CHRONIC WOUND. A chronic wound is a wound that fails to heal in a reasonable amount of time, given the wound's etiology, location, and tissue type. Prolonged or incomplete healing occurs as a consequence of a disruption in the normal process of acute wound healing, which leads to a poor anatomic and functional result. Most chronic wounds are slowed or arrested in the inflammatory or proliferative phases of healing and have marked increased levels of matrix metalloproteinases, which bind up or degrade the various cytokines and growth factors at the wound surface. Most often, there are definable causes of the failure of these wounds to heal, and treatment of these causes, along with maximal medical management of the patient's medical problems, leads to a restoration of more normal healing processes. Therefore, treating a patient with a chronic wound involves investigating the cause(s) of delayed healing and improving the intrinsic (within the wound itself) and extrinsic (systemic) patient factors that lead to poor wound healing.

A. **Intrinsic or local factors** are abnormalities within the wound that prevent normal wound healing. These factors include the presence of a foreign body, necrotic tissue, repetitive trauma, hypoxia/ischemia, venous insufficiency, infection, growth factor deficit, excessive matrix protein degradation, and radiation. Factors that can be controlled by the surgeon include the blood supply to the wound; the temperature of the wound environment; the presence or absence of infection, hematoma, or seroma; the amount of local tissue trauma; and the technique and suture material used to close the wound. It should be noted that the technique and suture material are important only after other local factors have been addressed.

   1. **Ischemia and hypoxia** are common contributing causes of nonhealing wounds. Atherosclerosis or local damage to vessels in the form of trauma or vasculitis causes ischemia and subsequent hypoxia in the wound. Hypoxia leads to impaired collagen synthesis, prevents fibroblast migration, and increases the susceptibility of the wound to infection. Essential to normal wound healing, molecular oxygen is needed for the hydroxylation reaction that cross-links collagen fibers. Molecular oxygen also contributes to the ability of the host's defense to kill pathogens. Sickle cell anemia may lead to vascular occlusion, with subsequent ischemia and tissue ulceration. Local wound edema can also limit small vessel blood flow and exacerbate deficiencies in oxygen and perfusion. Measurement of local wound hypoxia is possible with tissue concentration of oxygen measurements (TCOM) and may be diagnostic for not only local hypoxia needing adjunctive therapy such as hyperbaric oxygen, but also vascular disease amenable to percutaneous angioplasty or surgical bypass as well as systemic cardiopulmonary insufficiencies.

   2. **Infection** in the wound delays healing. Infection is considered to be present when the bacterial count of a quantitative tissue culture is greater than 10^5 organisms/g of tissue. The critical factors in determining the susceptibility to infection are concentration of organisms, virulence, and host resistance. The host's resistance can be impaired by diabetes, malnutrition, malignancy, steroids, or other immunosuppressive therapies. If there are allowed to persist, wound infections lead to increased tissue destruction and alter the effect of cytokines on wound healing. Clinical signs of infection are pyrexia, erythema, swelling, and purulence. Treatment must involve drainage, local débridement, and systemic antibiotics. Judicious use of properly collected tissue cultures may diagnose and direct treatment of wounds that are infected.

   3. The **presence of foreign bodies and necrotic tissue** can contribute to delayed wound healing. This bioburden can harbor infection and prolongs the inflammatory phase of wound healing. The combined presence of infection and a foreign body or devitalized tissue within the wound necessitates the removal of the latter by débridement before eradication of the infection can be achieved. Hematomas, seromas, devascularized bone, and sequestrum are all factors that can increase the susceptibility of a wound to infection.

   4. **Chronic venous insufficiency** leads to persistent venous hypertension and chronic edema in the lower extremities. These factors in turn lead to pericapillary fibrosis, tissue ischemia, and the liberation of superoxide radicals, which are thought to result in delayed wound healing in extremities with chronic venous insufficiency.

   5. **Ionizing radiation** to the wound leads to abnormal wound healing. Early manifestations include erythema, edema, and hyperpigmentation, but the chronic effects of tissue ischemia, atrophy, and fibrosis cause radiation-exposed wounds to enter a chronic course.

6. **Edema.** Acute swelling, especially around joints, can lead to skin breakdown and full-thickness skin loss. Chronic swelling often leads to fibrofatty tissue deposition in underlying skin, which develops verrucous changes and at times irregular crevices and folds. Such skin is prone to breakdown and to development of infection. Infection leads to further lymphatic blockage and obliteration, and the problem gets chronically worse. Patients need to adopt an aggressive program of limb elevation, external compression, and medical management of the edema.

7. The **microenvironment of the chronic wound** has been shown to be different from that of the acute wound in investigational settings. Studies have implicated a decrease in the endogenous levels of certain growth factors in wounds with impaired healing. Other studies have established that an imbalance in the synthesis and degradation of extracellular matrix proteins is central to the establishment and maintenance of chronic wounds. This occurs through inadequate synthesis of extracellular matrix proteins, increased degradative enzymes, decreased regulation of degradative enzymes, or a combination of these causes.

B. **Extrinsic or systemic factors** also contribute to abnormal wound healing. These factors are primarily linked to the underlying general health of the patient.

1. **Malnutrition** alters normal healing through the indirect and the direct effects of vitamin and mineral deficiency. An example is the patient with clinical or subclinical scurvy (vitamin C deficiency); such an individual produces inadequately hydroxylated collagen, and the healed wound becomes significantly weakened as a result.

2. **Diabetes mellitus** is believed to affect healing adversely at every level and in every phase of the healing process. The lack of insulin (and its poorly understood trophic effects on healing tissues), hyperglycemia (by adversely affecting the migratory and phagocytic functions of inflammatory cells and the proliferation of fibroblasts and endothelial cells), neuropathy, and the vascular disease that occurs in diabetic patients all contribute to poor healing.

3. **Steroids and antineoplastic drugs** can markedly diminish the speed and quality of the healing process. The exact effects of steroids are not understood. Vitamin A, by poorly understood mechanisms, seems to cause a partial reversal of the detrimental effects of steroids on healing. Chemotherapeutic agents alter wound healing by decreasing mesenchymal cell proliferation and inducing a leukopenic state that reduces the inflammatory cells available for wound healing. Immunosuppression from AIDS or other diseases may also affect various phases of wound healing.

4. **Smoking** contributes to delayed wound healing by causing cutaneous vasoconstriction, decreasing the oxygen-carrying capacity of hemoglobin, and contributing to atherosclerosis.

5. **Collagen vascular diseases** are often accompanied by a vasculitic component, which needs to be controlled before healing can begin. The medicines that are used to treat collagen vascular diseases may impair cell migration and collagen deposition. Adjustment of dose may lead to improved wound healing.

6. **Cleansing agents** such as chlorhexidine gluconate (Hibiclens) or povidone-iodine (Betadine) **or chemicals** may impair wound healing by affecting cell migration.

7. **Repetitive trauma,** intentional or otherwise, from shearing or pressure forces often leads to a failure in healing. Wound areas over pressure points often require stabilization of the overlying skin envelope with external taping or splinting.

8. Wounds in patients with **renal disease and liver disease** often heal more slowly due to chronic protein deficiencies and reduced capacities for protein synthesis.

9. **Hematopoietic disorders.** Sickle cell disease, with its high incidence of ankle wounds and leukoclastic and granulomatous processes, and mycosis fungoides are associated with poorly healing wounds. Maximal medical treatment for the underlying disorder is needed to effect meaningful healing.

II. **EVALUATION AND MANAGEMENT OF THE CHRONIC WOUND**

A. **History and physical examination.** Evaluation and management of a chronic wound must begin with a thorough history and physical examination.

1. In taking a **history,** one must establish whether the wound is new, recurrent, or chronic, how long it has been present, how it started, how quickly it developed, and whether it is improving or worsening. The patient must be questioned about existing comorbidities, with a focus on potential causes for immunosuppression (HIV, steroids, chemotherapy), undiagnosed diabetes mellitus, peripheral vascular disease, coronary artery disease, rheumatologic disorders, and radiation exposure. Smoking and alcohol use must also be documented.

2. The **physical examination** must evaluate the size, depth, and location of the wound and tissues that are involved. Signs of infection (erythema, purulence, tenderness, warmth, swelling, drainage, or odor) must also be evaluated, and a good vascular examination for extremity wounds must be performed. The patient's self-reported pain as well as the examiner's elicitation of any tenderness should be sought and treated. The wound and its tissue planes should be examined for exudates or excessive separation. The periwound should also be examined for maceration, infection, or other changes requiring treatment. Serum chemistries may aid with the diagnosis of diabetes and renal or hepatic dysfunction. A complete blood cell count may indicate infection with elevated white cell count or white cell abnormalities. Radiography can be performed to determine underlying bony pathology. Doppler evaluation of the extremities should be carried out for suspected arterial insufficiency.

B. **Management** of the chronic wound must focus on the optimization of host and local factors.

1. **Adequate nutrition** is necessary for appropriate wound healing. Sufficient calories, protein, vitamins, minerals, and water are necessary to aid in the healing. Patients who have severe malnutrition or whose gastrointestinal tract cannot be used should be placed on parenteral nutritional support.

2. **Underlying factors** that affect wound healing, such as chemotherapy, steroids, alcohol consumption, cigarette smoking, and blood glucose levels, must be modified as necessary to aid in the wound-healing process.

3. **Effective local wound care** is essential for the resolution of a chronic wound. Eradication of infection, aggressive débridement, and drainage of abscesses from the wound are important steps in local control.

4. **Antibiotics.** Systemic antibiotics should be administered to treat active infection such as cellulitis. Topical antibiotics applied to the wound are effective in lowering the bacterial count.

5. **Proper dressings** are an essential aspect of local care by helping to provide the appropriate environment for healing. Frequent wet-to-dry dressings are used when infection and drainage predominate. With the development of healthy granulation tissue, dressings should provide adequate protection and moisture to facilitate healing. Wounds with exudate should have this controlled by the dressing to protect the periwound from maceration.

6. **Edema control** is often necessary for wounds of the lower extremity due to venous insufficiency. Elevation and wrapping in an elastic bandage reduce edema and venous hypertension. Unna boot, Jobst compression garments, and pneumatic compression devices can also be used.

7. **Surgical therapy** may be necessary to aid in the healing of a chronic wound. This may occur through surgical débridement of infected or necrotic wounds and skin grafting on a healthy bed of granulation tissue. Revascularization procedures may be necessary to provide adequate blood flow to distal circulation that supplies a nonhealing/or chronic wound.

III. **SPECIAL CATEGORIES OF CHRONIC WOUNDS.** Chronic wounds are a heterogeneous group. Chronic wounds associated with diabetes, pressure necrosis, and radiation therapy are frequently encountered, cause great disability within the population, and place a great burden on the health care system.

A. **Diabetic foot ulcers**

1. **Differential diagnosis.** The three most common causes of lower-extremity ulcers are arterial insufficiency, venous stasis, and diabetes mellitus. Venous stasis ulcers most often occur on the medial aspect of the patient's lower leg or ankle (gaiter

distribution) and are associated with the chronic edema and hyperpigmentation seen with venous insufficiency. Arterial insufficiency ulcers tend to occur distally on the tips of the patient's toes, but they can also occur at or near the lateral malleolus. The surrounding skin exhibits the thin, shiny, hairless characteristics that have been well described in these patients, and these individuals typically relate symptoms of claudication or rest pain. Peripheral pulses are diminished or absent. Diabetic ulcers are believed to be secondary to the severe neuropathy seen in these patients and, to a lesser extent, vasculopathy. They are typically associated with very thick callus and most often occur on the patient's heels or on the plantar surface of the metatarsal heads.

2. **Causes**
   a. **Neuropathy**
      (1) **Peripheral neuropathy** is believed to be the most significant contributor to the development of lower-extremity ulcers in diabetic patients through impaired detection of injury from poorly fitting shoes or trauma. Diabetic motor neuropathy is also associated with abnormal weightbearing. The motor neuropathy results in abnormalities such as hammer toes or hallux valgus, which shifts weightbearing more proximally than normal on the metatarsal heads. Additionally, the dorsum of the toes at the posterior interphalangeal joints is often traumatized by ill-fitting shoes in patients with hammer toes.
      (2) **Autonomic neuropathy** leads to failure of sweating and inadequate lubrication of the skin. Dry skin leads to mechanical breakdown that initiates ulcer formation. Autonomic neuropathy also contributes to failure of autoregulation in the microcirculation; therefore, arterial blood will shunt past capillaries into the venous blood flow. This reduces the nutritive blood flow to the skin and predisposes to ulcer formation.
   b. **Ischemia.** The microvascular disease seen in diabetic patients also contributes to the development and progression of lower-extremity ulcers. These patients should be evaluated for proximal atherosclerotic disease, which may be amenable to intervention, thus improving the chances of healing of the ulcer or healing of an amputation.
3. **Evaluation and treatment**
   a. **Examination.** The quality of the peripheral circulation, the extent of the wound, and the degree of sensory loss should be assessed. Web spaces should be examined for evidence of mycotic infection, which may lead to fissuring of the skin and subsequent infection. Mal perforans ulcers occur on the plantar surface of the metatarsals and extend to the metatarsal head, leaving exposed cartilage. Osteomyelitis of the phalanx or metatarsal is common.
   b. **Treatment. Clean wounds** are treated with conservative débridement and dressing changes, with careful trimming of the calluses and nails. Close follow-up is essential. **Infected wounds** are diagnosed clinically; wound cultures are unreliable unless derived from actual tissue samples. Plain x-rays may show osteomyelitis or gas in the soft tissues. The progression of infectious processes in diabetic patients can occur with extreme rapidity, and thus these patients require hospitalization, aggressive wound care, and broad-spectrum antibiotics at initial presentation. Abscess cavities must be completely drained and all dead tissue débrided; daily whirlpool treatments help cleanse the wound mechanically. Absolute nonweightbearing is crucial.
   c. **Prevention** remains one of the most important elements in the management of the diabetic foot. Meticulous attention to hygiene and daily inspection for signs of tissue trauma prevent the progression of injury. Podiatric appliances or custom-made shoes are helpful in relieving pressure on weightbearing areas and should be prescribed for any patient who has had neuropathic ulceration.
B. **Leg ulcers**
   1. When **arterial ulcers** are suspected, a vascular evaluation should be instituted. Due to the tissue ischemia, antibiotics are indicated if there are signs of cellulitis.
   2. **Venous stasis ulcers** are among the most common types of leg ulcers and typically occur on the medial leg in the supramedial malleolar location. A patient

with a venous stasis ulcer typically has a history of ulceration and associated leg swelling or of deep venous thrombosis. The ulcer may appear as a relatively superficial and extremely painful wound with irregular borders and an inflamed wound bed that bleeds fairly easily or as a partial-thickness wound with a dense, whitish-yellow fibrotic base. There may be multiple wounds, and they may be surrounded with a varying degree of inflammatory dermatitis. Cleansing the wound, providing a dressing that absorbs the wound drainage, leg compression, and leg elevation are the mainstays of treatment. After excluding significant ischemia, which can be present in up to 15% of patients, one can often use a multilayered compression dressing (Unna boot). This is changed on a weekly or biweekly basis until the wound heals. Aggressive medical treatment is often required to control the peripheral edema, which can be quite marked. More advanced methods of wound management such as skin grafting or the use of skin substitutes can be used, but only after the leg edema is controlled. External leg compression pumps and massage therapy are also useful in some patients. Wounds that are present for some time and exhibit increased drainage or pain are often infected. Treatment of infected wounds requires systemic antibiotic therapy.

C. **Skin tears** are often seen in the elderly with skin that is markedly thinned and in the chronic steroid-using patient. The hypermobile skin, with its poor subcutaneous connections, is prone to rip under shearing forces, and patients often present with a flap of skin that is torn away from its wound bed. One should follow the principles outlined previously, with this exception: The skin flap should be trimmed of obvious necrotic portions, and the remaining flap should be secured in place over the wound bed only to the extent that it can be without tension. It is rare that such a wound should be sutured closed because the flap will most likely necrose under the tension of the swelling that occurs over the following 2 to 4 days. Topical management of the area that is intentionally left open is often easily achieved with a hydrogel dressing (see Section III.D).

D. **Pressure ulcers**
   1. **Pathophysiology.** Prolonged pressure applied to soft tissue over bony prominences, usually caused by paralysis or the immobility associated with severe illness, predictably leads to ischemic ulceration and tissue breakdown. Muscle tissue seems to be the most susceptible. The prevalence of pressure ulcers is 10% of all hospitalized patients, 28% of nursing home patients, and 39% of spinal cord injury patients (*JAMA* 2006;296:974). Pressure ulcers increase mortality rates more than twofold, and are the cause of death in 8% of paraplegics (*Am J Surg* 2004;188:9S). The particular area of breakdown depends on the patient's position of immobility, with ulcers most frequently developing in recumbent patients over the occiput, sacrum, greater trochanter, and heels. In immobile patients who sit for prolonged periods on improper surfaces without pressure relief, ulcers often develop under the ischial tuberosities. Pressure ulcers are described by stages (Table 6-1). Such wounds do not necessarily proceed through each one of these

TABLE 6-1	National Pressure Ulcer Advisory Panel Classification Scheme

Stage	Description
I	Nonblanchable erythema of intact skin; wounds generally reversible at this stage with intervention
II	Partial-thickness skin loss involving epidermis or dermis; may present as an abrasion, blister, or shallow crater
III	Full-thickness skin loss involving damage or necrosis of subcutaneous tissue but not extending through underlying structures or fascia
IV	Full-thickness skin loss with damage to underlying support structures (i.e., fascia, tendon, or joint capsule)

stages during formation but can present at the advanced stages. Likewise, as these wounds heal, they do not go backward through the stages despite their present depth (e.g., a nearly healed stage IV ulcer does not become a stage II ulcer but rather a healing stage IV ulcer, signifying that the tissues of the healing wound are abnormal). When a full-thickness injury to the skin has occurred, one cannot adequately stage the wound until the eschar is incised and the actual depth is determined. The examiner must also look for underlying bony breakdown, osteomyelitis, or an overall physiologic decline as the root cause of a "pressure" ulcer whose actual etiology may be multifactorial in nature, and any successful healing regimen must be equally multifactorial. The clinician must also consider whether such regimens are realistic and discuss assessments and care plans openly with the patient and family regarding realistic expectations and treatment goals.

2. Prophylaxis

   a. Skin care. The patient's skin should be inspected and cleansed at least daily with application of moisturizers and barrier creams as necessary. Patients need to have a complete skin assessment and risk assessment done at the time of admission. All patients should be placed on the optimal support surface. Pressure-reducing support can be classified as static or dynamic. Static systems include mattresses filled with air, water, gel, or foam; dynamic support systems include low–air-loss mattresses and air-fluidized beds. Maintain urinary and fecal continence to prevent maceration and skin breakdown.

   b. Nutrition. Nutritional deficits should be assessed and treated appropriately. Supplementation with vitamin C or vitamin A, or both, may be necessary if the patient is malnourished or is taking steroids.

   c. Mobility. Bedridden patients should be turned and repositioned with a minimum frequency of every 2 hours. Heel protectors, pillows, and foam wedges diffuse pressure from bony prominences across greater areas.

3. Treatment. Most pressure ulcers heal spontaneously when pressure is relieved. This remains the most important factor in their healing. The healing process may require up to 6 months. Unless the patient was only temporarily immobilized, recurrences are common. Surgical management may include simple closure, split-thickness skin grafting, or musculocutaneous flap, but these measures should be reserved for well-motivated patients in whom a real reduction of risk factors for recurrence is possible. Urinary and fecal diversion reduce soiling and maceration of perineal and sacral wounds, which facilitates healing of these wounds.

E. Ionizing radiation

   1. Although ionizing radiation is a useful mode of cancer therapy, it produces detrimental local effects on tissue in the field of radiation and impairs normal wound healing. Radiation injures target and surrounding cells by direct damage to DNA or indirectly through free radicals or reactive species. Radiation has a negative impact on wound healing by harming the cellular elements that play a prominent role in various phases of wound healing. For instance, radiation alters wound healing by decreasing the proliferative capacity of cells, particularly those of endothelial, mesenchymal, and epithelial origin. Radiation also harms wound healing by decreasing the vascularity of the wound, leading to the development of ischemia and hypoxia. Decreased vascularity occurs through the occlusion and thrombosis of small blood vessels and capillaries, and the mechanisms for angiogenesis are limited due to poor endothelial cell proliferation.

   2. The **early epithelial changes** that are characteristic of acute radiation injury include ulceration, edema, and sustained inflammation. Late changes include parenchymal degeneration, epithelial and dermal atrophy, decreased vascularity, fibrosis, and tissue necrosis. Like the healing wound, the skin has characteristic changes that are associated with radiation exposure. The skin is affected in a dose-dependent manner. Acute changes associated with the skin include erythema from dilation of blood vessels in the dermis, dry desquamation at moderate doses, or moist desquamation in conjunction with the eradication of the cells of the epidermis. Late manifestations include hyper- or hypopigmentation, fibrosis of the skin and subcutaneous tissues, telangiectasia, sebaceous and sweat gland dysfunction, alopecia, and necrosis.

3. The **timing of radiation therapy** as it relates to operative therapy has been an important aspect of oncologic care. The primary factors that determine the effects of preoperative radiation therapy on wound healing are the timing and the dose. These vary from tissue to tissue. Postoperative radiation therapy has no effect on healing if it is administered 1 week after wounding. The intentional (surgical) wounding of a previously irradiated wound needs careful planning and consideration. Many of the cells in such an area have been permanently damaged; therefore, their proliferative capacity is decreased. In addition, the wound has decreased vascularity, which creates a relative state of hypoxemia. Furthermore, the dermis of such a wound is more susceptible to bacterial invasion. The combined factors place a previously irradiated area at extreme risk for abnormal wound healing if it is subjected to surgical intervention.

4. It has long been realized for the foregoing reasons that **radiation-damaged skin and wounds heal poorly.** Local measures that must be undertaken with wounds affected by radiation follow the same principles of good wound care. These measures include infection control through aggressive débridement and systemic antibiotics, topical antibiotics to promote epithelialization, moist dressings, and lubrication of dry skin. Optimal nutritional status must also be emphasized. Other methods, such as hyperbaric oxygen, have been used to increase the oxygen tension of irradiated wounds. Experimental therapies are currently under investigation. The use of the growth factors transforming growth factor β (TGF-β) and platelet-derived growth factor (PDGF) has shown promise for treatment in radiation wound models in animals.

 PROPHYLACTIC SURGICAL WOUND CARE

I. PREOPERATIVE PREPARATION. Even though antibiotic prophylaxis and sterile surgical technique have gained widespread acceptance, surgical site infections (SSIs) persist, contributing to 3.7 million excess hospital days and more than $1.6 billion in patient and hospital costs (*Infect Control Hosp Epidemiol* 1993;14:73). Clean surgical operations typically result in SSIs from Gram-positive aerobes representing pathogens in common skin flora (*Curr Infect Dis Rep* 2004;6:426). Clean-contaminated, contaminated, or dirty operations usually result in polymicrobial infections with enteric Gram-negative and anaerobic bacteria along with skin flora pathogens. Over the last 10 years, there has been a rise in antibiotic resistance among both Gram-positive and Gram-negative organisms. The rate of *Staphylococcus aureus* resistance to methacillin, oxacillin, or nafcillin (MRSA) now approaches 60%, and the rate of *Klebsiella pneumoniae* resistance to cephalosporins is 50% (*Expert Rev Anti Infect Ther* 2006;4:223).

A. Patient factors. Whereas some characteristics, such as age, cannot be altered, other patient factors can be optimized.

1. Cigarette smoking is a known risk factor for SSI (*Plast Reconstr Surg* 2001; 107:342). A recent prospective, randomized trial demonstrated an 83% reduction in wound infections in the smoking cessation group compared to controls (*Lancet* 2002;359:114). The Centers for Disease Control and Prevention (CDC) recommends smoking cessation at least 30 days prior to elective surgery (*Am J Infect Control* 1999;27:97).

2. The impact of **nutrition** on wound healing depends on the wound type. Wounds closed by primary intention often heal even in emaciated patients as long as there are no wound infections (*Annu Rev Nutr* 2003;23:263). In contrast, wounds that heal by secondary intention are heavily dependent on the patient's nutritional status. Malnourished patients have increased rates of infection and delayed wound healing, and there is ample evidence that tailored preoperative nutritional repletion reduces these complications (*Plast Reconstr Surg* 2006;117:42S).

B. Operative factors

1. Chlorhexidine showers the night before surgery reduce bacterial counts when compared to placebo (*Am J Infect Control* 1993;21:205), but no studies have demonstrated reduced operative infection rates. Previous recommendations regarding showers as well as updates on other interventions as detailed in the following can be found on the CDC Web site.

2. **Shaving** is associated with an increased risk of surgical site infections. In a prospective randomized trial of more than 1,000 patients, **clipping** performed immediately before surgery was associated with significantly fewer infections than clipping the night before or shaving at either time (*Arch Surg* 1983;118:347).

3. **Prophylactic antibiotics** are indicated for some clean cases and most clean-contaminated cases. Antibiotics should be administered prior to the incision, with many regulatory groups recommending administration within 60 minutes (*Expert Rev Anti Infect Ther* 2006;4:223). Most guidelines recommend postoperative discontinuation of prophylactic antibiotics within 24 hours (*Surg Clin North Am* 2005;85:1115). Recently, large prospective, randomized trials have demonstrated no evidence to support the use of antibiotic prophylaxis in hernia surgery (*Ann Surg* 2004;240:955, *J Am Coll Surg* 2005;200:393).

II. PERIOPERATIVE

A. **Surgeon hand antisepsis** has traditionally been performed with a 5- to 10-minute scrub. Several studies have shown that a 2-minute scrub is as effective at reducing skin flora as a 10-minute scrub (*Br J Surg* 1991;78:685). Current guidelines include use of either (1) a traditional scrub with antimicrobial soap for 2 to 6 minutes or (2) a prewash of the hands and forearms with nonantimicrobial soap combined with use of an alcohol-based surgical hand scrub (*MMWR Recomm Rep* 2002;51(RR-16):1).

B. **Surgical site antisepsis** starts with cleansing and removing visible debris, followed by a prep of the intended incision site to the periphery in concentric circles using a sterile instrument (*Am J Infect Control* 1999;27:97). No conclusive differences have been found to recommend among 7.5% povidine-betadine foaming solution, 10% povidine-betadine paint, alcohol solutions, chlorhexidine/alcohol preparations, and alcohol-containing iodophor solutions. However, chlorhexidine is superior to iodophors for central venous catheter insertion (*Lancet* 1991;338:339).

C. **Active warming** to prevent intraoperative hypothermia has been demonstrated to reduce surgical infections in two separate prospective, randomized trials (*N Engl J Med* 1996;334:1209). Interestingly, one of the studies showed that local active warming to the incision site was equivalent to systemic warming in preventing infections, and that either was superior to nonwarming (*Curr Infect Dis Rep* 2004;6:428).

D. **Tight glycemic control** is recommended in the perioperative period, although the mechanisms explaining the detrimental effect of hyperglycemia remain largely unknown. In 2001, Van den Berghe reported a randomized, prospective study of 1,548 surgical patients in which stringent glycemic control between 80 to 110 mg/dL resulted in 34% decreased mortality versus maintenance of 180 to 200 mg/dL (*N Engl J Med* 2001;345:1359). In addition, continuous intravenous insulin infusion has been shown significantly to reduce the incidence of sternal wound infections when compared to sliding-scale insulin (*Ann Thoracic Surg* 1999;67:352). The American Diabetes Association and the American Association of Clinical Endocrinologists recommend glycemic targets between 80 to 110 mg/dL for critically ill patients in the intensive care unit. For patients with noncritical illness, a preprandial glucose of less than 110 mg/dL and a random glucose level of less than 180 mg/dL were recommended in the perioperative period (*Endocr Pract* 2004;10 (Suppl 2):4).

E. **Other controllable factors** include the length of operation, gentle tissue handling, and supplemental oxygen to diminish surgical site infections.

WOUND CLOSURE AND CARE

I. TIMING OF WOUND HEALING

A. **Primary intention** occurs when the wound is closed by direct approximation of the wound margins or by placement of a graft or flap. Direct approximation of the edges of a wound provides the optimal treatment on the condition that the wound is clean, the closure can be done without undue tension, and the closure can occur in a timely fashion. Wounds that are less than 6 hours old are considered in the "golden period" and are less likely to develop into chronic wounds. At times, rearrangement of tissues is required to achieve tension-free closure. Directly approximated wounds typically heal as outlined earlier, provided that there is adequate perfusion of the tissues and no infection. Primary intention also describes the healing of wounds created in the operating room that are closed at the end of the operative period. Epithelialization of surgical incisions occurs within 24 hours of closure. CDC guidelines dictate that a sterile dressing should be left in place during this susceptible period to prevent bacterial contamination (*Am J Infect Control* 1999;27:97).

  B. Secondary intention, or spontaneous healing, occurs when a wound is left open and is allowed to close by epithelialization and contraction. Contraction is a myofibroblast-mediated process that aids in wound closure by decreasing the circumference of the wound (myofibroblasts are modified fibroblasts that have smooth muscle cell–like contractile properties). This method is commonly used in the management of wounds that are treated beyond the initial 6-hour "golden period" or of contaminated infected wounds with a bacterial count of greater than 10^5 per/gram of tissue. These wounds are characterized by prolonged inflammatory and proliferative phases of healing that continue until the wound has either completely epithelialized or been closed by other means.

  C. Tertiary intention, or delayed primary closure, is a useful option for managing wounds that are too heavily contaminated for primary closure but appear clean and well vascularized after 4 to 5 days of open observation so that the cutaneous edges can be approximated at that time. During this period, the normally low arterial partial pressure of oxygen (PaO_2) at the wound surface rises and the inflammatory process in the wound bed leads to a minimized bacterial concentration, thus allowing a safer closure than could be achieved with primary closure and a more rapid closure than could be achieved with secondary wound healing.

II. WOUND CLOSURE MATERIALS AND TECHNIQUES

  A. Skin adhesives. Topical adhesives (e.g., Dermabond, Indermil) can be used to maintain skin edge alignment in wounds that are clean, can be closed without tension, and are in areas not subject to motion or pressure. When applied to an incision that has been closed by subcuticular sutures, it can provide a waterproof and antimicrobial barrier that prevents ingress of bacteria (*Infect Control Hosp Epidemiol* 2004;25:664). Infection rates with Dermabond are similar to those with traditional closure methods (*Neurosurgery* 2005;56(1 Suppl):147), with the advantages that there are no staples or sutures to remove and that patients may shower immediately.

  B. Steri-Strips. Skin tapes are the least invasive way to close a superficial skin wound; however, because they provide no eversion of wound edges, the cosmetic result may be suboptimal. In addition, skin tapes tend to loosen if moistened by serum or blood and therefore are seldom appropriate for all but the most superficial skin wounds in areas of minimal or no tension. Their most frequent use is in support of a skin closure after suture or staple removal.

  C. Suture

    1. Needles. Curved needles are designed for use with needle holders, whereas straight (Keith) needles can be used with or without a holder. Two types are in common use: circular (tapered, noncutting) and triangular (cutting). Cutting needles are preferable for closure of tough tissue, such as skin, and noncutting needles are preferable for placing sutures in delicate tissues, such as blood vessels or intestine.

    2. Suture material. Several characteristics differentiate the various suture materials. They include the following:

      a. Absorbable versus nonabsorbable. Among the absorbable materials, wide variability is found with regard to tensile strength, rate of absorption, and tissue reaction.

      b. Monofilament versus braided. Braided suture has better handling characteristics than monofilament suture, but the interstices between the braided strands that compose the suture are easily colonized by bacteria and thus pose an infection risk.

    c. Natural versus synthetic. Characteristics of commonly used suture materials are summarized in Tables 6-2 and 6-3.

  3. Staples allow for quick closure. In areas of lower cosmetic sensitivity, such as the thick skin of the back or anterior abdominal wall, staples may produce cosmetic results approximating those of sutures. They are particularly useful for closure of scalp wounds.

D. Skin suture technique

  1. Basic surgical principles apply: closure without tension, elimination of dead space, aseptic technique, and (when closing skin) eversion of the skin margins. A dog-ear occurs when unequal bites are taken on opposing sides of a wound or incision, causing the tissue to bunch up as the end of the wound is approached. This can be prevented by carefully aligning the wound at the time of deep tissue closure (elimination of dead space) with interrupted absorbable sutures and by taking equal bites of tissue on both sides of the wound.

  2. Suture removal. Suture scars occur when stitches are left in place too long, allowing epithelialization of the suture tracts. This complication can be minimized by timely suture removal. Facial sutures should be removed at days 3 to 5; elsewhere, days 7 to 10 are appropriate. These guidelines should be modified for the individual patient. Application of skin tapes after suture removal provides further support.

III. OPEN WOUND CARE OPTIONS (SEE TABLE 6-4). This brief review is not meant to be comprehensive or an endorsement of any product or product category. It remains an area of intense research, clinical, and commercial interest in which availability and indications of both established and new products can be expected to change during the publication cycle of this manual. The clinician would do well to weigh each patient's response to treatment, the indications and risks of any particular product, and need for further treatment.

A. Topical ointments. Petroleum-based ointments that contain one or several antibiotics prevent adherence of dressings to the wound and, by maintaining moisture of the wound environment, accelerate epithelialization and healing of primarily approximated wounds.

B. Impregnated gauze. Gauze that is impregnated with petrolatum is used for the treatment of superficial, partial-thickness wounds to maintain moisture, prevent excessive loss of fluid, and, in the case of Xeroform, provide mild deodorizing. It can also be used as the first layer of the initial dressing on a primarily closed wound. The use of this type of gauze is contraindicated when infection of the wound is suspected and inhibition of wound drainage would lead to adverse consequences.

C. Gauze packing. The practice of packing an open wound with gauze prevents dead space, facilitates drainage, and provides varying degrees of débridement. The maximum amount of débridement is seen when the gauze is packed into the wound dry and removed after absorption and evaporation have taken place, leaving a dry wound with adherent gauze, which on removal extracts superficial layers of the wound bed (dry-to-dry dressing). This dressing is seldom indicated. Wounds that are in need of great amounts of débridement usually benefit most from sharp débridement in the operating room or at the bedside; dry-to-dry dressings are painful and violate the principle of maintaining a moist environment for the wounds. Moist-to-dry dressings provide a much gentler débridement, are less painful, and can include sterile normal saline or various additives. Dakin solution [in full (0.5% sodium hypochlorite), half, or quarter strength] can be used to pack infected open wounds for a brief period when antimicrobial action is desirable. Due to toxic effects upon keratinocytes, the use of Dakin solution is not indicated except in infected wounds for a short period (*Adv Skin Wound Care* 2005;18:373). Improvement of the foul odor that often emanates from drained abscesses and other infected open wounds is an added benefit of using this additive.

D. Hydrogels. These water- or glycerin-based gels (e.g., IntraSite) can be used in shallow or deep, open wounds. The gel promotes healing by gently rehydrating necrotic tissue, facilitating its débridement, and absorbing exudate produced by the wounds, as well as maintaining a moist wound environment. A nonadherent, nonabsorbent

TABLE 6-2 Characteristics of Absorbable Suture Materials

Suture (trade name)	Manufacturing process	Effective strength (d)	Complete absorption (d)	Absorption profile		Application
				Tissue reactivity	Handling	
Surgical gut	Collagen from sheep intestine submucosa	4–10	70	High	Poor	Used for quick-healing mucosa
Chromic gut	Catgut treated with chromic acid	10–14	90	Moderate	Poor	Used for quick-healing mucosa
Polyglycolic acid (Dexon)	Synthetic monofilament or braided	14–21	60–120	Minimal	Good	Subcutaneous sutures, mucosa, ligation of vessels
Polyglactic acid (Vicryl)	Synthetic braided, lubricated with polyglactin 370; undyed or purple	20–30	60–90	Minimal	Excellent	Subcuticular and subcutaneous sutures
Polydioxane (PDS)	Monofilament polyester	40–60	180	Minimal	Good	Used for extended support
Polyglyconate (Maxon)	Synthetic monofilament	40–60	180–210	Minimal	Excellent	More supple than polydioxane

TABLE 6-3 Characteristics of Nonabsorbable Suture Materials

Suture (trade name)	Manufacturing process	Tissue reactivity	Handling	Application
Silk	Braided; derived from cocoon of silkworm larva	High	Excellent	Vessel ligation; high capillarity; should be avoided in areas prone to infection
Cotton	Braided	High	Excellent	Same as silk
Polyester	Braided terephthalate (Dacron), polyethylene (Mersilene), coated with Teflon (Tevdek), silicone (Ti-Cron), polybutilate (Ethibond)	Minimal	Good if uncoated; excellent if coated	Commonly used for fascia; uncoated sutures have excellent knot security; coated sutures require five throws for knot security
Nylon	Synthetic polyamide monofilament or braided (Nurolon, Surgilon)	Minimal	Good	Used for skin, fascia; requires five throws for knot security
Polypropylene (Prolene, Surgilene)	Plastic monofilament	Minimal	Good	High elasticity; commonly used for skin closure and vascular anastomoses; requires five throws
Polybutester (Novofil)	Plastic monofilament copolymer	Minimal	Good	Very high elasticity; used when tissue swelling is present
Steel	Alloy monofilament	None	Poor	Retention sutures, bone

TABLE 6-4   Wound and Skin Care Products

Product/trade name	Advantages	Limitations	Applications
Gauze Kerlix (roll gauze)	Débride mechanically Manages exudates by capillarity	May disrupt viable tissue during change May cause bleeding on removal	Moderately/heavily exudating wounds Partial- and full-thickness chronic wounds (stages II, III, IV)
Gauze sponges	Permeable to gases Fills deadspace Conformable Adaptable	May cause pain on removal Particulate matter may be left in wound Permeable to fluids and bacteria Limited thermal insulation May dehydrate wound bed (if allowed to dry) Wet to dry dressings contraindicated—Wound Ostomy Continence Nurses (WOCN) Society Standards of Care, 1992	Acute wounds Secondary dressing
Transparent adhesive dressings Tegaderm (3M)	Manages exudates by moisture vapor	Manage light exudates only	IV entry sites
Opsite (Smith & Nephew)	Impermeable to fluids and bacteria Permeable to gases Visualization of wound Conformable	May disrupt fragile skin Application may be difficult	Minor burns or lacerations Reduces surface friction in high-risk areas (stage I) Lightly exudating partial-thickness chronic wounds (stage II) Over eschar to promote autolytic débridement

Dressing		
Hydrocolloids	Low profile	Cover dressing
Restore Hydrocolloid (Hollister)	Forms moist gel in wound bed	Reduces surface friction in high-risk areas
DuoDerm (ConvaTec)	Impermeable to fluids and bacteria	Manages moderate exudates
Comfeel Ulcer Care Dressing (Coloplast)	Manages exudates by particle swelling	Impermeable to gases
Tegasorb (3M)		May traumatize fragile skin
		Partial- and full-thickness wounds
		Moderately exudating wounds
	Thermal insulation good	Do not use over eschar or puncture wounds
		Use with extreme caution on diabetic ulcers
	Conformable	Venous stasis ulcers in conjunction with Unna boot
		Contraindicated in third-degree burns
Wound fillers	Wound filler	Absorbs moderate to minimal exudate
AcryDerm strands		Not recommended in dry wounds or wounds with sinus tracts or tunnels
Absorbent Wound Dressing (AcryMed)	Absorbs exudate	May be used in combination with other wound dressing to increase absorption or fill shallow areas
Hydrogels	Forms moist wound bed	
Amorphous	Forms moist wound bed	May dehydrate
		Partial- and full-thickness chronic wound (stages II, III)
Restore Hydrogel (Hollister)	Conformable	Minimal absorption
IntraSite Gel (Smith & Nephew)	Manages exudates by swelling	Requires secondary dressing
		Partial- and full-thickness burns
		Diabetic ulcers
		Lightly exudating wounds

(continued)

TABLE 6-4 Wound and Skin Care Products (Continued)

Product/trade name	Advantages	Limitations	Applications
Enzymatic débriding agents			
Collagenase (Santyl, Smith & Nephew)	Liquefies necrotic tissue	Conditions with pH higher or lower than 6–8 decreases enzyme activity	Débridement of chronic dermal ulcers and severely burned areas
	Contributes toward formation of granulation tissue and epithelialization of wounds		
Accuzyme (Healthpoint)	Does not attack healthy tissue or newly formed granulation tissue		
Absorbent dressings			
Bard Absorption Dressing (Bard Medical)	Manages exudates by osmotic action	Permeable to fluids and bacteria	Heavily exudating wounds
	Cleans debris	May increase pH beyond physiologic levels	Full-thickness chronic wounds (stages III, IV)
	Reduces odor	May sting on application	Malodorous wounds
	Maintains moist wound bed	Requires secondary dressing	
	Permeable to gases		
	Molds to wound contour		
	Fills deadspace		
	Extends life of secondary dressing		
	Daily dressing change		
	Inexpensive		
Alginate			
Restore CalciCare (Hollister)	Forms moist gel in wound bed	Permeable to fluids and bacteria	Moderately/heavily exudating wounds
Sorbsan (Dow Hickman Pharmaceuticals)	Manages exudates by capillarity	May produce burning sensation on application	Partial- and full-thickness wounds (stages III, IV)
	Permeable to gases		

Kaltostat (Convatec)	Molds to wound contour	Requires irrigation before removal if allowed to dry out
	Fills deadspace	
	Irrigates easily from wound bed	
	Reduces wound pain	
	Fibers left in wound are absorbed	
	May be used on clinically infected wounds	
	Nonirritating	
		Partial-thickness burns
		Skin donor sites
Solutions		
0.9% Normal saline	Noncytotoxic solution for wound care	Wound dehydrates if allowed to dry out
		If dressing saturated, may macerate periwound skin
		Partial- and full-thickness wounds
		Dressing changes two to three times daily
Hydrogen peroxide	Chemical débridement of necrotic tissue when used as an irrigating solution	Cytotoxic to fibroblasts
		Has been documented to result in air embolus if instilled into wound cavities under pressure
		Wound irrigation—use only half-strength and always rinse wound with normal saline
Povidine-iodine (Betadine)	FDA has not approved for use in wounds	Cytotoxic to fibroblasts until diluted to 1:1,000
		May cause acidosis in burn patients
		Lasting systemic effects include cardiovascular toxicity, renal toxicity, hepatotoxicity, and neuropathy
		Impairs wound's ability to fight infection and increases potential for wound infection
		None for wound care

(continued)

TABLE 6-4 Wound and Skin Care Products *(Continued)*

Product/trade name	Advantages	Limitations	Applications
Antibacterial cream Silver sulfadiazine (Silvadene)	Broad-spectrum antibacterial (S. aureus, E. coli, P. aeruginosa, P. mirabilis, β-hemolytic streptococci)	Never approved by FDA for wound management Should not be used in presence of hepatic or renal impairment	Apply 1/8 in. to clean, débrided wound daily or twice daily
Platelet-derived growth factor Becaplermin (Regranex, Ortho-McNeil Pharmaceuticals)	May promote wound healing in otherwise recalcitrant neuropathic ulcer Very few side effects	Dressing protocol may be confusing Wound must have adequate blood supply Wound must be free of infection No osteomyelitis Wound must be free of necrotic tissue Complex dosing	Calculate dose by multiplying length by width of wound in cm and divide by 4 Wound is irrigated with NS Apply precise amount of drug to wound, cover with NS dressing Leave in place for 12 hr Then irrigate wound with NS Pack wound with NS dressing Leave in place for 12 hr

FDA, Food and Drug Administration; *E. coli, Escherichia coli*; NS, normal saline; *P. aeruginosa, Pseudomonas aeruginosa; P. mirabilis, Proteus mirabilis; S. aureus, Staphylococcus aureus*; IV, intravenous.
Adapted with permission from Rolstad BS, Ovington LG, Harris A. Wound care product formulary. In: Bryand RA, ed. *Acute and Chronic Wounds: Nursing Management*, 2nd ed. St. Louis: Mosby; 2000.

secondary dressing is applied over the gel; dressings should be changed every 8 hours to 3 days, depending on the condition of the wound.

E. Hydrocolloids. These occlusive, adhesive wafers provide a moist and protective environment for shallow wounds with light exudate. They can remain in place for 3 to 5 days and can be used under compression dressings to treat venous stasis ulcers.

F. Alginates. Complex carbohydrate dressings composed of glucuronic and mannuronic acid, derived from brown seaweed, are formed into ropes or pads that are highly absorbent (e.g., Kaltostat). Alginates are absorbable and are useful for the treatment of deep wounds with heavy exudate because they form a gel as they absorb wound drainage.

G. Adhesive films. These plastic membranes (e.g., Tegaderm) are self-adhering and waterproof, yet are permeable to oxygen and water vapor. They are appropriate for partial-thickness wounds, such as split-thickness skin graft donor sites or superficial abrasions. They can also be used as secondary dressings on wounds that are being treated with hydrocolloids or alginates.

H. Collagen-containing products. A number of collagen-containing products are available in powder, sheet, or fluid form. They are available as pure collagen, typically types 1 and 3, or combined with other materials such as calcium alginate (Fibracol). Some wounds respond better to collagen than to other dressing materials.

 I. Hydrofibers represent a newer dressing category of strands; they are some of the most absorptive materials available for packing in a heavily draining wound.

J. Growth factors. Human recombinant PDGF is the only U.S. Food and Drug Administration–approved clinically available growth factor. Topically applied to a granulating wound, it promotes granulation tissue formation, angiogenesis, and epithelialization. A saline-moistened gauze dressing is applied daily at midday to help keep the wound bed moist. Although initial approval was for the treatment of diabetic plantar foot ulcers, the drug is often used on other wound types. Epidermal growth factor (EGF) is in clinical trials for the treatment of venous stasis ulcers.

K. Skin substitutes. Numerous cultured, xenograft, or cadaveric-derived allograft skin substitutes are available, depending on desired indication and cost restrictions. Cultured dermis and epidermis are available clinically as 5-cm^2 circular sheets (Apligraft) for the treatment of diabetic foot ulcers and venous ulcers. Wounds must have a good granulating wound bed and low bacterial counts, and hemostasis must be meticulous. Dermagraft, a cryopreserved human fibroblast–derived dermal substitute composed of collagen, matrix proteins, growth factors, and cytokines in a bioabsorbable polyglactin mesh scaffold, was available for restoration of the dermal bed for full-thickness diabetic foot ulcers. Another biologic tissue substitute, Alloderm, is composed of decellularized freeze-dried human dermis. The resultant matrix retains vacated vascular channel and has been used in abdominal wall reconstruction, breast reconstruction, head/neck reconstruction, and grafting for wound coverage. A similar product, GRAFTJACKET, has been approved for use in diabetic foot ulcers. Finally, OASIS, derived from porcine small intestinal submucosa (SIS) material, is indicated for partial- and full-thickness wounds and skin-loss injuries.

L. Negative-pressure wound therapy. Negative pressure created by vacuum-assisted closure devices (Wound VAC or Blue Sky or institutionally created dressings) appears to stimulate capillary ingrowth and the formation of granulation tissue in open wounds while keeping a relatively clean wound environment. VAC therapy is effective in the management of wounds as diverse as diabetic foot wounds, sacral ulcers, mediastinal dehiscence, perineum wounds, and wounds including prosthetic mesh (*Plast Reconstr Surg* 2006;117:127S). Recently, VAC therapy has been reported to be successful in managing enterocutaneous fistulae (*J Wound Care* 2003;12:343) and over areas with exposed bone (*Wounds* 2005;17:137) or tendon (*J Burn Care Rehabil* 2002;23:167). VAC therapy is contraindicated when there are exposed major blood vessels, untreated osteomyelitis, or cancer within the wound, and it is relatively contraindicated in anticoagulated patients.

M. Hyperbaric oxygen. Capillary microthrombi at the wound periphery limiting the passage of red blood cells, diabetic and other microvascular disease, and local edema can all create a local wound hypoxia; however, at increased atmospheric pressure of at least 2 atm of oxygen, the dissolved oxygen in the plasma can meet 100% of the oxygen extraction rate of the skin (*Chronic Wound Care* 1997:260). Randomized clinical trials have demonstrated that hyperbaric oxygen treatment (HBOT) is successful in healing diabetic foot ulcers (*Diabetes Care* 1987;19:81), preventing diabetic amputations (*Diabetes Care* 1996;19:1338), and healing chronic ulcerations (*Plast Reconstr Surg* 1996;93:829). Standard treatment protocols are based on appropriate débridement and wound care in conjunction with 90 minutes/day at 2 atm of oxygen. In critical situations, treatments may be twice daily. It should be noted that the effects of HBOT are regional and systemic as well as at the location of the wound. The combined local, regional and systemic effects of hyperoxemia achieved at whole body exposure to pressure are the rationale for HBO. The criteria for appropriate treatment are available on the Undersea and Hyperbaric Medical Society Web site, http://www.UHMS.org, and should be consulted for consideration to initiate treatment.

N. Metallic silver–impregnated dressings. The antimicrobial properties of metallic silver have long been recognized (*Burns* 1999;26:117, *J Wound Care* 2002a;11:125). Although there are many forms of topical silver applications, silver-impregnated dressings have been shown to have greater efficacy against a broader range of bacteria than cream-based forms and were better tolerated and less irritating than silver nitrate solution (*Am J Infect Control* 1998;26:572). Silver-impregnated dressings have been used extensively for wound management in a variety of settings, including burn wounds (*Br J Plast Surg* 1993;46:582, *J Burn Care Rehabil* 2004;25:89), chronic leg ulcers (*J Wound Care* 2003;12:351), diabetic wounds (*Clin Infect Dis* 2004;39(Suppl 2):S100), and traumatic injuries. The form of silver contained in these dressings has varied from compounds of silver nitrate or sulfadiazine, to sustained silver-ion release preparations (*Br J Nurs* 2001;10(15 Suppl. 2):S3), to silver-based crystalline nanoparticles (*Proc Natl Acad Sci USA* 1999;96:13611). A variety of materials and forms have also been used for the dressing component, including nylon, mesh, hydrocolloid, and methylcellulose. They have also previously been used in impregnated biological skin such as allografts and xenografts (*Ann Plast Surg* 1984;13:482, *J Burn Care Rehabil* 1988;9:476). For commercial use, a wide range of silver-impregnated dressings is currently available. However, only recently have comparative analyses of the antimicrobial effect and efficacy of these dressings and their cost-effectiveness begun to appear in the literature (*J Pediatr Surg* 2007;42:211, *J Med Microbiol* 2006;55:59, *J Wound Care* 2006;15:199).

IV. CARE OF WOUNDS IN THE EMERGENCY ROOM

A. History and physical examination. A careful history and physical examination of the whole patient should be performed, with attention to the time and mechanism of injury, initial treatments given, and prior or associated injuries. Medical, surgical, and immunization history and all known medication allergies should be documented. It is critically important that all injuries be identified, with appropriate prioritization of administered treatment plans. Careful neurologic and vascular examination should be performed distal to the site of injury and before administration of any anesthetics that could limit a later assessment.

B. Anesthesia. Lidocaine (Xylocaine) in concentrations from 0.5% to 2% is generally chosen for its rapidity of action (1 to 2 minutes). If longer duration is desired, bupivacaine (Marcaine) can be used; however, it may require up to 10 minutes to full onset. A 1:1 mixture of 1% lidocaine and 0.25% bupivacaine provides a rapid and reasonably long acting local anesthetic to improve hemostasis and prolong the effect of the anesthetic. Mixtures containing epinephrine should not be used to treat wounds on distal extremities (nose, earlobes, fingers, toes, or penis) because the profound vasoconstriction may lead to ischemic tissue loss. Whenever local anesthetics are used, care should be taken to avoid intravascular injection by aspirating before infiltration. The maximum safe amount of anesthetic that can be administered to the patient should be calculated before starting treatment. Patients with an allergy to amide anesthetics should be treated with ester anesthetics. The addition of sodium bicarbonate to lidocaine in a 1:9 ratio adjusts the acidic pH of the anesthetic so that its administration is less painful.

C. **Wound cleansing.** After adequate anesthesia is administered, the wound and surrounding skin should be cleansed in a gentle fashion. This is best accomplished with a standard wound-cleansing solution (e.g., Saf-Clens, Shur-Clens). It should be remembered that many standard scrub solutions are extremely toxic to all living cells; thus, they should never be used to wash the wound itself. A good rule to follow is that one should never place a solution in a wound that one would not place in one's eye. Wounds are best irrigated with saline or lactated Ringer's solution with pressures of 8 to 15 psi. An 18- or 19-gauge intravenous catheter or needle on a 35- to 60-mL syringe provides 8-psi irrigating pressure, which is adequate to irrigate most wounds. Battery-powered irrigation systems, available for portable use, deliver pressures of up to 15 psi and are easier to use when irrigating a wound with several liters of fluid. Abrasions should be scrubbed carefully with a gloved hand during cleansing to remove foreign material that might lead to traumatic skin tattooing.

D. **Wound hemostasis and exploration.** Direct pressure, elevation, and even the use of a blood pressure cuff as a tourniquet are effective means of limiting blood loss in the emergency setting. Electrocautery, suture ligation, or hemostat clamping of a bleeding site is best done by a practitioner who is familiar with the anatomy of the area because major nerves often lie adjacent to major arteries and any imprecision can lead to an iatrogenic injury worse than the initial trauma. Wounds should be explored carefully for foreign bodies and to determine the extent of injury. Multiplane x-ray views of the soft tissues of the wounded area can prove to be useful in locating radiopaque objects. If the wound contains difficult-to-locate or numerous foreign bodies, it can best be explored in the operating room.

E. **Débridement.** Traumatic breaks of the skin are often irregular, and the force of impact leaves a zone of surrounding skin and underlying tissue injury that is often best treated by judicious sharp débridement. All foreign material and devitalized tissue must be removed before wound closure is attempted. The goal of débridement is to obtain a clean wound with a bleeding skin margin that overlies healthy, viable tissue.

F. **Wound closure.** The decision to close a wound depends largely on the amount of contamination present and the amount of time that the wound has been open. Wounds that are older than 6 to 8 hours, puncture wounds, human bites, and wounds with gross infection should not be closed, with the possible exception of facial wounds, for in these the superior vascular supply can often overcome otherwise major contamination. At a microscopic level, wounds with greater than 10^5 bacteria/g of tissue are considered too heavily contaminated to close safely. Dog and cat bites should be allowed to heal by secondary intention, or they may be closed primarily over wicks only after thorough irrigation and débridement, with administration of appropriate antibiotics.

G. **Additional considerations for wounds in the emergency room**
1. **Tetanus prophylaxis.** Tetanus is a potentially fatal disorder that is characterized by uncontrolled spasms of the voluntary muscles. It is caused by the neurotoxin of the anaerobic bacterium *Clostridium tetani*. A tetanus-prone wound has one or more of the following characteristics: (1) more than 6 hours old; (2) deeper than 1 cm; (3) contaminated by soil, feces, or rust; (4) stellate configuration (burst-type injury with marked soft-tissue injury); (5) caused by missile, crush, burn, or frostbite; (6) contains devitalized or denervated tissue; and (7) caused by an animal or human bite (*Emerg Med Clin North Am* 1992;10:531). Recommendations for tetanus prophylaxis are summarized in Table 6-5.
2. **Antibiotics.** Antibiotic use does not allow closure of a wound that would otherwise be left open to heal secondarily, and it is not a substitute for good wound cleansing and débridement. Antibiotics should be chosen based on the indication (prophylactic or therapeutic), the location and age of the wound, and the mechanism of injury. In addition, one should consider the likely pathogen(s) that are most involved under the circumstances. Prophylactic antibiotics are indicated for immunocompromised patients and those with prosthetic heart valves or other permanently implanted prostheses. Prophylactic antibiotics should also be used when intestinal or genitourinary tract contamination is present, when an infection

TABLE 6-5	Summary of Immunization Practices Advisory Committee Recommendations for Tetanus Prophylaxis in Routine Wound Management			
Tetanus	**Clean minor wounds**		**Tetanus-prone wounds**	
Immunization Unknown or less than three doses	Td[a] Yes	TIG[b] No	Td Yes	TIG Yes
Three doses or more	No (yes if >10 yr since last dose)	No	No (yes if >5 yr since last dose)	No

Td, tetanus-diphtheria toxoid (adult type); TIG, tetanus immune globulin.
[a]Adsorbed tetanus and diphtheria toxoids, 0.5 mL intramuscularly. For children <7 yr, diphtheria-polio-tetanus is recommended.
[b]TIG (human), 250 units intramuscularly, given concurrently with the toxoid at separate sites. Heterologous antitoxin (equine) should not be given unless TIG is not available within 24 hr and only if the possibility of tetanus outweighs the danger of adverse reaction.
Reprinted with permission from Centers for Disease Control and Prevention. Tetanus United States, 1987 and 1988. *MMWR* 1990;39(3):37.

is likely to develop, or when an infection has potentially disastrous consequences (*Surg Clin North Am* 1997;77:3). For wounds that are likely to become infected, obtaining good wound cultures at the time of injury helps to better target the specific organism(s) that failed to respond to initial broad-spectrum antibiotic treatment.

3. **Furuncles** are small boils or abscesses caused by an infection of the hair follicle that extends into the subcutaneous tissue. The usual causative organism is *S. aureus*, and the incidence and prevalence of skin abscesses has risen in parallel with the emergence of community-acquired MRSA (*Clin Infect Dis* 2005;41:1373). Furuncles manifest as firm, tender, erythematous nodules. Predisposing factors include diabetes, corticosteroid use, impaired neutrophil function, or increased friction or perspiration as occurs in athletes or obese individuals. Whereas initial treatment can include oral antibiotics and warm compresses to promote drainage, if the furuncle exhibits fluctuance, an incision-and-drainage procedure is required. Under local anesthesia and after site prep with chlorhexidine or an iodine-containing solution, the initial incision is made with a no. 11 scalpel with the blade oriented perpendicular to the skin and inserted into the area of maximum fluctuance. A cruciform or elliptical incision will help to prevent premature epidermal closure with recurrent cavity formation. A hemostat or blunt finger dissection is used to probe and break up any loculations within the abscess cavity. The cavity should be irrigated and packed with iodoform or plain gauze stripping, which will require regular packing change. The use of antibiotics after abscess drainage remains controversial and depends on appropriate clinical judgment. If antibiotics are administered and community-acquired MRSA is a possible cause of the infection, trimethoprim/sulfamethoxazole (TMP/SMX), doxycycline, clindamycin, or a third- or fourth-generation fluoroquinolone should be considered, and a 7-day course is generally sufficient (*Prim Care* 2006;33:697). Oral, perirectal, or genital abscesses should be considered multibacterial, and agents such as amoxicillin-clavulanate or third- or fourth-generation fluoroquinolones should be used to cover Gram-positive, Gram-negative, and anaerobic organisms. Some patients may require intravenous antibiotics. If oral or intravenous antibiotics are administered, a wound culture should be obtained from the abscess cavity prior to irrigation to determine whether the appropriate antibiotic has been selected. For all skin infections and drained abscesses, follow-up is extremely important.

4. **Carbuncles** are deep cutaneous infections of multiple hair follicles, characterized by the destruction of fibrous tissue septa and resulting in a series of loculated, interconnected abscesses. Carbuncles are diagnosed and treated in the same manner as furuncles. Because it is difficult to differentiate furuncles from carbuncles based

on the overlying epidermis, it is important to probe all abscess cavities for loculations.

H. Bites. The treatment of a bite wound beyond the basic treatment of copious irrigation and débridement is most dependent on the source of the bite.

1. **Human bites** typically occur during interpersonal conflict. Because the wound often seems relatively trivial, such as a small puncture wound or a laceration in a patient who is very upset or intoxicated, the patient may delay seeking treatment, which increases the likelihood of the wound to become infected. A particularly troublesome bite is a small skin injury that is seen over the metacarpophalangeal joint of a patient who punched someone else in the mouth and sustained a tooth cut of the skin overlying the fisted knuckle. Such injuries often require operative joint irrigation and parenteral antibiotics. Unintentional bites of the lip or tongue sustained in a fall or during a seizure may also occasionally come to the attention of a surgeon. The oral flora of humans includes *Staphylococcus* and *Streptococcus* species, anaerobic bacteria, *Eikenella corrodens*, and anaerobic Gram-negative rods; antibiotic coverage should be directed initially toward these organisms.

2. **Mammalian animal bites.** Because infection is the most common complication of domestic animal bites, these bites should be considered contaminated and their immediate closure deferred. Infections that are caused by dog bites are usually polymicrobial, and pathogens include viridans streptococci, *Pasteurella multocida,* and *Bacteroides, Fusobacterium,* and *Capnocytophaga* species. Because these wounds are often larger open lacerations, only about 5% of dog bites become infected. The oral flora of the domestic cat is believed to be less complex, with *P. multocida* found in up to 60% of wounds caused by cat bites. Because these are smaller puncture wounds, up to 80% of these will become infected. Local laws require the confinement of animals to ensure that they do not manifest rabies. Rabies, a routinely fatal disease of the central nervous system, is caused by the rabies virus, which is a member of the rhabdovirus group and contains a single strand of RNA. Thanks in large part to an intensive immunization program, the incidence of rabies in the United States has been reduced greatly, to approximately five cases/year. Today, the major risk comes from wild animal bites. The recommendations for rabies prophylaxis and treatment are summarized in Table 6-6.

TABLE 6-6   **Rabies Postexposure Prophylaxis Treatment Guide**

Species	Condition of animal	Treatment[a]
Domestic cat or dog	Healthy and available for at least 10 d of observation	None; however, treatment should be initiated at the first sign of rabies[b]
	Suspected rabid[b]	Immediate
	Unknown	Contact public health department
Wild skunk, bat, fox, coyote, raccoon, or other carnivore	Regard as rabid; animal should be killed and tested as soon as possible	Immediate; however, discontinue if immunofluorescence test is negative

[a](1) Human rabies immune globulin, 20 IU/kg [if feasible, infiltrate half of dose around the wound(s), the rest intramuscularly in gluteal area] and (2) human diploid cell vaccine (HDCV), 1 mL intramuscularly in deltoid area (never in gluteal area) on days 0, 3, 7, 14, and 28. If the patient has previously been immunized, give booster HDCV only on days 0 and 3.

[b]Any animal suspected of being rabid should be killed and its brain studied with a rabies-specific fluorescent antibody.

Adapted with permission from Immunization Practices Advisory Committee. Rabies Prevention United States, 1991. *MMWR* 1991;40(RR-3):1.

3. **Snake bites.** Ten percent of the snakes in the United States are venomous. Determining whether a venomous snake caused the bite is critical in the early management of bite injuries. Pit vipers usually leave two puncture wounds, whereas nonvenomous snakes generally leave a characteristic U-shaped bite wound. Poisonous snake venom contains many polypeptides that are damaging to human tissues, including phospholipase A, hyaluronidase, adenosine triphosphatase, 5-nucleotidase, and nicotinic acid dehydrogenase. The degree of envenomation and the time from injury determine the clinical manifestations. Immediate signs of envenomation include regional edema, erythema, and intense pain at the site of the bite. Systemic manifestations can ensue rapidly, especially with greater envenomation. The hematocrit and platelet count may fall, with concomitant elevation of the prothrombin time, partial thromboplastin time, and bleeding times. Without treatment, severe envenomation may lead to pulmonary edema, peripheral vascular collapse, direct cardiotoxicity, and acute renal failure. Coral snake venom is less toxic locally but can lead to profound neurologic sequelae. Early symptoms include nausea, euphoria, salivation, paresthesias, ptosis, and muscle weakness leading to respiratory arrest.

Treatment is most successful if administered promptly. Extremity wounds should be immobilized and a tourniquet applied proximal to the bite site to minimize the spread of the venom. Although small amounts of venom can be removed by suction through small incisions over the bite wound, a wider surgical excision of the bite removes even more, provided that it can be done in a timely fashion. Antivenom may help to neutralize the venom and should be administered intravenously as soon as possible after more severe bites or when systemic symptoms are noted. Earlier formulations of antivenom (including polyvalent antivenin) were limited by acute reactions in 20% to 25% of patients, and more than 50% developed serum sickness (*Arch Int Med* 2001;161:2030). A newer antivenom, CroFab, is a Fab-segment–based product that lacks antigenic Fc antibody fragments. The antibody is produced by injecting sheep with one of four pit viper species indigenous to the United States: western diamondback rattlesnake, eastern diamondback rattlesnake, Mojave rattlesnake, and cottonmouth. The venoms of different species vary in composition and potency, but they are similar enough that CroFab can neutralize venom from many species, including those not included in the production process (*Am J Trop Med Hyg* 1995;53:507). Indications for CroFab antivenom use are pit viper envenomation with worsening edema or any systemic symptom including coagulopathy. Relative contraindications include known hypersensitivity to CroFab, papain, or papaya (*Curr Opin Pediatr* 2005;17:234). Shock is treated with circulatory support. Broad-spectrum antibiotics and tetanus prophylaxis are also indicated.

4. **Spider bites**
   a. The **black widow spider (*Latrodectus mactans*)** is found throughout the United States and prefers to inhabit dry, dark crevices. The female is distinguished by her shiny black body and a red hourglass mark on the abdomen. The actual bite may cause little pain, and victims often do not recall the event. The venom, a neurotoxin, causes muscular rigidity. Chest pain from muscular contraction follows upper-extremity bites, whereas lower-extremity bites may cause rigidity of the abdominal wall. Patients who present with abdominal wall rigidity, which might typically suggest an acute abdominal emergency, lack associated abdominal tenderness. Intense muscular spasms and pain are usually self-limiting and require no specific treatment. Severe cases may progress to respiratory arrest, which, along with shock, accounts for the observed mortality of approximately 5%. Therapy consists of respiratory and circulatory support, broad-spectrum antibiotics, narcotic analgesia, and muscle relaxants. Antivenin (*L. mactans*) is indicated for the very young or old and for patients with severe illness.
   b. The **brown recluse spider (*Loxosceles reclusa*)** is found throughout the central and southern United States, most often inhabiting dark, moist environments. It is 10 to 15 mm long, with a light tan to brown color, a flat body, and a

violin-shaped band over the head and chest area of the back. Brown recluse venom is very locally toxic, containing hyaluronidase and other elements that lead to coagulation necrosis of the area around the wound. Systemically, hemolysis with hemoglobinuria, hemolytic anemia, and renal failure may develop. Pain at the time of the bite is an inconsistent symptom; however, several hours after the bite, a characteristic lesion is seen, with a central zone of pale induration surrounded by an erythematous border. By this time, pain is severe. After approximately 1 week, a black eschar develops, which soon sloughs, leaving an ulcer that may continue to enlarge, with extensive necrosis of the underlying fat and subcutaneous tissues. Systemic illness most often occurs in children, with fever, malaise, nausea, and vomiting. Therapy is supportive, and mortality is rare. Many of these wounds will heal spontaneously. If necessary, excision of the wound should be deferred until the ulcer is well demarcated; broad-spectrum antibiotics are recommended.

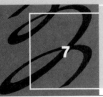

CRITICAL CARE

Emily B. Rivet and Craig M. Coopersmith

$\mathcal{P}$atients are admitted to intensive care units (ICUs) because of either the presence or the risk of organ dysfunction. This chapter focuses on routine monitoring of the critically ill patient, the three most common reasons for surgical ICU admissions (respiratory, circulatory, and renal failure), and sepsis. It also addresses adjunctive topics, including sedation and analgesia, prophylaxis against stress-induced upper gastrointestinal hemorrhage, and the role of transfusion and glucose control in the care of the critically ill.

I. MONITORING OF THE CRITICALLY ILL PATIENT

A. **Temperature monitoring.** Critically ill patients are at increased risk for temperature alterations as a result of debilitation and predisposition to infection. All critically ill patients should have their core temperatures measured at least every 4 hours. A rectal thermometer is the most accurate method of obtaining the core temperature.

B. **Electrocardiographic (ECG) monitoring.** Continuous ECG monitoring with computerized arrhythmia detection systems is standard in most ICUs. Continuous monitoring allows for rapid detection of dysrhythmias and assessment of heart rate and rhythm.

C. **Arterial pressure monitoring**
   1. Indirect arterial pressure measurement with a sphygmomanometer should be performed at least hourly.
   2. **Direct arterial pressure measurement** with intra-arterial catheters offers continuous measurement of arterial pressures and waveforms and easy, painless access for arterial blood gas (ABG) measurement. Arterial cannulation is warranted in patients with hemodynamic instability and in those who require frequent blood gas analysis. The most common site of insertion is the radial artery, which is chosen because of its accessibility and generally good collateral blood flow. If this is unavailable, alternatives include femoral and, less commonly, dorsalis pedis or axillary artery catheterization. These should be avoided in infants because occlusion may cause extremity ischemia and subsequent deformity. The extremity distal to the catheter should be assessed prior to insertion and frequently after insertion. The catheter should be removed immediately if there is evidence of distal ischemia. Rare infectious complications include local cellulitis and bacteremia, which may result from catheter colonization or contamination of the fluid-filled monitoring system.

D. **Central venous pressure (CVP) monitoring.** Central venous catheters provide access to measure CVP and to administer vasoactive drugs and total parenteral nutrition. For techniques of catheter insertion, refer to Chapter 37.

E. **Pulmonary artery (PA) catheterization.** PA (also called *Swan-Ganz*) catheters are used to determine cardiac filling pressures, cardiac output (CO), pulmonary artery pressures, systemic vascular resistance, and mixed venous saturation (SvO_2). They can be used in unstable patients with rapid changes in hemodynamic status to assess responses to treatment with fluid and cardioactive agents. It is important to note that the use of PA catheters has not been demonstrated to change mortality in prospective, randomized trials.
   1. **Continuous ECG and blood pressure monitoring and peripheral intravenous access** are required. An ECG must be checked prior to PA catheter

placement to rule out left-bundle-branch block because PA catheter placement can induce transient right-bundle-branch block. If a patient with left-bundle-branch block needs a PA catheter, a trancutaneous pacemaker should be placed prior to PA catheter placement.

2. **Complications** associated with central venous access are described in Chapter 37. PA catheter **balloon rupture** exposes the patient to the risk of air and balloon fragment emboli. Balloon rupture should be suspected when air inflated into the balloon does not return; the diagnosis is confirmed if blood can be aspirated from the balloon port. If either of these occurs, the catheter should be removed immediately. **PA perforation** presents with hemoptysis, typically after balloon inflation. Management of this serious complication includes placement of the patient with his or her involved side in the dependent position and emergent thoracic surgical consultation. Atrial and ventricular **arrhythmias** occur commonly during insertion of PA catheters and usually are self-limited. Most frequently, this is a catheter-induced right-bundle-branch block.

3. **Esophageal Dopplers** (CardioQ, Deltex Medical) have recently been introduced as a less invasive alternative to PA catheters. There has been no demonstration of improvement in outcomes associated with their use. However, their potential risk is much lower than with PA catheters.

F. **Respiratory monitoring**

1. **Pulse oximetry** should be used in all critically ill patients. It provides quantitative, continuous assessment of arterial oxygen saturation (SaO_2). Probe malposition, motion, hypothermia, vasoconstriction, and hypotension may result in poor signal detection and unreliable measurements. Nail polish, dark skin, and elevated serum lipids falsely lower the SaO_2 measurement, whereas elevated carboxyhemoglobin or methemoglobin falsely raises the measurements.

2. **Capnography** provides quantitative, continuous assessment of expired CO_2 concentrations, and the gradient between arterial CO_2 partial pressure ($PaCO_2$) and end-tidal CO_2 ($ETCO_2$) measurements can be used to follow trends. A rise in $ETCO_2$ can indicate a decrease in alveolar ventilation or an increase in CO_2 production, as seen with overfeeding, sepsis, fever, exercise, or acute increases in CO. A fall in $ETCO_2$ indicates either an increase in alveolar ventilation or an increase in dead space, as seen with massive pulmonary embolism or air embolism, endotracheal tube or main-stem bronchus obstruction, ventilator circuit leak, or a sudden drop in CO.

II. **SEDATION AND ANALGESIA.** Altered mentation, which can span the spectrum from delirium to coma, is a common manifestation of acute illness. Pain and emotional distress should be treated. Sedation allows critically ill patients to tolerate invasive supportive interventions such as intubation and mechanical ventilation. Titration of sedation is simplified by the use of an objective scoring system, such as the modified Ramsay scale (Table 7-1).

A. **Control of agitation.** The most frequently used agents are **benzodiazepines,** which are potent inducers of sedation, anxiolysis, and amnesia. The action of benzodiazepines appears to be mediated through γ-aminobutyric acid, an inhibitory

TABLE 7-1   Modified Ramsay Sedation Scale

Score	Characteristics
1	Anxious and agitated or restless, or both
2	Cooperative, oriented, and tranquil
3	Responds to commands only
4	Asleep, but responds to physical or auditory stimuli
5	Asleep, but responds sluggishly to physical or auditory stimuli
6	No response

neurotransmitter. Effective doses of benzodiazepines may be higher in tolerant patients (e.g., those who have taken similar agents previously or who consume alcohol regularly). Patients older than 50 years or those with preexisting cardiopulmonary, hepatic, or renal dysfunction are particularly susceptible to benzodiazepines and their metabolites. Initial doses should be reduced in these patients.

1. **Midazolam** has a short half-life (20 to 60 minutes) and a rapid onset (1 to 3 minutes) and offset of action. Although midazolam has a short half-life, when it is given as a continuous infusion for a prolonged period of time, metabolites accumulate, and patients may take a number of days to fully awaken.

2. **Lorazepam** has a longer half-life (10 to 20 hours) and a slower onset (10 to 20 minutes) of action. Unlike midazolam, lorazepam does not have active metabolites. However, similar to midazolam, the drug accumulates with prolonged use, and patients may remain sedated for a number of days after the agent is stopped. Midazolam and lorazepam are acceptable alternatives for long-term sedation in the critically ill patient.

3. **Propofol** is a nonbenzodiazepine sedative-hypnotic that has an extremely short onset and offset of action and is usually delivered as a continuous infusion. It does not accumulate to the same degree as benzodiazepines and thus results in a shorter length of sedation after discontinuation. A major side effect of propofol is hypotension, especially in hypovolemic patients. Although it is more expensive than benzodiazepines, propofol is preferred for short-term sedation (<2 days) because of its rapid elimination.

4. **Dexmedetomidine** is a new, relatively selective α_2-adrenoreceptor agonist that may be helpful for short-term sedation of mechanically ventilated patients. Patients treated with this agent are more easily arousable than those sedated with either propofol or benzodiazepine infusions. The main side effect is hypotension. Dexmedetomidine is approved for use for a maximum of 24 hours.

B. **Control of delirium**

1. **Haloperidol** is an antipsychotic medicine that can be used to treat delirium. The combination of haloperidol and a benzodiazepine can be effective and allow smaller doses of each agent to be used, thereby avoiding the extrapyramidal side effects of haloperidol. Major toxicities include hypotension, cardiac arrhythmias, and prolongation of the QT interval. Therefore, ECGs should be checked daily in patients on haloperidol.

C. **Control of pain.** Pain management is an important concern in the surgical ICU.

1. **Morphine** is administered most commonly for PRN (as-needed) and patient-controlled dosing because of its low cost and familiarity. Morphine should not be used in patients with renal failure.

2. **Fentanyl** is the most commonly used opiate for continuous drips. It has a half-life of 30 to 60 minutes due to its rapid redistribution. Unlike morphine, fentanyl does not cause histamine release and is therefore less likely to cause hypotension.

3. **Hydromorphone** is a viable option for patients who are allergic to morphine or fentanyl. Care should be used in patients with liver failure.

4. **Meperidine** is used least frequently because of its side effects. Patients with renal or hepatic dysfunction are at risk for accumulation of normeperidine, a metabolite, which can cause neurotoxic side effects including seizures.

5. **Methadone** is a narcotic with a long half-life (8 to 59 hours) that can be used for pain management and to facilitate withdrawal from other narcotics. Substantial variability between individuals with regard to its pharmacokinetic properties mandates close monitoring of patients during initiation of treatment and conversion from other opioids.

6. **Thoracic or lumbar epidural catheters** are usually well tolerated, decrease the need for intravenous narcotics, and can substantially improve compliance with respiratory therapy.

D. Regardless of which agents are used for sedation and analgesia, the presence of a **sedation protocol** decreases both length of stay in the ICU and the length of time a patient requires mechanical ventilation compared with physician-directed sedation.

E. For patients who require **long-term sedation and analgesia,** daily interruption of sedation to wakefulness produces decreased time on mechanical ventilation and shorter ICU stays, according to a prospective, randomized, controlled study (*N Engl J Med* 2000;342:1477). However, this study did not include surgical patients, who have higher analgesia requirements than typical medical ICU patients. Therefore, the applicability of a "daily wake-up" to surgical ICU patients is less clear.

III. RESPIRATORY FAILURE

A. Etiology. Respiratory failure results from inadequate exchange of oxygen and carbon dioxide. It may be caused by a failure of the gas-exchange mechanism [e.g., asthma, chronic obstructive pulmonary disease (COPD), acute respiratory distress syndrome (ARDS), pneumonia, pulmonary embolism, and pulmonary edema] and a consequent ventilation–perfusion mismatch. Alternatively, it may be caused by a failure of the mechanical ventilatory apparatus (e.g., neuromuscular disease, inspiratory muscle fatigue, and airway obstruction), which results in hypoventilation and thereby hypercapnia and hypoxemia. Although the etiology (possibly multifactorial) is important for longer-term treatment and prognosis, the early treatment of respiratory failure is similar regardless of the immediate cause.

B. Diagnosis. Signs or symptoms of respiratory impairment (e.g., tachypnea, dyspnea, or mental status changes) should prompt analysis of pulse oximetry and ABGs. Pulse oximetry monitoring results of less than 90% correspond to a partial arterial oxygen pressure (PaO_2) of greater than 60 mm Hg, which seriously compromises tissue oxygenation. An acute rise in $PaCO_2$ to greater than 50 mm Hg along with a pH of less than 7.35 (respiratory acidosis) implies a significant imbalance between carbon dioxide production and elimination (alveolar ventilation). **It is important to note that adequate oxygenation does not guarantee adequate ventilation.** A complete physical exam and portable chest x-ray are essential for figuring out the etiology of respiratory failure.

C. Treatment

1. Oxygen therapy. The objective of supplemental oxygen administration is to increase the relative concentration of oxygen in the alveoli. This is accomplished most commonly by delivering oxygen through a nasal cannula, simple facemask, or facemask with a reservoir (Table 7-2). The inspired oxygen concentration varies depending on the percentage of entrained air: The more air that is entrained (with an ambient oxygen concentration of 0.21), the lower the fraction of inspired oxygen (FiO_2). When the required FiO_2 is high (~0.60), a high–air-flow system with oxygen enrichment via a jet-mixing or Venturi apparatus is used, and the oxygen is delivered by a tight-fitting mask with a reservoir. Whenever possible, inspired oxygen should be humidified to prevent drying of the airways and respiratory secretions.

2. Airway management. Securing and maintaining a patent airway is the first priority in an unstable patient. The most common source of airway obstruction in a patient with an altered sensorium is the tongue. This is corrected easily by the chin-lift or jaw-thrust maneuver or by placing an oropharyngeal or nasopharyngeal airway. If uncertainty exists about whether the airway is patent or protected from aspiration, endotracheal tube (ET) intubation is indicated. In most cases, intubation is not urgent. **Unless the physician is skilled in the placement of an artificial airway, the appropriate maneuver is to give supplemental oxygen and to bag the patient if necessary until someone with airway expertise arrives.**

a. Oral and nasal ET intubation. The oral route is usually the most expeditious. The nasal route can be used only when the patient is breathing spontaneously; significant skill is needed to direct the tip of the ET tube blindly past the vocal cords and into the trachea. Once the tube is in the trachea, the adequacy of bilateral ventilation must be established using auscultation and a carbon dioxide indicator. A chest x-ray is used to document correct ET tube position.

b. Noninvasive ventilation. Biphasic positive airway pressure is a form of ventilation that is delivered by means of a tight-fitting mask (no ET tube), which

TABLE 7-2	Oxygen Delivery Systems	
Type	**Fio₂ capability**	**Comments**
Nasal cannula	24%–48%	At flow rates of 1–8 L/min; true F_{IO_2} uncertain and highly dependent on minute ventilation; simple, comfortable, and can be worn during eating or coughing
Simple facemask	35%–55%	At flow rates of 6–10 L/min
High-humidity mask	Variable from 28% to nearly 100%	Flow rates should be 2–3 times minute ventilation; levels >60% may require additional oxygen bleed-in; excellent humidification
Reservoir mask		
Nonrebreathing	90%–95%	At flow rates of 12–15 L/min; incorporates directional valves that reduce room air entrainment and rebreathing of expired air
Partial rebreathing	50%–80%	At flow rates of 8–10 L/min
Ventimask	Available at 24%, 28%, 31%, 35%, 40%, and 50%	Provides controlled F_{IO_2}; useful in chronic obstructive pulmonary disease patients to prevent depression of respiratory drive; poorly humidified gas at maximum F_{IO_2}

F_{IO_2}, fraction of inspired oxygen.

allows independent control of positive inspiratory and expiratory pressures. It is most useful as a bridge to aid respiratory efforts in patients with mild to moderate respiratory insufficiency of short duration (e.g., asthma or COPD exacerbations or pulmonary edema) and frequently can prevent the need for intubation in patients with rapidly reversible respiratory failure.

c. **Tracheostomy** should be considered in the presence of severe maxillofacial injury to ensure an adequate airway or if prolonged intubation is anticipated. Timing of tracheostomy has been found to be significantly correlated with length of mechanical ventilation, as well as duration of ICU and hospital stay (*Crit Care Med* 2005;33:2513). Tracheostomy provides a more secure airway, improves patient comfort and oral hygiene, increases patient mobility, and enhances secretion removal. **If a tracheostomy falls out before an adequate tract has formed, the patient should be reintubated orotracheally rather than subjected to a blind attempt to replace the tracheostomy.**

d. **Cricothyroidotomy** is useful in emergency situations when attempts to ventilate by bag-valve-mask and ET tube are unsuccessful. The technique is described in Chapter 37. Percutaneous cricothyoidotomy may also be performed if a kit is available and someone with expertise is present.

e. **Complications.** Immediate complications include passage of the ET tube into either the esophagus or the tissue surrounding the trachea. Either can lead to death if not promptly recognized. Of these, esophageal intubation is substantially more common. When an ET tube is placed in tissue surrounding the trachea (most common when attempting to replace a tracheostomy that has fallen out), it can lead to hemorrhage, pneumothorax, pneumomediastinum, subcutaneous emphysema, and injury to the recurrent laryngeal nerve. Delayed complications of ET intubation include hemorrhage, which results from erosion of the tube into a vessel (usually the brachiocephalic artery). Immediate orotracheal intubation, removal of the tracheostomy tube, insertion of the surgeon's finger into the tracheostomy site, and anterior compression of the brachiocephalic artery against the clavicle can be used treat the hemorrhage.

ET tube cuff pressures should be monitored frequently and kept below capillary filling pressures (i.e., <25 mm Hg) to prevent tracheal ischemia, which, if untreated, can lead to tracheomalacia or tracheal stenosis.

3. **Mechanical ventilation** is indicated for the treatment of respiratory failure. The goal of treatment is to improve alveolar ventilation and oxygenation and to reduce the work of breathing while other therapies are instituted to treat underlying disease processes.

   a. **Modes of mechanical ventilation** can be divided into volume-limited and pressure-limited modes. The key to understanding the differences between these modes lies in the relationship of pressure to volume [i.e., pulmonary compliance, in which compliance equals the change in volume divided by the change in pressure $(C = \Delta V / \Delta P)$]. The goal of volume-limited modes is to deliver a set tidal volume to the patient at a rate that ensures adequate alveolar ventilation; airway pressure varies depending on compliance. In contrast, the goal of pressure-limited modes is to deliver a set airway pressure; tidal volume varies depending on compliance.

   (1) Volume-limited modes

   (a) Assist-control (A/C) ventilation delivers a preset tidal volume at a set rate. As the machine senses each inspiratory effort by the patient, it delivers the set tidal volume. If the patient's respiratory rate is below the machine's set rate, ventilator-initiated breaths are delivered to make up the difference between the set rate and the patient's. A/C ventilation minimizes the work of breathing because the ventilator assists all breaths (hence, the term *full support*); however, for this reason, this mode is uncomfortable if the patient's breaths are dyssynchronous with those delivered by the ventilator. Respiratory alkalosis from hyperventilation may develop in agitated patients.

   (b) Intermittent mandatory ventilation (IMV), like A/C ventilation, delivers a preset tidal volume at a set rate. IMV does not assist spontaneous respiratory efforts; it is commonly used with pressure support.

   (2) Pressure-limited modes

   (a) Pressure-support ventilation delivers a preset inspiratory pressure but at no set rate. Constant inspiratory pressure continues until the inspiratory flow of gas falls below a predetermined level and the exhalation valve opens. Thus, tidal volumes are generated only when the patient is breathing spontaneously. This allows the patient to maintain control of inspiratory and expiratory time and thus tidal volume; as a result, this mode is the most comfortable for spontaneously breathing patients. The disadvantages of pressure-support ventilation are that (1) all ventilation depends on patient effort and (2) sudden increases in airway resistance decrease tidal volumes. Small amounts (5 to 8 cm H_2O) of pressure-support ventilation are used routinely to overcome the resistance to air flow caused by the ET tube and the inspiratory demand valves of the ventilator.

   (b) Pressure-control ventilation delivers a preset inspiratory pressure (as opposed to tidal volume) at a set rate. This mode is used in patients with poor (low) lung compliance who develop high inspiratory pressures when they are ventilated with the more traditional modes described previously. Thus, the advantage of this mode is that it allows the physician to set the airway pressure and thereby minimize barotrauma. The disadvantage is that the tidal volume varies depending on compliance. The sudden development of an increase in airway resistance (coughing, thick secretions, a kink in the ET tube, a Valsalva maneuver), for example, increases airway pressures and decreases tidal volumes to dangerously low levels.

   (3) BiLevel ventilation is a style of ventilator support that allows a patient to breathe spontaneously at two levels of positive end-expiratory pressure

(PEEP). The time at the lower PEEP level may be limited so that all breaths are taken at the upper PEEP level and the pressure is then released just long enough to allow the lung volume to decrease (airway pressure release ventilation). Alternatively, spontaneous breathing may occur at both levels. There is evidence to suggest that this improves patient comfort and synchrony with the ventilator.

(4) **High-frequency oscillatory ventilation** (HFOV) uses substantially faster rates (180 to 300/minute) and smaller tidal volumes than conventional modes. The result is a relative decrease in diaphragmatic excursion, lung movement, and airway pressures. The physical mechanisms responsible for gas movement are complex and incompletely understood. Although HFOV has not been demonstrated to improve survival, it is associated with a trend toward decreased mortality in ARDS in a recent prospective, randomized trial (52% vs. 37%, $p = 0.102$) and represents a viable "rescue" therapy for those failing with conventional ventilation (*Am J Respir Crit Care Med* 2002;166:801). HFOV may be considered when FIO_2 requirements exceed 70% and mean airway pressure is approaching 20 cm H_2O or higher or when there is a positive end-expiratory pressure of greater than 15 cm H_2O in ARDS. Patients do not always need to be paralyzed to undergo HFOV, but they do need to be deeply sedated (Ramsay 5 to 6).

b. **Ventilator management**

(1) **Choice of ventilator mode.** Patient needs should be matched with the appropriate ventilator mode by considering each mode's advantages and disadvantages.

(2) **FIO_2** should be adjusted to ensure adequate arterial oxygenation, which is a blood hemoglobin saturation of 92% in lighter-skinned individuals and 95% in darker-skinned patients. The lowest possible FIO_2 (ideally ≤0.40) should be used to achieve these levels of arterial saturation to prevent pulmonary oxygen toxicity.

(3) **Tidal volume.** There is no consensus on the optimal tidal volume for the postoperative patient who requires short-term mechanical ventilatory support. However, in ARDS, low tidal volumes are associated with improved survival. A recent multicenter, prospective, randomized trial demonstrated improved survival in patients who were ventilated with low tidal volumes (6 mL/kg ideal body weight) compared with high tidal volumes (12 mL/kg) (*N Engl J Med* 2000;342:1301). As a result of this important study, the tidal volume should be adjusted to as low as 4 mL/kg ideal body weight to maintain plateau pressures at less than 30 cm H_2O to minimize barotrauma but greater than 20 cm H_2O to minimize atelectasis.

(4) **Ventilatory rate.** Once the tidal volume has been determined, the rate is chosen (typically 8 to 16 breaths per minute) to provide adequate minute ventilation (the product of rate and tidal volume). The rate is adjusted to optimize arterial pH and $PaCO_2$; an end-tidal CO_2 monitor is useful in this regard.

(5) **Inspiratory-expiratory (I:E) ratio.** The normal I:E ratio is 1:2 to 1:3. Longer expiratory times allow patients with obstructive lung disease (high compliance) to exhale fully and prevent stacking of breaths. In contrast, longer inspiratory times, which decrease peak airway pressures, are useful in patients with low pulmonary compliance. Inverse-ratio ventilation takes advantage of breath stacking, using I:E ratios from 1:1 to 4:1. Used only in patients with severe consolidating lung disease, inverse ratio ventilation is believed to improve gas exchange by progressive alveolar recruitment (mean airway pressures are higher, keeping a larger number of alveoli open for a greater percentage of the respiratory cycle). Inverse-ratio ventilation is used most commonly with pressure-control ventilation.

(6) Positive end-expiratory pressure increases functional residual capacity, increases lung compliance, and improves ventilation–perfusion matching by opening terminal airways and recruiting partially collapsed alveoli. PEEP of 5 cm H_2O is considered physiologic; higher levels are used when hypoxemia is moderate to severe. PEEP significantly increases intrathoracic pressure and therefore decreases CO, reduces venous return to the heart, increases airway pressure, and alters pulmonary vascular resistance. PEEP levels of greater than 15 cm H_2O significantly increase the risk of barotrauma and spontaneous pneumothorax. PEEP applied to the spontaneously ventilating patient without inspiratory ventilatory support is called *continuous positive airway pressure (CPAP)*.

(7) Sedation and neuromuscular paralysis. Sedation is often necessary in mechanically ventilated patients to control anxiety, allow the patient to rest, and synchronize breathing. The need for paralysis is rare, except in patients with severe respiratory failure that benefit from increased pulmonary compliance due to decreased chest wall elastic recoil. If paralytics are necessary, they should be discontinued as soon as possible because long-term use is associated with paresis, which may last for weeks to months.

(8) Prone positioning is one of several techniques that may have benefit as "rescue" strategies in patients with severe acute lung injury or acute respiratory distress syndrome. Patients are placed in a prone position for a scheduled period of time on a daily basis; theoretical benefits include recruitment of dorsal lung units, improved mechanics, decreased ventilation–perfusion mismatch, and increased secretion drainage (*JAMA* 2005;294:2889). Although this therapy has been shown to benefit oxygenation, it has not been demonstrated to improve survival.

c. Complications

(1) ET tube dislodgment and patient self-extubation can produce a medical emergency characterized by life-threatening hypoxia and hypercarbia in those who are profoundly ill. For this reason, restraint of the patient's upper extremities is frequently required. If a patient does self-extubate, he or she should be closely observed because a surprising number of patients will be able to remain successfully extubated. If the patient shows any signs of respiratory distress, however, he or she should be immediately reintubated or placed on noninvasive ventilation, depending on the clinical scenario.

(2) ET tube cuff leaks should be suspected when there is an unexplained decrease in the returned expired volume associated with a fall in airway pressure. A cuff leak may indicate that the ET tube is at or partially above the vocal cords, and the tube may be advanced using a bronchoscope. A severe cuff leak should prompt change of the ET tube because there is increased risk of aspiration and decreased efficiency of ventilation.

(3) Respiratory distress may occur suddenly during mechanical ventilation due either to an acute change in the patient's status or to ventilator malfunction. The first priority is to disconnect the ventilator and switch to bag ventilation using 100% oxygen to ensure adequate ventilation and oxygenation. Increased airway pressures may indicate obstruction of the tube with secretions or a kink in the tube, bronchospasm, pneumothorax, or migration of the ET tube into a main-stem bronchus. Check the ET tube for patency and suction; if there is a partial obstruction, use large-volume saline lavage to clear the tube. If the obstruction is complete, remove the ET tube and reintubate the patient. Listen closely for any change in breath sounds consistent with a pneumothorax, new lung consolidation, or pleural fluid collection. A less common but important cause of respiratory distress is pulmonary embolism. **Check the ventilator's function** and, if it is normal, return the patient to the ventilator, making any needed changes in ventilator settings to ensure adequate ventilation and oxygenation. The results of an ABG and a chest x-ray are frequently helpful.

(4) Barotrauma from very high peak airway pressures (≥ 50 cm H_2O) can lead to subcutaneous emphysema, pneumomediastinum, and pneumothorax. Whereas subcutaneous emphysema and pneumomediastinum usually are benign, a pneumothorax that develops while a patient is on positive-pressure ventilation is at high risk for tension pneumothorax and is usually treated emergently with tube thoracostomy.

(5) Oxygen toxicity refers to levels of intra-alveolar oxygen high enough to cause lung damage. The precise mechanism is not known, but it probably involves oxidation of cell membranes and generation of toxic oxygen radicals. An FiO_2 of 0.40 or less is considered safe even for long periods. Although experimental data demonstrate that microscopic damage to alveoli occurs after only a few hours of an FiO_2 of 1 in animals, convincing studies in human patients are impossible to perform due to ethical consideration. It appears prudent, however, to keep the FiO_2 at less than 0.60 whenever possible, often using higher levels of PEEP (8 to 12 cm H_2O) to help reduce the FiO_2.

d. Weaning off mechanical ventilation. Although there are exceptions (e.g., immediate extubation of a healthy patient with normal lungs after general anesthesia), discontinuing mechanical ventilation may require weaning. In general, hemodynamic instability or high work of breathing (e.g., minute ventilation >15 L/minute) are contraindications to weaning. Reduction of the FiO_2 to 0.40 or less and of PEEP to 5 cm H_2O or less is accomplished first. The patient who has needed prolonged ventilatory support may require from several days to weeks to wean because of marginal respiratory muscle strength and the time required for the injured lungs to recover. The optimal strategy for weaning patients continues to be a topic of debate. The results of clinical trials indicate that the method of weaning from ventilator support is most likely of little consequence for patients who have been on mechanical ventilatory support for 2 weeks or less because the primary determinant of weaning success is simply resolution of the pathology that induced respiratory failure. At Washington University, patients are maintained on A/C ventilation with daily CPAP trials to assess their suitability for extubation. An acceptable alternative is to provide a high level of pressure support, which is decreased twice a day until the patient is ready for extubation. The presence of a weaning protocol decreases patient time on the ventilator compared with physician-directed weaning.

IV. CIRCULATORY FAILURE: SHOCK

A. Shock is defined by global tissue hypoxia; it occurs when either the supply of or the ability to use oxygen and other nutrients is insufficient to meet metabolic demands. Shock can be recognized functionally by hypotension. If left uncorrected, shock leads to the death of cells, tissues, organs, and, ultimately, the patient. Understanding the **pathophysiology of shock** depends on an appreciation of the relationship of blood pressure [specifically, mean arterial pressure (MAP)] to CO and systemic vascular resistance (SVR): MAP is directly proportional to CO and SVR. Because CO is equal to stroke volume times heart rate, and stroke volume is directly proportional to preload, afterload, and myocardial contractility, MAP is directly proportional to heart rate, preload, afterload, and contractility. Compensatory changes in response to systemic hypotension include the release of catecholamines, aldosterone, renin, and cortisol, which act in concert to increase heart rate, preload, afterload, and contractility.

B. Classification and recognition of shock (Table 7-3). The morbidity and mortality of circulatory shock are related not only to the underlying cause, but also to the depth and duration of circulatory compromise. Early recognition and prompt intervention are therefore critical.

| TABLE 7-3 | Clinical Parameters in Shock |

Shock classification	Skin	Jugular venous distention	Cardiac output	Pulmonary capillary wedge pressure	Systemic vascular resistance	Mixed venous oxygen content
Hypovolemic	Cool, pale	↓	↓	↓	↑	↓
Cardiogenic	Cool, pale	↑	↓	↑	↑	↓
Septic						
Early	Warm, pink	↑↓	↑	↓	↓	↑
Late	Cool, pale	↓	↓	↓	↑	↑↓
Neurogenic	Warm, pink	↓	↓	↓	↓	↓

1. **Hypovolemic shock** results from loss of circulating blood volume (usually at least 20%) caused by acute hemorrhage, fluid depletion, or dehydration; these three are frequently distinguishable from one another by history. These patients typically are peripherally vasoconstricted, tachycardic, and have low jugular venous pressure.

2. **Distributive shock** is characterized by a hyperdynamic state consisting of tachycardia, vasodilation (with decreased cardiac filling pressures), decreased SVR, and increased CO; however, some patients present with hypodynamic septic shock and have decreased CO and hypoperfusion. Patients with hyperdynamic distributive shock feel warm. The most common causes of distributive shock include sepsis, the systemic inflammatory response syndrome (SIRS), adrenal insufficiency, and liver failure.

3. **Obstructive shock** results from etiologies that prevent adequate CO but are not intrinsically cardiac in origin. This type of shock may be caused by pulmonary embolus, tension pneumothorax, or cardiac tamponade. Jugular venous pressure is often elevated in these patients.

4. **Cardiogenic shock** results from inadequate CO due to intrinsic cardiac failure (e.g., acute myocardial infarction, valvular stenosis, regurgitation or rupture, ischemia, arrhythmia, cardiomyopathy, or acute ventricular septal defect). These patients typically are peripherally vasoconstricted and tachycardic. Their jugular venous pressure typically is elevated.

5. **Neurogenic shock** results from interruption of the spinal cord at or above the thoracolumbar sympathetic nerve roots, which produces loss of sympathetic tone to the vascular system, causing vasodilation. The cardiovascular response is the same; patients are typically peripherally vasodilated (warm extremities) and tachycardic. Jugular venous pressure is usually low.

6. **Interventions common to all types of shock.** The goal of therapy is to ensure adequate delivery of oxygen to the peripheral tissues. Because oxygen delivery is the arithmetic product of arterial oxygen saturation (SaO_2), hemoglobin concentration, and CO, each of these parameters should be optimized.
   a. **SaO_2.** It is necessary to administer supplemental oxygen, secure or provide an adequate airway, and check for adequate bilateral ventilation. A pulse oximetry (SaO_2) level that exceeds 92% should allow adequate delivery of oxygen at the periphery; however, levels should be maximized in the acute setting.

b. **Hemoglobin concentration.** The hemoglobin concentration must be adequate to deliver oxygen to the tissues. One study indicated that for most critically ill patients, a transfusion trigger of 7 g/dL is appropriate, with the goal of keeping the hemoglobin concentration at 7 to 9 g/dL, except in patients with an ongoing myocardial infarction or severe ischemic cardiomyopathy (*N Engl J Med* 1999;340:409). An important caveat is early goal-directed therapy in septic patients with SvO$_2$ less than 70 and hemoglobin less than 10 (*N Engl J Med* 2001;345:1368).

c. **Cardiac output (CO).** The ECG tracing provides direct information about heart rate and several indirect clues about stroke volume. The atrial contraction provides approximately 25% of ordinary CO, so the atrioventricular dyssynchrony observed in atrial fibrillation or third-degree atrioventricular block causes impairment of CO. This is clinically relevant for patients who have decreased ejection fraction at baseline. Tachyarrhythmias decrease diastolic ventricular and coronary artery filling times. When it is severe (e.g., heart rate ~140 beats per minute), tachycardia predictably impairs preload, stroke volume, and CO. When treating tachycardia per se, it is imperative to distinguish between tachycardia as a compensatory response (e.g., sinus tachycardia secondary to hypovolemia) and tachycardia as a cause of shock (e.g., ventricular tachycardia). With the exception of the patient in pulmonary edema, *all* patients in circulatory shock should initially receive 10 to 20 mL/kg of a balanced salt solution, such as lactated Ringer's solution. The pace of volume infusion should reflect the depth of circulatory shock. To achieve rapid infusion rates, short, large-bore intravenous catheters (e.g., 14 or 16 gauge) in an antecubital vein are best. If this is not possible, an 8.5-French cordis (Swan-Ganz introducer) inserted into a central vein is effective. **A multilumen central line is NOT an effective access for rapid volume resuscitation.** The stopcocks should be removed from the venous lines to reduce flow resistance and deliver *warmed* fluids. Hypothermia is aggravated by rapid infusion of room-temperature crystalloid and refrigerated blood, impairing the ability to unload oxygen from hemoglobin in the periphery and compromising all enzymatic processes, especially coagulation.

d. To assess the adequacy of resuscitation, peripheral pulses and urine output should be evaluated. Palpable pedal pulses or urine output that exceeds 1 mL/kg per hour usually indicates a cardiac index of greater than 2 L/m^2 per minute. These two simple techniques can be used to estimate cardiac performance in many patients. Patients who do not improve with initial resuscitative measures may require invasive hemodynamic monitoring. All patients in shock should be monitored with an indwelling bladder catheter. Metabolic acidosis, identified by an ABG determination and serum electrolytes, can reflect the depth of circulatory compromise and the adequacy of resuscitation; however, this is not true in patients acidotic with preexisting renal failure. Infusion of sodium bicarbonate should be reserved for patients with a pH of less than 7.15 because the sodium bicarbonate may actually worsen intracellular pH as the bicarbonate is converted to CO$_2$ at the tissue level.

7. **Specific therapy**

a. **Hypovolemic shock.** Therapy focuses on control of ongoing volume loss and restoration of intravascular volume. External hemorrhage should be controlled by direct pressure. Internal hemorrhage may require further diagnostic tests and/or surgical intervention. The degree of volume deficit (Table 7-4) determines the type and volume of resuscitative fluid. Patients with blood losses of up to 20% of their circulating blood volume can be resuscitated using crystalloid solutions alone, typically lactated Ringer's solution. However, because salt solutions equilibrate with the interstitial space, volume replacement with these solutions alone requires three times the estimated volume deficit. Patients in whom diaphoresis, ashen facies, and hypotension develop have lost 30% or more of their blood volume and require urgent transfusion of blood. Individuals with severe dehydration often have profound metabolic

TABLE 7-4	Physiologic Changes in Hypovolemic Shock			
Blood loss (%)	<15	15–30	30–40	>40
Blood loss (mL)[a]	<750	750–1,500	1,500–2,000	>2,000
Heart rate (bpm)	Nl	>100	>120	>140
Blood pressure	Nl	SBP Nl	SBP↓	SBP↓↓
		DBP↑	DBP↓	DBP↓↓
Respiratory rate	Nl	↑	↑↑	↑↑↑
Urine output	Nl	↓	Oliguria	Anuria
Mental state	Minimal anxiety	Mild anxiety	Confusion	Lethargy

bpm, beats per minute; DBP, diastolic blood pressure; Nl, normal; SBP, systolic blood pressure.
[a]Based on a 70-kg male patient.

and electrolyte abnormalities. Fluid administration should be modified once laboratory analysis of serum electrolytes is completed. With adequate volume resuscitation, vasoconstrictors and vasoactive agents can usually be avoided.

b. Distributive shock

(1) Septic shock (see Section V.C).

(2) Adrenal insufficiency. The diagnosis and treatment of adrenal insufficiency in septic shock are evolving and controversial. There is a consensus that patients with primary adrenal insufficiency should be treated.

(3) SIRS may result from noninfectious causes of inflammation (e.g., necrotizing pancreatitis, burns). Treatment is supportive, with volume resuscitation, mechanical ventilation, and the administration of pressors as needed until the inflammatory process resolves.

c. Obstructive shock. Tension pneumo- or hemothoraces and pericardial tamponade require mechanical intervention. Tension pneumothorax is treated by needle decompression followed by tube thoracostomy. Hemothorax requires tube thoracostomy. Pericardial tamponade is treated by needle decompression, often with catheter placement for drainage. The treatment of pulmonary embolism varies based on the degree of hemodynamic compromise and must be individualized. Alternatives include systemic anticoagulation, thrombolysis, and surgical clot removal. Inferior vena cava (IVC) filters are used in patients who have a contraindication to systemic anticoagulation.

d. Cardiogenic shock. It is critical to distinguish shock caused by intrinsic myocardial dysfunction from extrinsic processes that interfere with venous return to the heart. Diagnosis may require echocardiography and cardiac catheterization. Management is directed toward maintaining adequate myocardial perfusion and CO with volume expansion and vasopressors, inotropes, or chronotropes (Table 7-5). Initial treatment is often guided by CVP measurements or, in severe cases, PA catheter data, while the precipitating cause of compromise is identified and treated. Mechanical support with intra-aortic balloon counterpulsation may be necessary before and during recovery from definitive surgical treatment (see Chapter 30).

e. Neurogenic shock. As with septic shock, the initial intervention in neurogenic shock is volume infusion. A peripheral vasoconstrictor, such as phenylephrine or norepinephrine, is administered centrally to increase vascular tone if hypotension is refractory to volume infusion alone. Dopamine is useful in patients with neurogenic shock and bradycardia. Because patients with spinal shock tend to equilibrate body temperature with their environment, fluids and ambient room temperature must be kept warm.

V. SEPSIS

A. Definition. Sepsis is defined as SIRS resulting from infection. There is a consensus clinical definition of SIRS: body temperature greater than 38°C or less than 36°C,

TABLE 7-5 Vasoactive Drugs and Their Specific Actions

Class and drug	Blood pressure	Systemic vascular resistance	Cardiac output	Heart rate	Inotrope Low-dose	Inotrope High-dose	Renal blood flow	Coronary blood flow	Mvo₂
Alpha only									
Phenylephrine	↑↑	↑↑↑↑	↓	↓	±	±	↓↓↓	± ↑↑	↑
Alpha and beta									
Norepinephrine	↑↑↑	↑↑↑↑	↑↑↑	± ↓	↑	↑	↓↓↓	↑↑	↑↑
Epinephrine	↑↑↑	↑↑↑↑	↑↑↑↑	↑↑↑	↑↑	↑↑↑	↓ ±	↑↑	↑↑↑
Dopamine	↑↑	↑↑	↑↑↑	↑↑	±	↑↑	↑↑↑	↑↑	↑↑
Beta only									
Dobutamine	±	↓↓↓	↑↑↑↑	↑↑	↑↑↑	↑↑↑	±	↑↑↑	↑↑↑
Beta-blocker									
Metoprolol	↓	↓	↓↓	↓↓↓	↓↓	↓↓↓	±	↓	↓
Other									
Nitroglycerine	± ↓	↓↓	↑↑	±	±	±	± ↑	↓	↓↓
Hydralazine	↓↓	↓↓↓	↑↑	↑↑	±	±	± ↑	↓	↓↓
Nitroprusside	↓↓↓	↓↓↓	↑↑↑	± ↑	±	±	↑↑	±	↓↓

Mvo₂, mixed venous oxygen saturation.

heart rate greater than 90 beats/minute, respiratory rate greater than 20/minute or PaCO$_2$ less than 32, and white blood cell count (WBC) greater than 12 or less than 4 or greater than 10% bands. Severe sepsis is multiple-organ dysfunction or hypoperfusion resulting from infection.

B. Diagnosis

    1. Appropriate cultures should be obtained as part of the initial evaluation. Two or more blood cultures are recommended, one of which should be drawn percutaneously.

    2. Additional radiologic imaging and diagnostic procedures should be performed as warranted.

C. Treatment

    1. Addressing the infection

        a. Antibiotic therapy

            (1) Broad-spectrum intravenous antibiotics should be initiated within the first hour after obtaining appropriate cultures. Failure to do so results in significantly increased mortality from severe sepsis (*Chest* 2000;118:146). The use of antifungal therapies and agents directed at highly resistant Gram-negative rods, methacillin-resistant *Staphylococcus aureus*, vancomycin-resistant enterococcus, and resistant pneumococcus should be guided by the clinical situation and local patterns of susceptibility.

                (a) The following increase a patient's risk for infection with resistant organisms:

                    (i) Prior treatment with antibiotics during the hospitalization.

                    (ii) Prolonged hospitalization.

                    (iii) Presence of invasive devices.

            (2) For pneumonias, the initial broad-spectrum antibiotic coverage should be narrowed to focus on the causative organism(s) identified on culture. For intra-abdominal infections, therapies remain broadly directed at the range of intra-abdominal organisms.

        b. Source control: drainage, débridement, or removal of the infectious source as appropriate, through surgical or other means.

    2. Circulatory support

        a. Early goal-directed therapy involves adjustments of cardiac preload, afterload, and contractility to balance oxygen delivery with oxygen demand before the patient even arrives in the ICU. A recent study demonstrated a hospital mortality of 30.5% for patients treated with early goal-directed therapy compared with 46.5% for patients treated with standard therapy (*N Engl J Med* 2001;345:1368).

        b. In the first 6 hours, the goals of resuscitation are as follows (*Intensive Care Med* 2004;30:536):

            (1) CVP 8 to 12 mm Hg.

            (2) MAP at least 65 mm Hg.

            (3) Urine output at least 0.5 mg/kg/hour.

            (4) Mixed venous saturation at least 70%.

        c. Vasoactive medications. To maintain CO, heart rate usually is increased. Septic patients who fail to achieve rapid hemodynamic stability with fluids and small doses of vasoconstrictors often undergo insertion of a PA catheter to optimize cardiac performance. Because PA catheters have not been demonstrated to improve outcome in either high-risk surgical patients or ARDS patients, placing this form of invasive monitoring should not be automatic but should be decided on an individual basis. If a PA catheter is placed, higher filling pressures are typically needed (pulmonary capillary wedge pressure of 14 to 18 mm Hg) to optimize performance in the dilated, septic heart.

            (1) Dopamine and levophed are both commonly used; however, phenylephrine is not beneficial in the setting of sepsis.

            (2) Circulatory concentrations of **vasopressin** increase initially, then decrease (*Crit Care Med* 2003;31:1752), and they are lower in septic shock than in cardiogenic shock. Low-dose vasopressin increases MAP, SVR, and urine output in septic patients who are hyporesponsive to catecholamines. This may spare patients from high-dose vasopressor requirements, although its impact on survival is unclear.

3. **Adjunctive treatments**

   a. **Activated protein C** has recently been demonstrated to reduce mortality in a large-scale prospective, randomized trial (*N Engl J Med* 2001;344:699–709). Although this drug clearly improves survival in patients with severe sepsis and has a very short half-life, it is associated with an increase in serious bleeding and must be used with caution in patients in the immediate postoperative setting. Activated protein C can be started 12 hours after an operative procedure and should be held for approximately 1 hour before and after minor interventions such as central venous catheter placement. Of note, activated protein C is approved for use in patients with Acute Physiology and Chronic Health Evaluation (APACHE) II scores of greater than 25 and has not been documented to help patients with less severe forms of sepsis.

VI. **UPPER GASTROINTESTINAL HEMORRHAGE PROPHYLAXIS.** Patients in the ICU are at increased risk for stress-induced mucosal ulceration and resultant GI hemorrhage. Risk factors include head injury (Cushing ulcers); burns (Curling ulcers); requirement for mechanical ventilation; previous history of peptic ulcer disease; use of nonsteroidal anti-inflammatory drugs or steroids; and the presence of shock, renal failure, portal hypertension, or coagulopathy. Strong data exist to support the use of drugs to maintain mucosal integrity in these patients at increased risk. In an evidence-based review of discordant meta-analyses, H_2-receptor antagonists (cimetidine, ranitidine, famotidine) were found to reduce significantly the incidence of clinically important GI bleeding in critically ill patients. Proton-pump inhibitors are useful in patients who bleed despite being on appropriate H_2-receptor antagonists, but they should not be used as first-line agents for GI prophylaxis in the ICU.

VII. **RENAL DYSFUNCTION**

A. **Etiology and diagnosis.** Renal dysfunction commonly presents as progressive oliguria in the setting of increased renal function indices [blood urea nitrogen (BUN) and serum creatinine]. This can progress to renal failure and anuria (urine output <100 mL/day), which require renal replacement therapy (approximately 5% of all ICU admissions). Renal insufficiency can also present as polyuria when decreased renal tubular function (fluid resorption) is not coupled with decreased glomerular filtration ("high-output" renal failure). Traditionally, the etiology of renal dysfunction has been divided into prerenal, intrarenal, and postrenal causes. A careful history and a review of the medical record are critical to making the correct diagnosis.

   1. **Prerenal.** The glomerular and tubular function of the kidneys is normal, but clearance is limited as a result of decreased renal blood flow. This is the most common cause of renal insufficiency in the surgical ICU, and it is usually the result of inadequate volume resuscitation. The rise in the BUN typically is greater than that of the serum creatinine (BUN/creatinine ratio >20). The concentrating ability of the kidneys is normal, and thus the urine osmolality (>500 mOsm) and the fractional excretion of sodium (FE_{Na} <1) are normal.

      a. **Abdominal compartment syndrome** results from massive tissue (bowel) edema within the abdominal compartment or retroperitoneal hemorrhage, frequently although not exclusively as a complication of severe trauma and massive resuscitation. Increased intra-abdominal pressure decreases renal perfusion and retards renal venous and urinary outflow, inducing renal injury by a combination of pre-, intra-, and postrenal insults. Assessment of urinary bladder pressure via a Foley catheter serves as an indirect but accurate measure of intra-abdominal pressure (*J Trauma* 1998;45:597). An acute increase in pressure greater than 25 cm H_2O demands intervention and typically surgical exploration (convert mm Hg to cm H_2O by multiplying mm Hg by 1.3).

   2. **Intrarenal.** Tubular injury is most often caused by ischemia or toxins. Nephrotoxins commonly encountered by ICU patients include aminoglycosides,

intravenous radiocontrast agents, amphotericin, and chemotherapeutic drugs. Patients with preexisting renal disease or diabetes are particularly susceptible. Intravenous hydration before and during the administration of nephrotoxins should be used to decrease the incidence of renal insufficiency in patients at risk. The concentrating ability of the tubules is compromised, so the urine osmolality is low (<350 mOsm) and the FE_{Na} is greater than 1. Urinalysis and microscopic analysis of the urinary sediment may yield additional information about tubular pathology.

    a. ***N*-Acetylcysteine,** an antioxidant, has recently been shown to prevent nephrotoxicity induced by intravenous dye (*N Engl J Med* 2000;343:180, *Am J Kidney Dis* 2004;43:1).

    b. A prospective, single-center, randomized trial demonstrated that hydration with sodium bicarbonate is more effective than hydration with sodium chloride for prophylaxis of contrast-induced renal failure. The protocol was an infusion of 3 mL/kg per hour of 154 mEq/L of sodium bicarbonate in dextrose and water for the hour prior to contrast exposure, then 1 mL/kg per hour during the exposure and for 6 hours after (*JAMA* 2004;291:2328).

  3. Postrenal. Bilateral obstruction of urinary flow can be caused by direct intraoperative injury or manipulation, prostatic hypertrophy, coagulated blood, or extrinsic compression (e.g., tumors). Urinary catheter malfunction must always be ruled out, typically by flushing the catheter with sterile saline. Ultrasound examination of the urinary system is used to rule out hydronephrosis.

B. Treatment

  1. Supportive measures. Initial therapy should be directed at minimizing ongoing renal injury by optimizing renal perfusion and discontinuing potentially nephrotoxic agents. Optimization of renal perfusion is usually accomplished by judicious volume resuscitation. If fluid resuscitation does not improve low urine output (<0.5 mL/kg per hour), measurement of CVP or pulmonary capillary wedge pressure can be used to guide fluid resuscitation and optimization of CO. Low-dose dopamine does not change progression to renal failure nor does it change mortality. **There is no role for "renal dose" dopamine in the ICU** (*Lancet* 2000;356:2139). The doses or medications to be eliminated by the kidney should be adjusted for the degree of renal insufficiency. Refer to Chapter 4 for the treatment of the electrolyte (hyperkalemia) and acid-base disorders (metabolic acidosis) that accompany renal failure.

  2. Renal replacement therapy. Indications include complications of renal dysfunction that fail medical management, including hypervolemia, severe acidemia, refractory hyperkalemia, and uremia (pericarditis or encephalopathy). Decisions about when and how to initiate renal replacement therapy are the subject of controversy and ongoing clinical trials.

    a. Intermittent. Because peritoneal dialysis is usually impractical in the surgical ICU, intermittent hemodialysis is the method of choice. Some hemodynamic impairment will ensue as a result of rapid, large shifts of fluid from the intravascular compartment through the dialysis filter. In healthy patients, this is usually well tolerated. However, hemodynamic deterioration (hypotension or dysrhythmias) can be induced in unstable patients due to decreased myocardial preload.

    b. Continuous venovenous hemodialysis (CVVHD) (*N Engl J Med* 1997; 336:1303) is used in patients with preexisting hemodynamic instability, usually in the setting of shock. CVVHD decreases the rate of fluid shifts and thus has less risk of hemodynamic compromise relative to HD. The disadvantage of this type of dialysis is that CVVHD requires constant systemic anticoagulation to prevent clotting of blood in the filter and continuous sophisticated nursing surveillance.

VIII. ANEMIA. It is not uncommon for patients in the ICU to receive multiple units of packed red blood cells during their critical illness. Concerns have arisen regarding morbidity from transfusion, most likely related to immunosuppression, and **transfusing all patients to a hemoglobin of 10 mg/dL either has no effect or may actually decrease survival in the critically ill** (*N Engl J Med* 1999;340:409). According to a recent

TABLE 7-6 Drugs Commonly Used in the Intensive Care Unit

Drug	Dilution (concentration)	Loading dose	Initial maintenance dose	Comments
Diltiazem	125 mg/125 mL 0.9% NaCl or D5W (1 mg/mL)	0.25 mg/kg (followed by 0.35 mg/kg if needed)	5–10 mg/hr (max 15 mg/hr)	May cause hypotension
Dobutamine	250 mg/100 mL 0.9% NaCl (2,500 μg/mL)		2 μg/kg/min (max 20 μg/kg/min)	Selective inotropic (beta) effect; may cause tachycardia and arrhythmias
Dopamine	400 mg/250 mL 0.9% NaCl or D5W (1,600 μg/mL)		Dopa, 1–3 μg/kg/min; alpha, 3–10 μg/kg/min; beta, 10–20 μg/kg/min	Clinical response is dose and patient dependent; may cause arrhythmias and tachycardia
Epinephrine	5 mg/500 mL 0.9% NaCl or D5W, or 4 mg/100 mL 0.9% NaCl or D5W		14 μg/min	Mixed alpha and beta effects; use central line; may cause tachycardia and hypotension
Esmolol	2.5 g/250 mL 0.9% NaCl or D5W (10 mg/mL)	500 μg/kg/min for 1 min (optional)	50 μg/kg/min (max 300 μg/kg/min)	Selective beta1-blocker; T1/2 9 min; not eliminated by hepatic or renal routes; may cause hypotension
Heparin	25,000 units/250 mL 0.45% NaCl (100 units/mL)	60 units/kg	14 units/kg/hr	Obtain PTT every 4–6 hr until PTT is 1.5–2 times control; may cause thrombocytopenia

Drug	Preparation	Dose	Notes
Lidocaine	2 g/500 mL D5W (4 mg/mL)	1 mg/kg (can repeat 2 times if needed)	Dose should be decreased in patients with hepatic failure, acute MI, CHF, or shock
Nitroglycerin	50 mg/250 mL D5W (200 μg/mL)	5–20 μg/min	Use cautiously in right-sided MI
Nitroprusside	50 mg/250 mL D5W (200 μg/mL)	0.25–0.50 μg/kg/min (max 10 μg/kg/min)	Signs of toxicity include metabolic acidosis, tremors, seizures, and coma; thiocyanate may accumulate in renal failure
Norepinephrine	8 mg/500 mL D5W (16 μg/mL)	2–10 μg/min	Potent alpha effects; mainly beta1 effects at lower doses; use central line
Phenylephrine	10 mg/250 mL 0.9% NaCl or D5W (40 μg/mL)	10–100 μg/min	Pure alpha effects; use central line; may cause reflex bradycardia and decreased cardiac output
Vasopressin	20 units/100 mL NS (0.2 units/mL)	0.04 units/min per infusion	Do not titrate; higher doses may cause myocardial ischemia.

CHF, congestive heart failure; D5W, 5% dextrose in water; max, maximum; MI, myocardial infarction; PTT, partial thromboplastin time; QTc, electrocardiographic QT interval; T1/2, terminal half-life.

report, patients started on recombinant erythropoietin on day 3 of ICU hospitalization were significantly less likely to undergo transfusion (*JAMA* 2002;288:2827), although whether this affects patient outcomes is unclear.

IX. BLOOD GLUCOSE CONTROL. A recent study of 1,548 surgical patients randomly assigned to tight glucose control with intensive insulin therapy (blood glucose between 80 and 110 mg/dL) versus conventional control (blood glucose between 180 and 200 mg/dL and treatment only above 215 mg/dL) showed nearly a twofold decrease in mortality in the tight-glucose-control group. Intensive insulin therapy also reduced overall in-hospital mortality, bloodstream infections, acute renal failure, the median number of red cell transfusions, and critical illness polyneuropathy *(N Engl J Med* 2001;345:1359). However, a follow-up study in medical patients did not demonstrate a benefit (*N Engl J Med* 2006;354:449). A goal blood sugar of less than 140 mg/dL seems safe and beneficial; further study will be required to determine the response of different patient populations to varying intensities of insulin therapy.

X. COMMONLY USED DRUGS. Table 7-6 lists commonly used ICU drugs and their doses.

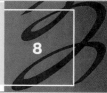

ESOPHAGUS

Rishindra M. Reddy and Bryan F. Meyers

8

STRUCTURAL AND FUNCTIONAL DISORDERS OF THE ESOPHAGUS

I. HIATAL HERNIA. The distal esophagus normally is held in position by the *phrenoesophageal membrane,* a fusion of the endothoracic and endoabdominal fasciae at the diaphragmatic hiatus. A hiatal hernia is present when a lax or defective phrenoesophageal membrane allows protrusion of the stomach up through the esophageal hiatus of the diaphragm.

A. Epidemiology. Hiatal hernia is the most common abnormality reported in upper gastrointestinal (GI) radiographic studies. An estimated 10% of the adult population in the United States has a hiatal hernia. The condition occurs most commonly in women in their fifth and sixth decades. Most hiatal hernias are asymptomatic; however, an estimated 5% of patients with a hiatal hernia have symptoms related to persistent gastroesophageal reflux (GER) disease.

B. The **type of hiatal hernia** is defined by the location of the gastroesophageal (GE) junction and the relationship of the stomach to the distal esophagus.

  1. In **type I** or **sliding** hiatal hernia, the phrenoesophageal membrane is intact but lax, thereby allowing the distal esophagus and gastric cardia to herniate through the esophageal hiatus and placing the GE junction above the diaphragm. This is the most common type and is usually asymptomatic.

  2. A **type II** or **paraesophageal** hiatal hernia occurs when a focal defect is present in the phrenoesophageal membrane, usually anterior and lateral to the esophagus, which allows a protrusion of peritoneum to herniate upward alongside the esophagus. The GE junction remains anchored within the abdomen, whereas the greater curvature of the stomach rolls up into the chest alongside the distal esophagus. Eventually, most of the stomach can herniate. Because the stomach is anchored at the pylorus and cardia, however, the body of the stomach undergoes a 180-degree organoaxial rotation, resulting in an upside-down intrathoracic stomach when it is herniated.

  3. **Type III** represents a **combination** of types I and II. This type is more common than a pure type II and is characterized by herniation of the greater curvature of the stomach and the GE junction into the chest.

  4. A **type IV** hiatal hernia occurs when abdominal organs other than or in addition to the stomach herniate through the hiatus. Typically, these hernias are large and contain colon or spleen in addition to the stomach within the chest.

C. Symptoms and complications in patients with **sliding (type I)** hiatal hernias are related to GE reflux (GER; see Section II). **Paraesophageal and combined (types II, III, and IV) hernias** frequently produce postprandial pain or bloating, early satiety, breathlessness with meals, and mild dysphagia related to compression of the distal esophagus by the adjacent herniated stomach. The herniated gastric pouch is susceptible to volvulus, obstruction, and infarction and can develop ischemic longitudinal ulcers (termed *Cameron ulcers*) with frank or occult bleeding.

D. Diagnosis and evaluation

  1. Chest x-ray. The finding of an air-fluid level in the posterior mediastinum on the lateral x-ray suggests the presence of a hiatal hernia. Differential diagnosis includes mediastinal cyst, abscess, or a dilated obstructed esophagus (as is seen in end-stage achalasia).

2. A **barium swallow** confirms the diagnosis and defines any coexisting esophageal abnormalities, including strictures or ulcers. It is the diagnostic study of choice. The positions of the GE junction and proximal stomach define the type of hiatal hernia.

3. **Esophagogastroduodenoscopy (EGD)** is indicated in patients with symptoms of reflux or dysphagia to determine the degree of esophagitis and whether a stricture, Barrett esophagus, or a coexisting abnormality is present. EGD also establishes the location of the GE junction in relation to the hiatus. A sliding hiatal hernia is present when greater than 2 cm of gastric mucosa is present between the diaphragmatic hiatus and the mucosal squamocolumnar junction.

4. **Esophageal manometry** to evaluate esophageal motility is warranted in patients who are being considered for operative repair.

E. **Management**

1. **Asymptomatic sliding hernias** require no treatment.

2. Patients with **sliding hernias** and **GER** with mild **esophagitis** should undergo an initial trial of medical management.

3. Patients who **fail** to obtain symptomatic relief with **medical therapy** or who have severe esophagitis should undergo esophageal testing to determine their suitability for an **antireflux procedure** (see Section II) **and hiatal hernia repair.**

4. Patients who do not experience reflux but have symptoms related to their hernia **(chest pain, intermittent dysphagia, or esophageal obstruction)** should undergo hiatal hernia repair.

5. All patients who are found to have a **type II, III, or IV hiatal hernia** and who are operative candidates should be **considered for repair.** The management of asymptomatic paraesophageal hernias is a controversial issue. Some surgeons believe that all paraesophageal hernias should be corrected electively, irrespective of symptoms, to prevent the development of complications. However, recent data suggest that observation of the asymptomatic patient, especially for those older than 65 years, may be the safest course (*Ann Surg* 2002;236:492). Operative repair, which can be performed using either an abdominal or thoracic approach, consists in reduction of the hernia, resection of the sac, and closure of the hiatal defect. In type III hiatal hernias, the esophagus frequently is shortened, and thus a thoracic approach may be preferred.

6. **Paraesophageal hiatal hernias** are associated with a 60% incidence of GER. Furthermore, the operative dissection may lead to postoperative GER in previously asymptomatic patients. Therefore, an antireflux procedure should be performed at the time of hiatal hernia repair. A recent prospective, randomized trial showed that the addition of a biologic mesh to reinforce the crural repair resulted in a decreased recurrence at 6 months (*Ann Surg* 2006;244:481).

II. **GASTROESOPHAGEAL REFLUX**

A. **Prevalence.** GER is a normal event after a meal and during belching. Symptoms of heartburn and excessive regurgitation are relatively common in the United States, occurring in approximately 7% of the population on a daily basis and in 33% at least once a month. Often, these individuals have x-ray evidence of a hiatal hernia. Reflux and hiatal hernia are not necessarily related, and each can occur independently.

B. **Pathophysiology** in GER relates to abnormal exposure of the distal esophagus to refluxed stomach contents. In 60% of patients, a mechanically defective lower-esophageal sphincter (LES) is responsible for the GER. The sphincter function of the LES depends on the integrated mechanical effect of the sphincter's intramural pressure and the length of esophagus exposed to intra-abdominal positive pressure. Other etiologies of GER are inefficient esophageal clearance of refluxed material, fixed gastric outlet obstruction, functional delayed gastric emptying, increased gastric acid secretion, and inappropriate relaxation of the LES.

C. The classic **symptom** of GER is posturally aggravated substernal or epigastric burning pain that is readily relieved by antacids. Additional common symptoms include regurgitation or effortless emesis, dysphagia, and excessive flatulence. Atypical symptoms may mimic laryngeal, respiratory, cardiac, biliary, pancreatic, gastric, or duodenal disease.

D. Diagnosis and evaluation

1. **Contrast radiography (upper GI)** demonstrates spontaneous reflux in only approximately 40% of patients with GER. However, it documents the presence or absence of hiatal hernia; can demonstrate some complications of reflux, such as esophageal stricture and ulcers; and is an appropriate initial study. The study should include a full view of the esophagus as well as a complete evaluation of the stomach, pylorus, and duodenum.

2. **EGD** is indicated in patients with symptoms of GER to evaluate for esophagitis and the presence of Barrett changes. **Esophagitis** is a pathologic diagnosis, but an experienced endoscopist can readily distinguish the more advanced stages. Four general grades of esophagitis occur.

   a. **Grade I:** normal or reddened mucosa

   b. **Grade II:** superficial mucosal erosions and some ulcerations

   c. **Grade III:** extensive ulceration with multiple, circumferential erosions with luminal narrowing; possible edematous islands of squamous mucosa present, producing the so-called cobblestone esophagitis

   d. **Grade IV:** fibrotic peptic stricture, shortened esophagus, columnar-lined esophagus

3. **Esophageal manometric testing** is appropriate in the patient with reflux symptoms once surgery is being considered. Manometry defines the location and function of the LES and helps to exclude achalasia, scleroderma, and diffuse esophageal spasm from the differential diagnosis. Characteristics of a manometrically abnormal LES are (1) a pressure of less than 6 mm Hg, (2) an overall length of less than 2 cm, and (3) an abdominal length of less than 1 cm. These values are abnormal, and a patient with one or more of these abnormal values has a 90% probability of having reflux. Manometry also assesses the adequacy of esophageal contractility and peristaltic wave progression as a guide to the best antireflux procedure for the patient.

4. **Esophageal pH testing** over a 24-hour period is regarded as the gold standard in the diagnosis of GER. It is now used mainly when the data from the remainder of the evaluation are equivocal and diagnosis of reflux is in doubt. Twenty-four-hour pH testing can be performed on an outpatient or ambulatory basis: The patient has an event button to record symptoms and keeps a diary of body position, timing of meals, and other activities. This allows correlation of symptoms with simultaneous esophageal pH alterations. A **Demeester score** is derived based on the frequency of reflux episodes and the time required for the esophagus to clear the acid. Score values that fall outside of two standard deviations from the mean of values obtained from normal volunteers are considered abnormal. This test has a 90% sensitivity and a 90% specificity for diagnosing or excluding reflux (*J Thorac Cardiovasc Surg* 1980;79:656).

5. A **gastric emptying study** can be useful in evaluating patients with reflux and symptoms of gastroparesis. It may be especially pertinent in patients considered for redo surgery when there is suspicion of vagus nerve injury.

E. Complications. Approximately 20% of patients with GER have complications, including esophagitis, stricture, or Barrett esophagus. Other, less common complications include acute or chronic bleeding and aspiration.

F. Treatment

1. **Medical treatment** aims to reduce the duration and amount of esophageal exposure to gastric contents and to minimize the effects on the esophageal mucosa.

   a. Patients are instructed to remain upright after meals, avoid postural maneuvers (bending, straining) that aggravate reflux, and sleep with the head of the bed elevated 6 to 8 inches.

   b. **Dietary alterations** are aimed at maximizing LES pressure, minimizing intragastric pressure, and decreasing stomach acidity. Patients are instructed to avoid fatty foods, alcohol, caffeine, chocolate, peppermint, and smoking and to eat smaller, more frequent meals. Obese patients are instructed to lose weight, avoid tight-fitting garments, and begin a regular exercise program. In addition, anticholinergics, calcium channel blockers, nitrates, beta-blockers, theophylline, alpha-blockers, and nonsteroidal anti-inflammatory medications may exacerbate reflux and should be replaced with other preparations or reduced in dose if possible.

c. Pharmacologic therapy is indicated in patients who do not improve with postural or dietary measures. The goal is to lower gastric acidity or enhance esophageal and gastric clearing while increasing the LES resting pressure.

(1) **Antacids** neutralize stomach acidity and thus raise intragastric pH.

(2) **H_2-receptor antagonists** lower gastric acidity by decreasing the amount of acid that the stomach produces.

(3) **Proton-pump inhibitors** act by selective noncompetitive inhibition of the H^+/K^+ pump on the parietal cell and are more effective than H_2 antagonists in healing esophagitis (*Aliment Pharmacol Ther* 1990;4:145).

(4) **Prokinetic agents,** such as metoclopramide (dopaminergic antagonist), can decrease GER by increasing the LES tone and accelerating esophageal and gastric clearance.

d. Transoral endoscopic suturing to plicate the gastroesophageal junction and endoscopic application of **radiofrequency energy** (Stretta procedure) to the lower esophagus are two novel endoluminal therapies that can be performed on an ambulatory basis and generally with the patient under light sedation. These therapies, approved by the Food and Drug Administration, have been evaluated in several small, non–placebo-controlled trials with limited posttreatment evaluation. Evidence of dysphagia, stricture, large hiatal hernia, and moderate to severe esophagitis generally has excluded patients from eligibility for inclusion in these two endoluminal trials. Other treatments being developed include injection of biocompatible prostheses into the LES to alter compliance. These options remain experimental and controversial.

2. Surgical treatment should be considered in patients who have symptomatic reflux, have manometric evidence of a defective LES, and fail to achieve relief with maximal medical management. Alternatively, surgical therapy should be considered in symptomatic patients who have achieved relief with medical therapy but to whom the prospect of a lifetime of medicine is undesirable (i.e., because of cost, side effects, inconvenience, or compliance). Surgical treatment consists of either a transabdominal or a transthoracic antireflux operation to reconstruct a competent LES and a crural repair to maintain the reconstruction in the abdomen.

a. A laparoscopic, transabdominal approach is preferred in most patients, except when a shortened esophagus is present. A shortened esophagus should be suspected when a stricture is present and in patients who have had a failed antireflux procedure. The transabdominal approach is recommended for patients with a coexisting abdominal disorder, a prior thoracotomy, or severe respiratory disorder.

(1) **Nissen fundoplication** is the most commonly performed procedure for GER. It consists of a 360-degree fundic wrap via open or laparoscopic technique. Long-term results in several series of open procedures are excellent, with 10-year freedom from recurrence of greater than 90%. Short-term results of the laparoscopic approach are as good as the open-repair results for relief of GER symptoms, with concomitant shorter hospital stay, better respiratory function, and decreased pain postoperatively (*Br J Surg* 2000;87:873). The complete fundoplication in this repair is very effective at preventing reflux but is associated with a slightly higher incidence of inability to vomit, gas bloating of the stomach, and dysphagia. During surgery, care must be taken to ensure that the wrap is short, loose, and placed appropriately around the distal esophagus to minimize the incidence of these complications.

(2) The **Hill posterior gastropexy** aims to anchor the GE junction posteriorly to the median arcuate ligament and creates a partial or 180-degree imbrication of the stomach around the right side of the intra-abdominal esophagus. In the original description, Hill recommended using intraesophageal manometry during placement of the sutures to achieve a pressure of 50 mm Hg in the distal esophagus.

(3) The **Toupet fundoplication** is a partial 270-degree posterior wrap, with the wrapped segment sutured to the crural margins and to the anterolateral esophageal wall. For patients in whom esophageal peristalsis is documented to be markedly abnormal or absent preoperatively, a partial wrap has often been used to lessen the potential for postoperative dysphagia.

b. A **transthoracic approach** is recommended in patients with esophageal shortening or stricture, coexistent motor disorder, obesity, coexistent pulmonary lesion, or prior antireflux repair.

(1) **Nissen fundoplication** can be done via a transthoracic approach, with results similar to those obtained with a transabdominal approach.

(2) The **Belsey Mark IV repair** consists of a 240-degree fundic wrap around 4 cm of distal esophagus. In cases of esophageal neuromotor dysfunction, it produces less dysphagia than may accompany a 360-degree (Nissen) wrap. Furthermore, the ability to belch is preserved, thereby avoiding the gas-bloat syndrome that may occur after a complete wrap. Careful 10-year follow-up demonstrates a good long-term result in 85% of patients (*J Thorac Cardiovasc Surg* 1967;53:33).

(3) **Collis gastroplasty** is a technique used to lengthen a shortened esophagus. To minimize tension on the antireflux repair, a gastric tube is formed from the upper lesser curvature of the stomach in continuity with the distal esophagus. The antireflux repair then is constructed around the gastroplasty tube. A gastroplasty should be considered preoperatively in patients with esophageal shortening, such as those with gross ulcerative esophagitis or stricture, failed prior antireflux procedure, or total intrathoracic stomach (*Ann Surg* 1987;206:473). However, in many of these patients, the esophagus can be adequately mobilized to allow more than 3 cm of intra-abdominal esophagus and thereby avoid the need to lengthen the esophagus. Development of an angled endoscopic stapler has made laparoscopic Collis gastroplasty technically feasible.

III. FUNCTIONAL ESOPHAGEAL DISORDERS comprise a diverse group of disorders involving esophageal skeletal or smooth muscle.

A. Motor disorders of esophageal skeletal muscle result in defective swallowing and aspiration. Potential causes can be classified into five major subgroups: neurogenic, myogenic, structural, iatrogenic, and mechanical. Most causes of oropharyngeal dysphagia are not correctable surgically. However, when manometric studies demonstrate that pharyngeal contractions, although weak, are still reasonably well coordinated, cricopharyngeal myotomy can provide relief.

B. Motor disorders of esophageal smooth muscle can be subdivided into primary dysmotilities and disorders that involve the esophagus secondarily and produce dysmotility.

1. Primary dysmotility

a. Achalasia is rare (1/100,000 population) but is the most common primary esophageal motility disorder. It typically presents between the ages of 35 and 45 years. Chagas disease, caused by *Trypanosoma cruzi* and seen primarily in South America, can mimic achalasia and produce similar esophageal pathology. Achalasia is a disease of unknown etiology, characterized by loss of effective esophageal body peristalsis and failure of the LES to relax with swallowing, resulting in esophageal dilatation. LES pressure is often (but not invariably) elevated. The characteristic pathology is alteration in the ganglia of Auerbach plexus.

(1) Symptoms include progressive dysphagia, noted by essentially all patients; regurgitation immediately after meals (>70%); odynophagia (30%); and aspiration, with resultant bronchitis and pneumonia (10%). Some patients experience chest pain due to esophageal spasms.

(2) The **diagnosis** is suggested by a chest x-ray, which often shows a fluid-filled, dilated esophagus and absence of a gastric air bubble. A **barium esophagogram** demonstrates tapering ("bird's beak") of the distal esophagus and a dilated proximal esophagus. The bird's-beak deformity is not specific for achalasia and can be seen in any process that narrows the distal esophagus (e.g., benign strictures or carcinoma). **Esophageal manometry** is the definitive diagnostic test for achalasia. Characteristic manometric findings include the absence of peristalsis, mirror-image contractions, and limited or absent relaxation of the LES with swallowing. Endoscopy should be performed to rule out benign strictures or malignancy, so-called pseudoachalasia.

(3) **Medical treatment** is aimed at decreasing the LES tone and includes nitrates, calcium channel blockers, and endoscopic injection of botulinum toxin (blocks acetylcholine release from nerve terminals) in the area of the LES.

(4) **Surgical treatment** with a **modified Heller esophagomyotomy** has been shown to produce excellent results in 95% of patients, compared with only 65% achieving excellent results using forceful **pneumatic bougienage** (*Gut* 1989;30:299). Many esophageal surgeons favor extending the myotomy onto the stomach and a concomitant antireflux procedure with the esophagomyotomy to avoid the two major causes of operative failure: (1) an incomplete myotomy due to inadequate mobilization of the esophagogastric junction and (2) late stricture due to GER disease caused by the incompetent LES combined with the inability of the aperistaltic esophagus to evacuate refluxed material. **Video-assisted thoracoscopic approaches** have been tried, with early results showing a higher incidence of postoperative GER than with the open procedure (*Ann Thorac Surg* 1993;56:680). More recently, **laparoscopic esophagomyotomy** combined with a partial fundoplication has been reported, and it is rapidly being adopted by most centers as the primary surgical option (*Surg Endosc* 2000;14:746).

b. *Vigorous achalasia* is a term used to describe a variant of achalasia in which patients present with the clinical and manometric features of classic achalasia and diffuse esophageal spasm. These patients have spastic pain and severe dysphagia, likely because of residual disordered peristalsis ineffective in overcoming the nonrelaxed LES. Treatment is the same as for classic achalasia, except that consideration should be given to performing a longer esophagomyotomy (to the aortic arch). With relief of the obstruction caused by the nonrelaxing LES, the pain usually disappears.

c. **Diffuse esophageal spasm** is characterized by loss of the normal peristaltic coordination of the esophageal smooth muscle. This results in simultaneous contraction of segments of the esophageal body.

(1) The primary **symptom** is severe spastic pain, which can occur spontaneously and at night. In addition, dysphagia, regurgitation, and weight loss are common.

(2) The **diagnosis** is confirmed with esophageal manometry, which usually demonstrates spontaneous activity, repetitive waves, and prolonged, high-amplitude contractions. Characteristic broad, multipeaked contractions with or without propagation are seen, and normal peristaltic contractions also may be present. Intravenous injection with the parasympathomimetic bethanechol (Urecholine) can provoke pain and abnormal contractions.

(3) **Treatment** with calcium channel blockers and nitrates can reduce the amplitude of the esophageal contractions but usually is not beneficial. Surgical treatment consists of a long esophagomyotomy, extending from the stomach to the aortic arch, and often a concomitant antireflux procedure.

    d. Nutcracker esophagus refers to a condition characterized manometrically by prolonged, high-amplitude peristaltic waves associated with chest pain that may mimic cardiac symptoms. Treatment with calcium channel blockers and long-acting nitrates has been helpful. Esophagomyotomy is of uncertain benefit.

  2. Secondary dysmotility represents the esophageal response to inflammatory injury or systemic disorders, such as scleroderma, multiple sclerosis, or diabetic neuropathy. Inflammation can produce fibrosis, which can lead to loss of peristalsis and esophageal contractility. The most common cause of secondary dysfunction is the reflux of gastric contents into the esophagus.

    a. Progressive systemic sclerosis, or scleroderma, produces esophageal manifestations in 60% to 80% of patients, and often the esophagus is the earliest site of GI involvement. It is characterized by atrophy of the smooth muscle of the distal esophagus, deposition of collagen in connective tissue, and subintimal arteriolar fibrosis. Normal contractions are present in the striated muscle of the proximal esophagus.

    b. In a subset of patients with severe long-standing GER disease, erosive esophagitis and stricture formation occur as a result of the combination of an incompetent LES and poor esophageal emptying secondary to low-amplitude, disordered peristaltic contractions. Intensive medical treatment of the reflux is essential before operation. Most surgeons prefer a Collis gastroplasty and a Belsey antireflux procedure for these patients because of the presence of esophageal shortening and impaired peristalsis.

IV. ESOPHAGEAL STRICTURES are either benign or malignant, and the distinction is critical. **Benign strictures** are either congenital or acquired.

  A. Congenital webs are the only true congenital esophageal strictures. They represent a failure of appropriate canalization of the esophagus during development and can occur at any level. An imperforate web must be distinguished from a tracheoesophageal fistula, although a perforate web may not produce symptoms until feedings become solid.

  B. Acquired strictures

    1. Esophageal rings or **webs** occur at all levels in relation to the etiology of the webbing process. An example is **Schatzki ring,** which occurs in the lower esophagus at the junction of the squamous and columnar epithelium. A hiatal hernia is always present, and the etiology is presumed to be GER. Esophagitis is rarely present. Treatment generally consists of medical management of reflux with periodic dilation for symptoms of dysphagia.

    2. Strictures of the esophagus can result from any esophageal injury, including chronic reflux, previous perforation, infection, or inflammation.

  C. Symptoms associated with a stricture consist of progressive dysphagia to solid food and usually begin when the esophageal lumen narrows beyond 12 mm.

  D. Evaluation and treatment of a stricture begins with the categorical **exclusion of malignancy.** The diagnosis usually is based on a barium swallow. Esophagoscopy is essential to assess the location, length, size, and distensibility of the stricture and to obtain appropriate biopsies or brushings. Because a peptic stricture secondary to reflux always occurs at the squamocolumnar junction, biopsy of the esophageal mucosa below a high stricture should demonstrate columnar mucosa. If squamous mucosa is found, the presumptive diagnosis of a malignant obstruction should be made, although strictures due to Crohn disease, previous lye ingestion, or monilial esophagitis are among alternative diagnoses. Most strictures are amenable to **dilation,** and this relieves the symptoms. Attention is then directed at correcting the underlying etiology. **Resection** can be required for recurrent or persistent strictures or if malignancy cannot be ruled out.

V. ESOPHAGEAL DIVERTICULA are acquired conditions of the esophagus found primarily in adults. They are divided into traction and pulsion diverticula based on the pathophysiology that induced their formation.

  A. A **pharyngoesophageal (or Zenker) diverticulum** is a pulsion diverticulum. It is the most common type of symptomatic diverticulum. **Symptoms** include progressive cervical dysphagia, cough on assuming a recumbent position, and spontaneous regurgitation of undigested food, leading to episodes of choking and aspiration. **Diagnosis** with a barium swallow should prompt surgical correction with cricopharyngeal myotomy and diverticulectomy or suspension. Notably, almost all patients with a pharyngoesophageal diverticulum have GER that is thought to produce cricopharyngeal dysfunction. **Endoscopic approaches** (i.e., stapling to produce a myotomy and/or diverticulectomy) are being developed but do not have the success rate of open myotomy.

B. A **traction or midesophageal or parabronchial diverticulum** occurs in conjunction with mediastinal granulomatous disease often due to histoplasmosis or tuberculosis. Symptoms are rare, but when they are present, they mandate operative excision of the diverticulum and adjacent inflammatory mass. On rare occasions, these diverticula present with chronic cough from an esophagobronchial fistula.

C. An **epiphrenic or pulsion diverticulum** can be located at almost every level but typically occurs in the **distal 10 cm** of the thoracic esophagus. Many patients are asymptomatic at the time of diagnosis, and in those who are symptomatic, it is difficult to determine whether the complaints stem from the diverticulum or from the underlying esophageal disorder.

   1. The **diagnosis** is made with a **contrast esophagogram;** however, endoscopic examination and esophageal function studies are essential in defining the underlying pathophysiology. In advanced disease, the diagnosis can be confused with achalasia owing to the dependency of the diverticulum and the lateral displacement and narrowing of the GE junction.

   2. Operative treatment is recommended for patients with progressive or incapacitating symptoms associated with abnormal esophageal peristalsis. Surgery consists of diverticulectomy or diverticulopexy, along with an extramucosal esophagomyotomy. The myotomy extends from the neck of the diverticulum down to the stomach. When the diverticulum is associated with a hiatal hernia and reflux, a concomitant nonobstructive antireflux procedure (Belsey Mark IV) is recommended. Any associated mechanical obstruction also must be corrected.

TRAUMATIC INJURY TO THE ESOPHAGUS

I. ESOPHAGEAL PERFORATION

A. Overall, perforation is associated with a 20% mortality rate. The **etiologies** may be broadly divided into intra- and extraluminal categories.

   1. Intraluminal causes

   a. Instrumentation injuries represent 75% of esophageal perforations and may occur during endoscopy, dilation, sclerosis of esophageal varices, transesophageal echocardiography, and tube passage. The most common sites are the anatomic sites of narrowing of the esophagus (e.g., at the cricopharyngeus and GE junction).

   b. Foreign bodies can cause acute perforation, or more commonly follow an indolent course with late abscess formation in the mediastinum or development of empyema.

   c. Ingested caustic substances, such as alkali chemicals, can produce coagulation necrosis of the esophagus.

   d. Cancer of the esophagus may lead to perforation.

   e. Barotrauma induced by external compression (e.g., Heimlich maneuver), forceful vomiting (Boerhaave syndrome), seizures, childbirth, or lifting can produce esophageal perforation. Almost all of these injuries occur in the distal esophagus on the left side.

   2. Extraluminal causes

   a. Penetrating injuries to the esophagus can occur from stab wounds or, more commonly, gunshot wounds.

    b. Blunt trauma may produce an esophageal perforation related to a rapid increase in intraluminal pressure or compression of the esophagus between the sternum and the spine.

    c. Operative injury to the esophagus during an unrelated procedure occurs infrequently but has been reported in association with thyroid resection, anterior cervical spine operations, proximal gastric vagotomy, pneumonectomy, and laparoscopic fundoplication procedures.

B. Esophageal perforations initially manifest with **dysphagia, pain,** and **fever** and progress to **leukocytosis, tachycardia, respiratory distress,** and **shock** if the perforation is left untreated. Cervical perforations may present with neck stiffness and subcutaneous emphysema, and an intrathoracic perforation should be suspected in patients with chest pain, subcutaneous emphysema, dyspnea, and a pleural effusion (right pleural effusion in proximal perforations, left effusion in distal perforations). Patients with intra-abdominal perforations usually present with **peritonitis.**

C. The **diagnosis** of esophageal perforation is suggested by pneumomediastinum, pleural effusion, pneumothorax, atelectasis, and soft-tissue emphysema on **chest x-ray** or mediastinal air and fluid on **computed tomography (CT) scan.** Rapid evaluation with water-soluble or dilute **barium contrast esophagography** is mandatory, although contrast studies carry a 10% false-negative rate for esophageal perforations. Because esophagoscopy is used primarily as an adjunctive study and can miss sizable perforations, any discoloration or submucosal hematoma should be considered highly suspicious for perforation after trauma to the posterior mediastinum. Whenever an esophageal perforation is suspected, diagnosis and treatment must be prompt because morbidity and mortality increase in direct proportion to the delay.

D. Principles of management include (1) adequate **drainage** of the leak, (2) intravenous **antibiotics,** (3) aggressive fluid **resuscitation,** (4) adequate **nutrition,** (5) **relief** of any distal obstruction, (6) **diversion** of enteric contents past the leak, and (7) **restoration** of GI integrity. Initially, patients are kept on nothing-by-mouth status, a nasogastric tube is placed carefully in the esophagus or stomach, and they receive intravenous hydration and broad-spectrum antibiotics.

E. Definitive management generally requires operative repair, although a carefully selected group of nontoxic patients with a locally contained perforation may be observed. Patients with an intramural perforation after endoscopic procedures or dilation have a characteristic radiographic finding of a thin collection of contrast material parallel to the esophageal lumen without spillage into the mediastinum. Management with a nasogastric tube and antibiotics almost always is successful in these patients.

    1. Cervical and upper thoracic perforations usually are treated by cervical drainage alone or in combination with esophageal repair.

    2. Thoracic perforations should be closed primarily and buttressed with healthy tissue, and the mediastinum should be drained widely. Even when perforations are more than 24 hours old, primary mucosal closure usually is possible. When primary closure is not possible, options include wide drainage alone or in conjunction with resection, or with exclusion and diversion in cases of severe traumatic injury to the esophagus.

    3. Abdominal esophageal perforations typically result in peritonitis and require an upper abdominal midline incision to correct.

    4. Perforations associated with intrinsic esophageal disease (e.g., carcinoma, hiatal hernia, or achalasia) require addressing the perforation as described previously and surgically correcting the associated esophageal disease concomitantly.

II. CAUSTIC INGESTION. Liquid alkali solutions (e.g., **Drano** and **Liquid-Plumr**) are responsible for most of the serious caustic esophageal and gastric injuries, producing coagulation necrosis in both organs. Acid ingestion is more likely to cause isolated gastric injury.

A. Initial management is directed at hemodynamic stabilization and evaluation of the airway and extent of injury.

    1. Airway compromise can occur from burns of the epiglottis or larynx and may require tracheostomy.

2. **Fluid** resuscitation and broad-spectrum **antibiotics** should be instituted.
3. **Vomiting should not be induced,** but patients should be placed on nothing-by-mouth status and given an oral suction device.
4. Steroids are of no proven benefit.

B. **Evaluation** with water-soluble **contrast esophagography** and gentle **esophagoscopy** should be done early to assess the severity and extent of injury and to rule out esophageal perforation or gastric necrosis.

C. **Management**
   1. Without perforation, management is supportive, with acute symptoms generally resolving over several days.
   2. **Perforation, unrelenting pain,** or **persistent acidosis** mandate surgical intervention. A transabdominal approach is recommended to allow evaluation of the patient's stomach and distal esophagus. If it is necrotic, the involved portion of the patient's stomach and esophagus must be resected, and a cervical esophagostomy must be performed. A feeding jejunostomy is placed for nutrition, and reconstruction is performed 90 or more days later.
   3. **Late problems** include the development of **strictures** and an increased risk of **esophageal carcinoma** (1,000 times that of the general population).

 ESOPHAGEAL TUMORS

I. **BENIGN ESOPHAGEAL NEOPLASMS** are rare, although probably many remain undetected. The most common lesions are mesenchymal tumors such as gastrointestinal stromal tumors and leiomyomas, followed by polyps. Less common lesions include hemangioma and granular cell myoblastoma.

A. **Clinical features** depend primarily on the location of the tumor within the esophagus. **Intraluminal** tumors, such as polyps, cause esophageal obstruction, and patients present with dysphagia, vomiting, and aspiration. **Intramural** tumors, such as leiomyomas, usually are asymptomatic, but if they are large enough, they can produce dysphagia or chest pain.

B. **Diagnosis** usually involves a combination of barium swallow, esophagoscopy, and perhaps CT scanning or magnetic resonance (MR) scan studies.

C. **Treatment** for all symptomatic or enlarging tumors is **surgical removal.** Intraluminal tumors can be removed successfully via endoscopy, but if they are large and vascular, they should be resected via thoracotomy and esophagostomy. Intramural tumors usually can be enucleated from the esophageal muscular wall without entering the mucosa. This is done via a video-assisted thoracoscopic or open thoracotomy approach. Laparoscopic resection may be appropriate for distal lesions.

II. **BARRETT ESOPHAGUS** is defined as a metaplastic transformation of esophageal mucosa resulting from chronic GER. Histologically, the metaplastic epithelium must demonstrate **intestinal-type metaplasia** characterized by the presence of goblet cells. The columnar epithelium of Barrett esophagus may replace the normal squamous epithelium circumferentially, or it may be asymmetric and irregular.

A. **Prevalence.** Barrett esophagus is diagnosed in approximately 2% of all patients undergoing esophagoscopy and in 10% to 15% of patients with esophagitis. Autopsy studies suggest that the actual prevalence is much higher because many patients are asymptomatic and remain undiagnosed. Most patients diagnosed with Barrett esophagus are middle-aged white men.

B. The **symptoms** of Barrett esophagus arise from longstanding gastric reflux. Approximately 50% of patients with endoscopically proven Barrett have associated heartburn, 75% have dysphagia, and 25% have bleeding (*Ann Surg* 1983;198:554).

C. **Diagnosis.** Barrett esophagus may be suggested on x-ray by the presence of a hiatal hernia (associated with 80% of cases of Barrett esophagus) with esophagitis and an esophageal stricture. Confirmation of the diagnosis requires endoscopy and careful correlation between the endoscopic and histologic appearances.

D. Complications
1. **Esophageal ulceration and stricture** are more likely to occur in patients with Barrett esophagus than in those with GER alone. This probably reflects the more severe nature of the GER in patients with Barrett esophagus.
   a. **Barrett ulcers** are distinctly different from the common erosions seen in esophagitis in that they penetrate the metaplastic columnar epithelium in a manner similar to that seen in gastric ulcers. They occur in up to 50% of patients with Barrett esophagus and, like gastric ulcers, can cause pain, bleed, obstruct, penetrate, and perforate.
   b. **A benign stricture** occurs in 30% to 50% of patients with Barrett esophagus. The stricture is located at the squamocolumnar junction, which may be found proximal to the GE junction. Strictures secondary to Barrett esophagus are located in the middle or upper esophagus, unlike the routine peptic strictures that usually occur in the distal esophagus.
2. **Dysplasia.** The metaplastic columnar epithelium of Barrett esophagus is prone to development of dysplasia that can be detected only by biopsy. Dysplasia is categorized as low or high grade, with high grade being pathologically indistinguishable from carcinoma *in situ.*
3. **Malignant degeneration** from benign to dysplastic to malignant epithelium has been demonstrated in Barrett esophagus. Low-grade dysplasia is present in 5% to 10% of patients with Barrett esophagus and can progress to high-grade dysplasia and malignancy.
4. **Adenocarcinomas** that arise within the esophagus above the normal GE junction are characteristic of malignant degeneration in Barrett esophagus. The risk of development of adenocarcinoma in Barrett esophagus is 50 to 100 times that of the general population. In several long-term series, the incidence of malignant degeneration in Barrett esophagus was estimated at between 1 in 50 and 1 in 400 patient-years of follow-up.

E. Treatment
1. Uncomplicated Barrett esophagus in **asymptomatic** patients requires no specific therapy, but endoscopic surveillance and biopsy should be performed at least annually. Neither medical nor surgical treatment of reflux has been demonstrated to reverse the columnar metaplasia of Barrett esophagus. However, elimination of reflux with an **antireflux procedure** may halt progression of the disease, heal ulceration, and prevent stricture formation.
2. Uncomplicated Barrett esophagus in **symptomatic** patients should be treated using the same principles that apply to patients with GER without Barrett esophagus. In addition, symptomatic patients should have annual surveillance endoscopy with biopsy. After laparoscopic antireflux surgery, patients with Barrett esophagus have symptomatic relief and reduction in medication use equivalent to non-Barrett patients. Absence of progression to high-grade dysplasia or adenocarcinoma suggests that laparoscopic surgery is an effective approach for the management of patients with Barrett esophagus (*Am J Surg* 2003;186:6).
3. **Barrett ulcers** usually heal with medical therapy. Frequently, 8 weeks of treatment with an H_2-receptor antagonist or proton-pump inhibitor are necessary to achieve complete healing. Recurrence of ulcers is common after discontinuation of therapy. Ulcers that fail to heal despite 4 months of medical therapy are an indication for rebiopsy and antireflux surgery.
4. **Strictures** associated with Barrett esophagus are managed successfully with periodic esophageal dilation combined with medical management. Recurrent or persistent strictures warrant an antireflux operation combined with intraoperative stricture dilation. After surgery, several dilations can be required to maintain patency during the healing phase. Rarely, undilatable strictures require resection.
5. **Dysplasia** on biopsy of Barrett esophagus indicates that the patient is at risk for the development of adenocarcinoma.
   a. **Low-grade dysplasia** requires frequent (every 3 to 6 months) surveillance esophagoscopy and biopsy. Medical therapy for GER is recommended in these patients, even when asymptomatic.

b. **High-grade dysplasia** is pathologically indistinguishable from carcinoma *in situ* and is an indication for esophagectomy. Patients who undergo esophagectomy for high-grade dysplasia have up to a 73% incidence of having a focus of invasive carcinoma present in the resected esophagus. Cure rates of nearly 100% can be expected in patients whose cancer is limited to the mucosa and who undergo esophagectomy (*J Thorac Cardiovasc Surg* 1994;108:813). Because of the morbidity and mortality associated with esophagectomy, other methods of treatment have been evaluated, such as photodynamic therapy. A recent randomized, phase III trial was performed comparing photodynamic therapy versus omeprazole alone for patients with Barrett and high-grade dysplasia. It showed that photodynamic therapy can reduce the incidence of esophageal adenocarcinoma (*Gastrointest Endosc* 2005;62:488).

6. **Adenocarcinoma** in patients with Barrett esophagus is an indication for esophagogastrectomy. Early detection offers the best opportunity to improve survival after resection, which overall is 20% at 5 years.

III. ESOPHAGEAL CARCINOMA

A. **Epidemiology.** Carcinoma of the esophagus represents 1% of all cancers in the United States and causes 1.8% of cancer deaths. The two principal histologies are adenocarcinoma and squamous cell carcinoma.

1. **Risk factors** for squamous cell esophageal cancer include African American race, alcohol and cigarette use, tylosis, achalasia, caustic esophageal injury, Plummer-Vinson syndrome, nutritional deficiencies, and ingestion of nitrosamines and fungal toxins. Geographic location also represents a risk factor, likely as a result of local dietary customs, with a high incidence noted in certain areas of China, South Africa, Iran, France, and Japan.

2. **Risk factors** for adenocarcinoma of the esophagus include white race, GER, Barrett esophagus, obesity, and cigarette smoking.

B. **Pathology**

1. **Squamous cell carcinoma** was previously the most common type of esophageal carcinoma. It tends to be multicentric and most frequently involves the middle third of the esophagus.

2. **Adenocarcinoma** now constitutes the majority of malignant esophageal tumors and is the carcinoma with the greatest rate of increase in the United States. It is less likely to be multicentric, but it typically exhibits extensive proximal and distal submucosal invasion. Adenocarcinoma most commonly involves the distal esophagus.

3. **Less common malignant esophageal tumors** include small-cell carcinoma, melanoma, leiomyosarcoma, lymphoma, and esophageal involvement by metastatic cancer.

C. Most patients with early-stage disease are asymptomatic or may have symptoms of reflux. Patients with esophageal cancer may complain of **dysphagia, odynophagia, and weight loss.** Symptoms that are suggestive of unresectability include hoarseness, abdominal pain, persistent back or bone pain, hiccups, and respiratory symptoms (cough or aspiration pneumonia suggesting possible esophagorespiratory fistula). Approximately 50% of presenting patients have unresectable lesions or distant metastasis, which is largely responsible for the generally poor prognosis.

D. The **diagnosis** is suggested by a barium swallow and confirmed with esophagoscopy and biopsy or brush cytology.

E. **Staging.** A system for staging esophageal cancer allows assignment of patients to groups with similar prognosis, helps to determine if local or systemic therapy is needed, and allows comparison of response to different types of therapy (Table 8-1). Evaluation for lymph node and distant-organ metastatic disease is performed by CT scanning, which can be combined with positron emission tomographic (PET) scanning to improve diagnostic accuracy. Endoscopic ultrasonography is more accurate than radiographic studies for determining the depth of wall invasion and the involvement of peritumoral lymph nodes. Upper esophageal and midesophageal lesions require bronchoscopy to evaluate the airway for involvement by tumor.

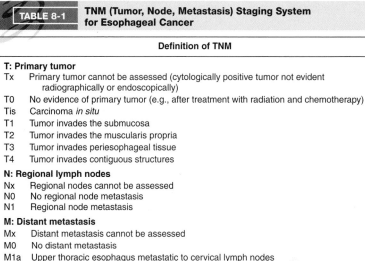

TABLE 8-1	TNM (Tumor, Node, Metastasis) Staging System for Esophageal Cancer

Definition of TNM

T: Primary tumor
Tx   Primary tumor cannot be assessed (cytologically positive tumor not evident radiographically or endoscopically)
T0   No evidence of primary tumor (e.g., after treatment with radiation and chemotherapy)
Tis   Carcinoma *in situ*
T1   Tumor invades the submucosa
T2   Tumor invades the muscularis propria
T3   Tumor invades periesophageal tissue
T4   Tumor invades contiguous structures

N: Regional lymph nodes
Nx   Regional nodes cannot be assessed
N0   No regional node metastasis
N1   Regional node metastasis

M: Distant metastasis
Mx   Distant metastasis cannot be assessed
M0   No distant metastasis
M1a   Upper thoracic esophagus metastatic to cervical lymph nodes
      Lower thoracic esophagus metastatic to celiac lymph nodes
M1b   Metastases to nonregional lymph nodes or other distant sites

Stage grouping			
Stage 0	Tis	N0	M0
Stage I	T1	N0	M0
Stage IIA	T2	N0	M0
	T3	N0	M0
Stage IIB	T1	N1	M0
	T2	N1	M0
Stage III	T3	N1	M0
	T4	Any N	M0
Stage IVA	Any T	Any N	M1a
Stage IVB	Any T	Any N	M1b

Adapted with permission from Greene FL, Fritz AG, Balch CM, et al., eds. *AJCC Cancer Staging Handbook*, 6th ed. New York: Springer-Verlag; 2002.

F. Treatment
   1. Surgical resection remains a mainstay of curative treatment for patients with localized disease. It offers the best opportunity for cure and provides substantial palliation when cure is not possible. The overall 5-year survival rate is 20% to 30%, with higher rates for patients with lower stages of disease (*J Thorac Cardiovasc Surg* 1993;105:265).
      a. Options for resection include a standard transthoracic esophagectomy, a transhiatal esophagectomy, or an en bloc esophagectomy. Total esophagectomy with a cervical esophagogastric anastomosis and subtotal resection with a high intrathoracic anastomosis have become the most common resections and produce the best long-term functional results as well as the best chance for cure. Esophagogastrectomy with anastomosis to the distal half of the esophagus is seldom used because troublesome postoperative reflux is common.
      b. Options for esophageal replacement include the stomach, colon, and jejunum.

2. **Neoadjuvant therapy** with preoperative chemotherapy or chemoradiotherapy has been evaluated in a number of trials. Although it may enhance local control and resectability, it does not appear to reduce the risk of systemic spread, and the survival benefit is unclear. However, a more recent prospective, randomized, controlled study evaluating preoperative treatment with epirubicin, cisplatin, and 5-fluorouracil and then surgery versus surgery alone showed an improved progression-free and overall survival rate. This study compared 250 patients in each arm and had a median follow-up of 4 years. It found an improved 5-year survival from 23% in the surgery-alone arm to 36% in the preoperative-chemotherapy-and-surgery arm (*N Engl J Med* 2006; 355:1).

3. **Radiotherapy** is used worldwide for attempted cure and palliation of patients with squamous cell esophageal cancer deemed unsuitable for resection. The 5-year survival rate is 5% to 10%. Palliation of dysphagia is successful temporarily in 80% of patients but rarely provides complete long-term relief. Combination therapy involving radiation and concurrent administration of 5-fluorouracil with mitomycin C or cisplatin has been suggested to improve results and has replaced radiation alone in most protocols.

4. The goal of **palliative treatment** is the relief of obstruction and dysphagia.
   a. **Radiotherapy and chemotherapy** work best in patients with squamous cell carcinoma, particularly when it is located above the carina. Adenocarcinoma is less responsive to radiation, and the acute morbidity (nausea and vomiting) of external-beam irradiation of the epigastric area is substantial.
   b. **Esophageal bypass procedures** have been largely abandoned due to excessive complication rates.
   c. **Intraluminal prostheses** have been developed to intubate the esophagus and stent the obstruction. Self-expanding wire-mesh stents, often with a soft silicone (Silastic) coating, have been used with greater ease of insertion and satisfactory results. None of these prostheses allows normal swallowing, and in most cases no more than a pureed diet can be tolerated. The two methods for insertion are (1) peroral (push technique) and (2) via a laparotomy (pull technique). Of these, the peroral route is associated with fewer complications. Potential complications include perforation, erosion or migration of the stent, and obstruction of the tube by food or proximal tumor growth.
   d. **Endoscopic laser techniques** can restore an esophageal lumen successfully 90% of the time, with only a 4% to 5% perforation rate.

IV. **COMPLICATIONS OF ESOPHAGEAL SURGERY.** Esophageal surgery is fraught with potential complications, and consistently good results require meticulous attention to operative technique.
   A. **Postthoracotomy complications** can include atelectasis and respiratory insufficiency, pneumonia, atrial fibrillation, wound infections, and persistent postoperative pain.
   B. **Complications related to an esophageal anastomosis** consist primarily of leaks and strictures.
      1. Management of an **anastomotic leak** is based on the size of the leak, the location of the anastomosis, and the clinical status of the patient.
         a. A **cervical** anastomotic leak usually can be managed by opening the incision to allow drainage. Occasionally, the leak tracks below the thoracic inlet into the mediastinum, necessitating wider débridement and drainage. If a major leak occurs, esophagoscopy should be performed to rule out a significant ischemic injury to the stomach. If present, the anastomosis should be taken down and a cervical esophagostomy should be performed. The necrotic portion of the stomach should be resected, and the remaining stomach should be returned to the abdomen, with placement of a gastrostomy and feeding jejunostomy. Reconstruction with residual stomach or the colon is done at a later date.
         b. **Intrathoracic** anastomotic leaks are associated with a high mortality rate. Small, well-drained leaks can be treated conservatively, but large or poorly drained leaks require operative exploration.

 2. **Strictures** usually are the result of a healed anastomotic leak, relative ischemia of the anastomosis, or recurrent cancer. Most can be dilated successfully.
C. **Complications of antireflux repairs** generally result from **preoperative** failure to recognize a confounding abnormality, such as poor gastric emptying or weak esophageal peristalsis, or **operative** miscalculations that result in too tight a fundoplication or excessive tension on the repair. Most of these complications require operative revision.
 1. **Postoperative dysphagia** can result from a fundoplication that is too long or tight, a misplaced or slipped fundoplication that is positioned around the stomach rather than the distal esophagus, or a complete fundoplication in the setting of poor esophageal contractile function. It also can result from operative distortion of the GE junction, excessive narrowing of the diaphragmatic hiatus, or disruption of the crural closure and herniation of an intact repair into the chest.
 2. **Persistent or recurrent reflux** after surgery suggests an inadequate or misplaced fundoplication, disruption of the fundoplication, or herniation of the repair into the chest (*Ann Surg* 1999;229:669).
 3. **Breakdown of an antireflux repair** usually is recognized by a gradual recurrence of symptoms and can be confirmed by a contrast esophogram. Most commonly, disruption of a repair is due to inadequate mobilization of the cardia and excessive tension on the repair.
 4. **Gas bloating** or gastric dilation can occur if the fundoplication is too tight or if there is unrecognized gastric outlet obstruction or delayed gastric emptying.

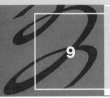

STOMACH

9

Sekhar Dharmarajan, Valerie J. Halpin, and William G. Hawkins

ANATOMY AND PHYSIOLOGY

The principal role of the stomach is to store and prepare ingested food for digestion and absorption through a variety of motor and secretory functions. The stomach can be divided into five regions based on external landmarks: the **cardia,** the region just distal to the gastroesophageal (GE) junction; the **fundus,** the portion of the stomach above and to the left of the GE junction; the **body,** or **corpus,** the largest portion of the stomach; the **antrum,** the distal 25% to 30% of the stomach, located between the incisa angularis and the pylorus; and the **pylorus,** a thickened ring of smooth muscle forming the distal boundary of the stomach. The arterial blood supply to the lesser curvature of the stomach is from the **left gastric** artery, a branch of the celiac axis, and the **right gastric** artery, a branch of the common hepatic artery. The greater curvature is supplied by the **short gastric** and **left gastroepiploic** arteries, branches of the splenic artery, and the **right gastroepiploic** artery, a branch of the gastroduodenal artery. Venous drainage of the stomach parallels arterial supply, with the left gastric (coronary) and right gastric veins draining into the portal vein, the left gastroepiploic vein draining into the splenic vein, and the right gastroepiploic draining into the superior mesenteric vein. The principal innervation to the stomach is derived from the right and left vagal trunks. Gastric physiology is covered in Chapter 2.

DISORDERS OF THE STOMACH

I. **PEPTIC ULCER DISEASE (PUD)** represents a spectrum of disease characterized by ulceration of the stomach or proximal duodenum due to an imbalance between acid secretion and mucosal defense mechanisms.
   A. **Epidemiology.** In the United States, there are approximately 500,000 new cases of PUD each year, with an annual incidence of 1% to 2% and a lifetime prevalence between 8% and 14%. Although there has been a steady decline in the incidence of peptic ulcer disease since the 1960s, ulcer-related mortality remains approximately 10,000 cases annually.
   B. **Pathogenesis.** Four etiologic factors are responsible for the vast majority of PUD.
      1. *Helicobacter pylori (H. pylori)* **infection** is associated with 90% to 95% of duodenal ulcers and 70% to 90% of gastric ulcers. Infection produces chronic antral gastritis, increased acid and gastrin secretion, and decreased mucosal resistance to acid.
      2. **Nonsteroidal anti-inflammatory drug (NSAID)** use confers an 8-fold increase in risk of duodenal ulcers and a 40-fold increase in risk of gastric ulcers due to suppression of prostaglandin production.
      3. **Cigarette smoking**
      4. **Acid hypersecretion** occurs in the majority of patients with duodenal ulcers.
   C. **Presentation** in uncomplicated ulcer disease is usually burning, gnawing intermittent epigastric pain that is relieved by food or antacid ingestion for duodenal ulcers but exacerbated by intake for gastric ulcers. Pain may be accompanied by nausea,

vomiting, and mild weight loss. **Differential diagnosis** is broad and includes gastroesophageal reflux disease, biliary colic and related biliary tract disease, inflammatory and neoplastic pancreatic disease, and gastric neoplasms.

D. **Diagnosis** can be made by barium contrast radiography or upper gastrointestinal endoscopy. **Esophagogastroduodenoscopy (EGD)** is more sensitive and specific than contrast examination for peptic ulcer disease (*Ann Intern Med* 1984;101:538). In addition, EGD offers therapeutic options (ligation of bleeding vessels) and diagnostic options (biopsy for malignancy, antral biopsy for *H. pylori*). Once the diagnosis of PUD is confirmed, further testing should be carried out to determine its etiology.

1. ***H. pylori* infection** can be detected noninvasively by radiolabeled **urea breath test** or **serologic antibody testing**. Antral tissue obtained during endoscopy can be subjected to direct **histologic examination** or rapid urease testing using the **cod liver oil (CLO) test**.

2. **Fasting serum gastrin levels** should be obtained in patients who have no history of NSAID use and are *H. pylori*-negative or who have recurrent ulcers despite adequate treatment, multiple ulcers, ulcers in unusual locations (such as the second and third portions of the duodenum), or complicated PUD (hemorrhage, perforation, obstruction). Such atypical presentations suggest the possibility of **Zollinger-Ellison syndrome**, a rare entity causing PUD in 0.1% to 1% of patients. This syndrome is discussed further in Chapter 21.

3. **Endoscopic biopsy of gastric ulcers** is mandatory to exclude malignancy.

E. **Treatment** of PUD has changed dramatically with the development of antisecretory drugs [histamine$_2$-receptor blockers and proton-pump inhibitors (PPIs)], and *H. pylori*–eradication regimens have greatly diminished the role of elective surgery for PUD.

1. **Medical therapy**

   a. ***H. pylori* eradication** is the cornerstone of medical therapy for PUD. Regimens typically consist of a PPI combined with two antibiotics administered for 10 to 14 days. These regimens are 85% to 90% effective in eradicating *H. pylori*. Antisecretory therapy is then continued until ulcer healing is complete.

   b. **NSAID-associated PUD** is treated by discontinuing the offending medication and initiating antisecretory therapy. If the NSAID must be continued, PPIs are most effective for facilitating ulcer healing.

   c. **Smoking cessation** greatly facilitates ulcer healing, but compliance rates are low.

   d. **Follow-up endoscopy** to ensure healing is essential for gastric ulcers because up to 3% harbor malignancy.

2. **Surgical therapy** for uncomplicated peptic ulcer disease is exceedingly rare. Indications for elective operation for PUD include failure of medical therapy and inability to exclude malignancy.

   a. **Duodenal ulcers** are treated by one of three acid-reducing operations: (1) truncal vagotomy with pyloroplasty, (2) truncal vagotomy with antrectomy and Billroth I (gastroduodenostomy) or Billroth II (gastrojejunostomy) reconstruction, or (3) highly selective vagotomy (HSV). Truncal vagotomy with antrectomy yields maximal acid suppression with lowest ulcer recurrence rates (1% to 2%) but carries the highest postoperative morbidity (15% to 30%) and mortality (1% to 2%) rates. HSV has the lowest postoperative morbidity (3% to 8%) and mortality rates but is technically demanding to perform and has higher recurrence rates (5% to 15%).

   b. **Gastric ulcers** are typically treated with either wedge excision or antrectomy with inclusion of the ulcer, depending on ulcer location. Concurrent truncal vagotomy is reserved for patients who are known to have refractory ulcer disease despite maximal medical management; this is rare today.

II. **COMPLICATED PEPTIC ULCER DISEASE** refers to PUD complicated by hemorrhage, perforation, or obstruction. These complications represent the most common indications for surgery in PUD. Although there has been a sharp decline in elective surgery for PUD, the rates of emergency surgery for complicated PUD have been stable over time.

A. **Hemorrhage** is the leading cause of death due to PUD, with associated 5% to 10% mortality. Evaluation and management begin with aggressive resuscitation and correction of any coagulopathy, followed by EGD. Although spontaneous cessation of bleeding occurs in 70% of patients, endoscopic therapy using thermal coagulation with or without epinephrine is warranted in individuals who present with hemodynamic instability, need for continuing transfusion, hematemesis or red stool, age greater than 60 years, and serious medical comorbidities, because these patients have a higher risk of recurrent bleeding. Endoscopic findings of a visible vessel or active bleeding also indicate high risk for rebleeding and require endoscopic hemostasis. **Indications for surgery** include repeated episodes of bleeding, continued hemodynamic instability, ongoing transfusion requirement of more than 6 units of packed red blood cells over 24 hours, and more than one unsuccessful endoscopic intervention.

1. **Bleeding duodenal ulcers** are usually located on the posterior duodenal wall within 2 cm of the pylorus and typically erode into the gastroduodenal artery. Bleeding is controlled by duodenotomy and oversewing of the bleeding vessel. In hemodynamically stable patients, consideration should be made for a concomitant acid-reducing procedure for those who have failed or are noncompliant with medical therapy. Postoperative *H. pylori* eradication is important to reduce the risk of recurrent bleeding.

2. **Bleeding gastric ulcers** present a diverse challenge because the patient's condition, comorbidities, and previous ulcer and medication history all play a role in surgical decision making. In unstable patients, biopsy followed by oversewing or wedge excision of the ulcer should be performed. Stable patients may be candidates for antrectomy and vagotomy.

B. **Perforated peptic ulcer** typically presents with sudden onset of severe abdominal pain but may be less dramatic, particularly in hospitalized, elderly, and immunocompromised patients. The resulting peritonitis is often generalized but can be localized when the perforation is walled off by adjacent viscera and structures. Examination reveals fever, tachycardia, and abdominal wall rigidity, and laboratory evaluation typically demonstrates leukocytosis. Abdominal x-ray reveals free subdiaphragmatic gas in 80% to 85% of cases. Aggressive fluid resuscitation and broad-spectrum antibiotics followed by prompt operative repair is indicated in the vast majority of patients with perforated PUD. **Nonoperative treatment of perforated duodenal ulcer** can be considered in poor operative candidates in whom the perforation has been present for more than 24 hours, the pain is well localized, and there is no evidence of ongoing extravasation on upper GI water-soluble contrast studies (*World J Surg* 2000;24:256).

1. **Perforated duodenal ulcers** are best managed by simple omental patching and peritoneal débridement, followed by *H. pylori* eradication. An acid-reducing procedure (preferably truncal vagotomy and pyloroplasty) should be added in stable patients who are known to be *H. pylori*-negative or have failed medical therapy.

2. **Perforated gastric ulcers** are best treated by simple wedge resection to eliminate the perforation and exclude malignancy. If wedge resection of the ulcer cannot be performed due to its juxtapyloric location, multiple biopsies of the ulcer are taken and omental patching is performed.

C. **Gastric outlet obstruction** can occur as a chronic process due to fibrosis and scarring of the pylorus from chronic ulcer disease or as a consequence of acute inflammation superimposed on previous scarring of the gastric outlet. In general, gastric outlet obstruction secondary to PUD has become exceedingly rare with modern medical antisecretory therapy. Patients present with recurrent vomiting of poorly digested food, dehydration, and hypochloremic hypokalemic metabolic alkalosis. Management consists in correction of volume and electrolyte abnormalities, nasogastric suction, and intravenous antisecretory agents. EGD is necessary for evaluating the nature of the obstruction and for ruling out malignant etiology, and **endoscopic hydrostatic balloon dilation** can be performed at the same time. This is feasible in up to 85% of patients, but fewer than 40% have sustained improvement at 3 months (*Gastrointest Endosc* 1996;43:98). **Indications for surgical therapy** include persistent obstruction after 7 days of nonoperative management and recurrent obstruction. Antrectomy to include the ulcer and truncal vagotomy is the ideal operation for most patients. In exceptional instances, truncal vagotomy with gastrojejunostomy may be preferred in those patients whose pyloroduodenal inflammation precludes safe management with Billroth I or II reconstructions.

III. **GASTRIC ADENOCARCINOMA** is the fourth-most common cancer worldwide and the tenth-most common malignancy in the United States. Its incidence has decreased dramatically over the last 60 years, perhaps secondary to improvements in refrigeration and diet. In addition, the anatomic pattern of gastric cancer is changing, with proximal or cardia cancers comprising a greater proportion of gastric cancers. Approximately one third of gastric cancers are metastatic at presentation. The overall 5-year survival rate is 15%.

A. The **etiology** of gastric cancer is complex and multifactorial, involving a combination of genetic, environmental, and infectious risk factors. **Risk factors** for gastric cancer include male gender, family history, polyposis syndromes, diets high in nitrates, salts, or pickled foods, adenomatous gastric polyps, previous gastric resection, Ménétrier disease, smoking, *H. pylori* infection, and chronic gastritis. Aspirin, fresh fruits and vegetables, selenium, and vitamin C may be protective against the development of gastric cancer.

B. **Classification.** Ninety-five percent of gastric cancers are adenocarcinomas arising from mucus-producing cells in the gastric mucosa. The **Lauren classification** system is most widely used and divides gastric cancers into two subtypes:

1. **Intestinal-type cancers** (30%) are glandular and arise from the gastric mucosa. Occurring more commonly in elderly men and in the distal stomach, they are associated with *H. pylori* and other environmental exposures that lead to chronic gastritis, intestinal metaplasia, and dysplasia.

2. **Diffuse-type cancers** (70%) arise from the lamina propria and are associated with an invasive growth pattern with rapid submucosal spread. They occur more commonly in young patients, females, and in the proximal stomach. Transmural and lymphatic spread with early metastases are more common, and diffuse-type cancers have worse overall prognosis.

C. **Presentation** of gastric cancer generally involves nonspecific signs and symptoms such as epigastric abdominal pain, unexplained weight loss, nausea, vomiting, anorexia, early satiety, and fatigue. Dysphagia is associated with proximal gastric cancers, whereas gastric outlet obstruction is more typical of distal cancers. Perforation and upper GI bleeding are the presenting manifestations in a minority of patients (1% to 4%) and generally portend advanced disease with poor prognosis. Classic physical findings in gastric cancer represent metastatic and incurable disease and include the following:

1. Enlarged supraclavicular nodes (Virchow's node).
2. Infiltration of the umbilicus (Sister Mary Joseph's node).
3. Fullness in the pelvic cul-de-sac (Blumer's shelf).
4. Enlarged ovaries on pelvic examination (Krukenberg's tumor).
5. Hepatosplenomegaly with ascites and jaundice.
6. Cachexia.

D. **Diagnosis** can be made by double-contrast upper GI barium contrast studies or by **EGD**. Endoscopy is generally the diagnostic method of choice because it permits direct visualization and biopsy of suspicious lesions. **Screening examination** by endoscopy or contrast studies is not cost-effective for the general U.S. population, given the low incidence, but may be warranted in high-risk individuals, such as patients more than 20 years post–partial gastrectomy, patients with pernicious anemia or atrophic gastritis, immigrants from endemic areas (Russia, Asia), and patients with familial or hereditary gastric cancer. Mass screening in Japan, a country with a high incidence of gastric cancer, resulted in an increase in the detection of gastric cancer confined to mucosa and led to improvements in 5-year survival rates.

E. Staging is important in determining prognosis and appropriate treatment. The American Joint Committee on Cancer and International Union against Cancer (AJCC/UICC) jointly developed a staging system that is most widely used worldwide (Table 9-1). The distribution of stage at presentation in the United States is 20% stage I, 19% stage II, 34% stage III, and 27% stage IV (*J Gastrointest Surg* 2005;9:718). Once the diagnosis of gastric cancer is established, **computed tomography (CT) and endoscopic ultrasonography (EUS)** are the primary modalities employed for staging.

    1. CT scan of the abdomen and pelvis is the best noninvasive modality for detecting metastatic disease in the form of malignant ascites or hematogenous spread to distant organs, most commonly the liver. Overall accuracy for tumor staging is 60% to 80% depending on the protocol used, but accuracy for determining nodal involvement is more limited and variable.

TABLE 9-1   **TNM (Tumor, Node, Metastasis) Staging of Gastric Cancer**

T: Primary tumor

T0	No evidence of primary tumor
Tis	Carcinoma *in situ*
T1	Invasion of lamina propria or submucosa
T2	Invasion of muscularis propria or subserosa
T3	Penetration of serosa
T4	Invasion of adjacent structures

N: Regional lymph nodes

N0	No regional node metastasis
N1	Involved perigastric nodes within 3 cm of tumor
N2	Involved perigastric nodes >3 cm from tumor edge or involvement of left gastric, splenic, celiac, or hepatic nodes

M: Distant metastasis

M0	No distant metastases
M1	Distant metastases present

Stage grouping		
Stage 0	Tis	N0	M0
Stage IA	T1	N0	M0
Stage IB	T1	N1	M0
	T2	N0	M0
Stage II	T1	N2	M0
	T2	N1	M0
	T3	N0	M0
Stage IIIA	T2	N2	M0
	T3	N1	M0
	T4	N0	M0
Stage IIIB	T3	N2	M0
	T4	N1	M0
Stage IV	T4	N2	M0
	Any T	Any N	Any M1

Adapted with permission from Fleming ID, Cooper JS, Henson DE, et al., eds. *AJCC Cancer Staging Manual,* 5th ed. Philadelphia: Lippincott Williams & Wilkins; 1998.

2. **EUS** adds to the preoperative evaluation of gastric cancer in several ways. It is superior to CT in delineating the depth of tumor invasion in the gastric wall and adjacent structures and identifying perigastric lymphadenopathy. EUS is the most accurate method available for T staging of gastric cancer, and accuracy for N staging approaches 70%. Addition of fine needle aspiration (FNA) of suspicious nodes increases accuracy even further and brings specificity to near 100%.

3. **Positron emission tomography (PET)/CT** combines the spatial resolution of CT with the contrast resolution of PET. It is most useful for its specificity in detecting nodal and distant metastatic disease not apparent on CT scan alone. Preliminary studies suggest that the use of PET/CT in staging patients with gastric cancer leads to upstaging in 6% and downstaging in 9% of patients.

4. **Laparoscopy** significantly enhances the accuracy of staging in patients with gastric cancer. Routine use of laparoscopy has been shown to detect small-volume peritoneal and liver metastases in 20% to 30% of patients believed to have locoregional disease, thereby avoiding unnecessary laparotomy in these patients (*Br J Surg* 1985;72:449, *Ann Surg* 1997;225:262). Although laparoscopic ultrasound enhances the accuracy of staging in other gastrointestinal cancers, its role in gastric cancer awaits further study. Laparoscopy is not indicated in patients with T1 and T2 lesions, given the low incidence of metastases with these tumors (*J Am Coll Surg* 2003;196:965).

F. **Treatment. Surgery** is the mainstay of curative therapy in the absence of disseminated disease.

1. **Extent of surgical resection** generally involves a wide resection to achieve negative margins with en bloc resection of lymph nodes and any structures involved by local invasion. In general, gross margins of 6 cm, confirmed to be negative intraoperatively with frozen section, are usually required to ensure microscopically negative margins on final histologic analysis.

   a. **Proximal tumors** of the stomach comprise up to half of all gastric cancers and can be resected by total gastrectomy or proximal subtotal gastrectomy. Total gastrectomy with Roux-en-Y esophagojejunostomy is generally the preferred option to avoid postoperative morbidity of reflux esophagitis and impaired gastric emptying associated with proximal subtotal gastrectomy. Tumors of the GE junction may require esophagogastrectomy with cervical or thoracic anastomosis.

   b. **Midbody tumors** comprise 15% to 30% of tumors and generally require total gastrectomy to achieve adequate margins.

   c. **Distal tumors** may be resected by distal subtotal gastrectomy or total gastrectomy with no difference in overall survival (*Ann Surg* 1989;209:162, *Ann Surg* 1994;220:176). However, nutritional status and quality of life are superior following subtotal gastrectomy, making it the preferred option when adequate margins can be obtained while maintaining an adequate gastric remnant (*Ann Surg* 1997;226:613, *Ann Surg* 1999;230:170).

   d. **Early gastric cancers,** defined as tumors confined to the mucosa, have limited propensity for lymph node metastasis and may be treated by limited gastric resections or **endoscopic mucosal resection**. Experience outside of Japan with early gastric cancers is limited.

   e. **Laparoscopic gastric resections** have been reported for the treatment of gastric cancer, with advantages of reduced pain, shorter hospitalization, and improved quality of life. Long-term outcome with respect to cancer recurrence awaits further study in a randomized, controlled fashion.

2. **Extent of lymphadenectomy** has long been a controversial issue in the surgical management of gastric cancer. Early retrospective Japanese studies showed improved survival with radical lymph node dissections. A standard (D1) lymphadenectomy entails removal of perigastric nodes, whereas an extended (D2) resection includes removal of nodes along the left gastric, hepatic, splenic, and celiac arteries. Although the results of major trials attempting to answer this question have yielded confounding results, it is generally agreed on that, at high-volume centers, D2 lymphadenectomies that preserve the distal pancreas

and spleen can be performed without increased morbidity, improve staging accuracy, and yield a survival advantage in patients with stage II and III gastric cancer.

3. **Adjuvant therapy** for gastric cancer is important because the majority of patients with locoregional disease (all patients except those with T1-2N0M0 disease) are at high risk for local or systemic recurrence following curative surgery.

   a. **Adjuvant combined modality therapy.** Although adjuvant chemotherapy or radiation therapy alone has not shown much benefit in studies, a recent landmark trial was able to demonstrate significant improvement in overall and disease-free survival rates in patients with completely resected gastric cancer treated postoperatively with 5-fluorouracil (5-FU)/leucovorin chemotherapy coupled with radiation therapy (*N Engl J Med* 2001;345:725).

   b. **Neoadjuvant chemotherapy** for gastric cancer has the potential for improving patient tolerance, resectability rates (downstaging) and overall patient survival. A recently reported European trial demonstrated significant improvement in 5-year survival rates in patients with gastric cancer who were treated with six cycles of chemotherapy (three preoperatively and three postoperatively) compared to surgery alone (*N Engl J Med* 2006;355:11). Chemotherapy regimen in this trial consisted of epirubicin, cisplatin, and 5-FU. Furthermore, preoperative chemotherapy improved curative resection rates.

4. **Palliative therapy** of gastric cancer is important due to overall low cure rates. Generally, patients with peritoneal disease, hepatic or nodal metastases, or other poor prognostic factors benefit most from endoscopic palliation. Laparoscopic or open palliative surgical resection can be considered in patients with better prognosis and good performance status to prevent bleeding, obstruction, and perforation in patients with metastatic or otherwise unresectable cancer. Palliative surgical resections appear to provide superior relief of symptoms compared to surgical bypass. Palliative chemoradiation therapy also prolongs survival in patients and improves symptoms and quality of life when it can be administered safely.

IV. **PRIMARY GASTRIC LYMPHOMA (PGL)** accounts for fewer than 5% of gastric neoplasms. However, PGL comprises two thirds of all primary GI lymphomas because the stomach is the most commonly involved organ in extranodal lymphoma. PGLs are usually B-cell, non-Hodgkin lymphomas. Most PGLs occur in the distal stomach.

   A. Patients typically present in their sixth decade with symptoms similar to those of gastric adenocarcinoma (epigastric pain, weight loss, anorexia, nausea, vomiting, and occult GI bleeding). Diagnosis is typically made using endoscopy, and staging to detect systemic disease is performed using CT of chest/abdomen/pelvis, bone marrow biopsy, and biopsy of enlarged peripheral lymph nodes.

   B. Therapy of PGL has been advanced by the recognition that low-grade PGLs have features resembling mucosa-associated lymphoid tissue (MALT) and that the majority of low-grade MALT lymphomas are associated with *H. pylori* infection. Thus, **first-line therapy for low-grade MALT lymphomas is use of antibiotics directed at *H. pylori* eradication**, which leads to complete remission rates of 70% to 100%. Chemoradiation therapy is used as salvage therapy for failure of antibiotics. High-grade or non-MALT lymphomas are generally treated with chemoradiation therapy alone, with surgical resection reserved for those who fail chemoradiation or in emergency cases of hemorrhage or perforation.

V. **BENIGN GASTRIC TUMORS** account for fewer than 2% of all gastric tumors. They are usually located in the antrum or corpus. Presentation can be similar to that of peptic ulcer or adenocarcinoma, and diagnosis is made by EGD or contrast radiography.

   A. **Gastric polyps** are classified by histologic findings. Endoscopic removal is appropriate if the polyp can be completely excised.

   1. **Hyperplastic polyps** are regenerative rather than neoplastic and constitute 75% of gastric polyps. Risk of malignant transformation is minimal.

2. **Adenomatous polyps** are the second-most-common gastric polyp and are neo-plastic in origin. The incidence of carcinoma within the polyp is proportional to its size, with polyps of greater than 2 cm having a 24% incidence of malignancy. Patients with familial adenomatous polyposis have a 50% incidence of gastro-duodenal polyps and require endoscopic surveillance. Surgical resection with a 2- to 3-cm margin of gastric wall can often be performed laparoscopically and is required if endoscopic excision is not possible.

VI. GASTROINTESTINAL STROMAL TUMORS (GISTs) comprise only 3% of all gastric malignancies and arise from mesenchymal components of the gastric wall. The me-dian age at diagnosis is 60 years, with a slight male predominance. GISTs frequently display prominent extraluminal growth and can attain large sizes before becoming symptomatic.

A. Presentation can be varied and includes asymptomatic masses found incidentally on physical exam or radiographic studies, vague abdominal pain and discomfort secondary to mass effect, and GI hemorrhage as a result of necrosis of overlying mucosa. Diagnosis is made by endoscopy and fine needle aspiration biopsy. GISTs are graded according to tumor size and histologic frequency of mitoses. Staging is accomplished by CT of abdomen/pelvis and chest x-ray.

B. Treatment is open or laparoscopic surgical resection with 2-cm margins of grossly normal gastric wall to ensure negative histologic margins. En bloc resection of any structures involved by local invasion should be attempted, although lymphadenec-tomy is not indicated because lymph node metastases are rare. Metastasis occurs by hematogenous route, and hepatic involvement is common, as is local recurrence af-ter resection. GISTs are not radiosensitive nor responsive to traditional chemother-apy. However, most GISTs express the **c-kit** receptor, a tyrosine kinase that acts as a growth factor receptor. **Imatinib mesylate (Gleevec™)** is a small-molecule inhibitor of the c-kit receptor that has become first-line therapy for metastatic or recurrent GIST. Approximately 60% of patients experience a partial response, and when maximal response is achieved, surgical therapy should be considered for patients in whom all gross disease can be removed.

VII. GASTRIC CARCINOIDS are rare neuroendocrine tumors accounting for less than 1% of all gastric neoplasms. Carcinoid tumors arise from enterochromaffin-like cells and can be secondary to hypergastrinemia associated with pernicious anemia or chronic at-rophic gastritis. Tumors tend to be small, multiple, and asymptomatic, although larger solitary tumors may cause ulceration of overlying mucosa and symptoms similar to PUD. EGD with biopsy generally provides diagnosis. Treatment of large (>2 cm), soli-tary tumors is gastrectomy because these have the highest invasive potential. Treatment for smaller, multifocal tumors is less clear, with options ranging from observation, gas-trectomy to include the tumors, and antrectomy without inclusion of tumors to reduce gastrin levels and induce tumor regression.

VIII. POSTGASTRECTOMY SYNDROMES are caused by changes in gastric emptying as a consequence of gastric operations. They may occur in up to 20% of patients who undergo gastric surgery, depending on the extent of resection, disruption of the vagus nerves, status of the pylorus, type of reconstruction, and presence of mechanical or functional obstruction. Clearly defining the syndrome that is present in a given patient is critical to developing a rational treatment plan (*World J Surg* 2003;27:725). Most are treated nonoperatively and resolve with time.

A. Nutritional disturbances occur in 30% of patients after gastric surgery, either as a result of functional changes or postgastrectomy syndromes. Prolonged **iron, folate, vitamin B$_{12}$, calcium, and vitamin D deficiencies** can result in anemia, neuropathy, dementia, and osteomalacia. These can be prevented with supplementation.

B. Dumping syndrome is thought to result from the rapid emptying of a high-osmolar carbohydrate load into the small intestine. Gastric resection leads to the loss of reservoir capacity and the loss of pylorus function. Dumping syndrome is most common after Billroth II reconstruction.

1. **Early dumping** occurs within 30 minutes of eating and is characterized by nau-sea, epigastric distress, explosive diarrhea, and vasomotor symptoms (dizziness, palpitations, flushing, diaphoresis). It is presumably caused by rapid fluid shifts

in response to the hyperosmolar intestinal load and release of vasoactive peptides from the gut. Symptoms are relieved by recumbence or saline infusion.

2. **Late dumping** symptoms are primarily vasomotor and occur 1 to 4 hours after eating. The hormonal response to high simple carbohydrate loads results in hyperinsulinemia and reactive hypoglycemia. Symptoms are relieved by carbohydrate ingestion.

3. **Treatment** is primarily nonsurgical and results in improvement in nearly all patients over time. Meals should be smaller in volume but increased in frequency, liquids should be ingested 30 minutes after eating solids, and simple carbohydrates should be avoided. Use of the long-acting somatostatin analog octreotide results in significant improvement and persistent relief in 80% of patients when behavioral modifications fail (*Clin Endocrinol* 1999;51:619). If reoperation is necessary, conversion to Roux-en-Y gastrojejunostomy is usually successful.

C. **Alkaline reflux gastritis** is most commonly associated with Billroth II gastrojejunostomy and requires operative treatment more often than other postgastrectomy syndromes. It is characterized by the triad of constant (not postprandial) epigastric pain, nausea, and bilious emesis. Vomiting does not relieve the pain and is not associated with meals. Endoscopy reveals inflamed, beefy-red, friable gastric mucosa and can rule out recurrent ulcer as a cause of symptoms. Bile reflux into the stomach is occasionally seen. Enterogastric reflux can be confirmed by hydroxy iminodiacetic acid (HIDA) scan. Mechanical obstruction is absent, distinguishing alkaline reflux gastritis from loop syndromes. **Nonoperative therapy** consists of frequent meals, antacids, and cholestyramine to bind bile salts but is usually ineffective. **Surgery** to divert bile flow from the gastric mucosa is the only proven treatment. The creation of a long-limb (45-cm) Roux-en-Y gastrojejunostomy effectively eliminates alkaline reflux and is the preferred option for most patients (*Gastroenterol Clin North Am* 1994;23:281).

D. **Roux stasis syndrome** may occur in up to 30% of patients after Roux-en-Y gastroenterostomy (*Am J Surg* 2003;186:269). It is characterized by chronic abdominal pain, nausea, and vomiting that is aggravated with eating. It results from functional obstruction due to disruption of the normal propagation of pacesetter potentials in the Roux limb from the proximal duodenum, as well as altered motility in the gastric remnant. Near-total gastrectomy to remove the atonic stomach can improve gastric emptying and is occasionally useful in patients with refractory Roux stasis. Use of an "uncut" Roux-en-Y reconstruction (*Am J Surg* 2001;182:52) may preserve normal pacemaker propagation and prevent the development of the syndrome.

E. **Loop syndromes** result from mechanical obstruction of either the **afferent** or **efferent** limbs of the Billroth II gastrojejunostomy. The location and etiology of the obstruction are investigated by plain abdominal x-rays, CT scan, upper GI contrast studies, and endoscopy. Relief of the obstruction may require adhesiolysis, revision of the anastomosis, occasionally bowel resection, or conversion of Billroth II to Roux-en-Y gastrojejunostomy.

1. **Afferent loop syndrome** can be caused acutely by bowel kink, volvulus, or internal herniation, resulting in severe abdominal pain and nonbilious emesis within the first few weeks after surgery. Lack of bilious staining of nasogastric drainage in the immediate postoperative period suggests this complication. Examination may reveal a fluid-filled abdominal mass, and laboratory findings may include elevated bilirubin or amylase. **Duodenal stump blowout** results from progressive afferent limb dilation, leading to peritonitis, abscess, or fistula formation. In the urgent setting, jejunojejunostomy can effectively decompress the afferent limb. A more **chronic form** of afferent loop syndrome results from partial mechanical obstruction of the afferent limb. Patients present with postprandial right upper quadrant pain relieved by bilious emesis that is not mixed with recently ingested food. Stasis can lead to bacterial overgrowth and subsequent bile salt deconjugation in the obstructed loop, causing **blind loop syndrome** (steatorrhea and vitamin B_{12}, folate, and iron deficiency) by interfering with fat and vitamin B_{12} absorption.

2. **Efferent loop syndrome** results from intermittent obstruction of the efferent limb of the gastrojejunostomy. Patients complain of abdominal pain and bilious emesis months to years after surgery, similar to the situation with regard to a proximal small bowel obstruction.

F. **Postvagotomy diarrhea** has an incidence of 20% after truncal vagotomy and is thought to result from alterations in gastric emptying and vagal denervation of the small bowel and biliary tree. The diarrhea is typically watery and episodic. Treatment includes antidiarrheal medications (loperamide, diphenoxylate with atropine, cholestyramine) and decreasing excessive intake of fluids or foods that contain lactose. Symptoms usually improve with time, and surgery is rarely indicated.

IX. **MORBID OBESITY** is a condition characterized by the pathologic accumulation of excess body fat. It is defined as a body mass index [BMI = weight (kg)/height (m^2)] equal to or greater than 40, which generally correlates with an actual body weight 100 lb greater than ideal body weight.

A. **Epidemiology.** Obesity is a disease process that has reached epidemic proportions worldwide, with the highest prevalence in the United States, where 5% of the adult population is morbidly obese (*Obes Surg* 2003;13:329, *JAMA* 1999;282:1519, *JAMA* 2002;286:1195). Obesity is also becoming increasingly prevalent in the pediatric population (*JAMA* 2002;288:1728).

B. The **etiology** of morbid obesity is poorly understood and thought to result from an imbalance in biologic, psychosocial, and environmental factors governing caloric intake and caloric expenditure. Risk factors for the development of morbid obesity include **genetic predisposition**, diet, and culture.

C. Most patients with morbid obesity present with one or more of a number of weight-related comorbidities. Patients with **central** obesity (android or "apple" fat distribution) are at higher risk for development of obesity-related complications than those with **peripheral** obesity (gynecoid or "pear" fat distribution). This is due to increased visceral fat distribution, producing increased intra-abdominal pressure and increasing fat metabolism (with subsequent hyperglycemia, hyperinsulinemia, and peripheral insulin resistance). Table 9-2 lists some of the medical complications associated with morbid obesity. In addition to the aforementioned comorbidities, obesity also increases mortality. One study showed a 12-fold increase in mortality among young morbidly obese men (*JAMA* 1980;243:443); a more recent study estimated that white males with a BMI of 45 or greater lose 13 years of life due to obesity, and black males with similar BMIs lose 20 years of life (*JAMA* 2003;289:187).

D. **Treatment** of morbid obesity is of paramount importance because of the many medical sequelae associated with obesity, nearly all are reversible on resolution of the obese state.

1. **Lifestyle changes** in diet, exercise habits, and behavior modification are first-line therapy for all obese patients. In combination, such changes can achieve 8% to 10% weight loss over a 6-month period, but losses are sustained at 1 year in only 60% of patients. However, certain comorbidities, such as diabetes, benefit from as little as 3% weight loss, and lifestyle changes alone may be sufficient in patients with BMI less than 27.

2. **Pharmacotherapy** is second-tier therapy used in patients with BMI greater than 27 and in combination with lifestyle changes. Currently, sibutramine, an appetite suppressant, and orlistat, a lipase inhibitor that reduces lipid absorption, are the only approved drugs for weight loss treatment. Weight loss with these agents is 6% to 10% at 1 year, but relapse rates after discontinuation of the drugs are high.

3. **Bariatric surgery** is the most effective approach for achieving durable weight loss in the morbidly obese. Multiple studies have confirmed the superiority of surgery to nonsurgical approaches in achieving and maintaining weight reduction in the morbidly obese (*N Engl J Med* 1984;310:352, *Int J Obes Relat Metab Disord* 2001;25(Suppl 1):S2). A National Institutes of Health Consensus Development Conference on morbid obesity established guidelines for the evaluation

TABLE 9-2	Complications of Morbid Obesity

Cardiac
  Hypertension
  Coronary artery disease
  Heart failure
  Arrythmias
Pulmonary
  Obesity hypoventilation syndrome
  Obstructive sleep apnea
  Respiratory insufficiency of obesity (pickwickian syndrome)
  Pulmonary embolism
Metabolic
  Type II diabetes
  Hyperlipidemia
  Hypercholesterolemia
  Nonalcoholic steatohepatitis
Musculoskeletal
  Degenerative joint disease
  Lumbar disc disease
  Osteoarthritis
Gastrointestinal
  Cholelithiasis
  Gastroesophageal reflux disease
  Hernias
Vascular
  Deep venous thrombosis
  Venous stasis ulceration
Infectious
  Fungal infections
  Necrotizing soft tissue infections
Genitourinary
  Nephrotic syndrome
  Stress urinary incontinence
Gynecologic
  Polycystic ovary syndrome
Neurologic/psychiatric
  Pseudotumor cerebri
  Depression
  Stroke
  Low self-esteem
Oncologic
  Cancers of uterus, breast, colon/rectum, and prostate

and treatment of morbidly obese patients with bariatric surgical procedures (*Ann Intern Med* 1991;115:956).

   a. **Indications.** Patients who have failed intensive efforts at weight control using medical means are candidates for bariatric surgery if they have a body mass index greater than 40 or greater than 35 with weight-related comorbidities.
   b. **Preoperative evaluation.** A bariatric multidisciplinary team including primary care physicians, dietitians, physical therapists, anesthesiologists, nurses, and psychiatrists or psychologists evaluates a patient's weight history, dietary

habits, motivation, social history, and comorbid medical conditions prior to surgery.

  c. **Benefits** of surgery are related to reversal of the disease processes associated with severe obesity. Hypertension completely resolves in 62% of patients and resolves or improves in 79%. Diabetes is completely resolved in 77% of patients and resolves or improves in 86%. Obstructive sleep apnea resolves or improves in 85% of patients and hyperlipidemia improves in 70% (*JAMA* 2004;292:1724). The quality of life is markedly better. Most importantly, recent studies demonstrate reduced mortality rates in morbidly obese patients undergoing bariatric surgery compared to matched controls (*J Am Coll Surg* 2004;199:543, *Ann Surg* 2004;240:416).

E. Bariatric surgical procedures can generally be divided into two types: **restrictive procedures**, which limit the amount of food that can be ingested, and **malabsorptive procedures**, which limit the absorption of nutrients and calories from ingested food by bypassing predetermined lengths of small intestine. The four standard operations used to produce weight loss in the morbidly obese include adjustable gastric banding and vertical banded gastroplasty (restrictive procedures), biliopancreatic diversion with and without duodenal switch (malabsorptive procedures), and Roux-en-Y gastric bypass (combination). Sleeve gastrectomy, the first component of a duodenal switch operation, increasingly is being performed alone as a restrictive procedure.

  1. **Vertical banded gastroplasty (VBG)** creates a small gastric pouch based on the lesser curvature. VBG can be performed through an open or laparoscopic approach. Although it produces an initial excess weight loss of 50% to 60%, a significant proportion of patients suffer late complications, require reoperations, and have difficulty maintaining weight loss. Overall perioperative morbidity is less than 10% and mortality is less than 1%. Early complications are rare, but late complications of stomal stenosis or staple line dehiscence can occur in up to 50% of patients. It is technically easier to perform than gastric bypass and results in minimal long-term metabolic or nutritional deficiencies. However, randomized trials have shown inferior weight loss compared to gastric bypass, and with the advent of adjustable gastric banding, VBG has largely fallen out of favor (*Obes Surg* 1995;5:55, *Ann Surg* 1994;220:784).

  2. **Adjustable gastric banding** (AGB) involves open or laparoscopic placement of a silicone band with an inflatable balloon around the proximal stomach at the angle of His. The band is connected to a reservoir that is implanted over the rectus sheath. The patient undergoes serial adjustments to inflate the band and create a small proximal gastric pouch. Excess weight loss is approximately 50%. Perioperative mortality is exceedingly low (0.05%), and overall complication rate is near 11%. Most complications are related to band slippage, which presents with obstructive symptoms or problems with the port (kinking or leaking of access tubing). Band erosion can occur but is far less frequent than the aforementioned complications. Advantages include safety, adjustability, and reversibility, whereas disadvantages include need for frequent postoperative visits.

  3. **Roux-en-Y gastric bypass (RYGBP)** is the most popular bariatric surgical procedure performed in the United States. A 30-mL proximal gastric pouch is created either by transection or by occlusion using a stapling device. A 1-cm-diameter anastomosis is then performed between the pouch and a Roux limb of small bowel. This results in a small reservoir, a small passage for pouch emptying, and bypass of the distal stomach, duodenum, and proximal jejunum. The length of the Roux limb directly correlates with the degree of postoperative weight loss, with a 75-cm limb used for standard gastric bypasses and a 150-cm limb used for the superobese. Gastric bypass results in weight loss superior to that achieved with restrictive procedures, with mean excess weight loss of 70%. Perioperative mortality is 1%, and despite aggressive prophylaxis, **pulmonary embolism** (PE) remains the most common cause of death after bariatric surgery. Anastomotic leak at the gastrojejunostomy is another serious early complication, occurring in approximately 2% of cases. Unexplained **tachycardia** is often

the only presenting sign of either complication in the perioperative period and warrants prompt investigation. Other early complications include wound infection (4% to 10%), gastric remnant dilation, and Roux limb obstruction. Late complications include incisional hernia (15% to 25%), stomal stenosis (2% to 14%), marginal ulcer (2% to 10%), bowel obstruction (2%), and internal hernia (1%). Early or late **bowel obstruction** after RYGBP can be a life-threatening complication and generally requires prompt reoperation because of its association with internal hernia and potential for bowel strangulation. **CT scan with oral contrast** is the best diagnostic test to evaluate for leak or obstruction after RYGBP. Nutritional complications include folate, vitamin B_{12}, iron, and calcium deficiency. Dumping syndrome occurs in many patients and may reinforce dietary behavior modification to avoid sweets and high-calorie foods. Laparoscopic RYGBP is a technically challenging but safe procedure when performed by surgeons with advanced laparoscopic skills. Laparoscopic RYGBP produces equal excess weight loss and has similar mortality and leak rates as the open procedure. Its main advantages are reduced postoperative pain, reduced length of stay, and significantly reduced wound-related complications, such as wound infections, dehiscence, and incisional hernias.

4. **Biliopancreatic diversion (BPD)** and **biliopancreatic diversion with duodenal switch (BPD-DS)** are two additional procedures for morbidly obese patients. BPD requires antrectomy with formation of a 200-cm alimentary channel and a 50- to 75-cm common channel. BPD-DS includes a sleeve gastrectomy, preservation of the pylorus, a 150-cm alimentary channel, and a 75- to 100-cm common channel. These procedures are done at select centers for the superobese and those who have failed to maintain weight loss following gastric bypass or restrictive procedures. Long-term outcomes indicate excess weight loss of 75% at 1 year, but nutritional deficiencies are more common than for RYGBP. Postoperative complications include anemia (30%), protein-calorie malnutrition (20%), dumping syndrome, and marginal ulceration (10%). These procedures are technically demanding and the applicability of these procedures to the obese population remains to be determined.

5. **Sleeve gastrectomy,** the first component of a duodenal switch operation, can be used alone as a purely restrictive procedure for the treatment of morbid obesity. It does not produce malabsorption and is technically easier to perform than BPD-DS or RYGBP. Preliminary reports have demonstrated 70% to 80% excess body weight loss at 1 year, but long-term outcomes and durability of this procedure remain unknown. It may be indicated as an initial procedure in the superobese population to induce enough weight loss to make BPD-DS or RYGBP technically more feasible.

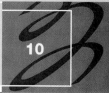

SMALL INTESTINE

Charles Robertson and David W. Dietz

10

I. EMBRYOLOGY

A. Origin. The small intestine forms during the fourth week of fetal development. The duodenum arises from the foregut, and the jejunum and ileum derive from the fetal midgut. The endoderm forms the absorptive epithelium and the secretory glands. The splanchnic mesoderm gives rise to the rest of the intestinal wall, including the musculature and the serosa.

B. Rotation. During the fifth week of fetal development, the intestine herniates through the umbilicus, rotating 90 degrees around the axis of the vitelline duct and the superior mesenteric artery. By the 10th week, the intestine returns to the abdominal cavity and rotates another 180 degrees. This rotation places the ligament of Treitz in the left upper quadrant and the cecum into the right upper quadrant. Around the fourth month, the cecum descends to the right lower quadrant.

C. Lumen formation. Between the fourth and seventh weeks, the small intestine is lined by cuboidal cells. Rapid proliferation occasionally occludes the lumen, particularly in the duodenum. Through apoptosis, the lumen regains patency by the 10th week.

II. ANATOMY

A. Gross anatomy. The small intestine begins at the pylorus and extends approximately 3 m to the ileocecal valve. The duodenum measures 20 cm. The first portion, the bulb, is intraperitoneal, with the remaining second, third, and fourth portions retroperitoneal. The second portion is particularly important because biliary and pancreatic secretions enter at the ampulla of Vater. The jejunum measures approximately 100 cm, and the ileum measures 150 cm. The jejunum and ileum can be differentiated by closely examining the mesenteric blood supply. Jejunal arcades are fewer and larger than ileal arcades, with longer vessels between the arcades and the bowel wall. Furthermore, the jejunum has many circumferential mucosal folds called plicae circularis.

B. Vascular supply. The pancreaticoduodenal arteries supply the duodenum, connecting the gastroduodenal and superior mesenteric arteries. The superior mesenteric artery (SMA) supplies the jejunum and ileum. The superior mesenteric vein runs parallel to the SMA and provides the venous drainage of the small bowel, joining with the splenic vein to form the portal vein.

C. Lymphatic drainage. The submucosal Peyer patches feed small lymphatics extending to the mesenteric lymph nodes. From there, drainage parallels the course of the named blood vessels and eventually accumulates at the subdiaphragmatic cysterni chyli before entering the thoracic duct.

D. Innervation. The vagus nerve is the origin for all abdominal parasympathetic fibers and plays an important role in regulating intestinal secretions and motility. These fibers cross mesenteric ganglia, particularly the celiac ganglion, and innervate the myenteric ganglion cells within the walls of the small intestine. Three sets of sympathetic nerves innervate the gut. They form a plexus around the superior mesenteric artery and modulate intestinal blood supply, secretion, and motility. Sympathetic nerves carry all pain signals from the intestine.

E. Anatomy of the intestinal wall is uniform from the duodenum to the ileocecal valve, consisting of four distinct tissue layers.

1. **Mucosa.** The epithelium, lamina propria, and muscularis mucosae compose the mucosa that lines the lumen of the gut.

   a. The **epithelium** has both villi and crypts. The *villi* are protrusions of the epithelial layer into the lumen that act to dramatically increase absorptive capacity. The *crypts* are the sites of pluripotent cells that give rise to the absorptive enterocytes (over 95% of the epithelial layer), *Paneth cells* secrete lysozyme, tumor necrosis factor, and cryptidins, which function in nonspecific immunity. *Goblet cells* secrete mucus. There are more than ten different subpopulations of *enteroendocrine cells*, which secrete a variety of hormones. Of note, the entire intestinal lining is replaced every 3 to 5 days.

   b. The **lamina propria** is a layer of loose connective tissue between the epithelial lining and the muscularis mucosae. Peyer patches, collections of lymphocytes that span the lamina propria and submucosa, are crucial for mucosal immunity.

   c. The **muscularis mucosa** is a layer of muscle separating the mucosa from the submucosa.

2. **Submucosa.** This layer of connective tissue adjacent to the mucosa is the strongest layer of the intestinal wall. Blood vessels and nerves run within this layer, including Meissner ganglion cells.

3. **Muscularis propria** consists of a thicker, inner circular layer and an outer longitudinal layer of smooth muscle cells. The Auerbach (myenteric) ganglion cells are located between those layers.

4. **Serosa** is a single layer of flat mesothelial cells composing the outermost layer of the small bowel. Serosa lines the extraluminal surface of the anterior duodenum and the entire jejunum and ileum.

F. **Enterocyte histology.** Two particular structures enhance the absorptive area of an enterocyte. Microvilli (tiny apical protrusions or folds projecting into the lumen) and a glycocalyx coating outside the cell membrane both increase absorptive capacity. Digestive enzymes, such as disaccharidases, and sodium-nutrient cotransporters are located in the apical membrane. In the lateral membrane, tight junctions prevent crossing of intraluminal contents across the epithelial layer. Intermediate junctions and desmosomes also help to maintain the barrier function of the intestinal epithelium. Na-K ATPases and passive nutrient transporters are located in the basal membrane.

III. **PHYSIOLOGY** of the small intestine involves a complex balance between absorption and secretion. The gut is also the largest endocrine organ in the human body.

A. **Absorption** is the principal function of the gastrointestinal (GI) tract.

   1. **Water.** Under normal circumstances, approximately 7 to 10 L of fluid enter the small intestine each day, but only 1 L reaches the colon. Of this fluid, 2 L are derived from oral intake, 1 L from saliva, 2 L from gastric secretion, 2 L from pancreatic secretion, 1 L from bile, and 1 L from small-intestinal secretion. Alterations in small-bowel permeability, tonicity of enteric substances, or rate of transit can result in diarrhea and large volume losses.

   2. The majority of **electrolyte** absorption occurs in the small intestine. The most important electrolytes absorbed are sodium, chloride, and calcium. Sodium absorption occurs through passive diffusion, countertransport with hydrogen, and cotransport with chloride, glucose, and amino acids. Chloride is absorbed in exchange for bicarbonate, which accounts for the alkalinity of the luminal contents. Calcium is actively absorbed in the proximal small intestine by a process that is stimulated by vitamin D. Emesis, diarrhea, obstruction, and small-bowel ostomy effluent can result in impaired small-bowel electrolyte absorption.

   3. **Bile salts** and **vitamin B_{12}–intrinsic factor** complexes are absorbed in the terminal ileum. Resection that leaves less than 100 cm of the ileum can result in bile acid deficiencies that limit absorption of the fat-soluble vitamins A, D, E, and K. Vitamin B_{12} deficiency can result in chronic megaloblastic anemia (pernicious anemia).

   4. **Nutrients.** The absorption of carbohydrates, proteins, and fat is discussed in Chapter 2 and in the next section.

B. Digestion. Macronutrient digestion by salivary, gastric, biliary, and pancreatic secretions is covered in Chapter 2. This section discusses digestion at the level of the
enterocyte.

1. Brush border peptidases and disaccharidases break down peptides and disac-
charides into simple amino acids and monosaccharides.

2. Active transport via Na-K ATPases in the basolateral membrane of enterocytes keeps the intracellular Na concentration very low. This sodium gradient
enables Na-nutrient cotransporters to move amino acids and monosaccharides
into enterocytes.

3. Passive transport. After digestion by pancreatic lipases, triglycerides and fatty
acids form micelles with bile salts. These micelles diffuse across the apical membrane and are reconstituted into chylomicrons, which subsequently enter submucosal lymphatics.

C. Motility

1. Types of contractions

a. Circular muscle contractions can temporarily segment the intestine for improved mixing of contents or they can propel food toward the colon if they
progress caudad.

b. When the **longitudinal muscle** contracts, sleeve contractions shorten the intestinal length, helping to propel food forward.

2. Neurohumoral effects. Vagal cholinergic input and hormones such as motilin
and cholecystokinin (CCK) stimulate contractions. Conversely, sympathetic neurons inhibit peristalsis.

3. During the **fasting state**, the migrating motor complex (MMC) performs the
housekeeping function of clearing the lumen of debris. After a period of rest,
random contractions of moderate strength are followed by several very strong
contractions.

4. During the **fed state**, contractions occur more frequently and last longer. Of
interest, multiple areas of the small bowel may contract at the same time. From
each site of contraction, peristalsis proceeds caudally for a varying distance.

D. Immunity. Tight junctions between the enterocyte apical membranes provide a
barrier function and prevent pathogens from crossing the epithelium. Mucosal
plasma cells secrete immunoglobulin A **(IgA),** which binds intraluminal pathogens
and targets them for destruction.

1. M cells are located in the epithelial layer over the Peyer patches. They facilitate
the conveying of antigens directly to macrophages and lymphocytes and help to
initiate acquired immunity to luminal pathogens.

2. $\gamma\delta$ T cells can be located within vacuoles of M cells and seem to have immunosuppressive effects. This may explain nonreactivity to ingested food.

E. Endocrine function is regulated by neural, hormonal (both autocrine and
paracrine), and anatomic mechanisms.

1. Cholecystokinin is produced by duodenal and jejunal I cells and enteric nerves
in response to intraluminal amino acids and fats. CCK induces gallbladder contraction, pancreatic enzyme secretion, and relaxation of the sphincter of Oddi.

2. Enteroglucagon from ileal and colonic L cells is produced in response to intraluminal fat and bile acids. Of note, inflammatory processes, such as Crohn
disease and celiac sprue, can dramatically increase enteroglucagon secretion.

3. Gastric inhibitory peptide (GIP), secreted by duodenal and jejunal K cells
in response to active transport of monosaccharides, long-chain fatty acids, and
amino acids, inhibits gastric acid and pepsinogen secretion and gastric emptying
but stimulates insulin release.

4. Duodenal G cells secrete **gastrin** in response to vagal stimulation and intraluminal peptides. Gastrin stimulates acid secretion by the gastric fundus and body
and increases gastric mucosal blood flow.

5. Motilin is produced by duodenal and jejunal M cells in response to duodenal
acid, vagal stimulation, and gastrin-releasing peptide. Motilin initiates phase III
of the MMC during the fasting state. Erythromycin is useful as a promotility
agent due to its action as a motilin agonist.

6. Duodenal and jejunal S cells release **secretin** in response to acid, bile salts, and fatty acids in the duodenum. Secretin increases bicarbonate and water secretion from pancreatic ducts. It inhibits gastric acid secretion and gastric motility.

7. **Somatostatin** broadly inhibits gut exocrine and endocrine function. Somatostatin and its analog, **octreotide,** are often used to decrease the volume of intestinal secretions in patients with enterocutaneous fistulas. Intestinal D cells and enteric neurons secrete somatostatin in response to intraluminal fat, protein, and acid.

8. **Vasoactive intestinal peptide (VIP)** is secreted throughout the small intestine in response to vagal stimulation. VIP increases mesenteric blood flow, intestinal motility, and pancreatic and intestinal secretions.

IV. SMALL-BOWEL OBSTRUCTION (SBO)

A. **Mechanical obstruction** can be partial, allowing some distal passage of gas or fluid, or complete, with total occlusion of the lumen. In a strangulated obstruction, the involved bowel has vascular compromise, which can ultimately lead to infarction and perforation of the intestinal wall. No clinical or laboratory values reliably differentiate simple from strangulated obstructions, although constant, as opposed to crampy, abdominal pain, fever, leukocytosis, and acidosis should raise the index of suspicion considerably. **Ileus** implies failure of peristalsis without mechanical obstruction. It can be caused by recent abdominal operations, electrolyte disturbances, peritonitis, systemic infections, bowel ischemia, trauma, or medications.

B. **Etiology**

1. **Adhesions are the most common cause of small-bowel obstruction in U.S. adults.** Most adhesions result from previous abdominal operations or inflammatory processes, although isolated congenital adhesions can occur as well.

2. **Incarcerated hernias** are the second-most-common cause of small-bowel obstructions in industrialized nations. They are the most common cause of SBO worldwide. In industrialized nations, they are the most common cause of SBO in children and in patients without prior abdominal surgery.

3. **Intussusception** occurs when one portion of bowel (the intussusceptum) telescopes into another (the intussuscipiens). Tumors, polyps, enlarged mesenteric lymph nodes, or even a Meckel diverticulum may serve as lead points of the telescoped segment. Unlike in children, intussusception in an adult should always prompt a workup for bowel pathology.

4. **Volvulus** is often caused by adhesions or congenital anomalies such as intestinal malrotation. It more commonly occurs in the colon.

5. **Strictures** secondary to ischemia, inflammation (Crohn disease), radiation therapy, or prior surgery may cause obstruction.

6. **Gallstone ileus** occurs as a complication of cholecystitis. Fistulization between the biliary tree and the small bowel allows gallstones to travel distally and become lodged, typically at the ileocecal valve.

7. **External compression** from tumors, abscesses, hematomas, or other masses can cause functional SBO.

8. **Foreign bodies** typically pass without incident. Items presenting with obstruction may require operation if they cannot be retrieved endoscopically. Pathology due to swallowing foreign bodies is more common in institutionalized patients.

C. **Diagnosis** of SBO incorporates the full range of history, exam, and radiographic findings.

1. **Signs and symptoms**

a. Proximal small-bowel obstructions present with early bilious **vomiting.** Distal obstructions present later, and vomit can be thick and feculent.

b. **Abdominal distention** typically increases the more distal the obstruction.

c. **Abdominal pain** is poorly localized and often characterized as crampy and intermittent (i.e., colicky).

d. **Obstipation,** complete absence of flatus and bowel movement, occurs after the bowel distal to a complete obstruction is evacuated.

e. With a persistent obstruction, **hypovolemia** progresses due to impaired absorption, increased secretion ("third spacing"), and vomiting.

    f. Bloody bowel movements suggest strangulation or a diagnosis other than obstruction.

2. **Physical examination**
   a. Abnormal **vital signs** are generally indicative of hypovolemia (e.g., tachycardia and hypotension).
   b. **Abdominal exam** may reveal distension, prior surgical scars, and hernias. Palpation should make note of any masses. Peritoneal signs mandate prompt surgical evaluation and treatment. Digital rectal examination may reveal the presence of an obstructing rectal tumor or impacted stool.

3. **Laboratory evaluation.** In early stages of a small-bowel obstruction, laboratory values may be normal. As the obstruction progresses, lab values reflect dehydration, most commonly demonstrating a contraction alkalosis with hypochloremia and hypokalemia. An elevated white blood cell count (WBC) may suggest strangulation (*Am Surg* 2004;70:40).

4. **Radiologic evaluation**
   a. Characteristic findings of SBO on **abdominal plain films** are dilated loops of small bowel, air-fluid levels, and paucity of colorectal gas. These findings may be absent in early, proximal, and/or closed-loop obstructions. Gas within the bowel wall (pneumatosis intestinalis) or portal vein is suggestive of a strangulated obstruction. Free intra-abdominal air indicates perforation of a hollow viscus. The findings of air in the biliary tree and a radiopaque gallstone in the right lower quadrant are pathognomonic of gallstone ileus. Paralytic ileus appears as gaseous distention uniformly distributed throughout the stomach, small intestine, and colon.
   b. **Contrast studies** (small-bowel follow-through [SBFT] or enteroclysis) can localize the site of obstruction and suggest an etiology. Barium can be used if subtle mucosal lesions are sought (i.e., lead point in a patient with recurring intussusceptions) but should be avoided in acute obstructions due to the risk of barium impaction. Water-soluble contrast agents are indicated in most instances because they will not worsen the situation and may actually be therapeutic in the case of adhesive partial obstruction.
   c. **Computed tomography (CT)** is an excellent imaging modality for diagnosing small-bowel obstruction. It has the ability to localize and characterize the obstruction as well as give information regarding the cause of obstruction and the presence of other intra-abdominal pathology. Evidence suggests that CT scanning can improve the preoperative diagnosis of strangulation, with negative and positive predictive values above 90% (*J Gastrointest Surg* 2005;9:690).

5. **Differential diagnosis**
   a. **Mesenteric vascular ischemia** can produce colicky abdominal pain, especially after meals. Acute occlusion often presents with marked leukocytosis and severe abdominal pain out of proportion to physical findings. Angiography confirms the diagnosis.
   b. **Colonic obstruction** can easily be confused with a distal small-bowel obstruction, especially if the ileocecal valve is incompetent. A water-soluble contrast enema can aid in diagnosis. In any event, the initial management and evaluation of large- and small-bowel obstructions are the same.
   c. **Paralytic ileus** is a common diagnosis in surgical patients. A thorough history, physical exam, and radiologic workup should differentiate ileus from obstruction. Narcotic and psychiatric medications, recent abdominal operations, and electrolyte abnormalities are common causes of ileus.
   d. As in paralytic ileus, radiography of primary **hypomotility** disorders reveals gas throughout the entire GI tract with particular distention of the small bowel. Treatment for these chronic diseases consists of prokinetic drugs and dietary manipulation.

D. **Treatment** of SBO has evolved over the last decade and now includes primary prevention at the time of initial laparotomy.

1. **Antiadhesion barriers may be beneficial in reducing the severity of adhesions after surgery.** These products are applied to the surface of the bowel at the end of an operation and act as a barrier to adhesion formation between adjacent loops of bowel and between bowel and the parietal peritoneum. Although randomized studies support a reduction in the number and severity of adhesions after major abdominal surgeries, the effect on bowel obstruction is less clear. A multicenter trial of 1,791 patients comparing Seprafil to no treatment (*Dis Colon Rectum* 2005;49:1) found no difference in the overall rate of SBO (12% in both groups). There was a very modest reduction in the risk of SBO *requiring operation* over a mean follow-up of 3.5 years (1.8% vs. 3.4%; absolute risk reduction of 1.6%, number needed to treat = 63).

2. **Nonstrangulated** obstructions can be treated expectantly if the patient is clinically stable. The cornerstone of treating any bowel obstruction is adequate fluid resuscitation to achieve a urine output of at least 0.5 mL/kg/hour. This resuscitation must meet maintenance fluid and electrolyte needs for a nothing-by-mouth (NPO) patient as well as replace prior and ongoing losses from nasogastric (NG) decompression. During any trial of nonoperative management, it is imperative that the patient undergo serial abdominal examinations every 4 to 6 hours. If the patient deteriorates (worsening abdominal exam, peritonitis, shock) or simply fails to improve within a few days, laparotomy is indicated. In patients with a bowel obstruction secondary to an incarcerated hernia, attempts to reduce the hernia can be made with mild sedation and gentle force. After successful reduction, the patient should be monitored carefully for evidence of bowel infarction or perforation. Inability to reduce the hernia requires urgent operation. Other situations that may warrant a trial of nonoperative therapy include early postoperative obstruction, multiple prior episodes of obstruction, a history of multiple previous abdominal operations with extensive adhesions, abdominal irradiation, Crohn disease, and abdominal carcinomatosis.

3. **Strangulated** obstructions and those with peritonitis require prompt operative intervention. Mortality associated with gangrenous bowel can approach 30% if operation is delayed beyond 36 hours. Once again, fluid/electrolyte resuscitation and tube decompression are crucial in the preoperative preparation of the patient.

4. **Fluid replacement** should begin with an isotonic solution. Serum electrolyte values, hourly urine output, and central venous pressure can be monitored to assess adequacy of resuscitation. Antibiotics should be given only as prophylaxis prior to surgery.

5. **Operative intervention** is generally performed via midline incision, but a standard groin incision can be used in the case of an incarcerated inguinal or femoral hernia. During the exploration, all adhesions are lysed, and the source of obstruction is identified. Any gangrenous bowel is resected. The viability of adjacent or compromised bowel must be determined, and a second-look operation within 24 to 48 hours should be planned if any doubt exists. If the obstructing lesion cannot be resected, it may be bypassed. Placement of a gastrostomy tube for postoperative decompression should be considered in select cases.

E. Prognosis. The postoperative mortality from nonstrangulating obstruction is very low. Obstructions that are associated with strangulated bowel carry a mortality of 8% if operation is performed within 36 hours of the onset of symptoms. Mortality can approach 30% if operation is delayed beyond 36 hours.

V. MECKEL DIVERTICULUM is the most common congenital anomaly of the gastrointestinal tract. It occurs from failure of the vitelline or omphalomesenteric duct to obliterate by the sixth week of fetal development. It is a true diverticulum that contains all layers of the bowel wall and is located on the antimesenteric border of the ileum. Half contain heterotopic gastrointestinal mucosa, usually gastric. A "rule of two" covers common facts: The incidence is 2%; the male/female ratio is 2:1; patients typically present before the age of 2 years; location is 2 ft from the ileocecal valve; and the base is typically 2 in. in width and often contains two types of mucosa.

A. Diagnosis. The vast majority of Meckel diverticula are **asymptomatic**.

1. **Bleeding** is the most common presenting symptom. It tends to be painless and episodic. The source is typically acid-secreting gastric mucosa in the diverticulum that causes a peptic ulcer of adjacent normal ileum.

2. **Intestinal obstruction** occurs due to volvulus of the small bowel around a fibrous band connecting the diverticulum to the anterior abdominal wall. Intussusception or incarcerated hernia (Littré hernia) is the second-most-common presentation.

3. **Meckel diverticulitis** occurs in 20% of symptomatic patients and is often mistaken for acute appendicitis. Intraluminal obstruction of the diverticulum leads to inflammation, edema, ischemia, necrosis, and perforation in a manner similar to appendicitis.

4. **Differential diagnosis** may include appendicitis, colonic diverticulitis, or Crohn disease.

B. Treatment

1. **Resection** is indicated in the symptomatic patient. For patients who present with obstruction, simple diverticulectomy can be performed. Segmental resections should be performed for acute diverticulitis, a wide-based diverticulum, volvulus with necrotic bowel, or bleeding.

2. **Incidental diverticulectomy** during surgery for other abdominal pathology is not indicated. Lifelong morbidity associated with the presence of a Meckel diverticulum is extremely low.

VI. SMALL-INTESTINAL BLEEDING

A. General. Upper and lower gastrointestinal bleeding are discussed in Chapters 9 and 12, respectively. Small-bowel lesions are the most common cause of "obscure gastrointestinal bleeding," defined as hemorrhage that persists or recurs after negative initial upper and lower endoscopies.

B. Diagnosis

1. **Enteroscopy**

   a. **Push enteroscopy** employs a 400-cm enteroscope to visualize well into the jejunum. Its efficacy is highly dependent on the skill of the endoscopist. It can perform biopsy and therapeutic maneuvers. Intraoperative push endoscopy can sometimes be useful; the scope is introduced through a small enterotomy distal to the ligament of Treitz following exploratory laparotomy.

   b. **Extended small-bowel enteroscopy** depends on peristalsis to move the scope distally; thus, the procedure may require up to 8 hours for completion. Furthermore, it has no biopsy or therapeutic capabilities. It may visualize as much as 70% of the small intestine and may be more sensitive than conventional enteroclysis.

   c. **Capsule endoscopy.** In 2001, the Food and Drug Administration approved a disposable "camera pill" that is swallowed and images the entire GI tract as it passes from mouth to anus. A recent meta-analysis suggests that capsule endoscopy is superior to push enteroscopy and barium small-bowel imaging for diagnosing obscure GI bleeding (*ACP J Club* 2006;144:76).

   d. **Double-balloon enteroscopy** is a novel method developed in Japan in the late 1990s. It uses two inflatable balloons on the tip of an endoscope to relatively quickly negotiate the small bowel. The technique can be used antegrade or retrograde and allows therapeutic intervention. Although indications and clinical applications are evolving, double-balloon enteroscopy offers the promise that the small bowel may be fully accessible to endoscopic diagnosis and treatment in the same manner as the rest of the GI tract. It also offers the intriguing possibility of endoscopic visualization and/or endoscopic retrograde cholangiopancreatography (ERCP) in segments of the bowel previously inaccessible due to surgery (i.e., the Roux limb and gastric remnant after gastric bypass).

2. **Imaging**

   a. A **tagged red-blood cell** nuclear medicine scan is highly sensitive for the detection of gastrointestinal bleeding, detecting rates of hemorrhage as low as 0.5 mL/second. However, it is of limited utility in direct resection of a bleeding small-bowel lesion because it lacks anatomic detail.

  b. Angiography has a better ability to localize a bleeding small-bowel lesion, although it is less sensitive than a nuclear medicine study (detects bleeding at 1 mL/second). The angiographer can embolize metal coils into the bleeding mesenteric vessel or leave a catheter in place to assist in intraoperative localization of the lesion. Methylene blue can also be selectively injected to stain the target segment of intestine.

  3. Effective **surgical therapy** hinges on successful preoperative **localization** of the bleeding lesion. Unlike the remainder of the GI tract, the small bowel cannot be resected en bloc for intractable bleeding. Preoperative localization of the lesion for segmental resection is strongly advised because it might be very difficult to identify intraoperatively. The angiographic techniques described previously are invaluable in this regard.

VII. ENTERIC FISTULAS represent a challenge to any surgeon. The definition of a fistula is a communication or tract between two epithelialized surfaces (e.g., bowel, skin, bladder, etc.). They may be categorized according to anatomy, output, and etiology. In general, a **high-output fistula** is defined as greater than 500 mL effluent/day.

  A. Anatomic considerations

  1. External fistulas are the most common fistulas and connect an internal organ system with the skin, for example, enterocutaneous fistula.

  2. Internal fistulas connect two hollow structures of the same or different organ systems, for example, colovesical fistula.

  3. Proximal fistulas are located in the duodenum or jejunum. They are usually associated with high outputs of 3 L/day or more. Profound dehydration, malnutrition, and electrolyte disturbances are common.

  4. Distal fistulas arise in the ileum. They are associated with fewer complications than proximal fistulas, and they more often close with nonoperative treatment.

  B. Pathophysiology. Fistula-associated complications may be life-threatening and require rapid intervention to avoid morbidity and mortality. The overall mortality for all enteric fistulas is 5% to 20%.

  1. Loss of GI contents

  a. Hypovolemia. High-output fistulas may discharge large volumes of fluid that cannot be adequately replaced by enteral means, leading to dehydration and intravascular volume depletion.

  b. Acid-base and electrolyte abnormalities. Loss of large fluid volumes and associated electrolytes results in metabolic derangement. Severity is directly correlated with the quantity of fistula output.

  2. Malnutrition is caused by caloric intake insufficient to meet increased metabolic demands associated with fistula formation, such as the demands related to sepsis. In addition, substantial portions of the GI tract may be functionally excluded. The ensuing malabsorption leads to vitamin and mineral deficiency, as well as alterations in carbohydrate, fat, and protein metabolism.

  C. Etiology

  1. Abdominal operations are the leading cause of fistula formation. The risk is greatest for operations performed for inflammatory bowel disease, ischemia, malignancy, or extensive intestinal adhesions. Dissection may result in unrecognized bowel perforation, devascularization, and serosal disruption. Anastomotic disruption, leaks, and perianastomotic abscesses also are common causes. Malnutrition and immunosuppression significantly increase the risk of fistula formation.

  2. Crohn disease of the small bowel is a common cause of enterocutaneous fistulas.

  3. Diverticular disease causes fistulas when localized abscesses drain into adjacent organs. Common examples include colovesical and colovaginal fistulas. Internal fistulas should be suspected in patients with diverticular disease who exhibit persistent and recurrent sepsis.

4. Fistulas can form when **malignancy** perforates or invades adjacent structures. Healing does not occur if cancer is present, and resection is the only means of cure.

5. **Radiation enteritis** predisposes to fistula formation after operation, regardless of the temporal proximity of exposure.

6. Fistula formation may occur after penetrating **trauma** to the abdomen or pelvis. Unrecognized enterotomies as well as injuries that are repaired amid contamination may be prone to fistula formation. Viscus rupture caused by blunt trauma may go unrecognized, and subsequent abscess formation and drainage into adjacent structures may result in fistula formation. This most commonly occurs after rupture of the duodenum, colon, or pancreas into the retroperitoneum.

7. Other causes of GI fistulas include presence of a foreign body, vascular insufficiency, and amebiasis.

D. Diagnosis

1. **Imaging.** Defining fistula anatomy via contrast radiography can help to determine prognosis and assist in the planning of operative repair. Fistulography may be performed in mature fistula tracts (usually after 10 days) and typically provides good visualization of all tracts and sites of enteral communication. Oral contrast studies can demonstrate contrast extravasation through the fistula and are most valuable for assessing internal fistulas and distal obstruction. Contrast enema is the study of choice for rectal or colonic fistulas. CT scanning is of limited value in assessing fistula anatomy.

2. **Endoscopy** aids in the assessment of coexistent disease in the organ from which the fistula arises, such as peptic ulceration, inflammatory bowel disease, and cancer. Fistula openings themselves are often difficult to identify by endoscopy.

E. Treatment

1. **Natural history.** Most fistulas that close spontaneously will do so within 4 to 6 weeks. The frequency of closure is not necessarily related to the quantity of initial fistula output. The difficult decision on how long to wait for spontaneous closure depends on individual circumstances and the complexity of the underlying illness. There has been a trend toward allowing longer periods for fistula closure because of improved home intravenous therapy, parenteral nutrition, and use of somatostatin analogs to control the volume of output. If spontaneous closure does not appear likely, operative therapy is indicated. It is advisable to wait at least 3 months from the time of last laparotomy before reoperating. This allows adhesions to attenuate and the patient to recover nutritional status and general health.

2. **Fluid resuscitation.** Once initial hypovolemia is corrected, accurate measurement of ongoing fluid losses and prompt replacement are essential. Intravenous fluid administration is typically necessary because attempts at enteral replacement result in increased fluid loss from the fistula due to stimulation of gastrointestinal secretions. Electrolyte and acid-base status must be followed closely. Fluid replacement composition depends on the site of the fistula in the GI tract and the quantity of fluid loss, and content must be tailored to meet the specific replacement demands (see Chapter 4, Table 4-1). Sending a sample of fistula output for a basic metabolic profile may help to direct fluid replacement in difficult cases.

3. **Complete bowel rest.** This may reduce fistula drainage and simplify the evaluation and stabilization of the patient. Nasogastric suction has not proved beneficial except in the presence of distal obstruction.

4. **Nutritional support.** Early, aggressive parenteral nutritional therapy has dramatically decreased mortality from fistulas (*Am J Surg* 1964;108:157).

   a. **Enteral feeding** is preferred if it does not increase fistula output. Patients with low-output colonic or distal small-bowel fistulas can be safely fed. Standard enteral formulas are sufficient in most cases; however, if the available bowel is short, elemental feeding may maximize absorption. In proximal fistulas, feeding can be given distal to the fistula if enteral access is available (e.g., feeding jejunostomy tube in a gastric fistula).

    b. Parenteral nutrition can provide adequate nutrition in cases in which enteral feeding is not possible. Indications include intolerance to enteral nutrition, jejunal and ileal high-output fistulas, and proximal fistulas if distal enteral access is not possible. Complications of parenteral nutrition include hepatic dysfunction, trace element deficiencies, and venous catheter–related difficulties.

5. Sepsis is the main determinant of mortality from a fistula. Sepsis accompanies a large percentage of fistulas and is caused by undrained enteric leaks. A septic focus diminishes the potential for healing.

    a. Intra-abdominal abscess should be excluded in every patient presenting with a GI fistula. A CT scan, typically with oral and intravenous contrast, can diagnose the abscess and guide percutaneous drainage.

    b. Intravenous antibiotics directed against bowel flora are indicated when infection is present. Continuous bacterial seeding from the GI tract is an indication for operation if uncontrolled with drainage and appropriate antimicrobial therapy.

    c. Infected wounds are adequately opened and packed to allow complete drainage, débridement, and healing by secondary intention. Frequent dressing changes may be required.

6. Control of fistula drainage. Dressings can be used for low-output fistulas to absorb drainage fluid. However, prolonged contact of enteric contents with surrounding skin may impede healing and cause skin breakdown. Intubation of matured fistula tracts may be beneficial. A suction or sump drainage system for high-output fistulas is preferred. The addition of somatostatin analogs has shown mixed results. Some studies have found decreased fistula output (*Lancet* 1987;2:672) and decreased time to closure; however, these results have not been uniformly replicated. H_2-receptor antagonists reduce gastric and duodenal fistula output and provide stress ulceration prophylaxis; however, their efficacy in reducing time to fistula closure has not been proven.

7. Skin protection. Irritation and excoriation of skin surrounding the site of fistula drainage can be very painful, complicate wound management, and promote secondary infection. Skin surrounding a fistula should be protected with a barrier device or powder. The skin should be examined and cleansed frequently. A vacuum-assisted wound closure device may help to control skin irritation and speed fistula closure. The early involvement of an enterostomal therapy nurse is critical in the management of fistula patients.

F. Operative treatment is indicated when fistulas fail to heal with nonoperative measures and when sepsis cannot be controlled. Common conditions under which fistulas fail to close can be remembered with the aid of the mnemonic FRIEND: foreign body, radiation, inflammation or infection, epithelialization, neoplasm, or distal obstruction. The goals of operation are to eradicate the fistula tract and to restore the epithelial continuity of the associated organ systems.

1. Gastric fistulas arise from anastomotic breakdown or ulcer perforation and require operative repair. Most low-output gastric fistulas close spontaneously, for example, gastrostomy closure after removal of gastrostomy tubes. In cases that do not close, primary repair or serosal patch placement is usually successful.

2. Duodenal fistulas typically close spontaneously with nonoperative management. When operative intervention is required, primary closure of small duodenal wall disruptions may be performed, but duodenal stricture is associated with primary closure of large defects. Close proximity of the defect to the ampulla may also prevent primary closure. In these cases, duodenal wall integrity may be restored by serosal patch using another segment of bowel. Alternatively, a Roux-en-Y duodenoenterostomy may be performed to divert duodenal output into the bowel.

3. Small-bowel fistulas are typically cured with bowel resection and primary reanastomosis. In rare severe cases, a temporary diverting enterostomy may be necessary. For internal fistulas, if the openings are in close proximity, the involved region can be resected en bloc.

4. **Large-bowel fistulas** are associated with high spontaneous closure rates. Fluid and electrolyte abnormalities are rare because outputs tend to be low. However, sepsis rates may be greater. If operative closure is required, an adequate mechanical bowel preparation is important. Primary closure, as opposed to resection with primary reanastomosis, depends on associated conditions, the nutritional status of the patient, and the location and complexity of the lesion. It is rarely appropriate.

5. **Enteral feeding tubes** placed at the time of definitive repair may facilitate postoperative management. Antibiotic therapy and nutritional support should continue into the postoperative period.

VIII. **SHORT-BOWEL SYNDROME.** In the adult, the length of the small bowel varies from 300 to 600 cm and correlates directly with body surface area. Several factors determine the severity of short-bowel syndrome, including the extent of resection, the portion of the GI tract removed, the type of disease necessitating the resection, the presence of coexistent disease in the remaining bowel, and the adaptability of the remaining bowel. Generally, resection resulting in less than 120 cm of intact bowel leads to short-bowel syndrome (<150 cm if ending in an ileostomy, <75 cm if colon remains). Infants may survive resection of up to 85% of bowel owing to the enhanced ability of the bowel to adapt and grow with the child. Because of its specialized absorptive function, resection of the ileum is usually not well tolerated. However, the entire jejunum can be resected without serious adverse nutritional sequela.

A. **Etiology and pathophysiology.** Short-bowel syndrome is characterized by dehydration, electrolyte derangements, acidic diarrhea, steatorrhea, malnutrition, and weight loss. Congenital anomalies leading to short-bowel syndrome include intestinal atresia, midgut volvulus with intestinal necrosis, and necrotizing enterocolitis. In middle-aged adults, inflammatory bowel disease and trauma are the leading causes of massive intestinal resection. In the elderly, prominent causes include mesenteric ischemia and strangulated hernia.

1. **Adaptation.** The distal small intestine has the greatest adaptive potential and can assume many of the absorptive properties of the proximal GI tract. Cellular hyperplasia and bowel hypertrophy occur over a 2- to 3-year period, increasing the absorptive surface area. Fat absorption is the metabolic process most likely to be permanently impaired; other functions adjust and normalize fairly well.

2. **Fluid and electrolyte response.** Of the 8 to 10 L of fluid presented daily to the small intestine, only 1 to 2 L are delivered into the colon. Significant quantities of electrolytes are absorbed in this process. With short-bowel syndrome, this physiology is altered. Strict intake and output records and close monitoring of serum electrolytes are critical in the early management of patients with short-bowel syndrome.

3. **Malabsorption and malnutrition**

   a. **Gastric hypersecretion,** seen early in the postoperative period, can persist for prolonged periods. Increased acid load may injure distal bowel mucosa, leading to hypermotility and impaired absorption. The severity of hypersecretion correlates directly with the extent of bowel resection. This generally is more pronounced after jejunal than after ileal resection. Loss of an intestinal inhibitory hormone has been implicated.

   b. **Cholelithiasis.** Altered bilirubin metabolism after ileal resection increases the risk of gallstones secondary to a decreased bile salt pool, which causes a shift in the cholesterol saturation index. Chronic total parenteral nutrition (TPN) also increases risk of cholelithiasis.

   c. **Hyperoxaluria and nephrolithiasis.** Excessive fatty acids within the colonic lumen bind intraluminal calcium. Unbound oxalate, normally made insoluble by calcium binding and excreted in the feces, is thus absorbed readily, resulting in hyperoxaluria and calcium oxalate urinary stone formation.

   d. **Diarrhea and steatorrhea.** Rapid intestinal transit, presence of hyperosmolar enteric contents in the distal bowel, disruption of the enterohepatic bile acid circulation, and bacterial overgrowth all promote diarrhea and steatorrhea. Fat absorption is most severely impaired by ileal resection. The delivery of bile acids into the colon produces a reactive watery diarrhea that may be severe. Unabsorbed fats in the colon further inhibit absorption and stimulate secretion of water and electrolytes.

   e. Intestinal microflora. Loss of the ileocecal valve permits reflux of colonic bacteria into the small bowel. Intestinal dysmotility further promotes bacterial colonization. Bacterial overgrowth and changes in the indigenous microbial population result in pH alteration and deconjugation of bile salts, with resultant malabsorption, fluid loss, and decreased vitamin B_{12} absorption. Infectious diarrhea (bacterial or viral) is a major cause of morbidity.

B. Acutely, the primary goal is to stabilize the metabolic, respiratory, and cardiovascular parameters related to the fluid shift and sepsis that frequently accompany massive small-bowel resection.

   1. Deranged motility patterns and changes in intraluminal milieu may produce a **prolonged ileus.** Parenteral nutrition should be provided until GI function resumes. If ileus persists for an unduly prolonged period, mechanical obstruction or sepsis may be the cause.

   2. Gastric hypersecretion requires H_2-receptor antagonists or proton-pump inhibitors to reduce the hypersecretion response and protect against peptic ulceration. Antacids neutralize acid on contact and should be administered for nasogastric aspirate pH of less than 5.

   3. Nutritional support should be instituted early to maintain positive nitrogen balance and to promote wound healing and adaptation of the remaining bowel. Enteral nutrition has a positive trophic effect on the bowel mucosa and should be started as soon as possible. Feeding tubes placed at laparotomy can be very helpful. Even if caloric goals are not met, enteral formula stimulates the remaining intestine and facilitates adaptation. Feeds should initially be low volume, low fat, and isosmotic.

C. Chronic Treatment

   1. Diarrhea has many causes in short-bowel syndrome. Frequently, dietary modification improves symptoms. H_2-receptor antagonists reduce acid production and the volume of enteric contents. Chelating resins, such as cholestyramine, reduce intraluminal bile salts and subsequent diarrhea but affect the available systemic bile salt pools. Antisecretory medications, such as loperamide and somatostatin analog, may be beneficial. Low-dose oral narcotics, such as diphenoxylate hydrochloride and atropine (Lomotil) or codeine, are efficacious but addictive. Bacterial overgrowth should be evaluated by stool culture and prophylactic antimicrobials administered as needed.

   2. Nutritional support with supplemental vitamins, trace elements and minerals, and essential fatty acids should be given parenterally until adequate enteral absorption is established. The absorption of fat-soluble vitamins A, D, E, and K is especially likely to be compromised. Vitamin B_{12} and calcium absorption are also affected by altered fat absorption and should be supplemented. If required, chronic TPN can be administered nightly to permit normal daytime activities.

   3. Late complications, mostly secondary to metabolic derangements, are common. Problems include nephrolithiasis, cholelithiasis, nutritional deficiency (e.g., anemia, bone disease, coagulopathy), liver dysfunction, TPN-related complications, and central venous catheter–related problems, for example, sepsis or thrombosis. Anastomotic leak, fistula, stricture, and obstruction can also occur well beyond the early postoperative period. Late obstruction (partial or complete) is fairly common, and reoperative rates are high.

D. Surgical therapy. Various surgical procedures have been described for the management of short-bowel syndrome, although they have not been widely adopted. Most important is the prevention of complications by minimizing the extent of initial bowel resection. Bowel transplantation is not widely performed but is an alternative in some patients, especially those with massive resection and virtually no remaining bowel.

IX. CROHN DISEASE is an idiopathic, chronic, granulomatous inflammatory disease that can affect any part of the GI tract from the mouth to the anus. It is an incurable, slowly progressive disease characterized by episodes of exacerbation and remission. The incidence is 4/100,000, with a bimodal age distribution among those 15 to 29 and 55 to 70 years old.

A. The **etiology** of Crohn disease is unknown but is believed to involve interplay between genetic and environmental factors. Pathogenesis likely relates to a defective mucosal barrier and/or dysregulated intestinal immunity, which leads to a chronic inflammatory reaction within the intestinal wall. The genetic component is strong: Crohn disease is 25 times more common among patients with a family history and has a concordance rate of 60% in monozygotic twins. Environmental factors such as smoking increase the risk of developing Crohn disease.

B. The **terminal ileum** is the most common site involved (75% of patients). Three "patterns" of disease have been described.

  1. Ileocolic disease involves the terminal ileum (and in some cases the cecum) and is the most common form, affecting 40% of patients.

  2. Small-bowel-only disease (30% of patients) is confined to the more-proximal small intestine.

  3. Colonic disease (30% of patients) affects only the large intestine. Perianal Crohn disease commonly coexists with these more proximal forms of the disease, especially when the colon is involved. Disease confined to the anorectum is rare (5%).

C. Grossly, diseased bowel is thickened, displays creeping fat and corkscrew vessels, and has a shortened fibrotic mesentery containing enlarged lymph nodes. The mucosal lesions include pinpoint hemorrhages, aphthous ulcers, deep linear fissures, and, ultimately, **cobblestoning**. It is common for these lesions to occur segmentally along the intestine rather than being contiguous.

  1. Crohn disease is characterized by full-thickness, **transmural inflammation** of the bowel wall. The inflammation begins adjacent to the crypts, leading to the development of crypt abscesses, aphthous ulcers, and linear fissures. The transmural involvement can produce sinus tracts and fistulas between crypt abscesses and adjacent segments of bowel.

  2. Granulomas are found in the bowel wall in 40% to 60% of patients, and they are detected in mesenteric lymph nodes in 25% of patients.

D. Clinical presentation of Crohn disease is highly variable. Patient history is important in narrowing the differential diagnosis. **Physical examination** is performed with special attention to the abdominal and anorectal areas. No physical signs are pathognomonic for Crohn disease, although the appearance of the perianal area described earlier is highly suggestive. Laboratory evaluation is nonspecific.

  1. Diarrhea occurs in almost all patients and usually is not bloody unless the colon is involved. Patients with ileal disease may be bile salt deficient, resulting in steatorrhea. Mucosal inflammation with decreased absorption and increased secretion also results in diarrhea.

  2. Abdominal pain typically is intermittent, crampy, worse after meals, relieved by defecation, and poorly localized. A mass caused by thickened bowel, a phlegmon, or an abscess may be palpable.

  3. Weight loss occurs as a result of decreased oral intake, malabsorption, protein-losing enteropathy, and steatorrhea. Children with Crohn disease develop vitamin and mineral deficiencies and growth retardation.

  4. Constitutional symptoms such as malaise and fever are common.

  5. Anorectal disease is a common finding and may precede intestinal symptoms by several years. Such lesions include recurrent nonhealing anal fissures, large ulcers, complex anal fistulas, perianal abscesses, large, fleshy tags, and bluish skin discoloration. They are characterized by a multiplicity of lesions, lateral fissures, deep ulcers of the perianal skin and anal canal, and anal stricture.

  6. Extraintestinal manifestations are numerous. The eyes may develop conjunctivitis, iritis, and uveitis. The skin may develop pyoderma gangrenosum, erythema nodosum multiforme, and aphthous stomatitis. Musculoskeletal manifestations include arthritis, ankylosing spondylitis, and hypertrophic osteoarthropathy. Finally, sclerosing cholangitis can lead to cirrhosis and liver failure.

E. **Imaging studies** are indicated when establishing the diagnosis of Crohn disease or when a complication develops that requires surgical intervention.

1. **Contrast radiographs,** which include small-bowel follow-through, enteroclysis, and water-soluble contrast enema, are very valuable in the diagnosis of Crohn disease. These studies usually reveal strictures or segments of ulcerated mucosa.

2. **Endoscopy** is most useful for obtaining biopsy material in patients with terminal ileal and colonic disease. As in patients with ulcerative colitis, those with long-standing (>10 years) Crohn colitis are at increased risk for adenocarcinoma, and colonoscopy is important for cancer surveillance. These patients also have an increased incidence of small-bowel cancer.

3. **CT** is useful for identifying abscesses, focal inflammation, and wall thickening. Abscesses can be drained percutaneously under CT guidance.

F. **Complications** include intestinal obstruction, stricture, fistula, perforation, intra-abdominal abscess, gastrointestinal bleeding, and perirectal abscess and fistula. Toxic colitis is a surgical emergency that can occur in these patients.

G. **Differential diagnosis** of Crohn disease includes other inflammatory bowel diseases, as well as common infectious abdominal conditions.

1. **Ulcerative colitis.** Patients with Crohn disease generally have less severe diarrhea, usually without gross blood. Perianal lesions, nonconfluent skip lesions, transmural involvement, large mucosal ulcers and fissures, involvement of small intestine, rectal sparing, and the presence of granulomas all help to differentiate Crohn disease from ulcerative colitis. Some patients who cannot be confidently diagnosed with either condition are labeled as having indeterminate colitis.

2. **Appendicitis.** Acute right-lower-quadrant abdominal pain due to Crohn ileitis can mimic acute appendicitis.

3. **Infectious ileitis** presents with pain and bloody diarrhea. The diagnosis is made by stool culture.

4. **Other** diseases that present similarly to Crohn disease include intestinal lymphoma, intestinal tuberculosis, ischemic enteritis, diverticulitis, pseudomembranous colitis, and irritable bowel syndrome.

H. **Treatment**

1. **Adequate nutrition** is essential both during and between disease flares, and enteral feeds should be continued whenever possible. A low-residue, high-protein, milk-free diet generally provides adequate nutrition. Vitamin and mineral supplementation may be necessary. Patients with severe or unresponsive disease should be started on TPN and placed on complete bowel rest.

2. **Medical management** is particularly important because Crohn disease has no cure. Therefore, treatment seeks to palliate symptoms, reduce bowel inflammation, and correct nutritional disturbances. Therapeutic recommendations depend on the disease location, severity, and complications. Mild to moderate disease can be treated with an oral aminosalicylates (sulfasalazine 3 to 6 g/day, or mesalamine 1 g four times a day). For ileal, colonic, or perianal disease, metronidazole, 500 mg three times a day, can be added. In patients with severe disease, steroid therapy should be initiated after active infection or abscess has been excluded. Prednisone, with initial daily doses of 40 to 60 mg orally, is a common outpatient treatment for acute flares; inpatients may receive hydrocortisone, 50 to 100 mg intravenously every 6 hours. Response to therapy should become evident within 7 days. Data have shown that infusions of infliximab (Remicade), a monoclonal antibody against tumor necrosis factor, is effective for Crohn flares and even Crohn fistulas (*N Engl J Med* 2004;350:876). Before receiving infliximab, the patient must have no active source of infection and be purified protein derivative (PPD)-negative. Infliximab is of particular use in poor surgical candidates who have otherwise failed medical management. After a patient has recovered from an acute flare, the medical regimen should be simplified to prevent long-term complications. In particular, steroids should be

tapered as soon as possible to prevent side effects such as osteopenia, avascular necrosis, psychosis, and weight gain. The addition of immunomodulators, such as 6-mercaptopurine, may allow patients with refractory disease to taper off of prednisone.

3. **Surgical therapy** is indicated for failure of medical therapy or to address acute complications of the disease, such as high-output fistulas, perforation, intra-abdominal abscess, severe colitis, bleeding, or obstruction from fibrotic strictures. Abdominal abscesses can usually be drained percutaneously with elective bowel resection thereafter. Most Crohn patients require operative treatment at some point in their life.

   a. At the time of operation, the most important principle is to correct the complication while **preserving bowel length** to prevent short-gut syndrome. Resection to histologically negative margins does not significantly reduce the likelihood of disease recurrence; therefore, grossly normal margins of 2 cm are accepted. In the absence of free perforation, large abscesses, massively dilated bowel, severe malnutrition, or high-dose immunosuppression, primary anastomosis is safe. Stapling should be avoided in thick-walled bowel; in this situation, a hand-sewn anastomosis is indicated. Recent series suggest that laparoscopic ileocolic resections are safe alternatives to open procedures, especially at the time of first operation (*Dis Colon Rectum* 2003;46:1129). Issues that require special consideration beyond the scope of this chapter are duodenal disease, multiple skip lesions, and chronic fibrotic strictures in the setting of short-bowel syndrome.

   b. **Appendectomy.** Patients who are being explored for presumed acute appendicitis and are found to have Crohn ileitis should have the appendix removed if the cecum is not inflamed. Conventional teaching has been that the terminal ileum should not be removed. This is controversial, however, given the low morbidity of ileocecal resection and the uncertainty of response to subsequent medical therapy.

   c. Surgical complications include anastomotic leaks, enterocutaneous fistulas, and sepsis related to intra-abdominal abscesses and wound infections.

I. **Prognosis.** Crohn disease is a chronic panintestinal disease that currently has no cure. It requires chronic, lifelong treatment, with operation reserved for severe complications. Recently, however, specific "susceptibility genes" (*NOD2/CARD15*) have been identified in patients with Crohn disease. Further study of the pathways involved may shed light on pathogenesis and lead to more effective medical treatments.

X. **NEOPLASMS** of the small bowel occur infrequently and account for fewer than 2% of all GI neoplasms. Tumors of the small intestine present insidiously with vague, nonspecific symptoms. Most benign tumors are diagnosed incidentally; however, they can act as lead points in an intussusception. On the other hand, the majority of malignant tumors eventually present with weight loss, abdominal pain, obstruction, perforation, or hemorrhage.

A. **Benign tumors** are much more common than malignant tumors.

   1. **Leiomyoma** is the most common benign neoplasm of the small intestine and arises from the mesenchymal cells of the small bowel. These tumors grow submucosally and project into the lumen of the small bowel. On a small-bowel contrast study, they appear as a smooth, eccentric filling defect with intact, normal-appearing mucosa. Histopathologic examination is needed to distinguish benign from malignant stromal tumors. Treatment consists of a segmental small bowel resection.

   2. **Adenomas** can occur sporadically as solitary lesions or in association with familial adenomatous polyposis syndrome (Gardner variant). When they are symptomatic, lesions can cause fluctuating pain secondary to intermittent obstruction, intussusception, or bleeding. The three types of small-bowel adenomas are simple tubular adenomas, Brunner gland adenomas, and villous adenomas. The duodenum is the most common site for all three types of adenomas. Tubular and Brunner gland adenomas have a low malignant potential and can be treated

with complete endoscopic polypectomy. Villous adenomas have significant malignant potential. If complete endoscopic resection is not possible, transduodenal excision with adequate margins is appropriate. Villous adenomas of the jejunum or ileum should be resected with a segmental bowel resection.

3. **Hamartomas** arise in patients with Peutz-Jeghers syndrome. This is an autosomal dominant inherited syndrome of mucocutaneous melanotic pigmentation and multiple gastrointestinal polyps. Operative therapy is indicated only for symptoms. At operation, all polyps larger than 1 cm should be resected. Due to an increased risk for de novo adenocarcinoma (arising separately from the hamartomatous polyps), patients need to be screened closely by endoscopy.

4. **Lipomas** occur most often in the ileum and have no malignant potential. On CT, they show fatty attenuation. **Hemangiomas** may be associated with Osler-Weber-Rendu disease and present with bleeding. Diagnosis can be made with enteroscopy, capsule endoscopy, or angiography. **Neurofibromas and fibromas,** less common tumors, can cause intussusception. **Endometriosis** can implant on the bowel, appearing as puckered, bluish-red, serosally based nodules. They can cause gastrointestinal bleeding or obstruction.

B. **Malignant tumors**

1. **Adenocarcinoma** is the most common malignant small intestinal tumor. Forty percent of these occur in the duodenum, and their frequency decreases distally through the small bowel.

   a. Risk factors for the development of adenocarcinoma include villous adenomas, polyposis syndromes, Crohn disease, and hereditary nonpolyposis colorectal cancer (HNPCC). Patients often remain asymptomatic for long periods of time, and most patients have distant metastases at diagnosis. The presenting symptoms depend on the location of the primary tumor. Periampullary tumors can present with painless jaundice, duodenal obstruction, or bleeding. More-distal tumors tend to present with abdominal pain and weight loss from progressive obstruction. Contrast studies, CT, and endoscopy with or without ERCP can be used to make the diagnosis.

   b. **Treatment** consists of segmental resection of the small bowel and its adjacent lymph node–bearing mesentery. Any adherent structures should be resected en bloc if possible. Tumors of the terminal ileum should be resected along with the right colon. For carcinomas of the duodenum, a pancreaticoduodenectomy is usually required. In completely resected duodenal adenocarcinoma, the 5-year survival rate is 56% for node-positive and 83% for node-negative disease, respectively (*Ann Surg Oncol* 2004;11:380). Distal lesions tend to present at a later stage. Patients with metastatic disease at the time of diagnosis rarely survive past 6 months. 5-Fluorouracil–based chemotherapy regimens have been tried, but data on their efficacy are lacking.

2. **Gastrointestinal stromal tumors** (GISTs) arise from mesodermal-derived components of the small intestine. They are equally distributed along the length of the small bowel. These tumors grow extraluminally and cause symptoms late in their course. Because of their vascular nature, when these tumors outgrow their blood supply and necrose, they may hemorrhage into either the peritoneum or the lumen of the bowel. Mutations of **c-kit** (CD117; a tyrosine kinase responsible for neoplastic growth) allow diagnosis by immunohistochemistry. The **treatment** for GI stromal tumors is resection. Wide en bloc resection to obtain tumor-free margins must be performed for curative therapy. Extensive lymph node resection is unnecessary because these tumors have a low potential for lymphatic spread. Traditional chemotherapy and radiation therapy are not effective in the treatment of metastatic GISTs. However, imatinib mesylate (Gleevec) is a recently developed medicine that may substantially change treatment of the disease. Imatinib targets the overactive tyrosine receptor c-kit found on all GIST cells. Inhibition of this receptor has been shown to lead to radiographic and histologic regression of metastatic lesions (*N Engl J Med* 2001;344:1052). Clinical trials are ongoing to address the use of imatinib after GIST resection. The benefit of resection of isolated pulmonary or hepatic lesions is unknown. Histologic grade

and tumor size are the most important predictors of survival. After complete resection, the overall 5-year survival rate is 50%. In low-grade tumors [<10 mitotic figures/high power field (mf/hpf)], the survival rate is 60% to 80%, whereas in high-grade tumors (>10 mf/hpf), the survival rate is less than 20%. With local recurrence, the median length of survival is 9 to 12 months. With metastatic disease, the median length of survival is 20 months (*Br J Surg* 2003;90:1178). However, imatinib mesylate treatment extends the 2-year survival rate to 78% for patients with metastatic disease (*Eur J Cancer* 2004;40:689).

3. **Primary small-bowel lymphomas** are most common in the ileum because it has the largest amount of gut-associated lymphoid tissue. Virtually all small-bowel lymphomas are non-Hodgkin, B-cell lymphomas. Lymphomas can arise de novo or in association with a preexisting systemic condition such as celiac disease, Crohn disease, or immunosuppression (iatrogenic, HIV, etc.). The presentation of these patients is highly variable. Imaging can help make a diagnosis, but operation is frequently required for histologic confirmation. Treatment of lymphoma localized to the small bowel involves wide resection of the affected segment of intestine and its associated mesentery. To stage the tumor accurately, the liver should be biopsied and the periaortic lymph nodes sampled. For widespread disease, resection of the affected small bowel should be performed to prevent complications. The role of adjuvant chemotherapy and radiotherapy remains controversial. The 5-year survival rate for patients with fully resected disease approaches 80%, but individuals with more advanced disease usually die within 1 year of operation.

4. **Carcinoid tumors** arise from the Kulchitsky or enterochromaffin cells of the intestinal crypts. Most intestinal carcinoids occur within 2 ft of the ileocecal valve. Small-bowel carcinoid tumors tend to be much more aggressive than their appendiceal or rectal counterparts. Patients rarely manifest signs or symptoms of the tumor until late in the course. Symptoms include local complications (intestinal obstruction, pain, or bleeding) or systemic symptoms of the carcinoid syndrome. Metastases are rare in tumors smaller than 1 cm in size; half of tumors between 1 and 2 cm metastasize, and almost all tumors larger than 2 cm spread.

   a. **Carcinoid syndrome** implies metastatic spread. Normally, hormones released by intestinal tumors are metabolized by the liver and produce no symptoms. However, hepatic metastases drain into the systemic circulation. Classic symptoms include **diarrhea** and **transient flushing** of the face, neck, and upper chest. Tachycardia, hypotension, bronchospasm, and even coma can also occur. In long-standing carcinoid syndrome, patients develop right heart endocardial and valvular fibrosis. The hormonal mediators responsible for carcinoid syndrome are not well understood. The diagnosis of carcinoid syndrome is confirmed by finding increased urinary excretion of 5-hydroxyindoleacetic acid, a metabolite of serotonin.

   b. The **treatment** of carcinoid tumors is operative. The entire small bowel should be inspected because in 30% of cases synchronous lesions are present. Jejunal and ileal tumors should be treated with segmental resection including the adjacent mesentery. Small tumors (<1 cm) that are located in the third or fourth portions of the duodenum can be either locally excised or included in a segmental resection. For large duodenal tumors and periampullary tumors, a pancreaticoduodenectomy should be performed. In the presence of locally advanced disease with involvement of adjacent organs or peritoneum, aggressive resection should be undertaken. This can help to delay the occurrence of mesenteric desmoplastic reaction, hepatic metastases, and carcinoid syndrome. Solitary and accessible liver lesions should be resected. Adjuvant cytotoxic chemotherapy and radiotherapy are of little benefit. The somatostatin analog **octreotide** offers excellent palliation of carcinoid syndrome in patients with unresectable disease. Octreotide decreases the concentration of circulating serotonin and urinary 5-hydroxyindoleacetic acid and can relieve diarrhea and flushing in 90% of patients.

    c. Carcinoids are slow-growing tumors, and **prognosis** depends on the stage of the tumor. The overall 5-year survival rate is 60%. Patients with local disease that is completely resected have a normal life expectancy. For patients with resectable node-positive disease, the median length of survival is 15 years. The median length of survival drops to 5 years with unresectable intra-abdominal disease, and it is 3 years for patients with hepatic metastases. Of note, there are outliers who survive for many years with metastatic disease.

5. Carcinomatosis is diffuse studding of the peritoneal, mesenteric, and bowel surfaces by tumor nodules. Many tumors can cause peritoneal carcinomatosis, including cancer of the pancreas, stomach, ovaries, appendix, and colon. Carcinomatosis has an extremely poor prognosis, and surgical treatment is palliative, usually for obstruction. The only exception is pseudomyxoma peritonei; patients with this low-grade malignancy may benefit from resection and intraperitoneal chemotherapy.

6. Metastases can spread to the small bowel. Palliative resection is appropriate if needed for symptom relief.

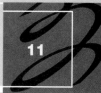

ACUTE ABDOMINAL PAIN AND APPENDICITIS

11

Li Ern Chen and Timothy G. Buchman

 ACUTE ABDOMINAL PAIN

Evaluation of the patient with acute abdominal pain requires a careful history and physical examination by a skilled physician in conjunction with selective diagnostic testing. Acute abdominal pain is the most common general surgical problem presenting to the emergency department. **Acute abdomen** is defined as a recent or sudden onset of abdominal pain. This can be new pain or an increase in chronic pain. The **differential diagnosis** includes both intra- and extraperitoneal processes. The acute abdomen **does not always** signify the need for surgical intervention; however, surgical evaluation is warranted.

I. PATHOPHYSIOLOGY. The abdomen is analogous to a box. Although this chapter focuses on pathophysiology inside the box, one must be cognizant of the fact that pathology on the surface of the box (e.g., rectus sheath hematoma) or even outside the box (e.g., testicular torsion) can present as abdominal pain. Abdominal pain arising from intra-abdominal pathophysiology originates in the peritoneum, which is a membrane comprising two layers. These layers, the visceral and parietal peritoneum, are developmentally distinct areas with separate nerve supplies.

A. Visceral pain
1. **Visceral peritoneum** is innervated bilaterally by the autonomic nervous system. The bilateral innervation causes visceral pain to be midline, vague, deep, dull, and poorly localized (e.g., vague periumbilical pain of the midgut).
2. Visceral pain is **triggered by inflammation, ischemia, and geometric changes** such as distention, traction, and pressure.
3. Visceral pain signifies **intra-abdominal disease** but not necessarily the need for surgical intervention.

B. Parietal pain
1. **Parietal peritoneum** is innervated unilaterally via the spinal somatic nerves that also supply the abdominal wall. Unilateral innervation causes parietal pain to localize to one or more abdominal quadrants (e.g., inflamed appendix producing parietal peritoneal irritation).
2. Parietal pain is **sharp, severe, and well localized.**
3. Parietal pain is **triggered by irritation of the parietal peritoneum** by an inflammatory process (e.g., chemical peritonitis from perforated peptic ulcer or bacterial peritonitis from acute appendicitis). It may also be triggered by mechanical stimulation, such as a surgical incision.
4. Parietal pain is **associated with physical examination findings of local or diffuse peritonitis** and frequently signifies the need for surgical treatment.

C. Embryologic origin of the affected organ determines the location of visceral pain in the abdominal midline.
1. **Foregut-derived structures** (stomach to the second portion of the duodenum, liver and biliary tract, pancreas, spleen) present with epigastric pain.
2. **Midgut-derived structures** (second portion of the duodenum to the proximal two thirds of the transverse colon) present with periumbilical pain.

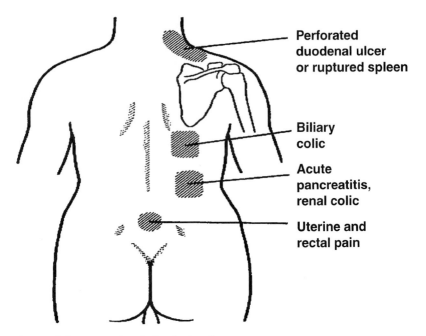

Figure 11-1. Frequent sites of referred pain and common causes.

3. **Hindgut-derived structures** (distal transverse colon to the anal verge) present with suprapubic pain.
D. **Referred pain** arises from a deep visceral structure but is superficial at the presenting site (Fig. 11-1).
   1. It results from **central neural pathways** that are common to the somatic nerves and visceral organs.
   2. Examples include **biliary tract pain** (referred to the right inferior scapular area) and **diaphragmatic irritation** from any source, such as subphrenic abscess (referred to the ipsilateral shoulder).
II. **EVALUATION** of the acute abdomen remains heavily influenced by patient history and physical exam findings. Ancillary imaging and lab tests can help to complete the diagnosis and guide treatment decisions.
   A. **History of present illness**
      1. **Onset and duration of pain**
         a. **Sudden onset of pain** (within seconds) suggests perforation or rupture [e.g., perforated peptic ulcer or ruptured abdominal aortic aneurysm (AAA)]. Infarction, such as myocardial infarction or acute mesenteric occlusion, can also present with sudden onset of pain.
         b. **Rapidly accelerating pain** (within minutes) may result from several sources.
            (1) **Colic syndromes,** such as biliary colic, ureteral colic, and small-bowel obstruction.
            (2) **Inflammatory processes,** such as acute appendicitis, pancreatitis, and diverticulitis.
            (3) **Ischemic processes,** such as mesenteric ischemia, strangulated intestinal obstruction, and volvulus.
         c. **Gradual onset of pain** (over several hours) increasing in intensity may be caused by one of the following:

(1) **Inflammatory conditions,** such as appendicitis and cholecystitis.

(2) **Obstructive processes,** such as nonstrangulated bowel obstruction and urinary retention.

(3) **Other mechanical processes,** such as ectopic pregnancy and penetrating or perforating tumors.

2. **Character of pain**

   a. **Colicky pain** waxes and wanes. It usually occurs **secondary to hyperperistalsis of smooth muscle** against a mechanical site of obstruction (e.g., small-bowel obstruction, renal stone).

   b. An important exception is **biliary colic,** in which pain tends to be constant.

   c. **Pain that is sharp, severe, persistent, and steadily increases in intensity** over time suggests an infectious or inflammatory process (e.g., appendicitis).

3. **Location of pain**

   a. Pain caused by **inflammation of specific organs** may be localized [e.g., right-upper-quadrant (RUQ) pain caused by acute cholecystitis].

   b. Careful attention must be given to the **radiation of pain.** The pain of renal colic, for example, may begin in the patient's back or flank and radiate to the ipsilateral groin, whereas the pain of a ruptured aortic aneurysm or pancreatitis may radiate to the patient's back.

4. **Alleviating and aggravating factors**

   a. Patients with **diffuse peritonitis** describe worsening of pain with movement (i.e., parietal pain); the pain is ameliorated by lying still.

   b. Patients with **intestinal obstruction** have visceral pain and usually experience a transient relief from symptoms after vomiting.

5. **Associated symptoms**

   a. **Nausea and vomiting** frequently accompany abdominal pain and may hint at its etiology. Vomiting that occurs after the onset of pain may suggest appendicitis, whereas vomiting before the onset of pain is more consistent with the diagnosis of gastroenteritis or food poisoning. The sequence as well as the character of the emesis should be documented. Bilious emesis suggests a process distal to the duodenum. Hematemesis may suggest a peptic ulcer or gastritis.

   b. **Fever or chills** suggests an inflammatory or an infectious process, or both.

   c. **Anorexia** is present in the vast majority of patients with acute peritonitis.

B. **Past medical history, surgical history, and organ-system review**

   1. **Pathologic medical conditions** may precipitate intra-abdominal pathology.

      a. Patients with **peripheral vascular disease or coronary artery disease** may have abdominal vascular disease (e.g., AAA or mesenteric ischemia).

      b. Patients with a history of **cancer** may present with bowel obstruction from recurrence.

      c. **Major medical problems** are important to recognize early in the patient and may call for urgent surgical exploration.

   2. A **thorough medical history and organ-system review** must be carried out to exclude various extra-abdominal causes of abdominal pain.

      a. **Diabetic** patients or patients with known **coronary artery disease or peripheral vascular disease** who present with vague epigastric symptoms may have myocardial ischemia as the cause of the abdominal symptoms.

      b. **Right-lower-lobe pneumonia** may present as RUQ pain in association with cough and fever.

   3. A **thorough menstrual history** must be obtained in women.

      a. **Pelvic inflammatory disease (PID)** typically occurs early in the cycle and may be associated with a vaginal discharge.

      b. **Ectopic pregnancy** must be considered in every woman of child-bearing age with lower abdominal pain, especially if accompanied by a history of amenorrhea.

      c. **Ovarian cysts** can cause sudden pain by enlarging, rupturing, or causing ovarian torsion. The timing in relation to the menstrual cycle is crucial. A ruptured follicular cyst pain occurs at midcycle (i.e., mittelschmerz), whereas the pain of a ruptured corpus luteum cyst develops around the time of menses.

  d. Abdominal pain that occurs monthly suggests **endometriosis.**

4. Previous abdominal surgery in a patient with colicky abdominal pain may suggest **intestinal obstruction** secondary to adhesions, incarceration of an incisional hernia, or recurrence or malignancy. These are generally accompanied by nausea and vomiting.

C. Medications

1. Nonsteroidal anti-inflammatory medications, such as aspirin or ibuprofen, place patients at risk for the complications of peptic ulcer disease, including bleeding, obstruction, and perforation.

2. Corticosteroids may mask classic signs of inflammation, such as fever and peritoneal irritation, making the abdominal examination less reliable.

3. Antibiotics consumed by patients may aid or hinder diagnosis.

  a. Patients with **peritonitis** may have decreased pain.

  b. Patients who have diarrhea and abdominal pain may have **antibiotic-induced pseudomembranous colitis** caused by *Clostridium difficile.*

  c. Be aware of the **elderly patient on immunosuppressants or antibiotics.**

D. Physical examination

1. Overall appearance should be assessed.

  a. Patients with diffuse peritonitis appear acutely ill and tend to lie quietly on their side with their knees drawn toward their chest.

  b. Patients with colic tend to be restless and unable to find a comfortable position. Patients with ureteral colic may writhe in pain or walk around the examination room.

  c. Patients who are jaundiced may have biliary obstruction.

  d. Patients who appear weak and lethargic may be septic.

2. Vital signs are important indicators of a patient's overall condition.

  a. Fever suggests the presence of inflammation or infection. Marked fever ($>39°C$) suggests an abscess, cholangitis, or pneumonia.

  b. Hypotension or tachycardia, or both, may indicate hypovolemia or sepsis.

3. The **abdominal examination** should be carried out thoroughly and systematically. Although opioid analgesia administered prior to physical examination may alter physical exam findings, this is not associated with a decrease in diagnostic accuracy (*Ann Emerg Med* 2006;48:150) or an increase in management errors (*JAMA* 2006;296:1764).

  a. The patient's abdomen should be inspected for **distention, surgical scars, bulging masses, and areas of erythema.**

  b. Auscultation may reveal the high-pitched, tinkling bowel sounds of obstruction or the absence of sounds due to ileus from diffuse peritonitis.

  c. Percussion may reveal the tympanitic sounds of distended bowel in intestinal obstruction or the fluid wave that is characteristic of ascites. Percussion is also useful in localizing tenderness and peritoneal irritation (deep palpation or rebound is usually unnecessary to determine peritoneal irritation).

  d. Palpation of the patient's abdomen should be performed with the patient in a supine position and with his or her knees flexed, if necessary, to relieve pain.

  (1) Begin the examination at a point remote from the reported site of pain.

  (2) Areas of tenderness and guarding should be noted. Rebound tenderness is not a very reliable sign of peritonitis. The presence of involuntary guarding (localized or diffuse) due to muscular rigidity from underlying peritoneal irritation is often a better sign of peritonitis. Peritonitis may also be elicited by rocking the patient's pelvis or shaking the bed to create friction between the abdominal wall and peritoneal viscera.

  (3) Pain out of proportion to physical examination findings suggests mesenteric ischemia.

  (4) Thoroughly search for **hernias** (incisional, ventral, umbilical, inguinal, femoral).

  (5) Any **palpable masses** should be noted.

e. Rectal examination should be performed routinely in all patients with abdominal pain.

   (1) Tenderness or a mass on the right pelvic side wall is sometimes seen in appendicitis.

   (2) A **mass in the rectum** may indicate obstructing cancer. Important details are the fraction of circumference involved, tumor mobility, and distance from the anal verge.

   (3) The presence of **occult blood in the stool specimen** may indicate GI bleeding from peptic ulcer disease.

f. Pelvic examination must be performed in all women of child-bearing age who present with lower abdominal pain.

   (1) Cervical discharge and overall appearance of the cervix should be noted.

   (2) Bimanual examination should be performed to assess cervical motion tenderness, adnexal tenderness, and the presence of adnexal masses.

g. Testicular and scrotal examination is essential in all males who complain of abdominal pain.

   (1) Testicular torsion produces a painful, swollen, and tender testicle that is retracted upward in the scrotum.

   (2) Epididymitis may coexist with urinary tract infection. The epididymis is swollen and tender, and the vas deferens may also be inflamed.

h. Specific physical examination findings should be sought in **the appropriate clinical setting.**

   (1) Murphy's sign is inspiratory arrest while continuous pressure is maintained in the RUQ. Seen in acute cholecystitis, Murphy's sign reflects the descent of an inflamed gallbladder with inspiration. When the inflamed gallbladder makes contact with the examiner's hand, the patient experiences pain, causing the inspiratory arrest. A sonographic Murphy's sign may be elicited during ultrasonographic examination of the gallbladder.

   (2) The **obturator sign** reflects inflammation adjacent to the internal obturator muscle (as is sometimes seen in appendicitis). It may also be present with an obturator hernia. While the patient is supine with the knee and hip flexed, the hip is internally and externally rotated. The test is positive if the patient experiences hypogastric pain during this maneuver.

   (3) The **iliopsoas sign** is seen when an adjacent inflammatory process irritates the iliopsoas muscle. It is classically observed in retrocecal appendicitis. The patient's thigh is usually already drawn into a flexed position for relief. The test is best performed with the patient lying on the left side. With the knee flexed, the thigh is hyperextended. The test is positive if the patient experiences pain on the right side with this maneuver.

   (4) Rovsing's sign may also be seen in acute appendicitis. Indicative of an inflammatory process in the right lower quadrant (RLQ), Rovsing's sign is RLQ pain resulting from percussion in the left lower quadrant (LLQ).

E. Laboratory evaluation

   1. A **complete blood count** with cell count differential is important in the assessment of surgical conditions and should be obtained in every patient with acute abdominal pain.

   a. White blood cell (WBC) count elevation may indicate the presence of an infectious source.

   b. Left shift on the differential to more immature forms is often helpful because this may indicate the presence of an inflammatory source even if the WBC count is normal.

   c. Hematocrit elevation may be due to volume contraction from dehydration. Conversely, a **low hematocrit** may be due to occult blood loss.

   2. An **electrolyte profile** may reveal clues to the patient's overall condition.

   a. Hypokalemic, hypochloremic, metabolic alkalosis may be seen in patients with prolonged vomiting and severe volume depletion. The hypokalemia reflects the potassium–hydrogen ion exchange occurring at the cellular level in an effort to correct the alkalosis.

      b. Elevation of the blood urea nitrogen or creatinine is also indicative of volume depletion.

  3. Liver enzyme levels may be obtained in the appropriate clinical setting.

      a. A mild elevation of transaminases (<2 times normal), **alkaline phosphatase, and total bilirubin** is sometimes seen in patients with acute cholecystitis.

      b. A **moderate elevation of transaminases** (>3 times normal) in the patient with acute onset of RUQ pain is most likely due to a common bile duct (CBD) stone. Elevation of the transaminases often precedes the rise in total bilirubin and alkaline phosphatase in patients with acute biliary obstruction.

      c. Markedly elevated transaminases (i.e., >1,000 IU/L) in the patient without pain are more likely due to hepatitis or ischemia.

  4. Pancreatic enzymes (amylase and lipase) should be measured if the diagnosis of pancreatitis is considered. It is important to note that the degree of enzyme elevation does not correlate with the severity of the pancreatitis.

      a. Mild degrees of hyperamylasemia may be seen in several situations, such as intestinal obstruction.

      b. Elevation of lipase usually indicates pancreatic parenchymal damage.

  5. Lactic acid level may be obtained when considering intestinal ischemia.

      a. Serum lactate is an indicator of tissue hypoxia.

      b. Mild lactic acidosis may be seen in patients with arterial hypotension.

      c. Ongoing elevation of serum lactate despite resuscitation is indicative of progression of tissue ischemia (e.g., mesenteric ischemia).

  6. Urinalysis is helpful in assessing urologic causes of abdominal pain.

      a. Bacteriuria, pyuria, and a positive leukocyte esterase usually suggest a urinary tract infection (UTI). Recurrent UTI in males is unusual and should always elicit an evaluation.

      b. Hematuria is seen in nephrolithiasis and renal and urothelial cancer.

  7. β-Human chorionic gonadotropin must be obtained in any woman of childbearing age. A positive urine result should be quantitated by serum levels.

      a. A **low level** (<4,000 mIU) is seen in ectopic pregnancy.

      b. Levels above 4,000 mIU indicate intrauterine pregnancy (i.e., one that should be seen on ultrasonography).

F. Radiologic evaluation of the patient with abdominal pain is a key element in the workup. However, its use should be very selective to avoid unnecessary cost and possible morbidity associated with some modalities.

  1. Plain abdominal x-rays often serve as the initial radiologic evaluation.

      a. X-rays should be obtained in the **supine and erect positions.**

      b. Free intraperitoneal air is best visualized on an **upright chest x-ray** with both hemidiaphragms exposed.

        (1) If the patient is unable to assume an upright position, a **left lateral decubitus x-ray** should be obtained.

        (2) Free air may not be detectable in up to 20% of cases of **perforated viscus.**

      c. The **bowel gas pattern** is assessed for dilation, air-fluid levels, and the presence of gas throughout the small and large intestine.

        (1) In **small-bowel obstruction,** one sees small-bowel dilation (valvulae conniventes) and air-fluid levels in the bowel proximal to the obstruction. There is a paucity of gas in the segment of bowel distal to the obstruction. The absence of air in the rectum suggests complete obstruction (beware of the presence of colonic gas following rectal examination).

        (2) A **sentinel loop** (i.e., a single, dilated loop of bowel) may be seen adjacent to an inflamed organ (as in pancreatitis) and is due to localized ileus.

      d. Calcifications should be noted.

        (1) The vast majority of **urinary stones** (90%) contain calcium and are visible on plain x-rays, whereas only 15% of **gallstones** are calcified.

        (2) Calcifications in the region of the pancreas may indicate chronic pancreatitis.

        (3) Fecalith in the RLQ may suggest appendicitis.

(4) Calcification in the wall of the aorta may suggest an AAA.

(5) The most common calcifications seen in the abdomen are **"phleboliths"** (benign calcifications of the pelvic veins). Phleboliths can be distinguished from renal stones by their central lucency, which represents the lumen.

e. The **presence of gas** in the portal or mesenteric venous systems, intramural gas in the GI tract, or gas in the biliary tree (in the absence of a surgical enteric anastomosis) is an ominous finding.

2. **Ultrasonography (US)** may provide diagnostic information in some conditions. Ultrasound is portable, relatively inexpensive, and free of radiation exposure. US visibility is limited in settings of obesity, bowel gas, and subcutaneous air.

a. **RUQ US** is particularly useful in biliary tract disease.

(1) Gallstones can be detected in up to 95% of patients.

(2) Findings suggestive of **acute cholecystitis** include gallbladder wall thickening of greater than 3 mm, pericholecystic fluid, a stone impacted at the neck of the gallbladder, or Murphy's sign.

(3) Dilation of the CBD (>8 mm, or larger in elderly patients) indicates biliary obstruction. Gallstones in the CBD may also be seen.

b. **US** can be used in the evaluation of RLQ pain.

(1) It may be helpful in the **diagnosis of appendicitis,** particularly in the pediatric population or in nonobese adults.

(2) Its utility and accuracy are operator dependent.

c. **Pelvic or transvaginal US** is particularly useful in women in whom ovarian pathology or an ectopic pregnancy is suspected.

d. **Testicular US** is adjunctive to physical exam in diagnosing testicular pathology (e.g., testicular torsion, epididymitis, orchitis).

3. **Contrast studies,** although rarely indicated in the acute setting, may be helpful in some situations.

a. In most instances, a **water-soluble contrast agent** (e.g., Hypaque) should be used to avoid possible barium peritonitis in the event of bowel perforation.

b. **Contrast enema** is particularly useful in differentiating adynamic ileus from distal colonic obstruction.

4. **Computed tomographic (CT) scanning** may provide a thorough evaluation of the patient's abdomen and pelvis relatively quickly. Oral and intravenous contrast should be administered if not specifically contraindicated by allergy, renal insufficiency, or patient hemodynamic instability. CT scanning is the best radiographic study in the patient with unexplained abdominal pain. It is of particular benefit in certain situations, including the following:

a. When **an accurate history cannot be obtained** (e.g., the patient is demented or obtunded or has an atypical history).

b. When a patient has **abdominal pain and leukocytosis and examination findings are worrisome but not definitive for peritoneal irritation.**

c. When a patient with a chronic illness (e.g., Crohn disease) experiences **acute abdominal pain.**

d. When **evaluating retroperitoneal structures** (e.g., in a stable patient with a suspected leaking AAA).

e. When evaluating patients with a history of **intra-abdominal malignancy.**

5. **Magnetic resonance imaging (MRI)**

a. MRI provides cross-sectional imaging while **avoiding ionizing radiation.**

b. Image acquisition **takes longer** than for CT scan; patients must be able to lie on their backs for a prolonged period of time and cannot be claustrophobic.

c. MRI has its greatest application in **pregnant women** with acute abdominal and pelvic pain (*AJR* 2005;184:452).

6. **Radionuclide imaging studies** have few indications in the acute setting.

a. **Biliary radiopharmaceuticals,** such as hepatic 2,6-dimethylimino-diacetic acid or di-diisopropyliminodiacetic acid, evaluate filling and emptying of the gallbladder. Nonfilling implies cystic duct obstruction and may indicate acute cholecystitis. This test is especially valuable in the diagnosis of acalculous cholecystitis and biliary dyskinesia.

TABLE 11-1	Differential Diagnosis for Acute Abdominal Pain	
Upper abdominal		Perforated peptic ulcer
		Acute cholecystitis
		Acute pancreatitis
Mid and lower abdominal		Acute appendicitis
		Acute diverticulitis
		Intestinal obstruction
		Mesenteric ischemia
		Ruptured AAA
Other	OB/GYN	PID
		Ectopic pregnancy
		Ruptured ovarian cyst
	Urological	Nephrolithiasis
		Pyelonephritis/cystitis
	Nonsurgical	Acute MI
		Gastroenteritis
		Pneumonia
		DKA

AAA, abdominal aortic aneurysm; DKA, diabetic ketoacidosis; MI, myocaridial infarction; OB/GYN, obstetric/gynecologic; PID, pelvic inflammatory disease.

    b. Radioisotope-labeled red blood cell (RBC) or WBC scans are sometimes helpful in localizing sites of bleeding or inflammation, respectively.

    c. Technetium-99m pertechnetate may be used to detect a Meckel diverticulum because this isotope is concentrated in the ectopic gastric mucosa that frequently lines the diverticulum.

  7. Invasive radiologic techniques may have a role in some situations, including angiographic diagnosis and therapeutic intervention for **mesenteric arterial occlusion and acute GI bleeding.**

III. DIFFERENTIAL DIAGNOSES. See Table 11-1.

APPENDICITIS

I. EPIDEMIOLOGY

  A. Appendectomy is the most common urgently performed surgical procedure.

  B. Lifetime risk of undergoing appendectomy is between 7% and 12%.

  C. The **maximal incidence** occurs in the second and third decades of life.

  D. The **male:female ratio** of approximately 2:1 gradually shifts after age 25 years toward a 1:1 ratio.

II. PATHOPHYSIOLOGY

  A. Appendiceal obstruction is the most common initiating event of appendicitis.

    1. Hyperplasia of the submucosal lymphoid follicles of the appendix accounts for approximately 60% of obstructions (most common in teens).

    2. In older adults and children, the **fecalith** is the most common etiology (35%).

  B. Intraluminal pressure of the obstructed appendiceal lumen increases secondary to continued mucosal secretion and bacterial overgrowth; the appendiceal wall thins, and lymphatic and venous obstruction occurs.

  C. Necrosis and perforation develop when the arterial flow is compromised.

III. DIAGNOSIS. The diagnosis of acute appendicitis is made by clinical evaluation. Although laboratory tests and imaging procedures can be helpful, they are of secondary importance.

A. Clinical presentation

1. **Classic presentation.** Appendicitis typically begins with progressive, persistent midabdominal discomfort caused by obstruction and distention of the appendix, stimulating the visceral afferent autonomic nerves (levels T8 to T10). Anorexia and a low-grade fever ($<38.5°C$) follow. As distention of the appendix increases, venous congestion stimulates intestinal peristalsis, causing a cramping sensation that is soon followed by nausea and vomiting. Symptoms include anorexia (90%), nausea and vomiting (70%), and diarrhea (10%). Once the inflammation extends transmurally to the parietal peritoneum, the somatic pain fibers are stimulated and the pain localizes to the RLQ. Peritoneal irritation is associated with pain on movement, mild fever, and tachycardia. One fourth of patients present with localized pain and no visceral symptoms. The onset of symptoms to time of presentation is usually less than 24 hours for acute appendicitis and averages several hours.

2. **Unusual presentations**
   a. When the appendix is **retrocecal or behind the ileum,** it may be separated from the anterior abdominal peritoneum, and abdominal localizing signs may be absent. Irritation of adjacent structures can cause diarrhea, urinary frequency, pyuria, or microscopic hematuria depending on location.
   b. When the appendix is **located in the pelvis,** it may simulate acute gastroenteritis, with diffuse pain, nausea, vomiting, and diarrhea. The diagnosis may be suspected if digital rectal examination produces pain.

3. **Pregnancy**
   a. Appendicitis is the most common nongynecologic surgical emergency during pregnancy. The **incidence of appendicitis** during pregnancy is 0.15 to 2.10/1,000 pregnancies (*Can Fam Physician* 2004;50:355); appendicitis occurs with a slightly lower frequency in the pregnant patient (*Int J Epidemiol* 2001;30:1281).
   b. Appendicitis must be suspected in any pregnant woman with **abdominal pain.** The gravid uterus displaces the appendix superiorly and laterally toward the RUQ (Fig. 11-2), thereby complicating diagnosis. Separation of the visceral and parietal peritoneum due to the enlarging uterus limits localization of the pain by decreasing the somatic component of the pain. In addition, nausea and vomiting can be incorrectly attributed to the morning sickness that is common in the first trimester.
   c. **Operation** is indicated in a pregnant patient as soon as the diagnosis of appendicitis is suspected. A negative laparotomy carries a risk of fetal loss of up to 3%, but fetal demise rates reach 35% in the setting of perforation and diffuse peritonitis.

B. Physical examination

1. The examination begins by **assessing the patient's abdomen** in areas other than the area of suspected tenderness. Location of the appendix is variable. However, the base is usually found at the level of the S1 vertebral body, lateral to the right midclavicular line at **McBurney's point** (two thirds of the distance from the umbilicus to the anterosuperior iliac spine). Rovsing's sign indicates peritoneal irritation. The degree of tenderness to direct right-lower-quadrant tenderness is appreciated. The degree of muscular resistance to palpation (guarding) parallels the severity of the inflammatory process. Cutaneous hyperesthesia is often present, overlying the region of maximal tenderness. Iliopsoas sign implies retrocecal appendicitis. A pelvic appendix may produce a positive obturator sign.

2. **Rectal examination** is performed to evaluate the presence of localized tenderness or an inflammatory mass in the pararectal area. It is most useful for atypical presentations suggestive of a pelvic or retrocecal appendix.

3. In women, a **pelvic examination** is performed to assess for cervical motion tenderness and adnexal pain or masses.

4. A **palpable mass in the RLQ** suggests a periappendiceal abscess or phlegmon.

C. Laboratory evaluation.
The following tests should be obtained preoperatively for patients with suspected appendicitis. A serum pregnancy test must be performed in all ovulating women.

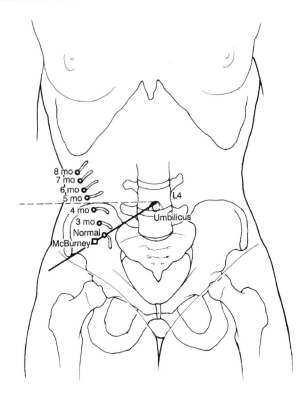

Figure 11-2. Changes in location and direction of the appendix during pregnancy. The normal and postpartum positions of the base of the appendix are medial to McBurney's point. At the fifth month, the appendix is at the level of the umbilicus and iliac crest. (Adapted from Baer JL, Reis RA, Arens RA. Appendicitis in pregnancy with changes in position and axis of normal appendix in pregnancy. *JAMA* 1932;98:1359.)

1. **Complete blood cell count.** A leukocyte count of greater than 10,000 cells/μL, with polymorphonuclear cell predominance ($>75\%$), carries a 77% sensitivity and 63% specificity for appendicitis (*Radiology* 2004;230:472). The total number of WBCs and the proportion of immature forms increase if there is appendiceal perforation. In older adults, the leukocyte count and differential are normal more frequently than in younger adults. Pregnant women normally have an elevated WBC count that can reach 15,000 to 20,000 as their pregnancy progresses.
   2. **Urinalysis** is abnormal in 25% to 40% of patients with appendicitis. Pyuria, albuminuria, and hematuria are common. Large quantities of bacteria suggest UTI as the cause of abdominal pain. A urinalysis showing more than 20 WBCs per high-power field or more than 30 RBCs per high-power field suggests UTI. Significant hematuria should prompt consideration of urolithiasis.
   3. **Serum electrolytes, blood urea nitrogen, and serum creatinine** are obtained to identify and correct electrolyte abnormalities caused by dehydration secondary to vomiting or poor oral intake.
   D. **Radiologic evaluation.** Diagnosis of appendicitis can usually be made without radiologic evaluation. In complex cases, however, the following can be helpful.
      1. **X-rays** are rarely helpful in diagnosing appendicitis. One study demonstrated an appendicolith on only 1.14% of the x-rays performed on patients with surgically

proven appendicitis. Other suggestive radiologic findings include a distended cecum with adjacent small-bowel air-fluid levels, loss of the right psoas shadow, scoliosis to the right, and gas in the lumen of the appendix. A perforated appendix rarely causes pneumoperitoneum.

2. **Ultrasound** is most useful in women of child-bearing age and in children because other causes of abdominal complaints can be demonstrated. Findings associated with acute appendicitis include an appendiceal diameter greater than 6 mm, lack of luminal compressibility, and presence of an appendicolith. An enlarged appendix seen on US has a sensitivity of 86% and specificity of 81% (*Radiology* 2004;230:472). The perforated appendix is more difficult to diagnose and is characterized by loss of the echogenic submucosa and the presence of loculated periappendiceal or pelvic fluid collection. In women, ovarian pathology may be identified or excluded. The quality and accuracy of US are highly operator dependent.

3. **CT scan,** originally recommended only in cases that were clinically complex or diagnostically uncertain, has emerged as the most commonly used radiographic diagnostic test. It is superior to US in diagnosing appendicitis, with a sensitivity of 94% and specificity of 95% (*Ann Intern Med* 2004;141:537). CT findings of appendicitis include a distended, thick-walled appendix with inflammatory streaking of surrounding fat, a pericecal phlegmon or abscess, an appendicolith, or RLQ intra-abdominal free air that signals perforation. CT scan is particularly useful in distinguishing between periappendiceal abscesses and phlegmon.

4. **MRI** is an alternative when one needs cross-sectional imaging that avoids ionizing radiation. It is particularly useful in a pregnant patient whose appendix is not visualized on US (*Radiology* 2006;238:891).

E. **Diagnostic laparoscopy** is most useful for evaluating ovulating women with an equivocal examination for appendicitis. In this subgroup, one third of women prove to have primary gynecologic pathology. The appendix may also be removed via the laparoscopic approach. Therefore, some surgeons advocate an initial laparoscopic approach in all ovulating women with suspected appendicitis.

F. **Differential diagnosis**
1. **Gastrointestinal diseases**
   a. **Gastroenteritis** is characterized by nausea and emesis before the onset of abdominal pain, along with generalized malaise, high fever, diarrhea, and poorly localized abdominal pain and tenderness. Although diarrhea is one of the cardinal signs of gastroenteritis, it can occur in patients with appendicitis. In addition, WBC count is often normal in patients with gastroenteritis.
   b. **Mesenteric lymphadenitis** usually occurs in patients younger than 20 years old and presents with middle, followed by RLQ, abdominal pain but without rebound tenderness or muscular rigidity. Nodal histology and cultures obtained at operation can identify etiology, most notably *Yersinia* and *Shigella* species and *Mycobacterium tuberculosis*. Mesenteric lymphadenitis is known to be associated with upper respiratory tract infections.
   c. **Meckel diverticulitis** presents with symptoms and signs indistinguishable from those of appendicitis, but it characteristically occurs in infants.
   d. **Peptic ulcer disease, diverticulitis, and cholecystitis** can present clinical pictures similar to those of appendicitis.
   e. **Typhlitis,** characterized by inflammation of the wall of the cecum or terminal ileum, is managed nonoperatively. It is most commonly seen in immunosuppressed patients undergoing chemotherapy for leukemia and in HIV-positive patients. It is difficult to distinguish preoperatively between typhlitis and appendicitis.
2. **Urologic diseases**
   a. **Pyelonephritis** causes high fevers, rigors, costovertebral pain, and tenderness. Diagnosis is confirmed by urinalysis with culture.
   b. **Ureteral colic.** Passage of renal stones causes flank pain radiating into the groin but little localized tenderness. Hematuria suggests the diagnosis, which

is confirmed by intravenous pyelography or noncontrast CT. Abdominal plain films frequently show renal stones.

3. Gynecologic diseases

a. Pelvic inflammatory disease can present with symptoms and signs indistinguishable from those of acute appendicitis, but the two often can be differentiated on the basis of several factors. Cervical motion tenderness and milky vaginal discharge strengthen a diagnosis of PID. In patients with PID, the pain is usually bilateral, with intense guarding on abdominal and pelvic examinations. Transvaginal US can be used to visualize the ovaries and to identify tubo-ovarian abscesses.

b. Ectopic pregnancy. A pregnancy test should be performed in all female patients of child-bearing age presenting with abdominal complaints. A positive test should prompt US investigation.

c. Ovarian cysts are best detected by transvaginal or transabdominal US.

d. Ovarian torsion. The inflammation surrounding an ischemic ovary often can be palpated on bimanual pelvic examination. These patients can have a fever, leukocytosis, and RLQ pain consistent with appendicitis. A twisted viscus, however, differs in that it produces sudden, acute intense pain with simultaneous frequent and persistent emesis. Ovarian torsion may be confirmed by Doppler US.

IV. TREATMENT

A. Preoperative preparation. Intravenous isotonic fluid replacement should be initiated to achieve a brisk urinary output and to correct electrolyte abnormalities. Nasogastric suction is helpful, especially in patients with peritonitis. Temperature elevations are treated with acetaminophen and a cooling blanket. Anesthesia should not be induced in patients with a temperature higher than 39°C.

B. Antibiotic therapy. Antibiotic prophylaxis is generally effective in the prevention of postoperative infectious complications (wound infection, intra-abdominal abscess). Preoperative initiation is preferred, although some suggest that it can be delayed (*Cochrane Database Syst Rev* 2005;20:CD001439). For acute appendicitis, coverage typically consists of a second-generation cephalosporin. In patients with acute nonperforated appendicitis, a single dose of antibiotics is adequate. Antibiotic therapy in perforated or gangrenous appendicitis should be continued for 3 to 5 days.

C. Appendectomy. With very few exceptions, the treatment of appendicitis is appendectomy. Patients with diffuse peritonitis or questionable diagnosis should be explored through a midline incision. The mortality after appendectomy is high in elderly patients. Equivocal diagnosis of appendicitis in this frail patient population warrants increased diagnostic efforts before emergent appendectomy (*Ann Surg* 2001;233:4). In most patients, a transverse incision (e.g., Rockey-Davis, Fowler-Weir) provides the best cosmetic appearance and allows easy extension medially for greater exposure. The external and internal oblique and transversus abdominis muscle layers may be split in the direction of their fibers. After entering the peritoneal cavity, obtain purulent fluid for Gram stain and culture. Once the cecum is identified, the anterior taenia can be followed to the base of the appendix. The appendix is gently delivered into the wound and any surrounding adhesions carefully disrupted. If the appendix is normal on inspection (5% to 20% of explorations), it is removed and appropriate alternative diagnoses are entertained. The cecum, sigmoid colon, and ileum are carefully inspected for changes indicative of diverticular (including Meckel diverticulum), infectious, ischemic, or inflammatory bowel disease (e.g., Crohn's disease). Evidence of mesenteric lymphadenopathy is sought. In women, the ovaries and fallopian tubes are inspected for evidence of PID, ruptured follicular cysts, ectopic pregnancy, or other pathology. Bilious peritoneal fluid suggests peptic ulcer or gallbladder perforation.

D. Laparoscopic appendectomy is an accepted alternative to traditional open approaches. It is most useful when the diagnosis is uncertain or when the size of the patient would necessitate a large incision. Although recent studies suggest that postoperative lengths of stay may be marginally briefer (*Surg Endosc* 2006;20:495), most patients undergoing routine appendectomy can be safely discharged from the hospital on the first postoperative day. Irrespective of the choice of approach, care must be taken to ensure secure ligation of the appendiceal stump.

E. **Drainage of periappendiceal abscess.** Management of appendiceal abscesses remains controversial. Patients who have a well-localized periappendiceal abscess and are initially seen when symptoms are subsiding can be treated with systemic antibiotics and considered for percutaneous US- or CT-guided catheter drainage, followed by elective appendectomy 6 to 12 weeks later (*Radiology* 1987;163:23). This strategy is successful in more than 80% of patients. The appendix must be removed because the patient has a 60% risk of developing appendicitis again within 2 years. Systemic antibiotics are administered for at least 5 days or until the patient is afebrile and leukocytosis resolves. A recent study comparing immediate appendectomy (antibiotics, surgery) with expectant management (antibiotics, percutaneous drainage, and interval appendectomy) in patients with appendiceal abscesses found that the immediate-appendectomy group had a higher complication rate and longer hospital stay (*Am Surg* 2003;69:829).

F. **Incidental appendectomy** is removal of the normal appendix at laparotomy for another condition. The appendix must be easily accessible through the present abdominal incision, and the patient must be clinically stable enough to tolerate the extra time needed to complete the procedure. Because most cases of appendicitis occur early in life, the benefit of incidental appendectomy decreases substantially once a person is older than 30 years. Crohn's disease involving the cecum, radiation treatment to the cecum, immunosuppression, and vascular grafts or other bioprostheses are contraindications for incidental appendectomy because of the increased risk of infectious complications or appendiceal stump leak.

V. COMPLICATIONS OF ACUTE APPENDICITIS

A. **Perforation** is accompanied by severe pain and fever. It is unusual within the first 12 hours of appendicitis but is present in 50% of appendicitis patients younger than 10 years and older than 50 years. Acute consequences of perforation include fever, tachycardia, generalized peritonitis, and abscess formation. Treatment is appendectomy, peritoneal irrigation, and broad-spectrum intravenous antibiotics for several days. During pregnancy, perforation substantially increases the risk of maternal mortality from negligible to 4%. Fetal death rates rises from 0% to 1.5% in uncomplicated appendicitis to 20% to 35% in the setting of perforation.

B. **Postoperative wound infection risk** can be decreased by appropriate intravenous antibiotics administered before skin incision. The incidence of wound infection increases from 3% in cases of nonperforated appendicitis to 4.7% in patients with a perforated or gangrenous appendix. Primary closure is not recommended in the setting of perforation (*Surgery* 2000;127:136). Wound infections are managed by opening, draining, and packing the wound to allow healing by secondary intention. Intravenous antibiotics are indicated for associated cellulitis or systemic sepsis.

C. **Intra-abdominal and pelvic abscesses** occur most frequently with perforation of the appendix. Postoperative intra-abdominal and pelvic abscesses are best treated by percutaneous CT- or US-guided drainage. If the abscess is inaccessible or resistant to percutaneous drainage, operative drainage is indicated. Antibiotic therapy can mask but does not treat or prevent a significant abscess.

D. **Other complications**

1. **Pyelephlebitis** is septic portal vein thrombosis caused by *Escherichia coli* and presents with high fevers, jaundice, and eventually hepatic abscesses. CT scan demonstrates thrombus and gas in the portal vein. Prompt treatment (operative or percutaneous) of the primary infection is critical, along with broad-spectrum intravenous antibiotics.

2. **Enterocutaneous fistulae** from a leak at the appendiceal stump closure occasionally require surgical closure, but most close spontaneously.

E. **Small-bowel obstruction** is four times more common after surgery in cases of perforated appendicitis than in uncomplicated appendicitis.

OTHER INTRA-ABDOMINAL ETIOLOGIES OF ACUTE ABDOMINAL PAIN

This section deals only with presentation and diagnosis. Readers are referred to the respective chapters in this manual for management of specific disease processes.

I. ACUTE CHOLECYSTITIS
  A. Presentation
   1. Most patients provide an **antecedent history of biliary colic** (i.e., epigastric or RUQ pain after consumption of a fatty meal).
   2. Typical presentation is **epigastric or RUQ pain, nausea, and emesis** 4 to 6 hours after consumption of a meal.
  B. Examination is characterized by RUQ tenderness and a positive Murphy's sign.
  C. Ancillary studies
   1. **Laboratory tests may** reveal leukocytosis and a slight elevation of liver enzymes.
   2. Helpful **radiographic studies** include US (looking for gallstones, gallbladder wall thickening, pericholecystic fluid, sonographic Murphy's sign, bile duct size) and diisopropyliminodiacetic acid scan (showing nonfilling of the gallbladder).
  D. It is important to consider the full spectrum of **biliary tract disease.**

II. ACUTE PANCREATITIS
  A. Etiology. The most common cause is **alcohol consumption. Gallstones** account for the majority of remaining cases. Other causes include endoscopic retrograde cholangiopancreatography, medications, and hypertriglyceridemia.
  B. Presentation and severity
   1. Typical presentation is **severe epigastric pain** radiating to the patient's back.
   2. Examination is characterized by **epigastric tenderness** and varying degrees of **tachycardia, fever, and hypotension,** depending on the severity of the attack.
   3. The spectrum of severity ranges from **mild edema** around the pancreas to **pancreatic necrosis with infection.**
  C. The **severity of the attack and the prognosis** may be estimated using various grading schemes [e.g., Ranson's criteria, Acute Physiology and Chronic Health Evaluation (APACHE) II score, Glasgow criteria].
  D. Ancillary studies
   1. **Laboratory examination** typically shows elevation of amylase, lipase, and serum transaminases, none of which correlates with severity.
   2. **Plain x-rays** may reveal a sentinel loop or pancreatic calcifications.
   3. **CT scan** with intravenous contrast is indicated in severe cases to identify pancreatic necrosis or fluid collection (optimal results are obtained after 3 days).

III. PERFORATED PEPTIC ULCER
  A. Duodenal ulcers are more common than **gastric ulcers.**
  B. Presentation
   1. Perforated peptic ulcer is associated with the **chronic use of nonsteroidal anti-inflammatory medications.**
   2. Most patients provide a **history compatible with peptic ulcer disease.**
   3. Perforated peptic ulcer typically presents as sudden onset of **severe epigastric pain** that progresses to peritonitis.
  C. Physical examination is remarkable for diffuse abdominal tenderness, rigidity, and peritoneal signs.
  D. Plain x-rays usually, but not always, reveal free intraperitoneal air.

IV. INTESTINAL OBSTRUCTION
  A. Small-bowel obstruction
   1. The most common cause is **adhesions from previous surgery;** others include hernias, cancer, intussusception, and volvulus.
   2. Usually presents as **sharp, crampy periumbilical pain** with intervening pain-free periods; associated symptoms include nausea and vomiting.
   3. **Examination** is marked by abdominal distention, high-pitched or tinkling bowel sounds, and a variable degree of abdominal tenderness.

4. **Plain x-rays** reveal dilated loops of small bowel, air-fluid levels, and paucity of gas in the colon. Proximal small-bowel obstruction may not be associated with dilated bowel loops on x-ray and often requires a contrast study for diagnosis.
   B. Large-bowel obstruction
   1. Causes include **cancer, diverticulitis, volvulus, and stool impaction.**
   2. Presenting symptoms include **constipation, abdominal distention, and varying degrees of abdominal pain.**
   3. Examination may reveal **abdominal distention or a mass** (the latter revealed by rectal examination).
   4. Plain x-rays may reveal **colonic distention.** A contrast enema is often necessary to rule out the presence of a mass (e.g., obstructing colon, or rectal cancer).
   5. The **risk of perforation** increases as the cecal diameter exceeds 12 cm.

V. MESENTERIC ISCHEMIA
   A. It results from **superior mesenteric artery thrombosis,** from severe vascular disease, or from superior mesenteric artery occlusion by embolus (e.g., in atrial fibrillation).
   B. It presents as **sudden onset of severe, constant abdominal pain** with associated emptying of bowel contents (vomiting and diarrhea).
   C. Examination may reveal **pain out of proportion to physical findings.**
   D. Laboratory studies reveal leukocytosis and acidosis (due to accumulation of lactate).
   E. Angiography may confirm the diagnosis; however, radiologic studies are not indicated if the patient has peritonitis on physical examination.

VI. RUPTURED AAA
   A. A ruptured AAA presents as **sudden onset of abdominal pain** with varying degrees of radiation to the patient's flank, back, or both.
   B. Patients with free intra-abdominal rupture rarely survive until hospital arrival; those with contained rupture or leak may present in shock.
   C. Examination is notable for the presence of a tender, pulsatile abdominal mass.
   D. Plain x-rays may reveal calcification in the aortic wall; CT scan is the gold standard for diagnosis (only performed in hemodynamically stable patients).
   E. Patients with **hypotension from a known aneurysm** should be taken emergently to the operating room without further workup. Anesthetic induction should be delayed until the patient is prepped and draped to avoid intubation-induced hypotension.

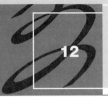

COLON, RECTUM, AND ANUS

12

Sean C. Glasgow and James W. Fleshman

COLORECTAL PHYSIOLOGY

I. NORMAL COLON FUNCTION

  A. Water absorption. Normal ileal effluent totals 900 to 1,500 mL/day, with stool water loss typically less than 200 mL/day. The right colon maximally can absorb 6 L of fluid/day, and only when large-bowel absorption is less than 2 L/day does an increase in fecal water content result in diarrhea.

  B. Electrolyte transport. Sodium and chloride absorption occur by active processes in exchange for potassium and bicarbonate in the right colon.

  C. Nutrition. Although absorption of nutrients is minimal in the colon, mucosal utilization of short-chain fatty acids (SCFAs) produced by colonic bacteria can account for up to 540 kcal/day. Chronic absence of SCFAs such as butyrate and proprionate results in "diversion colitis," a condition characterized by rectal bleeding and rare stricture formation. Subclinical diversion colitis occurs in almost all diverted patients and uniformly resolves following stomal closure.

  D. Motility patterns of the colon allow for mixing and elimination of intestinal contents. Factors influencing motility include emotional state, amount of exercise and sleep, amount of colonic distention, and hormonal variations.

   1. Retrograde movements occur mainly in the right colon. These contractions prolong the exposure of luminal contents to the mucosa and thereby increase the absorption of fluids and electrolytes.

   2. Segmental contractions, the most commonly observed motility pattern, represent localized simultaneous contractions of the longitudinal and circular colonic musculature in short colonic segments.

   3. Mass movements occur three to four times a day and are characterized by an antegrade, propulsive contractile wave involving a long segment of colon.

  E. Microflora. One third of the dry weight of feces is normally composed of bacteria. Anaerobic *Bacteroides* species are most prevalent (10^{11}/mL), whereas *Escherichia coli* has a titer of 10^9/mL. Bacteria produce much of the body's vitamin K. Endogenous colonic bacteria also suppress the emergence of pathogenic micro-organisms. Antibiotic therapy can alter the endogenous microflora, resulting in changes in drug sensitivity (warfarin) or infectious colitides due to pathogenic microbial overgrowth (*Clostridium difficile* colitis).

  F. Colonic gas (200 to 2,000 mL/day) is composed of (1) swallowed oxygen and nitrogen and (2) hydrogen, carbon dioxide, and methane produced during fermentation by colonic bacteria. Because hydrogen and methane are combustible gases that may explode when electrocautery is used for biopsy, adequate bowel cleansing is mandatory before using hot-snare techniques during colonoscopy.

II. DISORDERS OF COLONIC PHYSIOLOGY

  A. The term **constipation** is often used by patients to describe a number of different defecatory symptoms (infrequent bowel movements, difficult or painful movements, etc.). Constipation is generally defined clinically **as one or fewer spontaneous bowel movements or stools per week.**

   1. Etiologies include medications (narcotics, anticholinergics, antidepressants, calcium channel blockers), hypothyroidism, hypercalcemia, dietary factors (low fluid or fiber intake), decreased exercise, neoplasia, and neurologic disorders (e.g., Parkinson disease, multiple sclerosis). Abnormalities of pelvic floor function (obstructed defecation), such as paradoxical puborectalis muscle function or intussusception of the rectum (internal or external rectal prolapse), may result in constipation, as may idiopathic delayed transit of feces through the colon (dysfunction of the intrinsic colonic nerves or colonic inertia).

2. **Evaluation.** Change in bowel habits is a common presentation of colorectal neoplasia. The initial evaluation of constipation should include digital rectal exam and colonoscopy. If this workup is negative and the patient fails to respond to a trial of fiber supplementation and increased fluid intake, the next step is a **colonic transit time study.** On day 0, the patient ingests an enteric-coated capsule containing 24 radiopaque rings. Abdominal plain x-rays are obtained on days 3 and 5. Normal transit results in 80% of the rings in the left colon by day 3 and 80% of all the rings expelled by day 5. The persistence of rings throughout the colon on day 5 indicates colonic inertia. When the rings stall in the rectosigmoid region, functional anorectal obstruction (obstructed defecation) may be present. This may be evaluated with cine defecography, anorectal manometry, or both; the task is to look for nonrelaxation of the puborectalis muscle or internal intussusception of the rectum.

3. **Treatment** of colonic inertia initially includes laxatives (polyethylene glycol, 12 oz/day), fiber (psyllium 9 g/day), increased exercise, and avoidance of predisposing factors. In patients with long-standing, debilitating symptoms refractory to nonoperative measures, **total abdominal colectomy with ileorectal anastomosis** may prove curative. The risk of total intestinal inertia after surgery is significant, and the patient should understand this.

B. **Colonic pseudo-obstruction** (Ogilvie syndrome) is a profound colonic ileus without evidence of mechanical obstruction. It most commonly occurs in critically ill or institutionalized patients. Colonic obstruction or volvulus must be ruled out; Hypaque enema is often therapeutic as well as diagnostic. The initial management consists of nasogastric decompression, rectal tube placement, an aggressive enema regimen (e.g., cottonseed and docusate sodium enema), correction of metabolic disorders, and discontinuation of medications that decrease colonic motility. Neostigmine intravenous infusion (2 mg/hour) in a monitored setting has been shown to be useful in resistant cases (*N Engl J Med* 1999;341:137). Rapid cecal dilation or a cecal diameter greater than 12 cm on plain abdominal x-rays requires prompt colonoscopic decompression. This is successful in 70% to 90% of cases, with a recurrence rate of 10% to 30% (recurrence is usually amenable to repeat colonoscopic decompression). Laparotomy is reserved for patients with peritonitis, at which time a total abdominal colectomy with end ileostomy should be performed.

C. **Volvulus** is the twisting of an air-filled segment of bowel about its mesentery and accounts for nearly 10% of bowel obstruction in the United States.

1. **Sigmoid volvulus** accounts for 80% to 90% of all volvulus and is most common in elderly or institutionalized patients and in patients with a variety of neurologic disorders. It is an acquired condition resulting from sigmoid redundancy with narrowing of the mesenteric pedicle.

   a. **Diagnosis** is suspected when there is abdominal pain, distention, cramping, and obstipation. **Plain films** often show a characteristic **inverted-U,** sausage-like shape of air-filled sigmoid pointing to the right upper quadrant. If the diagnosis is still in question and gangrene is not suspected, water-soluble **contrast enema** usually shows a **bird's-beak deformity** at the obstructed rectosigmoid junction.

   b. In the absence of peritoneal signs, **treatment** involves **sigmoidoscopy,** with the placement of a rectal tube beyond the point of obstruction. The recurrence rate after decompressive sigmoidoscopy approaches 40%; therefore, elective sigmoid colectomy should be performed in acceptable operative candidates. If peritonitis is present, the patient should undergo laparotomy and **Hartmann procedure** (sigmoid colectomy, end-descending colostomy, and defunctionalized rectal pouch). An alternative in the stable patient without significant fecal soilage of the peritoneal cavity is sigmoidectomy, on-table colonic lavage, and colorectal anastomosis with or without proximal fecal diversion (loop ileostomy).

2. **Cecal volvulus** occurs in a younger population than does sigmoid volvulus, likely due to congenital failure of retroperitonealization of the cecum (in axial volvulus) or a very redundant pelvic cecum that flops into the left upper quadrant to kink the right colon (in bascule volvulus).

   a. **Diagnosis.** Presentation is similar to that of distal small-bowel obstruction, with nausea, vomiting, abdominal pain, and distention. Plain films show a **coffee bean–shaped,** air-filled cecum with the convex aspect extending into the left upper quadrant. A **Hypaque enema** may be performed, which shows a tapered (in axial volvulus) or linear cutoff (in bascule volvulus) of the ascending colon.

   b. **Management** involves urgent laparotomy and right hemicolectomy. Ileo-colostomy is preferred; otherwise, ileostomy and mucous fistula are performed if concern about patient stability or bowel viability exists. Cecopexy has an un-acceptably high rate of recurrent volvulus, and although cecectomy will prevent recurrence, it is technically more challenging than formal right hemicolectomy.

3. **Transverse volvulus** is rare and has a clinical presentation similar to that of sigmoid volvulus. Diagnosis is made based on the results of plain films (which show a dilated right colon and an upright, U-shaped, dilated transverse colon) and contrast enema or computed tomography (CT). Endoscopic decompression has been reported, but operative resection is usually required.

D. **Diverticular disease**

1. **General considerations.** Colonic diverticula are **false diverticula** in which mu-cosa and submucosa protrude through the muscularis propria. Outpouchings oc-cur along the mesenteric aspect of the antimesenteric taenia where arterioles pene-trate the muscularis. The **sigmoid colon** is most commonly affected, perhaps owing to decreased luminal diameter and increased luminal pressure. Diverticula are as-sociated with a low-fiber diet and are rare before age 30 years (<2%), but the **incidence increases with age** to a 75% prevalence after age 80 years. Right-sided diverticula are rare, comprising less than 10% of diverticular disease.

2. **Complications**

   a. **Infection (diverticulitis).** Microperforations can develop in long-standing di-verticula, leading to fecal extravasation and subsequent peridiverticulitis. Di-verticulitis develops in 10% to 25% of patients with diverticula.

   (1) **Presentation** is notable for left-lower-quadrant pain (which may radiate to the suprapubic area, left groin, or back), fever, altered bowel habit, and urinary urgency. Physical examination varies with severity of the disease, but the most common finding is localized left-lower-quadrant tenderness. The finding of a mass suggests an abscess or phlegmon.

   (2) **Evaluation** by CT scan and complete blood count (CBC) is the standard of care. CT findings may include segmental colonic thickening, focal extra-luminal gas, and abscess formation. Neither sigmoidoscopy nor contrast enema is recommended in the initial workup of diverticulitis because of the risk of perforation or barium or fecal peritonitis, respectively.

   (3) **Treatment** is tailored to symptom severity.

   (a) **Mild diverticulitis** can be treated on an outpatient basis with a clear liquid diet and broad-spectrum oral antibiotics for 10 days.

   (b) **Severe diverticulitis** is treated with complete bowel rest, intravenous fluids, narcotic analgesics, and broad-spectrum parenteral antibiotics (e.g., ciprofloxacin and metronidazole). If symptoms improve within 48 hours, a clear liquid diet is resumed, and antibiotics are given orally when the fever and leukocytosis resolve. A high-fiber, low-residue diet is resumed after 1 week of pain-free tolerance of a liquid diet. Fiber supplements and stool softeners should be given to prevent constipation. A colonoscopy or water-soluble contrast study must be performed after 4 to 6 weeks to rule out colon cancer, inflammatory bowel disease, or ischemia as a cause of the segmental inflammatory mass.

(4) The lifetime likelihood of **recurrence** is 30% after the first episode and more than 50% after the second episode of diverticulitis. Therefore, **resection** is considered 4 to 6 weeks after treatment of a complicated initial attack of diverticulitis or after treatment of the first recurrence. The belief that diverticulitis in young patients (<50 years) somehow is more virulent is largely anecdotal. Large retrospective reviews have demonstrated that young patients have the same risk of recurrent diverticulitis following an uncomplicated attack as their older counterparts (*Dis Colon Rectum* 2006;49:1341).

(5) Elective resection for diverticulitis usually consists of a sigmoid colectomy. The proximal resection margin is through uninflamed, nonthickened bowel, but there is no need to resect all diverticula in the colon. The distal margin extends to normal, pliable rectum, even if this means dissection beyond the anterior peritoneal reflection. Recurrent diverticulitis after resection is most frequently related to inadequate distal margin of resection.

b. Diverticular abscess is usually identified on CT scan. A **percutaneous drain** should be placed under **radiologic guidance.** This avoids immediate operative drainage, allows time for the inflammatory phlegmon to be treated with intravenous antibiotics, and turns a two- or three-stage procedure into a one-stage procedure. A low pelvic abscess may be drained into the rectum via a transanal approach.

c. Generalized peritonitis is rare and results if diverticular perforation leads to widespread fecal contamination. In most cases, resection of the diseased segment is possible **(two-stage procedure)**, and a Hartmann procedure is performed. The colostomy can then be reversed in the future. An alternative in the management of the stable patient undergoing urgent operation for acute diverticulitis without significant fecal contamination is sigmoidectomy, on-table colonic lavage, and colorectal anastomosis with or without proximal fecal diversion (loop ileostomy).

d. Fistulization secondary to diverticulitis may occur between the colon and other organs, including the bladder, vagina, small intestine, and skin. Diverticulitis is the most common etiology of colovesical fistulas. Colovaginal and colovesical fistulas usually occur in women who have previously undergone hysterectomy. Colocutaneous fistulas are uncommon and are usually easy to identify. Coloenteric fistulas are likewise uncommon and may be entirely asymptomatic or result in corrosive diarrhea.

(1) The presentation of **enterovesical fistula** includes frequent urinary tract infections and often is unsuspected until **fecaluria** or **pneumaturia** is noted. CT findings of air and solid material in a noninstrumented bladder confirm the diagnosis. Lower endoscopy, barium enema, intravenous pyelography, and cystoscopy often fail to demonstrate the fistula.

(2) A **colovaginal fistula** is usually suspected based on the passage of air or gas per vagina. The fistula may be difficult to identify on physical examination or the previously mentioned tests. The presence of methylene blue staining on a tampon inserted in the vagina following dye instillation in the rectum is diagnostic.

(3) Immediate treatment of the inflammatory mass adjacent to the bladder is as previously described for severe diverticulitis [Section II.D.2.a(3)(b)]. Colonoscopy is performed after 6 weeks to rule out other possible etiologies, including cancer or inflammatory bowel disease. Elective sigmoid resection is performed after preoperative placement of temporary ureteral catheters. Ureteral catheters can be very helpful in identifying the distal ureter in the inflammatory pericolonic mass, thereby shortening the operative time. Usually, the fistula tract can be broken using finger fracture, and the bladder defect can be repaired in a single layer. A Foley catheter is left in place for 7 to 10 days to allow this defect to heal. A colovaginal fistula is managed in a similar fashion. It may be helpful to interpose omentum between the colorectal anastomosis and the bladder or vaginal defect.

E. **Acquired vascular abnormalities and lower gastrointestinal (GI) bleeding** are more common in elderly patients than in younger individuals. Most cases of massive lower GI hemorrhage stop spontaneously, but surgery is required in 10% to 25% of cases.

1. **Etiologies** (with relative approximate incidence) of lower GI bleeding in industrialized nations include the following:

   a. **Diverticulosis (60%).** The media of the perforating artery adjacent to the colonic diverticulum may become attenuated and eventually erode. This arterial bleeding usually is bright red and is not associated with previous melena or chronic blood loss. Bleeding most commonly occurs from the left colon. Urgent resection of the affected colonic segment should be considered in patients with active ongoing bleeding [>6 units packed red blood cells (RBCs)/24 hours]. Elective resection of the affected colonic segment should be performed in patients with recurrent bleeding or need for long-term anticoagulation or in those in whom excessive blood loss may be poorly tolerated.

   b. **Inflammatory bowel disease (IBD) (13%).** Bleeding due to IBD tends to occur in a younger population; it is more commonly due to ulcerative colitis than Crohn disease.

   c. **Benign anorectal disease (11%)** is discussed later in this chapter.

   d. **Neoplasia (10%)** of the colon and rectum rarely presents with massive blood loss, but rather with chronic microcytic anemia and possible syncope. Hemorrhage following polypectomy can occur up to 1 month postprocedure and has an incidence of 3% in some series.

   e. **Angiodysplasias (<5%)** are small arteriovenous malformations composed of small clusters of dilated vessels in the mucosa and submucosa. An acquired condition, they rarely occur before age 40 years and are more common in the right colon (80%). Diagnosis can be made by colonoscopy or angiographic features (delayed filling of a dilated venule).

2. **Massive lower GI bleeding** is defined as hemorrhage distal to the ligament of Treitz that requires more than 3 units of blood in 24 hours. **Management** consists of simultaneously restoring intravascular volume and identifying the site of bleeding so that treatment may be instituted.

   a. **Resuscitation** is performed using a combination of isotonic crystalloid solutions and packed RBCs as needed, administered via short, large-bore peripheral intravenous catheters.

   b. **Diagnosing the site of bleeding** is more important initially than identifying the cause. Gastric lavage via a nasogastric tube must be performed to rule out an upper GI source of bleeding. Digital rectal exam can eliminate hemorrhoidal bleeding. The choice of localizing study depends on the estimate of bleeding rate.

      (1) **Nuclear scan** using technetium-99m sulfur colloid or tagged RBCs can identify bleeding sources with rates as low as 0.1 to 0.5 mL/minute. Tagged RBC scan can identify bleeding up to 24 hours after isotope injection, which may be important in patients who bleed intermittently. Although these scans can accurately demonstrate ongoing bleeding, they do not definitively identify the anatomic source of bleeding; hence, planning a segmental gastrointestinal resection based on this study is not entirely reliable. A rapidly positive scan indicates that angiography has a high likelihood of identifying the source.

      (2) **Mesenteric angiography** should be performed in the patient with a positive nuclear medicine bleeding scan with massive lower GI bleeding to definitively identify the anatomic source of bleeding. Angiography can localize bleeding exceeding 1 mL/minute and allows either therapeutic vasopressin infusion (0.2 unit/minute) or embolization, which together are successful in stopping the bleeding in 85% of cases. The advantage is that this can convert an emergent operation in an unstable patient with unprepared bowel to an elective one-stage procedure.

(3) Colonoscopy frequently fails to identify the source of massive lower GI bleeds. With slower bleeding after the administration of an adequate bowel preparation over 2 hours, colonoscopy offers the therapeutic advantages of injecting vasoconstrictive agents (epinephrine) or vasodestructive agents (alcohol, morrhuate, sodium tetradecyl sulfate) or applying thermal therapy (laser photocoagulation, electrocoagulation, heater probe coagulation) to control bleeding.

(4) In the rare **patients who continue to bleed with no source identified,** laparotomy should be considered. Intraoperative small-bowel enteroscopy may be performed if the source is not obvious at the time of exploration. If the source is still not identified, **total colectomy with ileorectostomy or end-ileostomy** is performed. This is associated with an incidence of recurrent bleeding of less than 10%, but the mortality rate for patients who rebleed is 20% to 40%. It is now rare for a patient to undergo resection for lower GI bleeding without preoperative localization.

3. **Ischemic colitis** results from many causes, including venous or arterial thrombosis, embolization, iatrogenic inferior mesenteric artery (IMA) ligation after abdominal aortic aneurysm repair, thromboangiitis obliterans, and polyarteritis nodosa. It is **idiopathic** in the majority of patients. Patients are usually elderly and present with lower abdominal pain localizing to the left and melena or hematochezia. The rectum often is normal on proctoscopy, owing to its dual vascular supply. Contrast enema may show thumbprinting that corresponds to submucosal hemorrhage and edema. Diagnosis depends on the appearance of the mucosa on colonoscopy. Although it may occur anywhere in the colon, disease is present most frequently at the watershed areas of the splenic flexure and sigmoid colon. In the presence of full-thickness necrosis or peritonitis, emergent resection with diversion is recommended. Patients without peritonitis or free air but with fever or an elevated white blood cell count may be treated with bowel rest, close observation, and intravenous antibiotics. Up to 50% of patients develop focal colonic strictures eventually. These are treated with serial dilations or segmental resection once neoplasm is ruled out.

4. **Radiation proctocolitis** results from pelvic irradiation for uterine, cervical, bladder, prostate, or rectal cancers. Risk factors include a dose of greater than 6,000 cGy, vascular disease, diabetes mellitus, hypertension, prior low anterior resection, and advanced age. The early phase occurs within days to weeks; mucosal injury, edema, and ulceration develop, with associated nausea, vomiting, diarrhea, and tenesmus. The late phase occurs within weeks to years, is associated with tenesmus and hematochezia, and consists of arteriolitis and thrombosis, with subsequent bowel thickening and fibrosis. Ulceration with bleeding, stricture, and fistula formation may occur. Medical treatment may be successful in mild cases, with the use of stool softeners, steroid enemas, and topical 5-aminosalicylic acid products. If these measures fail, transanal application of formalin 4% to affected mucosa may be efficacious in patients with transfusion-dependent rectal bleeding. Patients with stricture or fistula require proctoscopy and biopsy to rule out locally recurrent disease or primary neoplasm. Strictures may be treated by endoscopic dilation but often recur. Surgical treatment consists of a diverting colostomy and is reserved for medical failures, recurrent strictures, and fistulas. Proctectomy is rarely required and is usually associated with unacceptable morbidity and mortality.

ANORECTAL PHYSIOLOGY

I. NORMAL ANORECTAL FUNCTION

   A. The **rectum functions as a capacitance organ,** with a reservoir of 650 to 1,200 mL compared to an average daily stool output of 250 to 750 mL.

B. The **anal sphincter mechanism** allows defecation and maintains continence. The internal sphincter (involuntary) accounts for 80% of resting pressure, whereas the external sphincter (voluntary) accounts for 20% of resting pressure and 100% of squeeze pressure. The internal anal sphincter relaxes periodically to sample rectal contents but is contracted at rest. The puborectalis muscle is contracted at rest and relaxes only during defecation. It also maintains the anorectal angle. The external anal sphincter contracts in response to stimulation and relaxes during defecation.

C. **Defecation** has four components: (1) mass movement of feces into the rectal vault; (2) rectal-anal inhibitory reflex, by which distal rectal distention causes involuntary relaxation of the internal sphincter; (3) voluntary relaxation of the external sphincter mechanism and puborectalis muscle; and (4) increased intra-abdominal pressure.

D. **Continence** requires normal capacitance, normal sensation at the anorectal transition zone, puborectalis function for solid stool, external sphincter function for fine control, and internal sphincter function for resting pressure.

II. **INCONTINENCE** is the inability to prevent elimination of rectal contents (gas, liquid, or solid).

A. **Etiologies** include (1) **mechanical defects,** such as sphincter damage from obstetric trauma, treatment of abscess or fistula by anterior quadrant fistulotomy, and scleroderma affecting the external sphincter; (2) **neurogenic defects,** including spinal cord injuries, pudendal nerve injury due to birth trauma or lifelong straining, and systemic neuropathies such as multiple sclerosis; and (3) **stool content–related causes,** such as diarrhea and radiation proctitis.

B. **Evaluation** includes visual and digital examination observing for gross tone or squeeze abnormalities. **Anal manometry** quantitatively measures parameters of anal function, including resting and squeeze pressure (normal mean >40 and >80 mm Hg, respectively), sphincter length (2.5 cm in men, 2 cm in women), and minimal sensory volume of the rectum. Pudendal nerve terminal motor latency **(PNTML)** testing and endoanal ultrasound can further evaluate sphincteric physiology and anatomy, respectively.

C. **Treatment** depends on the type and severity of the defect. Neurogenic and minor mechanical anal sphincter defects are treated using dietary fiber to increase stool bulk and **biofeedback** to strengthen muscle and improve early sensation. Major defects require **anal sphincter reconstruction,** in which the external sphincter is circularized and then plicated to recreate the perineal body. Artificial anal sphincters may be used in patients without a reconstructible native anal sphincter. Severe denervations of an intact anal sphincter may be managed with sacral nerve stimulation, artificial sphincters, or palliative diverting colostomy.

III. **OBSTRUCTED DEFECATION** (pelvic floor outlet obstruction) presents with symptoms of chronic constipation and straining with bowel movements. Problems may include **fecal impaction** and **stercoral ulcer** (mucosal ulceration due to pressure necrosis from impacted stool); both are treated with enemas, increased dietary fiber, and stool softeners. Attempts at surgical correction of any of the following conditions without addressing the underlying pathology are doomed to failure.

A. **Physiologic evaluation** includes (1) **defecography** to evaluate maintenance of fixation of the posterior rectum to the sacrum as well as relaxation of the puborectalis and (2) **colonic transit study** to distinguish colonic inertia from anorectal malfunction.

B. **Anal stenosis** is a rare cause of obstructed defecation and presents with frequent thin stools and bloating. The most common etiologies include scarring after anorectal surgery (rare), chronic laxative abuse, radiation, recurrent anal ulcer, Crohn disease, and trauma. Initial treatment is anal dilation, although advanced cases are treated with advancement flaps of normal perianal skin.

C. **Nonrelaxation of puborectalis** results in straining and incomplete evacuation. Diagnosis requires a normal colonic transit time and persistent puborectalis distortion on defecography. Biofeedback is the treatment of choice.

D. **Descending perineum syndrome** occurs when chronic straining causes pudendal nerve stretch and subsequent neurogenic defect. **Rectocele** results from a weak, distorted rectovaginal septum that allows the anterior rectal wall to bulge into the vagina due to failure of the pelvic floor to relax during defecation.

IV. ABNORMAL RECTAL FIXATION leads to internal or external prolapse of the full thickness of the rectum.

    A. Internal intussusception (internal rectal prolapse) causes outlet obstruction with mucus discharge, hematochezia, tenesmus, and constipation. Proctoscopy demonstrates a **solitary rectal ulcer** at the lead point of the internal prolapse. **Treatment** consists of increased bulk, stool softeners, and glycerin suppositories. **Indications for surgery** are chronic bleeding, impending incontinence, and lifestyle-changing symptoms. Surgical options are controversial. The most frequent procedure is transabdominal rectopexy (suture fixation of the rectum to the presacral fascia) and anterior resection of the sigmoid colon if constipation is prominent among the patient's complaints. Chronic ischemia of the solitary rectal ulcer causes entrapment of mucin-producing cells, eventually resulting in **colitis cystica profunda.** Treatment is low anterior resection and rectopexy.

    B. External rectal prolapse is protrusion of full-thickness rectum through the anus. Symptoms include pain, bleeding, mucous discharge, and incontinence. Physical examination can distinguish rectal prolapse (concentric mucosal rings) from prolapsing internal hemorrhoids (deep radial grooves). **Risk factors** include increased age, female gender, institutionalization, antipsychotic medication, previous hysterectomy, and spinal cord injury. Evaluation includes **barium enema or colonoscopy** to rule out malignancy and **manometry and electromyography** to determine sphincter function. In general, abdominal procedures trade higher operative morbidity with lower recurrence rates relative to perineal-only operations. Continence improves in almost all patients, regardless of procedure.

        1. Sigmoid resection and rectopexy (Goldberg-Frykman procedure) is performed in patients able to tolerate a general anesthetic to shorten the redundant rectosigmoid colon and re-establish posterior sacral fixation. Prolapse recurs in less than 10% of patients following rectopexy with or without resection.

        2. Perineal proctectomy (modified Altemeier procedure) is an alternative for elderly or infirm patients. This is also an attractive procedure for the rare young man with external rectal prolapse in whom potency is a concern. Recurrence rate is generally around 20%, although lower rates have been reported in retrospective, single-institution studies (*Dis Colon Rectum* 2006;49:1052).

V. HEMORRHOIDS are vascular and connective tissue cushions that exist in three columns in the anal canal: right anterolateral, right posterolateral, and left lateral. **Internal hemorrhoids** are above the dentate line and thus covered with mucosa. These may bleed and prolapse, but they do not cause pain. **External hemorrhoids** are below the dentate line and covered with anoderm. These do not bleed but may thrombose, which causes pain and itching, and secondary scarring may lead to skin tag formation. Hard stools, prolonged straining, increased abdominal pressure, and prolonged lack of support to the pelvic floor all contribute to the abnormal enlargement of hemorrhoidal tissue. **Treatments** are based on grading and patient symptoms (Table 12-1); options include the following:

    A. Medical treatment for first-degree and most second-degree hemorrhoids includes increased dietary fiber and water, stool softeners, and avoidance of straining during defecation. Refractory second- and third-degree hemorrhoids may be treated in the office by **elastic ligation.** The ligation must be 1 to 2 cm above the dentate line to avoid pain and infection. One quadrant is ligated every 2 weeks in the office, and the patient is warned that the necrotic hemorrhoid may slough in 7 to 10 days with bleeding occurring at that time. Patients on anticoagulation should be treated with excisional hemorrhoidectomy instead of elastic ligation (see following section). Severe sepsis may occur after banding in immunocompromised patients or those who have had full-thickness rectal prolapse ligated by mistake. Patients present with severe pain, fever, and urinary retention within 12 hours of ligation. Patients with this life-threatening disorder should undergo examination under anesthesia, immediate removal of rubber bands, and débridement of any necrotic tissue, accompanied by broad-spectrum intravenous antibiotics.

    B. Excisional hemorrhoidectomy is reserved for large third- and fourth-degree hemorrhoids, mixed internal and external hemorrhoids, and thrombosed, incarcerated

TABLE 12-1	Classification and Treatment of Symptomatic Internal Hemorrhoids	

Grade	Description	Treatments
I	Palpable, nonprolapsing enlarged venous cushions	Dietary fiber, stool softeners
II	Prolapse with straining and defecation, spontaneously reduce	Dietary fiber, stool softeners, elastic ligation
III	Protrude spontaneously or with straining, require manual reduction	Dietary fiber, stool softeners, elastic ligation, excisional hemorrhoidectomy, stapled hemorrhoidectomy
IV	Chronically prolapsed and cannot be reduced, often with dentate line released from internal position	Dietary fiber, stool softeners, excisional hemorrhoidectomy, stapled hemorrhoidectomy

hemorrhoids with impending gangrene. The procedure is performed with the patient in the **prone flexed position,** and the resulting elliptical defects are completely closed with chromic suture (Ferguson hemorrhoidectomy). Complications include a 10% to 50% incidence of urinary retention, bleeding, infection, sphincter injury, and anal stenosis from taking too much mucosa at the dentate line.

C. **Stapled hemorrhoidectomy** is an alternative to traditional excisional hemorrhoidectomy for large prolapsing, bleeding third-degree hemorrhoids with minimal external disease. This procedure is performed by a circumferential excision of redundant rectal mucosa approximately 5 cm superior to the dentate line using a specially designed circular stapler. In the largest prospective, multicenter study comparing stapled with excisional hemorrhoidectomy, 156 patients were randomized to treatment and followed for 1 year (*Dis Colon Rectum* 2004;47:1824). Stapled hemorrhoidectomy resulted in significantly less perioperative discomfort, and no statistical difference in recurrence was detected. However, a subsequent Cochrane database analysis of 12 randomized, controlled trials including more than 530 patients found a significantly greater recurrence rate following stapled hemorrhoidectomy, particularly with longer follow-up intervals (*Cochrane Database Syst Rev* 2006;4:5393). The authors concluded that excisional hemorrhoidectomy remains the "gold standard."

D. **Acutely thrombosed external hemorrhoids** are treated by excision of the thrombosed vein outside the mucocutaneous junction, which can be done in the office or emergency room with the wound left open. If the thrombosis is more than 48 hours old, the patient is treated with nonsurgical management.

VI. **ANAL FISSURE** is a split in the anoderm. Ninety percent of anal fissures occur posteriorly and 10% occur anteriorly; location elsewhere should prompt exam under anesthesia and biopsy. Symptoms include tearing pain with defecation and severe anal spasm that lasts for hours afterward and blood (usually on the toilet paper). Manometry and digital rectal examination demonstrate increased sphincter tone and muscular hypertrophy in the distal one third of the internal sphincter. An external skin tag or "sentinel pile" may also be present. Differential diagnosis includes Crohn disease (fissure often in the lateral location), tuberculosis, anal cancer, abscess or fistula, cytomegalovirus, herpes simplex virus, chlamydia, and syphilis. **Ninety percent of patients heal with medical treatment** that includes increased fiber, steroid suppositories, stool softeners, and sitz baths. Topical nifedipine ointment (0.2%) or nitroglycerin also has been shown to promote healing. If surgery is required, **lateral internal sphincterotomy** is 90% successful. Recurrence and minor incontinence occur in fewer than 10% of patients.

INFECTIONS

I. COLITIS

A. Pseudomembranous colitis is an acute diarrheal illness resulting from toxins produced by overgrowth of *Clostridia difficile* after antibiotic treatment (especially the use of clindamycin, ampicillin, or cephalosporins). Antibiotics already have been discontinued in one fourth of cases, and symptoms can occur up to 6 weeks after even a single dose. **Diagnosis** is made by detection of toxin A in one of at least three stool samples. Proctoscopy demonstrates sloughing colonic mucosa or pseudomembranes, and CT often shows transmural colonic thickening. **Treatment** begins with stopping unnecessary antibiotics and starting oral or intravenous metronidazole. Oral (but not intravenous) vancomycin is an alternative but more expensive therapy. For severe cases in patients unable to take oral medications, vancomycin enemas (500 mg in 250 mL saline) may be useful. Rarely, pseudomembranous colitis presents with severe peritoneal irritation and colonic distention with **toxic megacolon** or **perforation.** Emergency laparotomy with total colectomy and end-ileostomy is required.

B. Amebic colitis results from invasive infection by the protozoan *Entamoeba histolytica,* which is spread by the fecal-oral route. It is most commonly encountered in patients who have traveled abroad. The cecum usually is affected with small ulcers that may perforate or form an inflammatory mass or **ameboma. Diagnosis** is made by examining stool for ova and parasites, which is 90% sensitive in identifying the trophozoites. **Treatment** is oral metronidazole and iodoquinol. Surgical treatment is reserved for perforation or for ameboma refractory to treatment.

C. Actinomycosis is an abdominal infection that most commonly occurs around the cecum after appendectomy owing to the anaerobic Gram-positive *Actinomyces israelii.* An inflammatory mass often is present with sinuses to the skin that can drain **sulfur granules. Diagnosis** is confirmed by anaerobic culture (the organism may take up to 1 week to isolate), and **surgical drainage** combined with penicillin or tetracycline is required.

D. Neutropenic enterocolitis after chemotherapy occurs most commonly in the setting of acute myelogenous leukemia after cytosine arabinoside therapy. It is also seen frequently in patients undergoing chemotherapy for stage III or IV colon cancer. Patients present with abdominal pain, fever, bloody diarrhea, distention, and sepsis. The cecum often dilates, and there may be pneumatosis. **Initial treatment** includes bowel rest, total parenteral nutrition, granulocyte colony–stimulating factor (G-CSF), and broad-spectrum intravenous antibiotics. Laparotomy with total colectomy and ileostomy is required only if peritonitis develops.

E. Cytomegalovirus colitis presents with bloody diarrhea, fever, and weight loss. It affects 10% of patients with acquired immunodeficiency syndrome (AIDS; homosexual men are more commonly affected) and is the most common cause for emergent abdominal surgery in patients with AIDS. Ganciclovir is the treatment of choice; emergent colectomy with ileostomy is reserved for toxic megacolon.

II. INFECTION OF THE ANORECTUM

A. Anorectal abscess

1. Cryptoglandular abscess results from infection of the anal glands in the crypts at the dentate line. The initial abscess occurs in the intersphincteric space. Infection then can spread (1) superficial to the external sphincter into the **perianal** space, (2) through the external sphincter into the **ischiorectal** space (which in turn may connect posteriorly via the deep postanal space, resulting in a horseshoe abscess), or (3) deep to the external sphincter into the **supralevator** space.

a. Diagnosis usually is obvious, with severe anal pain and a palpable, tender, fluctuant mass. An intersphincteric abscess yields only a painful bulge in the rectal wall and no external manifestations.

b. Treatment is surgical drainage, with the skin incision kept close to the anal verge to avoid the possible creation of a long fistula tract. Intersphincteric abscesses are drained by an internal sphincterotomy over the entire length of the abscess. Perianal and ischiorectal abscesses are drained through the perianal skin with a small mushroom-shaped catheter placed to keep the abscess unroofed. Antibiotic therapy is not necessary unless the patient (1) is immunocompromised, (2) is diabetic, (3) has extensive cellulitis, or (4) has valvular heart disease. Immunocompromised patients may present with anal pain without fluctuance because of the paucity of leukocytes. The painful indurated region must still be drained, and the underlying tissue must undergo biopsy and culture.

    c. **Outcome from drainage alone** shows that 40% of patients develop a chronic fistula. We do not advocate fistulotomy at the initial operation because the internal opening may not be evident and a complicated fistulotomy may result in sphincter injury.

  2. **Fistula-in-ano** represents the chronic stage of cryptoglandular abscess but also may be due to trauma, Crohn disease, tuberculosis, cancer, or radiation.

    a. Patients present with persistent fecopurulent **perianal drainage** from the external opening of the fistula. The location of the internal opening along the dentate line is approximated by using **Goodsall's rule**: Fistulas with external openings anterior to a transverse plane through the anal canal penetrate toward the dentate line in a radial direction, whereas fistulas posterior to that plane curve so that the internal opening is in the posterior midline.

    b. **Treatment** depends on the level of the fistula and preexisting sphincter function. Placement of a soft, noncutting seton permits resolution of surrounding inflammation while preserving sphincter musculature. **Fistulotomy,** dividing the overlying internal sphincter, may be performed for intersphincteric fistulas. **Fibrin glue injection** of the tract has a high failure rate but does not limit future options. A newer alternative is insertion of an **anal fistula plug** composed of lyophilized porcine submucosa to create a collagen scaffold to allow tract healing. Early pilot studies reported an 85% success rate at median 12-month follow-up; long-term data are lacking (*Dis Colon Rectum* 2006;49:1817). Definitive treatment of a posterior midline fistula is fistulotomy, whereas anterior fistulas require sliding flap repairs if less invasive options fail.

B. Necrotizing anorectal infection (Fournier gangrene) can result in massive, life-threatening tissue destruction. Patients present with systemic toxicity and perianal pain. There may be crepitance and extensive necrosis under relatively normal skin. Synergistic flora (including clostridial and streptococcal species) of anorectal and urogenital origin may be involved. Immediate wide surgical débridement of all nonviable tissue and intravenous antibiotics are mandatory. Early treatment is critical, but mortality still approximates 50%.

C. Pilonidal disease occurs secondary to infection of a hair-containing sinus in the postsacral intergluteal fold 5 cm superior to the anus. Patients present with pain, swelling, and drainage when the sinuses become infected. The disease is most prevalent in men in the second and third decades of life. Symptoms are distinguished from perianal abscess by the lack of anal pain, the more superior location of the fluctuant mass, and the presence of midline cutaneous pits. Treatment is incision, drainage, and curettage, with allowance for secondary closure when the sinus is acutely inflamed. The disease tends to recur, however, and once the active inflammation has resolved, the sinus can be excised electively, with primary closure and a higher chance of cure.

D. Hidradenitis suppurativa is an infection of the apocrine sweat glands and mimics fistula-in-ano except that involvement is external to the anal verge. The treatment of choice is wide incision of the involved skin.

E. Pruritus ani is a common symptom of hemorrhoids, fissure, rectal prolapse, rectal polyp, anal warts, Bowen disease, and Paget disease. Treatment is directed toward resolution of the underlying cause. Failure to find an underlying cause should prompt investigation of dietary factors (e.g., coffee, alcohol). Children should be evaluated for pinworms, which, if found, are treated with piperazine citrate.

F. Condyloma acuminatum is an anorectal and urogenital wart caused by infection with human papilloma virus. The disease is most commonly transmitted through anal intercourse and presents with visible perianal growth, often accompanied by pruritus, anal discharge, bleeding, and pain. Common treatments include topical trichloracetic acid, Aldara (imiquimod), or excision with electrocoagulation under local anesthesia. Smoke generated by coagulation contains viable organisms and must be completely evacuated. Anal canal warts must be destroyed at the same time as external warts.

INFLAMMATORY BOWEL DISEASE

I. GENERAL CONSIDERATIONS

A. Ulcerative colitis is an inflammatory process of the colonic mucosa characterized by alterations in bowel function, most commonly bloody diarrhea with tenesmus. It has a male predominance. The disease **always involves the rectum** and extends continuously variable distances in the proximal colon. Patients often have abdominal pain, fever, and weight loss. As the duration of the inflammation increases, pathologic changes progress. Initially, mucosal ulcers and crypt abscesses are seen. Later, mucosal edema and pseudopolyps (islands of normal mucosa surrounded by deep ulcers) develop, and the end-stage pathologic changes show a flattened, dysplastic mucosa. The lumen is normal in diameter. Cancer must be considered in any colonic stricture in a patient with ulcerative colitis.

B. Crohn disease is a transmural inflammatory process that can affect any area of the GI tract, from the mouth to the anus. It has a female predominance. The disease has a segmental distribution, with **normal mucosa interspersed between diseased areas of bowel.** Common symptoms include diarrhea, abdominal pain, nausea and vomiting, weight loss, and fever. There can be signs of an abdominal mass or perianal fistulas on physical examination. The **terminal ileum** is involved in up to 45% of patients at presentation. Common pathologic changes include fissures and fistulas, transmural inflammation, and granulomas. Grossly, the mucosa shows aphthoid ulcers that often deepen over time and are associated with fat wrapping and bowel wall thickening. As the disease progresses, the bowel lumen narrows, and obstruction or perforation may result. Over time, the areas of stricture may develop dysplastic or even neoplastic changes.

C. "Indeterminate colitis" is a term used for cases in which the pathologic pattern does not fall clearly into one or the other of the aforementioned patterns (10% to 15% of patients with IBD). The indeterminacy can be due either to inadequate tissue biopsy or to a truly indeterminate form of disease.

D. Extraintestinal manifestations of inflammatory bowel disease are common with ulcerative colitis and with Crohn disease. Patients with either disease can develop dermatologic conditions such as erythema nodosum and pyoderma gangrenosum, ocular inflammatory diseases, and arthritis/synovitis. These typically correlate with the degree of colonic inflammation. Ulcerative colitis patients also can develop sclerosing cholangitis.

II. ULCERATIVE COLITIS

A. Indications for surgery

1. Failure to respond to medical treatment. Inability to wean from high-dose steroids after two successive tapers prompts evaluation for surgery.

2. The **risk of malignancy** is related to the extent and duration of the disease but not the intensity of the disease. Colitis-associated cancer usually infiltrates submucosally and has signet-ring histology. The risk increases by 1%/year after 10 years of disease. Colonoscopy is performed 7 to 10 years after the diagnosis and every 1 to 2 years thereafter, with random biopsies every 10 cm and directed biopsies of mass lesions. Resection is recommended for dysplasia or stricture.

3. Severe bleeding that does not respond adequately to medical therapy requires resection for control.

4. Acute severe fulminant colitis [white blood cell count (WBC) >16,000, fever, abdominal pain, distention] initially is treated with bowel rest, antibiotics, steroids, and avoidance of contrast enemas, antidiarrheals, and morphine. If the patient develops worsening sepsis or peritonitis, abdominal colectomy with end-ileostomy is performed.

B. Surgical management aims at removing the colorectal mucosa while maintaining bowel function as much as possible. Because the disease is localized to the rectum and colon, curative resection is possible. Sphincter-sparing procedures are preferred to preserve the functions of continence and defecation. However, they are associated with higher postoperative complication risk. Anal sphincter function is assessed with manometry to ensure normal function before contemplation of a sphincter-sparing procedure in a patient medically able to undergo the operation.

1. **Restorative proctocolectomy (ileal pouch–anal anastomosis, IPAA)** maintains enteral continuity through the anal sphincter mechanism and is the operation of choice in most patients. A total proctocolectomy is carried out to the anal transition zone. The rectum is transected, leaving the sphincters and levators intact. A distal ileal pouch is constructed over a distance of 15 cm in a J configuration, pulled through the sphincters, and stapled or sutured to the rectal cuff. Stapled anastomoses leaving a 2-cm cuff of anal canal mucosa technically are easier but require long-term surveillance of the residual mucosa. A diverting loop ileostomy is constructed, then reversed 3 months later after healing of the distal anastomosis. **Complications** include increased stool frequency (five to seven times daily), nocturnal soiling (20%), pouch fistula (<10%), and pouchitis (28%), an intermittent inflammatory process that typically responds to metronidazole. Pouch capacity increases over time; eventually, the patient needs to empty the pouch an average of four to five times daily. The pouch procedure can be performed laparoscopically.

2. **Total proctocolectomy with end-ileostomy** is performed in patients who have perioperative sphincter dysfunction or incontinence and in high-risk patients who would not tolerate potential postoperative complications. Most patients do well with a well-placed **Brooke ileostomy** that has a spigot configuration and empties into a bag appliance in an uncontrolled fashion. A **Kock pouch** or continent ileostomy does not empty spontaneously, does not require a permanent appliance, and requires cannulation six to eight times daily. These are more difficult to construct and prone to obstruction. This alternative is occasionally offered to patients who desire continence or who have severe skin allergies, which make ileostomy appliances problematic.

III. CROHN DISEASE is a chronic disease that is not surgically curable. Surgery should be performed only for complications of the acute disease, such as perforation, fistulas, and phlegmon or when chronic disease results in stricture formation. When a patient presents with a complication requiring surgery, all attempts should be made to prepare the patient so that a single operation will suffice and as much intestine as possible can be preserved. Preparations often include parenteral nutrition, antibiotics, anti-inflammatory medications, and percutaneous drainage of abscesses.

A. Surgical management of Crohn disease is limited to resection of the diseased segment of intestine responsible for the complication. Resection is bounded by grossly normal margins; no attempt is made to obtain microscopically negative margins because outcome and recurrence are unaffected by this. If significant intra-abdominal infection or inflammation is encountered during surgery, a proximal ostomy is created to allow complete diversion of intestinal contents and resolution of the initial process. If no infection or inflammation is encountered, normal-appearing bowel can be primarily anastomosed. **Stricturoplasty** to preserve small-bowel length is favored by some groups, with single-institution retrospective reviews demonstrating comparable recurrence rates to resectional treatment (*J Am Coll Surg* 2001;192:330).

B. Small-intestinal Crohn disease is covered in Chapter 10.

C. Colonic Crohn disease often requires operation after a shorter duration of symptoms than is typical for patients with either small-intestinal or ileocolic Crohn disease. Perforation can occur without dilation of the colon secondary to thickening of the colonic wall. Surgical options include total abdominal colectomy with ileorectal anastomosis, total abdominal colectomy with an end-ileostomy and maintenance of the rectum as a Hartmann pouch, or total proctocolectomy with permanent end-ileostomy. Rarely, colonic strictures can occur in an isolated segment, causing obstruction. The risk of colon cancer with Crohn disease is 7% at 20 years; thus, any colonic stricture should be biopsied. Segmental resection is the treatment of choice for isolated segmental colonic Crohn disease; stricturoplasty has no role in colonic strictures. All efforts should be directed to preserving the rectum in colonic Crohn disease because restorative proctocolectomy is not an option.

D. Rectal Crohn disease rarely occurs in isolation. Once the rectum has become so fibrotic that it loses its reservoir capacity, proctectomy should be considered. Precise **intersphincteric** dissection along the rectal wall beginning at the anal verge should minimize complications.

E. Anal disease occurs in 35% of patients with Crohn disease, but only 2% present with disease confined exclusively to the perineum. Treatment of acute disease entails surgical drainage of perianal sepsis followed by medical therapy (steroids, bowel rest, antibiotics). **Infliximab,** an anti–tumor necrosis factor-α (TNF-α) antibody, also has a role in acute and chronic perianal fistulas to reduce local disease activity and allow for subsequent surgical therapy. The ACCENT II (A Crohn's disease Clinical study Evaluating infliximab in a New long-term Treatment regimen) study was a landmark multicenter, double-blind, randomized trial of more than 300 patients with fistulizing Crohn disease. Initial response was observed in 69% of patients treated with infliximab, and maintenance therapy (in responders) was shown to prolong time to recurrent fistulization (*N Engl J Med* 2004;350:876). However, both infusion reactions and infections occur in approximately 30% of patients, and prolonged treatment with azathioprine is necessary to maintain remission. Ultimately, proctectomy or diversion may be the only way to return quality of life to the patient.

NEOPLASTIC DISEASE

I. The **etiology** of colorectal neoplasia has genetic and environmental components.

A. Familial cancer syndromes account for 10% to 15% of colorectal cancers (Table 12-2).

B. Sporadic cancers account for approximately 85% of colorectal neoplasia. Although no inherited genetic mutation can be identified, first-degree relatives of patients with colorectal cancer have a three- to ninefold increase in the risk of developing the disease. Overwhelming evidence suggests that colorectal carcinomas develop from precursor adenomas and are associated with an increasing number of genetic mutations (the so-called **Vogelstein progression**). A single genetic mutation in the germline of a patient may cause an adenoma to develop. Further mutations in either tumor-suppressor genes or oncogenes are responsible for further development of the adenoma and eventually transformation to neoplasia. Genes implicated in this journey from normal epithelium to carcinoma include *K-ras, DCC,* and *p53.*

C. Environmental factors have also been proposed to play a significant role in the etiology of colorectal neoplasia. Dietary factors that have been shown to increase cancer risk include a diet high in unsaturated animal fats and highly saturated vegetable oils. Increased fiber decreases cancer risk in those on a high-fat diet. Epidemiologic studies indicate that people from less-industrialized countries have a lower risk of colorectal cancer, likely due to dietary differences. This survival benefit disappears in people who immigrate to the United States.

II. DETECTION. Surveillance is the periodic complete examination of a patient with known increased risk. **Screening** is the limited examination of a population with the goal of detecting patients with increased risk.

A. Screening of the general population is recommended starting at **age 50** years by the American Cancer Society, the American College of Gastroenterology, and the American Society of Colon and Rectal Surgeons. Screening entails either dual-contrast barium enema with sigmoidoscopy or total colonoscopy, and these should be repeated every 10 years if normal or if the patient is not at high risk for

TABLE 12-2 Hereditary Colorectal Cancer (CRC) Syndromes

Syndrome	% of total CRC burden	Genetic basis	Phenotype	Extracolonic manifestations	Treatment	Notes
Familial adenomatous polyposis (FAP)	<1%	Mutations in tumor suppressor gene APC (5q21)	<100 adenomatous polyps; near 100% with CRC by age 40 yr	CHRPE, osteomas, epidermal cysts, periampullary neoplasms	TPC with end-ileostomy or IPAA or TAC with IRA and lifelong surveillance	Variants include Turcot (CNS tumors) and Gardener (desmoids) syndromes
Hereditary nonpolyposis colorectal cancer (HNPCC)	5%–7%	Defective mismatch repair: MSH2 and MLH1 (90%), MSH6 (10%)	Few polyps, predominantly right-sided CRC, 80% lifetime risk of CRC	At risk for uterine, ovarian, small intestinal, pancreatic malignancies	Genetic counseling; consider prophylactic resections, including TAH/BSO	High microsatellite instability (MSI-H) tumors, better prognosis than sporadic CRC
Peutz-Jeghers (PJS)	<1%	Loss of tumor suppressor gene LKB1/STK11 (19p13)	Hamartomas throughout GI tract	Mucocutaneous pigmentation, risk for pancreatic cancer	Surveillance EGD and colonoscopy q3 yr; resect polyps >1.5 cm	Majority present with SBO due to intussuscepting polyp
Familial juvenile polyposis (FJP)	<1%	Mutated SMAD4/DPC (18q21)	Hamartomas throughout GI tract; >3 juvenile polyps; 15% with CRC by age 35 yr	Gastric, duodenal and pancreatic neoplasms; pulmonary AVMs	Genetic counseling; consider prophylactic TAC with IRA for diffuse disease	Presents with rectal bleeding or diarrhea

AVM, arteriovenous malformation; CHRPE, congenital hypertrophy of retinal pigmented epithelium; CNS, central nervous system; EGD, esophagogastroduodenoscopy; GI, gastrointestinal; IPAA, ileal pouch-anal anastomosis; IRA, ileal-rectal anastomosis; TAC, total abdominal colectomy; TAH/BSO, total abdominal hysterectomy and bilateral salpingo-oophorectomy; TPC, total proctocolectomy.

colorectal neoplasia. Colonoscopy has a perforation risk of 0.1%, hemorrhage incidence of 0.3%, and mortality of 0.01%. It offers the advantages of obtaining a tissue diagnosis of any abnormality (potentially therapeutic) and greater sensitivity over barium enema. CT colonography is available for those patients unfit or unable to undergo endoscopic evaluation.

B. High-risk individuals should be in a surveillance program. Previous cancer or polypectomy increases the risk of metachronous cancer by a factor of 2.7 to 7.7. Routine surveillance has been shown to reduce the incidence of metachronous cancer, although its influence on survival is unknown. High-risk patients are those with (1) ulcerative colitis of more than 10 years' duration, (2) Crohn or ulcerative colitis with stricture, (3) a history or family history of polyps or cancer, or (4) a family history of adenomatous polyposis (FAP) or hereditary nonpolyposis colorectal cancer (HNPCC). Our surveillance algorithm calls for initial or perioperative colonoscopy followed by yearly examination until no lesions are detected, followed by examination every 3 years until no lesions are detected, and then examination every 5 years.

III. POLYPS
A. Nonadenomatous polyps
1. **Peutz-Jeghers syndrome** is an autosomal dominant condition characterized by **hamartomatous polyps** of smooth muscle throughout the GI tract and mucocutaneous pigmentation. Symptoms include bleeding or obstruction secondary to intussusception. Although hamartomas are benign, patients with Peutz-Jeghers syndrome are at increased risk for gastrointestinal adenocarcinoma as well. Therefore, treatment for polyps greater than 1.5 cm in diameter is polypectomy. Surveillance colonoscopy and esophagogastroduodenoscopy (EGD) are recommended every 2 years, as well as periodic screening for breast, cervical, testicular, ovarian, and pancreatic cancer.
2. **Juvenile polyps** are cystic dilations of glandular structures in the lamina propria without malignant potential that may result in bleeding or obstruction. There are two peaks in incidence of isolated juvenile polyps: in infants and at age 25 years. They are the most common cause of GI bleeding in children and should be treated with polypectomy. **Multiple polyposis coli** (diffuse juvenile polyps) is an autosomal dominant syndrome characterized by multiple juvenile polyps and increased risk for GI malignancy. These patients are considered for total abdominal colectomy or proctocolectomy with IPAA.
3. **Hyperplastic polyps** show epithelial dysmaturity and hyperplasia and are the most common colorectal neoplasm (10 times more common than adenomas). They have no malignant potential. Most are less than 0.5 cm in diameter and rarely need treatment. However, those showing a mixed adenoma/hyperplastic histology carry the same risks as adenomatous polyps.

B. Adenomas are benign neoplasms with unrestricted proliferation of glandular epithelium within the colonic mucosa but with no invasion of the basement membrane. The degree of differentiation decreases as a polyp becomes more like a cancer. *Severe atypia* refers to malignant cells in a polyp that have not invaded the muscularis mucosae (formerly known as *carcinoma in situ*). Adenomatous polyps fall into three broad categories, based on the percentage of villous composition:
1. **Tubular adenomas** are usually pedunculated and account for roughly 85% of adenomas. They have a 5% risk of containing malignant cells.
2. **Tubulovillous adenomas** account for 10% of adenomas. They have a 22% risk of containing cancer.
3. **Villous adenomas** are usually sessile and account for 5% of adenomas. Both size and induration of the polyp reflect cancer risk. For example, a 4-cm sessile villous adenoma has a 40% risk of cancer, whereas the same polyp with induration has a 90% risk.

C. Treatment consists of colonoscopic removal. Pedunculated polyps have a stalk and can be removed using the cautery snare. Semisessile and sessile polyps may require piecemeal extraction. The site of incomplete removal should be marked with 0.1 mL of India ink for possible later intraoperative or repeat colonoscopic identification.

For sessile or large polyps (>3 cm) that cannot be removed endoscopically, surgical resection is required.

1. **The risk of metastatic cancer** in regional lymph nodes is 1% in a completely excised, pedunculated polyp in which cancer invades only the head of the polyp, unless there is lymphatic or vascular invasion. These cases may be treated with either colectomy or polypectomy with close follow-up. Invasion of the cancer down the stalk to the lower third requires colectomy.

2. **Sessile polyps** containing cancer require colectomy, even if completely excised, because the risk of local recurrence and lymph node metastasis is greater than 10% to 20%.

D. **Villous adenoma of the rectum** can present with watery diarrhea and hypokalemia. The risk of cancer in lesions greater than 4 cm with induration is 90%, and transrectal ultrasonography should be used to determine the depth of invasion before excision. Treatment of favorable lesions is by transanal, full-thickness local excision followed by closure of the defect with suture. The role of **transanal endoscopic microsurgery (TEM)** continues to evolve and has become an accepted approach to rectal villous adenomas. Accurate interpretation of the existing small series of patients with early rectal cancer undergoing TEM is difficult due to heterogeneous inclusion criteria, misstaging of rectal cancer, and varying surgeon experience. If the adenoma is large (>4 cm), circumferential, contains invasive cancer, or is located above the peritoneal reflection (generally 10 cm above the anal verge), a transabdominal proctectomy should be performed.

IV. COLON CANCER

A. The **incidence** of colorectal cancer in the United States has been stable since the 1950s, with 145,000 new cases (105,000 colon and 40,000 rectal) each year and 58,000 deaths each year. It is the third-most-lethal cancer in men and women, with a slight female predominance in colon cancer and male predominance in rectal cancer. There is a 5% lifetime risk; 6% to 8% of cases occur before age 40 years, and the incidence increases steadily after age 50 years.

B. **Clinical presentation** of colon cancer depends on the location of the lesion. Many tumors are asymptomatic and discovered on routine screening colonoscopy. **Right-colon** lesions occasionally cause hematochezia, but more often bleeding is occult, causing anemia and fatigue. **Left-colon** lesions more often cause crampy abdominal pain, altered bowel habit, or hematochezia. In less than 10% of cases, left-colon cancer presents as large-bowel obstruction with inability to pass flatus or feces, abdominal pain, and distention. Approximately 50% of patients with other symptoms complain of weight loss, but weight loss is almost never the sole manifestation of a colorectal tumor. Rarely, colon cancer presents as perforation with focal or diffuse peritonitis or as a fistula with pneumaturia or feculent vaginal discharge. These symptoms may be difficult to distinguish from those of diverticulitis. Metastatic disease is usually asymptomatic but may present with jaundice, pruritus, and ascites or with cough and hemoptysis.

C. **Diagnosis and staging**

1. **Once the diagnosis is suspected based on history, physical examination, or screening tests,** every attempt should be made to obtain biopsy of the primary lesion and rule out synchronous cancer (3% to 5%). Colonoscopy to the cecum or flexible sigmoidoscopy and barium enema are acceptable. In patients presenting with obstructive symptoms, water-soluble contrast enema is performed to assess the degree and level of obstruction and to "clear" the colon proximal to the obstruction.

2. **Staging studies** to look for distant metastases include chest x-ray and abdominal CT scan. CT identifies liver metastases as well as adrenal, ovarian, pelvic, and lymph node metastases. Serum carcinoembryonic antigen (CEA) is a useful prognostic and surveillance tumor marker in colorectal cancer. CEA should be obtained preoperatively as part of the staging evaluation. Recently, positron emission tomography (PET)-CT has been shown to have greater sensitivity for detecting metastatic disease than CT alone. It is routinely performed prior to concurrent colectomy and liver resection for hepatic metastases.

D. Surgical treatment

  1. Bowel preparation minimizes the titers of *Escherichia coli* and *Bacteroides fragilis* and facilitates bowel manipulation by reducing stool bulk. Mechanical cleansing with Fleets Phospho-Soda (mono and dibasic sodium phosphate) must be accompanied by ingestion of large volumes (24 oz) of clear liquids. Two 45-mL doses are given at 12 PM and at 6 PM the day before surgery. Patients with cardiac, hepatic, or renal dysfunction may experience severe fluid and electrolyte abnormalities after administration of this mechanical bowel preparation. An alternate mechanical bowel preparation for these patients includes an isotonic lavage solution (GoLYTELY). Early on the preoperative day, 4 L are given orally within a 4-hour period, accompanied by a clear liquid diet. All patients should receive preoperative intravenous antibiotics (typically cefoxitin or ciprofloxacin and metronidazole) within 1 hour of skin incision. We routinely administer prophylactic enoxaparin preoperatively to reduce the risk of deep venous thrombosis.

  2. Open operative technique begins with a thorough exploration that includes palpation of the liver. After mobilization of the involved segment, the main segmental vessels are then ligated and divided, and en bloc resection of colon and any adherent structure is carried out, including small bowel, ovaries, uterus, or kidney. If curative resection is not possible, palliative resection should be attempted, and if this cannot be done, bypass should be performed. For right-colon cancer, resection includes the distal 10 cm of terminal ileum to the transverse colon, taking the ileocolic, right colic, and right branch of the middle colic vessels. A transverse colon lesion is resected with either an extended right colectomy or a transverse colectomy, taking only the middle colic vessels. Left colon lesions require dividing the inferior mesenteric artery (IMA) at its origin. If multiple carcinomas are present, or if a colon carcinoma with multiple neoplastic polyps is present, then a subtotal colectomy is performed. The specimen margin is inspected in the operating room to ensure at least a 2-cm margin (5 cm for poorly differentiated tumors).

  3. Laparoscopic colectomy offers a shorter hospital stay and faster recovery for patients with colon cancer. Oncologically, it is guided by the same principles as open resection. The Clinical Outcomes of Surgical Therapy (COST) trial demonstrated noninferiority of the laparoscopic approach as compared to open surgery, with statistically similar times to tumor recurrence, wound implantation, and overall survival at 4.5 years (*N Engl J Med* 2004;350:2050). This multicenter trial of 872 patients is commendable for the strict requirement of surgeon credentialing prior to enrolling patients, including video review of operative technique by a panel of experts.

  4. Emergency operations are undertaken without bowel preparation and have a higher incidence of wound infection. For obstruction, right colectomy still can be performed with primary anastomosis and no diversion. Options with a left colon cancer include (1) resection with colostomy and either mucous fistula or Hartmann pouch, (2) resection with intraoperative lavage and primary anastomosis, (3) resection with primary anastomosis and proximal diverting ileostomy, (4) subtotal colectomy and ileosigmoidostomy, and (5) colostomy with staged resection of the tumor in an unstable patient with markedly dilated colon. In all but the subtotal colectomy, the proximal colon must be evaluated in the postoperative period for synchronous cancer.

E. Staging and prognosis. The American Joint Committee on Cancer TNM staging identifies the depth of invasion of the tumor (T), regional lymph node status (N), and presence of distant metastases (M). Stage I (T1 or T2, N0, M0) tumors do not involve the muscularis and have a 90% 5-year survival. Stage II (T3 or T4, N0, M0) tumors penetrate the muscularis and have a 60% to 80% 5-year survival. Stage III (Tx, N1 or N2, M0) tumors involve lymph nodes and have a 60% 5-year survival. Stage IV (Tx, Nx, M1) tumors have distant metastases and a 5-year survival of 10%. Unfavorable characteristics include poor differentiation, mucinous or signet-ring pathology, venous or perineural invasion, bowel perforation, aneuploid nuclei, and elevated carcinoembryonic antigen (CEA).

F. **Adjuvant chemotherapy** remains a standard treatment for stage III and IV colon cancer. Current regimens involve the combination of 5-fluorouracil/leucovorin with either irinotecan (FOLFIRI) or oxaliplatin (FOLFOX). The role of targeted therapy using vascular endothelial growth factor (VEGF) inhibitors (bevacizumab) or epidermal growth factor receptor (EGFR) inhibitors (cetuximab) is evolving. Patients with stage IIb tumors with poor prognostic factors may also benefit from adjuvant chemotherapy, although the risk-to-benefit ratio is not as great.

G. **Follow-up** is crucial in the first 2 years after surgery, when 90% of recurrences occur. Surveillance colonoscopy is recommended the first year after resection and then every 3 years until negative, at which time every 5 years is recommended. CEA should be checked in the first year, and rising levels should prompt a CT scan, a chest x-ray, and a PET scan to detect and stage recurrence.

V. RECTAL CANCER

A. The **pathophysiology** of rectal cancer differs from that of colon cancer because of several anatomic factors: (1) confinement of pelvis and sphincters, making wide excision impossible; (2) proximity to urogenital structures and nerves, resulting in high levels of impotency in men; (3) dual blood supply and lymphatic drainage; and (4) transanal accessibility.

B. **Diagnosis and staging**

1. **Local aspects.** Digital rectal examination can give information on the size, fixation, ulceration, local invasion, and lymph node status. Rigid sigmoidoscopy and biopsy are crucial for precisely measuring the distance to the dentate line and for obtaining a tissue diagnosis. Flexible sigmoidoscopy cannot accurately assess the length of the tumor from the dentate line (which in turn determines the operative procedure to be performed). In experienced hands, **transrectal ultrasonography** has an accuracy of approximately 75% for T stage and 65% for N stage; it should be an integral part of the staging of rectal tumors. T1 lesions are limited to the mucosa and submucosa, T2 lesions are limited to the muscularis propria, T3 lesions penetrate the rectal wall, and T4 lesions invade adjacent structures.

2. **Regional aspects.** Pelvic CT, magnetic resonance (MR) scan, and transrectal ultrasound can yield information on the local extension of the tumor toward the bony pelvis. Pelvic examination is necessary to assess the possible fixation of the tumor to adjacent genitourinary structures. Cystoscopy may be required in some men to evaluate extension into the prostate or bladder.

3. **Distant spread** is evaluated (as with colon cancer) with chest x-ray, abdominal CT, and serum CEA. PET scanning is frequently helpful in identifying recurrent disease or disease outside of the liver or lung.

C. **Surgical treatment goals** are to remove cancer with adequate margins and perform an anastomosis only if there is good blood supply, absence of tension, and normal anal sphincters. If any of these conditions cannot be met, the entire rectum must be removed and the patient left with a permanent colostomy.

1. **Bowel preparation** is the same as that for colon cancer.

2. The **stoma sites on the abdominal wall should be marked** for possible colostomy on the left side, avoiding bony prominences, belt lines, and scars and staying medial to the rectus muscle at the summit of a fat fold. The right lower quadrant should also be marked in the event that a temporary loop ileostomy is necessary. Stoma sites should be marked even if the surgeon is anticipating performing an anastomosis.

3. **Positioning and preparation.** If the patient has had previous pelvic surgery or the cancer is suspected to involve the bladder or ureter, ureteral stents should be placed after induction of anesthesia. The patient is placed in the dorsal lithotomy position, which gives access to the abdomen and perineum. A nasogastric tube, Foley catheter, and 34-French mushroom rectal catheter are placed, and the rectum is irrigated until clear with warm saline before instilling 100 mL of povidone-iodine (Betadine).

4. **Operative technique.** The patient's abdomen is explored through a midline incision. The left colon is mobilized through the splenic flexure using the embryonic fusion plane, reflecting the ureter and gonadal vessels posteriorly. The IMA is ligated at the aorta. The inferior mesenteric vein is ligated with the left colic artery or at the ligament of Treitz. The colon is transected at the descending and sigmoid junction with a purse-string suture, and an end-to-end anastomosis stapler anvil is placed in the proximal segment. Rectal dissection then proceeds posteriorly along the avascular presacral plane, laterally through the vascular lateral ligaments, and finally anteriorly, with preservation of the seminal vesicles or vagina. Dissection continues distally well beyond the tumor so that transection allows at least a 2-cm distal margin and a full removal of the rectal mesentery transected at a right angle at the level of the distal intestinal margin. The Dutch Rectal Cancer Trial demonstrated the value of this standardized surgical approach, **the total mesorectal excision (TME),** reporting a local recurrence rate of only 2.4% at 2-year follow-up in patients receiving preoperative short-course radiation and TME (*N Engl J Med* 2001;345:638).

5. **Surgical options** at this point depend on the height of the lesion, the condition of the sphincters, and the condition of the patient. An abdominoperineal resection is performed for tumors that cannot be resected with a 2-cm distal margin or if sphincter function is questionable. Low anterior resection using an intraluminal stapler is the operation of choice for tumors that can be resected with an adequate distal margin. A colonic J-pouch or coloplasty may also be constructed to recreate the reservoir function of the rectum. Generally, ultralow resections or those with marginal blood supply should be protected with a temporary diverting ileostomy. A hand-sewn coloanal anastomosis is required when the distal margin includes the anal transition zone.

6. **Complications**
   a. **Impotence** occurs in 50% of men and must be discussed preoperatively. The sites of nerve injury are the IMA origin, the presacral fascia, the lateral ligaments, and anteriorly at the level of the seminal vesicles. Prosthesis may be considered 1 year after surgery, once the pelvis is shown to be free of recurrence and the patient has had appropriate time to adapt to changes in body image.
   b. **Leakage** at the anastomosis occurs in up to 20% of patients, typically between postoperative days 4 and 7. Fever, elevated WBC count, increased or changed drain output, or abdominal pain during this period should prompt in-depth physical examination and CT scan evaluation. Intravenous antibiotics and bowel rest are usually sufficient, but laparotomy and fecal diversion are necessary for large leaks.
   c. **Massive presacral venous bleeding** can occur at the time of resection. This is controlled either with a pledget of abdominal wall muscle sutured to the sacrum or by packing the pelvis for 24 to 48 hours.

7. **Obstructive rectal cancer** requires emergent laparotomy on an unprepared bowel. The type of procedure depends on whether presurgical adjuvant therapy is considered. A decompressing transverse colostomy can be made through a small upper midline incision. This may be a blowhole type if the colon is massively dilated, or it may be a loop colostomy over a rod. If preoperative radiotherapy is not given, options include Hartmann resection, total colectomy with ileorectostomy, and low anterior resection protected by proximal diversion.

D. **Adjuvant therapy** for rectal cancer should routinely be considered to reduce local recurrence and possibly improve overall survival.
   1. **Preoperative radiotherapy** was shown in the Swedish Rectal Cancer Trial to increase the 5-year survival rate and decrease local recurrences in all stages in a multicenter, prospective, randomized trial performed before the widespread use of TME (*N Engl J Med* 1997;336:980). Preoperative radiation remains the standard of care, sometimes in conjunction with chemotherapy. Two dosing options that are biologically similar may be considered: (1) 2,000 cGy over 5 days preoperatively, followed by immediate operation, or (2) 4,500 cGy over 5 weeks,

followed by a 7-week waiting period to allow for tumor shrinkage. Postoperative therapy has been advocated by some if the adequacy of the resection is in doubt and the patient did not receive preoperative radiotherapy. Postoperative radiotherapy is associated with a higher risk of complications, including injury to the small intestine and the colorectal anastomosis.

2. **Neoadjuvant chemoradiation,** including chemotherapy with a 5-fluorouracil–based regimen, results in a modest survival benefit and decreased local recurrence over radiation therapy alone. It is generally reserved for patients with large, bulky tumors or evidence of nodal metastases.

E. **Nonresectional therapy** is indicated in some early-stage cancers, patients with poor operative risk, and patients with widespread metastases. Options include transanal excision, electrocoagulation, endocavitary radiation, and laser vaporization. Most recently, we have used combined external-beam and endocavitary radiation as the definitive treatment for favorable but invasive rectal cancers.

F. If the patient has **incurable cancer** and a life expectancy of less than 6 months, external beam radiation, with or without chemotherapy, combined with laser destruction, dilation, or stenting the rectum can prevent obstruction. If the life expectancy exceeds 6 months, resectional therapy is attempted.

G. The major cause of **locally recurrent rectal cancer** is a positive margin on the pelvic side wall (radial margin). Recurrences tend to occur within 18 months and grow back into the lumen, presenting with pelvic pain, mass and rectal bleeding, or a rising CEA level. Diagnosis is confirmed by examination and biopsy as well as CT or PET scan. Treatment is not highly satisfactory, and there is a 10% to 20% palliation rate. If chemoradiation has not been given previously, it is given at this point using intensity modulated radiation therapy (IMRT). If distant metastases are again ruled out, low anterior resection, abdominoperineal resection, or pelvic exenteration (resection of rectum and urinary bladder) is performed based on whether the sphincters and the genitourinary organs are involved.

VI. OTHER COLORECTAL TUMORS

A. **Lymphoma** is most often metastatic to the colorectum, but primary non-Hodgkin colonic lymphoma accounts for 10% of all GI lymphomas. The GI tract is also a common site of non-Hodgkin lymphoma associated with human immunodeficiency virus. The most common presenting symptoms include abdominal pain, altered bowel habit, weight loss, and hematochezia. Biopsies are often not diagnostic because the lesion is submucosal. The workup is similar to that for colon cancer but should include a bone marrow biopsy and a thorough search for other adenopathy. Treatment is resection with postoperative chemotherapy. Intestinal bypass, biopsy, and postoperative chemotherapy should be considered for locally advanced tumors.

B. **Retrorectal tumors** usually present with postural pain and a posterior rectal mass on physical examination and CT scan (*Dis Colon Rectum* 2005;48:1581).

1. The **differential diagnosis** includes congenital, neurogenic, osseous, and inflammatory masses. Chordomas are the most common malignant retrorectal tumor; they typically are slow growing but difficult to resect for cure.

2. **Diagnosis** is suspected based on CT scan and physical findings. Biopsy should not be performed. Formal resection should be undertaken.

C. Carcinoid tumor

1. **Colonic carcinoids** account for 2% of GI carcinoids. Lesions less than 2 cm in diameter rarely metastasize, but 80% of lesions greater than 2 cm in diameter have local or distant metastases, with a median length of survival of less than 12 months. These lesions are treated with local excision if small and with formal resection if greater than 2 cm.

2. **Rectal carcinoid** accounts for 15% of GI carcinoids. As with colonic carcinoids, lesions less than 1 cm in diameter have low malignant potential and are well treated with transanal or endoscopic resection. Rectal carcinoids greater than 2 cm in diameter are malignant in 90% of cases. Treatment of large rectal carcinoids is controversial, but low anterior resection or abdominoperineal resection is probably warranted.

VII. ANAL NEOPLASMS

A. Tumors of the anal margin

1. **Squamous cell carcinoma** behaves like cutaneous squamous cell carcinoma, is well differentiated and keratinizing, and is treated with wide local excision and chemoradiation if large.

2. **Basal cell carcinoma** is a rare, male-predominant cancer and is treated with local excision.

3. **Bowen disease** is intraepidermal squamous cell carcinoma. It is rare and usually slow growing. Treatment is wide local excision of all affected skin to the dentate line. Usually a rotational skin flap is used to fill the resulting defect.

B. Anal canal tumors

1. **Epidermoid carcinoma** is nonkeratinizing and derives from the anal canal up to 6 to 12 mm above the dentate line.

   a. **Epidermoid cancer** has a female predominance and usually presents with an indurated, bleeding mass. On examination, the inguinal lymph nodes should be examined specifically because spread below the dentate line passes to the inguinal nodes. Diagnosis is made by biopsy, and 30% to 40% are metastatic at the time of diagnosis.

   b. **Treatment** involves chemoradiation according to the **Nigro protocol:** 3,000-cGy external-beam radiation, mitomycin C, and 5-fluorouracil. Current regimens substitute cisplatin for mitomycin. Surgical treatment is reserved for locally persistent or recurrent disease only. The procedure of choice is abdominoperineal resection; perineal wound complications are frequent.

2. **Adenocarcinoma** is usually an extension of a low rectal cancer and has a poor prognosis.

3. **Melanoma** accounts for 1% to 3% of anal cancers and is more common in white in the fifth and sixth decades of life. Symptoms include bleeding, pain, and a mass, and the diagnosis is often confused with that of a thrombosed hemorrhoid. At the time of diagnosis, 38% of patients have metastases. Treatment is wide local excision, although the 5-year survival rate is less than 20%.

DRAINS AND OSTOMIES

I. ENTERIC DRAINS

A. Nasogastric (NG) tubes are commonly utilized in patients with small-bowel obstructions, prolonged or expected postoperative ileus, or surgical conditions that may be jeopardized if exposed to excessive gastric secretions (e.g., new duodenal closures).

1. Most standard NG tubes are **sump drains.** When the main channel is placed to negative pressure suction, the smaller secondary channel permits air to be drawn into the stomach. This allows continuous suction to be used while preventing gastric mucosa from being drawn into the suction ports. The sump port should never be plugged; frequent flushing with air will ensure a properly functioning tube. Typically, the NG is placed correctly when two of the four marker dots are outside of the nose. Although auscultation over the epigastrium is reassuring, placement should **always** be confirmed by plain radiograph, with the key finding being a radiopaque tube going below the diaphragm that ends in the body of the stomach.

2. **Routine nasogastric decompression** following abdominal surgery should be strongly discouraged. In a systematic review of 28 randomized, controlled trials with almost 4,200 patients, the authors determined that patients without NG tubes actually had faster return of bowel function while experiencing fewer pulmonary complications (*Br J Surg* 2005;92:673).

3. **Complications** of NG tubes include aspiration, posterior laryngeal irritation, gastritis resulting in upper GI bleeding, distal migration, inadvertent placement in the bronchial system, and nasopharyngeal hemorrhage. A particularly troublesome

complication is nasal septal cartilage or cutaneous pressure necrosis that occurs from draping the NG over the top of the face in an obtunded patient.

B. Rectal tubes. Rectal tubes are indicated in bedridden patients who have diarrhea or frequent loose stools to prevent maceration of the skin of the perineum. The tubes can be placed at the bedside and connected to gravity drainage. They are available with or without a balloon tip. The tubes should not be left in place for more than 1 week to prevent pressure necrosis. Long-rectal tubes placed using a colonscope are used to "stent" the colon following volvulus and for irrigation purposes in treating severe infectious colitis.

II. INTESTINAL STOMAS

A. Ileostomy creation and care was revolutionized with the description of the eversion technique by **Brooke** in 1952. Eversion eliminates the serositis reaction commonly observed from the proteolytic ileal effluent. Another advance has occurred with the widespread employment of trained nurse enterostomal therapists to educate and care for patients with ostomies.

1. **Physiology.** The small intestine adapts to ileostomy formation within 10 days postoperatively, with ileostomy output typically reaching a plateau between 200 and 700 mL/day. Because the effluent is highly caustic, it is crucial to maintain a stoma appliance that protects the surrounding skin and seals to the base of the ileostomy.

2. **Stoma construction** of either a loop ileostomy or end-ileostomy should include eversion of the functioning end to create a 2.5-cm spigot configuration. Stoma creation lateral to the rectus abdominis increases the risk of peristomal herniation. Precise apposition of mucosa and skin prevents serositis and obstruction. Preoperative marking of the planned stoma prevents improper placement near bony prominences, belt/pant lines, abdominal creases, and scars.

3. **Ileostomy care** requires special attention to avoid dehydration and obstruction. The patient is encouraged to drink plenty of fluids and to use antidiarrheal agents as needed to decrease output volume. Patients should be warned to avoid fibrous foods, such as whole vegetables and citrus fruits, because these may form a bolus of indigestible solid matter that can obstruct the stoma. Irrigating the ostomy with 50 mL of warm saline from a Foley catheter inserted beneath the fascia, in combination with intravenous fluids and nasogastric decompression, may relieve obstruction and dehydration. Alternatively, water-soluble contrast enema may be diagnostic as well as therapeutic.

4. **Reversal** of a loop ileostomy is relatively straightforward and rarely requires laparotomy. A double-stapled technique with a GIA stapler is utilized if enough intestinal length can be obtained; otherwise, the enterostomy is closed with sutures in two layers.

B. The **colostomy** construction technique depends on whether the goal is decompression or diversion. Ongoing surveillance of the remaining colon is necessary but often overlooked in patients with colostomies.

1. A **decompressing colostomy** vents the distal and proximal bowel limbs while maintaining continuity between the limbs. A blowhole is used for massively dilated colon. The anterior wall of the transverse colon is sewn in two layers to the abdominal fascia and the skin. Typically, blowhole colostomies are reserved for patient palliation.

2. **Diverting colostomies,** such as end-colostomy and mucous fistula, are used following distal resection or perforation so that the distal limb is completely separated from the fecal stream. All colostomies are matured in the operating room. If a stoma rod is used, it is removed 1 week after surgery.

3. **Complications** of colostomies include necrosis, stricture, and herniation. If the stoma becomes dusky, an anoscope is inserted. If necrosis does not extend below the fascia, it can be observed safely; otherwise, urgent revision is performed. **Parastomal hernias** are repaired only if they prevent application of a stomal appliance or cause small-bowel obstruction; these can be approached locally, although definitive treatment generally entails relocation of the stoma to a different site. Laparoscopic parastomal hernia repair has also been described.

4. **Colostomy closure** is not a trivial procedure, with a reported morbidity rate of 20 to 30% (bleeding, anastomotic leak, abscess) and a mortality rate of 3%. Tagging the rectal stump with long, nonabsorbable sutures and mobilizing the splenic flexure during the initial resection and placing preoperative ureteral stents can facilitate reanastomosis. Placement of adhesion barriers at the time of initial exploratory laparotomy may reduce adhesions enough to allow laparoscopic colostomy closure.

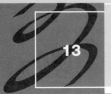

PANCREAS
13
Tricia A. Moo-Young and David C. Linehan

$\mathcal{T}$he pancreas is an entirely **retroperitoneal** structure lying posterior to the stomach and anterior to the mesenteric vessels, left kidney, and third portion of the duodenum. It is divided into four regions: the head/uncinate, neck, body, and tail. The body of the pancreas lies at the level of L2 and the tail extends toward the spleen. The pancreas receives its blood supply from both the celiac trunk and the superior mesenteric artery (SMA). The arterial supply of the pancreatic head is provided by the **inferior pancreaticoduodenal arteries** (from the SMA) and the superior pancreaticoduodenal arteries (from the gastroduodenal artery). The tail receives its arterial supply from branches of the splenic artery. Venous drainage is primarily by the pancreaticoduodenal veins, which ultimately drain into the portal vein. The main pancreatic duct is called the **duct of Wirsung.** It arises in the tail and runs the entire length of the pancreas to terminate at the papilla of Vater within the wall of the duodenum. The **duct of Santorini** is much smaller and arises from the lower part of the head, terminating separately at the lesser papilla.

I. **ACUTE PANCREATITIS** is an inflammatory process of variable severity. Most episodes of acute pancreatitis are self-limiting and associated with mild transitory symptoms that remit within 3 to 5 days. By contrast, up to 20% of patients develop a severe form of acute pancreatitis that is associated with a mortality rate as high as 40% (*Nat Clin Pract Gastroenterol Hepatol* 2005;2:473). The exact mechanism by which various etiologic factors induce acute pancreatitis and with such variable severity is unclear. However, the chain of events begins with **pancreatic acinar cell injury.** Afflicted acinar cells locally release activated pancreatic digestive enzymes that result in parenchymal autodigestion along with the recruitment of inflammatory cell mediators, eventually leading to a systemic inflammatory response.

A. **Etiology.** The two most common causes of acute pancreatitis in the United States are **gallstones** and **alcoholism,** collectively accounting for 80% of pancreatitis hospital admissions. Endoscopic retrograde cholangiopancreatography (ERCP)–induced pancreatitis causes another 5%. Other causes include the following:

1. **Drug induced** (definite association: isoniazid, estrogens; probable association: thiazides, furosemide, sulfonamides, tetracycline, corticosteroids).
2. **Hypertriglyceridemia** (especially types I and V).
3. **Hypercalcemia.**
4. **Infectious diseases** (mumps; orchitis; coxsackie virus B; Epstein-Barr virus; cytomegalovirus; rubella; hepatitis A, B, non-A, non-B; *Ascaris* species; and *Mycoplasma pneumoniae*).
5. **Tumors.**
6. **Trauma.**

B. **Diagnosis**

1. Patients typically present with **epigastric pain,** often radiating to the back. Tenderness is usually limited to the upper abdomen but may be associated with signs of diffuse peritonitis. Occasionally, irritation from intraperitoneal pancreatic enzymes results in impressive peritoneal signs, simulating other causes of an acute abdomen. Nausea, vomiting, and a low-grade fever are frequent, as are tachycardia and hypotension secondary to hypovolemia. Asymptomatic hypoxemia, renal failure, hypocalcemia, and hyperglycemia are evidence of severe systemic effects. Flank ecchymosis **(Gray-turner sign)** or periumbilical ecchymosis **(Cullen**

sign) are almost always manifestations of severe pancreatitis and have been associated with a 40% mortality rate. However, these signs are present in only 1% to 3% of cases and do not usually develop until 48 hours after the onset of symptoms.

2. **Laboratory studies**
   a. **Serum amylase** is the most useful test. Levels rise within 2 to 12 hours of symptoms and may return to normal over the following 2 to 5 days. Persistent elevations of levels for longer than 10 days indicate complications, such as pseudocyst formation. Normal levels can indicate resolution of acute pancreatitis, pancreatic hemorrhage, or pancreatic necrosis. There is no correlation between amylase level and etiology, prognosis, or severity. In addition, hyper-amlasemia can be found in a variety of other clinical conditions including renal failure, intestinal obstruction, gynecologic disorders, and malignancy.
   b. **Serum lipase** generally is considered more sensitive for pancreatic disease (95%), but its specificity varies from 55% to 95%.
   c. **Trypsin-activated peptide (TAP)** is elevated in the urine of patients with acute pancreatitis within 12 hours of symptom onset and has a sensitivity and specificity of 96% and 95%, respectively.
   d. **C-reactive protein (CRP)** is not specific for acute pancreatitis, but elevation of CRP is sensitive for severe acute pancreatitis.
   e. **Serum calcium** levels may fall as a result of complexing with fatty acids (saponification) produced by activated lipases.
   f. **Hepatic function panel** [aspartate aminotransferase (AST), alanine amino-transferase (ALT), bilirubin, alkaline phosphatase] should be checked to assess for concomitant biliary disease.

3. **Radiologic imaging** complements clinical history and exam because no single modality provides a perfect diagnostic index of pancreatitis severity.
   a. **Ultrasonography's** (US) specificity in pancreatitis can be greater than 95%, yet its sensitivity ranges between 62% and 95%. The pancreas is not visualized in up to 40% of patients due to overlying bowel gas and body habitus. The primary utility of US in acute pancreatitis is to determine whether gallstones or choledocholithiasis are present.
   b. **Computed tomography (CT)** is superior to ultrasonography in evaluating the pancreas and is not limited by bowel gas. The sensitivity and specificity of CT are 90% and 100%, respectively. Iodinated contrast enhancement is essential to detect the presence of pancreatic necrosis. CT may also be helpful in differentiating acute pancreatitis from conditions such as malignancy, small-bowel obstruction, or acute cholecystitis. CT findings include parenchymal enlargement and edema, necrosis, blurring of fat planes, peripancreatic fluid collections, bowel distention, and mesenteric edema. Every patient with a presumed diagnosis of acute pancreatitis does not require a CT scan. In general, patients who warrant further imaging include those in whom the diagnosis is not conclusive, any severely ill patient in whom necrosis is more likely (only after aggressive resuscitation so as not to induce contrast-associated nephropathy), and any patient who exhibits a deterioration in clinical course or fails to improve after 4 days of medical management.
   c. **Magnetic resonance imaging** (MRI) is a useful substitute for CT scan in patients allergic to iodinated contrast or in acute renal failure. In addition, MRI/MR cholangiopancreatography (MRCP) is better than CT at visualizing cholelithiasis, choledocholithiasis, and anomalies of the pancreatic duct.

4. **ERCP** is not routinely indicated for the evaluation of patients during an attack of acute pancreatitis. **Indications for ERCP** are as follows:
   a. **Preoperative evaluation** of patients with suspected traumatic pancreatitis to determine whether the pancreatic duct is disrupted.
   b. Patients with **suspected biliary pancreatitis and possible cholangitis** who are not clinically improving by 24 hours after admission should undergo endoscopic sphincterotomy and stone extraction. However, the literature is clear that early endoscopic intervention for gallstone pancreatitis does not

beneficially influence morbidity or mortality (*N Engl J Med* 1997;336:237, *Ann Surg* 2007;245:10).

  c. **Patients older than age 40 years with no identifiable cause** to rule out occult common bile duct stones, pancreatic, or ampullary carcinoma or other causes of obstruction.

  d. **Patients younger than age 40 years** who have had cholecystectomy or have experienced more than one attack of unexplained pancreatitis.

C. **Prognosis.** Because the associated mortality of severe acute pancreatitis approaches 40% and randomized studies have shown that early aggressive supportive care improves outcomes, attempts have been made to identify clinical parameters that predict patients at higher risk of developing severe outcomes.

  1. **Ranson's criteria** (Table 13-1) constitute the most frequently utilized predictor of mortality associated with acute pancreatitis. The limitation of this assessment tool is that a score cannot be calculated until 48 hours after admission.

  2. **CT Severity Index (CTSI)** is a prognostic scale based on CT findings, including peripancreatic fluid collections, fat inflammation, and extent of pancreatic necrosis.

  3. The **Glasgow** scoring, like Ranson's criteria, requires 48 hours to prognosticate patients and is based on clinical and laboratory values.

  4. The **Acute Physiology and Chronic Health Evaluation (APACHE) II** score was developed in 1985 for assessing critically ill patients and incorporates physiology, age, and chronic health. The major benefit of the APACHE II score is that it can be calculated at admission and updated daily to allow continual reassessment of prognosis.

D. **Complications**

  1. **Necrotizing pancreatitis** occurs in about 10% to 20% of acute pancreatitis cases, and its presence correlates with prognosis. It can be present at initial presentation or develop later in the clinical course. Necrosis is diagnosed on CT as failure to enhance with intravenous contrast.

  2. **Infected pancreatic necrosis** occurs in 5% to 10% of cases and is associated with mortality as high as 80%. Whether pancreas necrosis visualized on CT scan

---

TABLE 13-1   **Ranson's Criteria**

Admission	
Age	>55 yr
White blood cell count	>16,000/μL
Blood glucose	>200 mg/dL
Serum lactate dehydrogenase	>350 IU/L
Aspartate aminotransferase	>250 IU/L
Initial 48 hr	
Hematocrit decrease	>10%
Blood urea nitrogen elevation	>5 mg/dL
Serum calcium	<8 mg/dL
Arterial Po_2	<60 mm Hg
Base deficit	>4 mEq/L
Estimated fluid sequestration	>6 L

Mortality	
Number of Ranson's signs	**Approximate mortality (%)**
0–2	0
3–4	15
5–6	50
>6	70–90

is infected cannot be determined by imaging. The gold standard for diagnosing infected pancreatic necrosis is fine needle aspiration (FNA). However, a sudden deterioration of the clinical course and the presence of septic physiology strongly suggest infected pancreatic necrosis even without FNA. Gram-negative organisms are more common than Gram-positive organisms (typically *Pseudomonas, Escherichia coli, Klebsiella, Proteus, Enterobacter,* and *Staphylococcus* species).

3. **Acute pseudocyst** (see Section V).

4. **Visceral pseudoaneurysm** is a rare complication in pancreatitis. The incidence ranges between 4% and 10%, and it is most common among patients with necrotizing pancreatitis. Visceral pseudoaneurysm is believed to result from exposure of visceral arteries to the proteolytic pancreatic enzymes frequently extravasated during bouts of acute pancreatitis. The most common arteries involved are splenic and left gastric arteries. Detection of pseudoaneurysms usually occurs 3 to 5 weeks following the onset of acute pancreatitis, but hemorrhage can occur at any time. A ruptured pseudoaneurysm can be a surgical emergency and often presents with signs and symptoms associated with upper gastrointestinal bleeding. The optimal operative or endovascular treatment of pseudoaneurysms is controversial. If a source of hemorrhage can be identified by angiography, then it should be embolized. If operative treatment is required, distal pancreatectomy is superior to vessel ligation.

5. **Venous thrombosis** of the splenic, portal, or superior mesenteric vein has an overall incidence of 24%, with the largest incidence in the splenic vein and in patients with necrotizing pancreatitis. Although the thromboses can be temporary, progression can lead to collateralization and esophageal varices.

E. **Treatment.** One of the key predictors of poor outcome in acute pancreatitis is end-organ dysfunction resulting from circulatory collapse. Therefore, the initial approach to managing acute pancreatitis focuses on fluid resuscitation and close monitoring for evolving organ dysfunction.

1. **Supportive care**

a. **Volume resuscitation** with isotonic fluids is crucial; urinary output is monitored with a Foley catheter. Central hemodynamic monitoring (central venous pressure or pulmonary artery catheter) may be useful in guiding resuscitation. During the course of resuscitation, frequent monitoring of electrolytes, including calcium, is mandatory.

b. **Gastric rest with nutritional support.** Nasogastric decompression is performed to decrease neurohormonal stimulation of pancreatic secretion. Acute pancreatitis is a hypercatabolic state, and nutritional support has been shown to have a significant impact on outcomes in critically ill patients. Enteral feeding (beyond the ampulla of Vater) is generally preferred to parenteral nutrition. A large body of evidence suggests that early enteral feeding in patients with severe acute pancreatitis is associated with lower rates of infection, surgical intervention, and length of stay (*BMJ* 2004;328:1407).

c. **Analgesics** are required for pain relief.

d. **Respiratory monitoring** and arterial blood gases should be done every 12 hours for the first 3 days in severe pancreatitis to assess oxygenation and acid-base status. Hypoxemia is extremely common, even in mild cases of acute pancreatitis. Pulmonary complications occur in up to 50% of patients.

e. **Antibiotics.** The routine use of antibiotic prophylaxis in acute pancreatitis, especially in mild to moderate cases, is not supported in the literature. Conflicting data exist regarding antibiotics in severe cases, and there are small prospective, randomized trials demonstrating significantly lower rates of septic complications in patients receiving antibiotics (10.6% vs. 36.4%; *Ann Surg* 2006;243:154). However, a recent multicenter, double-blind, randomized, controlled trial evaluated early initiation of meropenem versus placebo in 100 patients with documented necrotizing pancreatitis (*Ann Surg* 2007;245:674). There were no differences in pancreatic infections, need for surgery, or mortality rate between the two groups. The authors surmised that prophylactic antibiotics are not indicated for severe pancreatitis, although they certainly should be used when infected necrosis is suspected.

2. **Surgical treatment** must be entertained for the small percentage of patients who continue to deteriorate despite aggressive supportive therapy. Although there is not a clear consensus of the indications for operative intervention, some of the incontrovertible indications include (1) diagnostic uncertainty in the face of clinical deterioration, (2) related life-threatening complications (i.e., intra-abdominal hemorrhage, viscus perforation, abdominal compartment syndrome), and (3) infected pancreatic necrosis.

   a. **Timing.** Because patients with severe necrotizing pancreatitis can rapidly progress to a critical condition, historically almost all patients were operated on within the first 72 hours of admission. Mortality rates in these patients, however, were reported as high as 80%. Subsequent studies have demonstrated decreased mortality with later débridement (*Am J Surg* 1997;173:71), and it is our policy to delay operative intervention for as long as possible without jeopardizing the patient.

   b. In necrotizing pancreatitis, **percutaneous drainage** can be an effective therapy in a very select group of patients (*Ann Surg* 2000;232:175). In rare cases, percutaneous drainage can be the only intervention necessary, particularly if the necrosis is well demarcated and liquefied to the extent that it is more consistent with a pancreatic abscess.

   c. Wide débridement **(necrosectomy)**, supplemented by either open packing or closed drainage, is the standard operative approach for managing infected necrotizing pancreatitis. At our institution, the preference is for wide débridement and packing with repeated débridement in the operating room. However, a positive correlation exists between repeated surgical interventions and morbidity, including fistula, gastric outlet obstruction, local bleeding, and incisional hernia. Marsupialization of the lesser sac allows rapid access to the pancreatic bed and facilitates daily dressing changes (usually done in the intensive care unit).

   d. **Pancreatic resection.** Because severe pancreatitis often leads to necrosis in large areas of the pancreas and peripancreatic fat, some have attempted to gain control of fulminant disease by resecting much or even the entire pancreas (partial or total pancreaticoduodenectomy). Radical resection procedures place greater stress on already severely ill patients; pancreaticoduodenectomy or total pancreatectomy is associated with very high mortality and is not recommended.

   e. **Gallstone-induced pancreatitis.** Ongoing choledocholithiasis is found in only 25% of biliary acute pancreatitis cases. Nonetheless, all patients with pancreatitis should be evaluated for the presence of gallstones because the etiology has specific therapeutic implications. Cholecystectomy should be carried out as soon as possible after recovery to prevent recurrent attacks of pancreatitis, typically just prior to patient discharge. During open or laparoscopic cholecystectomy, intraoperative cholangiography is recommended.

II. **CHRONIC PANCREATITIS** is caused by alcohol abuse in the majority of patients. Other etiologies include idiopathic or metabolic (hypercalcemia, hypertriglyceridemia, hypercholesterolemia, hyperparathyroidism, cystic fibrosis) factors, drugs, trauma, and congenital abnormalities (sphincter of Oddi dysfunction or pancreas divisum). A history of recurrent acute pancreatitis is present in some but not all patients with chronic pancreatitis.

A. **Pathophysiology.** Chronic pancreatitis is characterized by diffuse scarring and strictures in the pancreatic duct and often leads to endocrine or exocrine insufficiency, although substantial glandular destruction must occur before secretory function is lost. The islets of Langerhans have a greater resistance to injury than do the exocrine tissues; most patients who develop diabetes already have pancreatic exocrine insufficiency and steatorrhea. Based on ductal involvement and morphology, the disease is subclassified as either large-duct or small-duct disease.

B. **Diagnosis** is based on a complete history and examination, complemented by the appropriate investigative studies. **Upper midepigastric pain radiating to the back** is the cardinal symptom and is present in 95% of cases. Early episodes mimic acute pancreatitis and may last for several hours to days. As the disease progresses, the attacks tend to be more frequent and prolonged. Physical findings include weight loss proportional to the severity of anorexia, as well as steatorrhea. Tenderness of the upper abdomen is common. An enlarged pancreas occasionally is palpable, especially in a thin person, but a mass suggests the presence of a pseudocyst. Occasional findings include jaundice secondary to stricture of the common bile duct, enlarged spleen secondary to thrombosis of the splenic vein, or ascites secondary to a pancreaticoperitoneal fistula.

1. **Laboratory tests**
   a. **Amylase and lipase levels** are elevated in acute pancreatitis but rarely are useful in chronic pancreatitis.
   b. **Pancreatic secretin stimulation tests** have proven to be sensitive and specific test for the diagnosis of chronic pancreatitis, especially in small-duct disease, in which structural findings on imaging are less pronounced. Secretin testing is noted as abnormal when approximately 60% of the pancreas is damaged.
   c. **Pancreatic endocrine function.** Fasting and 2-hour postprandial blood glucose levels or glucose tolerance tests may be abnormal in 14% to 65% of patients with early chronic pancreatitis and in up to 90% of patients when calcifications are present.
   d. **A 72-hour fecal collection for estimation of daily fecal fat** is the most sensitive and specific stool test for exocrine insufficiency. Fat absorption has the most clinical significance, although fewer problems are associated with protein malabsorption. Carbohydrate malabsorption probably is unimportant.
2. **Radiologic studies**
   a. **Plain films** of the abdomen show diffuse calcification of the pancreas in approximately 30% of patients with relatively early stages of chronic pancreatitis and in 50% to 60% of cases of advanced disease.
   b. **CT** is 75% sensitive for the diagnosis of parenchymal or ductal disease. It is also useful for detecting complications or associated findings in patients presenting with epigastric abdominal pain, such as splenic aneurysms, pancreatic pseudocyst, or pancreatic cancer.
   c. **ERCP is essential** to define the extent of disease and optimize surgical management through evaluation of ductal anatomy. Brushings and biopsies of suspicious lesions can be performed as well as therapeutic interventions, including stenting and sphincterotomy.
   d. **MRI** is less sensitive than CT for detection of calcification. Falsely positive studies for filling defects can be caused by air in the duct, clips, and artifacts. MR pancreatography is more sensitive in visualizing a dilated duct and strictures but loses sensitivity relative to ERCP in evaluating side branch disease (i.e., small-duct disease). MR pancreatography is particularly useful in patients whose postsurgical anatomy makes ERCP technically unfeasible.
   e. **Ultrasonography- or CT-guided fine-needle biopsies** may be useful in cases in which chronic pancreatitis cannot be distinguished from pancreatic cancer. By itself, however, a single biopsy finding of inflammatory changes is not sufficient to rule out carcinoma. A normal biopsy may also result from sampling error.

C. **Complications**
   1. **Common bile duct obstruction** may result from transient obstruction from pancreatic inflammation and edema or from stricture of the intrapancreatic common bile duct. When present, **strictures** are often **long and smooth** (2 to 4 cm in length) and must be distinguished from pancreatic carcinoma.
   2. **Duodenal obstruction** can occur due to acute pancreatic inflammation, chronic fibrotic reaction, pancreatic pseudocyst, or neoplasm.
   3. **Pancreaticoenteric fistulas** result from spontaneous drainage of a pancreatic abscess cavity or pseudocyst into the stomach, duodenum, transverse colon, or biliary tract. They are often asymptomatic but may become infected or result in hemorrhage.

4. Pancreaticopleural fistulas often have communication from the distal duct traversing the esophageal hiatus.

5. Pseudocyst (see Section V.A).

6. Splenic vein thrombosis (see Section I.D.5).

7. Pancreatic carcinoma. Chronic pancreatitis has been suggested in some studies to increase the risk of pancreatic carcinoma by two- to threefold.

D. Treatment

1. Medical management

   a. Malabsorption or steatorrhea. There is some evidence that adequate oral pancreatic enzyme supplementation improves pain control.

   b. Diabetes initially is responsive to careful attention to overall good nutrition and dietary control; however, use of oral hypoglycemic agents or insulin therapy often is required. There is some propensity for hypoglycemic attacks. Diabetic ketoacidosis is not commonly seen except after major pancreatic resections.

   c. Narcotics usually are required for pain relief. Narcotic dependency is a frequent complication of therapy and correlates with higher mortality. In selected patients, tricyclic antidepressants and gabapentin may be effective.

   d. Abstinence from alcohol and withdrawal prophylaxis are of paramount importance.

   e. Cholecystokinin antagonists and somatostatin analogs have been considered for treatment of chronic pancreatitis, but early studies have shown disappointing or only short-lived effects.

   f. Tube thoracostomy or repeated paracentesis may be required for pancreatic pleural effusions or pancreatic ascites. Approximately 40% to 65% of patients respond to nonsurgical management within 2 to 3 weeks.

2. Endoscopic therapy. Endoscopic sphincterotomy, stenting, stone retrieval, and lithotripsy have all been used with moderate success in the management of patients with ductal complications from chronic pancreatitis. Currently, the outcome studies are all relatively small, and at least preliminarily there appears to be a high rate of symptoms relapse ($>30\%$).

3. Surgical principles

   a. Indications for surgery include severe intractable pain, multiple relapses, inability to rule out neoplasm, and complications of pancreatitis (pseudocyst, obstruction, fistula, infections, portal hypertension).

   b. Choice of procedure. The goals of surgical therapy are drainage and resection of the diseased pancreas. The choice of procedure is largely dependent on whether there is evidence of large- or small-duct disease. For large-duct disease, surgery is more effective long term than endoscopic treatment (*N Engl J Med* 2007;356:676); durable pain relief in surgical patients was achieved in 75% versus only 32% in those treated endoscopically. A drainage procedure is preferable to pure resection because it allows for preservation of pancreatic tissue and function. There may be a role for resection in small-duct disease, but the morbidity and mortality rates from resection are higher mainly due to the technical difficulty of the procedure and the poor performance status of these nutritionally deprived patients.

   c. Drainage-only procedures at our institution are uncommon because of poor relief of symptoms postoperatively.

      (1) Longitudinal side-to-side pancreaticojejunostomy (Partington-Rochelle) is indicated in patients with functionally significant strictures along the pancreatic duct (chain of lakes on pancreatograms) and with ducts at least 8 mm in diameter.

      (2) Puestow procedure includes a distal pancreatectomy with a distal pancreaticojejunostomy for drainage, with reported success in postoperative pain relief ranging between 61% and 90% (*Am J Surg* 1987;153:207). However, success is strongly associated with a minimum duct size of 7 mm or greater, thus restricting this operation to a small number of patients (*Gastrointest Surg* 1998;2:223).

d. Combined duct drainage-resection

  (1) Pancreaticoduodenectomy (Whipple procedure) is indicated in cases in which the pancreatitis disproportionately involves the head of the pancreas, the pancreatic duct is of small diameter, or cancer cannot be ruled out in the head of the pancreas. For chronic pancreatitis, the pylorus-preserving technique is advocated. The use of vagotomy is controversial.

  (2) The Beger procedure is a duodenum-preserving resection of a portion of the pancreatic head. This operation preserves a small amount of pancreatic tissue within the C-loop of the duodenum and also in front of the portal vein. The pancreas is then transected at the pancreatic neck. Reconstruction requires two pancreaticojejunostomies. A Roux jejunal loop is anastomosed to both the proximal (duodenal) stump and the larger distal stump of the remaining pancreas. This procedure should not be performed in the presence of cancer.

  (3) The Frey procedure is a modification of the Beger procedure consisting of a duodenum-sparing limited pancreatic head resection combined with a lateral pancreaticojejunostomy. In the Frey procedure, the pancreatic neck is not transected, but the pancreatic parenchyma is extensively cored out from the head to the extent of diseased segment distally. This is the most common procedure performed at our institution because postoperative morbidity has been shown to be lower in Frey patients than in those undergoing a pylorus-sparing Whipple procedure (19% vs. 53%). In addition, patient satisfaction indices were increased by 71% versus 43% in Whipple patients (*Ann Surg* 1998;228:771).

e. Pancreatectomy

  (1) Distal subtotal pancreatectomy is used for disease in the tail of the gland and in patients with previous ductal injury from blunt abdominal trauma with fracture of the pancreas and stenosis of the duct at the midbody level.

  (2) Total pancreatectomy is performed only as a last resort in patients whose previous operations have failed and who appear to be capable of managing an apancreatic state. Some centers have combined this procedure with islet cell transplantation.

f. Celiac plexus block. Although transiently effective in some cases, nerve ablation procedures more recently have been shown to have a beneficial role in the management of pain in patients with chronic pancreatitis. Methods for ablating the celiac ganglion include image-guided ethanol injection and surgery (ganglionectomy).

III. EXOCRINE PANCREATIC CANCER

A. Incidence and epidemiology. Pancreatic cancer is the fifth-leading cause of cancer-related mortality in the United States. Most patients have incurable disease at the time of diagnosis, and the overall 5-year survival is less than 5%. The median age at diagnosis is 65 years.

B. Risk factors. An increased risk of pancreatic cancer has been associated with smoking, alcoholism, hereditary disorders [familial adenomatous polyposis (FAP), van Hippel-Lindau disease (VHL), hereditary breast cancer, Gardner syndrome], and chronic pancreatitis. The association with alcohol-induced pancreatitis is related to concurrent chronic pancreatitis and the well-established hypothesis that chronic inflammation is a predisposing factor for malignancy. Inherited pancreatic cancers represent approximately 5% to 10% of all diagnoses of the disease. Palladin is a recently identified gene found to be mutated in certain forms of familial pancreas cancer (*PLOS* 2006;3:221).

C. Pathology. Approximately 80% of pancreatic carcinomas are ductal cell adenocarcinomas. Seventy percent of pancreatic cancers occur at the head, 20% in the body, and 10% in the tail. Other periampullary tumors, such as carcinomas of the distal bile duct, duodenum, and ampulla of Vater, are less common and constitute approximately one third of resectable periampullary cancers.

D. Diagnosis. The symptoms associated with pancreas cancer are almost always gradual in onset and are nonspecific.

1. **History and examination.** Patients complain of dull midepigastric pain, malaise, nausea, fatigue, and weight loss. Classically, the report of new-onset **"painless jaundice"** is believed to be pancreas cancer until proven otherwise. Pruritus may accompany obstructive jaundice. If obstructive jaundice is present, patients will also note darkening of the urine and "light-colored" stools. Finally, new-onset diabetes within the year prior to diagnosis is found in 15% of patients with pancreatic cancer. Jaundice, temporal wasting to suggest weight loss, and, in rare cases, a palpable abdominal mass all may result from pancreas cancer but are not universally present in patients with this disease. The so-called *Courvoisier sign* (painless jaundice with a palpable gallbladder) is an associated finding in patients with periampullary tumors and primary bile duct tumors. *Trousseau's sign* (migratory thrombophlebitis) has been associated with pancreas cancer.

2. **Laboratory tests.** None is singularly diagnostic for pancreatic cancer.
   a. Elevated serum bilirubin.
   b. Elevated alkaline phosphatase.
   c. Mild elevations of serum glutamic-oxaloacetic transaminase and serum glutamate pyruvate transaminase.
   d. Tumor markers. CA19-9 is useful in patients for whom the diagnosis is already highly likely as a means of confirmation and in follow-up for response to treatment, but it has no role in screening. In addition, elevation in CA19-9 is seen in nonmalignant conditions such as acute or chronic biliary disease. Carcinoembryonic antigen (CEA) is a common tumor marker in a variety of gastrointestinal malignances but has been found to be elevated in only 40% to 50% of patients with pancreas cancer.

3. **Radiologic studies**
   a. Plain films of the abdomen are of little benefit.
   b. Pancreatic cancer on **CT** appears as hypoattenuating indistinct mass that distorts the normal architecture of the gland, often paired with findings of a dilated pancreatic or biliary ductal system (the so-called "double-duct" sign). If there is pancreatic ductal obstruction, it is also possible that the remainder of the gland will be atrophied. The CT criteria used to define potential resectability are as follows:
      (1) Absence of distant metastasis.
      (2) Preserved fat plane between the mass and the superior mesenteric vein (SMV)/portal vein (PV).
      (3) Absence of tumor encasement of the hepatic, celiac, or superior mesenteric arteries.
   c. Percutaneous (CT- or ultrasonography guided) needle biopsies have a limited role. A percutaneous needle biopsy should be performed in patients who are not surgical candidates to obtain a tissue diagnosis. A negative biopsy does not rule out carcinoma and is unlikely to change management in patients felt to be radiographically resectable.
   d. The utility of positron emission tomography **(PET)** is limited to investigating for occult metastatic disease. A relatively high false-positive rate has been reported in pancreatitis when evaluating the pancreas for the diagnosis of cancer.
   e. Others. Ultrasonography is not as sensitive as CT and is limited by the presence of bowel gas. MRI may provide as much information as does CT but is costly, is limited in availability, and takes longer. Endoscopic ultrasonography can assess tumor size as well as portal and mesenteric vascular involvement and obtain tissue samples. Staging laparoscopy may be useful in identifying small liver metastasis and peritoneal implants.

E. Treatment
   1. Curative resection
      a. In selected patients, we advocate **staging laparoscopy** and biopsies to assess the resectability prior to laparotomy. Laparoscopy allows determination of the extent of local invasion, peritoneal implantation, and presence of regional metastases. The data suggest that this technique, combined with preoperative spiral CT scanning, can reduce the incidence of unresectable disease at

laparotomy to less than 10%. This is significant because palliation can often be accomplished endoscopically, thus avoiding an unnecessary laparotomy in patients with subclincal metastatic disease.

   b. **Pancreaticoduodenectomy (Whipple procedure)** consists of en bloc resection of the head of the pancreas, distal common bile duct, duodenum, jejunum, and gastric antrum. Pylorus-sparing pancreaticoduodenectomy has been advocated by some, but there are no data demonstrating improved survival or lower morbidity. Extended lymphadenectomy, including nodes from the celiac axis to the iliac bifurcation and nodes from the portal vein and superior mesenteric artery, has not been shown to affect survival but does increase morbidity (*Surg Oncol Clin North Am* 2007;16:157). There has been a sharp decline in morbidity and mortality in specialized centers, with a 30-day mortality of less than 5%.

2. **Palliative treatment.** If the disease is considered unresectable at the time of surgery, palliative treatment must be considered. The goals are to offer prevention or relief from the three major problems that present in advanced metastatic pancreas cancer: (1) obstructive jaundice, (2) gastric outlet obstruction, and (3) pain.

   a. **Surgical palliation** for obstructive jaundice and gastric outlet obstruction is achieved by performing a biliary internal drainage procedure such as choledochojejunostomy and gastrojejunostomy. Incapacitating pain is a common complaint of patients at the end stages of their disease. Chemical splanchnicectomy can be preformed by instilling 50% ethyl alcohol in the celiac nerve plexus just adjacent the aorta at the level of the celiac artery.

   b. **Endoscopic biliary stenting** can be used to temporize symptoms related to obstructive jaundice, and laparoscopic gastrojejunostomy tube placement has a possible role in patients with intestinal outlet obstructions. Endoscopic chemical splanchnicectomy can be done to help manage intractable pain.

3. **Postoperative considerations.** Delayed gastric emptying, pancreatic fistula, and wound infection are the three most common complications of the pancreaticoduodenectomy. Up to 10% of patients require a nasogastric tube for longer than 10 days, but delayed gastric emptying almost always subsides with conservative treatment. The incidence of delayed gastric emptying may be increased with pylorus-preserving procedures. The rate of pancreatic fistula has been demonstrated to be reduced to less than 2% by meticulous attention to the blood supply of the pancreaticoenteric duct-to-mucosa anastomosis (*J Am Coll Surg* 2002;194:746). Although many surgeons routinely place abdominal drains, a prospective, randomized study showed no benefit and possible increased complications due to the presence of drains. Randomized studies have not demonstrated that the perioperative use of octreotide (a somatostatin analog) decreases pancreatic fistulas in patients undergoing pancreaticoduodenectomy.

4. **Radiotherapy and chemotherapy.** The use of adjuvant therapy has been investigated in prospective fashion, and clear conclusions are not evident. Given the high recurrence rate after resection, most patients are considered for some form of adjuvant therapy. Current regimens consist of radiation and 5-flurouracil. Newer agents incorporating gemcitabine or immunomodulation therapy utilizing a combination of radiation, conventional chemotherapy, and interferon alpha are under study in randomized, controlled trials. The largest of these studies is the European Study Group for Pancreatic Cancer (ESPAC)-1 trial. Results of this study demonstrated a significant survival benefit for 5-fluorouracil chemotherapy and no survival benefit for adjuvant chemoradiotherapy (*Surg Oncol Clin North Am* 2004;4:567).

5. **Prognosis.** Surgical resection can increase survival. Overall 5-year survival rates are 5% to 20% for patients after resection. In patients with small tumors, negative resection margins, and no evidence of nodal metastases, the 5-year survival rate is as high as 40%. Mean length of survival for unresectable locally advanced disease is 3 to 10 months, and for hepatic metastatic disease it is 6 months.

IV. CONGENITAL ABNORMALITIES

A. Failure of the ventral and dorsal pancreatic buds to fuse during the sixth week of development results in **pancreatic divisum.** In this condition, the normally minor duct of Santorini becomes the primary means of pancreatic drainage from the larger mass of pancreatic tissue. The condition is detected by ERCP, and the incidence is estimated to be 5%. Approximately 25% of affected patients develop pancreatitis secondary to obstruction or stenosis. However, the association between pancreatitis and pancreas divisum is controversial. Open sphincteroplasty of the minor papilla forming the orifice of the minor duct of Santorini and cholecystectomy is the procedure of choice for symptomatic patients. One should exclude other etiologies of pancreatitis before embarking on surgical intervention for pancreas divisum.

B. Typical locations for **ectopic pancreatic tissues** include the stomach, duodenal or ileal wall, Meckel diverticulum, and umbilicus. Less common sites are the colon, appendix, gallbladder, omentum, and mesentery. Most ectopic pancreatic tissue is functional; islet tissue is most often present in the stomach and duodenum. Heterotopic pancreas may result in pyloric stenosis, disruption of peristalsis, peptic ulcers, or neoplasms.

C. Malrotation of the ventral primordium during the fifth week results in **annular pancreas:** a thin, flat band of normal pancreatic tissue surrounding the second part of the duodenum. The pancreatic tissue may be completely free from the duodenum or may invade the muscularis deeply. The annular pancreas usually contains a duct that connects to the main pancreatic duct. Annular pancreas may cause duodenal obstruction in utero, resulting in hydramnios. Approximately one half of affected patients do not have symptoms until late in adulthood, however, and complaints usually relate to duodenal obstruction. Treatment of choice is duodenoduodenostomy for symptomatic patients.

V. CYSTIC DISEASES

A. Pancreatic pseudocysts. It is important to distinguish pseudocysts from tumors and other fluid collections. An acute pancreatic fluid collection follows in approximately 25% of patients with acute pancreatitis. It is characterized by acute inflammation, cloudy fluid, a poorly defined cyst wall, and necrotic but sterile debris. This may resolve spontaneously, and in fact most "pseudocysts" that resolve are likely of this type. By definition, a fluid collection in the first 4 weeks is an *acute fluid collection*; after 4 weeks, it becomes an *acute pseudocyst*.

1. Causes. Pseudocysts develop after disruption of the pancreatic duct with or without proximal obstruction; they usually occur after an episode of acute pancreatitis. In children, most pseudocysts arise as a complication of blunt abdominal trauma.

2. Diagnosis

a. Clinical presentation. The most common complaint is recurrent or persistent upper abdominal pain. Other symptoms include nausea, vomiting, early satiety, anorexia, weight loss, and jaundice. Physical examination is significant for upper abdominal tenderness and occasionally reveals an abdominal mass.

b. Laboratory tests

(1) Amylase. Serum concentrations are elevated in approximately one half of cases.

(2) Liver function tests occasionally are elevated and therefore are not of diagnostic use.

(3) Cystic fluid analysis is discussed in Section V.B.2.

c. Radiologic studies

(1) CT is the radiographic study of choice for initial evaluation of pancreatic pseudocysts and is twice as sensitive as ultrasonography in detection of pseudocysts. CT scan findings that determine prognosis include the following:

(a) Pseudocysts **smaller than 4 cm** usually resolve spontaneously.

(b) Pseudocysts with **wall calcifications** generally do not resolve.

(c) Pseudocysts with **thick walls** are resistant to spontaneous resolution.

(2) **Ultrasonography** detects approximately 85% of pseudocysts. Its use is limited by obesity and bowel gases, but it may be used in follow-up studies once a pseudocyst has been identified by CT scan.

d. **ERCP** allows for the determination of pancreatic duct anatomy and influences therapeutic intervention. Approximately one half of pseudocysts have ductal abnormalities identified by ERCP, such as proximal obstruction, stricture, or communications with the pseudocyst. ERCP itself risks superinfection of a communicating pseudocyst.

3. **Complications**
   a. **Infection** is reported in 5% to 20% of pseudocysts and requires external drainage.
   b. **Hemorrhage** results from erosion into surrounding visceral vessels and occurs in approximately 7% of cases. The most common arteries are the splenic (45%), gastroduodenal (18%), and pancreaticoduodenal (18%) arteries. Immediate angiography has emerged as the initial treatment of choice.
   c. **Obstruction.** Compression can occur anywhere from the stomach to the colon. The arteriovenous system also can be subject to compression, including the vena caval and portal venous system. Hydronephrosis can result from obstruction of the ureters. Biliary obstruction can present as jaundice, cholangitis, and biliary cirrhosis.
   d. **Rupture** occurs in fewer than 3% of cases. Approximately one half of patients can be treated nonsurgically, with total parenteral nutrition and symptomatic paracentesis or thoracentesis. Rupture is occasionally associated with severe abdominal pain and presents as a surgical emergency.

4. **Treatment** depends on symptoms, age, pseudocyst size, and the presence of complications. **Pseudocysts smaller than 6 cm and present for less than 6 weeks have low complication rates.** The chance of spontaneous resolution after 6 weeks is low, and the risk of complications rises significantly after 6 weeks.
   a. **Nonoperative.** If the pseudocyst is new, asymptomatic, and without complications, the patient can be followed with serial CT scans or ultrasonography to evaluate size and maturation of the pseudocyst. The majority of pseudocysts larger than 6 cm require surgery.
   b. **Percutaneous drainage** can be considered for patients in whom the pseudocyst does not communicate with the pancreatic duct and for those who cannot tolerate surgery. External drainage is indicated when the pseudocyst is infected and without a mature wall. Simple aspiration is the least effective of the percutaneous interventions. The duration of drainage ranges from several days to several months (usually 3 to 4 weeks). The results are variable, and the rate of complications (e.g., fistulas) may be high.
   c. **Excision** may be necessary in patients with symptomatic immature pseudocysts associated with complications or in those with mature distal pancreatic pseudocysts. Resection can require a Whipple procedure (pancreaticoduodenectomy) for pseudocysts at the head of the pancreas (rarely indicated) or distal pancreatectomy for pseudocysts in the body or tail of the pancreas.
   d. **Internal drainage.** Cystoenteric drainage is the procedure of choice in uncomplicated pseudocysts requiring surgical treatment. Options include Roux-en-Y cystojejunostomy, loop cystojejunostomy, cystogastrostomy, and cystoduodenostomy. A biopsy of the cyst wall should be obtained to rule out cystic neoplasm. The recurrence rate after these procedures is approximately 10%. Endoscopic cystogastrostomy or cystoenterostomy has been performed in some centers. There is an increased risk of perforation with this procedure and an increased risk of recurrence due to inadequate drainage. At our institution, we favor the Roux-en-Y cystojejunostomy or cystogastrostomy in most patients.

B. **True pancreatic cysts**
   1. **Histopathologic classification.** Although several different histologic types of cystic pancreatic neoplasms (CPNs) have been described, the following are most common:

a. **Serous cystadenoma** are benign lesions and are usually asymptomatic. They are more common in women (65%), are located in the head of the pancreas, and account for 30% of all CPNs.

b. **Mucinous cystic neoplasms (MCNs)** are considered premalignant lesions and account for 35% of all CPNs. At presentation they can be symptomatic, are twice as likely to present in women, and anatomically are more commonly located in the body or tail. The cystic lesions do not communicate with the pancreatic ductal system.

c. **Intraductal papillary mucinous tumors (IPMTs)** account for 25% of all CPNs and have a slight male predominance. They can be symptomatic and do communicate with the pancreatitic ductal system. IPMTs carry a very high malignant potential, up to 40% in some series. They are more commonly located in the head of the pancreas and can involve the ampulla of Vater.

d. **Other rare cystic pancreatic neoplasms** (remaining 10%) include cystadenocarcinoma, acinar cell cystadenocarcinoma, cystic choriocarcinoma, cystic teratoma, and angiomatous neoplasms.

2. When a cystic pancreatic lesion has been identified by imaging, **cyst fluid analysis** is an essential part of the diagnostic workup. The most important finding is the presence of **mucin.** During ERCP, mucin egress from the bulging papilla can be highly suggestive of IPMT. If mucin is present on ERCP or cyst fluid analysis, the lesions is either premalignant or malignant and therefore requires resection. Analysis for the following may also prove useful:

a. **Carcinoembryonic antigen** is elevated in both MCNs and IPMTs but most markedly in MCNs. It is low in serous cysts and pseudocysts.

b. **CA 19-9** can be elevated in malignant cyst neoplasms.

c. **CA 72-4** is low in pseudocysts and serous tumors. Levels are elevated in benign mucinous cystadenomas and very high in the setting of cystic malignancy.

d. **Amylase** and **lipase** generally are high in pseudocysts and low in cystic tumors.

e. **Fluid viscosity** is elevated in mucinous tumors and low in pseudocysts and serous cystic tumors.

f. **Percutaneous cytology** is useful in determining malignant tumors but limited in discriminating between pseudocysts and cystic cystadenoma.

g. **Percutaneous wall biopsy** allows for discrimination between pseudocysts (which lack epithelial lining) and cystic neoplasms. It also can discriminate between serous (cuboidal epithelium) and mucinous (tall columnar epithelium and goblet cells). However, neoplastic cysts may have areas of cyst wall denuded of epithelium, which mimic pseudocysts.

3. **Treatment**

a. **Serous cystic neoplasms** are benign lesions for which radiographic observation is sufficient. Indications for operative management are lesions that are symptomatic or distal disease for which there is some diagnostic uncertainty.

b. **Mucinous cystic neoplasms** have malignant potential, and therefore surgical resection is warranted. However, lesions less than 2 cm in size rarely have malignant foci and can be followed. With curative resection, patients with mucinous cystadenocarcinoma have 5-year survival rates over 95%.

c. **IPMT** warrants resection. The type of resection is dictated by the anatomic location of the lesion and its relation to the pancreatic ductal system. So-called "branched duct disease," typically involving the head, requires a localized resection, most commonly a pylorus-sparing Whipple procedure. However, in "main duct disease," the process can be either localized or multifocal. Traditionally, the approach to this disease pattern was to perform a distal pancreatectomy with immediate frozen-section analysis of the proximal ductal margin. More recently, a consensus statement established that histologic interpretation of frozen section margins is not as straightforward as had been previously believed. IPMT requires long-term follow-up and carries a 75% 5-year survival rate.

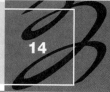

SURGICAL DISEASES OF THE LIVER
Marcus Tan and William C. Chapman

14

RESECTION OF THE LIVER

I. RESECTION of up to 80% of the liver is possible because the remaining liver regenerates rapidly to a normal liver volume in the noncirrhotic patient. By the third postoperative week, liver function tests such as albumin, bilirubin, and prothrombin time usually reflect restored physiology.

II. NOMENCLATURE. A standard nomenclature for hepatic structures and resections was introduced by the International Hepato-Pancreato-Biliary Association (*HPB* 2000;2:333). This system is predicated on the surgical anatomy of the liver, with the internal hepatic divisions delineated by the arterial and biliary anatomy.

   A. Internal anatomy: first division. The liver is divided into two almost equally sized *hemilivers*. The plane between the hemilivers is the *midplane* of the liver and runs from the gallbladder fossa to the inferior vena cava. Each hemiliver is supplied by one hepatic arterial branch, one bile duct, and one portal vein; those of the right hemiliver, for example, are referred to as the *right hepatic artery, right bile duct,* and *right portal vein,* respectively. A resection of a hemiliver is termed a *hepatectomy* or *hemihepatectomy* (e.g., right hepatectomy).

   B. Internal anatomy: second division. Further divisions of the liver are based on the internal course of the hepatic artery and bile duct. These structures retain a high order of bilateral symmetry, whereas the portal vein does not. Its asymmetry results from retained portions from the fetal circulation. The liver is thus divided into four nearly equal **sections:** the right anterior and posterior sections and the left medial and lateral sections. A vessel supplying a section is a sectional vessel (e.g., the right anterior sectional artery).

   C. Internal anatomy: third division. The liver is further subdivided into segments numbered I to VIII. These are the same as originally described by Couinaud. Resection of a segment is termed a *segmentectomy.*

III. OPERATIVE CONDUCT for major liver resection usually consists of wide exposure through a bilateral subcostal incision, with a midline extension to the xiphoid process as needed **(chevron incision).** The ipsilateral vascular pedicles are isolated. The hepatic vein(s) draining the part of the liver to be resected are similarly isolated. During transection, maintenance of a low central venous pressure (<5 mm Hg) and placement of the patient in the Trendelenburg position reduce blood loss. A small amount of positive end-expiratory pressure (5 cm H_2O) is used to prevent air embolism. Vascular control can be augmented by intermittent occlusion of all hepatic inflow **(Pringle maneuver)** or total vascular exclusion. Postoperatively, frequent blood sugar measurements should be obtained. Monitoring and supplementation of phosphorous levels is important to support liver regeneration. Hyperbilirubinemia is unusual but may occur and persist for days to weeks. Prolongation of the International Normalized Ratio (INR) may develop but usually is not severe; if necessary, fresh-frozen plasma is infused to keep the INR less than 2. Due to decreased clearance of hepatically metabolized drugs posthepatectomy, the dose of pain medications should be adjusted and monitored. The most common complication from liver resection is intra-abdominal abscess. Bile leaks from the cut surface of the liver or a damaged biliary duct may also occur. These manifest as a bile fistula or a *biloma,* a localized collection of bile. This can usually be managed by percutaneous drainage. Liver failure may result from insufficient residual functional hepatic parenchyma after extensive resections.

 DISEASES OF THE LIVER

I. HEPATIC NEOPLASMS

A. Benign neoplasms of the liver

1. **Hemangioma is the most common benign liver tumor,** with the prevalence (estimated from autopsy series) ranging from 3% to 20%. The majority are diagnosed in middle-aged women, and there is a female-to-male ratio of 5 to 6:1. The pathogenesis of hemangiomas is poorly understood. They are thought to represent hamartomatous outgrowths of endothelium rather than true neoplasms. Some of these tumors express estrogen receptors, and accelerated growth has been associated with high-estrogen states, such as puberty, pregnancy, and when oral contraceptives and androgens are used.

   a. **Pathology.** Hemangiomas are usually less than 5 cm in diameter, but they can reach 20 cm or larger. Their blood supply is derived from the hepatic artery. Macroscopically, they are spherical, well-circumscribed, soft, and easily compressible. Microscopically, the tumor consists of multiple large vascular channels lined by a single layer of endothelial cells supported by collagenous walls. Malignant degeneration does not occur.

   b. Most hemangiomas are **asymptomatic** and are identified incidentally during imaging examinations for unrelated reasons. Patients with large lesions (>5 cm) occasionally complain of nonspecific abdominal symptoms such as upper abdominal fullness or vague abdominal pain. Intermittent symptoms may occur when there is necrosis, infarction, or thrombosis of the tumor. Life-threatening hemorrhage is extremely uncommon even in large tumors but can be precipitated by needle biopsy. Kasabach-Merritt syndrome is a rare consumptive coagulopathy resulting from sequestration of platelets and clotting factors in a giant hemangioma.

   c. **Diagnosis.** Laboratory abnormalities are rare. Because of the possibility of severe hemorrhage from attempts at biopsy, diagnosis relies on imaging investigations. On ultrasound, hemangiomas appear as well-defined, lobulated, homogeneous, hyperechoic masses, although there may be hypoechoic regions representing hemorrhage, fibrosis, and/or calcification. Compressibility of the lesion is pathognomonic. Ultrasound is highly sensitive but not specific, with an estimated overall accuracy of 70% to 80%. Multiphasic (contrast) computed tomography (CT) scans reveal a low-density area with characteristic **peripheral enhancement in the early phase.** Subsequently, contrast enhancement progresses toward the center of the lesion until, in the delayed enhanced images, the tumor appears uniformly enhanced. The best imaging study is magnetic resonance imaging (MRI), with specificity and sensitivity approximately 85% and 95%, respectively. These tumors appear bright on T2-weighted images, with a similar pattern of enhancement as seen with multiphasic CT. Single photon emission CT (SPECT) with technetium-labeled red blood cells has similar accuracy to MRI, but only if the lesion is larger than 3 cm and close to the surface. Due to these limitations, SPECT is only used as an adjunctive test. Hemangiomas can also be differentiated from other tumors by tagged red blood cell scan.

   d. Most hemangiomas are treated safely with **observation.** Indications for intervention include symptoms, complications, and inability to exclude malignancy. In these select patients, the preferred treatment is surgical extirpation. Hemangiomas can usually be enucleated under vascular control (intermittent Pringle maneuver). Formal anatomic resection (e.g., right hepatectomy) is used when the tumor has largely replaced a distinct anatomic unit. Regression after low-dose radiation therapy or embolization in select cases has been described but should be reserved for large, unresectable lesions or for a patient unfit for surgery. In the very rare case of spontaneous hemorrhage, control with vascular embolization provides temporary help until a definitive operative approach can be safely implemented.

2. **Focal nodular hyperplasia (FNH)** is the second-most-common benign hepatic tumor, constituting about 8% of cases. The pathogenesis of FNH is a matter of debate. In the past, it was thought to be either a hamartoma or a neoplasm. Currently, it is thought to represent a nonneoplastic, hyperplastic response to a congenital vascular malformation. FNH is found predominantly in women of child-bearing age, with a female-to-male ratio of 6 to 8:1. Although an association with oral contraceptives has been suggested, the correlations are much lower than are those for hepatic adenomas.

   a. **Pathology.** The lesions usually are solitary and small and often are located near the edge of the liver. Grossly, they are well circumscribed and lobulated but unencapsulated. Histologically, they are characterized by a dense, **central stellate scar** with septa radiating outward, thereby dividing the tumor into nodules. The parenchyma between the septa has the appearance of normal hepatic cords composed of hepatocytes, sinusoids, and Kupffer cells.

   b. **Clinical manifestations** of FNH are rare. Epigastric or right-upper-quadrant pain with a palpable mass is present only in a small minority of patients. Spontaneous rupture with hemorrhage is extremely rare. Malignant degeneration has not been reported, but it is critical to distinguish FNH from the fibrolamellar variant of hepatocellular carcinoma (HCC), a malignant lesion with a similar central scar. It is important to note that the latter's scar is usually large and eccentric, with broad fibrous bands and calcifications.

   c. **Diagnostic studies.** Although ultrasound is often the imaging study that first detects focal hepatic lesions, it does not discriminate FNH from other pathology well. FNH lesions have an echogenicity very similar to that of surrounding normal liver. However, distinguishing characteristics on multiphasic CT can be readily identified. In the late arterial phase, FNH has a bright homogeneous enhancement with a **hypodense central scar.** Delayed-phase images may show hyperattenuation of the central scar. Occasionally, the radiating septa may also be visualized. When MRI is employed, the central scar appears hyperintense on T2-weighted images, and when contrast is used, the enhancement pattern is similar to that seen on CT. Superparamagnetic iron oxide (SPIO) is an MR contrast agent that undergoes phagocytosis by the reticuloendothelial system (RES) (the Kupffer cells in the liver). On SPIO-enhanced T2-weighted images, FNH is hypointense but with a bright central scar. On hepatic scintigraphy with 99m Tc-sulfur colloid, FNH has variable colloid uptake compared with the normal liver. However, intense colloid uptake (10% of cases, related to the number of Kupffer cells present) is a very specific finding for FNH. In combination, use of different imaging modalities, especially MRI, yields a precise diagnosis of FNH in 70% to 90% of cases. When the diagnosis remains in doubt, histologic examination is indicated.

   d. **Treatment.** Elective resection is not indicated in asymptomatic patients when studies differentiate FNH from adenoma or malignant lesions. When the lesion is unresectable, it can be treated with transarterial embolization. Oral contraceptives should be stopped. There is no contraindication to pregnancy with this lesion, but close observation for tumor growth during pregnancy and the postpartum period is prudent.

3. **Hepatic adenoma (HA)** is the benign proliferation of hepatocytes. It is not to be confused with the term "hepatoma," which refers to hepatocellular carcinoma. HA is found in young women and has a 4:1 female-to-male ratio. There is a **strong association** with all synthetic estrogen and progesterone preparations (*Toxicol Environ Health* 1979;5:231). The incidence of adenomas markedly increased in the 1960s and 1970s with the widespread use of oral contraceptive medications. It has stabilized since that time, probably due to the decreased estrogen content

of these medications. In addition, anabolic steroids may drive the growth of these lesions.

    a. Pathology. Adenomas are usually solitary (70% to 80%), round, well-circumscribed lesions. Although they are unencapsulated, there is often a pseudocapsule formed by compression of normal surrounding tissue. Microscopically, they are made up of monotonous sheets of hepatocytes separated by dilated sinusoids. HA does not contain bile ductules, a key histologic finding distinguishing it from FNH.

    b. HA is of clinical importance because of its tendency to **spontaneous rupture and hemorrhage.** About one third of patients present with intraperitoneal bleeding, and others present with abdominal pain without rupture. More often, these lesions present with vague symptoms such as fullness or discomfort in the right upper quadrant or are detected incidentally. These lesions are **premalignant,** with large or multiple tumors carrying a greater risk of malignant degeneration. Rupture may occur during pregnancy due to rapid growth under the influence of estrogens.

    c. Diagnostic studies. Ultrasonography can identify lesions but cannot differentiate an adenoma from a malignant lesion. Unlike FNH, HA frequently appears heterogeneous on CT due to intratumor hemorrhage, necrosis, and fat. On multiphasic CT, HA demonstrates **early enhancement,** often first in the periphery with centripetal progression. The relative lack of Kupffer cells in HA compared to FNH allows SPIO-enhanced MRI and scintigraphy with 99m Tc-sulfur colloid to distinguish between these two entities.

    d. Because of the risk of spontaneous rupture and malignant transformation, HA must be identified and treated promptly. Small (<4 cm), asymptomatic lesions occasionally regress with cessation of oral contraceptives. Although radiofrequency ablation may be an option when there are multiple adenomas, resection of HA remains the standard therapy. **Indications** for operative intervention include the following:

      (1) Patients with lesions that are 5 cm or greater in diameter.

      (2) Tumors that do not shrink after discontinuation of oral contraceptives (OCPs).

      (3) Patients who medically cannot stop OCP use.

      (4) Women who are planning pregnancy.

  4. Bile duct hamartomas are the most common liver lesions seen at laparotomy. They are usually peripherally located and firm, smooth, and white in appearance. Typically, lesions are 1 to 5 mm in diameter, but they may be larger. Distinguishing them from miliary metastatic lesions (especially those from colorectal cancer or cholangiocarcinoma) may be difficult. Where there is uncertainty, biopsy should be performed.

B. Malignant neoplasms of the liver are either primary (such as hepatocellular carcinoma and cholangiocarcinoma) or secondary. The latter are far more common in Western countries.

  1. Hepatocellular carcinoma (HCC, also known as hepatoma)

    a. Demographics. The annual incidence in the United States is approximately 2.4/100,000. The incidence is rising rapidly due in large part to the hepatitis C epidemic. There is a 2 to 3:1 male-to-female predominance. The incidence in African American men is almost twice that in white men. HCC is diagnosed mainly in the fifth and sixth decades.

    b. Major risk factors for cirrhosis in the United States include hepatitis C, alcohol, autoimmune phenomena such as primary biliary cirrhosis and autoimmune hepatitis, and hereditary metabolic disorders. From 70% to 85% of HCC arises in the setting of cirrhosis. Malignant tumors of the liver occur in 4.5% of cirrhotic patients and in up to 10% when hemochromatosis is the inciting factor.

    c. Pathology. Gross patterns of HCC include the nodular type (aggregate of clusters of nodules), the massive type (single large mass), and the diffuse type (widespread fine nodular pattern). The right hemiliver is involved more frequently than the left. Microscopically, the formation of giant cells is a feature of HCC. HCC cells frequently invade venous branches, causing vascular dilation, which contributes to the nodular appearance of the liver.

d. Clinical manifestations. Eighty percent of patients experience **weight loss and weakness.** Approximately 50% have abdominal pain that is dull, persistent, and occurs in the epigastrium or right upper quadrant. Acute severe abdominal pain infrequently has been associated with intraperitoneal hemorrhage due to rupture of a necrotic nodule or erosion of a blood vessel.

e. Diagnostic studies

(1) In cirrhotic patients, HCC may be associated with abnormal liver function tests due to hepatitis. Elevated **serum α-fetoprotein** (AFP) occurs in 75% of affected African patients but in only 30% of patients in the United States. AFP is also often elevated in chronic hepatitis and cirrhosis. A level greater than 200 ng/mL (normal <20 ng/mL) is suggestive of HCC, even in the cirrhotic patient.

(2) Radiologic studies

(a) Ultrasonography can be highly accurate in the detection of HCC, especially when coupled with concomitant AFP elevations.

(b) MR scan can be useful in differentiating other small nodular masses from HCC. This is the most accurate imaging modality for distinguishing HCC from dysplastic or regenerative nodules in the cirrhotic patient.

(c) Multiphasic CT scan with arterial and portal venous phase contrast imaging can distinguish among different types of liver masses. **HCC enhances in the arterial and not usually in the portal venous phase.** Washout of contrast in the delayed (portal venous) phases of enhancement is an additional characteristic of HCC. Washout is defined as hypointensity of a nodule in the delayed phase compared with surrounding liver parenchyma. It is thought to be due to greater arterial neovascularization in HCC lesions than in the adjacent normal parenchyma; thus, in the portal venous phase, there is early venous drainage. A mass in a cirrhotic liver that manifests arterial enhancement with washout has a sensitivity of about 80% with specificity of 95% to 100%. The sensitivity of CT may also be enhanced with lipiodol (a lipid lymphographic agent that is selectively retained in HCC) when this is injected 2 hours before the imaging examination.

(3) When required, laparoscopic or image-guided percutaneous biopsies may be used to obtain a tissue diagnosis. However, **a tissue diagnosis is not required before therapeutic intervention** (including surgical extirpation and liver transplantation) if other diagnostic modalities favor HCC as the diagnosis. Unresectable tumors likewise usually do not require biopsy to confirm the diagnosis because imaging and laboratory studies allow a definitive diagnosis in the majority of cases.

f. Staging. Several staging systems for HCC have been proposed. The most commonly used in the United States is the TNM classification. The individual TNM (tumor, nodes, and metastases) stages are grouped into overall stages: T1 to T4 with N0M0 correspond to stages I, II, IIIA, and IIIB, respectively, whereas N1M0 with any T stage is stage IIIC, and M1 disease is designated stage IV.

g. Treatment

(1) Surgical resection is the treatment of choice for noncirrhotic patients who have HCC. However, this constitutes only 5% of HCC patients in the United States and up to 40% of those in Asian countries. A macroscopic margin of 1 cm generally is regarded as adequate. Overall 5-year survival rates for patients with HCC treated with resection is 40% to 50%, with recurrence rates of around 40% to 50%. The most important predictors of recurrence are microvascular invasion and multinodular tumors. Repeat hepatic resection for recurrence has been demonstrated to be safe and effective in selected lesions.

(2) **Orthotopic liver transplantation** (OLT) is theoretically the best treatment option for HCC because it removes the tumor together with the entire diseased liver, thus eliminating the risk of de novo or recurrent disease. Initial results of OLT for HCC were dismal. However, Mazzaferro and colleagues (*N Engl J Med* 1996;334:693) demonstrated that when OLT is restricted to patients with a single tumor 5 cm or less or patients with up to three tumors with the largest less than 3 cm in size (with no vascular invasion on imaging and absence of nodal and distant metastases), the 4-year actuarial survival rate was 75%, with recurrence-free survival of 83%. These so-called **"Milan criteria"** have subsequently been adopted by the United Network for Organ Sharing (UNOS). Recent reports (e.g., *J Am Coll Surg* 2006;203:411) suggest that even more-advanced stage III patients who are downstaged with pretransplant therapy have results similar to those with stage I and II HCC.

(3) **Local ablation** is the best treatment option for patients who have early-stage HCC and are not suitable for resection or OLT. In addition, these therapies may serve as bridges to OLT for those on the transplant waiting list. Indeed, downstaging tumors improves survival of HCC patients who subsequently undergo OLT. Ablation may be accomplished by chemical (100% ethanol) or physical (radiofrequency, cryoablation) techniques. **Percutaneous ethanol injection** has been shown to be effective for small tumors; the necrosis rate for HCC less than 2 cm is 90% to 100%, but declines to 50% in larger tumors. However, multiple sessions may be required to achieve complete necrosis of each tumor. This technique is rarely used in the United States today. **Radiofrequency ablation (RFA)** has emerged as the procedure of choice in most centers. A needle electrode is placed into the tumor, destroying tissue by heating it to temperatures of 60°C to 100°C. RFA may be performed intraoperatively or percutaneously under imaging guidance. Extendable electrodes within the needle allow larger tumors to be ablated compared to ethanol injection, as well as allow the specific volume of tissue for ablation to be varied. **Transarterial chemoembolization (TACE)** involves selective intra-arterial administration of chemotherapeutic agents followed by embolization of the major tumor artery. HCC preferentially derives its blood supply from the hepatic artery rather than from a combination of the hepatic artery and portal vein as for normal hepatic parenchyma. TACE has a survival benefit for select patients with unresectable tumors, Child class A cirrhosis, and tumors less than 5 cm. The procedure rarely may be complicated by hepatic failure due to infarction of adjacent normal liver. For this reason, it should not be used in decompensated (Child class C) cirrhosis. An emerging therapy is **local radiation therapy with yttrium-90,** a beta-particle-emitting radioisotope. Yttrium-90 microspheres are selectively injected into the hepatic artery or one of its branches, causing tumor destruction through a combination of radiation and embolization.

(4) **Systemic chemotherapy and external beam radiation** have had poor results. Toxicity may lead to decompensation of liver disease. Combining chemotherapy with surgical resection preoperatively or postoperatively has no benefit in terms of patient survival.

h. Without treatment, HCC has a very poor prognosis, with a median length of survival of 3 to 6 months after the diagnosis.

i. **Fibrolamellar hepatocellular carcinoma (FLC)** is a rare histologic variant of HCC. However, there is considerable evidence that FLC is distinct from HCC in its epidemiology, biology, and prognosis. Males and females are equally affected, commonly at a younger age (20 to 40 years old). It is uncommon for FLC to be associated with underlying liver disease such as cirrhosis. The histology of FLC strongly resembles that of focal nodular hyperplasia, but any etiologic association between them remains unproven. FLC appears as a hypoattenuated, well-defined, solitary mass on nonenhanced CT scan. On contrast-enhanced CT, the cellular portion enhances homogeneously; the central scar usually does not enhance, unlike the scar of FNH. FLC is best treated with complete surgical resection, which is possible in 80% of patients. Compared with standard HCC, FLC is associated with a better prognosis: Patients with resectable FLC have a greater 5-year survival rate (>70%) than noncirrhotic patients who have resectable nonfibrolamellar HCC. Late recurrence is common (more than two thirds of cases), and repeat resection of local disease should be considered (*Cancer* 2006;106:1331). Liver transplantation is an option for unresectable but nonmetastatic lesions.

2. **Metastatic disease to the liver** represents the most common malignancy of the liver in the United States. The liver is a common site of metastasis from gastrointestinal cancers because it is the first organ drainage site of venous blood from the gastrointestinal tract.

   a. **Colorectal cancer metastatic to the liver** is the prototype disease treated by partial hepatectomy. Approximately 50% of all patients with colorectal cancer develop metastases, and of these, about one third have disease limited to the liver. Without treatment, hepatic metastasis has a dismal prognosis, with a medial survival of 6 to 12 months. In contrast, numerous studies have shown that resection of hepatic metastases is associated with a 25% to 35% 5-year survival rate and a 20% 10-year survival rate. As a result, operative resection has been established as the most effective therapy for patients with isolated colorectal liver metastases.

      (1) **Staging.** The purpose of preoperative evaluation is to exclude the presence of extrahepatic disease and to identify all the metastatic lesions in the liver that require treatment. An abdominal/pelvic CT scan with oral and intravenous contrast is performed, along with chest x-ray. There should be a colonoscopy within the last 6 months to document absence of anastomotic recurrence or a metachronous colorectal cancer. Whole-body positron emission tomography (PET) after administration of ^{18}F-flurodeoxyglucose (FDG) is valuable for the detection of occult metastases, both intra- and extrahepatic. On MRI, hepatic metastases appear as low-intensity lesions on T1-weighted images and intermediate intensity on T2-weighted images. MRI also provides greater visualization of vascular structures such as the hepatic veins and the inferior vena cava (IVC).

      (2) **Partial hepatectomy.** Formal anatomic liver resection produces greater local disease control than nonanatomic, wedge resection of tumors. In the case of synchronous liver metastasis, the primary colonic tumor and the secondary liver tumor may be resected simultaneously or sequentially. Combined resection avoids a second laparotomy and reduces the overall complication rate without changing operative mortality. When the colorectal and liver resections are both extensive (e.g., extended hepatic lobectomy and low anterior resection), then a staged approach may be preferable. Factors predictive of poor prognosis after resection of hepatic colorectal metastases include node positivity of the primary tumor, multiple metastases, and size of the largest metastasis greater than 5 cm.

      (3) **Postoperative follow-up** consists of serial physical examination, serum CEA level, and abdominal/pelvic CT scans every 3 to 4 months for the first 2 years, then every 6 months for the subsequent 3 years. Unfortunately, disease recurrence is common, but when cancer is isolated to the liver, repeat resection can provide additional survival benefit.

      (4) For **unresectable hepatic colorectal metastases,** multidrug systemic chemotherapy (e.g., oxaliplatin plus infusional 5-flurouracil/leucovorin, also known as FOLFOX) with or without bevacizumab, an anti-VEGF antibody, is offered to patients with adequate performance status. Hepatic arterial infusion (HAI) of the 5-fluorouracil derivative fluorodeoxyuridine (FUDR) has not been shown to offer better survival than systemic therapy.

(5) Local ablation with RFA should be considered in patients unfit for operative resection or who have unresectable disease. In those patients with multiple scattered tumors, a combined approach of resection of the dominant or larger tumors with RFA of the remaining lesions may be feasible.

b. Other liver metastases

(1) Gastrointestinal neuroendocrine tumors. There are a number of reasons supporting resection of neuroendocrine hepatic metastases. These include their relatively long tumor doubling time, lack of effective chemotherapy, and the ability of metastatectomy to provide symptom palliation and long-term survival. For those patients with unresectable disease, hepatic artery embolization may provide symptom relief.

(2) There is limited experience with liver resection for **noncolorectal and nonneuroendocrine metastasis.** Liver resection may provide the only chance for long-term survival. In a study at Memorial Sloan-Kettering Cancer Center of 96 patients with noncolorectal, nonneuroendocrine metastatic tumors of the liver, liver resection was associated with an overall actuarial survival of 37% at 5 years, with a median survival of 32 months (*Surgery* 1997;121:625). The presence of liver metastasis from melanoma or cancer of the breast or stomach should be viewed as a marker of disseminated disease, and liver resection in these contexts is not recommended (*Annu Rev Med* 2005;56:139).

II. HEPATIC ABSCESS. Liver abscesses may originate from bacterial, parasitic, or fungal pathogens. Bacterial abscesses predominate in the United States, whereas amebic (parasitic) abscesses are more common in younger age groups and in endemic areas.

A. Pyogenic abscesses in the liver occur secondary to other sources of bacterial sepsis. Up to 60% of cases arise from direct spread of bacteria from biliary infections such as empyema of the gallbladder or cholangitis. Ruptured appendicitis or diverticulitis are other potential sources for bacterial seeding to the liver.

1. Pathogenesis. For liver abscesses arising from an intra-abdominal infection, it is important to note that hematogenous seeding is *not* the usual pathway for the development of the abscess; rather, the mechanism of spread of infection to the liver is along channels within the peritoneal cavity. For unknown reasons, liver abscesses are usually found in the right lobe of the liver.

2. Microbiology. The bacteria cultured from pyogenic liver abscesses reflect the origin of the infectious process. Most commonly, **mixed species** are isolated, with one third of cultures containing anaerobes. When the biliary tree is the source, enteric Gram-negative bacilli and enterococci are common isolates. When the abscess develops from hematogenous seeding, there is most likely a single organism responsible, such as *Staphylococcus aureus* or *Streptococcus milleri*. Fungal abscesses have been associated with patients who are recovering from chemotherapy. There should be suspicion of amebic abscesses in patients who are from or have recently traveled to an endemic area in the last 6 months.

3. Fever and abdominal pain are the most common symptoms, whereas nonspecific symptoms such as anorexia, weight loss, chills, and malaise may also be present.

4. Laboratory findings are usually nonspecific, such as leukocytosis and elevated serum alkaline phosphatase. A chest x-ray may demonstrate new elevation of the right hemidiaphragm, an infiltrate at the right lung base, or a right-sided pleural effusion. Definitive diagnosis is by CT scanning.

5. Treatment consists in identifying the infectious source as well as managing the liver abscess. **Pyogenic liver abscesses require drainage and systemic antibiotic therapy.** Drainage can be performed percutaneously in most cases, but an operative procedure is recommended when there are multiple, large, loculated abscesses and in patients who otherwise require laparotomy for the underlying cause of the abscess. Drains are usually left in place until drainage becomes minimal, typically 7 days. Empirical antibiotic treatment should include coverage for bowel flora (e.g., metronidazole plus ciprofloxacin or monotherapy with piperacillin/tazobactam). Once identification has been made of the causative organism(s), antibiotic therapy should be modified to reflect their sensitivities. Aggressive antibiotic therapy should continue for at least 1 week beyond clinical recovery and resolution of the abscess on follow-up imaging.

B. Amebic abscess should be considered in *every* case of solitary hepatic abscess. Amebiasis is caused by the protozoan *Entamoeba histolytica*. This parasite exists in two forms: an infective cyst stage and a trophozoite stage, which is the form that causes invasive disease. Amebic liver abscess is the most common extraintestinal manifestation of amebiasis. Infection occurs by hematogenous spread from the gut via the portal venous system.

   1. Epidemiology. Amebic liver abscesses are 7 to 10 times more frequent in adult men, despite an equal sex distribution of intestinal amebic disease. An abscess can develop after travel exposures of just 4 days.

   2. Clinical symptoms are classically **persistent fever and right-upper-quadrant pain.** The presence of diarrhea (reflecting concurrent intestinal amebiasis) is more variable. Presentation usually occurs with 4 months after return from endemic areas. On examination, patients have hepatomegaly and point tenderness over the liver. Rupture of the abscess may cause peritonitis.

   3. Diagnosis. Serologic tests for amebic infestation are positive in nearly 100% of affected patients. Ultrasound and CT are the most useful imaging modalities.

   4. Treatment requires systemic **metronidazole** (750 mg orally three times a day, or 500 mg intravenously every 6 hours, for 7 to 10 days). Needle aspiration should be considered if there is no response to initial therapy or if there is doubt about the diagnosis. The material aspirated contains proteinaceous debris and an "anchovy paste" fluid of necrotic hepatocytes. After completion of the course of metronidazole, the patient should be treated with an intraluminal agent, even if stools are negative for amebas. Intraluminal agents include paromomycin, iodoquinol, and diloxanide furoate. Complications can include bacterial superinfection, erosion into surrounding structures, or free rupture into the peritoneal cavity. Although mortality is infrequent in uncomplicated cases, complicated cases may carry a considerable mortality (as high as 20%).

III. HEPATIC CYSTS can be divided into nonparasitic cysts and echinococcal cysts.

   A. Nonparasitic cysts generally are benign. They can be solitary or multiple and often are identified incidentally on imaging for other symptoms.

   1. Asymptomatic cysts require no treatment regardless of size. Large cysts may be symptomatic because of increased abdominal girth or compression of adjacent structures. Bleeding, infection, or obstructive jaundice can occur but are infrequent.

   2. Symptomatic cysts can be unroofed operatively by either an open approach or, more recently, by laparoscopy. Infected cysts are treated in a similar manner to hepatic abscesses. If the cyst contains bile, communication with the biliary tree is assumed. It should be excised, enucleated, or drained, with closure of the biliary communication.

   3. Polycystic kidney disease sometimes is accompanied by **polycystic liver disease,** which usually is asymptomatic. Symptoms generally are attributable to hepatomegaly from numerous cysts. Liver function is rarely impaired by the gross displacement of parenchyma by these massive cystic cavities. Symptomatic polycystic liver disease has been treated by drainage of the superficial cysts into the abdominal cavity and fenestration of deeper cysts into the superficial cyst cavities. Liver resection and retention of the least-cystic areas of hepatic parenchyma may be more effective. Neoplastic cystic lesions such as cystadenoma or cystadenocarcinoma rarely occur in the liver. These lesions are distinguished from simple cysts by the presence of a mass or septa. They are treated by resection or enucleation (in the case of cystadenoma) to completely remove cyst epithelium.

   B. Echinococcal cysts are the most common hepatic cystic lesions in areas outside the United States. Approximately 80% of hydatid cysts are single and in the right liver. The most common presenting symptoms and signs are right-upper-quadrant abdominal pain and palpable hepatomegaly. Imaging by nuclear medicine scan, ultrasonography, CT scan, or MR scan can demonstrate the abnormality. The **cyst should not be aspirated** as an initial test because aspiration can cause spillage of the organisms and spread the disease throughout the abdominal compartment. A peripheral **eosinophilia** is often detected. Serologic tests include indirect hemagglutination and Casoni skin test, each of which is 85% sensitive. **Treatment** is primarily operative, although percutaneous drainage after antihelminthic treatment is increasingly utilized in many centers in endemic regions. The abdomen is explored, and before unroofing, the cyst cavity is aspirated with a closed system. If there is no evidence of bile in the cyst aspirate, a scolecidal agent is instilled into the cavity. Choices include hypertonic saline, 80% alcohol, or 0.5% cetrimide. A second cycle is performed after 5 minutes. In patients with biliary communication, only hypertonic sodium chloride (10% to 20%) or 0.5% sodium hypochlorite should be used as a scolecidal agent because other agents may damage communicating bile ducts. Pericystectomy is excision of the cyst in the plane between the host pericyst and liver tissue. The advantage of this technique is that there is no residual cavity. Formal hepatectomy is rarely necessary except for large and/or multiple cysts. For those cysts with demonstrated communication with a biliary radical, drainage should be achieved with a Roux-en-Y hepaticoenterostomy. Postoperative therapy with mebendazole or albendazole has been advocated to prevent recurrence.

IV. PORTAL HYPERTENSION (PH) is defined as a chronic increase in portal pressure due to mechanical obstruction of the portal venous system. It is an almost unavoidable consequence of cirrhosis and is responsible for many of the lethal complications of chronic liver disease, including bleeding from gastroesophageal varices, ascites, and hepatic encephalopathy.

    A. The most common cause of portal hypertension in the United States is *intrahepatic* obstruction of portal venous flow from **cirrhosis** (most commonly due to alcohol and/or hepatitis C); intrahepatic portal venous obstruction can also be due to hepatic fibrosis from hemochromatosis, Wilson disease, and congenital fibrosis. *Prehepatic* portal venous obstruction due to congenital atresia or portal vein thrombosis is far less common. Posthepatic obstruction may occur at any level between the liver and the right heart. This includes thrombosis of the hepatic veins (Budd-Chiari syndrome), congenital IVC malformations (web, diaphragm), IVC thrombosis, and constrictive pericarditis.

    B. The clinical manifestations of liver disease with portal hypertension result from hepatic insufficiency and the mechanical effects of portal venous hypertension.

        1. Hepatic encephalopathy (HE) is the spectrum of neuropsychiatric abnormalities in patients with advanced chronic liver disease. It results from portosystemic shunting of neurotoxins usually cleared by the liver. In addition to the usual signs of severe hepatic dysfunction (jaundice, ascites, spider telangiectasias, etc.), manifestations characteristic of encephalopathy include disrupted sleep–wake cycles (insomnia and hypersomnia), asterixis, and hyperreflexia. There are a number of conditions that can precipitate HE, including hypovolemia, hypoxia, gastrointestinal bleeding, electrolyte and acid-base disorders, sedatives, hypoglycemia, and infection. An elevated ammonia level is the best-described neurotoxin associated with HE, but other agents not adequately cleared by the diseased liver have also been implicated, such as γ-aminobutyric acid, mercaptans, and short-chain fatty acids. HE is a clinical diagnosis, and the utility of measuring ammonia levels remains controversial. Treatment is directed at the precipitating cause and reduction of ammoniagenic substrates using lactulose, with second-line therapy including oral antibiotics such as neomycin and rifaximin.

        2. Portosystemic shunting. Increased blood flow through the portal vein leads to increased flow through collateral venous beds that bypass the liver, thereby connecting the portal circulation directly to the systemic circulation. The most clinically significant sites are those at the gastroesophageal junction connecting the left gastric vein (a part of the portal circulation) to the esophageal veins (systemic circulation). Other common collaterals develop when a recanalized umbilical vein collateralizes to the abdominal wall veins or a superior hemorrhoidal vein collateralizes to middle and inferior hemorrhoidal veins. Left-sided **(sinistral)** portal hypertension can be caused by isolated splenic vein thrombosis. This is most often caused by adjacent pancreatitis. Thrombosis results in increased pressure in the splenic vein at the distal end of the pancreas and the development of collaterals through the short gastric vessels and gastric mucosa back to the liver. This segmental area of PH typically causes gastric varices without esophageal varices.

3. The **mechanisms of ascites and edema** are salt and water retention by the kidneys, decreased plasma oncotic pressure, and increased lymphatic flow from increased portal venous hydrostatic pressure. Although the ascites can be massive, it is rarely life-threatening unless complications occur, such as erosion or incarceration of an umbilical hernia, respiratory compromise, and spontaneous bacterial peritonitis. The diagnosis of spontaneous bacterial peritonitis is made by paracentesis and is likely when ascitic fluid contains more than 250 polymorphonuclear leukocytes per microliter and if a single organism is cultured. The most common organisms are *Escherichia coli*, pneumococci, and streptococci. Frequently, however, it is not possible to obtain a positive culture, and so the diagnosis relies on ascitic fluid cell count and differential.

C. **Diagnosis.** Formal measurement of portal pressure by catheterization of the portal vein is seldom performed. Indirect evaluation by measurement of the hepatic wedge pressure after hepatic vein catheterization is considered the gold standard for diagnosis and monitoring PH. The hepatic venous pressure gradient (HVPG) is the difference between the wedged and free hepatic venous pressures. **PH is considered present when the HPVG is 8 mm Hg or greater.** Varices do not develop until the HVPG reaches 10 to 12 mm Hg. Reduction in the HVPG below 12 mm Hg is accepted as the therapeutic target for treating PH.

D. **Management of portal hypertension**

1. **Prophylaxis of variceal bleeding** includes both the prevention of variceal hemorrhage in patients who have never bled (primary prophylaxis) and preventing rebleeding in patients who have survived a bleeding episode (secondary prophylaxis). Every cirrhotic patient should be screened endoscopically for varices at time of diagnosis. Those without varices at this time should have endoscopy repeated after 2 to 3 years, whereas monitoring every 1 to 2 years is recommended when varices are present. **Propranolol** or nadolol therapy has been shown to markedly reduce risk of variceal bleeding, as well as slow the progression of small varices into larger ones. The dose should be titrated to the maximal tolerable dose and maintained indefinitely. For prevention of recurrent bleeding, endoscopic band ligation versus combination pharmacologic therapy (beta-blocker plus isosorbide mononitrate) have equivalent results. Transjugular intrahepatic portosystemic shunting **(TIPS)** has been shown to be superior to either endoscopic or pharmacologic therapies at reducing the rate of rebleeding. However, its use does not improve mortality, has been associated with a greater risk of encephalopathy, and is more costly than endoscopic procedures. Thus, it is limited to situations in which endoscopic therapy has failed or in patients who would not tolerate a rebleed such as those with Child class C cirrhosis (*Eur J Gastroenterol Hepatol* 2006;18:1167).

2. **Management of active variceal hemorrhage.** Up to one third of patients with hemorrhage from gastroesophageal varices die during the initial hospitalization for gastrointestinal (GI) bleeding. All patients with known or suspected esophageal varices and active GI bleeding should be admitted immediately to an intensive care unit for resuscitation and monitoring. Endotracheal intubation to protect the airway, prevent aspiration, and facilitate the safe performance of endoscopy and other procedures is nearly always indicated. Vascular access via short, large-bore peripheral lines should be secured. Recombinant activated factor VII (rFVIIa) may be useful for correcting the prothrombin time in cirrhotics. Infection is a strong prognostic indicator in acute variceal hemorrhage, and use of antibiotics has been shown to reduce both the risk of rebleeding and mortality. Once stabilized, the patient should have emergent upper endoscopy to document the source of hemorrhage. Because up to 50% of patients with known esophageal varices have upper GI hemorrhage from an alternative source, such as gastric or duodenal ulcer, a thorough endoscopy is required. Recommendations for specific

therapy are (1) early administration of vasoactive drugs, even if active bleeding is only suspected, and (2) endoscopic band ligation after initial resuscitation.

a. The pharmacologic treatment of choice for active variceal bleeding in the United States is **octreotide** (intravenous bolus, then infusion for 5 days). It has been shown to be more effective for controlling bleeding than placebo or vasopressin, as well as have fewer side effects than vasopressin. Terlipressin is not available in the United States but is the only pharmacologic treatment associated with a reduction in mortality.

b. Endoscopic therapy is the definitive therapy for active variceal hemorrhage. Two forms of treatment are available: sclerotherapy and variceal band ligation (EBL). A meta-analysis found that EBL is superior to sclerotherapy in the initial control of bleeding and is associated with fewer adverse events and improved mortality (*Semin Liver Dis* 1999;19:439). Emergent endoscopic therapy fails to control bleeding in 10% to 20% of patients. If a second attempt at endoscopic hemostasis fails, then more definitive therapy must be enacted immediately.

c. Balloon tamponade is useful as a temporary remedy for severe variceal bleeding while more definitive therapy is planned. The specially designed balloon catheters include the Sengstaken-Blakemore tube, the Minnesota tube, and the Linton-Nachlas tube. Each has a gastric balloon; the Sengstaken-Blakemore and Minnesota tubes also have an esophageal balloon. For safe and effective use of these devices, the balloons must be carefully placed according to the manufacturer's directions. The position of the gastric balloon in the stomach must always be confirmed radiographically before inflation because inflation of the larger gastric balloon in the esophagus can be disastrous. The pressure of the esophageal balloon must be maintained as directed by the manufacturer to avoid the complications of mucosal ulceration and necrosis. Balloon tamponade achieves bleeding control in 60% to 90% of cases, but should be used only when there is massive bleeding and for a short period of time (<24 hours) until definitive therapy is instituted.

d. TIPS can be used in the acute management of patients with variceal bleeding. It involves the intrahepatic placement of a stent between branches of the hepatic and portal venous circulation. Technical success rates approach 95%, with short-term success in controlling acute variceal hemorrhage observed in more than 80% of patients. The TIPS procedure can provide acute decompression of portal pressure and thus control refractory variceal bleeding. TIPS stenoses require careful follow-up and revision procedures in a significant percentage of patients. Use of polytetrafluoroethylene (PTFE) stents rather than bare metal stents has dramatically decreased the rate of TIPS dysfunction, clinical relapses, and the need for interventions.

e. Emergency portacaval shunt generally is reserved for patients in whom other measures have failed and is almost never performed today. This operation carries significant in-hospital mortality and risk of hepatic encephalopathy, particularly because the patients undergoing the operation typically have failed other measures and have advanced liver disease. Only the technically simpler central portacaval shunts (end to side or side to side) should be used in the emergency setting because other shunts require more dissection and operative time.

3. Management of ascites must be gradual to avoid sudden changes in systemic volume status that can precipitate hepatic encephalopathy, renal failure, or death.

a. Salt restriction is the initial treatment. Sodium intake should be limited to 1,000 mg/day. Stricter limitations are unpalatable.

b. Diuretic therapy should be gradually applied in patients in whom ascites is not controlled by salt restriction. Weight loss should rarely be more than 500 g/day to avoid significant side effects. **Spironolactone** is the initial diuretic of choice at 25 mg orally twice per day. This dose may be increased to a maximum of 400 mg/day in divided doses. Furosemide (20 mg orally/day initially) may be added if spironolactone fails to initiate diuresis. Volume status must be monitored closely by daily weight check and frequent examinations during initial furosemide treatment.

c. Paracentesis is useful in the initial evaluation of ascites, when spontaneous bacterial peritonitis (SBP) is included in the differential diagnosis, and to provide acute decompression of tense ascites. Up to 10 L of ascites can be removed safely if the patient has peripheral edema, the fluid is removed over 30 to 90 minutes, and oral fluid restriction is instituted to avoid hyponatremia. Paracentesis can be used to provide acute relief of symptoms of tense ascites, including respiratory compromise, impending peritoneal rupture through an ulcerated umbilical hernia, or severe abdominal discomfort.

d. TIPS can be used for refractory ascites. Complete resolution of ascites has been reported in 57% to 74% of patients and partial response in another 9% to 22%.

e. A **peritoneovenous shunt,** which reinfuses ascites into the vascular space, is now rarely used for ascites refractory to medical therapy. The LeVeen shunt is placed with one end in the peritoneal cavity and the other end in the subclavian vein. The Denver shunt is a modification that includes a subcutaneous manual pump that can be used to transfer ascites intermittently from the abdomen to the subclavian vein. These shunts are particularly useful in patients with tense ascites and umbilical hernias because they provide decompression of the ascites during the perioperative period of the hernia repair. The main complication of peritoneal venous shunting is disseminated intravascular coagulation, which can be fulminant after shunt placement and requires shunt occlusion. This rarely occurs if the peritoneal cavity is lavaged first. Shunts are **contraindicated** in patients with bacterial peritonitis, recent variceal hemorrhage, liver failure, advanced hepatorenal syndrome, or existing severe coagulopathy. The shunts tend to occlude with time and are used very rarely today.

4. Control of hepatic encephalopathy requires the limitation of dietary protein intake and the use of lactulose and oral antibiotics.

a. Dietary changes should be initiated first. Dietary protein should be eliminated while adequate nonprotein calories are administered. After clinical improvement, a 20-g/day protein diet may be administered, with increasing protein allowances of 10 g/day every 3 to 5 days if encephalopathy does not recur.

b. If the encephalopathy is not controlled by diet alone, **oral agents** can be added.

   (1) Lactulose is a nonabsorbed synthetic disaccharide that produces an osmotic diarrhea, thus altering intestinal flora. The oral dosage is 15 to 45 mL two to four times a day. The dose then is adjusted to produce two to three soft stools daily. Alternatively, a lactulose enema can be prepared with 300 mL of lactulose and 700 mL of tap water administered two to four times a day.

   (2) Useful oral antibiotic preparations include neomycin (1 g orally every 4 to 6 hours or 1% retention enema every 6 to 12 hours) and metronidazole (250 mg orally every 8 hours). The oral antibiotics are used as second-line agents to lactulose because, although they are equally effective, neomycin carries some risk of ototoxicity and nephrotoxicity, and metronidazole carries some risk of neurotoxicity.

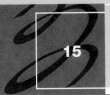

BILIARY SURGERY
Richard A. Pierce and Steven M. Strasberg

15

I. CHOLELITHIASIS

A. The **incidence** of cholelithiasis increases with age. At age 60 years, approximately 25% of women and 12% of men in the United States have gallstones. In some countries (e.g., Sweden, Chile) and ethnic groups (e.g., Pima Indians), the incidence of gallstones may approach 50%.

B. Pathogenesis and natural history. Patients can be divided into three clinical stages: asymptomatic, symptomatic, and those with complications of cholelithiasis. There is generally a stepwise progression from stage to stage. Annually, only 1% to 2% of those with asymptomatic disease progress to the symptomatic stage. It is unusual (<0.5% per year) for an asymptomatic patient to develop complicated gallstone disease without first suffering symptoms.

  1. Cholesterol gallstones (85% of stones, radiolucent) are associated with increasing age, obesity, female gender, and Western diet. The female-to-male ratio is 2:1, and the increased incidence among women is in part related to pregnancy and/or oral contraceptive use. Obesity is an independent factor, increasing the prevalence of cholesterol gallstones by a factor of 3. Western diet is closely related, and these stones are rare in vegetarians.

  2. Pigment gallstones (15% of stones, radiopaque, two distinct types)

    a. Black gallstones are hard, spiculated, and brittle, and are composed of calcium bilirubinate, calcium phosphate, and calcium carbonate. Risk factors include hemolytic disorders, cirrhosis, and ileal resection.

    b. Brown gallstones are soft, associated with biliary stasis and infection (especially *Klebsiella* species), and are composed of bacterial cell bodies, calcium bilirubinate, and calcium palmitate.

C. Asymptomatic gallstones

  1. Diagnosis. Asymptomatic gallstones are usually discovered on routine imaging studies or incidentally at laparotomy for unrelated problems. Common abdominal symptoms such as dyspepsia, bloating, eructation, or flatulence *without associated pain* are probably not caused by gallstones.

  2. Management. There is no role for prophylactic cholecystectomy in most patients with asymptomatic gallstones, with a few exceptions.

    a. Patients with a **porcelain gallbladder** should undergo cholecystectomy due to a high risk of malignancy. Prophylactic cholecystectomy may be warranted in patients with asymptomatic gallstones who have other risk factors for gallbladder cancer as outlined in Section VI.C.1.

    b. Children with gallstones have a relative indication for cholecystectomy due to the general difficulty of declaring and interpreting symptoms in this population.

    c. In adult patients with **diabetes mellitus, spinal cord trauma,** and **sickle cell anemia,** prophylactic cholecystectomy is generally *not* indicated for *asymptomatic* or uncomplicated gallstone disease. Even after cholecystectomy, sickle cell patients may still develop bile duct stones.

    d. Management of **gallstones discovered at laparotomy** remains controversial because the literature is conflicting with regard to the incidence of biliary symptoms after surgery in patients in whom the gallbladder is not removed.

D. Symptomatic gallstones (biliary colic)

1. **Diagnosis** largely depends on correlating symptoms with the presence of stones on imaging. Differential diagnosis includes acute cholecystitis, liver diseases, peptic ulcer disease, renal colic, gastroesophageal reflux, irritable bowel syndrome, and diseases based in the chest, including inferior wall myocardial ischemia/infarct or right-lower-lobe pneumonia. Appropriate testing is dictated by clinical suspicion of these entities.

   a. **Symptoms.** Biliary colic is the main symptom and is initiated by impaction of a gallstone in the outlet of the gallbladder, as characterized by the following:

      (1) **Periodicity.** The pain comes in distinct attacks lasting 30 minutes to several hours.

      (2) **Location.** The pain occurs in the epigastrium or right upper quadrant.

      (3) **Severity.** The pain is steady and intense and may cause the patient to restrict breathing. Frequently, it is so severe that immediate care is sought and narcotics are necessary for control.

      (4) **Timing.** The pain occurs within hours of eating a meal, often awakening the patient from sleep.

      (5) **Other symptoms** include back pain, left-upper-quadrant pain, nausea, and vomiting. These *usually* occur in addition to, rather than in place of, the pain as described.

   b. **Physical signs** include mild right-upper-quadrant tenderness, although there may be few abdominal findings during an attack. Jaundice is not caused by impaction of a stone in the cystic duct without inflammation. If jaundice is present, another cause should be sought.

   c. **Diagnostic imaging.** Ultrasound diagnosis is based on the presence of echogenic structures having posterior acoustic shadows. There is usually little or no associated gallbladder wall thickening or other evidence of cholecystitis. Bile ducts must be assessed for evidence of dilation or choledocholithiasis (gallstones in the common bile duct).

2. **Laparoscopic cholecystectomy** (LC) is the appropriate treatment for the vast majority of patients with symptomatic gallstones (see Section I.F.1).

E. Complications of cholelithiasis

1. **Acute calculous cholecystitis** is initiated by obstruction of the cystic duct by an impacted gallstone. Persistence of stone impaction leads to inflammation of the gallbladder. Although the onset and character of the resulting pain resemble those of biliary colic, the pain is unremitting. Severe complications including empyema, gangrene, or contained or free gallbladder perforation with abscess formation may develop in some cases.

   a. **Diagnosis** depends on the constellation of symptoms and signs and the demonstration of characteristic findings with diagnostic imaging.

      (1) The **symptoms** of acute cholecystitis are similar to but more severe and persistent than those of biliary colic. As the inflammatory process spreads to the parietal peritoneum, tenderness develops in the right upper quadrant or even more diffusely, and movement becomes painful. Systemic complaints such as anorexia, nausea, and vomiting are common. Fever may or may not be present. Elderly patients tend to have mild symptoms and may present only with reduced food intake. **Murphy's sign** (inspiratory arrest during deep palpation of the right upper quadrant) is characteristic of acute cholecystitis and is most informative when the acute inflammation has subsided and direct tenderness is absent. Mild jaundice may be present, but severe jaundice is rare and suggests the presence of common bile duct (CBD) stones, cholangitis, or obstruction of the CBD caused by external compression from a stone impacted in an inflamed Hartmann's pouch **(Mirizzi syndrome).**

      (2) **Laboratory abnormalities** may include leukocytosis (typically 12,000 to 15,000 cells/μL), although often the white blood cell count is normal. Complications, such as gangrene, perforation, or cholangitis, are suggested by an extremely high white blood cell count (>20,000 cells/μL).

Liver function tests (LFTs), including serum bilirubin, alkaline phosphatase, alanine transaminase (ALT), aspartate transaminase (AST), and serum amylase, also may be abnormal.

(3) Diagnostic imaging

(a) Ultrasonography is the most commonly used test for diagnosing acute cholecystitis and any associated cholelithiasis. Findings indicative of acute cholecystitis include gallbladder wall thickening, pericholecystic fluid, and a **sonographic Murphy sign** (tenderness over the gallbladder when compressed by the ultrasound probe). In one meta-analysis, the sensitivity and specificity of ultrasonography for diagnosing gallstones were 0.84 and 0.99, respectively. For the diagnosis of acute cholecystitis, the sensitivity was 0.88 and the specificity was 0.80 (*Arch Int Med* 1994;154:2573).

(b) Radionuclide cholescintigraphy can be useful as an adjunct in the diagnosis of acute cholecystitis; however, the test's sensitivity and specificity for gallstones are lower than those for ultrasound. Scintigraphic scanning with hepatic 2,6-dimethyliminodiacetic acid (HIDA) enables visualization of the biliary system. The radionuclide is concentrated and secreted by the liver, allowing visualization of the bile ducts and the gallbladder normally within 30 minutes. Because the test depends on hepatic excretion of bile, it may not be useful in jaundiced patients. Nonfilling of the gallbladder *after* 4 hours is good evidence of acute cholecystitis. Administration of morphine may enhance the test by causing spasm of the sphincter of Oddi and thereby stimulating gallbladder filling.

(c) Computed tomographic (CT) scanning is now frequently performed to evaluate the patient with acute abdominal pain. CT can demonstrate gallstones, although it is less sensitive for these than ultrasonography. Other signs of acute cholecystitis on CT include gallbladder wall thickening, pericholecystic fluid, edema, and emphysematous cholecystitis (air in the gallbladder wall).

b. Management

(1) Initial management for patients with acute cholecystitis includes hospitalization, intravenous fluid resuscitation, and parenteral antibiotics (e.g., piperacillin/tazobactam). Separate coverage for enterococci is not necessary because they are rarely the solitary pathogen.

(2) Acute cholecystitis often resolves with nonsurgical initial management. However, the patient must be **reassessed frequently** with respect to fever, symptomatology, physical signs of inflammation, and laboratory values. If the patient is not improving, alterations in management must be made. These include changing the antibiotic regimen, percutaneous cholecystostomy, or operative cholecystectomy or cholecystostomy.

(3) Patients with acute cholecystitis should have **cholecystectomy as definitive treatment.** Although cholecystectomy may be performed in either an early or a delayed fashion, evidence now leans heavily toward an early procedure for those patients that present within an appropriate time frame (symptoms <72 hours in duration).

(a) Early cholecystectomy has the advantage of resolving the illness more quickly than delayed cholecystectomy. The operation is best performed within 48 hours after the onset of symptoms, when there is less gallbladder inflammation. Cholecystectomy performed during an episode of acute cholecystitis (vs. symptomatic cholelithiasis) increases the conversion rate from laparoscopic to open surgery from less than 1% to approximately 5%.

(b) If presentation is delayed (>3 days of symptoms) or the patient has a palpable gallbladder and leukocytosis greater than 18,000 cells/μL, **delayed cholecystectomy** ("interval cholecystectomy") is usually indicated to allow surrounding inflammation to subside before the operation.

  (c) **Several prospective, randomized trials** have compared early versus delayed (6 weeks) LC for acute cholecystitis. Four recent meta-analyses of the existing literature showed no significant differences in early versus delayed procedures with regard to mortality, conversion rate, bile duct injury, and perioperative complications. However, these studies almost universally showed, in the early group, significantly fewer readmissions for interval complications (due to failure of conservative therapy in ~20% of patients) and a significantly reduced hospital length of stay (*Cochrane Database Syst Rev* 2006;4:CD005440, *Surg Endosc* 2006;20:82, *Surg Today* 2005;35:553, *Am J Gastroenterol* 2004;99:147). Nonetheless, controversy still exists about the relationship between operation in the acute phase of inflammation and bile duct injury. A large registry series from Connecticut reported that when LC is performed for acute cholecystitis, the incidence of injury is three times higher (0.51%) than for elective LC and twice as high as for open cholecystectomy (*Arch Surg* 1996;131:382).

  (4) Tube cholecystostomy should be performed in patients who have acute cholecystitis and who are failing systemic therapy but are not candidates for cholecystectomy because of severity of illness or concomitant medical problems. Although surgical cholecystostomy can be performed operatively, these patients usually benefit from the less invasive percutaneous approach (percutaneous cholecystostomy). Drainage of the gallbladder almost uniformly resolves the episode of acute cholecystitis, and the indwelling catheter allows for performance of interval cholangiography. After resolution of the acute episode, the patient can eventually undergo either cholecystectomy or percutaneous stone extraction and removal of the cholecystostomy tube. Such nonoperative stone removal as definitive treatment is reasonable in very elderly or debilitated patients who cannot have a general anesthetic.

2. **Choledocholithiasis** generally is due to gallstones that originate in the gallbladder and pass through the cystic duct into the common duct. In Western countries, stones rarely originate in the hepatic or common ducts, although these "primary" stones, usually brown pigment stones, are more prevalent in Asia.

  a. **Diagnosis.** The most common manifestation of uncomplicated choledocholithiasis is **jaundice,** with bilirubin typically between 3 and 10 mg/dL. Biliary colic is common and is similar to that previously described (see Section I.D). On examination, signs may be limited to icterus. Ultrasonography usually demonstrates gallbladder stones and bile duct dilation. Due to obscuring gas in the duodenum, ductal stones are visible in only about 50% of cases. The diagnosis may be confirmed by endoscopic retrograde cholangiopancreatography (ERCP) or percutaneous transhepatic cholangiography (PTC), which can opacify the biliary tree and demonstrate the intraductal stones. Occasionally, the diagnosis of choledocholithiasis is confirmed by intraoperative cholangiography (IOC) at the time of cholecystectomy.

  b. **Management** depends on available expertise and clinical situation.

    (1) In patients with choledocholithiasis who also have cholelithiasis, standard management consists of LC and IOC, possibly followed by laparoscopic CBD exploration if stones are seen. Intraoperative measures to clear the CBD of stones include administration of intravenous (IV) glucagon, use of irrigation, blind passage of balloon catheters or stone baskets, or passage of these devices via choledochoscope. If the bile duct cannot be cleared of stones by laparoscopic exploration, open bile duct exploration or postoperative ERCP may be required, but this is uncommon.

    (2) In some cases, choledocholithiasis should be handled by ERCP or PTC. **ERCP with sphincterotomy and stone removal** is used in patients who are not surgical candidates or have had prior cholecystectomy. It is also used in patients who are jaundiced (these patients may have tumors as opposed to choledocholithiasis), including all patients with acute cholangitis. Patients with intrahepatic stones and those with many CBD stones are also usually treated with ERCP. ERCP with sphincterotomy carries a less than 1% risk of mortality and a 5% to 10% risk of morbidity, principally acute pancreatitis. An intraoperative cholangiogram should be performed at the time of surgery even when preoperative ERCP has been done because residual stones may be present in a small percentage of patients.

3. **Biliary pancreatitis** is caused by blockage of pancreatic secretions by passage of a gallstone into the common biliary-pancreatic channel. The greatest risk is carried by small (~2 mm) stones. Once the acute episode of pancreatitis has resolved, the gallbladder should be removed as expeditiously as possible to avoid recurrent pancreatitis. A longer delay may be justified in patients who have had severe pancreatitis and in whom local inflammation or systemic illness contraindicates surgery. An IOC should *always* be done at the time of the cholecystectomy to confirm that the bile duct is free of stones. In patients in whom cholecystectomy is contraindicated, endoscopic sphincterotomy (ES) may be protective against further attacks of pancreatitis.

4. **Cholangitis is often caused by choledocholithiasis (see Section II.B).**

5. **Gallstone ileus (bowel obstruction caused by a gallstone)** is an uncommon complication that results from a gallstone eroding through the wall of the gallbladder into the adjacent bowel (usually duodenum). Usually the stone migrates until it lodges in the narrowest portion of the small bowel, just proximal to the ileocecal valve. Patients present with symptoms of bowel obstruction and air in the biliary tree (from the cholecystoenteric fistula). Treatment is exploratory laparotomy and removal of the obstructing gallstone by milking it back to an enterotomy made in healthy intestine. The entire bowel should be searched diligently for other stones, and cholecystectomy should be performed if the patient is stable and the inflammation is not too severe.

F. **Surgical management of symptomatic cholelithiasis and acute cholecystitis**

1. **Laparoscopic cholecystectomy** has a low complication rate, and the patient's recovery and return-to-work times are excellent.

   a. **Indications.** Approximately 95% of patients with cholelithiasis are candidates for the laparoscopic approach. Contraindications include generalized peritonitis, cholangitis, concomitant diseases that prevent use of a general anesthetic, and the patient's refusal of open cholecystectomy should urgent conversion be required. Local inflammation in the triangle of Calot can prevent complete visualization of the appropriate structures and increases the risk of injury to the bile ducts or hepatic arteries.

   b. **Technique.** Because misidentification of the cystic duct is the commonest cause of biliary injury, the surgeon must use a technique to provide conclusive identification of the cystic duct and artery.

      (1) In the **Critical View of Safety Technique** pioneered at our institution, the triangle of Calot is dissected free of fat, fibrous, and areolar tissue, and importantly, the lower end of the gallbladder must be dissected off of the liver bed (*J Am Coll Surg* 1995;180:101). A complete dissection demonstrates two and *only* two structures (the cystic duct and artery) entering the gallbladder, constituting the "critical view of safety."

      (2) **Intraoperative cholangiography** may be used as the sole method of ductal identification. In addition, an absolute indication is the need to confirm the ductal anatomy during LC whenever the critical view is not achieved. IOC is also indicated in patients with known choledocholithiasis, a history of jaundice, a history of pancreatitis, a large cystic duct and small gallstones, any abnormality in preoperative LFTs, or dilated biliary ducts on ultrasonography. **Laparoscopic ultrasound** as an alternative method for the detection of CBD stones is highly accurate and has decreased operative time and cost in experienced hands (*Surg Clin North Am* 2000;80:1151).

c. **Complications.** LC appears to be associated with a higher incidence (~2.5/1,000) of major bile duct injury than open cholecystectomy. The serious problems include both misidentification injuries and technical problems such as cautery-induced damage (*J Hepatobiliary Pancreat Surg* 2002;9:543). In addition, there are also risks to other structures, including the hepatic artery and the bowel. Unretrieved gallstone spillage can be the source of infrequent but serious long-term complications such as abscess and fistula formation. Factors associated with an increased rate of conversion to an open procedure include emergent cholecystectomy, male sex, age greater than 60 years, obesity, gallbladder inflammation (acute cholecystitis), choledocholithiasis, and prior upper abdominal surgery.

2. **Open cholecystectomy** is performed in the minority of patients who have contraindications to LC, in patients who require conversion from LC because of inability to complete the laparoscopic procedure, or when necessary in conjunction with a laparotomy for another operation (e.g., Whipple procedure).

3. **Medical dissolution** of gallstones can sometimes be achieved with oral bile acid therapy, but given the proven effectiveness of LC, there is virtually no current application of medical dissolution. Development of gallstones after gastric bypass for morbid obesity is very common and may largely be prevented by bile acid therapy. The current optimal bile acid therapy for dissolution of gallstones is ursodeoxycholic acid (10 to 15 mg/kg/day).

II. ACALCULOUS CHOLECYSTITIS AND OTHER BILIARY TRACT INFLAMMATIONS

A. **Acalculous cholecystitis** typically occurs in severely ill hospitalized [i.e., intensive care unit (ICU)] patients, especially those with a history of hypotension. It is also associated with prolonged nothing-by-mouth (NPO) status and dependence on parenteral nutrition, with episodes of systemic sepsis, or during multiple-organ-system failure. Mortality rate is high, ranging from 10% to 50%.

1. A high index of suspicion is required to make the **diagnosis.**

   a. **Presentation** depends largely on the patient's concurrent medical conditions. Alert patients typically complain of right-upper-quadrant or diffuse upper abdominal pain and tenderness. However, many of these patients may not be alert, and therefore pain and tenderness are absent in up to 75% of patients. Unexplained deterioration in severely ill patients should lead to suspicion of this diagnosis.

   b. In sedated patients, **laboratory data,** although variable, may be the only indication of acalculous cholecystitis.

   c. Diagnostic **imaging** is essential for establishing the diagnosis because a false-positive result may lead to an unnecessary intervention in a critically ill patient.

      (1) **Ultrasonography** can be done at the bedside in the critically ill patient. Typical findings are similar to those of acute calculous cholecystitis. Limitations include overlying bowel gas, concomitant abdominal wounds or dressings, and the fact that gallbladder abnormalities are often seen in the ICU population (e.g., congestive heart failure may lead to gallbladder wall thickening), even in those patients not suspected of having acute cholecystitis.

      (2) **Hepatobiliary scintigraphy** (HIDA) can also be done at the bedside and represents a valuable adjunct to ultrasound in the diagnosis of acalculous cholecystitis. In 2000, a study of 107 consecutive patients found scintigraphy to be superior to ultrasonography in terms of sensitivity, specificity, and positive and negative predictive value for the diagnosis of acute cholecystitis. The accuracy of the two tests in all patients was 92% for scintigraphy and 77% for ultrasonography, but this margin widened to 91% versus 61% when only surgically treated patients were considered (*Surgery* 2000;127:609). In addition, a more recent retrospective review of 132 patients with acute cholecystitis demonstrated a sensitivity of only 48% for ultrasound compared to 86% for cholescintigraphy and 90% when both modalities were employed (*J Am Coll Surg* 2001;193:609).

Similar conclusions were reached in a large meta-analysis of all English-language articles dealing with tests used to diagnose biliary tract disease from 1966 through 1992 (*Arch Intern Med* 1994;154:2573).

(3) **CT scan** is as sensitive as ultrasonography for acalculous cholecystitis and has the advantage of providing more complete imaging of the abdominal cavity from the lung bases to the pelvis. However, CT requires transfer of the patient to the radiology suite, which may be a prohibitive risk in the critically ill.

(4) In difficult cases, **percutaneous cholecystostomy** may be both diagnostic and therapeutic because an infected gallbladder can be decompressed and inciting stones extracted via the tube.

(5) **The choice of imaging** depends largely on the clinical picture, and a high index of suspicion is often necessary to make the diagnosis in sedated or unresponsive ICU patients. Due to its portability and low cost, ultrasound is almost universally the first test of choice, but if the diagnosis is in doubt, then scintigraphy can be added significantly to improve the diagnostic index. CT can be used to evaluate other potential sources of abdominal pathology, whereas percutaneous cholecystostomy may avoid a trip to the operating room for patients who are unable to tolerate surgery.

2. **Management** of acalculous cholecystitis must be tailored to the individual patient, but at the minimum involves systemic antibiotics, NPO status, and treatment of any comorbidities. Primary treatment involves decompression of the gallbladder, typically with a percutaneously placed tube. The definitive treatment is interval cholecystectomy.

B. **Acute cholangitis** is a potentially life-threatening bacterial infection of the biliary tree typically associated with partial or complete obstruction of the ductal system. Although acute cholangitis is often associated with cholelithiasis and choledocholithiasis, other causes of biliary tract obstruction and infection, including benign and malignant strictures of the bile ducts or at biliary-enteric anastomoses, parasites, and indwelling tubes or stents, also have a causative relationship. ERCP without concomitant stenting in the presence of a stricture may lead to cholangitis above the stricture. Therefore patients should routinely be pretreated with antibiotics in case a stent cannot be placed.

1. Diagnosis

a. Patients present with a spectrum of disease severity, ranging from subclinical illness to acute toxic cholangitis. Greater than 90% of patients with cholangitis present with fever. **Charcot's triad** (fever, jaundice, and right-upper-quadrant pain) remains the hallmark of this disease but is present in only a minority of patients. The advanced symptoms of **Reynold's pentad** (Charcot's triad with hemodynamic instability and mental status changes) are seen on presentation in up to 10% of patients, especially in the elderly, and suggest a more toxic or suppurative course of cholangitis.

b. **Laboratory data** supportive of acute cholangitis include elevations of the white blood cell count and LFTs.

c. Investigation of the biliary tree is mandatory to demonstrate and relieve the underlying etiology of the obstruction. Ultrasonography or CT scan may reveal gallstones and biliary dilatation, but **definitive diagnosis is made by ERCP or PTC.** These studies are both diagnostic and therapeutic because they demonstrate the level of obstruction and allow culture of bile, removal of stones or indwelling foreign bodies, and placement of drainage catheters if necessary.

2. Management

a. Initial management of cholangitis includes **intravenous antibiotics** appropriate for the coverage of the most commonly cultured organisms: *Escherichia coli, Klebsiella pneumoniae,* enterococci, and *Bacteroides fragilis.* In patients with acute toxic cholangitis or in patients who fail to respond to antibiotic therapy, **emergent decompression of the biliary tree** via ERCP or PTC is required. If decompression by these means is not available or possible, operative intervention to decompress the biliary tree is indicated, though it should usually be limited to extraction of obvious stones and insertion of a T tube in the CBD.

    b. Cholangitis in patients with indwelling tubes or stents generally requires **stent removal and replacement.**

    c. Definitive operative therapy for benign or malignant biliary tract strictures should be deferred until a later date.

C. Oriental cholangiohepatitis, also known as **recurrent pyogenic cholangitis,** is endemic to the Far East. It is usually due to infestation of the biliary tree with parasites such as *Opisthorchis* species (Thailand) and *Clonorchis* species (China) that cause stasis, bacterial overgrowth, and brown stone formation. Typical findings include multiple intrahepatic and extrahepatic biliary ductal stones, strictures, and repeated bacterial infections of the biliary tract. **Management** involves palliation of biliary strictures and the provision of wide biliary drainage, usually using a choledochoduodenostomy or Roux-en-Y hepaticojejunostomy above the level of the strictured CBD.

III. BILIARY DYSKINESIA is seen in patients with *typical* symptoms of biliary colic but without evidence of gallstones. These patients require extensive workup to exclude other causes of right-upper-quadrant pain. Cholecystokinin–technetium-HIDA scan is useful in evaluation: After the gallbladder has filled with the labeled radionuclide, cholecystokinin is administered, and a gallbladder ejection fraction is calculated 20 minutes later. An ejection fraction of less than 35% is suggestive of biliary dyskinesia. The definitive treatment is cholecystectomy, and greater than 85% of patients report postoperative improvement or relief of symptoms.

IV. PRIMARY SCLEROSING CHOLANGITIS (PSC) is a cholestatic disorder characterized by a progressive fibrous obliteration of the bile ducts. An underlying autoimmune process is thought to be the cause. Almost 70% of patients are men, predominantly in the fifth decade of life. An association with inflammatory bowel disease exists because PSC is present in 1% to 5% of those with IBD. However, the incidence of IBD in patients with PSC is greater, between 25% and 75%. PSC is a risk factor for cholangiocarcinoma, which may occur in 4% to 20% of patients.

A. Pathology. Liver biopsy most commonly shows periductal concentric fibrosis around the macroscopic bile ducts. Obliterative fibrous cholangitis, or concentric fibrosis with obliteration of the small ducts, is virtually diagnostic but is seen in less than 10% of cases. Additional findings may include cholestasis, inflammation (with accumulation of plasma cells, lymphocytes, and polymorphonuclear leukocytes), and secondary biliary sclerosis. Findings may be either diffuse or segmental, and both intrahepatic and extrahepatic ductal segments are generally involved. The hepatic duct bifurcation is typically the area most severely involved.

B. Diagnosis is based on a combination of findings.

    1. There are **no pathognomonic signs** of PSC. Although patients can be asymptomatic for up to 15 years, prolonged disease ultimately leads to progressive hepatic failure. The condition is characterized by relapses and remissions, with quiescent periods. Jaundice with pale (acholic) stools and dark urine forms the initial clinical picture. With advanced disease, pain in the right upper quadrant, pruritus, fatigue, and weight loss often accompany the jaundice. Cholangitis with fever and rigors may ultimately occur. Physical exam commonly reveals jaundice, hepatomegaly, and splenomegaly.

    2. Diagnostic imaging. The procedure of choice is ERCP, and PTC may be complementary if the intrahepatic biliary tree is not well visualized. The most common finding is a diffuse and irregular narrowing of the entire biliary tree, with short, annular strictures giving a beaded appearance. In progressive disease, the strictures become confluent, and diverticula of the ducts appear. Although cholangiography is the gold standard, scintigraphy, sonography, and CT scan also are useful in making the diagnosis.

    3. Laboratory data. The alkaline phosphatase level is almost always elevated, usually out of proportion to the bilirubin. Serum transaminases may be mildly elevated. Most patients are negative for hepatitis B surface antigen.

C. **Management.** Symptomatic improvements have been reported with the use of various drugs aimed at reversing the presumed autoimmune etiology, including corticosteroids, immunosuppressive agents, methotrexate, and D-penicillamine. However, none of these alters the natural history of the disease. PSC has been effectively palliated with endoscopic or percutaneous dilation of strictures. Although operative intervention is required for most patients, placement of stents after dilation can be a valuable preoperative adjunct.

1. **Resection or bypass of localized strictures.** The role of nontransplant surgery in this disease is limited. Rarely, surgery is indicated when the disease is located only in the extrahepatic bile ducts and a dominant stricture exists that can be excised or bypassed by hepaticojejunostomy.

2. Extensive, diffuse stricture disease with end-stage cirrhosis is an indication for orthotopic **liver transplantation.** If the patient has undergone a previous decompressive operation, transplantation is technically more challenging but not contraindicated.

3. Because PSC is a risk factor for cholangiocarcinoma, **close surveillance** of patients is needed. The diagnosis is difficult because cholangiocarcinomas also masquerade as strictures. A dominant biliary stricture or elevated carbohydrate antigen 19-9 level should raise the suspicion of cholangiocarcinoma in a PSC patient and suggests the need for further evaluation.

D. **Prognosis.** Many patients have a course that progresses to cirrhosis and liver failure despite early palliative interventions. Liver transplantation likely improves survival and quality of life, and early referral for liver transplantation is indicated to decrease the risk of developing cholangiocarcinoma. Overall, the median length of survival from diagnosis to death or liver transplantation is 10 to 12 years.

V. **CHOLEDOCHAL CYSTS** are congenital dilations of the biliary tree that may occur in any bile duct but characteristically involve the common hepatic and common bile ducts. They are more frequently identified in women (3:1 ratio) and those of Asian descent. Sixty percent are diagnosed in patients under the age of 10 years. Diagnosis and treatment are essential because the cysts predispose to choledocholithiasis, cholangitis, portal hypertension, and cholangiocarcinoma, which develop in up to 30% of cysts and usually present in the fourth decade of life.

A. **An anatomic classification scheme** has identified five distinct types. Type I cysts are fusiform dilations of the CBD and are the most common (65% to 90%). Type II cysts are rare, isolated saccular diverticula of the CBD. Type III cysts, also termed *choledochoceles*, are localized dilations within the intraduodenal part of the CBD. Most lesions thought to be choledochoceles are in fact duodenal duplications. Type IV cysts are characterized by multiple cystic areas of the biliary tract, both inside and outside of the liver. Type V cysts are single or multiple lesions based only in the intrahepatic portion of the tract (Caroli disease).

B. **Diagnosis.** The classic triad of jaundice, a palpable abdominal mass, and right-upper-quadrant pain mimicking biliary colic is present only a minority of the time. Neonates frequently present with biliary obstruction, whereas older youths suffer from jaundice and abdominal pain. Rarely, pancreatitis or duodenal obstruction can be caused by a choledochocele. Initial diagnosis is often made with ultrasonography and/or CT. Further evaluation of the cyst should be obtained with specific biliary imaging such as ERCP.

C. **Treatment** is primarily surgical. Cyst excision with a Roux-en-Y hepaticojejunostomy is the treatment of choice for types I and IV. Simple excision of the rare type II cyst has been performed. Local endoscopic cyst unroofing plus sphincteroplasty is usually effective for type III disease. Caroli disease can be treated with hemihepatectomy when it is confined to one side of the liver. More often, bilateral disease is present with associated liver damage and mandates orthotopic liver transplantation.

VI. **TUMORS OF THE BILE DUCTS**

A. **Benign tumors of the bile ducts,** usually adenomas, are rare and arise from the ductal glandular epithelium. They are characteristically polypoid and rarely are larger than 2 cm. Most are found adjacent to the ampulla, with the CBD being the next-most-common site. The malignant potential of these uncommon lesions is unclear.

1. Most patients present with **intermittent obstructive jaundice,** often accompanied by right-upper-quadrant pain. This presentation may be confused with choledocholithiasis.

2. **Treatment** should involve complete resection of the tumor with a margin of duct wall. High recurrence rates have been reported after simple curettage of the polyps. Lesions situated at the ampulla can usually be managed by transduodenal papillotomy or wide local excision.

B. **Cholangiocarcinoma** arises from the bile duct epithelium and can occur anywhere along the course of the biliary tree. Cholangiocarcinoma is an uncommon malignancy, with an incidence in the United States of approximately 0.85/100,000 population and representing about 2% of all cancers (approximately 5,000 new cases per year). Tumors tend to be locally invasive, and when they metastasize, they usually involve the liver and the peritoneum. They characteristically spread along the bile ducts microscopically for long distances beyond the palpable end of the tumor. The median age of onset is approximately 65 years. Predisposing conditions include male gender, PSC, choledochal cysts, intrahepatic stones, parasitic infestations such as *Opisthorchis* and *Clonorchis* species, and exposure to the radiocontrast agent Thorotrast (historical).

1. **Classification.** Cholangiocarcinoma has been classified according to anatomic location and growth pattern. The anatomic location classification includes three main types: intrahepatic (20%), extrahepatic upper duct (also called *hilar* or *Klatskin tumor,* 40%), and extrahepatic lower duct (40%). Tumor morphology is also divided in three primary types: (1) a mass-forming (or MF) type that grows in a nodular fashion and projects into both the bile duct lumen and the surrounding tissues; (2) a periductal infiltrating (PI) type characterized by a cicatrizing growth pattern that infiltrates the walls of the bile ducts and grows both within them and along their exterior surfaces; and (3) an intraductal growing (IG) type that displays a polypoid or sessile pattern that forms intraductal excrescences of tumor that may grow along the inside of, but do not penetrate, the wall of the duct (also commonly referred to as "papillary subtype"). The specific anatomic location and growth pattern of perihilar tumors are further described by the Bismuth-Corlette classification scheme as shown in Table 15-1.

2. **Staging** is currently based on the TNM (tumor, nodes, and metastases) system of the sixth edition of the American Joint Committee on Cancer (AJCC) Guidelines. Intrahepatic malignancies are staged along with those of primary hepatic origin, whereas extrahepatic lesions have their own set of criteria (see Tables 15-2 and 15-3).

3. **Diagnosis**

   a. **Jaundice,** followed by weight loss and pain, are the most frequently encountered signs and symptoms at presentation.

   b. **Serum markers.** Numerous serum tumor markers are currently in use and/or being evaluated for their utility in the diagnosis of cholangiocarcinoma.

   (1) **Carbohydrate antigen 19-9 (CA19-9)** is a carbohydrate antigen that is traditionally associated with pancreatic cancer but is also the most commonly used marker in the diagnosis of cholangiocarcinoma. Sensitivity

TABLE 15-1	Bismuth-Corlette Classification of Hilar Cholangiocarcinoma
Type I	Tumor remains below the confluence of the right and left hepatic ducts
Type II	Tumor involves the confluence of the right and left hepatic ducts
Type III	Tumor involves *either* the right *or* the left hepatic duct and extends to secondary radicals
Type IV	Tumor involves secondary radicals of *both* the right *and* left hepatic ducts

TABLE 15-2	American Joint Committee on Cancer TNM (Tumor, Nodes, and Metastases) Staging for Extrahepatic Cholangiocarcinoma

TX	Primary tumor cannot be assessed	**NX**	Regional lymph nodes cannot be assessed
T0	No evidence of primary tumor	**N0**	No regional lymph node involvement
Tis	Carcinoma *in situ*	**N1**	Regional lymph node involvement
T1	Tumor confined to bile duct histologically		
T2	Invades beyond the wall of the bile duct	**MX**	Distant metastases cannot be assessed
T3	Invades liver, gallbladder, pancreas, and/or unilateral branches of portal vein or hepatic artery	**M0**	No distant metastases
T4	Invades any of the following: main portal vein or bilateral branches, common hepatic artery, adjacent structures such as colon, stomach, duodenum, or abdominal wall	**M1**	Distant metastases

and specificity vary depending on the threshold used and on coexisting conditions such as inflammation and cholestasis. For example, two large studies encompassing over 300 patients each showed sensitivities and specificities of 73% to 76% and 63% to 74%, respectively, when a cutoff value of 37 U/mL was applied in a patient population without cholangitis. However, the specificity dropped to approximately 42% when patients with cholangitis were included (*Am J Gastroenterol* 1999;64:1941, *Br J Cancer* 1991;63:636). In two other studies of 55 and 74 patients with PSC, higher CA19-9 cutoffs of 180 and 100 U/mL gave improved specificities of 98% and 91%, respectively, whereas sensitivities were comparable to those of other series—67% and 60%, respectively (*Gastrointest Endosc* 2002;56:40, *Gastroenterology* 1995;108:865). Thus, whereas a CA19-9 cutoff of around 40 U/mL is likely to be adequate in patients without any evidence of cholangitis or cholestasis, a higher value (probably in the 150-U/mL range) should be used for those patients with either of these concurrent conditions.

(2) **Carcinoembryonic Antigen (CEA).** Although most commonly used for the diagnosis of colorectal cancer, CEA has also demonstrated some elevation in patients with malignancies of biliary origin.

c. **Diagnostic imaging**

(1) **Magnetic resonance cholangiopancreatography (MRCP)** can be used for an all-purpose investigation of cholangiocarcinoma. It provides

TABLE 15-3	American Joint Committee on Cancer TNM (Tumor, Nodes, and Metastases) Staging for Extrahepatic Cholangiocarcinoma and Gallbadder Cancer

Stage	TNM status	Gallbladder cancer 5-year survival (%)
0	Tis N0 M0	81
IA	T1 N0 M0	50
IB	T2 N0 M0	29
IIA	T3 N0 M0	7
IIB	T1–3 N1 M0	9
III	T4 Nany M0	3
IV	Tany Nany M1	2

cholangiography, demonstrates the tumor and its relationship to key vessels, and detects intrahepatic metastases.

(2) Ultrasonography can demonstrate bile duct masses and dilation and provide rudimentary information on the extent of tumor involvement within the liver. Reports indicate that ultrasonography is more than 80% accurate in predicting portal vein involvement.

(3) CT may be helpful in delineating the mass and defining its relation to the liver, especially for those patients in whom magnetic resonance imaging (MRI) is contraindicated or unable to be tolerated.

(4) Positron emission tomography (PET) may be helpful in the diagnosis of cholangiocarcinoma; however, it is currently incompletely studied and not yet part of the standard diagnostic workup.

(5) ERCP is the most valuable diagnostic tool for cholangiography of lower duct tumors. Distal lesions may be indistinguishable from small pancreatic carcinomas on preoperative evaluation, and the distinction is often not made until final pathologic analysis. It is also valuable for upper duct tumors, but if obstruction is complete, the upper limit of the tumor cannot be delineated. Since the advent of MR cholangiography, ERCP is increasingly being used for preoperative **therapeutic decompression** of the biliary tree. Preoperative decompression of the biliary tree has the advantage of improving liver function prior to resection but has the risk of cholangitis and increased postoperative infection. It is not usually performed unless the bilirubin is greater than 10 mg/dL. When used, only the less-affected hemiliver should be decompressed so that it will hypertrophy while the undrained side (the side to be resected) atrophies. The side to be resected should be drained only if cholangitis is present.

ERCP carries the potential added benefit of obtaining cellular material for **cytologic analysis,** either via ductal brushing, fine needle aspiration (FNA), or forceps biopsy. In an attempt to increase diagnostic yields, new molecular techniques have been applied to biopsy samples, including digital image analysis (DIA) and fluorescence *in situ* hybridization (FISH). These tests can detect genetic aneuploidy and chromosomal rearrangements as indicators of malignancy.

(6) PTC has been used when ERCP and MRI cannot precisely delineate the upper limit of a tumor. Under PTC guidance, FNA cytology can also provide a tissue diagnosis in many of patients. If a tumor is resectable, prolonged efforts to obtain a tissue diagnosis before resection are not indicated.

(7) Endoscopic ultrasound (EUS) with FNA represents an important development in the investigation of *lower* bile duct strictures and masses. It is useful as an alternative to ERCP for obtaining tissue to establish a cytologic diagnosis, especially if a primary pancreatic mass is suspected. A recent study demonstrated that EUS-FNA has a sensitivity, specificity, positive predictive value (PPV), negative predictive value (NPV), and accuracy of 86%, 100%, 100%, 57%, and 88%, respectively, for the diagnosis of extrahepatic cholangiocarcinoma (both hilar and distal CBD), and the test results positively changed the management of 84% of the study participants (*Clin Gastroenterol Hepatol* 2004;2:209). The potential value of such a biopsy needs to be weighed against risks such as bleeding and potentially seeding the traversed peritoneal cavity with malignant cells (*Am J Gastroenterol* 2004;99:45).

4. **Assessment of tumor resectability and treatment.** Resection remains the primary treatment for cholangiocarcinoma, although only 15% to 20% are resectable at presentation. Adjuvant radiation and chemotherapy have been attempted, but clinical trials are limited by the paucity of eligible patients.

   a. Intrahepatic tumors are best treated with hepatic resection. Resectability is assessed as for other primary tumors or secondary metastases, with a goal of 1-cm tumor-free margins and retention of at least 30% of functioning liver mass. If resection of more than 60% of the hepatic parenchyma is required, preoperative portal vein embolization can be used to cause atrophy of the affected hemiliver and hypertrophy of the unaffected liver segments.

b. **Extrahepatic upper duct (hilar) tumors.** Because hilar lesions are generally not as easily biopsied, resection is often undertaken based on the clinical assessment and radiographic demonstration of a mass lesion at the ductal bifurcation. With the rare exception of low-lying Bismuth I tumors in which a negative common hepatic duct margin may be obtained, resection of hilar tumors includes the bile duct bifurcation and the caudate lobe, and ipsilateral hemihepatectomy is often required to obtain an R0 resection. Biliary reconstruction is performed as a Roux-en-Y hepaticojejunostomy. Pancreaticoduodenectomy may be necessary in some cases to obtain negative lower margins of the CBD. Vascular involvement is not an absolute contraindication to resection because portal venous resection and reconstruction may be possible. Resection is usually excluded by the following:

(1) Bilateral intrahepatic ductal spread.

(2) Extensive involvement of the main trunk of the portal vein.

(3) Bilateral involvement of hepatic arterial and/or portal venous branches.

(4) A combination of vascular involvement with evidence of contralateral ductal spread.

(5) Lymph node involvement or distant spread.

c. Some lesions situated in the **middle of the extrahepatic bile duct** may be approached with an excision of the supraduodenal extrahepatic bile duct, cholecystectomy, and portal lymphadenectomy. However, most malignant strictures in the mid CBD are due to local invasion of a gallbladder cancer rather than cholangiocarcinoma.

d. **Extrahepatic lower duct tumors.** The considerations are the same as for carcinoma of the head of the pancreas, although vascular involvement is much less common. In contrast to more-proximal tumors, approximately 80% of lower duct tumors are resectable by pancreaticoduodenectomy, and 5-year survival rates range from 17% to 39%. Tumors derived from the bile duct have a slightly better prognosis than those of pancreatic origin in the same region, probably reflecting a more favorable biologic behavior.

e. **Adjuvant therapy** has traditionally consisted of 5-fluorouarcil (5-FU) for advanced cholangiocarcinoma, but this has demonstrated minimal benefit (survival $\leq$15%). Combining 5-FU with other agents such as leucovorin, cisplatin, and interferon α has shown some additional benefit (response rates up to 35%). Gemcitabine-based therapies have shown response rates between 25% and 50% and median survival times of up to 14 months when used in combination with either cisplatin or oxaliplatin (*Future Oncol* 2006;2:509).

5. **Palliation** for patients with unresectable disease involves surgical, radiologic, or endoscopic biliary decompression. When unresectability is demonstrated preoperatively or at staging laparoscopy, the first choice for biliary decompression is via endoscopic or percutaneous internal stenting. When encountered at laparotomy, internal biliary drainage is best achieved by choledochojejunostomy for lower duct lesions.

6. **Prognosis** is highly dependent on resectability of the tumor at presentation. Patients with resectable cholangiocarcinoma with microscopically negative margins and negative lymph nodes have a 5-year survival of approximately 35%, whereas median survival for patients with unresectable cholangiocarcinoma is only 3 to 6 months. An R0 resection is necessary for any chance of a cure because the condition almost universally recur within 5 years in patients with R1 resections. Other factors associated with increased survival include papillary phenotype, lower tumor grade, unaffected local lymph nodes, and a lack of vascular involvement.

C. **Gallbladder cancer** is the most common cancer of the biliary tract and the sixth-most-common cancer of the gastrointestinal (GI) tract, representing about 9,000 new cases per year in the United States. It is more aggressive than cholangiocarcinoma, has a poor prognosis, and accounts for approximately 6,000 deaths yearly.

The incidence peaks at 70 to 75 years, with a 3:1 female-to-male ratio. There is a strong correlation with gallstones (95%). Histologically, nearly all gallbladder cancers are adenocarcinomas, and concomitant cholecystitis is frequently present. Tumors spread primarily by direct extension into liver segments IV and V adjacent to the gallbladder fossa, but also via lymphatics along the cystic duct to the CBD. Due to its generally late stage at presentation, only a small percentage of patients with a preoperative diagnosis of gallbladder cancer are resectable for potential cure.

1. **Risk factors**
   a. **The presence of gallstones** is the most common risk factor, and up to 75% of patients with this malignancy are noted to have cholelithiasis. Longer duration of cholelithiasis and larger stone size seem to further increase the risk, with reported cancer development odds ratios of up to 10 for stones 3 cm or greater (*JAMA* 1983;250:2323).
   b. **Polyps** 1.5 cm or greater in diameter have a 46% to 70% prevalence of cancer, whereas those in the 1- to 1.5-cm range have an 11% to 13% incidence. In those less than 10 mm in size, the cancer incidence is less than 5%. Cancerous polyps also tend to be sessile in nature and echopenic on ultrasound, and prophylactic cholecystectomy should be considered for lesions greater than 1 cm in size or meeting morphologic criteria.
   c. **Anomalous junction of the pancreatobiliary duct (AJPBD)** has been noted in approximately 10% of patients with gallbladder cancer, and up to 40% of patients with this anomaly develop a biliary tract malignancy. The anomaly represents a union of the pancreatic and biliary ducts outside of the duodenal wall, resulting in a long common channel. Subsequent reflux of pancreatic juice into the biliary system is thought to be the initiator of carcinogenesis.
   d. **Porcelain gallbladder** is a condition characterized by calcification of the gallbladder wall. Although the overall incidence of carcinoma associated with porcelain gallbladder has been estimated at approximately 20%, studies have shown that gallbladders with diffuse intramural calcification rarely harbor cancer. Conversely, the selective mucosal calcification variant has been associated with malignancy in 7% to 42% of cases. Regardless, prophylactic cholecystectomy is generally recommended for any finding of gallbladder wall calcification on imaging studies.
   e. **Other risk factors** include PSC, gallbladder infection with *E. coli* and/or *Salmonella* species, and exposure to certain industrial solvents and toxins.
2. **Diagnosis.** Approximately one third of these tumors are diagnosed incidentally during cholecystectomy, and **cancer is found in 0.3% to 1%** of all cholecystectomy specimens. Symptoms of stage I and II gallbladder cancer are often directly caused by gallstones rather than the cancer, whereas stage III and IV cancers present with weight loss and symptoms typical of CBD obstruction. Suggestive ultrasound findings include thickening or irregularity of the gallbladder, a polypoid mass, or diffuse wall calcification indicative of porcelain gallbladder.
3. **Staging** is similar to that of cholangiocarcinoma, as shown in Tables 15-3 and 15-4. PET scanning and combined PET/CT have proven useful in detecting distant metastases in these patients.
4. **Treatment**
   a. **Mucosal disease** confined to the gallbladder wall (Tis and T1a tumors) is often identified after routine LC. Because the overall 5-year survival rate is as high as 80%, cholecystectomy alone with negative resection margins (including the cystic duct margin) is adequate therapy. Patients with a preoperative suspicion of gallbladder cancer should undergo open cholecystectomy because port site recurrences and late peritoneal metastases (associated with bile spillage) have been reported even with *in situ* disease.
   b. **Early disease** involving T1b and T2 tumors may be treated by radical cholecystectomy that includes the gallbladder, the gallbladder bed of the liver, as well as the hepatoduodenal ligament, periduodenal, peripancreatic, hepatic artery, and celiac lymph nodes.

TABLE 15-4	American Joint Committee on Cancer TNM (Tumor, Nodes, and Metastases) Staging for Gallbadder Cancer

TX	Primary tumor cannot be assessed	NX	Regional lymph nodes cannot be assessed
T0	No evidence of primary tumor	N0	No regional lymph node involvement
Tis	Carcinoma *in situ*	N1	Regional lymph node involvement
T1a	Invades lamina propria		
T1b	Invades muscular layer	MX	Distant metastases cannot be assessed
T2	Invades perimuscular connective tissue	M0	No distant metastases
T3	Through serosa or involving adjacent organ	M1	Distant metastases
T4	Invasion into portal vein, hepatic artery, or multiple adjacent organs		

   c. **Stage II or III disease** with invasion of adjacent organs or the presence of lymph node metastases requires more radical resection. Depending on the extent of local invasion, extirpation may range from wedge resection of the liver adjacent to the gallbladder bed to resection of 75% of the liver. Dissection of the portal, paraduodenal, and hepatic artery lymph nodes should accompany the liver resection. Survival advantages have been demonstrated after radical resection. Because of the aggressive nature of this malignancy, adjuvant chemoradiation is often recommended, but no proof of efficacy is available.
   d. Most gallbladder cancers have invaded adjacent organs, extend into the porta hepatis, or distantly metastasized before clinical diagnosis. **Extensive liver involvement or discontiguous metastases** preclude surgical resection as a reasonable option. Jaundice may be palliated by percutaneous or endoscopically placed biliary stents. Duodenal obstruction can be surgically bypassed if present. Radiotherapy can decrease tumor bulk and temporarily relieve obstruction, but no survival benefits have been demonstrated.
  5. **Prognosis** is stage dependent, and the respective 5-year survival rates are shown in Table 15-3. The median survival for stage IB cancers is less than 2 years, and for stage II lesions, it is less than 1 year. With stage II disease or higher, fewer than 20% of patients are alive at 2 years.
VII. **BENIGN STRICTURES AND BILE DUCT INJURIES** occur in association with a number of conditions, including pancreatitis, choledocholithiasis, Oriental cholangiohepatitis, PSC, prior hepatic transplantation, trauma, or iatrogenic injury after instrumentation or surgery. These benign strictures may masquerade as a biliary malignancy. Attempts to differentiate between the two etiologies should be made prior to surgery because the patient may not be a candidate for a curative resection if an advanced stage of cancer is found. Laparoscopic cholecystectomy is by far the leading cause of iatrogenic bile duct injuries and subsequent benign strictures.
   A. **Risk factors.** Numerous studies elucidate those factors that contribute to a more challenging surgical procedure and increase the likelihood of bile duct injury. These are divided into three major categories of risk factors: (1) patient-related factors, (2) procedure-related factors, and (3) surgeon/hospital-related factors (*J Hepatobiliary Pancreat Surg* 2002;9:543).
      1. **Patient-related factors**
         a. **Inflammation**
            (1) **Acute inflammation,** such as that seen in acute cholecystitis, may cause the inflamed gallbladder, cystic duct, and CBD to appear as a single mass (*J Am Coll Surg* 2000;191:661). This can lead to misidentification of the CBD as the cystic duct with subsequent clipping and transection.
            (2) **Severe chronic inflammation** and dense scarring may result from repeated bouts of cholecystitis and/or choledocholithiasis, effectively obliterating the triangle of Calot and leaving a shrunken, contracted

gallbladder densely adherent to the common hepatic duct and/or right hepatic artery.

b. Congenital Abnormalities

   (1) Aberrant right hepatic ducts are present in about 2% of patients and are well-recognized risk factors for biliary injury.

   (2) Parallel union of the cystic duct with the common bile duct occurs in approximately 20% of individuals. Injury to the CBD occurs when the two apposed ducts appear as one.

   (3) Aberrant insertion of the cystic duct may occur at almost any point along the biliary tree, with the most hazardous location being direct insertion into the right hepatic duct.

   (4) Congenital adhesions between the gallbladder and the common hepatic duct can obliterate the triangle of Calot, making dissection difficult.

   (5) Abnormal length or diameter of the bile ducts may lead to misidentification and transection of the improper duct.

   (6) An intrahepatic gallbladder is difficult to grasp and may prevent proper exposure of the cystic duct.

   (7) Intrahepatic ducts connecting directly with the gallbladder (ducts of Luschka) are usually less than 1 mm in diameter and are generally transected while taking the gallbladder off its liver bed. Their injury often goes unrecognized at the time of cholecystectomy.

c. Large, impacted gallstones may prevent proper retraction of the gallbladder and can obscure the anatomic relationships between the cystic duct and surrounding structures.

d. Obesity can contribute to a difficult operation due to both intra-abdominal and extra-abdominal fat and loss of intra-abdominal domain during laparoscopy.

2. Procedure-related factors

a. Operative technique likely represents the most important factor contributing to the risk of inadvertent bile duct injury because it is this aspect of the surgical procedure that is the most within the surgeon's control. Various techniques are associated with an unacceptably high incidence of CBD injury when used with the laparoscopic approach and should be avoided, especially in the setting of acute inflammation.

b. Intraoperative cholangiography can be extremely helpful in the avoidance of potentially devastating bile duct injury.

c. Technical problems frequently arise secondary to other risk factors such as inflammation but may also occur even in the absence of a specific predisposing condition.

   (1) Inadvertent injury to a bile duct during the course of dissection most commonly results form the injudicious use of electrocautery, although sharp dissection and excessive traction on the gallbladder or adjacent structures may also contribute to this type of injury.

   (2) Failure to securely close the cystic duct may be due to a poorly placed or incompletely closed surgical clip, usually in the setting of a thickened fibrotic cystic duct or increased biliary pressure secondary to retained CBD stones. If there is any concern for incomplete closure, a **laparoscopic loop ligature** should be used, either alone or combined with previously placed clips.

   (3) Tenting injuries occur when the CBD or common hepatic duct is clipped after being elevated due to excessive traction on the gallbladder and cystic duct.

3. Surgeon/hospital-related factors

a. The learning-curve effect may be due to a lack of sufficient operator experience with safe techniques for performing cholecystectomy, either laparoscopically or open.

b. Surgeon mindset, often characterized by a sense of infallibility even when faced with adversity, may result in biliary injury.

    c. Laparoscopic equipment must be regularly maintained in excellent working condition. Loss of insulation from electrocautery instruments may be particularly hazardous, and preventative systems should be employed.

  4. The difficult cholecystectomy. In an attempt to preoperatively identify what factors might contribute to a "difficult cholecystectomy," 22,953 cases of LC performed in Switzerland were studied. Those factors associated with an increase in all intraoperative complications (not limited to only bile duct injury) included the presence of acute cholecystitis [odds ratio (OR) = 1.86], male gender (OR = 1.18), patient age (OR = 1.12 per 10 years), increased body weight (OR = 1.34 for >90 kg vs. <60 kg), and surgeon experience (OR = 1.36 for 11 to 100 cases vs. >100 cases). Multivariate analysis also showed an increase in complications for each additional 30 minutes of operative time, with OR = 1.68 (*J Am Coll Surg* 2006;203:723). In general, conversion to an open operation in the face of a difficult laparoscopic procedure should never be viewed as a surgical failure or complication but rather as a way to avoid potential injury to the patient.

B. Classification. A widely accepted classification scheme has been developed in this institution (*J Am Coll Surg* 1995;180:101). Type A injuries are cystic duct leaks or leaks from small ducts in the liver bed. Type B and C injuries involve an aberrant right hepatic duct. Type B represents an occluded segment, whereas type C involves open drainage from the proximal draining duct not in continuity with the common duct. Type D injuries are *lateral* injuries to the extrahepatic bile ducts. Type E injuries (subtypes 1 to 5) are derived from the Bismuth classification and represent circumferential transections or occlusions at various levels of the CBD.

C. Diagnosis

  1. Presentation depends on the type of injury. Approximately 25% of major bile duct injuries are recognized at the time of the initial procedure. Intraoperative signs of a major ductal injury include unexpected bile leakage, abnormal IOC, and delayed recognition of the anatomy after transection of important structures. If an injury is not recognized intraoperatively, the patient usually presents with symptoms within 1 week and almost always within 3 to 4 weeks after the initial procedure. Patients with a bile leak often present with right-upper-quadrant pain, fever, and sepsis secondary to biloma and may have bile drainage from a surgical incision. Patients with occlusion of the CBD without a bile leak present with jaundice. Occasionally, a delayed presentation of months or years is seen.

  2. Diagnostic imaging. CT scan is the best imaging test to demonstrate an intraabdominal bile collection, which should then be percutaneously drained. Ongoing bile leaks can also be diagnosed by HIDA scan. ERCP is also useful to demonstrate biliary anatomy, and therapeutic stent placement is often possible for ductal leaks. In the case of occlusion of the CBD, PTC can demonstrate the proximal biliary anatomy, define the proximal extent of the injury, and be used for therapeutic decompression of the biliary tree. MRI with MRCP can demonstrate the bile ducts both above and below an obstruction and is now often used for the initial investigation.

D. Management depends on the type and timing of the presentation.

  1. If the injury is identified at the time of the initial procedure, the surgeon should proceed directly to open exploration and repair only if qualified and comfortable with complex techniques in hepatobiliary surgery or to control life-threatening hemorrhage. If the surgeon is not prepared to perform a definitive repair, a drain should be placed in the right upper quadrant and the patient immediately **referred to a specialist hepatobiliary center.**

  2. Immediate management. Many of the simpler injuries can be successfully managed with ERCP and sphincterotomy, stenting, or both. Occlusive lesions require decompression of the proximal system via PTC. In general, if an injury requires operative repair and the patient is stable, the repair should be done within the first few days after the initial procedure while inflammation is at a minimum. If this is not possible due to delayed diagnosis, longer-term temporization (at least 8 weeks) is required to allow the acute inflammation to resolve. In addition, if there is a concern about a vascular injury along with the bile duct injury, definitive repair should be delayed to more easily identify areas of ductal ischemia, which should not be incorporated in the repair.

3. Control of sepsis, percutaneous drainage, and adequate nutrition should be **optimized before definitive repair.**

4. **Operative repair,** when indicated, is best achieved by means of a Roux-en-Y hepaticoenterostomy, in which the bile duct is débrided back to viable tissue. All bile ducts must be accounted for, and an adequate blood supply must be apparent for each. A tension-free mucosa-to-mucosa anastomosis constructed with fine absorbable suture is desired. Excellent long-term outcomes have been described, with anastomotic stricture the most common, yet infrequent, complication (*Arch Surg* 1999;134:604).

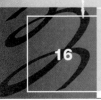

SPLEEN 16

T. Elizabeth Robertson and L. Michael Brunt

 SPLENIC ANATOMY AND PHYSIOLOGY

I. SPLENIC ANATOMY

A. Macroscopic anatomy

1. The spleen is located in the **left upper quadrant of the abdomen** beneath the 9th to 11th ribs. The costodiaphragmatic recess of the left pleural cavity extends as far as the inferior border of a normal spleen.

2. The **normal spleen** is approximately 12 cm long, 7 cm wide, and 4 cm thick and weighs 100 to 150 g.

3. The spleen is **intimately related** to the splenic flexure of the colon, the greater curvature of the stomach, the left kidney, and the pancreatic tail. The tail of the pancreas extends laterally to within 1 cm of the splenic hilum in most patients and is in direct contact with the spleen in up to 30% of patients.

4. **Peritoneal reflections** in the region surrounding the spleen form the fibrous suspensory "ligaments" through which most of the principal vascular structures course. These ligaments are the splenocolic, splenorenal, gastrosplenic, and splenophrenic. Their division is one of the keys to splenectomy. The pancreas is partially invested in the leaves of the splenorenal ligament, just inferior to the contained splenic artery and its branches.

5. The **splenic artery** is a branch of the celiac trunk and follows a serpiginous path along the superior border of the pancreas. The terminal branching pattern into the spleen is most commonly distributive in which the main trunk arborizes into multiple arterial branches that enter the hilum broadly over its surface. Less commonly, the arterial supply has a magistral configuration, with one dominant splenic artery entering over a narrow and compact area.

6. **Accessory spleens** occur in 10% to 20% of patients and are most commonly found at the splenic hilum, the gastrosplenic omentum, along the tail of the pancreas, and in the retroperitoneum posterior to the spleen. However, accessory splenic tissue can be found throughout the abdomen and pelvis.

B. Microscopic anatomy

1. The **spleen consists** of red pulp with interspersed areas of white pulp.

    a. The **red pulp** is highly vascular and is composed of large, branching, thin-walled sinuses, with intervening areas filled with phagocytic cells and blood cells, known as splenic cords.

    b. The **white pulp** has three components: periarteriolar lymphoid sheaths (T cells), lymphoid nodules (B cells), and the marginal zone.

II. SPLENIC FUNCTION. In its normal physiologic state, the spleen has two major functions. It is a part of the reticuloendothelial system and is also a component of the immune system.

A. Reticuloendothelial/filtration system

1. The red pulp serves as a **mechanical filter** for the removal of senescent erythrocytes (*culling*) and the remodeling of healthy red cells, including removal of nuclear remnants, denatured hemoglobin, and iron granules (*pitting*).

2. A minor hematologic function of the spleen is to serve as a **reservoir for platelets.** In certain disease states (e.g., myelofibrosis), the adult spleen becomes a major site of **extramedullary hematopoiesis.**

B. Immune system

1. The white pulp is a **nonspecific filter** and removes blood-borne pathogens (e.g., bacteria and viruses) that are coated with complement.

2. The spleen also participates in the **specific immune response** by producing anti-body, plasma cells, and memory cells in response to specific trapped antigens.

3. **Encapsulated bacteria** are also effectively removed from the circulation, likely via prolonged contact with macrophages in the splenic parenchymal cords.

4. The spleen also **manufactures opsonins,** namely, properdin and tuftsin.

 INDICATIONS FOR SPLENECTOMY

I. GENERAL INDICATIONS

A. The initial therapy for most hematologic disorders of the spleen is medical. In general, splenectomy is warranted only after failure of medical therapy, as an adjunct to medical therapy, for diagnostic reasons, or in some cases as primary therapy for an underlying malignancy.

B. The **goals of splenectomy** can be broadly classified into one of the following groups:

1. Cure or palliation of hematologic disease. Idiopathic (immune) thrombocytopenic purpura (ITP) and hemolytic anemias are the most common indications for splenectomy. Splenectomy may also be used to palliate other disease states [e.g., chronic lymphocytic leukemia (CLL), hairy cell leukemia, Felty syndrome], primarily via the control of cytopenias.

2. Palliation of hypersplenism. Patients with refractory cytopenias due to hypersplenism that require frequent transfusion or significantly limit the delivery of cytotoxic therapy may benefit from splenectomy.

3. Relief from symptomatic splenomegaly. Patients with a massively enlarged spleen can develop early satiety, abdominal pain, and weight loss from mass effect.

4. Diagnosis of splenic pathology. Solid mass lesions in the spleen can be an indication for splenectomy, particularly if a malignant diagnosis is suspected. Splenectomy may be used to establish a diagnosis of lymphoma in the absence of more easily accessible tissue but is no longer indicated for staging lymphomas.

5. Control of splenic hemorrhage. Although splenic injury is increasingly managed nonoperatively, splenectomy is the definitive treatment for patients with ongoing traumatic splenic hemorrhage. Splenic hemorrhage may also rarely occur spontaneously in disease states such as infectious mononucleosis.

II. SPECIFIC INDICATIONS (see Table 16-1)

A. Hematologic splenic pathology

1. Thrombocytopenias

a. Idiopathic (immune) thrombocytopenic purpura (ITP) is the most common indication for elective splenectomy. It is an acquired disorder in which autoantibodies are produced against a platelet glycoprotein. The spleen is the major site for the production of antiplatelet antibodies and also serves as the principal site of platelet destruction.

(1) Children usually present with acute ITP, often associated with a recent viral syndrome. In 90% of cases, the disease spontaneously remits within 6 to 12 months. Only refractory cases require splenectomy.

(2) Adults typically present with a more chronic form of ITP that is much less likely to spontaneously remit. Asymptomatic patients with platelet counts greater than 50,000/mm^3 may simply be followed. Symptomatic patients or those with counts less than 30,000/mm^3 should be treated with oral

TABLE 16-1	Indications for Splenectomy

Hematologic splenic pathology
  Thrombocytopenias
    Immune thrombocytopenic purpura (ITP)
    Thrombotic thrombocytopenic purpura (TTP)
  Anemias
    Hereditary hemolytic anemias (hereditary spherocytosis)
    Acquired warm autoimmune hemolytic anemias
    Congenital hemoglobinopathies (sickle cell anemia)
  Myeloproliferative and myelodysplastic disorders
    Chronic myelogenous leukemia
    Polycythemia vera
    Myelofibrosis or myeloid metaplasia
    Essential thrombocytosis
    Myeloproliferative disorder not otherwise specified
  Lymphoproliferative disorders
    Chronic lymphocytic leukemia
    Hairy-cell leukemia
    Non-Hodgkin lymphoma
    Hodgkin lymphoma
  Neutropenias
    Felty syndrome
Nonhematologic splenic disorders
  Splenic abscess
  Splenic cyst/pseudocyst
  Storage diseases
Other disorders
  Trauma
  Incidental splenectomy
  Vascular problems (splenic artery aneurysm, splenic vein thrombosis)

glucocorticoids. Greater than 50% of patients respond to glucocorticoids. In refractory cases, or in patients with bleeding, intravenous immunoglobulin (IVIG) is used, although the effects are transient (*Mayo Clin Proc* 2004;79:504). Indications for splenectomy are failure to respond to medical therapy and intolerable side effects from steroid administration.

(3) Indications for more urgent splenectomy in patients with ITP include need for other emergency surgery or a life-threatening bleed, including central nervous system (CNS) hemorrhage. The majority of patients who respond to splenectomy do so within the first 10 postoperative days.

(4) A recent systematic review of 135 case series spanning 58 years found a complete remission in two thirds of patients. Either a complete or partial response was observed in 88% of patients. Complete response was defined as achievement of a platelet count of at least 100×10^9/L. A partial response included a platelet count response of at least 30×10^9/L. Variables associated with a response to splenectomy include younger age and response to IVIG therapy. Mortality rates of 0.2% to 1% are similar to mortality due to medically treated severe ITP over 5 to 10 years (0.4% to 1.6%). Surgical complication rates range from 10% to 13% (*Blood* 2004;104:2623).

(5) Patients who fail splenectomy or relapse after an initial response should be investigated for **accessory splenic tissue.** A peripheral smear and magnetic resonance imaging (MRI) or nuclear medicine studies with technetium (Tc)-99m–labeled heat-damaged red cells are indicated. If accessory splenic tissue is found, re-exploration should be considered, although long-term response to removal of an accessory spleen is uncommon (*N Engl J Med* 2002;346:995).

b. Thrombotic thrombocytopenic purpura (TTP) is characterized by the pentad of hemolytic anemia, consumptive thrombocytopenia, mental status changes, renal failure, and fever, although only hemolytic anemia and thrombocytopenia (without other obvious cause) are required to initiate therapy. Symptoms result from multiorgan microvascular thrombosis.

(1) First-line therapy for TTP is medical, with plasmapheresis. A randomized, controlled trial with 102 patients demonstrated significantly improved initial response (47% vs. 25%) and 6-month survival (78% vs. 63%) for plasmapheresis as compared to plasma infusion (*N Engl J Med* 1991;325:393). Glucocorticoids, in addition to plasmapheresis, are prescribed in the rare case of relapse.

(2) Splenectomy is indicated in patients who do not respond to medical therapy or those with chronically relapsing disease. A recent 20-year retrospective review of 33 patients found that those who were continuously dependent on plasmapheresis and underwent splenectomy had a postoperative relapse rate of 0.07 per patient-year. In those patients who were not continuously dependent on plasmapheresis, splenectomy reduced the relapse rate from 0.74 to 0.10 per patient-year (*Br J Heme* 2005;130:768).

2. Anemias

a. Hemolytic anemias constitute a group of disorders in which splenectomy is almost universally curative.

(1) Hereditary spherocytosis is an autosomal dominant disorder in which there is a defect in *spectrin*, a red blood cell (RBC) membrane protein. This defect leads to small, spherical, relatively rigid erythrocytes that are unable to deform adequately to traverse the splenic microcirculation. This results in their sequestration and destruction in the splenic red pulp. In addition to anemia, patients may have jaundice from the hemolytic process and splenomegaly from RBC destruction in the spleen. Splenectomy is indicated in nearly all cases, but should be delayed to age 6 years in children to minimize the risk of overwhelming postsplenectomy sepsis. An exception is if the child is transfusion dependent. Prior to splenectomy, patients should have a right-upper-quadrant ultrasound, and if gallstones are present (usually pigment stones from hemolysis), a cholecystectomy can be performed concomitantly.

(2) Hereditary elliptocytosis is an autosomal dominant disorder in which an intrinsic cytoskeletal defect causes the RBCs to be elliptical. The majority of patients have an asymptomatic and mild anemia that does not need specific treatment. Patients with symptomatic anemia should undergo splenectomy to prolong RBC survival.

b. Acquired autoimmune hemolytic anemias are characterized as either warm or cold, depending on the temperature at which they interact with antibody.

(1) Warm autoimmune hemolytic anemia results from splenic sequestration and destruction of RBCs coated with autoantibodies that interact optimally with their antigens at 37°C. Anti-immunoglobulin G (IgG) antiserum causes agglutination of the patient's RBCs (positive direct Coombs test). Etiologies include CLL, non-Hodgkin lymphoma, collagen vascular disease, and drugs, although most cases are idiopathic. Primary treatment is directed against the underlying disease. If this is unsuccessful, therapy is corticosteroids. Nonresponders or patients requiring high steroid doses respond to splenectomy in 60% to 80% of cases.

(2) Cold autoimmune hemolytic anemia is characterized by fixation of C3 to IgM antibodies that bind RBCs with greater affinity at temperatures approaching 0°C and cause Raynaud-like symptoms combined with anemia. Hemolysis occurs either immediately by intravascular complement–mediated mechanisms or via removal of C3-coated RBCs by the liver.

Treatment is usually successful with use of increased protective clothing. Splenectomy has no therapeutic benefit.

c. Congenital hemoglobinopathies

(1) Sickle cell anemia is due to the homozygous inheritance of the S variant of the hemoglobin β chain. The disease is usually associated with autosplenectomy due to repeated vaso-occlusive crises, but splenectomy may be required for those patients with acute splenic sequestration crisis, evidence of hypersplenism, splenic abscess, and symptomatic splenomegaly.

(2) Thalassemias are hereditary anemias caused by a defect in hemoglobin synthesis. β-Thalassemia major is primarily treated with iron chelation therapy, but splenectomy may be required to treat symptomatic splenomegaly or pain from splenic infarcts.

3. Myeloproliferative and myelodysplastic disorders

a. Chronic myelogenous leukemia (CML) is a myelodysplastic disorder characterized by the *bcr-abl* fusion oncogene, known as the *Philadelphia chromosome*. This oncogene results in a continuously active tyrosine kinase.

(1) First-line therapy is medical with imatinib mesylate (Gleevec), which targets the tyrosine kinase protein. Alternative chemotherapies are used in cases of intolerance or suboptimal response. Stem cell transplantation is used for cases of treatment failure in eligible patients (*Blood* 2006;108:1809).

(2) In 1984, the Italian Cooperative Study Group prospectively randomized 189 patients in the early phase of CML to splenectomy plus chemotherapy or chemotherapy alone. Splenectomy had no effect on survival or disease progression, but it did increase the rate of thrombosis and vascular accidents (*Cancer* 1984;54:333). Splenectomy is indicated only for palliation of symptomatic splenomegaly or hypersplenism that significantly limits therapy.

b. Polycythemia vera and essential thrombocytosis are chronic diseases of uncontrolled red blood cell and platelet production, respectively. These diseases are treated medically, but splenectomy can be required to treat symptomatic splenomegaly or pain from splenic infarcts. Splenectomy can result in severe thrombocytosis, causing thrombosis or hemorrhage, which requires perioperative antiplatelet, anticoagulation, and myelosuppressive treatment. A recent case series demonstrated success in surgical management of severe, symptomatic splenomegaly in patients with polycythemia vera with no long-term complications (*Am J Surg* 2004;188:94).

c. Myelofibrosis and myeloid metaplasia are incurable myeloproliferative disorders that usually present in patients older than 60 years. The condition is characterized by bone marrow fibrosis, leukoerythroblastosis, and extramedullary hematopoiesis, which can result in massive splenomegaly. Indications for splenectomy include symptomatic splenomegaly and transfusion-dependent anemias. Although the compressive symptoms are effectively palliated with splenectomy, the cytopenias frequently recur. In addition, these patients are at increased risk for postoperative hemorrhage and thrombotic complications after splenectomy.

4. Lymphoproliferative disorders

a. Chronic lymphocytic leukemia (CLL), a B-cell leukemia, is the most common of the chronic leukemias and is characterized by the accumulation of mature but nonfunctional lymphocytes. Primary therapy is medical, with splenectomy reserved for those patients with symptomatic splenomegaly and severe hypersplenism. Although the use of splenectomy in such cases is controversial, data from one retrospective study demonstrated that early splenectomy (the majority of which were for hypersplenism or cytopenias) in some patient subgroups was associated with improved survival (*J Am Coll Surg* 1997;185:237).

b. The **non-Hodgkin lymphomas** are a diverse group of disorders with a wide range of clinical behaviors, ranging from indolent to highly aggressive. As with other malignant processes, splenectomy is indicated for palliation of hypersplenism and cytopenias or for diagnosis in patients with suspected persistent or recurrent disease after systemic therapy. Splenectomy plays an important role in the diagnosis and staging of patients with isolated splenic lymphoma (known as *malignant lymphoma with prominent splenic involvement*). In these cases, improved survival has been shown in patients undergoing splenectomy (*Cancer* 1993; 71:207).

   c. **Hodgkin lymphoma.** Splenectomy has a limited role in the diagnosis and treatment of Hodgkin lymphoma due to refinements in imaging techniques and progress in the methods of treatment. Indications for surgery are similar to those for non-Hodgkin lymphoma.

   d. **Hairy cell leukemia** is a rare disease of elderly men that is characterized by B lymphocytes with membrane ruffling. Splenectomy was previously regarded as the primary therapy for this disease, but improvements in systemic chemotherapy have reduced the role of splenectomy, which is now reserved for patients with massive splenomegaly or refractory disease.

 5. **Neutropenias**
   a. **Felty syndrome** is characterized by rheumatoid arthritis, splenomegaly, and neutropenia. The primary treatment is steroids, but refractory cases may require splenectomy to reverse the neutropenia. Patients with recurrent infections and significant anemia may benefit from splenectomy. The clinical course of the arthritis is not affected.

B. **Nonhematologic splenic disorders**
 1. **Splenic cysts** are uncommon and can be parasitic or nonparasitic. Most are located in the lower pole in a subcapsular position.
   a. **Parasitic cysts** make up more than two thirds of splenic cysts worldwide but are rare in the United States. The majority are hydatid cysts caused by *Echinococcus* species. They are typically asymptomatic but may rupture or cause symptoms due to splenomegaly. The primary treatment is splenectomy, with careful attention not to spill the cyst contents. The cyst may be aspirated and injected with hypertonic saline prior to mobilization if concern about rupture exists.
   b. **Nonparasitic cysts** can be true cysts or pseudocysts, but this differentiation is difficult to make preoperatively.
      (1) **True cysts** (or primary cysts) have an epithelial lining, and are most often congenital. Other rare true cysts include epidermoid and dermoid cysts.
      (2) **Pseudocysts** (or secondary cysts) lack an epithelial lining and make up more than two thirds of nonparasitic cysts. They typically result from traumatic hematoma formation, and subsequently resorb.
      (3) **Treatment.** Splenic cysts are typically asymptomatic, but they may present with left upper abdominal or shoulder pain. Those smaller than 5 cm can be followed with ultrasonography and often resolve spontaneously. Larger cysts risk rupture and require cyst unroofing or splenectomy. Percutaneous aspiration is associated with infection and reaccumulation and is not indicated. A recent small retrospective study of 15 patients over 12 years demonstrated that laparoscopic management of splenic cysts yields shorter hospital length of stay and fewer complications with no adverse effects (*Surg Endosc* 2007;21:206).
 2. **Splenic abscesses** are rare, with less than 600 cases reported in the literature, but they are potentially lethal if untreated. Approximately two thirds are due to seeding from a distant bacteremic focus, most commonly endocarditis or urinary tract infection. Fever is present in nearly all cases, and abdominal discomfort and splenomegaly occur in one half of patients. Associated conditions include sickle cell anemia.
   a. **Computed tomography (CT) scanning and ultrasonography** are the best diagnostic modalities for splenic abscess. CT scanning typically shows an area of low homogeneous density with edges that do not intensify with intravenous contrast.
   b. **Antibiotic therapy** should be instituted immediately after blood cultures are obtained. Greater than 60% of identified infectious agents are aerobes, with

one half being *Staphylococcus* and *Streptococcus* species. A minority of splenic abscesses involve fungal organisms, which can be cured with antifungal agents alone.

    c. Surgical therapy. Unilocular abscesses may be amenable to treatment by percutaneous drainage. Splenectomy, open or laparoscopic, in combination with postoperative antibiotics is the definitive therapy.

C. Other forms of splenic pathology

    1. Trauma to the adult spleen has historically been managed with laparotomy (most children have been successfully managed nonoperatively). With imaging advances, grading of this solid organ injury and conservative management in the stable adult patient have been made possible. The common grading system for splenic injury is listed in Table 16-2. Management depends on stability and age (adult vs. child) of the patient and associated injuries. Grade of the injury and amount of hemoperitoneum can also be considered. A recent analysis of the National Trauma Data Bank found that only 16% of identified splenic injuries were severe (grade IV or V). From 1996 to 2003, 3,085 adult patients were recorded with severe injuries, and 40% of these had nonoperative management attempted. Of these, 50% failed nonoperative management (*J Trauma* 2006;61:1113).

    2. *En bloc* oncologic resections for colon, pancreatic, or gastric cancers may require splenectomy if the tumor invades the spleen.

    3. Incidental splenectomy occurs when the spleen is injured iatrogenically during another abdominal operation. This can occur either by damage from a retractor in the left upper quadrant or from mobilization of the splenic flexure in colon resection. Capsular tears can often be treated with topical hemostatic agents or even with use of the argon beam coagulator, but if significant hemorrhage results and cannot be controlled expeditiously, splenectomy is indicated.

    4. Splenic artery aneurysm is the most common visceral artery aneurysm and has a particular tendency to affect women, with increased incidence of rupture during pregnancy. Asymptomatic aneurysms less than 2 cm in size in patients in whom pregnancy is not anticipated can be followed closely with serial imaging. Operative management is warranted for larger or symptomatic aneurysms, those in whom pregnancy is anticipated, and pseudoaneurysms associated with inflammation. Percutaneous management such as transcatheter embolization and laparoscopic excision are good options in selected patients.

TABLE 16-2	American Association for the Surgery of Trauma Spleen Injury Scale (1994 Version)	
Grade[a]		**Injury description**
I	Hematoma	Subcapsular, <10% surface area
	Laceration	Capsular tear, <1 cm parenchymal depth
II	Hematoma	Subcapsular, 10%–50% surface area; intraparenchymal, <5 cm in diameter
	Laceration	1–3 cm parenchymal depth that does not involve a trabecular vessel
III	Hematoma	Subcapsular, <5% surface area or expanding ruptured subcapsular or parenchymal hematoma
		Intraparenchymal hematoma >5 cm or expanding
	Laceration	>3 cm parenchymal depth or involving trabecular vessels
IV	Laceration	Laceration involving segmental or hilar vessels producing major devascularization (>25% of spleen)
V	Laceration	Completely shattered spleen
	Vascular	Hilar vascular injury that devascularizes spleen

[a]Advance one grade for multiple injuries up to grade III.
With permission from Moore EE, Cogbill TH, Jurkovich GJ, et al. Organ injury scaling: spleen and liver (1994 revision). *J Trauma* 1995;38(3):323–324.

a. For proximal and middle-third aneurysms, the aneurysms may be simply excluded with distal ligation, with the splenic blood supply then coming predominantly from the short gastric vessels.

b. For distal-third aneurysms, resection with splenectomy is usually performed.

PREOPERATIVE CONSIDERATIONS IN SPLENECTOMY

I. VACCINATIONS

   A. Polyvalent pneumococcal vaccine (Pneumovax) covers 85% to 90% of pneumococcal types and should be administered at least 2 to 3 weeks before splenectomy to all patients older than 2 years. The vaccine should be repeated every 5 to 7 years.

   B. Meningococcal vaccine is a one-time vaccination for patients older than 2 years.

   C. *Haemophilus influenzae* **type B** conjugate vaccine should be considered if the patient was not vaccinated in infancy.

II. CONSIDERATIONS FOR TRANSFUSION

   A. Patients with hematologic disease, particularly those with autoimmune disorders, often have autoantibodies and are difficult to cross-match. Thus, blood should be typed and screened at least 24 hours prior to the scheduled operative time. Patients with splenomegaly should have 2 to 4 units of packed red blood cells cross-matched and available for surgery.

   B. Patients with severe thrombocytopenia (particularly those with counts $<10,000/\mu L$) should have platelets available for transfusion, but these should be withheld until the splenic artery is ligated so they will not be quickly consumed by the spleen. Most patients with thrombocytopenia from ITP can be safely managed with splenectomy even with very low platelet counts and do not often require platelet transfusion perioperatively.

III. PREOPERATIVE IMAGING

   A. Either **ultrasound or CT** may be necessary in patients with malignancy or suspected splenomegaly to determine spleen size and to evaluate for the presence of splenic hilar adenopathy that may complicate a laparoscopic approach.

   B. Right-upper-quadrant ultrasound is indicated preoperatively for those who are at high risk for developing gallstones (hemolytic anemias, sickle cell anemia) so that cholecystectomy may be performed concomitantly if indicated.

IV. OTHER CONSIDERATIONS

   A. If the **patient has been receiving steroids** in the preoperative period, perioperative stress-dose steroids should be considered. The patient should be continued on his or her oral steroid dose and gradually tapered only after he or she has shown a hematologic response to splenectomy.

   B. Patients who are to undergo a laparoscopic splenectomy should be counseled preoperatively about the possibility of **conversion to open splenectomy or a hand-assisted approach** and should be prepared identically to those patients for whom an open procedure is planned.

OPERATIVE APPROACH

I. OPEN SPLENECTOMY

   A. The incision used is either an upper midline or a left subcostal incision. When significant splenomegaly is present, a midline incision is usually preferred.

   B. A drain is not routinely required unless it is suspected that the pancreatic tail may have been injured during the hilar dissection.

   C. A search for **accessory splenic tissue** should be conducted, particularly if the patient has a hematologic indication for splenectomy.

II. LAPAROSCOPIC SPLENECTOMY has become the preferred method for elective splenectomy for all but the most difficult or largest spleens. It is now increasingly used for selected patients with splenomegaly.

TABLE 16-3	Contraindications to Laparoscopic Splenectomy

Absolute contraindications	Difficult cases
Massive splenomegaly (>30 cm length)	Moderate splenomegaly (>20–25 cm)
Portal hypertension	Severe uncorrectable cytopenia
Splenic trauma, unstable patient	Splenic vein thrombosis
	Splenic trauma, stable patient
	Bulky hilar adenopathy
	Morbid obesity

A. **Contraindications** to laparoscopic splenectomy are presented in Table 16-3.

B. **Splenomegaly** increases the complexity of the laparoscopic approach because of the difficulty of manipulating the organ atraumatically and achieving adequate exposure of the ligaments and hilum. Large spleens are also more difficult to place in an entrapment bag using a strictly laparoscopic approach.

   1. Although the size limits for attempting laparoscopic or laparoscopic-assisted splenectomy are evolving, most moderately enlarged spleens (<1,000 g weight or 15 to 20 cm in length) can be removed in a minimally invasive fashion, often without a hand-port device.

   2. For spleens larger than 20 cm in longitudinal length or those that weigh between 1,000 and 3,000 g, the use of a hand port should be considered. The use of a hand port in this setting has been associated with reduced operative times, less blood loss, and lower rates of conversion to open operation (*Arch Surg* 2006:141:755).

   3. In general, spleens greater than 30 cm in craniocaudal length (and weighing >3,000 g) should be approached in an open fashion because of the reduced working space and increased difficulty in manipulating the spleen.

C. **Outcomes of laparoscopic splenectomy.** Several large series of laparoscopic splenectomy have been published with excellent results. In a recent meta-analysis of 51 reports including 2,940 patients (*Surgery* 2003;134:647), laparoscopic splenectomy was associated with significantly fewer complications overall, primarily as a result of fewer wound and pulmonary complications.

COMPLICATIONS OF SPLENECTOMY

I. INTRAOPERATIVE COMPLICATIONS

A. Clinical evidence of **pancreatic injury** occurs in 0% to 6% of splenectomies, whether done open or laparoscopically. A retrospective review of one center's experience with laparoscopic splenectomy found pancreatic injury in 16% of patients; half of these were isolated instances of hyperamylasemia (*Surg Endosc* 2001;15:1273). If one suspects that the pancreatic parenchyma has been violated during laparoscopic splenectomy, a closed suction drain should be placed adjacent to the pancreas, and a drain amylase obtained prior to removal after the patient is eating a regular diet.

B. **Vascular injury.** The most common intraoperative complication is hemorrhage, which can occur during the hilar dissection or from a capsular tear during retraction. The incidence of this complication is 2% to 3% during open splenectomy but is nearly 5% using the laparoscopic approach. Bleeding during laparoscopic splenectomy may necessitate conversion to a hand-assisted or open procedure.

C. **Bowel injury**

   1. **Colon.** Because of the close proximity of the splenic flexure to the lower pole of the spleen, it is possible to injure the colon during mobilization. Some surgeons have advocated bowel preparation because of this potential complication, but that has not been our practice, and colon injury should be extremely rare.

2. **Stomach.** Gastric injuries can occur by direct trauma or can result from thermal injury during division of the short gastric vessels. Use of energy devices too close to the greater curvature of the stomach can result in a delayed gastric necrosis and perforation.

D. **Diaphragmatic injury** has been described during the mobilization of the superior pole, especially with perisplenitis, and is of no consequence if recognized and repaired. In laparoscopic splenectomies, it may be more difficult to recognize the injury given the pneumoperitoneum, but careful dissection of the splenophrenic ligament can minimize its occurrence. The pleural space should be evacuated under positive-pressure ventilation prior to closure to minimize the pneumothorax.

II. EARLY POSTOPERATIVE COMPLICATIONS

A. **Pulmonary complications** develop in nearly 10% of patients after open splenectomy, and these range from atelectasis to pneumonia and pleural effusion. Pulmonary complications are significantly less common with the laparoscopic approach.

B. **Subphrenic abscess** occurs in 2% to 3% of patients after open splenectomy but is uncommon after laparoscopic splenectomy (0.7%). Treatment usually consists of percutaneous drainage and the intravenous antibiotics.

C. **Wound problems** such as hematomas, seromas, and wound infections occur commonly (4% to 5%) after open splenectomy because of the underlying hematologic disorders. Wound complications after laparoscopic splenectomy are usually minor and occur less frequently (1.5%).

D. **Thrombocytosis and thrombotic complications** can occur after either open or laparoscopic splenectomy. The presumed causes of thrombosis after splenectomy may relate to the occurrence of thrombocytosis, alterations in platelet function, and a low-flow stasis phenomenon in the ligated splenic vein. Symptomatic portal vein thrombosis occurs more commonly than expected (8% to 10%) and can result in extensive mesenteric thrombosis if not recognized promptly and treated expeditiously. Massive splenomegaly and myelofibrosis are the two main risk factors for portal vein thrombosis (*Am J Surg* 2002;184:631).

E. **Ileus** can occur after open splenectomy, but a prolonged postoperative ileus should prompt the surgeon to search for concomitant problems such as a subphrenic abscess or portal vein thrombosis (*Surgery* 2003;134:647).

III. LATE POSTOPERATIVE COMPLICATIONS

A. **Overwhelming postsplenectomy infection (OPSI)** is a rare, late complication that may occur at any point in an asplenic or hyposplenic patient's lifetime. Patients present with nonspecific flulike symptoms rapidly progressing to fulminant sepsis, consumptive coagulopathy, bacteremia, and ultimately death within 12 to 48 hours. Encapsulated bacteria, especially *Streptococcus pneumoniae, H. influenzae* type B, and *Neisseria meningitidis,* are the most commonly involved organisms. Successful treatment of OPSI requires early supportive care and high-dose third-generation cephalosporins. Daily prophylactic antibiotics have been recommended after operation in all children younger than 5 years and in immunocompromised patients because these patients are unlikely to produce adequate antibody in response to pneumococcal vaccination. All patients who have had splenectomy should be educated about the risk of OPSI and the need for early physician consultation in the event that fever or other prodromal symptoms should occur. In 1997, a survey of U.K. microbiologists was published, with 42 cases of OPSI recalled from 1992 to 1996. All but one patient was an adult. In most of these 42 cases, OPSI occurred greater than 10 years since splenectomy, with a range of 24 days to 59 years (*J Infect* 1997;35: 289).

B. **Splenosis** is the presence of disseminated intra-abdominal splenic tissue, which usually occurs after splenic rupture. Splenosis does not appear to be more common after laparoscopic splenectomy, but care should be taken during splenic morcellation to avoid bag rupture and spillage of splenic tissue.

17

CEREBROVASCULAR DISEASE AND VASCULAR ACCESS

Christopher Chambers and Gregorio A. Sicard

 EXTRACRANIAL CEREBROVASCULAR DISEASE

Atherosclerotic occlusive disease of the extracranial carotid artery is a major risk factor for stroke, the primary cause of disability, and the third-most-common cause of death in the United States. More than 600,000 new strokes occur annually, with an estimated cost of more than $30 billion. The initial mortality from stroke is between 20% and 30%. Of patients who survive the initial event, one third function normally, one third recover with mild deficits, and one third recover with significant deficits. Furthermore, approximately 50% of survivors die of recurrent stroke within 5 years. Carotid bifurcation disease is responsible for 25% to 35% of ipsilateral cerebrovascular events.

I. PRESENTATION

    A. The clinical presentation of patients with symptomatic occlusive disease is a **neurologic deficit.** However, many patients have an asymptomatic stenosis that is identified by a health care provider based on auscultation of carotid bruits or screening Doppler study.

    B. Lateralizing ischemic events can result in aphasia (expressive or receptive), combined sensory and motor deficits, and various visual disturbances. Deficits such as these are usually associated with the anterior cerebral circulation (i.e., the internal carotid artery and its branches).

        1. Transient ischemic attacks (TIAs) are transient hemispheric neurologic deficits that may last from several seconds to hours but fewer than 24 hours. TIAs that occur in rapid succession, interspersed with complete recovery but with progressively smaller intervals between attacks, are termed **crescendo TIAs** and carry a high risk of progression to a permanent neurologic deficit; emergent evaluation is mandatory.

        2. Amaurosis fugax (temporary monocular blindness), often described as a shade coming down over one eye, results from emboli lodging in the ophthalmic artery. Fundoscopic examination demonstrates Hollenhorst plaques.

        3. A **reversible ischemic neurologic deficit** is a longer-lasting neurologic deficit that can last for up to 7 days but ultimately resolves completely.

        4. If the neurologic deficit is fixed and persists beyond 7 days, it is considered a **completed stroke.** In addition, some patients may present with a neurologic deficit that fluctuates, gradually worsening over a period of hours or days while the patient is under observation. This situation is considered a stroke in evolution and, like crescendo TIAs, needs prompt treatment.

    C. Global ischemic events are manifested by symptoms such as vertigo, dizziness, perioral numbness, ataxia, or drop attacks. These usually are associated with interruption posterior circulation supplying the brainstem (i.e., the vertebrobasilar system).

II. PATHOPHYSIOLOGY AND EPIDEMIOLOGY. Ischemic events in patients with extracranial vascular disease can be the result of emboli or a low-flow state. Although it can cause clinical symptoms, disease of the vertebral arteries typically remains asymptomatic. On the other hand, even when it is asymptomatic, significant occlusive carotid arterial disease carries with it a doubling of baseline stroke risk. Once a significant carotid lesion results in an ipsilateral lateralizing cerebral event, the risk of stroke may be as high as 26% over 2 years.

III. DIAGNOSIS. A careful neurologic examination is performed before obtaining any diagnostic studies. Furthermore, the presence of a carotid bruit warrants diagnostic evaluation. Imaging of the carotid arterial system attempts to classify the degree of stenosis, which is useful for determining prognosis. Due to methodologic differences in calculating the percentage of stenosis encountered in different studies, there is some disagreement about exact cutoff percentages. However, four levels of stenosis are typically described: mild (<50%), moderate (50% to 79%), severe (80% to 99%), and occluded (100%). A variety of noninvasive and invasive diagnostic studies are available.

A. Color-flow duplex scanning uses real-time B-mode ultrasound and color-enhanced pulsed Doppler flow measurements to determine the extent of the carotid stenosis. **This is the initial screening test for carotid disease.** The reliability of this study depends in large part on the abilities of the vascular technicians; when using an established laboratory, treatment of most carotid lesions can be instituted based on ultrasound duplex scanning alone.

B. Arteriography remains the gold standard for the diagnosis of cerebrovascular disease. Unlike duplex scanning, however, arteriography is an invasive procedure with inherent risks, such as contrast allergy, renal toxicity, and stroke (2% to 4% of patients). Because of these risks and improvements in duplex ultrasonography, carotid arteriography is generally limited to patients with technically inadequate duplex ultrasonography, planning for carotid artery stenting, or for verification of carotid occlusion.

C. Although **magnetic resonance (MR) angiography** is a highly sensitive technique for the evaluation of patients for symptomatic cerebrovascular disease, its precision remains inferior to that of conventional angiography. Recently, computed tomography (CT) angiography has been introduced as an alternative to arteriography.

IV. MANAGEMENT

A. Medical therapy. It is important to make every effort to modify risk factors to prevent progression of carotid occlusive disease. Control of hypertension, cessation of smoking, management of lipid disorders, attainment of ideal body weight, and regular exercise should be undertaken. No drug therapy has been shown to reduce the risk of stroke in patients with asymptomatic carotid disease. Medical management in symptomatic patients is focused primarily on the use of antiplatelet agents, specifically aspirin. Aspirin is effective in reducing stroke and stroke-related deaths. In a meta-analysis of more than 8,000 patients, the risk of major vascular events was reduced by 22% in patients receiving aspirin (*Br Med J* 1988;296:320). Low doses (81 mg/day) are as efficacious as higher doses (325 mg/day). Other antiplatelet agents, such as dipyridamole and ticlopidine (250 mg orally twice a day), are no better than aspirin alone. Recently, clopidogrel (Plavix) has been introduced as a potent antiplatelet agent, but it has not been evaluated as part of medical therapy compared to carotid endarterectomy (CEA). Anticoagulation with heparin sodium is beneficial in patients who have cardiac emboli. In addition, heparin may be useful in preventing progression of thrombus in evolving nonhemorrhagic strokes. The major contraindication to heparinization is a recent hemorrhagic brain infarct; therefore, a CT scan of the brain should be obtained before heparin is given.

B. Surgical/endovascular management is the treatment of choice for extracranial cerebrovascular disease and has been documented to reduce stroke.

1. Indications for carotid endarterectomy have been extensively studied in both asymptomatic and symptomatic patients, comparing surgical treatment to best medical therapy. Two commonly cited studies include the Asymptomatic Carotid Atherosclerosis Study (ACAS) (*JAMA* 1995;273:1421), and the North American Symptomatic Carotid Endarterectomy Trial (NASCET) (*NEJM* 1991;325:445). In the ACAS trial, the ipsilateral 5-year stroke rate in asymptomatic patients with at least 60% stenosis was 5.1% in patients undergoing a CEA versus 11% receiving best medical therapy. For symptomatic patients with at least 70% stenosis in the NASCET trial, the 2-year ipsilateral stroke rate was 9% versus 26% in the

CEA and best medical therapy groups, respectively. Based largely on these two definitive trials, current indications for CEA include the following:

a. Asymptomatic patients with greater than 70% stenosis.

b. Symptomatic patients with greater than 50% stenosis.

c. Symptomatic patients with greater than 50% stenosis who have an **ulcerated lesion** or whose **symptoms persist** while they are on **aspirin** or other antiplatelet therapy.

d. Selected patients with stroke in evolution. Surgery is performed to restore normal blood flow to allow recovery of ischemic brain tissue that is nonfunctional yet metabolically alive. Surgical candidates have mild to moderate neurologic defects and no evidence of hemorrhage on CT scan. The timing of surgery in these cases is controversial.

e. Selected patients with completed strokes. Interventions in these patients are performed in the hope of reducing stroke recurrence, which is 7% to 8% per year with nonsurgical therapy. Candidates for surgery include patients with a mild deficit and (1) greater than 70% stenosis or (2) greater than 50% stenosis and an ulcerated plaque, and patients with a moderate deficit and a lesion greater than 70% with an occluded contralateral carotid artery. The timing of surgery in these cases is debatable; however, surgery traditionally has been delayed to reduce the risk of perioperative hemorrhagic stroke. One early study showed a significantly increased risk of stroke if CEA was performed before as opposed to after 5 weeks from the initial event (5/27 for early group vs. 0/22 for delayed group; *J Vasc Surg* 1985;2:250). On the other hand, a 4.9% 30-day risk of stroke was seen in the medically treated arm of the NASCET trial. A prudent approach is to wait 4 to 6 weeks postinfarction to minimize the risk of intracranial hemorrhage.

f. Rarely, endarterectomy is performed on patients with **completely occluded carotid arteries.** Candidates for surgery include those who have:

(1) Recent endarterectomy with immediate postoperative thrombosis.

(2) Bruit disappear while under observation while remaining asymptomatic.

(3) Recent occlusion with fluctuating or progressive symptoms.

(4) New internal carotid occlusion that can be operated on within 2 to 4 hours of the onset of symptoms.

2. Carotid endarterectomy has been performed for more than 50 years and is the most commonly performed vascular operation. A beneficial outcome depends on meticulous technique. The use of such technique can keep the perioperative adverse event rate (stroke and death) below 3%.

a. Anesthesia for carotid endarterectomy can be general endotracheal anesthesia, regional cervical block, or local anesthesia. The choice of anesthesia depends on a combination of patient factors and surgeon expertise. No single method of anesthesia has been demonstrated superior.

b. During **exposure and mobilization** of the common carotid artery and its branches, it is important to proceed with gentle dissection and minimal manipulation of the carotid bulb to prevent embolization from the atherosclerotic plaque.

c. After **systemic heparinization** of the patient, the internal, external, and common carotid arteries are clamped, and a longitudinal arteriotomy is made from just proximal to the plaque in the common carotid artery to just beyond the distal extent of the plaque in the internal carotid artery.

d. Placement of tubing to **shunt** blood from the common carotid artery around the operative field to the internal carotid artery during endarterectomy is a controversial practice. Adequate cerebral perfusion without shunting occurs in 85% to 90% of patients. Intraoperative neurologic assessment of the awake patient under local anesthesia can be as simple as having the patient squeeze a noise toy in the contralateral hand and answering a few simple questions after carotid occlusion. **Awake assessment** is the most sensitive and specific method of determining the need for shunt placement (*J Vasc Surg* 2007;45:511). Patients that develop weakness or changes in mental status should be shunted.

For patients under general anesthesia, an alternative method of cerebral perfusion is required, although some surgeons simply choose routinely to shunt these patients. Stump pressure and intraoperative electroencephalogram (EEG) monitoring are commonly used alternative methods for the determination of cerebral perfusion and subsequent need for shunting. Shunting can be performed safely without an increased risk of stroke (*Ann Vasc Surg* 2006; 20:482).

e. The **plaque** is carefully separated from the media and removed. The carotid endarterectomy is closed using a running suture. A recent meta-analysis of multiple small trials reviewed the outcomes of patients with primary closure versus patch angioplasty, as well as results of patch angioplasty with autologous vein, polytetrafluoroethylene (PTFE), or Dacron (*J Vasc Surg* 2004;40:1126). Although interpretation is difficult because of variations among trials, patch angioplasty may be associated with significantly reduced risk for stroke, death, and arterial occlusion during the perioperative period. Patch angioplasty also decreased recurrent stenosis during long-term follow-up, especially in patients with small internal carotid arteries. Determining differences in the material for patch angioplasty requires further study.

f. **Postoperative care**
   (1) Immediately after endarterectomy, **neurologic function and blood pressure (BP) alterations** should be monitored. Hypertension and hypotension are common after endarterectomy and may cause neurologic complications. The extremes of BP should be treated with either sodium nitroprusside or phenylephrine (Neo-Synephrine) to keep the systolic BP between 140 and 160 mm Hg (slightly higher in chronically hypertensive patients). The wound should be examined for hematoma formation. Aspirin is resumed in the immediate postoperative period. Some advocate the use of dextran-40 (up to 20 mL/kg/day for up to 72 hours) as an additional antithrombotic agent, which can be started intraoperatively and continued into the early postoperative period.
   (2) **Patient follow-up.** A baseline duplex scan is obtained 3 months after the procedure and again at 12 months. After that, patients can be followed yearly. Patients who can tolerate aspirin are given 325 mg/day.

g. **Complications**
   (1) **Stroke rates** must be low (3%) to make operative management of cerebrovascular disease reasonable, especially in asymptomatic patients.
   (2) **Myocardial infarction** remains the most common cause of death in the early postoperative period. As many as 25% of patients who undergo endarterectomy have severe, correctable coronary artery lesions. The timing of coronary intervention relative to CEA is under debate.
   (3) **Cranial nerve injuries** occur in 5% to 10% of patients who undergo carotid endarterectomy. The most commonly injured nerve is the marginal mandibular, followed by the recurrent laryngeal, superior laryngeal, and hypoglossal nerves.
   (4) **Recurrent carotid stenosis** has been reported to occur in 5% to 10% of cases, although symptoms are present in fewer than 3%. Two types of lesions have been characterized. A myofibroblastic lesion that occurs early (within 3 years) results from uncontrolled proliferation of the medial smooth muscle cells and extracellular matrix. Recurrent atherosclerosis also may cause restenosis. The presence of symptoms is an indication for treatment of a recurrent lesion. Frequently, these lesions do not lend themselves to endarterectomy and are best treated by carotid artery stenting.

3. **Carotid artery stenting**
   a. The **indications** for carotid artery stenting (CAS) are the same as those for a carotid endarterectomy; however, this technique is under intense investigation. Several studies have been completed or are underway to examine the efficacy of CAS compared to CEA, particularly in high-risk patients. Outcomes have

varied, especially as device technology and operator experience improve. The SAPPHIRE (Stenting and Angioplasty with Protection in Patients and High Risk for Endarterectomy) trial demonstrated at 36 months that the incidence of stroke was virtually identical for both CAS and CEA (7.1% for CAS and 6.7% for CEA, $p = 0.945$) (N Engl J Med 2004;351:1565). However, a more recent trial, the EVA-3S (Endarterectomy Versus Angioplasty in Patients with Severe Symptomatic Carotid Stenosis), demonstrated that the 30-day risk of stroke or mortality was significantly increased in the stenting group compared with the endarterectomy group (9.6% vs. 3.9%, respectively; $p = 0.01$) (N Engl J Med 2006;355:1660). The results of current ongoing investigations including the CREST trial (Carotid Revascularization Endarterectomy vs. Stent Trial) will likely help to elucidate the role of CAS, especially in the normal-risk patient.

(1) Because CEA is well tolerated and has a very low risk of complications, CAS is commonly reserved for **high-risk patients,** including patients with the following conditions:

  (a) Severe cardiac disease.

  (b) Severe chronic obstructive pulmonary disease (COPD).

  (c) Severe renal insufficiency or end-stage renal disease (ESRD) requiring hemodialysis.

  (d) Prior ipsilateral neck surgery.

  (e) Prior neck radiation.

  (f) Contralateral vocal cord paralysis.

  (g) Surgically inaccessible lesion.

(2) **Relative contraindications** to carotid artery stenting include the following:

  (a) Severe tortuosity of common and internal carotid artery.

  (b) Complex aortic arch anatomy (increasing difficulty as great vessels arise from ascending rather than transverse aortic arch).

  (c) Severe calcification or extensive thrombus formation.

  (d) Near-complete or complete occlusion.

b. Carotid artery stenting has evolved and is commonly performed in the following basic steps. Meticulous technique is critical for reducing the incidence of stroke. Special attention must be taken to avoid catheter and wire manipulation of the lesion prior to cerebral protection device deployment and to ensuring removal of all air bubbles within the angiography tubing.

c. Embolization of plaque debris has been shown to occur with almost any endovascular manipulation of a carotid artery lesion. Consequently, **embolic protection devices** have been developed that significantly reduce the risk of stroke during CAS. The typical device used today is a filterlike device that is advanced across the lesion and then opened in the distal internal carotid artery (ICA) prior to angioplasty and stent deployment. A more recent device under investigation provides protection through reversal of flow in the internal carotid artery. Flow reversal is created after balloon occlusion of the external carotid artery (ECA) and common carotid artery (CCA), thus eliminating the need to cross the lesion and possibly decreasing the risk of stroke.

d. Complications

(1) **Embolic stroke** is the most common complication of CAS. Risk factors include lack of a cerebral protection device, long or multiple lesions, and age older than 80 years. Thrombolysis may be a successful treatment option, especially if the source of emboli is an acute thrombus. When an embolus is composed of atheroma or chronic thrombus, however, mechanical removal of emboli may become necessary to restore flow.

(2) **Hemodynamic instability** may occur during manipulation and angioplasty of the carotid bifurcation. Bradycardia should be anticipated and treated with atropine prior to dilation of the carotid bifurcation. Postoperatively, as with CEA, patients should be monitored to avoid extremes of blood pressure.

(3) Restenosis occurs in approximately 5% of patients at 12 to 24 months and is typically secondary to intimal hyperplasia. These lesions are often amenable to repeat angioplasty.

e. Follow-up using duplex ultrasound is important to identify patients with restenosis and is usually performed at baseline following CAS and then at 3, 6, and 12 months and every year thereafter. Significant elevation of peak systolic velocity from baseline should prompt further evaluation with angiography.

 VASCULAR ACCESS FOR DIALYSIS

The success of hemodialysis depends on the rate of blood flow through the dialyzer. Flow rates of between 350 and 450 mL/minute are required to provide adequate dialysis within a reasonable time frame (3 to 4 hours). The dialysis access is a port or site in the body that provides the necessary blood flow for dialysis. The access should be easy to cannulate and last for years with minimal maintenance. The incidence of complications, such as infection, stenosis, pseudoaneurysm formation, thrombosis, and outflow deterioration, should also be low. To date, no vascular access fulfills all of these criteria.

I. INDICATIONS

  A. Temporary hemodialysis access provided with short- or intermediate-term central venous access device (CVAD) is indicated when acute short-term dialysis is needed, as in (1) acute renal failure, (2) overdose or intoxication, (3) end-stage renal disease needing urgent hemodialysis without available mature access, (4) peritoneal dialysis patients with peritonitis, and (5) transplant recipients needing temporary hemodialysis during severe rejection episodes.

  B. Permanent hemodialysis access is created using subcutaneous conduits having high blood flows when long-term hemodialysis is needed, as in (1) long-term treatment of chronic renal failure and (2) patients awaiting renal transplantation.

II. DIALYSIS ACCESS CATHETERS

  A. Nontunneled central venous catheters. Short-term dialysis access includes percutaneous catheters in internal jugular, subclavian, or femoral veins. The **Quinton catheter** provides access for short-term hemodialysis in acute renal failure. Noncuffed, double-lumen catheters can be percutaneously inserted at the bedside and provide acceptable blood flow rates (250 mL/minute) for temporary hemodialysis— no more than 3 weeks for internal jugular or 5 days for femoral catheters due to considerations of infection and dislodgement.

  B. Tunneled central venous silicone dialysis catheters. Tunneled catheters [e.g., **Tesio, Ash Split** (Bard Access Systems) and **Duraflow catheters** (AngioDynamics)] have cuffs that anchor them to the subcutaneous tissues. Tunneled, cuffed venous catheters should be placed preferentially in the right internal jugular vein because this site offers a more direct route to the cavoatrial junction and a lower risk of complications than other potential catheter insertion sites. Advantages of tunneled catheters include the ability to insert into a variety of sites, no maturation time requirement, no hemodynamic consequences, ease and cost of catheter placement and replacement, and a life span of the access of months to years. Disadvantages of tunneled, cuffed venous catheters include potential morbidity due to thrombosis, infection, risk of permanent central venous stenosis or occlusion, and lower blood flow rates than for atrioventricular grafts and fistulas.

  C. Catheter complications

  1. Early dysfunction usually occurs secondary to either malposition or intracatheter thrombosis. Almost all catheters inserted into a central vein develop a fibrin sleeve after insertion, resulting in **late dysfunction.** They are usually clinically silent until they obstruct the ports at the distal end of the catheter. They also serve as a nidus for infection.

  2. Central vein stenosis, thrombosis, or stricture. Central vein stenosis arises from endothelial injury at the site of catheter–endothelial contact. Incidence increases with the use of nonsilicone catheters, with the use of a subclavian approach, and with a history of prior catheter-related infections. Removal of the CVAD may not improve the underlying problem and, by definition, sacrifices the access. Systemic anticoagulation remains the primary therapy.

III. ARTERIOVENOUS (AV) ACCESS NOMENCLATURE

A. Conduit. An **autogenous AV access** (also known as an **AV fistula**, a **native vein fistula**, and a **primary fistula**) is an access created by connecting a native vein to an adjacent artery. A **nonautogenous AV access** (also known as an **AV graft** or a **graft fistula**) uses grafts that are either synthetic or biologic. **Synthetic grafts** include expanded polytetrafluoroethylene (ePTFE, e.g., Gore-Tex or Impra) and polyester (e.g., Dacron) grafts. **Biologic grafts** include bovine heterografts, human umbilical veins, and cryopreserved allogeneic human vein grafts.

B. Configuration. A **direct access** often connects a native vein to an adjacent artery. An **indirect access** uses an autogenous or prosthetic material placed subcutaneously between the artery and vein. The course of the subcutaneous prosthesis may be **looped** (loop graft) or **straight** (straight graft).

IV. PREOPERATIVE EVALUATION

A. Timing. Ideally, any patient with renal insufficiency should be referred for surgical evaluation approximately 1 year before the anticipated need for dialysis. This point is reached when the creatinine clearance is less than 25 mL/minute or the serum creatinine rises above 4 mg/dL. This allows ample opportunity for appropriate access planning, and efforts can be instituted to ensure preservation of the native veins for later AV fistula creation.

B. Preservation of access sites. All ESRD patients should protect their forearm veins from venipuncture and intravenous catheters. Likewise, hospital staff should be instructed to avoid damaging these essential veins. The nondominant arm is preferred for initial access creation. Subclavian vein cannulation should be avoided at all costs because this may induce central venous stenosis, which could preclude later use of an entire arm.

C. History. A detailed assessment for the presence of peripheral vascular disease, diabetes mellitus, cardiopulmonary disease, and coagulation disorders best determines the type of vascular access needed for a particular patient. Any conditions that suggest stenosis or occlusion of the venous or arterial system should be elicited because these may limit options for dialysis access. These include prior central venous line; transvenous pacemaker; previous surgery; trauma; or radiation treatment to the chest, neck, or arm. Evidence of early cardiac dysfunction or volume overload indicates a patient at risk for congestive heart failure following fistula creation due to increased preload. Comorbid conditions that limit life expectancy, such as severe coronary artery disease or malignancy, may render a cuffed catheter the best option.

D. Physical examination

1. Pulse examination. The axillary, brachial, radial, and ulnar artery pulses are carefully palpated in both upper extremities, and, when indicated, the femoral, popliteal, and pedal arteries are palpated. Residual scars from previous central venous catheters or surgery should also be carefully assessed.

2. Cardiovascular status. Evaluation involves determining capillary refill, the presence of edema, unequal extremity size, and collateral veins on the chest wall. A tourniquet, gravity, and gentle percussion are used to distend the forearm and upper arm veins. Their patency and continuity can be addressed by palpation and detection of a fluid thrill.

3. Segmental blood pressure measurements. Discrepancies between the two upper extremities should be noted.

4. Allen test. This is intended to assess the integrity of the palmar circulatory arches and allow assessment of the dominant blood supply to the hand.

E. Duplex ultrasound scanning can determine the diameter of the artery and the adequacy of the superficial and deep veins. For venous evaluation, tourniquets are placed on the patient's midforearm and upper arm. Details of the venous lumen, such as webs, sclerosis, and occlusion, can be visualized. Doppler venous studies may also identify suitable veins for AV fistula creation that are not readily visible on the surface anatomy, especially in heavier patients.

F. **Diagnostic imaging.** History or physical findings suggestive of central venous stenosis or previous complicated vascular access warrant further diagnostic imaging.

1. **Contrast venography** is the gold standard for determining the patency and adequacy of the superficial and deep venous systems, particularly the central veins.

2. **Conventional arteriography** also remains the gold standard for the evaluation of a suspected arterial inflow stenosis or occlusion. When in doubt as to the adequacy of the donor artery or the runoff, it is advisable to obtain an arteriogram that shows the entire arterial system from the origin of the subclavian artery to the distal branches. **Magnetic resonance angiography** can also be used for the same purpose and is particularly useful when severe contrast allergy, vascular disease, or poor renal function precludes arteriography.

G. **Laboratory studies.** Hyperkalemia and acidosis are the most common electrolyte abnormalities seen in ESRD patients. Therefore, preoperative testing should include evaluation of serum electrolytes and glucose to avoid possible procedural or anesthesia-related complications.

V. NATIVE VEIN AV FISTULAS

A. **Characteristics.** Native vein fistulas are created by connecting a vein to the adjacent artery, usually the radial or brachial artery. These are the safest and longest-lasting permanent means of vascular access, with the highest 5-year patency rates and minimum requirements for intervention. Disadvantages include a long maturation time of weeks to months to provide a flow state adequate to sustain dialysis. Revision of the outflow vein and hand exercises to increase flow to the extremity can accelerate fistula maturation. The patient's arterial and venous anatomy remains the most significant limitation because diseased vessels (e.g., due to diabetes or atherosclerosis) can hinder normal maturation or may preclude the creation of a fistula altogether. Of the ESRD population in the United States, approximately 30% have AV fistulas as their permanent dialysis access (*Kidney Int* 2000;58:2178). The Kidney Disease Outcomes Quality Initiative (K/DOQI) guidelines recommend a 50% fistula placement rate for first-time access in ESRD patients.

B. **Location.** The Brescia-Cimino fistula at the wrist (creating an end-to-side anastomosis between the cephalic vein and radial artery) and the Gratz fistula at the elbow (i.e., anastomosing the cephalic vein to the brachial artery) are the two most commonly performed autogenous AV fistulas. Flow of arterial blood under pressure distends the outflow vein to produce the subcutaneous conduit. Peripheral sites should be used first, moving to more-central sites as the former sites fail.

C. **Construction.** Most procedures can be performed on an outpatient basis, using only conscious sedation administered intravenously and local anesthetics. The end of a superficial vein, usually the cephalic, is anastomosed to the side of the artery. A side-to-side anastomosis can result in venous hypertension and swelling in the distal extremity due to higher venous pressures. An end-to-end anastomosis performed in a radial artery fistula has the advantage of providing limited flow, thereby reducing a hypercirculatory state. The disadvantage is that the anastomosis is technically challenging and carries the risk of hand ischemia. This risk is particularly high in elderly and diabetic patients. The length (diameter) of the anastomosis dictates the blood flow in fistulas based on larger arteries (e.g., the brachial artery), making it an important determinant in the development of vascular steal symptoms in distal extremity.

VI. AV GRAFT

A. **Characteristics.** AV grafts consist of biologic or synthetic conduits that connect an artery and a vein and are tunneled under the skin and placed in a subcutaneous location. PTFE allows in-growth of host tissue and formation of a pseudointimal lining, which resists infection and self-seals after needle puncture. The advantages of AV grafts over AV fistulas include (1) large surface area, (2) easy cannulation, (3) short maturation time, and (4) easy surgical handling. However, the long-term patency of AV grafts remains inferior to that of AV fistulas, despite a fourfold increase in salvage procedures. Synthetic grafts require 3 to 6 weeks before they can be used; this period allows sufficient time for the material to incorporate into the surrounding subcutaneous tissues and for the inflammation and edema to subside.

B. **Location.** AV grafts are typically placed between the brachial artery and the cephalic or brachial vein in the antecubital fossa and arranged in a loop configuration in the forearm. Upper-arm grafts can also be created between the brachial artery and basilic or axillary veins. When all upper-extremity sites are exhausted, attention is turned to the lower extremity, where loop grafts typically connect the superficial femoral artery and femoral or saphenous veins.

C. **Placement.** AV grafts are placed under local anesthesia with conscious sedation. Prophylactic antibiotics (e.g., second-generation cephalosporins) are commonly administered immediately prior to the surgery.

VII. **COMPLICATIONS OF AV ACCESS** account for 19% of all hospitalizations in hemodialysis patients, and their management requires a multidisciplinary approach (*Kidney Int* 1993;43:1091).

A. **Stenosis.** Pseudointimal hyperplasia within a synthetic graft or neointimal hyperplasia in a native AV fistula or outflow vein of a graft constitutes the most common cause of dysfunction. Approximately 85% of graft thromboses result from hemodynamically significant stenosis (*J Vasc Surg* 1997;26:373). Arterial inflow lesions are less common but can lead to low flow as well as elevated recirculation, making it more difficult to distinguish them from outflow lesions. Elevated venous pressures, increased recirculation, or recurrent thrombosis necessitates a fistulogram and treatment of any underlying lesion(s) by angioplasty or surgical revision. Stenoses in long segments (>30% after angioplasty) or those that recur within a short interval require surgical intervention.

B. **Thrombosis.** Thrombosis occurring within a month of placement is often due to anatomic or technical factors, such as a narrow outflow vein, misplaced suture, or graft kinking. Early thrombosis of native vein fistulas often results in permanent loss of the access. Prolonged hypotension during and after dialysis occasionally precipitates thrombosis, as can trauma from needle puncture or excessive compression after needle removal following hemostasis. By 24 months, 96% of grafts require thrombectomy, angioplasty, or surgical revision. Prosthetic AV shunt thrombosis can be managed by pharmacologic thrombolysis, mechanical maceration, or surgical thrombectomy, either separately or in combination. Fistulography at the time of treatment usually reveals the precipitating cause, allowing immediate intervention. Surgical thrombectomy should be followed by fistulography to detect stenosis not fully appreciable during standard balloon thrombectomy. The rate of secondary graft patency after intervention reaches only 65% at 1 year and 51% at 2 years (*Am J Kidney Dis* 2000;36:68).

C. **Infection.** Infection and bacteremia in dialysis patients are usually caused by *Staphylococcus aureus*. The type of access constitutes the major risk factor for infection, with a relative risk of 1.29 for grafts in comparison to primary fistulas and 7.64 for catheters (*ASAIO J* 2000;46:S6). AV fistula infections usually respond to a prolonged course (6 weeks) of antibiotic therapy. If septic embolization occurs, the fistula should be revised or taken down. AV graft infections occur in approximately 5% to 20% prosthetics placed and present a more challenging problem. Antibiotic treatment should cover Gram-positive organisms (including enterococci) as well as Gram-negative organisms (e.g., *Escherichia coli*). A superficial skin infection not involving the graft may respond to antibiotics alone. Focal graft infections can be salvaged with resection of the infected portion of the graft, but extensive infections and those that involve newly constructed, unincorporated grafts should be managed with complete excision. Evidence of bacteremia, pseudoaneurysm formation, or local hemorrhage should prompt graft removal, with placement of a new access at a different site.

D. **Pseudoaneurysm formation.** Pseudoaneurysms result from destruction of the vessel wall and replacement by biophysically inferior collagenous tissue, usually after repetitive puncture of the same vessel segment. A downstream stenosis predisposes to upstream aneurysm formation. Major complications include rupture, infection (which is promoted by intra-aneurysmal thrombus), and, rarely, antegrade or retrograde embolization. Prior to any intervention, imaging is indispensable for identification of thrombus and assessment of the venous anastomosis and outflow. Aneurysmal dilations of AV fistulae often can be treated by surgical correction, including partial or complete resection of the aneurysmal sac, repair of accompanying stenoses, and reconstruction of an adequate lumen. Aneurysm in an AV graft calls for replacement of the weakened graft segment.

   E. Arterial "steal" syndrome. All AV accesses divert or "steal" blood from the distal circulation to a certain extent. A clinical syndrome resulting from this decrease in distal circulation occurs when the various local compensatory mechanisms fail; this syndrome is reported to occur in approximately 1% of patients with distal AV accesses (*Surgery* 1991;110:664). The clinical presentations of arterial insufficiency in the tissues distal to the fistula may include ischemic pain, neuropathy, ulceration, and gangrene. Patients with diabetes, prior AV access, or atherosclerotic disease are at a higher risk. Patients with mild ischemia complain of subjective coldness and paresthesias without sensory or motor loss and can be managed expectantly with increasing exercise tolerance. Failure of these symptoms to improve may require surgical correction with banding or ligation. Severe ischemia requires immediate surgical intervention to avoid irreversible nerve injury.

   F. Venous hypertension. Venous hypertension can be caused by the presence or development of outflow vein obstruction. It manifests as swelling, skin discoloration, and hyperpigmentation in the access limb. In chronic cases, ulceration and pain may develop. Management consists of correction of stenosis and disconnecting the veins that are responsible for retrograde flow and pressure transmission.

   G. Congestive heart failure. Venous return to the heart, cardiac output, and myocardial work can significantly increase after AV fistula or graft placement, leading to cardiomegaly and congestive heart failure in some patients. Hypercirculation ensues if the outflow resistance is too low and the anastomosis is too wide. This problem is more common with ePTFE grafts and brachial artery fistulas. Correction involves narrowing the proximal shunt or graft with either a prosthetic band or suture ligature. Occasionally, a new access must be constructed using a smaller-diameter conduit or tapered prosthetic material.

VIII. VASCULAR ACCESS MONITORING

   A. Angiography (fistulogram) remains the gold standard for the evaluation of access problems. However, the need for frequent evaluations and the invasive nature of angiography prevent it from being a practical option for routine surveillance.

   B. Doppler ultrasound measures access flow and correlates with the presence and severity of stenoses detected by angiography. Blood flow below a critical level (350 mL/minute) or a reduction in flow over time (>15%) predicts the presence of stenosis and the development of thrombosis.

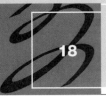

THORACOABDOMINAL VASCULAR DISEASE
Rochus K. Voeller and Luis A. Sanchez

*T*he vast majority of aortic diseases are secondary to atherosclerotic changes of the arterial wall. This is primarily a progressive disease, influenced to a degree by genetic predisposition. However, the evolution of the disease for most individuals can be modified by changes in environmental factors, particularly diet and exercise. The arterial wall is composed of the intima, media, and adventitia. Endothelium lines the intima. The media contains layers of smooth muscle cells and an extracellular matrix (ECM) of elastin, collagen, and proteoglycans. The adventitia is made of loose connective tissue and fibroblasts. An arterial aneurysm is a weakness of the arterial wall resulting in a permanent localized dilation greater than 50% of the normal vessel diameter. All three layers are dilated, but the majority of degeneration occurs in the media. Occlusive arterial disease (i.e., renal artery stenosis and mesenteric ischemia), on the other hand, is caused by atherosclerotic change of the arterial intima.

I. **ABDOMINAL AORTIC ANEURYSMS** (AAAs) are the most common type of arterial aneurysm, occurring in 3% to 10% of people older than 50 years of age in the Western world (*Br J Surg* 1998;85:155). They are five times more common in men than in women and 3.5 times more common in whites than in African Americans.
   A. **Pathophysiology.** Ninety percent of AAAs are believed to be degenerative in origin, whereas 5% are inflammatory and the remainder are idiopathic (*J Vasc Surg* 2003;38:584). Matrix metalloproteinases (MMPs) have been documented to have increased activity in aneurysmal tissues. Infection and possible autoimmune processes may play a role in AAA formation. *Chlamydia pneumonia,* B-type lymphocytes, plasma cells, and large amounts of immunoglobulin have been found in the walls of AAAs. Familial clustering of AAAs has been noted in 15% to 25% of patients undergoing aneurysm surgery. The risk of rupture correlates with wall tension in accordance with Laplace's law, such that the risk of aneurysm rupture increases exponentially with aneurysm diameter (Fig. 18-1). Ninety-five percent of AAAs are infrarenal, 25% involve the iliac arteries, and 2% involve the renal or other visceral arteries (*J Cardiovasc Surg* 1991;32:636). Four percent are associated with peripheral (e.g., femoral or popliteal) aneurysms.
   B. **Diagnosis**
      1. **Clinical manifestations.** Seventy-five percent of AAAs are asymptomatic and are found incidentally. Aneurysm expansion or rupture may cause severe back, flank, or abdominal pain and varying degrees of shock. Distal embolization, thrombosis, and duodenal or ureteral compression can produce symptoms. Fifty percent of AAAs are identifiable on physical examination as a pulsatile mass at or above the umbilicus. The differential diagnosis includes a tortuous aorta or an abdominal mass lying adjacent to the normal aorta that might transmit aortic pulsations (e.g., lymphoma, pancreatic pseudocysts or carcinoma, mesenteric masses). AAA rupture may mimic renal colic, peritonitis, duodenal perforation, pancreatitis, degenerative spine disease, acute disk herniation, or myocardial infarction.
      2. **Radiologic evaluation**
         a. **Abdominal cross-table lateral films.** In 75% of patients with an AAA, arterial wall calcification suggests the presence of an aneurysm and permits a gross estimation of aneurysm diameter.

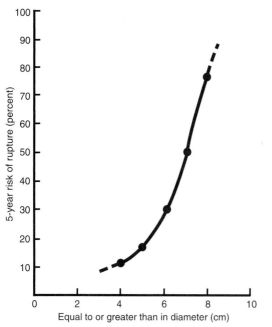

Figure 18-1. The 5-year risk of rupture is plotted against aneurysm size, showing the sharp increase in risk of rupture beyond a diameter of 6 cm. (With permission from Hollier L, Rutherford RB. Infrarenal aortic aneurysms. In: Rutherford RB, ed. *Vascular Surgery,* 3rd ed. Philadelphia: WB Saunders; 1989:912.)

   b. **Ultrasonography and computed tomography (CT) scanning** demonstrate AAAs with an accuracy of 95% and 100%, respectively, and are useful for serial examinations of small aneurysms. **CT angiography** is rapidly becoming the gold standard for evaluating AAAs because it allows operative planning for endovascular approaches.

   c. **Magnetic resonance (MR) scan** is comparable to CT but avoids radiation exposure and is useful in patients with intravenous contrast contraindications.

   d. **Aortography** is **not** sensitive for the diagnosis of AAA because it may underestimate the aneurysm size or fail to reveal the aneurysm owing to the presence of mural thrombus. However, aortography is indicated to evaluate suspected renal or mesenteric artery stenosis and lower-extremity occlusive disease (*Ann Vasc Surg* 1990;4:419).

C. **Elective management of abdominal aortic aneurysm.** The risk of aneurysm rupture correlates best with aneurysm size (Fig. 18-1) (*Ann Surg* 1966;164:678). However, even small aneurysms can rupture.

   1. **Medical management.** Patients with small aneurysms (<4.5 cm in diameter) without risk factors for rupture can be followed using ultrasound or CT scan yearly, and patients with larger ones are followed more frequently. Smoking cessation, control of hypertension, and treatment of chronic pulmonary obstructive disease are very important (*J Vasc Surg* 2002;35:72). Doxycycline is being investigated as an agent that may retard aneurysm growth, based on its MMP-inhibiting properties (*J Vasc Surg* 2001;34:606).

   2. **Elective surgical treatment.** Operative mortality ranges from less than 5% for uncomplicated AAA to greater than 50% for ruptured AAA (*Br J Surg* 1998;85:1624). Five-year survival after elective repair of AAA is no different from that for age-matched patients without AAA. Associated cardiovascular disease, hypertension, decreased renal function, chronic obstructive lung disease, and morbid obesity increase operative risk (*Arch Intern Med* 1995;155:1998). Table 18-1 outlines the cardiac evaluation of patients with an AAA. Indications

TABLE 18-1	Schemes of Cardiac Evaluation in Patients with Abdominal Aortic Aneurysms (AAAs)

I	Asymptomatic cardiac status → AAA repair
II	Mild, stable cardiac symptoms → noninvasive cardiac study (dobutamine echocardiogram or dipyridamole-thallium stress test) Study positive → coronary angioplasty Study negative → AAA repair
III	Significant cardiac symptoms → coronary angioplasty Significant CAD → CABG Insignificant CAD → AAA repair
IV	Very elderly, LVEF <20%, small AAA → observe Unreconstructible CAD → AAA repair with cardiac support

CABG, coronary artery bypass grafting; CAD, coronary artery disease; LVEF, left ventricular ejection fraction.
With permission from Hollier L, Rutherford RB. Infrarenal aortic aneurysms. In: Rutherford RB, ed. *Vascular Surgery*, 3rd ed. Philadelphia: WB Saunders; 1989:915.

for **surgical management** for AAAs include the following:
   a. Symptomatic aneurysms of any size.
   b. Aneurysms exceeding 5 cm diameter.
   c. Increase in diameter by more than 0.5 cm/year (*J Vasc Surg* 2003;37:1106).
   d. Saccular aneurysms (due to potential for active infection).
   e. Relative indications for repair of smaller AAAs include poorly controlled hypertension (diastolic blood pressure ≥100 mm Hg) and significant chronic obstructive pulmonary disease (1-second forced expiratory volume <50% of predicted value) (*Ann Surg* 1999;230:289).
   f. Relative contraindications to elective repair include recent myocardial infarction, intractable congestive heart failure, unreconstructible coronary artery disease, life expectancy of less than 2 years, and incapacitating neurologic deficits after a stroke.
   3. Operative technique. In the standard repair, the aneurysm is approached through a midline abdominal incision and exposed by incising the retroperitoneum. Alternatively, a left retroperitoneal approach is advantageous in obese patients, those with chronic pulmonary obstructive disease, and patients with previous intraabdominal surgery. In addition, proximal control of the aorta at the mesenteric level or above is more easily achieved via this approach. Next, the duodenum and left renal vein are dissected off the aorta in the transabdominal approach. After heparinization, the aorta and iliac arteries are cross-clamped. Aortotomy is then made and extended longitudinally to the aneurysm "neck," where the aorta is either transected or cut in a T fashion. The aneurysm is opened, thrombus is removed, and bleeding lumbar arteries are suture ligated. The proximal anastomosis is performed to nonaneurysmal aorta using a tube or bifurcation graft. The distal anastomosis is completed at the aortic bifurcation (tube graft) or at the iliac or femoral arteries (bifurcation graft), as the disease dictates. After the clamps have been removed and hemostasis is ensured, the aneurysm wall is closed over the graft.
D. Management of ruptured abdominal aortic aneurysm
   1. Preoperative management. Unstable patients with a presumed diagnosis of a ruptured aneurysm (hypotension, abdominal or back pain, and a pulsatile abdominal mass or history of aneurysmal disease) are gently resuscitated with fluids (crystalloid, colloid, or blood) to maintain organ perfusion pressure. Hypertension is avoided to lessen further bleeding. Unstable patients are transferred immediately to the operating room for exploration, whereas those who are stable should undergo emergency CT scanning to confirm the diagnosis.

2. **Operative management** is aimed at rapidly controlling the aorta. Anesthetic induction is delayed until the surgeon is ready to make the abdominal incision. Through a midline incision, the aorta is cross-clamped or compressed at the diaphragmatic hiatus. The retroperitoneal hematoma is opened, and the proximal neck of the aneurysm is identified and cross-clamped. Distal vessel dissection continues, and management is similar to repair of an elective AAA. Bifurcation grafts should be avoided in favor of the more expeditious tube graft techniques if possible. Heparin should also be avoided in these patients due to the high risk of intraoperative and postoperative bleeding. Some centers are now approaching ruptured AAAs with endovascular techniques by deploying an occlusive balloon inserted through the femoral artery as a means of controlling the aorta above the aneurysm.

E. **Complications** from open AAA repair
   1. **Arrhythmia, myocardial ischemia, or infarction** may occur.
   2. **Intraoperative hemorrhage** can be reduced by clamping the aorta proximal to the aneurysm and the iliac arteries distally. Once the aneurysm is opened, retrograde bleeding from lumbar arteries must be controlled rapidly with transfixing ligatures. Blood should be salvaged in the operating room and autotransfused to the patient.
   3. **Aortic cross-clamping shock,** which may occur on release of the aortic cross-clamp, may be obviated by adequate hydration and slow release of the aortic cross-clamp.
   4. **Renal insufficiency** may be related to intravenous contrast, inadequate hydration, hypotension, a period of aortic clamping above the renal arteries, or embolization of the renal arteries.
   5. **Lower-extremity ischemia** may result from embolism or thrombosis, especially in emergency operations for which heparin might not be used. Embolism to the lower extremities can be prevented by minimizing manipulation of the aneurysm prior to clamping and by perfusing the hypogastric arteries before perfusing the external iliac arteries at the time of unclamping. Use of a Fogarty catheter to remove a clot from lower-extremity vessels is indicated when leg ischemia is identified in the operating room.
   6. **Microemboli** arising from atherosclerotic debris can cause cutaneous ischemia ("trash foot"), which is usually treated expectantly as long as the major vessels are patent. Amputation may be required if significant necrosis results.
   7. **Gastrointestinal complications** consist of prolonged paralytic ileus, anorexia, periodic constipation, or diarrhea. This problem is diminished by using the left retroperitoneal approach. A more serious complication, ischemic colitis of the sigmoid colon, is related to ligation of the inferior mesenteric artery in the absence of adequate collateral circulation. Symptoms include leukocytosis, significant fluid requirement in the first 8 to 12 postoperative hours, fever, and peritoneal irritation. Diagnosis is made by sigmoidoscopy to 20 cm above the anal verge. Necrosis that is limited to the mucosa may be treated expectantly with antibiotics and bowel rest. Necrosis of the muscularis causes segmental strictures, which may require delayed segmental resection. Transmural necrosis requires immediate resection of necrotic colon and construction of an end colostomy.
   8. **Paraplegia,** a rare complication of infrarenal aneurysm surgery, may occur after repair of a ruptured AAA due to spinal cord ischemia. Supraceliac cross-clamping and prolonged hypotension increase the risk of paraplegia. Obliteration or embolization of important spinal artery collateral flow via the internal iliac arteries or an abnormally low origin of the accessory spinal artery (artery of Adamkiewicz) can result in paraplegia.
   9. **Sexual dysfunction** and retrograde ejaculation result from damage to the sympathetic plexus during dissection near the aortic bifurcation, especially around the proximal left common iliac artery.

F. **Endovascular management** of AAAs has dramatically decreased the acute morbidity of open surgery. It is important to note that the **indications** for endovascular treatment of AAA are no different than those for traditional open operative repair.

1. The most important **selection criterion** for endovascular treatment of an AAA is aortoiliac anatomy. Assessment of the AAA on preoperative CT angiogram includes the following factors:

   a. Length and diameter of nondilated and healthy infrarenal aorta (the neck). Most devices require a proximal neck that is 1.5 cm long, and some devices allow suprarenal attachment with an open stent segment. Current endograft dimensions at the proximal end are up to 36 mm in diameter.

   b. Angle between the neck and aneurysm. Significant angulation between the neck and adjacent aneurysm (>45 degrees) makes proximal graft deployment technically difficult and is associated with a higher risk of treatment failure.

   c. Presence of intraluminal thrombus. Significant mural thrombus or atheroma in the proximal neck can prevent adequate sealing of an endograft and therefore represents a relative contraindication for endovascular treatment.

   d. Shape of the aortic neck. The proximal neck segment geometry is also important in that a cone-shaped neck or reverse taper (i.e., widens more distally) precludes adequate apposition of the endograft to the aortic wall.

   e. All currently approved endovascular grafts are bifurcated and extend to the iliac arteries. Iliac artery tortuosity, calcification, and luminal narrowing, in combination with the profile of the delivery system, are critical for successful endograft delivery and deployment without complication.

   f. Patent aortic branches may influence the decision as to whether to proceed with endograft placement. A renal artery or large accessory renal artery arising from the proximal neck or the presence of a horseshoe kidney with multiple renal arteries is often a contraindication for endograft placement. Patent lumbar arteries arising from the aneurysm do not preclude endograft placement. A patent inferior mesenteric artery (IMA) associated with large mesenteric collaterals (e.g., meandering mesenteric artery) or a large patent IMA suggests abnormal mesenteric blood supply and risk of large-bowel ischemia with endograft coverage of the IMA orifice. Therefore, these vascular patterns are contraindications to endograft placement.

2. **Technique.** All current aortic endovascular grafts are usually introduced through direct femoral artery exposure. Percutaneous techniques for graft deployment are under development. Most endovascular grafts are bifurcated, and many devices are modular (consisting of two or more components). Endografts typically have a full-length stent skeleton that prevents graft kinking. The deployment is mostly by unsheathing of self-expanding stents. Oversized stent grafts (by 10% to 15%) are selected based on preoperative assessment of arterial diameter to ensure adequate graft apposition to the aortic wall. If necessary, graft length can be tailored by means of overlapping extension segments in modular devices. Positioning of the iliac limbs in bifurcated unibody aortic stent grafts is performed by using guidewires and pullwires placed across the aortic bifurcation. Modular aortic stent grafts include a bifurcated portion with short and long limbs. After deployment of the bifurcated main graft, a separate wire is placed through the opposite limb in a retrograde fashion from the contralateral femoral artery to guide deployment of an appropriate limb extension. The hypogastric artery is identified by intraoperative angiography, and the distal attachment site of the stent graft is positioned proximal to the hypogastric artery. An ipsilateral extension is added if necessary in similar fashion.

3. **Complications of endograft repairs of AAAs**

   a. Early complications include **branch occlusion, distal embolization, graft thrombosis, and arterial injury** (especially external iliac artery avulsion at the common iliac bifurcation in patients with small, calcified, diseased iliac arteries). These complications are often corrected endovascularly but may require emergent conversion to open repair.

   b. **Arterial dissection** may occur with device introduction, but this may not require additional treatment if the endograft spans the segment of dissection. Additional stents can be used to treat the dissected vessel if necessary.

c. As with open surgical AAA repair, **bowel ischemia** may occur postoperatively secondary to embolization or hypoperfusion, but it is rare. **Renal dysfunction** may occur because of the nephrotoxicity of the contrast agent used for intra-operative angiography or because of direct injury due to embolization or renal artery occlusion.

d. **Graft migration** occurs in 1% to 6% of patients, is associated with challenging arterial anatomy and poor graft placement, and can typically be treated with secondary endovascular procedures.

e. **Endoleak** is defined as failure to exclude the aneurysmal sac fully from arterial blood flow, potentially predisposing to rupture of the aneurysm sac (*J Endovasc Surg* 1997;4:152). Management strategies for endoleaks discovered on follow-up imaging studies are evolving. For any endoleak that is associated with aneurysm sac enlargement, intervention is required. Endoleaks are usually corrected by endovascular means but may require conversion to open surgical repair.

(1) In general, endoleaks from the proximal or distal attachment sites **(type I)** warrant intervention because these are frequently associated with increasing aneurysm sac size. Proximal endoleaks may be sealed with angioplasty, placement of a stent, or an endovascular graft component.

(2) **Type II** endoleaks are due to collateral flow (IMA, lumbar arteries) and are generally closely observed. Type II endoleaks may be treated with embolization through collateral vessels (via the hypogastric artery for lumbar branch bleeding, via the superior mesenteric artery for IMA bleeding) or directly through the aneurysm sac via a translumbar approach, which is usually the most successful strategy.

(3) **Type III** endoleaks are usually due to component separation, and they should be corrected as soon as they are diagnosed.

(4) **Type IV** endoleaks are due to porosity of the graft material and are usually self-limiting.

4. **Results.** Relative to open surgical repair, endovascular treatment of AAA is associated with a reduction in perioperative morbidity, shorter duration of hospitalization (*J Vasc Surg* 2003;37:262), and reduction of perioperative mortality (*J Vasc Surg* 2000;31:134). The short- and mid-term results are encouraging and are similar to results seen with open repair, but long-term results are not yet available. Close follow-up with CT scanning every 6 months initially and yearly after the first year is essential to understand the behavior of these devices. Future fenestrated and branched devices may allow treatment of pararenal and other more complex AAAs.

II. **THORACIC AORTIC ANEURYSMS** are primarily a disease of the elderly. Ascending and transverse arch aneurysms each comprise 25% of thoracic aortic aneurysms (TAAs). The remaining 50% occur in the descending aorta (thoracic or thoracoabdominal). Most descending TAAs begin just distal to the left subclavian artery.

A. **Pathophysiology.** TAAs are divided into five main types: ascending, transverse, descending, thoracoabdominal, and traumatic. Ascending aortic aneurysms are usually caused by medial degeneration. Transverse, descending, and thoracoabdominal aortic aneurysms are related to atherosclerosis. Hypertension contributes to their expansion.

B. **Diagnosis**

1. **Clinical manifestations** are usually absent; most nontraumatic TAAs are detected as incidental findings on chest films obtained for other purposes. A minority of patients may present with chest discomfort or pain that intensifies with aneurysm expansion or rupture, aortic valvular regurgitation, congestive heart failure, compression of adjacent structures (recurrent laryngeal nerve, left-mainstem bronchus, esophagus, superior vena cava, porta hepatis), erosion into adjacent structures (esophagus, lung, airway), or distal embolization.

2. **Radiologic evaluation. Chest films** may reveal a widened mediastinum or an enlarged calcific aortic shadow. Traumatic aneurysms may be associated with skeletal fractures. **MR or CT scanning** with intravenous contrast provides precise

estimation of the size and extent of these aneurysms and facilitates the planning of surgical therapy. **Echocardiography** is useful in evaluating aneurysms involving the aortic arch. **Aortography** demonstrates the proximal and distal extent of the aneurysm and the vessels arising from it.

C. **Surgical management** depends on the type and location of the TAA. Repair of proximal arch aneurysms requires cardiopulmonary bypass and circulatory arrest. Preclotted woven polyethylene terephthalate **(Dacron)** is the graft of choice. The ascending and transverse arches are repaired through a median sternotomy incision. The descending and thoracoabdominal aortas are approached through a left posterolateral thoracotomy incision. Intraoperative management of patients undergoing thoracotomy is facilitated by selective ventilation of the right lung using a double-lumen endobronchial tube. Cerebrospinal fluid drainage during and after surgery for descending and thoracoabdominal aneurysms can lower the incidence of postoperative paraplegia.

1. **Ascending aortic arch aneurysms**
   a. **Indications** for surgical repair include symptomatic or rapidly expanding aneurysms, aneurysms greater than 7 cm in diameter, ascending aortic dissections, mycotic aneurysms, and asymptomatic aneurysms greater than 5.5 cm in diameter in patients with Marfan syndrome (*Coron Artery Dis* 2002;13:85).
   b. **Operative management.** An aneurysm arising distal to the coronary ostia is replaced with an interposition graft. A proximal aneurysm resulting in aortic valve incompetency is replaced with a composite valved conduit **(Bentall procedure)** or a supracoronary graft with separate aortic valve replacement. Ascending arch aneurysms due to Marfan syndrome or cystic medial necrosis are repaired with aortic valve replacement owing to the high incidence of valvular incompetence associated with aneurysmal dilation of the native aortic root. When a composite graft is used, the coronary arteries are anastomosed directly to the conduit.

2. **Transverse aortic arch aneurysms**
   a. **Indications** for repair include aneurysms greater than 6 cm in diameter, aortic arch dissections, and ascending arch aneurysms that extend into the transverse arch.
   b. **Operative management.** After opening the aorta under hypothermic circulatory arrest, the distal anastomosis is performed using a beveled graft, followed by anastomosis of an island of the brachiocephalic vessels to the superior aspect of the graft. The proximal anastomosis is constructed to the supracoronary aorta (if the aortic valve is not involved) or to a segment of composite valved conduit interposed to complete the arch reconstruction. Involvement of the transverse arch and its branch vessels requires interposition grafting to the involved vessels.

3. **Descending thoracic aortic aneurysms**
   a. **Indications** for repair include symptomatic aneurysms and asymptomatic aneurysms greater than 6 cm in diameter.
   b. **Operative management.** Before cross-clamping, the anesthesiologist pharmacologically controls proximal blood pressure. After the distal clamp is applied, a proximal clamp is placed just distal to the left subclavian artery or between the left common carotid and left subclavian arteries. Selected intercostal branches are reattached to the aortic interposition graft. Use of left heart partial bypass is a valuable adjunct, and catheter-based drainage of cerebrospinal fluid may reduce the incidence of postoperative paraplegia.

4. **Thoracoabdominal aneurysms**
   a. **Indications** for repair include symptomatic aneurysms and aneurysms greater than 6 cm in diameter.
   b. **Operative management** consists of tube graft replacement along with anastomosis of major branches to the graft. Aneurysms involving the thoracic and proximal abdominal aortic segments may be approached through a left posterolateral thoracotomy extended to the umbilicus. Left heart partial bypass (atriofemoral) is often used, both to protect the heart from overdistention and

to provide distal blood flow while the aorta is clamped. Sodium nitroprusside may be given before cross-clamping to reduce proximal blood pressure, and cerebrospinal fluid drainage is used as an adjunct to decrease the incidence of postoperative paraplegia. The thoracic aorta is clamped and opened to perform the proximal anastomosis while visceral perfusion is maintained retrograde. The aorta is clamped distally opening the remaining aneurysm. The orifices of all major aortic branches are occluded with balloon catheters or vascular clamps. Temporary perfusion can be maintained to those branches during aneurysm repair by using balloon catheters connected to the atriofemoral bypass. The anastomoses of significant aortic branches to the graft are performed as an island patch or separate bypasses. The clamp is moved to the graft below the renal arteries to reperfuse all visceral vessels in a prograde fashion. The distal anastomosis is made either to the uninvolved aorta or to the iliac arteries.

   5. Traumatic aortic aneurysms
      a. Indications. Urgent repair is indicated, except when precluded by more compelling life-threatening injuries or major central nervous system trauma.
      b. Operative management. Using proximal and distal control, these aneurysms may be repaired by primary aortorrhaphy, aneurysmectomy, and end-to-end reanastomosis or by interposition grafting. Endovascular techniques have also been reported.

D. Possible **complications** of thoracic aortic surgery include arrhythmia, myocardial infarction, intraoperative hemorrhage, stroke, aortic cross-clamp shock, renal insufficiency, lower-extremity ischemia, microemboli, and disseminated intravascular coagulopathy. The incidence of paraplegia may be as high as 30% with some types of TAAs (*Ann Thorac Surg* 2007;83:S856). This risk can be reduced by multimodal therapies implemented to prevent or minimize spinal cord ischemia: distal aortic perfusion, intercostal and lumbar artery reimplantation, preoperative or intraoperative localization of spinal blood supply, hypothermia, cerebrospinal fluid drainage, and pharmacotherapy.

E. Endovascular management of thoracic aortic aneurysm
   1. Indications and technique. Because of the considerable morbidity and mortality associated with surgical repair of descending thoracic aneurysms, the endovascular approach to aneurysm exclusion is particularly attractive. The decision to proceed with endovascular graft placement is based on similar anatomic considerations as for AAA: adequate length (2 cm) and diameter (20 to 37 mm) of the proximal and distal aneurysm necks, absence of significant mural thrombus within the neck, and aortic and iliofemoral anatomy amenable to device introduction. In situations in which the proximal neck length is too short, seating of the proximal graft end over the origin of the left subclavian artery has been performed successfully with or without an adjunctive left carotid-left subclavian transposition or bypass. Only one device, the TAG graft (W. L. Gore and Associates, Flagstaff, Arizona), is approved in the United States for the treatment of thoracic aortic aneurysms at this time, with other devices on the horizon.
   2. Results and complications. Early results for the use of endovascular devices are encouraging. Various studies have suggested low morbidity and mortality and high rates of aneurysm exclusion (*J Vasc Interv Radiol* 2004;15:361, *J Vasc Surg* 2005;42:1063, *Ann Thorac Surg* 2006;81:1570). Future fenestrated and branched devices may allow endovascular treatment of more complex arch and thoracoabdominal aneurysms, but this technology is in the developmental phase.

III. OTHER ARTERIAL ANEURYSMS
A. Renal artery aneurysms occur in approximately 0.1% of the general population and constitute approximately 1% of all aneurysms (*Semin Vasc Surg* 2005; 18:202).
   1. Pathophysiology. These aneurysms can be either extrarenal (85%) or intrarenal (15%). Extrarenal renal artery aneurysms are subdivided into saccular (most common), fusiform, and dissecting. Saccular aneurysms classically occur near the bifurcation of the renal artery (*Semin Vasc Surg* 1996;9:236). Fusiform aneurysms

are poststenotic dilations associated with renal artery stenosis. Renal artery dissections are associated with renal artery fibroplasias. Intrarenal aneurysms may be congenital, traumatic, or related to collagen vascular disease.

2. **Diagnosis**
   a. Clinical manifestations are usually absent until complications arise. Rupture and dissection may produce flank pain or hematuria (intrarenal aneurysms).
   b. Physical examination commonly reveals **hypertension and an abdominal bruit.** A palpable mass occurs in fewer than 10% of cases.
   c. Laboratory tests may reveal anemia or hematuria.
   d. Abdominal films may demonstrate **ring-shaped calcifications** in the renal hilum in patients with calcific saccular aneurysms. CT scan may reveal an incidental renal artery aneurysm. Arteriography confirms the diagnosis and details the anatomy of the renal branches.

3. **Operative management** is indicated for aneurysms that rupture, are associated with dissection, or produce renal artery stenosis leading to hypertension. Saccular aneurysms are repaired in pregnant women owing to an increased risk of rupture. Small aneurysms at the bifurcation can be treated with aneurysmectomy and reconstruction of the bifurcation. Aneurysmectomy with aortorenal or splenorenal bypass is advised for large aneurysms or stenotic lesions. Polar renal artery aneurysms can be excised with end-to-end arterial reanastomosis. Ruptured renal artery aneurysms are usually treated with nephrectomy.

B. **Infected aneurysms** have risen in incidence with the increased prevalence of immunocompromised patients and invasive transarterial procedures.

1. **Pathophysiology.** Infected aneurysms can be divided in to four types: mycotic aneurysm, microbial arteritis with aneurysm, infection of preexisting aneurysm, and posttraumatic infected false aneurysm. The clinical characteristics of each type are summarized in Table 18-2. *Staphylococcus aureus* is the most common pathogen, although *Salmonella* species (arteritis), *Streptococcus* species, and *Staphylococcus epidermidis* (preexisting aneurysms) also may occur. The risk of rupture for Gram-negative exceeds that for Gram-positive infections.

2. **Diagnosis**
   a. Clinical manifestations may be absent or include fever, tenderness, or sepsis. Physical examination may demonstrate a **tender, warm, palpable mass** in an

---

TABLE 18-2   Clinical Characteristics of Infected Aneurysm

	Mycotic aneurysm	Microbial arteritis	Infection of existing aneurysms	Posttraumatic infected false aneurysm
Etiology	Endocarditis	Bacteremia	Bacteremia	Narcotic addiction; trauma
Age (yr)	30–50	>50	>50	<30
Incidence	Rare	Common	Unusual	Very common
Location	Aorta; visceral; intracranial; peripheral	Atherosclerosis; aortoiliac; intimal defects	Infrarenal aorta	Femoral; carotid; injection sites
Bacteriology	Gram-positive cocci	*Salmonella* spp.; others	*Staphylococcus* spp.; *Escherichia coli*; others	*Staphylococcus aureus*; polymicrobial
Mortality (%)	25	75	90	5

With permission from Wilson SE, Van Wagenen P, Passaro E Jr. Arterial infection. *Curr Probl Surg* 1978; 15:11.

extremity aneurysm. Laboratory tests may reveal leukocytosis. Aerobic and anaerobic blood cultures should be obtained, but only 50% of cultures are positive.

b. **Abdominal plain films** may demonstrate vertebral body erosion suggesting infection. **MR or CT scanning** can demonstrate an aneurysm and verify its rupture. **Angiography** delineates the characteristics of the aneurysm. Aneurysms that are saccular, multilobed, or eccentric with a narrow neck are more likely a result of infection.

3. **Management**

a. **Preoperative.** Broad-spectrum antibiotics should be administered intravenously after aerobic and anaerobic blood cultures have been obtained.

b. **Intraoperative.** Goals of surgery include (1) controlling hemorrhage; (2) obtaining arterial specimens for Gram's stain, aerobic and anaerobic cultures, and drug sensitivities; (3) resecting the aneurysm with wide débridement and drainage; and (4) reconstructing major arteries through uninfected tissue planes. Extra-anatomic bypass may be necessary to avoid contamination of the graft. Inline reconstructions with antibiotic-impregnated grafts, cryopreserved vein grafts, or native veins are alternatives that can be used for arterial reconstructions depending on the location of the aneurysm and the extent of the infection.

c. **Postoperative.** Adequate drainage of the aneurysm cavity and long-term antibiotic therapy for at least 6 weeks typically are required.

IV. **RENOVASCULAR DISEASE.** Stenosis or occlusion of the renal arteries may result in hypertension, ischemic nephropathy, or both. **Renovascular hypertension is the most common form of surgically correctable secondary hypertension.** However, because of the predominance of primary hypertension and difficulties in clinical diagnosis of renovascular hypertension, its exact prevalence is difficult to assess.

A. A high index of suspicion is necessary to distinguish patients with potentially correctable renovascular hypertension from the majority of patients with primary hypertension. There are several clinical features that may be used to identify patients with potential renovascular hypertension:

1. The presence of **severe hypertension** in a child or young adult or an adult older than age 50 years.

2. The **sudden development** or **worsening** of hypertension at any age.

3. **Hypertension and unexplained impairment of renal function.**

4. Hypertension that is **refractory** to appropriate multidrug therapy.

5. **Hypertension** in a patient with **extensive coronary disease, cerebral vascular disease, or peripheral vascular disease.**

6. **Worsening of renal function.** Up to 15% of elderly patients hospitalized for the treatment of renal failure are ultimately diagnosed with ischemic nephropathy.

B. On **physical examination,** these patients may have an epigastric, subcostal, or flank bruit. The finding of a unilateral small kidney on any imaging study is a possible indicator.

C. **Pathophysiology**

1. Renal arterial stenosis is perceived by the ipsilateral kidney as a hypovolemic state and as such activates the **renin-angiotensin-aldosterone system.** Typical renovascular hypertension results from unilateral renal artery stenosis (renin-dependent hypertension): Renin release by the affected kidney remains high, and the resulting increase in intravascular volume is eliminated by the unaffected contralateral kidney. Bilateral renal artery stenosis (volume-dependent hypertension) results in an initial rise in renin; once the intravascular volume increases, however, feedback mechanisms return renin levels to near normal.

2. Even in the **absence of hypertension,** a significant renal artery stenosis may be present and may lead to renal failure.

a. In **acute renal failure,** renal arterial stenosis should be considered in the differential diagnosis if the urinary sediment is unremarkable and there are no signs of acute tubular necrosis, glomerulonephritis, or interstitial nephritis. Acute ischemic nephropathy may occur within 2 weeks of starting an angiotensin-converting enzyme (ACE) inhibitor or other antihypertensive or diuretic.

 b. Renal artery stenoses may account for up to 20% of **unexplained chronic renal failure** in patients older than 50 years of age. The diagnosis is more likely in those with generalized atherosclerosis or uncontrolled hypertension.

 c. Isolated unilateral renal artery stenosis generally **does not** cause an increase in the serum creatinine.

3. **Atherosclerosis** causes approximately two thirds of all renovascular lesions in adults and usually affects the ostia and proximal 2 cm of the renal artery. Associated extrarenal atherosclerosis occurs in 15% to 20% of patients.

4. The second-most-common renovascular lesion is **fibromuscular dysplasia,** most commonly medial fibroplasia. These lesions are multifocal, have a characteristic **string-of-beads** appearance on angiography, and typically occur in young and middle-aged women.

D. Diagnosis. Testing for clinically significant renal artery disease must evaluate the **anatomic and physiologic changes.** Anatomic lesions of the renal arteries by themselves correlate poorly with physiologic effect. More important, they also correlate poorly with treatment response.

 1. **Arteriography** remains the best test for making the diagnosis of anatomic renal artery stenosis. However, the usual caveats regarding the risks of arteriography, especially the nephrotoxic effects of the contrast agent, are important to consider.

 2. In patients with a relative contraindication to arteriography, **duplex scanning** is useful for screening. However, this procedure is highly technician dependent.

 3. **MR angiography** with gadolinium-based intravenous contrast is an excellent test for evaluating kidney and main renal artery morphology without nephrotoxins. It may also be useful for evaluating the functional significance of renal artery stenoses. Limitations include imaging of distal renal artery stenoses and patients with implanted devices, morbid obesity, or claustrophobia.

 4. The two most commonly used tests to determine the functional significance of a renal artery lesion are **captopril renal scintigraphy** and **selective renal vein renin measurement.** These tests can be complicated to perform and interpret, especially in patients with bilateral disease or in those taking ACE inhibitors or beta-blockers.

E. Management of fibromuscular disease

 1. Renal artery stenoses resulting from fibromuscular dysplasia rarely causes renal failure, and endovascular treatment of the lesions is frequently successful in treating the hypertension.

 2. **Endovascular techniques (angioplasty) have a high success rate for the treatment of this arterial pathology.** For failure of endovascular treatment (see Section F.3), surgical therapy may be employed, including *ex vivo* repair for complex disease as described in Section F.2.b(4).

F. Management of atherosclerotic disease has a dual purpose: to control target organ damage from hypertension and to avoid progressive ischemic renal failure. However, even with functional studies, response to therapy is difficult to predict because the hypertension may be primarily essential and the renal failure due to hypertensive glomerulosclerosis. No careful clinical studies exist comparing best medical therapy to surgical or endovascular intervention.

 1. **Medical therapy** with antihypertensive drugs is often successful in the management of patients with renovascular hypertension. A combination of beta-blockers and a calcium channel blocker, an ACE inhibitor, or an angiotensin II–receptor inhibitor is commonly used as first-line therapy. ACE inhibitors are often effective, but they should be used cautiously when the entire renal parenchymal mass is at risk, as occurs in renovascular hypertensive patients who have bilateral disease or a solitary kidney. Diuretics should be reserved for second-line therapy.

 2. **Surgical therapy**

  a. The **indications** for intervention are evolving. Classically, surgery usually has been reserved for patients with uncontrollable hypertension refractory to maximal medical therapy. Evidence is accumulating that revascularization may be more important as a means of maintaining renal mass. Consideration should also be given to renal revascularization in patients undergoing aortic surgery for aneurysmal or occlusive disease and concomitant renal stenoses.

b. **Procedures**

(1) **Aortorenal bypass** is the classic open treatment for renal revascularization. The stenotic renal artery is isolated with a segment of infrarenal aorta, and bypass is accomplished using saphenous vein, autologous hypogastric artery (in children), or prosthetic graft.

(2) **Renal endarterectomy** is also an excellent choice for renal revascularization and often is used for bilateral orificial lesions. Most commonly, a transverse arteriotomy is made over the orifices of both renal arteries. Distal endpoints and adequacy of endarterectomy can be assessed intraoperatively using duplex scanning.

(3) **Alternative bypass procedures** are available for patients who are not good candidates for aortorenal bypass due to prior aortic surgery, the presence of severe aortic disease, or unfavorable anatomy. Grafts can be taken from the supraceliac aorta or the superior mesenteric, common hepatic, gastroduodenal, splenic, or iliac arteries. Results for these procedures are comparable to those for direct aortic reconstruction but with less morbidity and mortality.

(4) *Ex vivo* **renal artery reconstruction** with renal autotransplantation is useful in patients with complex lesions that require microvascular techniques and for whom exposure *in situ* is inadequate. These procedures are time consuming, and adequate hypothermic protection from ischemic renal injury may be difficult with the kidney *in situ*. In general, operations requiring more than two branch artery reconstructions or anastomoses should be considered for *ex vivo* repair. Once repair is accomplished, the kidney can be transplanted orthotopically or heterotopically to the ipsilateral iliac fossa.

(5) **Nephrectomy** may be required in patients who have renal infarction, severe nephrosclerosis, severe renal atrophy, noncorrectable renal vascular lesions, failed revascularizations, or a normal contralateral kidney and who are high-risk surgical candidates.

c. **Postoperative care**

(1) **Immediately after operation,** patients should be kept well hydrated to maintain adequate urine output. Concern about the patency of the reconstruction may be addressed by a renal or duplex scan.

(2) **Patient follow-up** should consist of routine blood pressure monitoring, a renal scan, and creatinine determination at 3 months, 12 months, and then yearly. Any recurrence of hypertension or deterioration in renal function should prompt arteriography. Duplex scanning is also a useful test for following reconstructions.

d. **Complications** of renal revascularization include persistent hypertension, acute renal failure, renal artery restenosis, thrombosis, aneurysm formation, and distal embolization.

3. **Endovascular management of renal artery stenosis**

a. **Indications** for angioplasty of renal artery stenosis include the failure of medical management of renovascular hypertension in the absence of any clear indications for open aortic surgery. Balloon angioplasty is the treatment of choice for clinically significant fibromuscular dysplastic lesions of the renal artery. Angioplasty of renal artery atherosclerotic lesions has less favorable results but entails significantly less procedure-related morbidity than surgical bypass or endarterectomy. Surgical therapy also may be preferred in cases of long-segment disease or occlusions or when atherosclerosis is severe and widespread (i.e., to avoid the risk of atheroembolic complications with intra-arterial instrumentation). Renal artery stents are routinely used for restenosis after previous angioplasty, treatment of procedural complications (e.g., dissection), and the treatment of atherosclerotic ostial lesions.

    b. Technique. Intravascular access to the renal artery may be obtained from the femoral, brachial, or axillary arteries (access from the upper extremity may be preferable in cases of caudally angled renal arteries). In patients at high risk for renal failure (e.g., type II diabetes, preexisting renal insufficiency), nephrotoxic contrast may be avoided and angiography can be performed using gadolinium or carbon dioxide. Technical success for renal artery angioplasty is defined as a less than 30% residual stenosis and a pressure gradient across the lesion of less than 10 mm Hg.

    c. Results. Patients with fibromuscular dysplasia respond favorably to percutaneous transluminal angioplasty, with cure rates of greater than 50%. Patients with atherosclerotic disease respond less favorably in the long term, although immediate technical success is seen in almost all patients. Improvements in blood pressure are observed in approximately two thirds of patients; however, only 15% of patients with renal insufficiency demonstrate improved excretory renal function. In addition, up to 15% of patients exhibit decreased renal excretory function following intervention. Angiographic restenosis occurs in 15% to 20% of patients within 1 year of treatment, most commonly in small renal arteries (<4 mm). Based on these data, percutaneous angioplasty with stenting of atherosclerotic disease of the renal artery yields blood pressure, renal function, and anatomic results that are slightly inferior but comparable to contemporary surgical results. Percutaneous intervention is, however, associated with lower morbidity and mortality rates than open surgical procedures.

V. MESENTERIC ISCHEMIA can be a difficult diagnosis to make because most patients are asymptomatic until late in the disease process. Although considerable advances have been made in perioperative care as well as in the diagnosis and treatment of intestinal ischemia, mortality remains greater than 80% due to delays in diagnosis (*Eur J Surg* 1998;64:611).

    A. Acute occlusion

      1. Patients with acute mesenteric ischemia often have multiple risk factors, including significant cardiac disease (frequently atrial fibrillation) and severe atherosclerotic disease of nonmesenteric vessels, and may have a history consistent with chronic intestinal ischemia.

        a. Abdominal pain usually is sudden in onset and intermittent at first, progressing to continuous severe pain. It is often described as **pain out-of-proportion to the degree of abdominal tenderness.** These patients may also have bloody diarrhea before or after the onset of pain.

        b. Mesenteric venous thrombosis presents with varying manifestations, ranging from an asymptomatic state to catastrophic illness. Patients usually complain of prolonged, generalized abdominal pain that develops somewhat less rapidly than with acute mesenteric arterial occlusion. These patients may have occult gastrointestinal bleeding but no frank hemorrhage.

      2. Pathophysiology. Ischemia may result from either an embolus to or thrombosis of the superior mesenteric artery. Bowel ischemia also can result from portomesenteric venous thrombosis.

      3. Diagnosis

        a. The mainstay of diagnosis is **angiography** of the mesenteric circulation, including lateral views of the celiac axis and superior mesenteric artery. Modern **helical CT scans** can often detect proximal mesenteric thrombosis.

        b. Other laboratory findings can include an elevated white blood cell count with a left shift, persistent metabolic acidosis, an elevated lactate level, and an unexplained elevated serum potassium level.

        c. Abdominal plain radiographs are of limited utility. After acute arterial occlusion, the abdominal plain x-ray appears relatively normal. After venous thrombosis, x-rays may show small-bowel wall thickening or air in the portal venous system.

4. Surgical therapy

a. If an embolus or thrombosis is demonstrated, an **emergent embolectomy** should be performed. If a proximal stenosis is present in the superior mesenteric artery, a mesenteric bypass is indicated.

   (1) Assessment of bowel viability at laparotomy is made based on the gross characteristics of the bowel. The bowel is likely viable if it appears pink and if arterial pulsations are present in the adjacent vascular arcades. A number of other techniques have been described, including the use of fluorescein dye, Doppler studies, and tissue oximetry, but these are not substitutes for experienced clinical judgment.

   (2) Second-look procedures are prudent when bowel viability is questionable. Whether to perform a second operation 24 to 48 hours after initial exploration is decided at the time of initial laparotomy, and that decision should not be changed even if the patient's condition improves. This approach is especially important in patients who have extensive bowel involvement and in whom resection of all questionable areas could result in short-bowel syndrome.

b. For **venous occlusion,** surgical intervention rarely is helpful, although anecdotal reports suggest that portomesenteric venous thrombectomy may be beneficial. Similarly, the role of lytic therapy in the treatment of this disorder is unclear. It is imperative to begin systemic anticoagulation as soon as the diagnosis is made to limit progression of the thrombotic process. Frequently, the diagnosis is made at laparotomy. If the diagnosis is made before exploration, however, operation should be reserved until evidence of bowel infarction exists.

5. Perioperative care usually requires maximal medical support; these patients frequently are hemodynamically unstable and develop multiple organ system failure. Admission to the intensive care unit, prolonged endotracheal intubation, parenteral nutrition, and broad-spectrum antibiotic therapy are typically required.

B. Chronic intestinal ischemia

1. Patients with chronic intestinal ischemia present with **intestinal angina,** which is pain related to eating, usually beginning within an hour after eating and abating within 4 hours. Such patients experience significant weight loss related to the decreased ability to absorb food and decreased intake secondary to recurrent pain. The diagnosis usually is made from history alone because the only physical finding may be the presence of an abdominal bruit. In patients with a low-cardiac-output state and chronic intestinal angina, persistent shock may result from acute thrombosis and intestinal necrosis. This can occur in the absence of major vessel occlusion on angiography, and the mortality associated with it is as high as 90%.

2. Surgical therapy. Elective revascularization of the superior mesenteric and celiac arteries using autologous or prosthetic grafts from the aorta or iliac arteries is the treatment of choice. Aortic endarterectomy in patients with aortic and orificial disease is an alternative. The orificial nature of most of these lesions contributed in the past to the poor success of balloon angioplasty, but the addition of balloon-expandable stents has increased the use of these techniques in patients that are poor candidates for open surgical reconstructions.

3. Perioperative care. These patients often are malnourished. Some advocate parenteral nutrition for 1 to 2 weeks before surgery, which is continued postoperatively. Some patients develop a revascularization syndrome consisting of abdominal pain, tachycardia, leukocytosis, and intestinal edema. Concern about the adequacy of revascularization should prompt angiography.

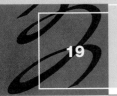

19

PERIPHERAL ARTERIAL OCCLUSIVE DISEASE
Jack R. Oak and Patrick J. Geraghty

*T*he vast majority of occlusive disease is secondary to **atherosclerotic change of the arterial intima.** Major risk factors for developing atherosclerosis include **cigarette smoking, diabetes, dyslipidemia, hypertension, and hyperhomocysteinemia.** Some of these risk factors may be influenced to a degree by genetic predisposition. However, the evolution of the disease for most individuals can be modified by changes in environmental factors, particularly diet and exercise. Atherosclerotic disease is a systemic illness, and although symptomatic disease may predominate in one organ, subclinical disease, particularly of the coronary arteries, is generally present. In fact, 50% of the mortality associated with peripheral arterial reconstructions for atherosclerotic disease is cardiac in nature. Other, less common causes of occlusive disease include fibromuscular dysplasia, radiation-induced vascular injury, and the vasculitides (e.g., Takayasu arteritis and Buerger disease).

 ACUTE ARTERIAL OCCLUSION OF THE EXTREMITY

Symptoms of acute arterial insufficiency occur abruptly. The presentation generally includes the **five Ps** of acute ischemia: **pain, pallor, pulselessness, paresthesias, and paralysis;** patients also may develop poikilothermy, the inability to thermoregulate. The level of occlusion may be localized by the absence of pulses and the level of coolness of the limb. If adequate collateral circulation is not present, irreversible changes may appear as early as 4 to 6 hours after onset. Therefore, priority must be given to restoration of blood flow within this time period. Once the occlusive process has begun, regardless of its cause, vasospasm and propagation of thrombus distal to the site of initial occlusion can contribute to further ischemia.

I. ETIOLOGY
   A. The most common cause of acute arterial insufficiency is **embolization.**
      1. Cardiac sources account for more than 70% of emboli and usually are the result of mural thrombi that develop due to cardiac aneurysms following myocardial infarction or arrhythmias such as atrial fibrillation. Other cardiac sources of emboli include valvular heart disease, prosthetic heart valves, bacterial endocarditis, and atrial myxoma.
      2. Arterial-arterial emboli can result from ulcerated atheroma or aneurysms, although embolization from abdominal aortic aneurysms is distinctly rare. *The blue toe syndrome* occurs in patients with microemboli from unstable proximal arterial plaques and is characterized by the presence of intact pulses and painful ischemic lesions in the distal extremity. Atheroemboli in the lower extremity secondary to plaque disruption by catheters can occur. The severely diseased distal aorta in some of these patients is evident on computed tomography (CT) scan and arteriography and has been termed *shaggy aorta.*
      3. Venous-arterial emboli (paradoxical emboli) can result from an intracardiac shunt (e.g., patent foramen ovale) or intrapulmonary arteriovenous malformations (e.g., Osler-Weber-Rendu syndrome).
      4. Occasionally, it is difficult to discern whether a person with advanced atherosclerotic disease has had an embolus or whether an already compromised vessel has

undergone acute thrombosis. This is particularly true in patients without arrhythmias or prior myocardial infarction. The presence of contralateral pulses and the absence of a history of claudication may help in making this differentiation.

B. Direct arterial trauma is frequently obvious but may initially be occult. Arterial stenosis or occlusion occurs only after an intimal flap or arterial wall hematoma progresses sufficiently to cause symptoms. Arterial compromise can also occur in the setting of compression by joint dislocations (e.g., knee), bone fragments (e.g., tibial plateau fracture), or compartment syndrome.

C. Other causes of acute ischemia include arterial thrombosis, aortic dissection, venous outflow occlusion, and low-flow state.

II. DIAGNOSIS AND EVALUATION

A. If history and physical examination demonstrate clear evidence of embolization, **definitive therapy** should not be delayed. If there is a concern that the occlusive process may be thrombotic, however, **arteriography** may be indicated. Angiographically, embolic occlusions can be distinguished from thrombotic occlusions by their occurrence just distal to vascular bifurcations and by the concave shadow formed at the interface with the contrast. In select cases, thrombolysis may be a useful adjunct for defining underlying occlusive disease. In general, patients with acute ischemia unrelated to trauma should be considered to have coexistent cardiac disease. All patients should have an electrocardiogram and chest x-ray performed. After limb revascularization, a transesophageal echocardiogram can be useful in diagnosing a cardiac source.

B. Patients who present with penetrating **trauma,** long-bone fractures, or joint dislocations may have vascular injuries. In certain situations, duplex scan of the injured area can be useful in the diagnosis of intimal flap, pseudoaneurysm, or arterial or venous thrombi. Patients with penetrating injuries who display "hard" signs of arterial injury need urgent surgical intervention without preoperative angiography. **Hard signs** of arterial injury include the following:

1. Diminished or absent pulses distal to an injury.

2. Ischemia distal to an injury.

3. Visible arterial bleeding from a wound.

4. A bruit at or distal to the site of injury.

5. Large, expanding, or pulsatile hematomas.

6. Soft signs of injury include the anatomic proximity of a wound to a major vessel, injury to an anatomically related nerve, unexplained hemorrhagic shock, or a moderately sized hematoma. In those with only soft signs, a careful documentation of pulses by **Doppler pressure** distal to the injury should be undertaken, along with comparison with the contralateral limb. A difference of greater than 10% to 20% suggests the need for arteriography or exploration.

III. MANAGEMENT

A. Once a diagnosis of acute arterial ischemia due to emboli or thrombi is made, **heparin** should be administered immediately. An intravenous bolus of 80 units/kg followed by an intravenous infusion of 18 units/kg/hour is usually satisfactory. Partial thromboplastin time (PTT) should be maintained between 60 and 80 seconds.

1. Surgical therapy, such as embolectomy, should be performed urgently in patients with an obvious embolus and acute ischemia. Embolectomy can be done under local anesthesia if the patient cannot tolerate general anesthesia. Once the artery is isolated, a Fogarty catheter is passed proximally and distally to extract the embolus and associated thrombus. In some cases, intraoperative thrombolysis may be necessary because distal vessels may be thrombosed beyond the reach of the Fogarty catheter. Distal patency can be proved with an intraoperative arteriogram, depending on the status of distal vessels and pulses after embolectomy. In the leg, if adequate distal perfusion is not established and an angiogram demonstrates distal thrombus, the distal popliteal artery and tibial arteries may be explored via angiographic or surgical approach. In conjunction with steerable guidewires, Fogarty catheters can be used to select the anterior tibial, posterior tibial, and peroneal arteries to retrieve distal thrombus. When angiographic approaches fail, popliteal artery cutdown can allow direct access to these vessels. The arteriotomy can be closed with a patch graft if there is arterial narrowing. Bypass grafting may also be required if significant preexisting arterial disease in the affected segment is discovered.

2. **Thrombolytic therapy** may be useful in patients with clearly viable extremities in whom thrombosis is the likely underlying cause of their acute ischemia. In general, the fresher the thrombus, the more successful thrombolysis can be. Thrombolysis and follow-up angiography frequently identify an underlying stenosis that may be treated by balloon angioplasty/stent or by surgical means.

   a. Lytic agents are instilled through an intra-arterial catheter placed as close to the thrombus as possible. **Urokinase** was the agent of choice until 1999, when the U.S. Food and Drug Administration withdrew the drug from the market because of production concerns. Dosing varies from 60,000 to 120,000 units/hour, with an optional loading dose of approximately 200,000 units. **Reteplase** (0.5 to 0.75 units/hour) and **alteplase** (t-PA, 0.5 to 1 mg/hour) are also in use and are administered with subtherapeutic heparin (approximately 400 units/hour intravenously). Complication rates of less than 10% have been reported for thrombolysis. Repeat arteriography is performed 6 to 18 hours after initiation of treatment to gauge the results. Duration of therapy is generally between 4 and 16 hours but may extend for as long as 30 hours.

   b. During thrombolysis, the patient is usually monitored in the **intensive care unit (ICU).** Thrombin time, fibrinogen level, fibrin degradation product level, PTT, and complete blood count are followed closely to limit the risk of hemorrhage. In general, the likelihood of serious hemorrhagic complications increases when fibrinogen levels drop below 100 mg/dL and the PTT rises above three to five times normal. Once the artery is open, the patient can be managed either with systemic anticoagulation or with surgical intervention (i.e., operative arterial reconstruction, balloon angioplasty).

3. Percutaneous mechanical thrombectomy may prove useful as an adjunct to thrombolysis by decreasing clot volume without the need for lytic agents. Various devices are available for use, with the AngioJet system (Possis Medical, Minneapolis, MN) garnering the most clinical experience to date.

B. In the setting of **trauma,** operative exploration should be performed in any limb that is ischemic or if arteriography demonstrates a significant intimal flap or other pathology. In the presence of coexistent neurologic or orthopedic injuries, it is essential to re-establish arterial flow first, by direct repair, bypass grafting, or temporary shunting. At the conclusion of the orthopedic repair, the arterial repair should be re-examined to ensure that it has not been disrupted and has been correctly fashioned to the final bone length. In cases of joint dislocation, reduction of the dislocation should be accomplished first because this may alleviate the need for arterial reconstruction.

   1. Intraoperatively it is essential to **obtain proximal and distal control** of the injured artery before exploring the hematoma or wound. When repairing an artery, an end-to-end anastomosis is preferable. A few centimeters of the artery can usually be mobilized proximally and distally to accomplish reapproximation. However, the uninjured leg or other potential vein harvest site should be prepared in case a conduit is required. It is preferable to use autologous tissue in this setting. If concomitant venous injuries are identified, these should be repaired as well. A completion angiogram can help to document distal flow. This is especially important if significant spasm is present and distal pulses are not readily palpable.

   2. In general, injuries to the subclavian, axillary, brachial, femoral, superficial femoral, profunda femoral, and popliteal arteries should be repaired. The radial or ulnar artery may be ligated if the other vessel is intact and functioning. Similarly, isolated injuries to the tibial arteries may be ligated if one or more of the tibial arteries remain intact.

IV. COMPLICATIONS

A. **Reperfusion injury** occurs after re-establishment of arterial flow to an ischemic tissue bed and may lead to further tissue death. It results from the formation of oxygen free-radicals that directly damage the tissue and cause white blood cell accumulation and sequestration in the microcirculation. This process prolongs the ischemic interval because it impairs adequate nutrient flow to the tissue, despite the restoration of axial blood flow. There is no proven therapy that limits reperfusion injury.

B. Rhabdomyolysis following reperfusion releases the by-products of ischemic muscle, including potassium, lactic acid, myoglobin, and creatinine phosphokinase. The electrolyte and pH changes that occur can trigger dangerous arrhythmias, and precipitation of myoglobin in the renal tubules can cause pigment nephropathy and ultimately acute renal failure. The likelihood that a patient will develop these complications relates to the duration of ischemia and the muscle mass at risk. In an attempt to ameliorate this, some surgeons clamp the femoral vein prior to revascularization and perform a transverse venotomy after lower-extremity arterial inflow is re-established. The first 250 to 500 mL of blood are discarded or aspirated to an autotransfusion system, thereby removing the hyperkalemic and acidotic plasma. **Aggressive hydration,** diuresis promotion with mannitol (25 g intravenously), and intravenous infusion of bicarbonate to alkalinize the urine are also accepted methods of mitigating renal impairment secondary to rhabdomyolysis.

C. Compartment syndrome results when prolonged ischemia and delayed reperfusion cause cell membrane damage and leakage of fluid into the interstitium. The edema can result in extremely high intracompartmental pressures, particularly in the lower extremity. Additional muscle and nerve necrosis occurs when the intracompartmental pressures exceed capillary perfusion (generally >30 mm Hg). A four-compartment fasciotomy should be performed when there is concern about the possible development of leg compartment syndrome. **Fasciotomy should be routine** in any patient with more than 6 hours of lower-extremity ischemia or in the presence of combined arterial and venous injuries. Leg fasciotomies usually are performed through two incisions, one anterolateral and another posteromedial. The skin is left open, to be closed either secondarily or by skin graft at a later time.

D. Catheter-related complications can occur early or late. Early complications result from arterial wall trauma and include arterial perforation and rupture, intimal dissection, development of arteriovenous fistulae, and pseudoaneurysm formation. A late catheter-related complication is the development of accelerated atherosclerosis in the embolectomized vessel, probably due to endothelial denudation and medial injury.

V. Follow-up care usually is directed at treating the underlying cause of the obstruction. Patients with mural thrombi or arrhythmias require long-term anticoagulation. The in-hospital mortality rate associated with embolectomy is as high as 30%, mostly due to coexistent cardiac disease.

CHRONIC ARTERIAL OCCLUSIVE DISEASE OF THE EXTREMITY

The lower extremities are most frequently affected by chronic occlusive disease, although upper-extremity disease can occur. The principal early symptom of arterial occlusive disease is **claudication,** which is usually described as a cramping pain or heaviness in the affected extremity that occurs after physical exertion. Claudication is relieved by rest but recurs predictably with exercise. Lower-extremity occlusive disease is subdivided into three anatomic sections based on symptoms and treatment options. Aortoiliac occlusive disease, or "inflow disease," affects the infrarenal aorta and the common and external iliac arteries. Femoral-popliteal occlusive disease, or "outflow disease," affects the common femoral, superficial femoral, and popliteal arteries. Finally, tibial-peroneal disease, or "runoff disease," affects the vessels distal to the popliteal artery.

I. CLINICAL PRESENTATION

A. Aortoiliac disease presents with **symptoms of lower-extremity claudication,** usually of the **hip, thigh, or buttock.** It may coexist with femoral-popliteal disease, contributing to more distal symptoms as well. The symptoms usually develop gradually, although sudden worsening of symptoms suggests acute thrombosis of a diseased vessel. Patients ultimately develop incapacitating claudication but not rest pain unless distal disease is present as well. *Leriche syndrome* (sexual impotence, buttock and leg claudication, leg musculature atrophy, trophic changes of the feet, and leg pallor) is a constellation of symptoms in men that results from the gradual occlusion of the terminal aorta. In contrast to the male predominance in chronic peripheral vascular disease (PVD), isolated aortoiliac disease afflicts women and men equally.

B. Patients with **femoral-popliteal** and **tibial disease** present with claudication of the lower extremity, usually most prominent in the **calves.** More severe impairment of arterial flow can present as rest pain. **Rest pain** is a burning pain in the distal foot, usually worse at night or when the leg is elevated and often relieved by placing the leg in a dependent position. Examination findings of the chronically ischemic extremity include the following:

1. Decreased or absent distal pulses.

2. Dependent rubor.

3. Trophic changes that include thickening of the nails, loss of leg hair, shiny skin, and ulceration at the tips of the toes.

C. Symptomatic arterial occlusive disease of the **upper extremity** is relatively rare.

1. The proximal subclavian artery is most commonly affected by **atherosclerotic disease,** followed by axillary and brachial arteries. These patients typically present with arm claudication or finger–hand ischemia or necrosis. Occasionally, ulcerated plaques of the innominate or subclavian arteries can be a source of embolization to the hand.

2. Most patients with proximal subclavian lesions are completely asymptomatic. **Subclavian steal** can result when an occlusive subclavian artery lesion is located proximal to the origin of the vertebral artery. With exercise of the affected limb, the arm's demand for blood is supplied by retrograde flow in the ipsilateral vertebral artery, shunting blood from the posterior cerebral circulation and resulting in drop attacks, ataxia, sensory loss, or diplopia.

II. DIAGNOSIS of chronic arterial occlusive disease is concerned with determining the presence of **significant flow-limiting lesions** and distinguishing the disease from those that may mimic it, such as arthritis, gout, and neuromuscular disorders.

A. For patients presenting with **lower-extremity symptoms,** it is essential to examine the femoral and distal pulses at rest and after exercise. The absence of femoral pulses is indicative of aortoiliac disease, although some patients with aortoiliac disease have palpable pulses at rest that are lost after exercise. Bruits may also be appreciated over the lower abdomen or femoral vessels. It is also important to differentiate ulcers that arise from arterial insufficiency versus those generated by venous insufficiency and neuropathy.

1. Arterial insufficiency ulcers are usually painful and have an irregular appearance.

2. Neuropathic ulcers are painless and usually occur over bony prominences, particularly the plantar aspect of the metatarsophalangeal joints.

3. Venous stasis ulcers are located on the malleolar surface ("gaiter" distribution) and are dark and irregular in shape.

B. Noninvasive testing can quantify flow through larger vessels and tissue perfusion.

1. Segmental arterial Doppler readings with waveforms should be performed in all patients with suspected symptomatic arterial disease. The **ankle-brachial index (ABI)** (the ratio of the systolic blood pressure in the leg to that in the arm) allows one to quantify the degree of ischemia. In general, patients without vascular disease have an ABI of greater than 1, patients with claudication have an ABI of less than 0.8, and patients with rest pain and severe ischemia have an ABI of less than 0.4. Waveform changes help to localize the site of significant disease. Patients with history of claudication and normal resting waveforms need postexercise ABI measurements.

2. Transcutaneous measurement of **local tissue oxygenation** has been developed to attempt to quantify the physiologic derangements of ischemia. However, the usefulness of this test in the general vascular patient has not been validated.

C. **Digital subtraction arteriography** is the **gold standard** for evaluating the arterial tree before planned revascularization. Typical digital subtraction arteriography of the lower extremities includes images of the infrarenal aorta and the renal, iliac, femoral, tibial, and pedal vessels. Noninvasive angiography using imaging modalities such as magnetic resonance or computer tomography has been gaining widespread use as the technology improves for both. **Magnetic resonance angiography (MRA)** is an excellent imaging modality for assessing PAD and is useful for selecting patients who are endoluminal candidates. However, MRA does have a tendency to overestimate the degree of stenosis and may be inaccurate in stented arteries. **CT angiography** produces high-resolution images of the vascular tree and gives other information about soft tissues that may be associated with PAD, such as aneurysms, popliteal entrapment, or cystic adventitial disease. However, diffuse calcifications may make interpretation of CT angiography images difficult. In addition, CT angiography does require iodinated contrast, which may adversely affect patients with renal insufficiency.

III. MANAGEMENT

A. Intermittent claudication by itself is not an indication for surgical intervention because it has a benign course in most patients. In patients presenting with claudication alone, 70% to 80% remain stable or improve and 10% to 20% worsen over the ensuing 5-year period. Only 5% to 10% of patients develop gangrene and are at risk for limb loss. Therefore, first-line treatment for patients with claudication should be medical therapy, with emphasis on risk factor modification.

Indications for surgical intervention include the following:

1. **Limb salvage** is the goal of surgery in patients with ischemic rest pain or tissue loss, including frank distal gangrene. Multilevel femoral-popliteal-tibial disease is the typical distribution in these patients. When significant aortoiliac disease and distal disease are jointly present in a patient with a threatened limb, however, an inflow (aortoiliac) procedure should be performed first.

2. **Prevention of further peripheral atheroembolization** from aortoiliac ulcerated plaques, even if there is little or no history of claudication, is an indication for exclusion and bypass or endarterectomy of the aortoiliac system.

3. **Incapacitating claudication** that jeopardizes a patient's livelihood or influences his or her quality of life indicates disease likely to respond well to treatment. These patients should adhere to a program of risk factor reduction as well.

B. **Medical therapy** is available for those patients with symptoms who are not candidates for surgical intervention. However, no medical therapy is available to reverse significantly the changes of advanced atherosclerotic disease.

1. **Risk factor modification** is the most important intervention for reducing the impact of advanced atherosclerotic disease. Control of hypertension and serum glucose, cessation of smoking, management of lipid disorders, attainment of ideal body weight, and regular exercise should be the goals.

   a. **Lipid reduction** is imperative in patients with PAD because the majority of the morbidity associated with PAD is related to cardiac events. Based on the Heart Protection Study involving statins, it is recommended to keep the low-density-lipoprotein (LDL) level of patients with PAD less than a 100 mg/dL to help reduce the likelihood of morbidity associated with cardiac events (*J Vasc Surg* 2007;45:645).

   b. **Antihypertensives** should be administered to normalize blood pressure. Medications such as beta-blockers or angiotensin-converting enzyme inhibitors have been shown in several studies to help reduce mortality-associated cardiovascular disease.

2. Because many of these patients have concomitant coronary artery or cerebrovascular disease, daily **aspirin** therapy (81 or 325 mg) is indicated to reduce the risk of myocardial infarction or stroke.

3. **Clopidogrel** is an **antiplatelet agent** that has been shown to reduce vascular morbidity and death in some recent studies in patients with systemic atherosclerosis. Clopidogrel is routinely administered following percutaneous coronary interventions, given its proven efficacy in reducing subacute and midterm thrombotic

complications. Although rigorous proof of its utility following peripheral arterial interventions is lacking, clopidogrel is frequently prescribed following these procedures.

4. **Pentoxifylline** is a **rheologic agent** thought to reduce blood viscosity and allow for improved flow through small arterioles and stenotic arteries. Although the drug is frequently prescribed, its benefit is unpredictable and generally small. It may be best suited for patients with severe disease not amenable to reconstruction.

5. **Cilostazol** is a type III **phosphodiesterase inhibitor** and the newest agent available for treatment of claudication. Cilostazol inhibits platelet aggregation and causes vasodilation. Given at 50 mg or 100 mg twice daily, it increases walking distances when compared with placebo and pentoxifylline. Early studies suggest that the drug is safe in most patients, although **its use is contraindicated in those with class III or IV heart failure** due to the toxicity of phosphodiesterase inhibitors in these patients.

C. **Preoperative care** of patients with PVD includes a complete arterial evaluation. In addition to angiographic evaluation of the symptomatic arterial tree, patients generally undergo screening for associated cardiac, renal, cerebrovascular, and pulmonary disease so that any correctable lesions can be addressed. Myocardial complications account for the majority of early and late deaths; therefore, patients with questionable myocardial function may require more extensive cardiac evaluation. Screening for carotid disease should also be performed, including a history of stroke or transient ischemic attack (TIA) and carotid auscultation.

D. **Open surgical therapy**

1. **Aortoiliac occlusive disease**

   a. **Aortobifemoral grafting** is the treatment of choice in low-risk patients with diffuse aortoiliac stenoses and occlusions. Aortobifemoral bypass may be performed through a transperitoneal or a retroperitoneal approach. Distal endarterectomy may be performed in conjunction with a bypass to improve outflow. Results are excellent, with reported patency rates of up to 95% at 5 years.

   b. **Femorofemoral, ilioiliac, or iliofemoral bypasses** are alternatives in high-risk patients with unilateral iliac disease. The patency rates are lower than those achieved with aortobifemoral grafts.

   c. **Axillobifemoral bypass** is an alternative for high-risk patients who need revascularization. This bypass avoids an intra-abdominal procedure and the need for cross-clamping the aorta. The patency rates are significantly poorer than those achieved with aortobifemoral bypass, although it may be a reasonable alternative for patients with short life expectancy (<5 years).

   d. **Aortoiliac endarterectomy** may be considered for patients who have disease localized to the distal aorta and common iliac vessels, although its use is becoming increasingly uncommon. Advantages include the avoidance of prosthetic material and preservation of antegrade flow into the hypogastric arteries. This procedure should not be done in patients with aneurysmal changes of the aorta, a completely occluded aorta to the level of the renal arteries, or extension of disease into the external iliac vessels.

2. **Femoral, popliteal, and tibial occlusive disease**

   a. In patients with above-knee occlusion, an **above-knee femoral-popliteal bypass** may be constructed. In patients who have disease below the knee, a **distal bypass** may be performed to the below-knee popliteal, posterior tibial, anterior tibial, or peroneal arteries. If all tibial vessels are occluded, pedal vessels may serve as suitable outflow vessels. These grafts usually originate from the common femoral artery, although a more distal vessel may be used if the inflow into that vessel is unobstructed.

   b. The best results are obtained with the use of **autologous vein** as a conduit. The greater saphenous is the vein of choice, but the lesser saphenous vein or the arm veins provide suitable alternatives. These autologous grafts can be used either *in situ* or reversed. The advantages of the *in situ* bypass are that (1) the vein's nutrient supply is left intact and (2) the vein orientation allows for a better size match (the large end of the vein is sewn to the large common femoral artery, and the small end is sewn to the distal vessel). The advantage of the reversed-vein bypass is that endothelial trauma is minimized because valve lysis is not necessary.

c. When autologous vein is not available, polytetrafluoroethylene **(PTFE) grafts** and **cryopreserved vein grafts** can be used. Patency rates for PTFE above-knee grafts approach those achieved with venous conduit, but use of PTFE for more distal bypass procedures is associated with substantially lower patency and is reserved for patients with critical limb ischemia who lack venous conduit. An alternative technique when performing PTFE bypass is the use of a small cuff of vein (Miller cuff) or patch angioplasty (Taylor patch) at the distal anastomosis. These modifications are believed to improve prosthetic graft patency by improving compliance match at the distal anastomosis. Cryopreserved vein graft patency also compares poorly to native autologous conduit, but it may prove useful when bypass is required in an infected field.

d. **Endarterectomy** as the sole procedure in an extremity is rarely performed. Endarterectomy may have a role in patients with limited vein availability or in the presence of an infected field.

e. **Sympathectomy** sometimes is used as an adjunct to vascular reconstructions and involves division of the sympathetic chain and L3–5 ganglia. With the development of percutaneous alcohol ablation of the sympathetic ganglia, performance of surgical sympathectomy is increasingly rare. Although it does not increase blood supply to the muscles, it results in maximal dilation of small arterioles and collaterals, providing increased blood flow to the skin and subcutaneous tissues. The effect lasts only 4 to 6 weeks.

f. **Amputation** is reserved for patients with gangrene or persistent painful ischemia not amenable to vascular reconstruction. These patients often have severe coexistent vascular and cardiovascular disease, and the survival rate for patients undergoing major amputations is approximately 50% at 3 years and 30% at 5 years.

  (1) The **level of amputation** is determined clinically. Important factors include the necessity of removing all the infected tissue and the adequacy of the blood supply to heal the amputation. A general principle is to preserve as much length of the extremity as safely possible because this improves the patient's opportunity for rehabilitation. In some cases, revascularization before amputation enables a more distal amputation to heal adequately.

  (2) **Digital amputations** are performed commonly in diabetic patients who develop osteomyelitis or severe foot infections.

  (3) **Transmetatarsal amputations** usually are performed when several toes are involved in the ischemic process or after previous single-digit amputations.

  (4) **Syme amputation** involves the removal of the entire foot and calcaneus while preserving the entire tibia. It is rarely appropriate for PVD.

  (5) **Below-knee amputation (BKA)** is the most common type of amputation performed for patients with severe occlusive disease.

  (6) **Above-knee amputation (AKA)** heals more easily than BKA and is useful in older patients who do not ambulate.

  (7) **Hip disarticulation** rarely is performed for PVD.

3. Upper-extremity occlusive disease

  a. For proximal subclavian disease, the **choice of bypass procedure** depends primarily on the patency of the ipsilateral common carotid artery.

  b. If the ipsilateral common carotid artery is patent, **carotid-subclavian bypass** is performed through a supraclavicular approach using a prosthetic graft (vein grafts are to be avoided). Subclavian artery transposition to ipsilateral carotid artery is an excellent alternative if anatomically feasible.

  c. If the ipsilateral carotid artery is occluded, **subclavian-subclavian bypass** may be performed. This is an extra-anatomic approach using a longer-segment prosthetic graft, with reduced patency.

4. **Intraoperative anticoagulation** is employed during most vascular reconstructions. Generally, unfractionated heparin (100 to 150 units/kg) is administered intravenously shortly before cross-clamping and supplemented as necessary until the cross-clamps are removed. Anticoagulation can be monitored intraoperatively by following activated clotting time (ACT) levels. The anticoagulant effect of heparin can be reversed with protamine administration.

E. **Postoperative care**

1. For open aortic procedures, early postoperative care is usually administered in the ICU, where frequent hemodynamic and hematologic measurements are performed. Assessment of distal pulses should be done intraoperatively, immediately after reconstruction and regularly thereafter. In uncomplicated cases, the patients usually are extubated on the day of surgery or on postoperative day 1. Patients are kept well hydrated for the first 2 postoperative days, after which third-space fluid begins to mobilize and diuresis ensues. Fluid management may be guided by central pressure monitoring. Antibiotics are continued for 24 hours postoperatively. A nasogastric tube is kept in place until return of bowel function. Patients are instructed not to sit with the hips flexed at greater than 60 degrees for the first 72 hours after graft placement, although ambulation as early as possible is encouraged.

2. For distal bypass grafts, **pulses should be assessed frequently** for the first 24 hours and then several times a day. Antibiotics are continued for 48 hours postoperatively or longer if infected ulcers warrant such treatment. Early ambulation is encouraged in patients without tissue necrosis. In patients who are unable to ambulate immediately, physical therapy can help to increase strength in the limb and prevent contracture. Sitting with the hips flexed to 90 degrees is discouraged in any patient with a femoral anastomosis. Patients should be instructed to elevate their legs while resting because this will mitigate the edema that develops in the revascularized extremity. Staples are left in place for 2 to 3 weeks because these patients frequently have delayed wound healing.

3. **Perioperative antithrombotic therapy** should include aspirin (81 to 325 mg/day) for all infrainguinal reconstructions. In patients sensitive to aspirin, clopidogrel (75 mg/day) may be substituted.

4. Postoperative oral anticoagulation has a more limited role. Owing in part to the increased risk of hemorrhage, anticoagulation with warfarin (international normalized ratio 2 to 3) is generally limited to grafts considered to be at a high risk for thrombosis. There may be some benefit to be gained from the administration of dextran 40 (0.5 mL/kg/hour intravenously) for up to 72 hours postoperatively in high-risk grafts.

5. Following major amputations, weightbearing is delayed for 4 to 6 weeks. Some advocate the use of compressive wraps to aid in the maturation of the stump. In all cases, early consultation with a physical therapist is recommended. Physical therapy is essential for maintaining strength in the limb, preventing contractures, and rehabilitating the patient once a prosthesis is fitted. In addition, as soon as the patient is ready, he or she should be fitted with a prosthetic limb and ambulation training should begin. Rehabilitation rates (ability to walk without assistance) for patients undergoing unilateral BKA or AKA are 60% and 30%, respectively. For those with bilateral amputations, rehabilitation rates drop to 40% for patients with bilateral BKA and 10% for patients with bilateral AKA.

6. **Long-term follow-up** for distal bypass grafts consists of arterial Doppler examinations every 3 months for the first 18 months, then every 6 months for a year, and then yearly. Less frequent follow-up is necessary for aortoiliac bypasses. Significant reductions in the ABIs or flow velocities predict pending graft failure, and such grafts should be studied further by arteriography. Intervention to repair or revise stenosed grafts results in much higher long-term patency than repairing or replacing occluded grafts.

F. **Complications**

1. Early complications occur in approximately 5% to 10% of patients after aortic surgery and frequently relate to preoperative comorbid disease. Myocardial

infarction, congestive heart failure, pulmonary insufficiency, and renal insufficiency are most common. Complications related directly to the aortic reconstruction include hemorrhage, embolization or thrombosis of the distal arterial tree, microembolization, ischemic colitis, ureteral injuries, impotence, paraplegia, and wound infection. Late complications include anastomotic pseudoaneurysm or graft dilation, graft limb occlusion, aortoenteric erosion or fistula, and graft infections.

2. In distal revascularizations, most of the early complications are also related to comorbid conditions. Early graft thrombosis (within 30 days of surgery) most often results from technical errors, hypercoagulability, inadequate distal runoff, and postoperative hypotension. **Technical errors** are responsible for more than 50% of early graft failures and include graft kinks, retained valve leaflets, valvulotome trauma, intimal flaps, significant residual arteriovenous fistulas, and the use of an inadequate conduit (i.e., small vein).

G. Endovascular options

1. Aortoiliac occlusive disease

a. Indications. Balloon angioplasty and intravascular stent placement of aortoiliac occlusive lesions produce excellent results. These procedures are indicated for symptomatic stenotic lesions (i.e., emboligenic lesions or lesions causing hypoperfusion) and in cases of distal bypass graft construction to improve graft inflow. Short-segment stenoses (<3 cm length) of the common iliac or external iliac artery display excellent long-term patency rates when treated with angioplasty alone or with stent placement. Angioplasty failure is an indication for arterial stenting; such failure manifests as residual luminal diameter reduction of 30% or more, greater than 10 mm Hg mean blood pressure gradient across the lesion, intimal flap, or medial dissection. Other indications for iliac stenting include eccentric stenotic lesions, recanalized iliac occlusions, restenosis after previous angioplasty, and ulcerated emboligenic lesions.

b. Technique. Intra-arterial access for iliac artery angioplasty and stenting is generally via the femoral arteries. For balloon angioplasty, the guidewire-mounted angioplasty balloon is positioned across the stenosis under fluoroscopy. When the occlusive lesion is in the distal aorta or proximal common iliac artery close to the aortic bifurcation, angioplasty should be performed using two balloons, one in each iliac artery and both partially projecting into the distal aorta ("kissing balloons"). The rationale for this is that lesions in proximity to the aortic bifurcation typically involve the distal aorta and both common iliac arteries. Unilateral balloon dilation may cause plaque fracture and dissection and narrowing of the contralateral vessel. Stenting may produce a more favorable result if postangioplasty dissection or lesion recoil is noted. Balloon-expandable and self-expanding stents are generally oversized 10% to 15% relative to the adjacent normal artery to ensure satisfactory stent apposition to the vessel wall. Balloon angioplasty is also commonly performed after deployment of self-expanding stents.

c. Complications include arterial wall dissection, vessel occlusion (either from thrombosis or dissection), arterial rupture, and distal embolization.

d. Results. Early balloon angioplasty failure can result from elastic recoil of atherosclerotic plaque or arterial wall dissection. These complications are potentially amenable to stent placement. Cases of late failure are due to intimal hyperplasia or progressive atherosclerosis. Iliac artery balloon angioplasty 2-year patency rates of between 60% and 70% have been reported. Reports on iliac artery stenting demonstrate 4-year patency rates as high as 85%. The results in general are better for common iliac artery lesions than for external iliac artery lesions and better for short-segment disease than for long-segment disease. Poor distal runoff also is associated with decreased patency.

2. Infrainguinal occlusive disease

a. Indications. Balloon angioplasty and stenting of infrainguinal occlusive lesions have had poorer results than surgical bypass procedures. A growing body of literature exists regarding infrainguinal application of other endovascular techniques, such as the use of cutting balloons, directional atherectomy, lasers, and cryoplasty. **None of these techniques provides the patency offered by surgical bypass,** yet the less invasive nature of endovascular treatment may be of benefit in certain circumstances. When limb-threatening ischemia occurs in patients without sufficient autologous conduit or in patients at high operative risk, angioplasty and stenting may allow limb salvage despite poor long-term patency. Stenting may be useful in cases of unsuccessful angioplasty (residual stenosis, intimal flap, dissection) or recurrent stenosis after previous angioplasty. Cutting balloon angioplasty has been proposed for treatment of focal (<1.5 cm) infrainguinal vein bypass graft stenoses. Although surgical revision has been the treatment of choice, endovascular treatment is reasonable for certain high-risk patients in whom reoperation is deemed difficult, risky, or both.

b. Results. The results of femoral-popliteal artery angioplasty and stenting are rapidly improving. Early data suggest that stent placement in the femoro-popliteal area is associated with a 30% to 50% primary patency rate at 2 years. Factors associated with higher patency following endovascular treatment include lesion characteristics (large-diameter vessel, short length of lesion, stenosis rather than occlusion, and absence of heavy calcification) as well as patent tibial runoff vessels. Two-year patency rates as high as 66% have been reported after balloon angioplasty of vein graft stenoses.

VENOUS DISEASE, THROMBOEMBOLISM, AND LYMPHEDEMA

20

Scott J. Ziporin and Brian Rubin

VENOUS ANATOMY

Venous anatomy is divided into the superficial, deep, and perforator components. In the lower extremity, the major superficial veins are the greater saphenous vein formed from the union of the dorsal vein of the great toe and the dorsal venous arch, then ascending anterior to the medial malleolus, passing posterior to the medial femoral condyle, and traveling medially to the fossa ovalis in the groin; the lesser saphenous vein formed from the joining of the dorsal vein of the fifth toe and the dorsal venous arch coursing posterior to the lateral malleolus, then posterolaterally to the popliteal fossa; and the posterior arch vein, also called *Leonardo's vein*, beginning in the medial ankle and joining the greater saphenous vein below the knee. The deep veins in the leg are named according to their paired arteries. The deep veins of the calf typically are duplicated as venae comitantes with numerous communicating branches. The posterior tibial and peroneal veins also communicate with the soleal sinusoids. In the thigh, the deep venous system includes the superficial and deep femoral veins that join approximately 4 cm below the inguinal ligament. The superficial and deep systems are connected by perforating veins (direct and indirect). Most blood flows from the superficial to the deep system via the direct perforators, but indirect perforators (small superficial veins draining into muscles that connect to the deep system via intramuscular veins) are also important. Venous return from the lower extremities toward the heart depends largely on compression of the deep veins by the *triceps surae* (gastrocnemius, soleus) during walking. Flow is unidirectional due to a series of one-way valves. Of surgical interest, when treating chronic venous insufficiency, five groups of direct medial calf perforators join either the greater saphenous vein or the posterior arch vein to the posterior tibial vein (*J Vasc Surg* 1996;24:800). They are named **Cockett** or **paratibial perforators.** The saphenous nerve travels medially, close to the saphenous vein near the ankle, making it susceptible to injury during stripping of the lower saphenous vein.

CHRONIC VENOUS INSUFFICIENCY

Chronic venous disease includes cosmetically undesirable telangiectasias, varicose veins, venous ulceration, and claudication. Advances in duplex scanning and minimally invasive surgical techniques such as subfascial endoscopic perforating vein surgery (SEPS) and radiofrequency (RF) ablation are used to tailor medical and surgical therapies, resulting in marked improvement in clinical outcomes and patient satisfaction.

I. PATHOPHYSIOLOGY
  A. Etiology
    1. Congenital (although it may present later in life), primary (cause undetermined), or secondary (postthrombotic, posttraumatic, or other).
    2. Risk factors
      a. Obesity.
      b. Tobacco use.
      c. Multiparity.
      d. Hormone therapy.

    e. Obstruction within a proximal segment (e.g., from adenopathy, arterial compression, or pregnancy).

    f. History of deep venous thrombosis (DVT). DVT accounts for most secondary cases and may be responsible for a significant number of other cases because many deep vein thrombi are asymptomatic.

  B. Reflux disease from venous valvular incompetence accounts for most (>80%) chronic venous disease.

    1. Valve malfunction can be inherited or acquired through sclerosis or elongation of valve cusps.

    2. May also result from dilation of the valve annulus despite normal valve cusps.

    3. Varicose veins may represent superficial venous insufficiency in the presence of competent deep and perforator systems, or they may be a manifestation of perforator or deep disease.

    4. Valvular disease below the knee appears to be more critical in the pathophysiology of severe disease than does deep valvular disease above the knee.

    5. The perforator veins are frequently implicated when venous ulcers exist, but any component of the venous system, either alone or in combination, may be incompetent.

    6. All of the above components need evaluation in the workup of chronic venous insufficiency (CVI) (*Am J Surg* 1995;169:572).

  C. Obstructive physiology is a less common cause of venous pathology, with reflux often being present simultaneously.

II. DIFFERENTIAL DIAGNOSIS

  A. Arterial disease

    1. Ulcers with discrete edges and pale bases; more painful than venous ulcers.

    2. Poor pulses.

    3. Dependent rubor.

    4. Pallor with elevation.

    5. Claudication.

  B. Lymphedema

    1. Pitting edema without pigmentation and ulceration.

    2. Less responsive to elevation, usually requiring several days to improve.

  C. Squamous cell carcinoma

  D. Trauma

  E. Arteriovenous malformation

  F. Orthostatic edema

III. NOMENCLATURE

  A. CEAP classification

    1. Based on the conclusions of an international consensus committee.

    2. Standardized nomenclature of chronic venous disease (*J Vasc Surg* 1995;21:635).

    3. CEAP: clinical signs, **e**tiology, **a**natomic distribution, and **p**athophysiology (Tables 20-1 and 20-2).

    4. Useful in defining clinical severity of disease and subsequent management strategies.

    5. Assessing response to therapy over time with the system proves difficult.

  B. Venous Clinical Severity Score (VCSS)

    1. Proposed by the American Venous Forum; expands the existing system.

    2. Ten clinical descriptors: pain, varicose veins, venous edema, skin pigmentation, inflammation, induration, number of active ulcers, duration of active ulceration, size of ulcer, and compressive therapy use.

    3. Better assesses ongoing response to therapy.

    4. Recent studies to validate the VCSS demonstrate low intraobserver and interobserver variation in accessing treatment outcomes for venous disease (*J Vasc Surg* 2002,36:889).

IV. DIAGNOSIS

  A. History

    1. A history of any DVT or trauma.

    2. Family history of varicose veins or CVI.

| TABLE 20-1 | Classification of Chronic Lower-Extremity Venous Disease |

Classification	Definition
C	Clinical signs (grade 0–6),[a] supplemented by (A) for asymptomatic or (S) for symptomatic presentation
E	Etiologic classification (congenital, primary, or secondary)
A	Anatomic distribution (superficial, deep, or perforator; alone or in combination)
P	Pathophysiologic dysfunction (reflux or obstruction; alone or in combination)

[a]See Table 20-2.
With permission from Porter JM, Moneta GL. Reporting standards in venous disease: an update. International Consensus Committee on Chronic Venous Disease. *J Vasc Surg* 1995;21:635.

3. Complaint of lower-extremity edema, aching, skin irritation, or varicose veins. Leg pain is described as a dull ache, worsening at the end of the day, and often relieved with exercise or elevation.

4. Individuals can experience acute, bursting pain with ambulation **(venous claudication).** Prolonged rest and leg elevation (20 minutes) are needed to obtain relief.

B. Physical examination

1. Ankle edema.

2. Subcutaneous fibrosis.

3. Hyperpigmentation (brownish discoloration secondary to hemosiderin deposition).

4. Lipodermatosclerosis.

5. Venous eczema.

6. Dilation of subcutaneous veins, including telangiectasias (0.1 to 1 mm), reticular veins (1 to 4 mm), and varicose veins (>4 mm).

7. Ultimately, ulcers develop, typically proximal to the medial malleolus.

8. Any signs of infection should be noted.

9. Arterial pulses should be examined and are usually adequate.

C. Noninvasive studies

1. Duplex scanning

a. B-mode ultrasound imaging combined with Doppler frequency shift display.

b. Invaluable in assessing valvular incompetence and obstruction.

c. With the individual standing, cuffs are placed on the thigh, calf, and foot and inflated; then the cuffs are rapidly deflated in an attempt to create retrograde venous blood flow in segments of valvular incompetence.

| TABLE 20-2 | Clinical Classification of Chronic Lower-Extremity Venous Disease |

Grade	Characteristics
0	No visible or palpable signs of venous disease
1	Telangiectasias, reticular veins, or malleolar flare
2	Varicose veins
3	Edema without skin changes
4	Skin changes ascribed to venous disease (e.g., pigmentation, venous eczema, or lipodermatosclerosis)
5	Skin changes as defined above and healed ulceration
6	Skin changes as defined above and active ulceration

Adapted with permission from Porter JM, Moneta GL. Reporting standards in venous disease: an update. International Consensus Committee on Chronic Venous Disease. *J Vasc Surg* 1995;21:635.

   d. Competent valves generally take no more than 0.5 to 1 second to close.
   e. Detailed mapping of valve competence of each segment of the venous system is possible, including the common femoral, superficial femoral, greater saphenous, lesser saphenous, popliteal, posterior tibial, and perforator veins.
   f. Has a predictive value of 77% for diagnosing reflux leading to severe symptoms.
2. **Descending phlebography** has a predictive value of 44%, previously considered the gold standard (*J Vasc Surg* 1992;16:687). Descending phlebography is limited by its inability to study valves distal to a competent proximal valve.
3. **Continuous-wave Doppler**
   a. Easily performed in the office using a handheld probe.
   b. Helpful for screening for reflux at the saphenofemoral and saphenopopliteal junctions.
   c. Limited due to inability to quantitate reflux and to provide precise anatomic information.
4. **Trendelenburg test**
   a. Largely replaced by the much more accurate duplex imaging studies.
   b. Patient's leg is elevated to drain venous blood. An elastic tourniquet is applied at the saphenofemoral junction, and the patient then stands.
   c. Rapid filling (<30 seconds) of the saphenous system from the deep system indicates perforator valve incompetence.
   d. When tourniquet is released, additional filling of the saphenous system occurs if the saphenofemoral valve is also incompetent.

V. NONSURGICAL TREATMENT
A. Infected ulcers
1. Necessitate treatment of the infection first.
2. *Staphylococcus aureus, Streptococcus pyogenes,* and *Pseudomonas* species are responsible for most infections.
3. Usually treated with local wound care, wet-to-dry dressings, and oral antibiotics.
4. Topical antiseptics should be avoided.
5. Severe infections require intravenous antibiotics.
B. Leg elevation can temporarily decrease edema and should be instituted when swelling occurs. This should be done before a patient is fitted for stockings or boots.
C. Compression therapy is the primary treatment for CVI.
1. Elastic compression stockings
   a. Fitted to provide a compression gradient from 30 to 40 mm Hg, with the greatest compression at the ankle.
   b. Donned on arising from bed and removed at bedtime.
   c. Effective in healing ulcers but can take months to obtain good results.
   d. Study of 113 patients treated with initial bedrest, local wound care, and elastic compression stockings demonstrated a 93% ulcer healing rate in a mean of 5.3 months (*Surgery* 1991;109:575).
   e. Stockings do not correct the abnormal venous hemodynamics and must be worn after the ulcer has healed to prevent recurrence.
   f. Principal drawback is patient compliance.
   g. Recurrence for compliant patients in the same study was 16% at a mean follow-up of 30 months.
2. Unna boots
   a. Paste gauze compression dressings that contain zinc oxide, calamine, and glycerin.
   b. Used to help prevent further skin breakdown.
   c. Provide nonelastic compression therapy.
   d. Changed once or twice a week.
   e. Healing time for ulcers is less than that of elastic compression alone, with 70% of ulcers healed by 7 versus 11 weeks (*J Am Acad Dermatol* 1985;12:90).
3. Pneumatic compression devices
   a. Provide dynamic sequential compression.
   b. Used primarily in the prevention of deep vein thrombi in hospitalized patients.

c. Also used successfully to treat venous insufficiency.

d. A prospective study comparing local wound care and gradient compression stockings with or without sequential pneumatic compression for 4 hours a day showed an ulcer healing rate of 2.1% of the ulcer area per week without dynamic compression compared with 19.8% with dynamic compression (*Surgery* 1990;108:871).

D. Topical medications

1. Largely ineffective as a stand-alone therapy for venous stasis ulcers.
2. Topical therapy is directed at absorbing wound drainage and avoiding desiccation of the wound.
3. Antiseptics can be counterproductive. Hydrogen peroxide, povidone-iodine, acetic acid, and sodium hypochlorite are toxic to cultured fibroblasts and should be used for the shortest duration necessary to control ulcer infection.

E. Sclerotherapy

1. Effective in treating telangiectasias, reticular varicosities, and small varicose veins.
2. If saphenous reflux is present, it should be corrected first.
3. Contraindications include arterial occlusive disease, immobility, acute thrombophlebitis, and hypersensitivity to the drug.
4. Sclerosing agents
   a. 1% or 3% sodium tetradecyl sulfate.
   b. Sodium morrhuate (rarely used because of anaphylactic reactions).
   c. Hypertonic saline.
   d. Polidocanol (not currently Food and Drug Administration approved in the United States).
5. Varices are marked while the patient is standing. A 25-gauge needle is used to inject 0.25 to 0.50 mL of sclerosant slowly into the lumen of larger veins. A 30-gauge needle is used for sclerosing reticular veins and telangiectasias in supine patients.
6. Compression stockings are applied at the end of the procedure and are worn for several days to 6 weeks. Patients should walk for 30 minutes after the procedure.
7. Complications include cutaneous necrosis, hyperpigmentation, telangiectatic matting (new, fine, red telangiectasias), thrombophlebitis, anaphylaxis, and allergic reaction (*Dermatol Surg* 1995;21:19).

VI. SURGICAL THERAPY is indicated for severe disease refractory to medical treatment and for patients who cannot comply with the lifelong regimen of compression therapy. Surgical therapy includes skin grafting, saphenous vein stripping, endovenous radiofrequency obliteration of the saphenous vein, varicose vein stab avulsion, SEPS, and valvuloplasty.

A. Preoperative evaluation

1. Consists primarily of duplex imaging in a reliable vascular laboratory.
2. All components of the venous system should be studied and the precise location of pathology noted.
3. Surgical therapy is directed at the component or components found to have pathology.
4. For valve reconstruction, ascending or descending phlebography may be useful.

B. Skin grafting

1. Occasionally used to speed healing of large ulcers.
2. Ulcer bed should be dry and free of infection.
3. Fenestrated split-thickness skin graft is preferred to allow for serous drainage.
4. Bedrest is recommended until the ulcer has healed completely.
5. Recurrence is common unless the underlying venous pathology is corrected or conservative support (elastic compression) is initiated and maintained after skin grafting.
6. Cultured skin substitutes are now commonly used to minimize patient discomfort and avoid possible donor-site complications.

C. Stripping the greater saphenous vein

1. One of the classic treatments for varicose veins.
2. The vein should be stripped only in the regions where pathology occurs.

3. If the entire vein is involved, one incision is made anterior to the medial malleolus and another just below the inguinal crease. A stripper is inserted into the vein lumen at one site and run through the lumen to the other site.
4. High ligation of the vein is done at the saphenofemoral junction, including all tributaries.
5. Reconnection of the saphenous to the femoral system via multiple tributaries near the saphenofemoral junction is thought to be the major cause of recurrent varices.
6. Compressive bandages are applied to reduce hematoma formation, and compression stockings are worn for several weeks.
7. Complications include ecchymosis, DVT, and saphenous nerve injury.
8. Stripping only the thigh portion is probably the most important aspect of the procedure (*Lancet* 1996;348:210).
9. Not stripping the calf eliminates much of the risk to the saphenous nerve because this nerve is closely associated with the saphenous vein from the knee to the ankle; this also allows the portion of the vein below the knee to be used for arterial bypass if needed in the future. The same technique can be applied to the lesser saphenous vein.
10. Because the goal of stripping is to stop reflux down the involved venous segment, removal of a limited portion of the saphenous system is now widely accepted. Ligation alone, however, is associated with high rates of recanalization and is therefore not adequate therapy.

D. **Endovenous radiofrequency or laser obliteration** of the greater saphenous vein
1. This was shown to effectively treat saphenous reflux and associated varicose veins with less morbidity than saphenectomy (*J Vasc Surg* 2003;38:207).
2. A probe is inserted into the greater saphenous vein under ultrasound guidance. The probe emits either laser or radiofrequency energy, which coagulates and coapts the vein walls, causing complete obliteration of the lumen.
3. Potential complications
   a. Skin burns.
   b. Deep venous thrombosis.
   c. Pulmonary thromboembolism.
   d. Vein perforation and hematoma.
   e. Paresthesias.
   f. Phlebitis.
4. Reported outcomes achieved with endovenous radiofrequency and laser obliteration are comparable to those resulting from saphenectomy (*J Vasc Surg* 2002;35:1190, *J Vasc Interv Radiol* 2003;14:991). Incomplete obliteration and recanalization occurs in a small percentage of patients.
5. A contraindication to endovenous obliteration is saphenous vein thrombosis.

E. The **stab avulsion technique** allows a cosmetically acceptable surgical approach to varicose veins.
1. Preoperatively, the patient's varicose veins are carefully marked with indelible ink while the patient is standing. Some authors consider this to be the most important technical step in the procedure (*Am J Surg* 1996;172:278).
2. Incision (2 to 3 mm) is made next to the markings. The vein is pulled out of the incision with a small vein hook, and the two arms of the vein are pulled taut and avulsed. This can be repeated many times to remove large clusters of veins. The small incisions can be closed with Steri-Strips. The patient's leg is covered with compression stockings for several days to weeks. This technique is often used in conjunction with saphenous stripping to provide optimal results. Alternatively, the greater saphenous vein can be removed by sequential avulsion instead of stripping. This has been shown prospectively to decrease pain and bruising (*Br J Surg* 1996;83:1559).

F. **Additional procedures**
1. For severe CVI, **more extensive surgery** is required, usually directed at correction of saphenous reflux and ligation of incompetent medial calf perforators.

2. Even in the presence of combined superficial and deep incompetence, treatment of only the superficial and perforator incompetence can significantly improve clinical symptoms and hemodynamics (*J Vasc Surg* 1996;124:711) by disrupting continued transmission of high deep venous pressure to the skin.

3. **Open surgical subfascial ligation** (the Linton procedure)
   a. Traditionally, treatment of perforator reflux.
   b. Requires an incision through diseased skin and extensive subcutaneous dissection.
   c. Wound complications have limited the acceptance of this procedure.

4. **Subfascial endoscopic perforating vein surgery**
   a. This is associated with decreased morbidity and has gained recognition as an alternative treatment option.
   b. Performed by making small port incisions in unaffected skin in the calf and fascia of the posterior superficial compartment. Various types of endoscopes (laparoscopic, arthroplastic, or bronchoscopic) can be used for visualization. Carbon dioxide insufflation in the subfascial space may or may not be used. A balloon expander can expand the subfascial space to improve visualization. Typically, 3 to 14 perforators are identified and ligated.
   c. Most patients are discharged within 24 hours of surgery.
   d. In a recent study using subfascial balloon dissection and routine posterior, deep compartment fasciotomy with subsequent interruption of incompetent perforating veins (usually in conjunction with greater saphenous vein ligation and stripping), 92% of patients exhibited significant improvement or resolution of venous stasis ulcers within 4 to 14 weeks. In 8% of patients, no benefit was achieved from SEPS (*J Vasc Surg* 2003;37:545).

5. **Valvuloplasty**
   a. This can be done using an open or closed technique (*J Vasc Surg* 1999;16:694).
   b. The open procedure involves a venotomy made above the valve, with cusps sutured until competence is achieved.
   c. Alternatively, an angioscope can be inserted through a tributary, and repair of the valve can be viewed directly without a venotomy.
   d. To correct an incompetent superficial femoral vein, transfer of a valved vein segment is performed using end-to-end anastomosis either to the proximal saphenous vein or to the deep femoral vein, thus providing a competent proximal valve.
   e. Autotransplantation of a segment of axillary or brachial vein into the proximal popliteal vein has also been used with variable success.

 VENOUS THROMBOEMBOLISM

I. EPIDEMIOLOGY. Venous thromboembolism, which includes DVT and pulmonary embolism (PE), is a common cause of death. The true incidence of DVT is difficult to determine because its clinical diagnosis can be inaccurate and often occurring in the setting of other critical illnesses. One recent study demonstrated an annual incidence of venous thromboembolism to be one to two events per 1,000 of the general population. Greater than 50% of these cases are DVT, with 75% occurring as first episodes. An equal incidence between men and women has been observed, with the likelihood of a thromboembolic event doubling with each decade of life after 40 (*Circulation* 2003;107:1). Venous thromboembolic disease represents a significant problem, with 250,000 hospitalizations for DVT/PE annually. From 50% to 60% of DVT episodes are asymptomatic. Of those patients with DVTs, 30% will have a symptomatic PE with a mortality of 17.5% if untreated. DVT and PE occur in approximately 20% to 30% of general surgical patients without perioperative prophylaxis (*N Engl J Med* 1998;339:93, *Arch Intern Med* 2001;161:2215;, *Am J Respir Crit Care Med* 1999;159:1).

II. PATHOPHYSIOLOGY. DVT starts as a platelet nidus, usually in the venous valves of the calf. The thrombogenic nature of the nidus activates the clotting cascade, leading to platelet and fibrin accumulation. The fibrinolytic system is subsequently activated, with thrombus growth if thrombogenesis predominates over thrombolysis. A thrombus can detach from the endothelium and migrate into the pulmonary system, becoming a PE; alternatively, it can also organize and grow into the endothelium, resulting in venous incompetency and phlebitis. Thrombi localized to the calf have less tendency to embolize than thrombi that extend to the thigh veins (*Am Rev Respir Dis* 1990;141:1). Approximately 20% of cases of calf DVT propagate to the thigh, and 50% of cases of thigh or proximal DVT embolize.

III. RISK FACTORS FOR VENOUS THROMBOEMBOLISM

A. Malignancy

1. Tumor cell activation of the clotting cascade can occur directly through interactions with factors VIIa, X, and tissue factor (TF).
2. Indirect clotting activation can occur through stimulation of mononuclear cells to produce TF or factor X activators and stimulation of macrophages to produce TF activators.
3. **Reactive thrombocytosis** can occur in patients, especially those with advanced disease of the lung, colon, stomach, or breast; it is caused by spontaneous clumping of platelets or increased levels of thrombopoietin, a glycoprotein regulating the maturation of megakaryocytes.

B. Endothelial injury

1. Adhesion of tumor cells to endothelium can lead to disruption of endothelial intracellular junctions and expose the highly thrombogenic subendothelial surface.
2. Chemotherapeutic drugs, such as bleomycin, carmustine, vincristine, and doxorubicin (Adriamycin), can also cause vascular endothelial cell damage.

C. Venous stasis

1. This is caused by immobility, venous obstruction, increased venous pressure, and increased blood viscosity.
2. Venous stasis promotes thrombus formation by reducing clearance of activated coagulation factors and by causing endothelial hypoxia, leading to reduced levels of surface-bound thrombomodulin and increased expression of TF.
3. Two very common causes of immobility leading to DVT formation are surgery and critical illness. Major chest surgery, abdominal/pelvic surgery, and lower-extremity surgery have all been associated with increased risk of DVT development. Similarly, a prolonged nonambulatory state, such as fracture of the hip, pelvis, or leg; multisystem trauma; neurologic injury; or other critical injury requiring bedrest can increase DVT risk.

D. Oral contraceptives (OCPs) and estrogen hormone replacement therapy

1. These have been linked to increased risk of venous thrombus formation. Many studies have found an odds ratio of 3 to 5 for risk of DVT in patients taking OCPs compared to non–OCP-using patients.
2. An increased risk is still found with patients using third-generation OCPs containing new progestins.

E. Hypercoagulable states

1. Primary hypercoagulable states are inherited conditions that can lead to abnormal endothelial cell thromboregulation.
   a. Decreased thrombomodulin-dependent activation of protein C (Factor V Leiden mutation).
   b. Impaired heparin binding of antithrombin III.
   c. Downregulation of membrane-associated plasmin production.
   d. Increased serum prothrombin levels (G20210A prothrombin gene mutation).
   e. Decreased thrombogenic inhibitors (e.g., antithrombin III, protein C, protein S).
2. Secondary hypercoagulable states are states in which endothelial activation by cytokines leads to an inflammatory, thrombogenic vessel wall.
   a. Antiphospholipid syndrome.
   b. Venous trauma.
   c. Surgery.

   d. Hyperhomocysteinemia.
   e. Heparin-induced thrombopathy.
   f. Myeloproliferative syndromes.
   g. Cancer.
   h. Chemotherapy agents: cyclophosphamide, methotrexate, and 5-fluorouracil, cause a decrease in the plasma levels of proteins C and S.

IV. DIAGNOSIS

A. Initial evaluation

1. Approximately 75% of patients with suspected DVT or PE turn out not to have these conditions.
2. Assessment of risk factors (see Section III).
3. Clinical presentation
   a. Extremity pain.
   b. Increased circumference with respect to contralateral extremity.
   c. Dilation of superficial veins of the suspected extremity only.
   d. Calf pain on dorsiflexion of the ankle.
   e. Phlegmasia alba dolens represents a more severe manifestation of DVT in which the deep venous channels of the extremity are affected while sparing collateral veins and therefore maintaining some degree of venous return. Patients present with blanching of the extremity, edema, and discomfort.
   f. Phlegmasia cerulea dolens occurs with extension of thrombus into the collateral venous system, resulting in limb pain and swelling, accompanied by cyanosis, a sign of arterial ischemia.

B. Suspected DVT

1. Compression ultrasonography of the femoral, popliteal, and calf trifurcation veins is highly sensitive (>90%) in detecting thrombosis of the proximal veins (femoral and popliteal) but less sensitive (50%) in detecting calf vein thrombosis.
2. It represents the preferred diagnostic modality because it is less invasive than the reference standard of venography and is more sensitive than impedance plethysmography.
3. Approximately 2% of patients with initial normal ultrasound results have positive results on repeat tests performed 7 days later. Delayed detection rate is attributed to extension of calf vein thrombi or small, nonocclusive proximal vein thrombi.

C. Assessment of PE

1. **Contrast-enhanced spiral computed tomography (CT)** has sensitivity (70% to 90%) comparable to that of pulmonary angiography. Spiral CT is preferable to angiography (less invasive and less expensive).
2. Chest CT can be combined with CT angiography of pelvic and deep thigh veins to detect DVT as well as PE.
3. Patients with significant contrast allergy or renal insufficiency are not candidates for CT scanning.
4. Radionucleotide ventilation and perfusion lung imaging (V/Q scan) has been replaced by chest CT as the initial imaging test for suspected PE. V/Q scanning is used in situations in which CT is deemed not feasible. A V/Q scan result of "high probability" strongly suggests the presence of PE. However, more than 50% of patients have "intermediate probability" results. Because approximately 25% of these patients have PE, further evaluation or initiation of empiric treatment must be considered.
5. **Pulmonary angiography,** the reference test, is reserved for patients whose diagnosis is still uncertain.

V. PREVENTION AND TREATMENT OF VENOUS THROMBOEMBOLISM. See also Chapter 1 for a detailed description.

A. Low-dose unfractionated heparin

1. This is given subcutaneously at 5,000 units 2 hours before surgery and every 8 or 12 hours postoperatively.
2. Low-dose heparin reduces the risk of venous thromboembolism by 50% to 70% (*N Engl J Med* 1988;318:18) and does not require laboratory monitoring. Because

of the potential for minor bleeding, it should not be used for patients undergoing cerebral, ocular, or spinal surgery.

B. Graduated compression stockings
1. These are effective in preventing DVT formation by reducing venous stasis.
2. In surgery patients, the combination of graduated compression stockings and low-dose heparin is significantly more effective than low-dose heparin alone (*Br J Surg* 1985;72:7).
3. Graduated compression stockings are relatively inexpensive and should be considered for all high-risk patients, even when other forms of prophylaxis are used. Furthermore, the early use of either over-the-counter or custom-fit stockings following diagnosis of DVT results in a reduction in the incidence of postthrombotic syndromes (*Lancet* 1997;349:759, *Ann Intern Med* 2004;141:249).

C. Intermittent pneumatic compression of the extremities
1. This enhances blood flow in the deep veins and increases blood fibrinolytic activity through upregulation of thrombomodulin and fibrinolysin.
2. For patients with significant bleeding risk with anticoagulation, pneumatic compression is an effective alternative.
3. Compression devices should not be placed on an extremity with known DVT.
4. In the case of known bilateral lower-extremity DVT, the compression devices can be placed on the upper extremity.
5. Pedal compression devices are also effective in patients whose body habitus does not allow conventionally sized devices to fit around the thighs or calves.

D. Low–molecular-weight heparins (LMWHs)
1. Several advantages over unfractionated heparin, with longer half-lives, a more predictable dose–response curve, a lower risk of heparin-induced thrombocytopenia (HIT), the possibility of ambulatory treatment at home and in laboratory animals, fewer bleeding complications with equivalent anticoagulation effects.
2. In large randomized trials of patients with DVT, outpatient treatment with a LMWH was as safe and effective as inpatient treatment with intravenous unfractionated heparin.

E. Newer medications such as the direct thrombin inhibitors (DTIs) and fondaparinux represent a possible alternative to the unfractionated and LMWHs in the prevention of thromboembolic disease. The univalent DTI Argatroban as well as the bivalent DTIs (binding to both the active site and an additional accessory site on the thrombin molecule) lepirudin, bivalirudin, hirudin, and desirudin, administered by intravenous, intramuscular, or subcutaneous injection, offer an alternative to the heparins, particularly in situations in which heparin is contraindicated such as heparin-induced thrombocytopenia. These medications, however, are less suitable for long-term treatment (*N Engl J Med* 2005;353:2827). Fondaparinux, the first synthetic pentasaccharide, blocks thrombin generation by accelerating the rate of factor IIa, VIIa, IXa, Xa, XIa, and XIIa inactivation by antithrombin. The agent possesses almost complete bioavailability after subcutaneous injection, with clearance by the kidneys in unaltered form (*Curr Opin Anaes* 2006;19:52). In one study comparing fondaparinux given once daily to 2,205 patients with known DVT versus LMWH, as well as an additional study evaluating the drug against unfractionated heparin in 2,213 patients with pulmonary embolism, fondaparinux was found to be of equivalent safety and effectiveness in the treatment of DVT and PE (*Ann Intern Med* 2004;140:867, *N Eng J Med* 2003;349:1695).

F. Caval interruption with intracaval filters
1. Absolute indications
   a. DVT or PE with contraindication to anticoagulation therapy, including the following:
      (1) Prior hemorrhagic stroke.
      (2) Recent neurosurgical procedure or other major surgery.
      (3) Multiple or major trauma.
      (4) Active internal bleeding.
      (5) Intracranial neoplasm.

(6) Bleeding diathesis (thrombocytopenia, idiopathic thrombocytopenic purpura, etc.).

(7) Pregnancy.

(8) Patients with unsteady gait or tendency to fall.

b. DVT or PE in patients with a complication related to anticoagulation therapy.

c. Failure of anticoagulation therapy.

d. Free-floating iliofemoral or caval thrombus.

2. Relative indications

   a. Prior history of chronic pulmonary hypertension or marginal cardiopulmonary reserve.

   b. Morbidly obese patients with a body mass index greater than 55 undergoing gastric bypass surgery (*Curr Treat Options Cardiovasc Med* 2005;7:149, *J Vasc Surg* 2006;44:1301).

3. Several studies have reviewed the incidence of pulmonary embolism and DVT recurrence following placement of inferior vena cava (IVC) filters. In one study, 400 patients with identified proximal DVT judged to be at high risk for pulmonary embolism were divided into two groups: those undergoing IVC filter placement and those placed on unfractionated heparin or enoxaparin followed by a vitamin K antagonist. All patients did not have a contraindication to anticoagulation. V/Q scans performed within 48 hours of admission and again 8 to 12 days later demonstrated a significantly lower incidence of PE in the filter group. Follow-up over an interval of 8 years again demonstrated a lower incidence of symptomatic PE in those in the filter-recipient group; however, DVT was significantly more common in these individuals. Of note, overall long-term mortality was similar in the two groups (*N Engl J Med* 1998;338:409). An additional study demonstrated a twofold increase in the relative hazard of subsequent DVT in filter recipient patients with initial PE. The time to recurrent pulmonary embolism was similar in filter recipients and nonrecipients (*Blood Rev* 2005;19:179). A third set of studies examined an important long-term complication of IVC filter placement: the thrombotic occlusion of the IVC, occurring in 6% to 30% of cases (*Abdom Imaging* 1996;21:368, *Clin Chest Med* 1995;16:295). These studies do not account for the current practice of extended-duration anticoagulation in patients at high risk for recurrence, both in those with initial contraindication to anticoagulation and in patients immediately receiving anticoagulation on diagnosis of DVT with continuation following discharge. Recently, several retrievable vena cava filters have become available for patients with temporary contraindications to anticoagulation. The Gunther Tulip (Cook Medical, Bloomington, IN), Recovery (Bard, Tempe, AZ), and OptEase (Cordis, Miami, FL) filters are retrievable filters approved for use in North America. Outcome data related to the efficacy of retrievable filters relative to the standard, permanent type in the form of prospective studies or randomized control trials are pending.

4. Nonferromagnetic and therefore magnetic resonance imaging (MRI)–safe filters include the titanium Greenfield (Boston Scientific, Natick, MA), Vena Tech-LGM and Vena Tech-LP (B. Braun, Bethlehem, PA), Simon Nitinol and Recovery (Bard, Tempe, AZ), TrapEase and OptEase (Cordis, Miami, FL), and Gunther Tulip (Cook Medical, Bloomington, IN) filters.

G. The **choice of prophylaxis method** depends on the risk of venous thromboembolism compared with the risk of anticoagulation. See Chapter 1 for a detailed description.

H. Catheter-directed thrombolysis of acute DVT with or without mechanical thrombectomy devices has been advocated to avoid sequelae of DVT. The goals are to restore venous flow, preserve venous valve function, and eliminate the possibility of thromboembolism. Technical success and early clinical benefit have been reported, but long-term data are unavailable. In patients with migration of DVT resulting in severe pulmonary embolism and hemodynamic instability, potentially life-saving thrombolytics should be considered (*Curr Opin Anaes* 2006; 19:52).

LYMPHEDEMA

I. PATHOPHYSIOLOGY

A. Primary lymphedema is the result of congenital aplasia, hypoplasia, or hyperplasia of lymphatic vessels and nodes that causes the accumulation of a protein-rich fluid in the interstitial space. Swelling of the patient's leg initially produces pitting edema, which progresses to a nonpitting form and may lead to dermal fibrosis and disfigurement.

1. Primary lymphedema is classified according to age at presentation.

a. Congenital primary lymphedema (present at birth) represents 10% to 15% of all cases, which can be hereditary (Milroy disease) or nonhereditary.

b. Praecox (early in life) or Meige disease represents 70% to 80% of cases.

(1) It is seen in female patients 80% to 90% of the time.

(2) It presents during the second and third decades of life, typically with localized swelling of the foot and ankle. Such swelling is worsened by prolonged standing.

(3) A single lower extremity is affected in 70% of patients.

c. Tarda (late in life) primary lymphedema, representing 10% to 15% of cases, is seen equally in men and women and presents after the third or fourth decade.

B. Secondary lymphedema results from impaired lymphatic drainage secondary to a known cause. Surgical or traumatic interruption of lymphatic vessels (often from an axillary or groin lymph node dissection), carcinoma, infection, venous thrombosis, and radiation are causes of secondary lymphedema. Secondary lymphedema in the context of filariasis, caused by the parasite *Wuchereria bancrofti,* represents the most common worldwide presentation of the disease.

II. DIAGNOSIS

A. Clinical presentation

1. Symptoms

a. Early lymphedema is characterized by unilateral or bilateral arm or pedal swelling that resolves overnight. With disease progression, the swelling increases and extends up the extremity, producing discomfort and thickened skin. With more advanced disease, swelling is not relieved overnight. Significant pain is unusual.

b. Secondary lymphedema patients commonly present with repeated episodes of cellulitis secondary to high interstitial protein content.

2. Physical examination

a. Edema of the affected extremity is present.

b. When a lower extremity is involved, the toes are often spared.

c. With advanced disease, the extremity becomes tense, with nonpitting edema.

d. Dermal fibrosis results in skin thickening, hair loss, and generalized keratosis.

B. Imaging studies

1. Lymphoscintigraphy is the injection of radiolabeled (technetium-99m) colloid into the web space between the patient's second and third toes or fingers. The patient's limb is exercised periodically, and images are taken of the involved extremity and the whole body. Lymphedema is seen as an abnormal accumulation of tracer or as slow tracer clearance along with the presence of collaterals. For the diagnosis of lymphedema, the study has a sensitivity and specificity of 92% and 100%, respectively (*J Vasc Surg* 1989;9:683).

2. CT and MR scan are able to exclude any mass obstructing the lymphatic system. MR scan has been able to differentiate lymphedema from chronic venous edema and lipedema (excessive subcutaneous fat and fluid).

3. Lymphangiography involves catheter placement and injection of radiopaque dye directly into lymphatic channels; it has largely been replaced by lymphoscintigraphy and CT. A decreased total number of lymphatic channels and structural abnormalities can be seen. Lymphangiography can demonstrate the site of a lymphatic leak in postsurgical or traumatic situations. Complications include lymphangitis and hypersensitivity reaction to the dye.

III. DIFFERENTIAL DIAGNOSIS includes all other causes of a swollen extremity.
  A. Trauma.
  B. Infection.
  C. Arterial disease.
  D. Chronic venous insufficiency.
  E. Lipedema.
  F. Neoplasm.
  G. Radiation effects.
  H. Systemic diseases, such as right ventricular failure, myxedema, nephrosis, nephritis, and protein deficiency. These causes must be excluded before invasive study.
IV. TREATMENT
  A. Medical management is limited by the physiologic and anatomic nature of the disease. The use of diuretics to remove fluid is not effective because of the high interstitial protein concentration. Development of fibrosis and irreversible changes in the subcutaneous tissue further limit options. The objectives of conservative treatment are to control edema, maintain healthy skin, and avoid cellulitis and lymphangitis.
    1. Combination of physical therapies (CPT) is the primary approach recommended in a consensus document by the International Society of Lymphology Executive Committee (*Lymphology* 1995;28:113). CPT involves gentle manual manipulation of tissues to direct lymph flow, physical therapy exercises, and compression bandages. It is followed by the wearing of custom-made compression garments. In a study of 119 patients with 3-year follow-up, CPT reduced lymphedema by 63% (*Oncology* 1997;11:99).
    2. Sequential pneumatic compression has been shown to improve lymphedema. Several designs have been used with various degrees of success. Elastic stockings or sleeves should be fitted and worn afterward to maintain results. Extremity elevation may also help.
    3. Skin care and good hygiene are important. Topical hydrocortisone cream may be needed for eczema.
    4. Benzopyrones (such as warfarin) have been effective in reducing lymphedema due to filariasis. Their action is believed to derive from enhanced macrophage activity and extralymphatic absorption of interstitial proteins.
    5. Cellulitis and lymphangitis should be suspected when sudden onset of pain, swelling, or erythema of the leg occurs. Intravenous antibiotics should be initiated to cover staphylococci and β-hemolytic streptococci. Broad-spectrum penicillins, cephalosporins, or vancomycin usually are adequate. Limb elevation and immobilization should be initiated, and warm compresses can be used for symptomatic relief. Topical antifungal cream may be needed for chronic infections.
  B. Surgical options. Only 10% of patients with lymphedema are surgical candidates, and surgery is directed at reducing limb size. Indications for operation are related to function because cosmetic deformities persist postoperatively. Results are best when surgery is performed for severely impaired movement and recurrent cellulitis. A paucity of recent publications on surgical therapy for lymphatic disease suggests that this approach is being largely abandoned.
    1. Total subcutaneous excision is performed for extensive swelling and skin changes. Circumferential excision of the skin and subcutaneous tissue from the tibial tuberosity to the malleoli is performed. The defect is closed with a split- or full-thickness skin graft from the resected specimen or a split-thickness skin graft from an uninvolved site. Recurrent lymphedema and hyperpigmentation occur more frequently when split-thickness skin grafts are used.
    2. Closure of disrupted lymphatic channels.
    3. Omental transposition.
    4. Lymphatic transposition includes direct (lymphovenous bypass, lymphatic grafting) and indirect (mesenteric bridge, omental flap) procedures. Lymphatic grafting is performed for upper-extremity or unilateral lower-extremity lymphedema. Good results have been reported in 80% of patients (*Plast Reconstr Surg* 1990;85:64). A mesenteric bridge is formed by suturing a segment of mucosa-stripped ileum with intact blood supply to transected distal iliac or inguinal nodes.

An omental flap placed in a swollen limb is believed to improve lymphatic drainage through spontaneous lympholymphatic anastomoses. Due to their complexity and associated complications, indirect procedures are not widely used.

5. Microsurgical lymphovenous anastomosis bypass the obstructed lymphatic system in patients with chronic lymphedema. With improved microvascular techniques, patency rates of 50% to 70% can be expected many months after surgery (*J Vasc Surg* 1986;4:148).

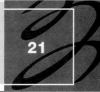

THYROID

I. EMBRYONIC DEVELOPMENT AND PHYSIOLOGY provide the basis and rationale for many aspects of thyroid surgery. The thyroid gland develops from the endoderm of the primitive foregut, arises in the ventral pharynx in the region of the base of the tongue, and descends into the neck. This course of descent of the thyroid is the embryologic reason for the pyramidal lobe and findings such as thyroglossal duct cysts and undescended thyroid at the base of the tongue. The parafollicular cells, or C cells, are derived from the neural crest and migrate to the thyroid. The thyroid is stimulated to release thyroid hormone in response to thyroid-stimulating hormone (TSH) from the anterior pituitary gland, which is stimulated by thyrotropin-releasing hormone (TRH) from the hypothalamus. Thyroid hormone synthesis begins when dietary iodide is ingested, actively transported into the thyroid gland, and then oxidized by thyroid peroxidase into iodine. Iodinization of tyrosine results in monoiodotyrosine (MIT) and diiodotyrosine (DIT). Iodine coupling of MIT and DIT results in the formation of triiodothyronine (T_3) and thyroxine (T_4), which are bound to thyroglobulin while in the thyroid. On release into plasma, the majority of T_3 and are bound to thyroid-binding globulin (TBG). Only the unbound or "free" hormones are active (i.e., available to tissues).

II. EVALUATION OF THYROID DISORDERS

A. Clinical features of hyperthyroidism reflect increased catabolism and excessive sympathetic activity caused by excess circulating thyroid hormones. Symptoms of hyperthyroidism include weight loss despite normal or increased appetite, heat intolerance, excessive perspiration, anxiety, irritability, palpitations, fatigue, muscle weakness, and oligomenorrhea. Signs of hyperthyroidism include goiter, sinus tachycardia or atrial fibrillation, tremor, hyperreflexia, fine or thinning hair, thyroid bruit, muscle wasting, and weakness, particularly of the proximal thigh musculature. The presentation of hyperthyroidism can vary considerably with age: Young patients usually present with hypermetabolism, whereas older patients may present primarily with tachyarrhythmias or cardiac failure. Rarely, elderly patients experience only wasting, apathy, confusion, or depression (apathetic hyperthyroidism). **Clinical features of hypothyroidism** include cold intolerance, weight gain, constipation, edema (especially of the eyelids, hands, and feet), dry skin, dry and thinning hair, weakness, somnolence, and menorrhagia.

B. Biochemical thyroid function testing confirms clinically suspected abnormalities in thyroid function; however, test results must be interpreted in the context of clinical findings. Measurement of serum TSH level and free T_4 (FT_4) is the best and most efficient combination of blood tests for diagnosis of most patients with thyroid disorders.

1. Measurement of **TSH** (0.3 to 5 mIU/L) by a second-generation sensitive TSH (sTSH) test is the most useful biochemical test in the diagnosis of thyroid illness. **In most ambulatory and hospitalized patients without pituitary disease, increased TSH signifies hypothyroidism, suppressed TSH suggests hyperthyroidism, and normal TSH reflects a euthyroid state.** Of note, critically ill, hospitalized patients, especially those receiving drugs such as dopamine or glucocorticoids, may have transient changes in TSH (usually elevated) without true abnormalities in thyroid function.

2. Assessment of T_4 concentration corroborates identified abnormalities in TSH and provides an index of severity of thyroid dysfunction. **Total T_4** (3 to 12 $\mu g/dL$) measurements quantify bound and unbound hormone and do not directly reflect the small "free" or active T_4 fractions. Factors that increase the thyroxine-binding globulin (TBG) concentration (estrogens, pregnancy, liver disease) may elevate the total T_4 or triiodothyronine (T_3) despite a normal free hormone concentration and a euthyroid state. Androgens, severe hypoproteinemia, chronic liver disease, and acromegaly result in decreased TBG.

3. **The FT_4 index** [FT_4I = total T_4 × RT_3U (RT_3U is the resin T_3 uptake)] (0.85 to 3.5) correlates more closely with the level of FT_4, eliminates ambiguity introduced by altered thyroglobulin levels, and is the preferred test for estimating FT_4.

4. **The resin T_3 uptake (RT_3U)** (20% to 40%) test measures unoccupied thyroid hormone–binding sites on TBG by allowing radiolabeled T_3 to compete for binding between TBG and a resin. This assay provides an indirect measure of FT_4. In patients with hyperthyroidism, the resin uptake is elevated because most of the sites on TBG are occupied by T_4 so that more radioactive T_3 binds to the resin. The RT_3U is directly related to the FT_4 fraction and inversely related to the TBG binding sites.

5. **Measurement of T_3** (80 to 200 ng/dL) is unreliable as a test for hypothyroidism. This test is useful in the occasional patient with suspected hyperthyroidism, suppressed sTSH, and normal FT_4I (T_3 thyrotoxicosis).

6. **Antithyroid microsomal antibodies** are found in the serum of patients with autoimmune thyroiditis (Hashimoto thyroiditis), and measurement of these antibodies is helpful for diagnosing this common cause of hypothyroidism. **Anti-TSH receptor antibodies,** which stimulate the TSH receptor, are detectable in more than 90% of patients with autoimmune hyperthyroidism (Graves disease); however, their measurement is not often needed in the diagnosis of this disease.

7. A useful **thyroid function test algorithm** (*Clin Lab Med* 1993;13:673) includes TSH assay as the initial test. If this is normal, no further tests are needed. If TSH is elevated, FT_4I and microsomal antibodies are measured to confirm hypothyroidism, which is often autoimmune. If TSH is suppressed, FT_4I is measured to confirm primary hyperthyroidism. If TSH is low and FT_4I is normal, T_3 is measured to diagnose T_3 thyrotoxicosis.

C. **Thyroid imaging** is most often accomplished with radionuclide scanning or ultrasound; other imaging modes, including computed tomography (CT) and magnetic resonance (MR) scan, are useful in special circumstances.

1. **Thyroid ultrasonography** with high-frequency (7.5 to 10 MHz) transducers accurately determines gland volume, as well as the number and character of thyroid nodules (*Am J Med* 1995;99:642). Although they are not completely reliable, features suggestive of malignancy on ultrasound include hypoechoic pattern, incomplete peripheral halo, irregular margins, and microcalcifications. Ultrasound is useful for guiding fine needle aspiration (FNA) biopsy and cyst aspiration. Cysts seen on ultrasound, especially those larger than 3 cm, are malignant in up to 14% of cases. Ultrasound followed by FNA of abnormalities larger than 1 cm is the most common imaging and diagnostic algorithm.

2. **Technetium thyroid scanning** can be useful in differentiating solitary functioning nodules from multinodular goiter or Graves disease. Hypofunctioning areas (cyst, neoplasm, or suppressed tissue adjacent to autonomous nodules) are "cold," whereas areas of increased synthesis are "hot." Thyroid scans cannot differentiate benign from malignant lesions and therefore are not generally useful in the routine workup of a thyroid nodule. **Radioactive iodine scanning** 4 to 24 hours after administration of oral iodine-131 (^{131}I) is useful for identifying metastatic differentiated thyroid tumors and for both confirming a diagnosis of Graves disease and predicting a response to ^{131}I radioablation.

3. **CT scanning and MR scan** of the thyroid are costly and generally are reserved for assessing substernal or retrosternal masses suspected to be goiters.
4. **Antithyroglobulin antibodies, antimicrosomal antibodies.**

III. SPECIFIC THYROID DISORDERS

A. Autoimmune diffuse toxic goiter (**Graves disease**) is the most common cause of hyperthyroidism and may be caused by stimulating immunoglobulins directed against the TSH receptor. Graves disease may be treated with antithyroid drugs, ablation with radioactive iodine (RAI), or surgery, depending on the clinical situation.

1. **Ablation with RAI is the treatment of choice for most patients with Graves disease.** A dose of 5 to 10 mCi of ^{131}I is given orally and is 75% effective after 4 to 12 weeks. In the 25% of patients with persistent thyrotoxicosis after 12 weeks, double the initial dose is repeated. After treatment, there is a high incidence (70%) of eventual permanent hypothyroidism, which is managed easily by replacement therapy. There are virtually no other long-term side effects of RAI (i.e., no significantly increased risk of thyroid cancer, leukemia, or teratogenicity). Contraindications to radiotherapy include pregnant women, newborns, patients who refuse, and patients with low RAI uptake (<20%) in the thyroid. Treatment of children or young adults (<30 years) with RAI is controversial because of presumed long-term oncogenic risks.

2. **Thyroidectomy for Graves disease** may be indicated for children and adolescents, pregnant women (late second or early third trimester), patients unresponsive to or noncompliant with medical therapy, and patients who refuse RAI. Opinions differ on whether bilateral subtotal thyroidectomy, in which a 1- to 2-g vascularized cuff of thyroid is left on each side, or total thyroidectomy is a better option. The long-term incidence of recurrent hyperthyroidism after surgery is approximately 10% but depends on amount of tissue left behind. Total thyroidectomy usually results in hypothyroidism. Risks of surgery are extremely small (<1%) in experienced hands but include hypoparathyroidism and injury to the recurrent laryngeal nerve. Patients with recurrent hyperthyroidism after thyroidectomy should be considered for treatment with RAI because reoperation carries a somewhat higher risk of complication.

3. Thionamide drugs, such as **propylthiouracil (PTU) or methimazole,** are used for antithyroid drug therapy. PTU (100 to 300 mg orally three times daily) is given for 4 to 6 weeks until the patient becomes euthyroid; then the dose usually is decreased (100 mg orally three times daily). The patient is then treated empirically for 6 to 18 months, at which time the drugs are withdrawn. Clinical features that favor remission include small gland size and mild hyperthyroidism. However, overall, long-term remission is achieved in less than 20% to 30% of patients. Antithyroid drugs also are used to prepare thyrotoxic patients for surgery or ablative therapy. PTU may be given during pregnancy at reduced doses, especially if thyroidectomy is necessary in the second trimester. Minor adverse reactions occur infrequently and include rash, hepatitis, arthralgias, and a lupuslike syndrome. Patients may also be treated throughout pregnancy with medication and have definitive treatment after delivery. Agranulocytosis is a rare (0.5%) but serious side effect of thionamide therapy.

B. In **multinodular goiter,** a large goiter or retrosternal extension can compress the trachea. Subtotal or total thyroidectomy is the treatment of choice if there are symptoms of compression, suspicion of malignancy, or questionable nodules or if the gland is cosmetically bothersome.

C. **Toxic adenoma** is an autonomously functioning thyroid nodule that produces hyperthyroidism and is treated by surgical excision (thyroid lobectomy) or RAI.

D. **Rare causes** of hyperthyroidism include self-administration of excessive thyroid hormone (factitious hyperthyroidism), iodine-induced hyperthyroidism, pituitary TSH-secreting adenoma, trophoblastic tumors secreting chorionic gonadotropin (which has TSH-like activity), struma ovarii, and thyroiditis.

IV. HYPOTHYROIDISM is almost always caused by primary hypofunction of the thyroid gland. Clinically, hypothyroid patients should be separated into those without goiter (primary atrophy), those with goitrous hypothyroidism (i.e., Hashimoto thyroiditis,

drug-induced hypothyroidism, iodine deficiency, and congenital causes of dyshormono-genesis), and those with postablative hypothyroidism (after thyroidectomy or treatment with RAI). Postablative hypothyroidism and Hashimoto thyroiditis are the most important causes of hypothyroidism encountered by the surgeon. Diagnosis rests on the characteristic clinical features and laboratory findings of an elevated TSH (usually 15 units/mL) and a decreased FT_4 level. A low TSH in association with low T_4 suggests pituitary or hypothalamic failure.

V. THYROIDITIS represents a diverse group of autoimmune and inflammatory disorders characterized by infiltration of the thyroid with inflammatory cells and subsequent fibrosis of the gland.

A. Hashimoto thyroiditis is a chronic autoimmune disorder characterized by destructive lymphocytic infiltration of the thyroid. The disease is 15 times more common in women, and more than 90% of patients have circulating antibodies directed against thyroid microsomes and thyroglobulin. Although patients initially are euthyroid, hypothyroidism may occur later. A firm symmetric or asymmetric goiter is palpable and usually (but not always) nontender. Cervical lymphadenopathy is uncommon. Euthyroid patients may not require treatment. Thyroid hormone is given to hypothyroid patients both as replacement therapy and to suppress TSH. Thyroidectomy is indicated for compressive symptoms, a dominant nodule suspicious for malignancy, or cosmetic preference.

B. Acute suppurative thyroiditis is rare and is caused by infection with *Streptococcus* or *Staphylococcus* species. Treatment consists of appropriate antibiotic therapy and surgical drainage of abscesses.

C. Subacute (de Quervain) thyroiditis is a rare condition that occurs in young women, often after a viral upper respiratory tract infection. Symptoms of fatigue, weakness, and painful thyroid enlargement radiating to the patient's jaw or ear are treated with nonsteroidal anti-inflammatory drugs or with steroids. The condition almost always remits spontaneously within a few weeks. Thyroidectomy may be indicated in rare cases of persistent thyroiditis after months of unsuccessful steroid treatment.

D. Riedel thyroiditis is a rare, progressive inflammatory condition of the entire thyroid gland, strap muscles, and other neck structures. Its cause is unknown, and it can be associated with other fibrotic processes, including retroperitoneal fibrosis, sclerosing cholangitis, and fibrosing mediastinitis. The lymphocytic infiltrate and dense fibrous tissue reaction in the thyroid result in a firm, nontender goiter with a woody texture. Riedel's thyroiditis may require surgical excision to exclude malignancy or relieve compressive symptoms.

VI. A SOLITARY THYROID NODULE commonly occurs (4% to 7% of adults) and is usually a benign lesion. Such nodules may be associated with a goiter or with an otherwise normal thyroid. The malignant potential of the newly discovered thyroid nodule is of justifiable concern to both physician and patient, and the goal of diagnostic testing is to separate the relatively few patients with thyroid malignancy from the larger group of patients with benign thyroid nodules. Surgical intervention is appropriate for all malignant or suspicious thyroid nodules and for all large (>3 or 4 cm) nodules. The frequency of cancer in surgically excised nodules is 8% to 17% (*N Engl J Med* 1993;328:553).

A. History and physical examination are invaluable in the management of the thyroid nodule. Nodules in the very young and very old (especially men) are more likely to be malignant. Exposure to ionizing radiation is a well-recognized risk factor for the development of thyroid carcinoma. A family history of thyroid malignancy, familial polyposis, or other endocrine disease also increases the risk of cancer. Rapid nodule growth, pain, compressive symptoms, or hoarseness of voice increase the likelihood of malignancy but are nonspecific. Physical findings of a solitary nodule with firm or irregular texture or with fixation to surrounding structures suggest malignancy. Similarly, the presence of enlarged cervical lymph nodes is extremely important because this finding is associated with thyroid cancer. Malignancy is uncommon in hyperfunctioning nodules, and all patients should have a serum TSH measured to exclude clinical or subclinical thyrotoxicosis.

B. FNA is the initial diagnostic test of choice for the euthyroid patient with a solitary thyroid nodule. This procedure is safe, inexpensive, and easy to perform, and it allows better selection of patients for operation than does any other technique (*Ann Intern Med* 1993;118:282).

   1. The technique of FNA involves palpation of the nodule, aspiration of sufficient material, and adequate preparation and staining of a smear of the aspirated cells. The equipment required includes a 25-gauge hypodermic needle, a syringe (3 to 10 cc), and a syringe holder (e.g., Cameco Ltd., London), which allows operation with a single hand. The thyroid gland is palpated with the patient supine and his or her neck slightly extended. The operator immobilizes the nodule between the index and middle fingers of his or her nondominant hand. The overlying skin is cleansed with povidone-iodine or alcohol. No local anesthetic is required. The needle is introduced into the nodule, and then either the piston of the syringe is retracted to create suction or material is allowed to pass into the syringe by passive action to minimize blood in the specimen. The needle tip can be gently angled in multiple directions within the nodule, again in an attempt to avoid excess trauma and bloody specimen. Before removing the needle, the suction is released to prevent aspiration of the needle contents into the syringe. Then the needle is detached, and air is introduced into the syringe before aspirated cells are expressed onto a slide. The smear is air-dried and stained using the May-Grünwald-Giemsa method, or it is alcohol-fixed and stained using the Papanicolaou method. Usually, two or three passes are made to limit sampling error. Ultrasound-guided FNA is useful when lesions are small or difficult to palpate.

   2. Cytologic **results of FNA** can be benign, malignant, or indeterminate, provided that an adequate specimen is obtained (an adequate specimen has at least ten groups of well-preserved follicular cells, with ten cells per group, obtained from two separate needle passes). The accuracy of the results ranges from 70% to 90% and is highly dependent on the skill and experience of the cytopathologist. The false-negative rate of FNA is low (<6%), and patients with negative (i.e., not cancerous, not indeterminate) cytology can be followed safely (*Surgery* 1989;106:980). Indeterminate aspirations pose difficult management decisions because carcinoma occurs in 10% to 30% of these cases. Follicular and Hürthle cell neoplasms and the follicular variant of papillary cancer account for many indeterminate results, whereas papillary, medullary, and undifferentiated thyroid carcinomas usually have distinctive cytopathologic features. Diagnostic thyroid lobectomy is indicated for all FNA-indeterminate and FNA-positive thyroid nodules and for all nodules, regardless of FNA result, in patients with a history of radiation exposure. An inadequate FNA biopsy is obtained in up to 20% of cases; half of these can be diagnosed with repeated aspiration. The management of nodules with persistently inadequate FNA should be guided by clinical criteria.

C. Ultrasonography and radionuclide thyroid scans cannot distinguish benign from malignant nodules and therefore are not essential in the workup of a thyroid nodule. Ultrasonography is commonly used to direct FNA biopsy and is a sensitive method for determining whether a lesion is solid or cystic. Although thyroid cysts have a lower likelihood of being malignant, larger carcinomas can undergo cystic degeneration. Cysts may disappear after FNA, but those that persist, recur, or yield insufficient material for interpretation should be excised. The role of radionuclide thyroid scanning in the workup of a thyroid nodule is limited.

D. Thyroid lobectomy is indicated for (1) nodules with malignant or indeterminate aspiration cytology, (2) nodules in children, (3) nodules in patients with either a history of neck irradiation or a family history of thyroid cancer, and (4) symptomatic or cosmetically bothersome nodules.

VII. THYROID NEOPLASMS

A. Differentiated (papillary and follicular) thyroid cancer is among the most curable of human cancers (*N Engl J Med* 1998;338:297). These cancers are rare in children and increase in frequency with age; the female-to-male ratio is approximately 2.5:1. The cause of these cancers is unknown, but childhood exposure to radiation (10 to 1,500 cGy) is the best-known etiologic factor. Approximately 30% of exposed children develop thyroid nodules, and of these, an estimated 30% are malignant. The appropriate initial procedure for a solitary thyroid nodule suspected of being malignant is a total lobectomy and isthmectomy. Controversy exists about the extent of surgery (lobectomy vs. total thyroidectomy) that should be performed for patients with proven differentiated thyroid cancer, principally because these patients have a good prognosis irrespective of the surgical treatment. The prognosis depends mostly on the patient's age as well as the extent and histologic subtype of the disease. Several prognostic index systems have been developed, including the MACIS (*m*etastasis, *a*ge, *c*ompleteness of resection, *i*nvasion, and *s*ize) and the tumor, node, metastasis classification (TNM) adjusted for patient age. In all, 85% to 90% of patients fall into a low-risk category with favorable prognosis.

1. **Papillary thyroid carcinoma (PTC)** represents 85% of thyroid carcinomas. PTC is often multifocal and frequently metastasizes to cervical lymph nodes. Occult, clinically insignificant foci of microscopic PTC are found in 4% to 28% of autopsies or in thyroidectomy specimens for benign diseases. A young age at diagnosis is a favorable prognostic factor, and even involvement of cervical nodes does not affect the prognosis adversely.

   a. **Total thyroidectomy** is appropriate for patients with gross evidence of bilateral disease, multifocal PTC, or a history of neck irradiation. Total thyroidectomy is arguably the treatment of choice for unilateral tumors larger than 1 to 1.5 cm. Advantages of total thyroidectomy include the ability to treat extrathyroidal metastases or recurrences with RAI and to use serum thyroglobulin to monitor therapy. Retrospective studies also show a decreased risk of recurrence or death. Complications of total thyroidectomy include hypoparathyroidism and recurrent laryngeal nerve (RLN) injury, which occur in less than 1% of cases. Patients with clinically evident lymph node involvement should undergo ipsilateral central or lateral neck dissection at the time of thyroidectomy. We use preoperative ultrasound on the day of surgery to identify suspicious lymph nodes whose sites are marked on the skin. The role of routine central neck dissection in patients without palpable lymph nodes is controversial. Sywak et al. presented data from the University of Sydney comparing 56 patients with differentiated thyroid cancer who underwent central neck dissection at the time of thyroidectomy with 391 who underwent thyroidectomy alone. They found that patients undergoing central neck dissection had lower overall thyroglobulin levels and were more likely to have undetectable thyroglobulin levels (a biochemical surrogate for cure) than patients who underwent thyroidectomy alone, with similar morbidity (*Surgery* 2006;140:1000).

   b. **Radioablation** of metastatic or residual cancer and residual thyroid tissue is performed with 75 to 100 mCi of ^{131}I at 4 weeks after total thyroidectomy while the patient is hypothyroid (i.e., **TSH 30 μIU/mL** on no replacement of T_4). Ablation may be repeated at higher doses if residual disease is detected on follow-up scans.

   c. Lifelong long-term **suppression** of TSH therapy with thyroid hormone replacement decreases recurrences and may improve survival.

2. **Follicular thyroid carcinoma** (10% of thyroid carcinomas) is rare before age 30 years and has a slightly worse prognosis than PTC. Unlike PTC, follicular thyroid cancer has a propensity to spread hematogenously to bone, lung, or liver. Small (<1 cm), unilateral follicular carcinomas with limited invasion of the tumor capsule may be treated with thyroid lobectomy, whereas larger tumors (>1 cm), multicentric tumors, and tumors with more extensive capsular and vascular invasion or distant metastases are treated with total thyroidectomy. Radioablation is indicated after total thyroidectomy, followed by lifelong thyroid hormone suppression.

B. **Medullary thyroid carcinoma (MTC)** arises from the thyroid C cells that derive from the neural crest and secrete calcitonin. MTC may occur sporadically or may be inherited, either alone or as a component of multiple endocrine neoplasia (MEN) type 2A or 2B. Sporadic MTC usually is detected as a firm, palpable, unilateral nodule with or without involved cervical lymph nodes. Patients with hereditary MTC develop bilateral, multifocal tumors and often are diagnosed on the basis of family screening. MTC should be suspected if tumor calcification is noted on plain x-rays or if the patient has profuse diarrhea and episodic flushing (caused by excess calcitonin release). MTC spreads early to cervical lymph nodes and may metastasize to liver, lungs, or bone. All patients with suspected or known MTC should have a careful family history taken, be tested biochemically for pheochromocytoma before thyroidectomy, and be genetically tested for DNA mutations in the tyrosine kinase receptor *RET* proto-oncogene (*Hum Mol Genet* 1993;2:851). MTC can be detected biochemically by measurement of an elevated plasma calcitonin level. **Treatment** of MTC is total thyroidectomy with removal of the lymph nodes in the central zone of the patient's neck (from the sternal notch to the hyoid bone and laterally to the carotid sheaths). A modified neck dissection is indicated for clinically involved ipsilateral cervical lymph nodes. Of patients with persistently elevated calcitonin levels after initial thyroidectomy, 28% had normalized early postoperative calcitonin levels after a subsequent meticulous bilateral microdissection of cervical lymph nodes (*Surgery* 1993;114:1090). There are no proven systemic chemotherapy options for MTC; however, in vitro research has demonstrated inhibition of MTC cell growth and RET tyrosine kinase activity by tyrosine kinase inhibitors (*Surgery* 2004:132:960), and clinical trials using multiple new agents are being carried out.

C. **Undifferentiated or anaplastic thyroid carcinoma** (1% to 2% of thyroid carcinomas) carries an extremely poor prognosis, usually presents as a fixed, sometimes painful goiter, and usually occurs in patients older than 50 years. Invasion of local structures, with resultant dysphagia, respiratory compromise, or hoarseness due to recurrent laryngeal nerve involvement can preclude curative resection. External irradiation or chemotherapy may provide limited palliation.

D. **Primary malignant lymphoma of the thyroid** often is associated with Hashimoto thyroiditis. Surgical resection is usually not indicated once a diagnosis is made.

VIII. **POSTOPERATIVE THYROID HORMONE REPLACEMENT** is necessary after total or near total thyroidectomy or ablation with radioiodine. Oral levothyroxine is begun before discharge at an average dose of 100 μg/day (0.8 μg/lb/day). Adequacy of thyroid hormone replacement is assessed by measuring T_4 and TSH at 6 to 12 weeks after surgery. Adjustments to the dose should not be more frequent than monthly in the absence of symptoms and should be cautious (12.5- to 25-μg increments).

IX. **MANAGEMENT OF COMPLICATIONS AFTER THYROIDECTOMY**

A. **Hemorrhage** is a rare but serious complication of thyroidectomy that usually occurs within 6 hours of surgery. Management can require control of the airway by endotracheal intubation and, rarely, can require urgent opening of incision and evacuation of hematoma before return to the operating room for wound irrigation and ligation of the bleeding point.

B. **Transient hypocalcemia** commonly occurs 24 to 48 hours after thyroidectomy but infrequently requires treatment. Patients who are markedly symptomatic or who have serum calcium below 7 mg/dL are given one to two ampules (10 to 20 mL) of 10% calcium gluconate intravenously over 1 to 2 minutes, followed by temporary oral calcium carbonate (500 mg orally three times a day). More prolonged intravenous replacement is achieved by mixing six ampules of 10% calcium gluconate (540 mg of elemental calcium) in dextrose 5% in water (D5W), 500 mL, for infusion at 1 mL/kg/hour. Permanent hypoparathyroidism is uncommon after total thyroidectomy. Normal parathyroid tissue removed or devascularized at the time of total thyroidectomy must be minced into 1 × 3-mm fragments and autotransplanted into individual muscle pockets in the sternocleidomastoid muscle to maximize the chances that the patient will not develop postoperative hypoparathyroidism (*Ann Surg* 1996;223:472).

C. **Recurrent laryngeal nerve injury** is a devastating complication of thyroidectomy that should occur rarely (<1%). Unilateral RLN injury causes hoarseness, and bilateral injury compromises the airway, necessitating tracheostomy. Repeat neck exploration, thyroidectomy for extensive goiter or Graves disease, and thyroidectomy for fixed, locally invasive cancers are procedures particularly prone to RLN injury. Intentional (as with locally invasive cancer) or inadvertent transection of the RLN can be repaired primarily or with a nerve graft, although the efficacy of these repairs is not known. Temporary RLN palsies can occur during thyroidectomy, and these usually resolve over a period of 4 to 6 weeks. The **external branch of the superior laryngeal nerve** may be injured if it is not identified during ligation of the superior thyroid pole vascular bundle. This injury results in weakness of the patient's voice at high pitch. The best prevention of these injuries is a thorough understanding of the anatomy of these nerves.

PARATHYROID

I. **HYPERPARATHYROIDISM (HPT)** refers to hypercalcemia caused by inappropriate parathyroid hormone (PTH) release from the parathyroid glands. Primary HPT results from autonomous release of PTH from parathyroid adenoma or hyperplastic parathyroid glands. Secondary HPT results from a defect in mineral homeostasis (e.g., renal failure), with a compensatory increase in parathyroid function. Tertiary HPT results from the development of autonomous, calcium-insensitive parathyroids after prolonged secondary stimulation (e.g., prolonged renal failure).

A. **Primary HPT**

1. **Incidence.** Primary HPT has an incidence of 0.25 to 1 per 1,000 population in the United States and is especially common in postmenopausal women. It most often occurs sporadically, but it can be inherited alone or as a component of familial endocrinopathies, including MEN types 1 and 2A.

2. The more common **clinical findings associated with HPT** include nephrolithiasis, osteoporosis, hypertension, and emotional disturbances. The widespread use of the multichannel autoanalyzer has led to more patients being diagnosed with **"asymptomatic" hypercalcemia** or with earlier symptoms, such as muscle weakness, polyuria, anorexia, and nausea. When they are carefully questioned, many patients with HPT turn out to be symptomatic.

3. **Differential diagnosis of hypercalcemia** includes HPT, malignancy, granulomatous disease (e.g., sarcoidosis), immobility, hyperthyroidism, milk-alkali syndrome, and familial hypocalciuric hypercalcemia (FHH). Patients with hypercalcemia and suspected HPT at a minimum should have their serum calcium, phosphate, creatinine, and PTH measured. The diagnosis of HPT is biochemical and requires demonstration of hypercalcemia (serum calcium 10.5 mg/dL) and an elevated PTH level. **The assay of choice for PTH is the highly sensitive and specific intact PTH level radioimmunoassay.** Free calcium level (ionized calcium) is a more sensitive test of physiologically active calcium. Hypercalcemia without an elevated PTH can be due to a variety of causes (especially malignancy, Paget disease, sarcoidosis, and milk-alkali syndrome) that must be excluded. FHH commonly causes a mild hypercalcemia and elevated PTH, as seen in HPT. FHH is caused by loss-of-function mutations in the calcium-sensing receptor, which leads to loss of feedback inhibition of PTH secretion by the parathyroids. FHH can generally be distinguished from HPT by measurement of the renal calcium/creatinine clearance ratio. A ratio less than 0.01 suggests FHH; the ratios seen in HPT are generally much higher. Parathyroidectomy is ineffective for FHH. Elevated PTH promotes bicarbonate excretion, causing hyperchloremic metabolic acidosis; the chloride-to-phosphate ratio exceeds 33 in 96% of patients with HPT (*Ann Intern Med* 1974;80:200). Radiographic features of HPT are seen in advanced cases and include decreased bone density, osteitis fibrosa cystica, and the pathognomonic sign of subperiosteal bone resorption on the radial aspect of the phalanges of the second or third digits of the hand.

4. **Preoperative localization** of parathyroid adenomas is generally not necessary before a careful neck exploration by an experienced endocrine surgeon, as stated

by the 1991 National Institutes of Health (NIH) consensus conference. However, current practice makes use of several techniques to facilitate limited neck exploration to ensure a high success rate in the outpatient setting. These techniques include radio- and/or image-guided exploration (sestamibi or ultrasound guided), videoscopic exploration, and intraoperative intact PTH-level monitoring (*Surgery* 1997;122:1107). The most frequently applied approach is preoperative sestamibi scanning, followed by direct excision of the identified gland and confirmation of cure by intraoperative PTH measurement. This intraoperative test requires the availability of a rapid assay of intact PTH, which confirms the success of the surgery immediately if the PTH level falls more than 50% at 10 minutes after the apparent source of PTH has been removed. If the preoperative localization scan is not informative, then a standard four-gland exploration is appropriate.

5. **Parathyroidectomy is indicated** for all patients with symptomatic HPT. Nephrolithiasis, bone disease, and neuromuscular symptoms are improved more often than renal insufficiency, hypertension, and psychiatric symptoms. Parathyroidectomy for asymptomatic HPT is somewhat controversial. A recent large prospective study of patients with asymptomatic HPT found that 27% developed symptoms of hypercalcemia with 10-year follow-up (*N Engl J Med* 1999;341: 1249). A consensus conference organized by the NIH in 1990 attempted to define a rational basis for recommending parathyroidectomy for asymptomatic patients. A follow- up conference of the NIH and the National Institute of Diabetes and Digestive and Kidney Diseases in 2002 recommended parathyroidectomy for the following patients: (1) those younger than 50 years of age, (2) those who cannot participate in appropriate follow-up, (3) those with a serum calcium level greater than 1 mg/dL above the normal range, (4) those with urinary calcium greater than 400 mg per 24 hours, (5) those with a 30% decrease in renal function, and (6) those with complications of primary HPT, including nephrocalcinosis, osteoporosis [T score <2.5 standard deviations (SD) at the lumbar spine, hip, or wrist], or a severe psychoneurologic disorder (*J Bone Miner Res.* 2002; 17(Supp2):N57).

6. **Neck exploration and parathyroidectomy** for HPT result in normocalcemia in more than 95% of patients when performed by an experienced surgeon without any preoperative or intraoperative localization studies. A thorough, orderly search and identification of all four parathyroid glands are the cornerstones of the standard surgical management of HPT. In the current era, preoperative localization studies are used in conjunction with rapid intraoperative PTH measurement to enable "minimally invasive parathyroidectomy," which generally means directed unilateral neck exploration and/or local/monitored anesthesia care (MAC) anesthesia. Most often, a single adenomatous gland is found and resected; normal parathyroid glands should be left in place. Intraoperative measurement of PTH demonstrating a 50% decrease and return to the normal level after resection of the adenoma is highly indicative of cure. In the event that an abnormally enlarged parathyroid or all four parathyroids cannot be found, a thorough exploration for ectopic or supernumerary glands should be performed. Embryonic development should inform this search: Superior parathyroid glands develop from the fourth pharyngeal pouch and most commonly are located dorsally along the middle or upper thyroid lobe, near the intersection of the inferior thyroid artery and recurrent laryngeal nerve, dorsal and superior to the nerve. Ectopic superior glands may be found posterior and deep to the thyroid, in the tracheoesophageal groove, posterior to the inferior thyroid vessels, between the carotid artery and the esophagus. Undescended or incompletely descended glands may be found cranial to the superior thyroid pole, and excessive caudal migration may result in a gland residing in the middle mediastinum. Inferior parathyroid glands develop in conjunction with the thymus from the third pharyngeal pouch, and are more variable in position than are the superior glands. They are usually located medial and ventral to the recurrent laryngeal nerve at the inferior pole of the thyroid lobe within the thyrothymic ligament. Ectopic inferior glands are most likely found embedded

in the thymus in the anterior mediastinum. Undescended inferior glands may be found in the superior neck between the carotid and the larynx. Occasionally, multiple parathyroid adenomas are found, which should be removed, leaving at least one normal parathyroid behind. Four-gland parathyroid hyperplasia is rare, and its management is controversial. Acceptable options include total parathyroidectomy with parathyroid autotransplantation or 3.5-gland parathyroidectomy. **The dictation of a clear, factual operative note detailing the identification and position of each parathyroid gland is essential.** This information is invaluable in the unlikely event of reoperation for persistent or recurrent HPT.

7. **Familial primary HPT** may occur alone or as a component of MEN type 1 and type 2A. HPT in these syndromes is primarily chief cell hyperplasia and variable enlargement of all four glands. These patients have a higher incidence of recurrent or persistent hypercalcemia after parathyroidectomy.

B. Hypercalcemia from **secondary and tertiary HPT** is treated initially with dietary phosphate restriction, phosphate binders, and vitamin D supplementation. Patients with medically unresponsive, symptomatic HPT (e.g., bone pain and osteopenia, ectopic calcification, or pruritus) may be surgically treated with total parathyroidectomy and heterotopic autotransplantation, or subtotal parathyroidectomy. Controversy exists as to what type of surgery is best and what postoperative level of parathyroid hormone is necessary to prevent adynamic bone disease after such procedures.

II. **REOPERATIVE PARATHYROID SURGERY** may be necessary for persistent or recurrent HPT. In all cases, HPT must be reconfirmed biochemically, and 24-hour urinary calcium should be obtained to exclude FHH. Preoperative localization is mandatory and includes careful review of the operative note from the initial surgery and concordant noninvasive studies. Approximately 70% to 80% of patients undergoing re-exploration after an initial failed operation have a missed gland that is accessible through a cervical incision. Reoperative parathyroid surgery carries a substantially higher risk of injury to the recurrent laryngeal nerve and of hypocalcemia due to postoperative scarring and disruption of normal tissue planes.

A. **Preoperative localization** should include ^{99m}Tc-sestamibi scintigraphy and ultrasound or CT scanning. These noninvasive studies are successful in localizing the missed gland in 25% to 75% of cases (*Radiology* 1987;162:133). With combined use of CT scan, ultrasonography, and scintigraphy, at least one imaging study identifies the tumor in more than 75% of patients. Noninvasive localizing studies must be interpreted in the context of the operative note. Invasive imaging tests, including angiography, are associated with greater morbidity and measurable mortality; they should be reserved for complex cases with negative or equivocal noninvasive studies. The success of these tests in localizing the concealed tumor is highly dependent on the skill and experience of the radiologist (*Radiology* 1987;162:138). Invasive studies are most helpful for identifying rare glands located outside the patient's neck (e.g., mediastinum).

B. **Operative strategy.** The goal of re-exploration is to perform an orderly search based on the information gained from the initial operation and from localization studies.

1. **Missed parathyroid glands** are found either in the usual position or in ectopic sites, as determined by the embryology of parathyroid development. Rarely, a parathyroid gland is intrathyroidal (especially in patients with multinodular goiter), and intraoperative thyroid ultrasound followed by thyroid lobectomy can be performed if an exhaustive search fails to identify the parathyroid adenoma. If four normal glands have been located, the adenoma is likely to represent a supernumerary (fifth) gland. Intraoperative ultrasound is an effective tool for localizing parathyroid glands.

2. **Mediastinal adenomas** within the thymus are managed by resecting the cranial portion of the thymus by gentle traction on the thyrothymic ligament or by a complete transcervical thymectomy using a specialized substernal retractor (*Ann Surg* 1991;214:555). Median sternotomy carries a higher morbidity and increased postoperative pain, and the possibility of these should be discussed with the patient preoperatively.

III. PARATHYROID AUTOTRANSPLANTATION

A. Indications for **total parathyroidectomy and heterotopic parathyroid autotransplantation** include HPT in patients with renal failure, in patients with four-gland parathyroid hyperplasia, and in patients undergoing neck re-exploration in which the adenoma is the only remaining parathyroid tissue. The site of parathyroid autotransplantation may be the sternocleidomastoid muscle or the brachioradialis muscle of the patient's nondominant forearm. Parathyroid grafting into the patient's forearm is advantageous if recurrent HPT is possible (e.g., MEN type 1 or 2A). If HPT recurs, localization is simplified, and the hyperplastic parathyroid tissue may be excised from the patient's forearm under local anesthesia.

B. **Technique.** Freshly removed parathyroid gland tissue is cut into fine pieces approximately 1 mm × 1 mm × 2 mm and placed in sterile iced saline. An incision is made in the patient's nondominant forearm, and separate intramuscular beds are created by spreading the fibers of the brachioradialis with a fine forceps. Approximately four to five pieces are placed in each site, and a total of approximately 100 mg of parathyroid tissue are transplanted. The beds are closed with a silk suture to mark the site of the transplanted tissue. Transplanted parathyroid tissue begins to function within 14 to 21 days of surgery.

C. **Cryopreservation of parathyroid glands** is performed in MEN patients and all patients who may become aparathyroid after repeat exploration. Cryopreservation may be performed by freezing approximately 200 mg of finely cut parathyroid tissue in vials containing 10% dimethyl sulfoxide, 10% autologous serum, and 80% Waymouth medium. Cryopreserved parathyroid tissue can be used for autotransplantation in patients who become aparathyroid or in patients with failure of the initial grafted parathyroid tissue. Viable cryopreservation and subsequent thawing must be performed in a Food and Drug Administration (FDA)–approved GMP (good medical practice) facility.

IV. POSTOPERATIVE HYPOCALCEMIA

A. **Transient hypocalcemia** commonly occurs after total thyroidectomy or parathyroidectomy and requires treatment if it is severe (total serum calcium <7.5 mg/dL) or if the patient is symptomatic. Chvostek sign (twitching of the facial muscles when the examiner percusses over the facial nerve anterior to the patient's ear) is a sign of relative hypocalcemia but is present in up to 15% of the normal population. This sign is not necessarily an indication for calcium replacement.

B. Patients with **persistent hypocalcemia** after total thyroidectomy or after parathyroid autotransplantation can require continued supplementation for 6 to 8 weeks postoperatively. Usually, patients are given calcium carbonate, 500 to 1,000 mg orally three times per day, and 1,25-dihydroxyvitamin D_3, 0.25 μg orally per day.

C. **Hypocalcemic tetany** is a medical emergency that is treated with rapid intravenous administration of 10% calcium gluconate or calcium chloride until the patient recovers. Specifically, one to two ampules (10 to 20 mL) of 10% calcium gluconate are given intravenously over 10 minutes, and the dose may be repeated every 15 to 20 minutes, as required. Subsequently, a continuous infusion of 10% calcium gluconate (90 mg of elemental calcium/10 mL), 60 mL in 500 mL D5W (1 mg/mL), is initiated at 0.5 to 2 mg/kg/hour to maintain the serum calcium at 8 to 9 mg/dL. Patients with severe hypocalcemia also must have correction of hypomagnesemia.

V. PARATHYROID CARCINOMA is rare and accounts for less than 1% of patients with HPT. Approximately 50% of these patients have a palpable neck mass, and serum calcium levels may exceed 15 mg/dL.

A. **Diagnosis** is made by the histologic finding of vascular or capsular invasion, lymph node or distant metastases, or gross invasion of local structures.

B. **Surgical treatment** is radical local excision of the tumor, surrounding soft tissue, lymph nodes, and ipsilateral thyroid lobe when the disease is recognized preoperatively or intraoperatively. Reoperation is indicated for local recurrence in an attempt to control malignant hypercalcemia.

C. Patients with parathyroid carcinoma and some patients with benign HPT may develop **hyperparathyroid crisis.** Symptoms of this acute, sometimes fatal illness include profound muscular weakness, nausea and vomiting, drowsiness, and confusion.

Hypercalcemia (16 to 20 mg/dL) and azotemia are usually present. Ultimate treatment of "parathyroid crisis" is parathyroidectomy; however, hypercalcemia and volume and electrolyte abnormalities should be addressed first. Treatment is warranted for symptoms or a serum calcium level greater than 12 mg/dL. First-line therapy is infusion of 300 to 500 mL/hour of 0.9% sodium chloride (5 to 10 L/day intravenously) to restore intravascular volume and to promote renal excretion of calcium. After urinary output exceeds 100 mL/hour, furosemide (80 to 100 mg intravenously every 2 to 6 hours) may be given to promote further renal sodium and calcium excretion. Thiazide diuretics impair calcium excretion and should be avoided. Hypokalemia and hypomagnesemia are complications of forced saline diuresis and should be corrected. If diuresis alone is unsuccessful in lowering the serum calcium, other calcium-lowering agents may be used. These include the **bisphosphonates** pamidronate (60 to 90 mg in 1 L of 0.9% saline infused over 24 hours) and etidronate (7.5 mg/kg intravenously over 2 to 4 hours daily for 3 days); **mithramycin** [25 μg/kg intravenously over 4 to 6 hours daily for 3 to 4 days (malignant hypercalcemia only)]; and salmon **calcitonin** (initial dose, 4 IU/kg subcutaneously or intramuscularly every 12 hours, increasing as necessary to a maximum dose of 8 IU/kg subcutaneously or intramuscularly every 6 hours). Orthophosphate, gallium nitrate, and glucocorticoids also have calcium-lowering effects.

 ENDOCRINE PANCREAS

Pancreatic islet cell tumors are rare tumors that produce clinical syndromes related to the specific hormone secreted. Insulinomas are the most common of these tumors, followed by gastrinoma, then the rarer VIPoma (vasoactive intestinal polypeptide–secreting tumor), glucagonoma, and somatostatinoma. Recognition of **characteristic syndromes** is key to the diagnosis, which **must be confirmed biochemically.** Islet cell tumors are often occult, and their localization may be difficult, especially for small, multifocal, or extrapancreatic tumors. Islet cell tumors may occur sporadically or as a component of MEN type 1 or von Hippel-Lindau disease (nearly always multifocal). Islet cell tumors may be benign or malignant, although prediction may be based on the hormone produced rather than the tumor size.

I. INSULINOMA

    A. Clinical features. Patients with insulinoma develop profound hypoglycemia during fasting or after exercise. The clinical picture includes the signs and symptoms of neuroglycopenia (anxiety, tremor, confusion, and obtundation) and the sympathetic response to hypoglycemia (hunger, sweating, and tachycardia). These bizarre complaints initially may be attributed to malingering or a psychosomatic etiology unless the association with fasting is recognized. Many patients eat excessively to avoid symptoms, causing significant weight gain. **Whipple triad** refers to the clinical criteria for the diagnosis of insulinoma: (1) hypoglycemic symptoms during monitored fasting, (2) blood glucose levels less than 50 mg/dL, and (3) relief of symptoms after administration of intravenous glucose. Factitious hypoglycemia (excess exogenous insulin administration) and postprandial reactive hypoglycemia must be excluded.

    B. A supervised, in-hospital **72-hour fast** is required to diagnose insulinoma. Patients are observed for hypoglycemic episodes and have 6-hour measurement of plasma glucose, insulin, proinsulin, and C peptide. The fast is terminated when symptoms of neuroglycopenia develop. Nearly all patients with insulinoma develop neuroglycopenic symptoms and have inappropriately elevated plasma insulin (>5 μU/mL) associated with hypoglycemia (glucose <50 mg/dL). Elevated levels of C peptide and proinsulin usually are present as well (*Curr Probl Surg* 1994;31:79).

    C. Localization. Insulinomas typically are small (<2 cm), solitary, benign tumors that may occur anywhere in the pancreas. Rarely, an insulinoma may develop in extrapancreatic rests of pancreatic tissue. Dynamic CT scanning at 5-mm intervals with oral and intravenous contrast is the initial localizing test for insulinoma, with success in 35% to 85% of cases. Endoscopic ultrasound is also effective but is operator dependent (*N Engl J Med* 1992;326:1721). The effectiveness of indium-111 (^{111}In)–octreotide scintigraphy for localizing insulinoma (approximately 50%) is less than for other islet cell tumors because insulinomas typically have few somatostatin receptors. Selective arteriography with observation of a tumor "blush" is the best diagnostic study for the primary tumor and hepatic metastases. If a tumor is still not identified, regional localization to the head, body, or tail of the pancreas can be accomplished by portal venous sampling for insulin or by calcium angiography. Calcium angiography involves injection of calcium into selectively catheterized pancreatic arteries and measurement of plasma insulin through a catheter positioned in a hepatic vein.

D. Treatment of insulinoma is surgical in nearly all cases. Surgical management of insulinomas consists in localization of the tumor by careful inspection and palpation of the gland after mobilization of the duodenum and the inferior border of the pancreas. Use of intraoperative ultrasonography greatly facilitates identification of small tumors, especially those located in the pancreatic head or uncinate process. Most insulinomas can be enucleated from surrounding pancreas, although those in the body or tail may require resection. In general, blind pancreatectomy should not be performed when the tumor cannot be identified. Approximately 5% of insulinomas are malignant and 10% are multiple (usually in association with MEN type 1). Medical treatment for insulinoma with diazoxide, verapamil, or octreotide has limited effectiveness but may be used in preparation for surgery or for patients unfit for surgery.

II. GASTRINOMA

A. Patients with **gastrinoma and the Zollinger-Ellison syndrome** (ZES) have severe peptic ulcer disease (PUD) due to gastrin-mediated gastric acid hypersecretion. Most patients present with epigastric pain, and 80% have active duodenal ulceration at the time of diagnosis. Diarrhea and weight loss are common (40% of patients). ZES is uncommon (0.1% to 1% of PUD cases), and most patients present with typical duodenal ulcer. Gastrinoma and ZES should be considered in any patient with (1) PUD refractory to treatment for *Helicobacter pylori* and conventional doses of H_2 blockers or omeprazole; (2) recurrent, multiple, or atypically located (e.g., distal duodenum or jejunum) peptic ulcers; (3) complications of PUD (i.e., bleeding, perforation, or obstruction); (4) PUD with significant diarrhea; and (5) PUD with HPT, nephrolithiasis, or familial endocrinopathy. All patients considered for elective surgery for PUD should have ZES excluded preoperatively.

B. Diagnosis of ZES requires demonstration of fasting hypergastrinemia and basal gastric acid hypersecretion. A fasting serum gastrin level of 100 pg/mL or greater and a basal gastric acid output (BAO) of 15 mEq/hour or more (>5 mEq/hour in patients with previous ulcer surgery) secure the diagnosis of ZES in nearly all cases. Fasting hypergastrinemia without elevated basal gastric acid output is seen in atrophic gastritis, in renal failure, and in patients taking H_2-receptor antagonists or omeprazole. Fasting hypergastrinemia with elevated basal gastric acid output is seen in retained gastric antrum syndrome, gastric outlet obstruction, and antral G-cell hyperplasia. A **secretin stimulation test** is used to distinguish ZES from these conditions. This test is performed by measuring fasting serum gastrin levels before and 2, 5, 10, and 15 minutes after the intravenous administration of secretin (2 units/kg). Eighty-five percent of patients with ZES have an increase in gastrin levels (>200 pg/mL over baseline) in response to a secretin stimulation test, whereas patients with other conditions do not. This test is most useful when ZES is suspected in patients who have had prior gastric surgery and in patients with moderately increased fasting gastrin levels (100 to 1,000 pg/mL).

C. Localization of gastrinoma should be performed in all patients considered for surgery. Approximately 80% of gastrinomas are located within the "gastrinoma triangle," which includes the duodenum and head of the pancreas. Gastrinomas are often malignant, with spread to lymph nodes or liver occurring in up to 60% of cases. Approximately 20% of patients with ZES have familial MEN type 1; these patients often have multiple, concurrent islet cell tumors. Dynamic CT scanning, ^{111}In-octreotide scintigraphy, endoscopic ultrasound, and MR scan are useful non-invasive tests for localizing gastrinoma; however, preoperative localization is un-successful up to 50% of the time. Selective angiography with or without secretin injection of the gastroduodenal, superior mesenteric, and splenic arteries and mea-surement of hepatic vein gastrin can localize occult gastrinoma in up to 70% to 90% of cases.

D. In cases of ZES, **medical treatment** of gastric hyperacidity with H_2-histamine-receptor antagonists and omeprazole is highly effective. These medications are indi-cated preoperatively in patients undergoing operation for cure and in patients with unresectable or metastatic gastrinoma. Increased doses of oral histamine-receptor antagonists can be required and often are given at 6-hour intervals. Starting doses (cimetidine, 300 mg orally every 6 hours; ranitidine, 150 mg orally every 6 hours; famotidine, 20 mg orally every 6 hours) are increased until the gastric acid secretion is less than 10 mEq/hour before the next dose. Alternatively, a continuous intravenous infusion can be initiated (e.g., ranitidine, 0.5 mg/kg/hour) and increased until control of gastric acid secretion is achieved. Omeprazole is given by mouth or nasogastric tube at 20 mg/day or twice a day.

E. Surgical management of ZES is indicated in all fit patients with nonmetastatic, sporadic gastrinoma. Goals of surgery include precise localization and curative re-section of the tumor. Resection of primary gastrinoma alters the malignant progres-sion of tumor and decreases hepatic metastases in patients with ZES. Intraoperative localization of gastrinomas is facilitated by extended duodenotomy and palpation, intraoperative ultrasonography, or endoscopic duodenal transillumination. Gastri-nomas within the duodenum, pancreatic head, or uncinate process are treated by enucleation, whereas tumors in the body or tail of the pancreas can be removed by distal or subtotal pancreatectomy. Immediate cure rates are 40% to 90% for resec-tions by experienced surgeons; however, half of patients initially cured according to biochemical tests experience recurrence within 5 years. **Gastric acid hypersecre-tion is controllable with H_2 blockers or omeprazole in most patients with ZES, rendering gastrectomy unnecessary.** If a gastrinoma cannot be localized intraoper-atively, a parietal cell vagotomy may be performed. Surgical debulking of metastatic or unresectable primary gastrinoma facilitates medical treatment and prolongs life expectancy in select patients. Patients with ZES and MEN-1 most often cannot be cured surgically and usually are treated medically.

III. UNUSUAL ISLET CELL TUMORS

A. VIPomas secrete vasoactive intestinal peptide and cause profuse secretory diar-rhea (fasting stool output of >1 L/day), hypokalemia, and either achlorhydria or hypochlorhydria (watery diarrhea, hypokalemia, and achlorhydria are the symp-toms of Verner-Morrison syndrome). Hyperglycemia, hypercalcemia, and cutaneous flushing may be seen. Other, more common causes of diarrhea and malabsorption must be excluded. A diagnosis of VIPoma is established by the finding of elevated fasting serum vasoactive intestinal peptide levels (>190 pg/mL) and secretory di-arrhea in association with an islet cell tumor. Octreotide (150 g subcutaneously every 8 hours) is highly effective as a means of controlling the diarrhea and cor-recting electrolyte abnormalities before resection. Most VIPomas occur in the dis-tal pancreas and are amenable to distal pancreatectomy. Metastatic disease is com-monly encountered (50%); nevertheless, surgical debulking is indicated to alleviate symptoms.

B. Glucagonomas secrete excess glucagon and result in type II diabetes, hy-poaminoacidemia, anemia, weight loss, and a characteristic skin rash, necrolytic migratory erythema. Diagnosis is suggested by symptoms and by biopsy of the skin rash but is confirmed by elevated plasma glucagon levels (usually $>1,000$ pg/mL). Tumors are large and are readily seen on CT scan. Resection is indicated in fit patients after nutritional support, even if metastases are present.

C. Somatostatinomas are the rarest of the islet cell tumors and cause a syndrome of diabetes, steatorrhea, and cholelithiasis. These tumors are frequently located in the head of the pancreas and are often metastatic at the time of presentation.

D. Other rare islet cell tumors include pancreatic polypeptide-secreting, neurotensin-secreting, and adrenocorticotropic hormone (ACTH)–secreting tumors, as well as nonfunctioning islet cell tumors. These tumors usually are large and often are malignant. Treatment is surgical resection.

 ## ADRENAL-PITUITARY AXIS

I. ADRENAL CORTEX

A. Cushing syndrome results from exogenous steroid administration or excess endogenous cortisol secretion. The clinical manifestations of Cushing syndrome include hypertension, edema, muscle weakness, glucose intolerance, osteoporosis, easy bruising, cutaneous striae, and truncal obesity (buffalo hump, moon facies). Women may develop acne, hirsutism, and amenorrhea as a result of adrenal androgen excess.

1. Pathophysiology

   a. The most common cause of Cushing syndrome is **iatrogenic,** namely, the administration of exogenous glucocorticoids or ACTH.

   b. Hypersecretion of ACTH from the anterior pituitary gland (**Cushing disease**) is the most common pathologic cause (65% to 70% of cases) of endogenous hypercortisolism. The adrenal glands respond normally to the elevated ACTH, and the result is bilateral adrenal hyperplasia. Excessive release of corticotropin-releasing factor by the hypothalamus is a rare cause of hypercortisolism.

   c. Abnormal secretion of cortisol from a primary adrenal adenoma or carcinoma is the cause of hypercortisolism in 10% to 20% of cases. **Primary adrenal neoplasms** secrete corticosteroids independent of ACTH and usually result in suppressed plasma ACTH levels and atrophy of the adjacent and contralateral adrenocortical tissue.

   d. In approximately 15% of cases, Cushing syndrome is caused by **ectopic secretion of ACTH** or an ACTH-like substance from a small-cell bronchogenic carcinoma, carcinoid tumor, pancreatic carcinoma, thymic carcinoma, medullary thyroid cancer, or other neuroendocrine neoplasm. Patients with ectopic ACTH-secreting neoplasms can present primarily with hypokalemia, glucose intolerance, and hyperpigmentation but with few other chronic signs of Cushing syndrome.

2. Diagnosis of Cushing syndrome is biochemical. The goals are to first establish hypercortisolism and then identify the source. However, all of the available tests are complicated by a lack of specificity and an overlap in the biochemical responses of patients with the different disease states.

   a. Establishing the presence of hypercortisolism

   (1) The best **screening test for hypercortisolism** is a 24-hour measurement of the urinary excretion of free cortisol. Urinary excretion of more than 100 μg/day of free cortisol in two independent collections is virtually diagnostic of Cushing syndrome. Measurement of plasma cortisol level alone is not a reliable method of diagnosing Cushing syndrome due to overlap of the levels in normal and abnormal patients.

   (2) An **overnight dexamethasone suppression test** (dexamethasone, 1 mg orally at 11 PM and measurement of plasma cortisol at 8 AM) is used to confirm Cushing syndrome, especially in obese or depressed patients who may have marginally elevated urinary cortisol. Patients with true hypercortisolism have lost normal adrenal-pituitary feedback and usually fail to suppress the morning plasma cortisol level to less than 5 μg/dL.

   b. Localization of the cause of hypercortisolism

   (1) Determination of basal ACTH by immunoradiometric assay is the best method of determining the cause of hypercortisolism. Suppression of the absolute level of ACTH below 5 pg/mL is nearly diagnostic of adrenocortical neoplasms. ACTH levels in Cushing disease may range from the upper limits of normal (15 pg/mL) to 500 pg/mL. The highest plasma levels of ACTH (1,000 pg/mL) have been observed in patients with ectopic ACTH syndrome.

(2) Standard **high-dose dexamethasone suppression testing** is used to distinguish a pituitary from an ectopic source of ACTH. Normal individuals and most patients with a pituitary ACTH-producing neoplasm respond to a high-dose dexamethasone suppression test (2 mg orally every 6 hours for 48 hours) with a reduction of urinary free cortisol and urinary 17-hydroxysteroids to less than 50% of basal values. Most patients with a primary adrenal tumor or an ectopic source of ACTH production fail to suppress to this level. However, this test does not separate clearly pituitary and ectopic ACTH hypersecretion because 25% of patients with the ectopic ACTH syndrome also have suppressible tumors.

(3) Additional tests that may be useful include the **metyrapone test** (an inhibitor of the final step of cortisol synthesis) and the **corticotropin-releasing factor infusion test.** Patients with pituitary hypersecretion of ACTH respond to these tests with a compensatory rise in ACTH and urinary 17-hydroxysteroids, whereas patients with a suppressed hypothalamic-pituitary axis (primary adrenal tumor, ectopic ACTH syndrome) usually do not have a compensatory rise.

3. **Imaging tests** are useful for identifying lesions suspected on the basis of biochemical testing. Reliance on radiologic studies to diagnose the cause of Cushing syndrome should be discouraged.

a. Patients with ACTH-independent hypercortisolism require thin-section **CT scan or MRI scan of the adrenal gland,** both of which identify adrenal abnormalities with more than 95% sensitivity. Patients with ACTH-dependent hypercortisolism and either markedly elevated ACTH or a negative pituitary MRI scan should have **CT scan of the chest** to identify a tumor producing ectopic ACTH.

b. **Gadolinium-enhanced MRI scan** of the sella turcica is the best imaging test for pituitary adenomas suspected of causing ACTH-dependent hypercortisolism.

c. Bilateral **inferior petrosal sinus sampling** can delineate unclear cases of Cushing disease from other causes of hypercortisolism. Simultaneous bilateral petrosal sinus and peripheral blood samples are obtained before and after peripheral intravenous injection of 1 μg/kg of corticotropin-releasing hormone. A ratio of inferior petrosal sinus to peripheral plasma ACTH of 2 at basal or of 3 after corticotropin-releasing hormone administration is 100% sensitive and specific for pituitary adenoma.

4. **Surgical treatment of Cushing syndrome** involves removing the cause of cortisol excess (a primary adrenal lesion or pituitary or ectopic tumors secreting excessive ACTH). Transsphenoidal resection of an ACTH-producing pituitary tumor is successful in 80% or more of cases of Cushing disease. Treatment of ectopic ACTH syndrome involves resection of the primary lesion, if possible. Primary adrenal causes of Cushing syndrome are treated by removal of the adrenal gland containing the tumor. All patients who undergo adrenalectomy for primary adrenal causes of Cushing syndrome require perioperative and postoperative glucocorticoid replacement because the pituitary-adrenal axis is suppressed.

B. **Primary aldosteronism** (Conn syndrome) is a syndrome of hypertension and hypokalemia caused by hypersecretion of the mineralocorticoid aldosterone. This uncommon syndrome accounts for less than 1% of unselected patients with hypertension. An aldosterone-producing adrenal adenoma (APA) is the cause of primary aldosteronism in two thirds of cases and is one of the few surgically correctable causes of hypertension. Idiopathic bilateral adrenal hyperplasia (IHA) causes 30% to 40% of cases of primary aldosteronism. Adrenocortical carcinoma and autosomal dominant glucocorticoid-suppressible aldosteronism are rare causes of primary aldosteronism. **Secondary aldosteronism** is a physiologic response of the renin-angiotensin system to renal artery stenosis, cirrhosis, congestive heart failure, and normal pregnancy. In these conditions, the adrenal gland functions normally.

1. **Diagnosis.** Aldosterone-mediated retention of sodium and excretion of potassium and hydrogen ion by the kidney causes **hypokalemia and moderate diastolic hypertension.** Edema is characteristically absent. Laboratory diagnosis of primary aldosteronism requires demonstration of hypokalemia (<3.5 mEq/L), inappropriate kaliuresis (>30 mEq/day), and elevated aldosterone (>15 ng/dL) with normal cortisol. Upright plasma renin activity (PRA) of less than 3 ng/mL/hour corroborates the diagnosis. A ratio of plasma aldosterone (ng/dL) to PRA (ng/mL/hour) of greater than 20 to 25 further suggests primary hyperaldosteronism. Confirmation of primary aldosteronism involves determination of serum potassium and PRA and a 24-hour urine collection for sodium, cortisol, and aldosterone after 5 days of a high-sodium diet. Patients with primary hyperaldosteronism do not demonstrate aldosterone suppressibility (>14 μg/24 hours) after salt loading. Alternatively, plasma aldosterone and PRA can be measured before and 2 hours after oral administration of 25 mg of captopril. Failure to suppress plasma aldosterone to less than 15 ng/dL is a positive test. Before biochemical studies, all diuretics and antihypertensives are discontinued for 2 to 4 weeks, and a daily sodium intake of at least 100 mEq is provided. **Differentiation between adrenal adenoma and IHA is important because unilateral adenomas are treated by surgical excision, whereas bilateral hyperplasia is treated medically.** Because suppression of the renin-angiotensin system is more complete in APA than in IHA, these two disorders can be distinguished imperfectly (with approximately 85% accuracy) by measuring plasma aldosterone and PRA after overnight recumbency and then after 4 hours of upright posture. Patients with IHA usually have an increase in PRA and aldosterone in response to upright posture, but patients with adenoma usually show continued suppression of PRA, and their level of aldosterone does not change or falls paradoxically. In practice, this test usually is not necessary because, after a biochemical diagnosis of primary hyperaldosteronism, sensitive imaging tests are used to localize the lesion or lesions.

2. **Localization.** High-resolution adrenal CT scan should be the initial step in localization of an adrenal tumor. CT scanning localizes an adrenal adenoma in 90% of cases overall, and the presence of a unilateral adenoma larger than 1 cm on CT scan and supportive biochemical evidence of an aldosteronoma are generally all that is needed to make the diagnosis of Conn syndrome. Uncertainty regarding APA versus IHA after biochemical testing and noninvasive localization may be definitively resolved by bilateral adrenal venous sampling for aldosterone and cortisol. Simultaneous adrenal vein blood samples for aldosterone and cortisol are taken: The ratio of aldosterone to cortisol is greater than 4:1 for a diagnosis of aldosteronoma and less than 4:1 for a diagnosis of IHA.

3. **Treatment.** Surgical removal of an APA through a posterior or laparoscopic approach results in immediate cure or substantial improvement of hypertension and hyperkalemia in more than 90% of patients with Conn syndrome. The patient should be treated with spironolactone (200 to 400 mg/day) preoperatively for 2 to 3 weeks to control blood pressure and to correct hypokalemia. Patients with IHA should be treated medically with spironolactone (200 to 400 mg/day). A potassium-sparing diuretic, such as amiloride (5 to 20 mg/day), and calcium channel blockers have also been used. Surgical excision rarely cures bilateral hyperplasia.

C. **Acute adrenal insufficiency** is an emergency and should be suspected in stressed patients with a history of either adrenal insufficiency or exogenous steroid use. Adrenocortical insufficiency is most often caused by acute withdrawal of chronic corticosteroid therapy but can result from autoimmune destruction of the adrenal cortex, adrenal hemorrhage (Waterhouse-Friderichsen syndrome), or, rarely, infiltration with metastatic carcinoma. Recently, adrenal insufficiency in acutely ill patients has been elucidated as being multifactorial and difficult to diagnose clinically. However, its diagnosis and prompt treatment can be of significant benefit in acutely ill patients (*N Engl J Med* 2003;20;348:727).

1. **Signs and symptoms** include fever, nausea, vomiting, severe hypotension, and lethargy. Characteristic laboratory findings of adrenal insufficiency include hyponatremia, hyperkalemia, azotemia, and fasting or reactive hypoglycemia.
2. **Diagnosis:** A rapid ACTH stimulation test is used to test for adrenal insufficiency. Corticotropin (250 μg), synthetic ACTH, is administered intravenously, and plasma cortisol levels are measured on completion of the administration and then 30 and 60 minutes later. Normal peak cortisol response should exceed 20 μg/dL. The most benefit from adrenocortical hormone replacement in critically ill septic patients is reported in those whose cortisol levels rose less than 9 μg/dL from baseline in response to corticotropin stimulation (*N Engl J Med* 2003;20;348:727).
3. **Treatment of adrenal crisis must be immediate, based on clinical suspicion,** before laboratory confirmation is available. Intravenous volume replacement with normal or hypertonic saline and dextrose is essential, as is immediate intravenous steroid replacement therapy with **4 mg of dexamethasone.** Thereafter, 100 mg of hydrocortisone is administered intravenously every 6 to 8 hours and is tapered to standard replacement doses as the patient's condition stabilizes. Subsequent recognition and treatment of the underlying cause, particularly if it is infectious, usually resolves the crisis. Mineralocorticoid replacement is not required until intravenous fluids are discontinued and oral intake resumes.
4. **Prevention.** Patients who have known adrenal insufficiency or have received supraphysiologic doses of steroid for at least 1 week in the year preceding surgery should receive 100 mg of hydrocortisone the evening before and the morning of major surgery, followed by 100 mg of hydrocortisone every 8 hours during the first postoperative 24 hours.

II. ADRENAL MEDULLA: PHEOCHROMOCYTOMA

A. **Pathophysiology.** Pheochromocytomas are neoplasms derived from the chromaffin cells of the sympathoadrenal system that result in unregulated, episodic oversecretion of catecholamines. Most pheochromocytomas secrete predominantly norepinephrine and smaller amounts of epinephrine. Rarely, epinephrine is secreted predominantly or exclusively.

B. **Clinical features.** Approximately 80% to 85% of pheochromocytomas in adults arise in the adrenal medulla, whereas 10% to 15% arise in the extra-adrenal chromaffin tissue, including the paravertebral ganglia, posterior mediastinum, organ of Zuckerkandl, and urinary bladder. Symptoms of pheochromocytoma are related to excess sympathetic stimulation from catecholamines and include paroxysms of pounding frontal headache, diaphoresis, palpitations, flushing, or anxiety. The most common sign is episodic or sustained hypertension, but pheochromocytoma accounts for only 0.1% to 0.2% of patients with sustained diastolic hypertension. Uncommonly, patients present with complications of prolonged uncontrolled hypertension (e.g., myocardial infarction, cerebrovascular accident, or renal disease). Pheochromocytomas can occur in association with several hereditary syndromes, including MEN types 2A and 2B and von Hippel-Lindau syndrome. Tumors that arise in familial settings frequently are bilateral.

C. The **biochemical diagnosis** of pheochromocytoma is made by demonstrating elevated plasma metanephrines or 24-hour urinary excretion of catecholamines and their metabolites (metanephrines, vanillylmandelic acid). If possible, antihypertensive medications (especially monoamine oxidase inhibitors) should be discontinued before the 24-hour urine collection, and creatinine excretion should be measured simultaneously to assess the adequacy of the sample.

D. **Radiographic tests** are used to demonstrate the presence of an adrenal mass.
1. **CT scanning** is the imaging test of choice and identifies 90% to 95% of pheochromocytomas larger than 1 cm. MR scan can also be useful because T2-weighted images have a characteristic high intensity in patients with pheochromocytoma and metastatic tumor compared with adenomas.
2. **Scintigraphic scanning** after the administration of ^{131}I-meta-iodobenzylguanidine (MIBG) provides a functional and anatomic test of

hyperfunctioning chromaffin tissue. MIBG scanning is very specific for both intra- and extra-adrenal pheochromocytomas.

E. **The treatment of benign and malignant pheochromocytomas is surgical excision.**

1. **Preoperative preparation** includes administration of an α-adrenergic blocker to control hypertension and to permit re-expansion of intravascular volume. Phenoxybenzamine, 10 mg orally twice a day, is initiated and increased to 20 to 40 mg orally twice a day until the desired effect or prohibitive side effects are encountered. Postural hypertension is expected and is the desired endpoint. β-Adrenergic blockade (e.g., propranolol) may be added if tachycardia or arrhythmias develop but only **after complete α-adrenergic blockade.** Patients with cardiopulmonary dysfunction may require a pulmonary artery (Swan-Ganz) catheter perioperatively, and all patients should be monitored in the surgical intensive care unit in the immediate postoperative period.

2. **The classic operative approach** for familial pheochromocytomas is exploration of both adrenal glands, the preaortic and paravertebral areas, and the organ of Zuckerkandl through a midline or bilateral subcostal incision. In patients with MEN type 2A or 2B and a unilateral pheochromocytoma, it is acceptable to remove only the involved gland (*Ann Surg* 1993;217:595). In patients with a sporadic, unilateral pheochromocytoma localized by preoperative imaging studies, adrenalectomy may be performed by an anterior or posterior approach or (increasingly) by laparoscopic adrenalectomy. Intraoperative labile hypertension can occur during resection of pheochromocytoma. This can be prevented by minimal manipulation of the tumor but can be controlled most effectively with intravenous sodium nitroprusside (0.5 to 10 μg/kg/minute) or phentolamine (5 mg).

III. **ADRENOCORTICAL CARCINOMA** is a rare but aggressive malignancy; most patients with this cancer present with locally advanced disease. Syndromes of adrenal hormone overproduction may include rapidly progressive hypercortisolism, hyperaldosteronism, or virilization. Large (>6 cm) adrenal masses that extend to nearby structures on CT scanning likely represent carcinoma. **Complete surgical resection of locally confined tumor is the only chance for cure of adrenocortical carcinoma.** Definitive diagnosis of adrenocortical carcinoma requires operative and pathologic demonstration of nodal or distant metastases. Any adrenal neoplasm weighing more than 50 g should be considered malignant. Often, patients with adrenocortical carcinoma present with metastatic disease, most often involving the lung, lymph nodes, liver, or bone. Palliative surgical debulking of locally advanced or metastatic adrenocortical carcinoma may provide these patients with symptomatic relief from some slow-growing, hormone-producing cancers. Chemotherapy with mitotane may be somewhat effective. Overall, the prognosis for patients with adrenocortical carcinoma is poor.

IV. **INCIDENTAL ADRENAL MASSES** are detected in 0.6% to 1.5% of abdominal CT scans obtained for other reasons. Most incidentally discovered adrenal masses are benign, nonfunctioning cortical adenomas of no clinical significance. The **NIH consensus state-of-the-science statement** from 2002 on adrenal incidentalomas recommends that patients with an incidentaloma should have a 1-mg dexamethasone suppression test and a measurement of plasma-free metanephrines. Patients with coexisting hypertension should also be evaluated for primary aldosteronism. Surgery should be considered in all patients with clinically apparent functional adrenal cortical tumors and pheochromocytomas. Tumors greater than 6 cm should be surgically removed. Tumors less than 4 cm should be monitored clinically and radiologically. Either open or laparoscopic adrenalectomy is acceptable. Laparoscopic adrenalectomy has been associated with shorter hospitalization and faster recovery. Its use is generally limited to malignant lesions less than 5 cm in diameter and benign-appearing lesions up to 8 to 10 cm in diameter.

CARCINOID TUMORS

Carcinoid tumors are classified according to their embryologic origin: foregut (bronchial, thymic, gastroduodenal, and pancreatic), midgut (jejunal, ileal, appendiceal, right colic), and hindgut (distal colic, rectal). Depending on the site of origin, carcinoids secrete hormones differently and have different clinical features. Carcinoid tumors most frequently occur in the gastrointestinal tract. Bronchial and thymic carcinoids occur less commonly. In general, the diagnosis of carcinoid rests on the finding of elevated circulating serotonin or urinary metabolites [5-hydroxyindoleacetic acid (5-HIAA)] and localizing studies. The best biochemical test is an elevated urinary 5-HIAA (normal, 2 to 8 mg/day). Rectal or jejunoileal tumors may be visualized by contrast studies, whereas bronchial carcinoids can be identified on chest x-rays, CT scans, or bronchoscopy. Abdominal or hepatic metastases are best identified by CT scanning, ultrasonography, or angiography. As with other neuroendocrine tumors, some carcinoids can be detected with metaiodobenzylguanidine (^{131}I-MIBG) scanning, and most are detectable by ^{111}In-octreotide scintigraphy.

I. CARCINOID OF THE APPENDIX is by far the most common carcinoid tumor and is found in up to 1 in 300 appendectomies. The risk of lymph node metastases and the prognosis of appendiceal carcinoids depend on the size: Tumors less than 1 cm never metastasize, tumors 1 to 2 cm have a 1% risk of metastasis, and tumors larger than 2 cm have a 30% risk of metastasis (*World J Surg* 1996;20:183). Extent of surgery for appendiceal carcinoid is based on size: simple appendectomy for tumors less than 1 cm, right hemicolectomy for tumors larger than 2 cm, and selective right hemicolectomy for tumors 1 to 2 cm. Prognosis for completely resected appendiceal carcinoid is favorable, with 5-year survival of 90% to 100%.

II. SMALL-INTESTINAL CARCINOID TUMORS usually present with vague abdominal symptoms that uncommonly lead to preoperative diagnosis. Most patients are operated on for intestinal obstruction, which is caused by a desmoplastic reaction in the mesentery around the tumor rather than by the tumor itself. Extended resection, including the mesentery and lymph nodes, is required, even for small tumors. Meticulous examination of the remaining bowel is mandatory because tumors are multicentric in 20% to 40% of cases, and synchronous adenocarcinomas are found in up to 10% of cases. An almost linear relationship exists between size of tumor and risk of nodal metastases, with a risk of up to 85% for tumors larger than 2 cm. Prognosis depends on the size and extent of disease; overall survival is 50% to 60%, which is substantially decreased if liver metastases are present. Small-bowel carcinoids have the highest propensity to metastasize to the liver and produce the carcinoid syndrome.

III. RECTAL CARCINOIDS are typically small, submucosal nodules that are often asymptomatic or produce one or more of the nonspecific symptoms of bleeding, constipation, and tenesmus. These tumors are hormonally inactive and almost never produce the carcinoid syndrome, even when spread to the liver occurs. Treatment of small (<1 cm) rectal carcinoids is endoscopic removal. Transmural excision of tumors 1 to 2 cm can be done locally. Treatment of 2-cm and larger tumors or invasive tumors is controversial but may include anterior or abdominoperineal resection for fit patients without metastases.

IV. FOREGUT CARCINOIDS include gastroduodenal, bronchial, and thymic carcinoids. These are a heterogeneous group of tumors with variable prognosis. They do not release serotonin and may produce atypical symptoms (e.g., violaceous flushing of the skin) related to release of histamine. Gastroduodenal carcinoids may produce gastrin and cause ZES. Resection is advocated for localized disease.

The **carcinoid syndrome** occurs in less than 10% of patients with a carcinoid and develops when venous drainage from the tumor gains access to the systemic circulation, as with hepatic metastases. The classic syndrome consists of flushing, diarrhea, bronchospasm, and right-sided cardiac valvular fibrosis. Symptoms are paroxysmal and may be provoked by alcohol, cheese, chocolate, or red wine. Diagnosis is made by 24-hour measurement of urinary 5-HIAA or of whole-blood 5-hydroxytryptamine. Surgical cure usually is not possible with extensive abdominal or hepatic metastases; however, debulking of the tumor may alleviate symptoms and improve survival when it can be performed safely. Hepatic metastases also have been treated with chemoembolization using doxorubicin, 5-fluorouracil, and cisplatin. **Carcinoid crisis** with severe bronchospasm and hemodynamic collapse may occur perioperatively in patients with an undiagnosed carcinoid. Prompt recognition is crucial because administration of octreotide (100 μg intravenously) can be lifesaving.

HEREDITARY ENDOCRINE TUMOR SYNDROMES

I. MULTIPLE ENDOCRINE NEOPLASIA SYNDROMES

A. **Multiple endocrine neoplasia type 1 (MEN-1).** MEN-1 is an autosomal dominant syndrome characterized by tumors of the parathyroid glands, pancreatic islet cells, and pituitary gland. Hyperparathyroidism occurs in virtually all patients. Clinical evidence of pancreatic islet cell and pituitary tumors develops in 50% and 25% of patients, respectively. Lipomas, thymic or bronchial carcinoid tumors, and tumors of the thyroid, adrenal cortex, and central nervous system (CNS) may also develop. The gene responsible for MEN-1, *MENIN*, is located on chromosome 11q13 and appears to act through transcription factors (*Science* 1997;276:404). Genetic testing is available in many centers, but if it is not available, screening of family members should begin in their early teens, including yearly determinations of plasma calcium, glucose, gastrin, fasting insulin, vasoactive intestinal polypeptide, pancreatic polypeptide, prolactin, growth hormone, and β-human gonadotropin hormone.

1. **Hyperparathyroidism.** Because HPT is frequently the first detectable abnormality in patients with MEN-1, yearly calcium screening of asymptomatic kindred members is recommended. Patients with HPT and MEN-1 usually have generalized (four-gland) parathyroid enlargement. Surgery should consist of 3.5-gland parathyroidectomy or a total parathyroidectomy with autotransplantation of parathyroid tissue to the forearm. This method achieves cure in more than 90% of cases and results in hypoparathyroidism in less than 5%. Graft-dependent recurrent HPT, however, is seen in up to 50% of cases. It is managed by resecting a portion of the autografted material (*Ann Surg* 1980;192:451).

2. **Pituitary tumors** occur in up to 40% of MEN-1 patients and most commonly are benign prolactin-producing adenomas. Growth-hormone, adrenocorticotropic hormone–producing, and nonfunctioning tumors are also seen. Patients may present with headache, diplopia, or symptoms referable to hormone overproduction. Bromocriptine inhibits prolactin production and may reduce tumor bulk and obviate the need for surgical intervention. Transsphenoidal hypophysectomy may be necessary if medical treatment fails.

3. **Pancreatic islet cell tumors** pose the most difficult clinical challenge and account for most of the morbidity and mortality of the syndrome. Gastrinomas (Zollinger-Ellison syndrome) are most common, but vasoactive intestinal polypeptide–secreting tumors, insulinomas, glucagonomas, and somatostatinomas are also encountered. The pancreas is usually diffusely involved, with islet cell hyperplasia and multifocal tumors. Tumors may be found in the proximal duodenum and peripancreatic areas (gastrinoma triangle), and these are virtually always malignant. The treatment goal is relief of symptoms related to excessive hormone production and cure or palliation of the malignant process. Patients frequently require medical and surgical therapy. Before surgical exploration, the patient should be evaluated for an adrenal tumor by measuring urinary excretion rates of glucocorticoids, mineralocorticoids, sex hormones, and plasma metanephrines.

II. MULTIPLE ENDOCRINE NEOPLASIA TYPE 2 (MEN-2).

MEN-2 is characterized by medullary thyroid carcinoma (MTC) and includes MEN-2A, MEN-2B, and familial, non-MEN MTC [familial MTC (FMTC)]. These autosomal dominant syndromes are caused by gain-of-function mutations in the *RET* proto-oncogene, which encodes a transmembrane tyrosine kinase receptor. Mutations in *RET* lead to constitutive activation (tyrosine phosphorylation) of the RET protein, which drives tumorigenesis. Genetic testing should be performed on all suspected individuals.

Because MTC occurs universally in all MEN-2 variants, prophylactic thyroidectomy is indicated for all RET-mutation carriers. Two recent series demonstrated an age-related increase in the incidence of MTC in RET-mutation carriers. Machens et al. reported a series of 207 RET-mutation carriers who underwent thyroidectomy before age 20 years. The majority of these patients were codon-634-mutation carriers (the most common MEN-2A–causing mutation). They found an age-specific progression from C-cell hyperplasia to medullary thyroid cancer to nodal metastases. Twelve of 16 patients with 634 mutations who underwent thyroidectomy before age 5 years were found to have MTC. No nodal metastases were noted prior to age 14 years (*N Engl J Med* 2003;349:1517). Skinner et al. reported a series of 50 patients under age 19 years who underwent prophylactic thyroidectomy on discovery of a germline MEN-2A causing RET mutation. Forty-four of 50 (88%) had no evidence of recurrence (including biochemical evidence) at least 5 years following resection. All 22 patients undergoing resection prior to age 8 years had no evidence of recurrence at least 5 years following resection (*N Engl J Med* 2005;353:1105.) These data and others form the basis for prophylactic thyroidectomy in RET-mutation carriers. Current guidelines call for thyroidectomy in the first year of life for MEN-2B–mutation carriers and thyroidectomy before age 5 years in MEN-2A–mutation carriers (*J Clin Endocrinol Metab* 2001;86:5658). Genetic counseling for parents of affected children is crucial prior to prophylactic surgery.

In more than 50% of patients with medullary thyroid carcinoma, the cancer recurs after primary surgical resection. Although reoperation is advocated for local recurrence, there is no accepted adjuvant regimen for effectively treating metastatic disease. Investigational therapies and clinical trials with targeted inhibitors of RET tyrosine kinase activity are being evaluated (*Surgery* 2002;132:960).

A. MEN-2A. All patients with MEN-2A will develop MTC, whereas pheochromocytomas arise in approximately 40% to 50% of patients, and hyperplasia of the parathyroid glands arises in approximately 25% to 35%. Patients with MEN-2A also develop gastrointestinal manifestations, including abdominal pain, distention, and constipation as well as Hirschsprung disease (*Ann Surg* 2002;235:648). On genetic analysis, patients with MEN-2A and Hirschsprung disease (MEN-2A-HD) share common mutations in either codon 609, 618, or 620 of exon 10 of the *RET* proto-oncogene. MTC occurs generally occurs earlier than pheochromoctyoma or hyperparathyroidism. Nonetheless, biochemical testing to exclude pheochromocytoma is mandatory in all MEN-2 and MTC patients prior to thyroidectomy.

B. MEN-2B is a variant of MEN-2 in which patients develop MTC and pheochromocytomas but not hyperparathyroidism. Patients also develop ganglioneuromatosis and a characteristic physical appearance, with hypergnathism of the midface, marfanoid body habitus, and multiple mucosal neuromas. MTC is particularly aggressive in these patients. MEN-2B patients also demonstrate multiple gastrointestinal symptoms and megacolon.

C. FMTC is characterized only by the hereditary development of MTC without other endocinopathies. MTC is generally more indolent in these patients.

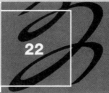

TRAUMA SURGERY
Kevin McConnell and Douglas J.E. Schuerer

22

Injury is a leading cause of death and disability around the world. This chapter outlines an overall approach to trauma care, provides a framework for therapy, and highlights critical aspects of decision making and interventions. The Eastern Association for the Surgery of Trauma (EAST) Web site (http://www.east.org) provides evidence-based clinical guidelines and can be referred to for additional detail.

TRAUMA CARE

I. PREHOSPITAL CARE. Field professionals are responsible for performing the three major functions of prehospital care: (1) assessment of the injury scene, (2) stabilization and monitoring of injured patients, and (3) safe and rapid transportation of critically ill patients to the appropriate trauma center. The observations and interventions performed are important in guiding the resuscitation of an injured patient. The MVIT (*m*echanism, *v*ital signs, *i*njury inventory, *t*reatment) system of reporting is one method of communicating data to the trauma team in an efficient, fast, and organized manner.

A. The **mechanism of a trauma** partially determines the pattern and severity of injuries sustained in the event.

1. Front-end car collisions can cause direct contact between the driver's knees and the dashboard. Such trauma can result in combination patellar fracture, posterior knee dislocation (with popliteal artery injury), femoral shaft fracture, and posterior rim fracture of the acetabulum.

2. Feet-first falls from significant heights cause axial loading and a possible combination of calcaneal fracture, lower-extremity long-bone fracture, acetabular injury, and lumbar spine compression fracture.

3. Adult pedestrians struck by motor vehicles often have a pattern of three distinct injuries: (1) injury to the tibia and fibula from striking the bumper, (2) injury to the head from striking the windshield or hood after being swept from the ground, and (3) injury to the upper extremity from falling to the pavement.

4. Young children struck by a motor vehicle should be assessed for Waddell triad: (1) femur fracture from striking the bumper, (2) abdominal solid-organ injury (liver or spleen) from striking the fender, and (3) opposite-side head injury from landing on the pavement.

B. **Vital signs,** including level of consciousness and voluntary movement, give insight into the clinical trajectory of the patient and are a key element in leveling trauma. Emergency medical service (EMS) providers typically measure and report these values, often in less than ideal conditions. Deterioration of vital signs en route to the trauma center suggests the existence of life threats requiring immediate intervention. Improvement in vital signs en route may reflect transient compensatory responses by the patient. They may, however, also reflect human error in obtaining data in difficult circumstances.

C. The **injury inventory** consists of the description of injuries as observed by the EMS personnel. Important prehospital observations include whether the patient was trapped in a vehicle, was crushed under a heavy object, or suffered significant exposure secondary to prolonged extrication. Such findings alert the trauma team to critical secondary injuries, including rhabdomyolysis, traumatic asphyxia, and hypothermia.

D. Prehospital treatment is aimed at stabilization of the injured patient and involves securing an airway, providing adequate ventilation, assessing and supporting circulation, and stabilizing the spine. EMS caregivers fulfill these goals through various therapies that include (but are not limited to) administration of oxygen and intravenous fluids, prevention of heat loss, and immobilization of the spine with a backboard and properly fitting hard cervical collar. All such interventions need to be taken into account during the initial evaluation, including immediate confirmation of any prehospital airway.

II. INITIAL HOSPITAL CARE. Trauma deaths have a **trimodal distribution**: (1) immediate death occurring at the time of injury due to devastating wounds; (2) early death occurring within the first few hours of injury due to major intracranial, thoracic, abdominal, pelvic, and extremity injuries; and (3) late death occurring days to weeks after the initial injury due to secondary complications (sepsis, acute respiratory distress syndrome, systemic inflammatory response syndrome, or multiple organ dysfunction and failure). Initial hospital care usually takes place in the emergency department and has two main components: the primary and secondary surveys.

A. Primary survey. The primary survey is a systematic, rapid evaluation of the injured patient following the **mnemonic ABCDE (airway, breathing, circulation, disability, exposure).** On completion of the survey, the patient should have an established airway with cervical spine control, adequate ventilation and oxygenation, proper intravenous access and control of hemorrhage, and an inventory of the patient's neurologic status and disability, and the patient should have undergone complete exposure with environmental control. During the survey, a rudimentary history is obtained, if possible. This history follows the acronym **AMPLE** (*a*llergies, *m*edications, *p*ast medical history, *l*ast meal, *e*vents surrounding the injury).

1. Airway. Establishing a patent airway is the highest priority in the care of a trauma patient because, without one, irreversible brain damage from hypoxia can occur within minutes. The airway should always be secured under cervical spine control. Engaging the patient in conversation on arrival at the emergency department allows for immediate evaluation of the airway. A patient who is able to respond verbally has a patent airway. A patient who cannot respond verbally must be assumed to have an obstructed airway until proven otherwise. Every trauma patient initially should have oxygen administered (via nasal cannula or bag valve facemask) and an oxygen saturation monitor (i.e., pulse oximeter) placed. An oximeter device is helpful, but it is important to remember that its output readings can be misleading in certain clinical situations (e.g., patients with severe anemia, carbon monoxide poisoning, insufficient pulse pressure, hypothermia, or burns with inhalation injury).

a. Basic maneuvers to alleviate obstruction

(1) Simple suctioning. This removes obstructions caused by vomitus, phlegm, or other debris in the oropharynx.

(2) Jaw-thrust maneuver. The tongue itself can occlude the airway. A jaw thrust can successfully displace the tongue anteriorly from the pharyngeal inlet, relieving the obstruction.

(3) Nasopharyngeal airway. In the semiconscious patient, this can provide a conduit for ventilation, but it may result in emesis if it is used in fully conscious patients.

(4) Oropharyngeal airway. Mechanically displace the tongue anteriorly, securing airway patency. Because of their strong induction of the gag reflex and emesis, these devices should be used only in unconscious patients.

b. Tracheal intubation is indicated in any patient in whom concern for airway integrity exists (unconscious or semiconscious patients, patients with mechanical obstruction secondary to facial trauma or debris, combative and hypoxic patients). The emergent tracheal intubation of an uncooperative trauma patient is a high-risk undertaking. The most skilled operator available should secure the airway by the most expeditious means possible. The preferred method of intubation is via the orotracheal route using **rapid-sequence induction (RSI).** Nasotracheal intubation should be discouraged. Rapid-sequence intubation follows a systematic protocol to ensure successful provision of an airway. The patient is first **spontaneously ventilated with 100% oxygen.** During this time, a team member provides in-line cervical spine stabilization to prevent unintentional manipulation as the hard cervical collar is removed anteriorly. Another team member provides anterior pressure on the cricoid cartilage to occlude the esophagus (Sellick maneuver). This pressure helps to prevent aspiration during intubation. Following preoxygenation, a **short-acting sedative or hypnotic medication is administered** via a functioning intravenous line with a stopcock. The choice of medication depends on the clinical situation. In general, etomidate, 0.3 mg/kg intravenously, or a short-acting benzodiazepine, such as midazolam, 1 to 2.5 mg intravenously, is used because these medications tend to have minimal effects on the cardiovascular status of the patient. In addition, midazolam provides anterograde amnesia. Opiates, such as fentanyl citrate, 2 μg/kg intravenously, should be used only in patients who are adequately perfused because their mild cardiac depressant activity can cause unexpected cardiovascular decompensation in hypoxic, hypoperfused patients. Sodium thiopental, 2 to 5 mg/kg intravenously, is exclusively reserved for the well-perfused patient with a seemingly isolated head injury because it diminishes the transient elevation in intracranial pressure (ICP) associated with tracheal intubation. A **paralytic agent is administered immediately after the sedative.** Succinylcholine, 1 to 1.25 mg/kg intravenously, is the paralytic of choice because, as a depolarizing muscle relaxant, it has a rapid onset (fasciculations within seconds) and a short half-life (recovery within 1 to 2 minutes). Contraindications in the acute trauma setting are limited to patients with known pseudocholinesterase deficiency or previous spinal injury. Succinylcholine can be used safely in patients with acute burns or spinal trauma. Rocuronium, 0.60 to 0.85 mg/kg intravenously, is an alternative paralytic, but as a nondepolarizing relaxant, it has a slower onset (up to 90 seconds) and a longer half-life (recovery after 40 minutes) than succinylcholine. **After onset of paralysis, the endotracheal tube (the largest for patient size and airway) is inserted through the vocal cords under direct vision** with the assistance of a laryngoscope and with the balloon inflated. The tube position is usually around 21 cm from the incisors in women and 23 cm from the incisors in men. Proper positioning of the tube in the trachea should be confirmed by exhalation of carbon dioxide over several breaths (using a litmus paper device or capnometer). **Adequacy of ventilation** should be verified by bilateral auscultation in each axilla. A chest x-ray should be taken within the next few minutes and checked to ensure proper endotracheal tube position. Tracheal intubation should secure an airway within 90 to 120 seconds (about three attempts). If it is unsuccessful, an airway placed directly through the cricoid membrane is often necessary.

c. **Cricothyrotomy** is the method of choice for establishing a surgical airway in adults in instances in which orotracheal intubation is not possible (unsuccessful orotracheal attempts or massive facial trauma). The cricoid membrane is easily palpated between the cricoid cartilage and the larynx. Because it is both superficial and relatively avascular, it provides rapid, easy access to the trachea. A 1.5-cm transverse skin incision is made over the trachea, and a scalpel is used to poke a hole through the membrane. Care is taken to avoid exiting through the trachea posteriorly, injuring the esophagus. Next, the scalpel handle, a tracheal spreader, or a similar surgical instrument is used to expand the hole. Finally, a 6-mm endotracheal or tracheostomy tube is inserted into the trachea through the cricothyrotomy. Historically, a cricothyrotomy would eventually require revision to a tracheostomy to decrease the risk of tracheal stenosis, but this has been challenged, and many institutions now use the cricothyrotomy site as a tracheostomy site. Cricothyrotomy is contraindicated in children younger than 12 years of age because of the anatomic difficulty in performing the procedure. In this situation, percutaneous transtracheal ventilation is an alternative. Laryngeal Mask Airway (LMA) and Combitube are appropriate alternatives to cricothyrostomy when cricothyrostomy expertise is limited (Guidelines For Emergency Tracheal Intubation Immediately Following Traumatic Injury, 2002, http://www.east.org).

  d. Percutaneous transtracheal ventilation can provide a temporary airway until a formal surgical airway can be supplied, especially in young children in whom cricothyrotomy is not possible. A small cannula (usually a 14-gauge intravenous catheter) is placed through the cricoid membrane. The cannula is connected to oxygen tubing containing a precut side hole. Temporary occlusion of the side hole provides passage of oxygen into the lungs via the cannula. Exhalation occurs passively through the vocal cords. Through this means, alveolar oxygen concentrations can be maintained for up to 30 to 45 minutes.

B. Breathing. Once an airway is established, attention is directed at assessing the patient's breathing (i.e., the oxygenation and ventilation of the lungs). A patent airway does not ensure adequate breathing because the trachea can be ventilated without successfully ventilating the alveoli. One hundred percent oxygen is administered through the secured airway. The chest is then examined, and important life-threatening abnormalities involving the thorax are identified and treated. The following are potentially fatal conditions that require immediate attention and treatment. (See Chapter 37 for a description of the **technique of tube thoracostomy.**)

  1. Tension pneumothorax
  a. Diagnosis: absence of breath sounds, hyperresonance, tracheal deviation away from the side of the abnormality, and associated hypotension due to decreased venous return.
  b. Treatment: immediate decompressive therapy (a chest x-ray should not delay treatment) via placement of a 14-gauge intravenous catheter in the second intercostal space in the midclavicular line, immediately followed by tube thoracostomy.

  2. Pneumothorax or hemothorax
  a. Diagnosis: Absent or decreased breath sounds without tracheal deviation usually indicate a simple pneumothorax or hemothorax on the affected side. A chest x-ray can usually confirm these conditions.
  b. Treatment: tube thoracostomy (32 Fr. or larger for hemothorax), connected to an underwater seal-suction device adjusted to –20 cm water suction.

  3. Flail chest
  Diagnosis: paradoxical chest wall motion with spontaneous respirations (three or more contiguous ribs with two or more fractures per rib). Pulmonary contusion often accompanies such an injury. Chest x-ray often reveals the extent of fractures and underlying lung injury.
  a. Treatment: adequate pain control (often with epidural analgesia), aggressive pulmonary toilet, and respiratory support. Many patients require early mechanical ventilatory support.

  4. Open pneumothorax
  a. Diagnosis: A chest wound communicating with the pleural space that is greater than two thirds the diameter of the trachea will preferentially draw air into the thorax ("sucking chest wound").
  b. Treatment: Cover with a partially occlusive bandage secured on three sides (securing all four sides can result in a tension pneumothorax and should be avoided), preventing air from entering the thorax but allowing it to exit via the wound if necessary. Prompt tube thoracostomy should follow placement of the partially occlusive dressing.

  5. Tracheobronchial disruption
  a. Diagnosis: Severe subcutaneous emphysema with respiratory comprise is suggestive; bronchoscopy is diagnostic.
  b. Treatment: Tube thoracostomy placed on the affected side will reveal a large air leak, and the collapsed lung may fail to re-expand. The patient is stabilized by intubation of the unaffected bronchus until operative repair can be performed (see Section V.D.2).

TABLE 22-1	Estimated Blood Loss by Initial Hemodynamic Variables			
	Class I	Class II	Class III	Class IV
Blood loss (mL)	Up to 750	750–1,500	1,500–2,000	>2,000
Blood loss (% blood volume)	Up to 15%	15%–30%	30%–40%	>40%
Pulse rate	<100	>100	>120	>140
Blood pressure (mm Hg)	Normal	Normal	Decreased	Decreased
Pulse pressure (mm Hg)	Normal or increased	Decreased	Decreased	Decreased
Urinary output (mL/hr)	>30	20–30	5–15	Negligible

C. **Circulation.** The goal of this portion of the primary survey is to identify and treat the presence of shock. Initially, all active external hemorrhage is controlled with direct pressure, and obvious fractures are stabilized. The pulse and blood pressure are obtained. The skin perfusion is determined by noting skin temperature and evaluating capillary refill. Over time, end-organ perfusion during a trauma resuscitation is estimated using mental status and urine flow as markers. Shock is defined as the inadequate delivery of oxygen and nutrients to tissue. The etiologies of shock can be divided into three broad categories: hypovolemic, cardiogenic, and distributive. The trauma team must be familiar with the manifestations and therapy of each category of shock because any of the three may be encountered in the injured patient.

1. **Hypovolemic shock** is the most common type of shock seen in trauma patients and occurs as a result of decreased intravascular volume, most commonly secondary to acute blood loss. It is divided into four classes (Table 22-1). In its severe form, it can manifest as a rapid pulse, decreased pulse pressure, diminished capillary refill, and cool, clammy skin. Therapy is restoration of the intravascular volume. Thus, the patient should have **two large-bore intravenous lines placed (14 or 16 gauge). The antecubital veins are the preferred sites.** If a peripheral intravenous catheter cannot be placed secondary to venous collapse, an 8.5-French cannula (Cordis catheter) should be placed via the Seldinger technique into the **femoral vein.** The subclavian and internal jugular veins should be reserved for those patients in whom major venous intra-abdominal injury or pelvic fractures prevent effective use of a femoral approach. Short, wide intravenous catheters are used to maximize the flow of resuscitation fluids into the circulation (the rate of fluid flow is proportional to the cross-sectional area of a conduit and inversely proportional to the fourth power of its radius). A blood specimen should be simultaneously obtained for cross-matching and for any other pertinent labs. Resuscitation should consist of an **initial bolus of 2 L of crystalloid solution** (children should receive an initial bolus of 20 mL/kg). All fluids administered should be warmed to prevent hypothermia. If time has not allowed proper cross-matching (as is frequently the case), type O blood should be used. Premenopausal women should receive Rh− blood. Men and postmenopausal women can receive either Rh− or Rh+ blood. In the setting of penetrating torso injury involving a large blood vessel, less aggressive resuscitation [keeping blood pressure (BP) around 90 mm Hg] until formal surgical control of the bleeding site is obtained has been shown to have some benefit in diminishing blood loss (*N Engl J Med* 1994;331:1105). Resuscitative thoracotomy is sometimes indicated for severe cardiopulmonary collapse (see Section VI.A.1).

2. **Cardiogenic shock** occurs when the heart is unable to provide adequate cardiac output to perfuse the peripheral tissues. In the trauma setting, such shock can occur in one of two ways: (1) **extrinsic compression** of the heart leading to decreased venous return and cardiac output or (2) **myocardial injury** causing inadequate myocardial contraction and decreased cardiac output. Patients in cardiogenic shock secondary to extrinsic compression of the heart usually present

with cool, pale skin, decreased BP, and distended jugular veins. They often respond transiently to an initial fluid bolus, but more definite therapy is always needed. Tension pneumothorax is the most common etiology. Cardiac tamponade is a less common cause. It usually occurs in the setting of a penetrating injury near the heart. Rapid diagnosis can be obtained with the use of ultrasound. Therapy consists of pericardial drainage and repair of the injury, usually a proximal great vessel or cardiac wound (see Sections V.D.5.a and V.D.6.a). Resuscitative thoracotomy may be required. Patients in cardiogenic shock secondary to myocardial injury can also present with cool skin, decreased BP, and distended jugular veins. Acute myocardial infarction can manifest in this way. Often, it is responsible for the traumatic event, but it can also occur as a result of the stress following an injury. Diagnosis of a myocardial infarction is via electrocardiogram (ECG) and troponin levels. Therapy should follow Advanced Cardiac Life Support guidelines, keeping in mind that anticoagulants may need to be avoided early until active bleeding related to the trauma has been excluded. Severe blunt cardiac injury is another manifestation. It usually occurs in the setting of high-speed motor vehicle crashes. An ECG and possibly an echocardiogram are essential. Therapy ranges from close monitoring with pharmacologic support in an intensive care unit (ICU) to operative repair (see Section V.D.6.b).

3. **Distributive shock** occurs as a result of an increase in venous capacitance leading to decreased venous return. Neurogenic shock secondary to acute quadriplegia or paraplegia is one type. Loss of peripheral sympathetic tone is responsible for the increased venous capacitance and decreased venous return. These patients present with warm skin, absent rectal tone, and inappropriate bradycardia. They often respond to an initial fluid bolus but often require pharmacologic support. Phenylephrine or norepinephrine can be used to restore peripheral vascular resistance. Chronotropic agents such as dopamine are sometimes used for bradycardic patients. Of note, the leading cause of shock in a trauma patient is hypovolemia, and thus neurogenic shock is usually a diagnosis of exclusion.

D. **Disability.** The goal of this phase of the primary survey is to identify and treat life-threatening neurologic injuries, and priority is given to evaluating level of consciousness and looking for lateralizing neurologic signs. The level of consciousness is quickly assessed using the **AVPU system** (ascertaining whether the patient is **a**wake, opens eyes to **v**oice, opens eyes to **p**ainful stimulus, or is **u**narousable). The pupils are examined, and their size, symmetry, and responsiveness to light are noted. Focal neurologic deficits are noted. Signs of significant neurologic impairment include inability to follow simple commands, asymmetry of pupils or their response to light, and gross asymmetry of limb movement to painful stimuli. Both intracranial and spinal injuries require urgent evaluation.

1. **Intracranial injuries.** Head injury remains a leading cause of trauma fatality in the United States. **Herniation (either uncal or cerebellar)** is often the final common pathway leading to death. Vigilance on the part of the trauma team can sometimes trigger interventions before such an event becomes irreversible. Acute therapy of severe intracranial injuries focuses on **maximizing cerebral perfusion pressure (CPP)** to provide an adequate supply of glucose and oxygen to the injured tissue. CPP is defined as the difference between mean arterial pressure (MAP) and ICP: CPP = MAP – ICP. Maximization of CPP therefore involves manipulating both MAP and ICP, and this is achieved when the BP is adequate (MAP >70 to 80 mm Hg) and the ICP is normal (<10 to 15 mm Hg in adults). A CPP of more than 60 to 70 mm Hg is the goal.

a. **Mean arterial pressure.** Maintaining an adequate MAP is very important in the patient with head trauma because hypotension is a major risk factor for poor outcome. Pharmacologic support may be used as necessary to maintain an adequate BP. Extreme hypertension should be avoided. Hypoxia is especially detrimental in traumatic head injuries, and all efforts to maintain adequate oxygenation should be made during trauma resuscitations.

b. **Intracranial pressure** is defined according to the modified Monro-Kellie hypothesis, which states that the intracranial contents are contained in a rigid sphere (skull). The three major constituents—brain, blood, and cerebrospinal fluid (CSF)—are distributed in a constant volume. An increase in the volume occupied by one constituent therefore must be accompanied by a decrease in the volume occupied by one of the remaining constituents or there will be a rise in pressure. In the trauma setting, early and rapid delineation of intracranial injuries by computed tomography (CT) scan is important because it allows decisions regarding the need for ICP monitoring to be made early. Usually reserved for the ICU or operating room, ICP monitoring is usually accomplished via the placement of a **subarachnoid pressure monitor ("bolt").** An **intraventricular catheter** placed in the nondominant lateral ventricle can also be used. This placement has the advantage of providing a means of draining CSF when necessary. General measures used to prevent an increase in the ICP include head elevation to 30 to 45 degrees, sedation, and prevention of jugular venous outflow obstruction. If ICP remains elevated, pharmacologic diuretic therapy to reduce the volume of both the CSF and the brain can be used. **Mannitol, 0.25 to 1 g/kg,** is the preferred agent, but hypertonic saline is also used. Sedation and therapeutic paralysis can acutely lower ICP, but they have the disadvantage of obscuring ongoing clinical neurologic examination. Although once advocated as an initial means of lowering ICP, hyperventilation is no longer recommended as a first-line therapy because of its adverse ischemic effects (it decreases ICP by causing intracranial vasoconstriction secondary to inducing hypocarbic alkalosis). It may be used in an acute setting with impending herniation until pharmacologic agents are available, and if it is used, the partial pressure of carbon dioxide (Pco_2) should be closely monitored and kept at a level of 30 to 35 mm Hg.

2. **Spinal cord injuries.** Acute injury to the spinal cord can result in neurogenic shock, which should be treated appropriately (see Section II.C.3). In addition, spinal cord trauma produces debilitating neurologic loss of function. The appropriate acute management of such deficits is very controversial. A multicenter trial showed that high-dose infusion of methylprednisolone immediately after blunt injuries to the spinal cord (complete or incomplete) resulted in modest but statistically significant functional preservation (*N Engl J Med* 1990;322:1405). This study has been followed by several other prospective trials that did not show benefit from steroid administration. Some trauma centers continue to administer an intravenous bolus dose of methylprednisolone at 30 mg/kg over 1 hour, followed by a 23-hour infusion of the same drug at a rate of 5.4 mg/kg/hour, in all patients presenting with blunt spinal trauma **within 8 hours of injury and without significant risk of infection.** Patients presenting with penetrating spinal trauma or being treated more than 8 hours after blunt spinal trauma should not receive any regimen. Patients treated longer than 24 hours trend toward increased pneumonia, sepsis, and higher mortality in a recent trial (NASCIS III) (*Crit Care Clin* 2004;20:25).

3. **Neurosurgical consultation.** A neurosurgeon should be consulted immediately in all patients with severe neurologic injuries. Early radiologic evaluation of the CNS to exclude evacuable intracranial mass lesions is also critical (see Section III.D.3).

E. **Exposure.** The last component of the primary survey is exposure with environmental control. Its purpose is to allow for complete visual inspection of the injured patient while preventing excessive heat loss. The patient is first completely disrobed, with clothing cut away so as not to disturb occult injuries. The patient then undergoes visual inspection, including logrolling to examine the back, splaying of the legs to examine the perineum, and elevation of the arms to inspect the axillae. The nude patient loses heat rapidly to the environment unless specific countermeasures are undertaken. The resuscitation room should be kept as warm as possible. Any cold metal backboard should be removed as quickly as possible, and all soggy clothing or bedclothes should be taken off expeditiously. All resuscitation fluid should be warmed. Finally, the patient should be covered with warm blankets or a "hot air" heating blanket.

III. COMPLETION OF THE PRIMARY SURVEY. The completion of the primary survey should be followed by a brief assessment of the adequacy of the initial resuscitation efforts.

A. Monitoring. Appropriate monitoring is essential to determine the clinical trajectory of the injured patient. If not already in place, **ECG leads and a pulse oximeter** should be applied. A manual blood pressure should be taken in all patients. An **automatic cuff** should be placed for subsequent serial BP measurements, although it should be kept in mind that such measurements can be inaccurate in a patient with a systolic blood pressure less than 90 mm Hg. Finally, an **indwelling urinary catheter** should be placed. Before insertion of the catheter, however, the urethral meatus should be inspected and found free of blood (the labia and scrotum should not harbor a hematoma). In addition, all male patients require palpation of the prostate to ensure that it is in the normal position, not displaced superiorly ("high riding"). If any genitourinary structures are abnormal, a retrograde urethrogram is necessary. If it is normal, the catheter may be passed. If urethral injuries are present, immediate consultation with a urologist is required before attempting to pass the catheter.

B. Laboratory values. After placement of two intravenous catheters, blood should be sent for laboratory studies. The most important test to obtain is the cross-match. Other studies include blood chemistries, hematologic analysis, coagulation profile, blood gas with base deficit, toxicologic analysis (with ethanol level), urinalysis, and β-human chorionic gonadotropin level if the patient is a woman of child-bearing age. The hematocrit value is the most commonly misinterpreted measure because it is not immediately altered with acute hemorrhage. It should not, therefore, be considered to be an indicator of circulating blood volume in the trauma patient. (Serial hematocrit values, however, may give an indication of ongoing blood loss.)

C. Adequacy of resuscitation. The adequacy of resuscitation can best be determined by using urine output and blood pH. Resuscitation, therefore, should strive for a blood pH of 7.4 and a urinary output of 0.5 to 1 mL/kg/hour in adults (1 to 2 mL/kg/hour in children). Base deficit and lactic acid levels are also used as markers of adequate resuscitation and have been shown to have prognostic value.

D. Radiographic investigations. Essential radiographic investigations are ordered during this period. These tests can provide critical data regarding injuries sustained in a trauma, but their performance should not get in the way of ongoing physical examinations and interventions.

1. Plain radiography

a. Blunt trauma. Patients who have sustained blunt trauma with major energy transfer require **chest and pelvic radiographs.** If time permits and the patient is stable, a formal three-view cervical spine series should be obtained (if not clinically cleared). If there is not any evidence of spinal or pelvic injury, an upright chest x-ray should be obtained because it provides crucial information with regard to hemothorax, pneumothorax, mediastinal widening, and subdiaphragmatic gas that sometimes cannot be gleaned from a supine film. Finally, plain radiographs should be obtained of any area of localized blunt trauma, especially if fractures are suspected on the basis of physical exam.

b. Penetrating trauma. Patients who have sustained penetrating injuries require regional plane radiographs to localize foreign bodies and exclude perforation of gas-filled organs (e.g., intestines, lungs). When these films are being obtained, all entrance and exit sites should be identified with a radiopaque marker. This technique gives insight into the trajectory of the penetrating object and the potential organs injured.

2. Trauma ultrasonography. Many trauma centers now use **focused abdominal sonography for trauma (FAST)** as an initial radiographic screening evaluation for all trauma following the primary survey. As the name implies, it is a focused examination designed to identify free intraperitoneal fluid and/or pericardial fluid. An ultrasound machine is used to take multiple views of six standard areas on the torso: **(1) right paracolic gutter, (2) Morison pouch, (3) pericardium, (4) perisplenic region, (5) left paracolic gutter, and (6) suprapubic region.** Free fluid in the abdomen and within the pericardium appears anechoic. FAST has many advantages: It is portable, rapid, inexpensive, accurate, noninvasive, and repeatable. Its disadvantages include operator variability as well as difficulty of use in morbidly obese patients or those with large amounts of subcutaneous air. It is most useful in evaluating patients with blunt abdominal trauma, especially those who are hypotensive. It may not be as useful in evaluating children or patients with penetrating trauma. It is important to note that if a FAST exam is negative, it does not exclude major intra-abdominal injury. Finally, some trauma centers use sonography to evaluate the thorax for traumatic effusions and pneumothoraces.

3. **Computed tomography.** The care of injured patients has been significantly changed by the use of CT scanning. Unnecessary laparotomy is associated with significant morbidity and cost. Because of CT, an increasing amount of both blunt and penetrating trauma has been safely managed nonoperatively. Triple-contrast CT (oral, intravenous, rectal) has been shown accurately to predict the need for laparotomy in patients with penetrating trauma, decreasing the incidence of unnecessary laparotomy (EAST Guidelines, 2007; http://www.east.org). The availability of high-resolution multislice scanners has reduced scan time to 1 to 4 minutes, prompting the development of protocols in some centers that call for early integration of complete-body (i.e., head, cervical spine, chest, abdomen, and pelvis) CT scanning of selected trauma patients. In this setting, the initial evaluation (including CT scan) averaged 13 minutes from time of arrival and obviated the need for preliminary radiologic studies (*Injury* 2007;38:552). Radiology investigation protocols for the trauma setting continue to evolve rapidly but remain dependent on the availability of equipment and skilled technicians or radiologists in any particular institution.

IV. SECONDARY SURVEY. The secondary survey follows the primary survey. It is a complete head-to-toe examination of the patient designed to inventory all injuries sustained in the trauma. Thoroughness is the key to finding all injuries, and a systematic approach is required. Only limited diagnostic evaluation is necessary for making decisions about subsequent interventions or evaluations. A review of important aspects of the secondary survey according to anatomic region follows. This review emphasizes only highlights and is not to be considered exhaustive.

A. Head. The patient should be evaluated for best motor and verbal responses to graded stimuli so that a **Glasgow Coma Score (GCS)** can be calculated. The GCS is highly reproducible and exhibits little interobserver variability. Severity of head trauma can be stratified according to the score obtained. Any patient with a GCS of 8 or below is considered to have severe neurologic depression and should be intubated to protect the airway. Inspection and palpation of the head are used to identify obvious lacerations and bony irregularities. All wounds require specific evaluation for evidence of depressed skull fractures or devitalized bone. Signs suggestive of basal skull fractures should be sought. These include periorbital hematomas ("raccoon eyes"), mastoid hematomas ("battle sign"), hemotympanum, and CSF rhinorrhea and otorrhea.

B. The face should be inspected for lacerations, hematomas, asymmetry, and deformities. The cranial nerves should be evaluated. The bones should be palpated in a systematic fashion to search for evidence of tenderness, crepitus, or bony discontinuity. In particular, the presence of a midfacial fracture should be sought by grasping the maxilla and attempting to move it. The nares should be examined for evidence of a septal hematoma. The oral cavity should be illuminated and inspected for evidence of mucosal violation (commonly seen in mandibular fractures). All dentures and/or displaced teeth should be removed to prevent airway occlusion. The conscious patient should be asked to bite down to determine whether abnormal dental occlusion is present (highly suggestive of a maxillary or mandibular fracture). The eyes should be examined for signs of orbital entrapment and the pupils re-examined. Finally, a nasogastric tube (contraindicated if there is a question of trauma to the midface) or orogastric tube (in patients who have midfacial fractures or are comatose) should be placed to decompress the stomach.

C. The neck should be inspected and palpated to exclude cervical spine, vascular, or aerodigestive tract injury.

1. **Cervical spine evaluation.** Assessing the status of the cervical spine is an important aspect of the secondary survey. Signs of cervical spine injury include midline cervical spine tenderness or vertebral step-off on palpation. Excluding the presence of a cervical injury can often be challenging. The proper algorithm is often dictated by the overall condition of the patient.

   a. **Awake, unimpaired patient.** In the awake, unimpaired, neurologically intact patient, the cervical spine should be palpated for signs of injury (e.g., midline cervical spine tenderness, vertebral step-off). If positive findings are present, the stabilizing cervical collar should remain in place, and a formal three-view cervical spine x-ray series should be obtained. If the physical examination is normal, the patient may be allowed, under supervision, to move the neck through the full range of motion. If there is not any cervical spine pain during this movement, the likelihood of a cervical spine injury is very low, and the stabilizing cervical collar can be removed. If any cervical spine pain is elicited during this movement, the stabilizing cervical collar should remain in place, and a formal cervical spine x-ray series should be obtained. If these x-rays are interpreted as normal, then the possibility of ligamentous injury should be entertained, and the patient should undergo supervised flexion-extension radiographs of the neck. If these films are interpreted as normal, the likelihood of cervical spine injury is low, and the stabilizing cervical collar can be removed (a soft collar may be placed for comfort). If the patient is unable to undergo the 30 degrees of excursion, the collar should be replaced and repeat films obtained at a later time.

   b. **Unconscious or impaired patient.** In the unconscious or impaired (e.g., acutely intoxicated) patient, the cervical spine should be considered to be unstable until a reliable clinical examination can be performed because significant ligamentous instability can exist with a normal three-view cervical spine x-ray series. The stabilizing cervical collar, therefore, should remain in place until the patient is fully awake and unimpaired. The patient then can be evaluated as previously described (see Section IV.C.1.a). A CT or MR scan of the cervical spine is a useful adjunct in patients who are unlikely to regain consciousness for extended periods of time.

2. **Vascular/aerodigestive evaluation.** In addition to evaluating the cervical spine, the neck should be inspected for active hemorrhage and palpated for local tenderness, hematomas, and evidence of subcutaneous air. Wounds should be classified according to their depth and their location. A wound is considered superficial if it does not penetrate the platysma; it is considered deep if the platysma is penetrated. The neck is divided anatomically into three zones: **Zone I** covers the thoracic inlet (manubrium to cricoid cartilage), **zone II** encompasses the midneck (cricoid cartilage to angle of the mandible), and **zone III** spans the upper neck (angle of mandible to base of skull).

D. **Thorax.** Significant pulmonary, cardiac, or great vessel injury may result from both penetrating and blunt trauma. In all cases, examination of the thorax includes inspection, palpation, percussion, and auscultation. Particular attention should be directed at observing the position of the trachea, checking for symmetric excursion of the chest, palpating for fractures and subcutaneous emphysema, and auscultating the quality and location of breath sounds. Two points bear further comment. First, thoracic extra-anatomic air (subcutaneous air, pneumomediastinum, or pneumopericardium) is frequently noted on physical examination or chest radiography in trauma patients (*Surg Clin North Am* 1996;76:725). Such a finding should alert the trauma team to four potential etiologies: (1) pulmonary parenchymal injury with occult pneumothorax (most common cause), (2) tracheobronchial injury, (3) esophageal perforation, and (4) cervicofacial trauma (usually self-limiting). Second, symmetric breath sounds are not a guarantee of adequate ventilation and oxygenation. End-tidal carbon dioxide, oxygen saturation, and arterial blood gas values must be monitored to ensure that breathing is intact.

E. **The abdomen** extends from the diaphragm to the pelvic floor, corresponding to the space **between the nipples and the inguinal creases** on the anterior aspect of the torso. When examining the abdomen during the secondary survey, the primary goal is to determine the presence of an intra-abdominal injury rather than to characterize its exact nature. Detecting those patients with occult injuries of the abdomen requiring operative intervention remains a diagnostic challenge. The mechanism of injury, however, often provides important clues.

1. **Penetrating trauma.** Stab wounds to the abdomen can be divided into thirds: One third do not penetrate the peritoneal cavity, one third penetrate the peritoneal cavity but do not cause any significant intra-abdominal injury, and one third penetrate the peritoneal cavity and do cause significant intra-abdominal damage. As a result, the ability to exclude penetration of the peritoneal cavity in the patient with a stab wound to the abdomen has important therapeutic implications. In the stable patient without obvious signs of intra-abdominal injury (e.g., peritonitis), **local wound exploration** remains a viable screening option. It is a well-defined procedure that entails preparing and draping the area of the wound, infiltrating the wound with local anesthetic, and extending the wound as necessary to follow its track. If the track terminates without entering the peritoneum (as occurs in approximately one half of the patients who undergo the procedure), the injury can be managed as a deep laceration. Otherwise, penetration of the peritoneum is assumed, and significant injury must be excluded by further diagnostic evaluation. Options include laparoscopy or celiotomy, CT, FAST, diagnostic peritoneal lavage, and admission with observation. Gunshot wounds within the surface markings of the abdomen have a high probability of causing a significant intra-abdominal injury and have therefore been taken to require immediate celiotomy, but this imperative has recently been challenged for those patients with stable hemodynamics and no peritoneal signs on physical examination. In a large retrospective study of patients with abdominal gunshot wounds, selective nonoperative management was reported to result in a significant decrease in the percentage of unnecessary laparotomies (*Ann Surg* 2001;234:395). Current recommendations for nonoperative management of penetrating trauma include the use of triple-contrast CT (accurately predicts the need for laparotomy) and serial examination. The majority of these patients can be discharged after 24 hours of observation (EAST Guidelines, 2007, http://www. east.org).

2. **Blunt trauma.** In the patient sustaining blunt abdominal trauma, physical signs of significant organ involvement are often lacking. As a result, a number of algorithms have been proposed to exclude the presence of serious intra-abdominal injury.

   a. **In the awake, unimpaired patient** without abdominal complaints, combining hospital admission and serial abdominal examinations is a cost-effective strategy for excluding serious abdominal injury as long as the patient is not scheduled to undergo an anesthetic that would interfere with observation. However, such patients are rare in the trauma setting.

   b. **Unstable patient with abdominal injury.** An unstable patient with injuries confined to the abdomen requires immediate celiotomy.

   c. **Unstable patient with multiple injuries.** If an unstable patient has multiple injuries and there is uncertainty about whether the abdomen is the source of shock, a FAST exam may be useful. If a patient is fairly stable and access to CT is readily available, head and abdomen/pelvis CT scans can be obtained. Diagnostic peritoneal lavage (DPL) may be useful in patients with head injuries requiring immediate operative therapy. In many large centers, a CT scan can be obtained as readily as the performance of a DPL.

   d. **Stable patient with multiple injuries.** If a stable patient has multiple injuries and the abdomen may harbor occult organ involvement that is not immediately life-threatening, a CT evaluation is necessary (see Section VI.C.2). In addition to identifying the presence of intra-abdominal injury, CT scanning can provide information helpful for determining the probability that a celiotomy will be therapeutic. Laparoscopy has also been proposed as an adjunct in this situation.

F. The pelvis should be assessed for stability by palpating (not rocking) the iliac wings. Signs of fracture include scrotal hematoma, unequal leg length, and iliac wing hematomas. Careful inspection for lacerations (and possible open fracture) is undertaken.

G. The back should be inspected for wounds and hematomas, and the spine should be palpated for vertebral step-off or tenderness. If there are positive signs of spinal injury, CT scan should be obtained.

H. The genitalia and perineum should be inspected closely for blood, hematoma, and lacerations. In particular, signs of urethral injury should be sought (see Section III.A). A rectal examination is mandatory to assess rectal tone and to look for the presence of gross blood in the rectum.

I. The extremities should be inspected and palpated to exclude the presence of soft tissue and orthopedic, vascular, or neurologic injury. Inspection should look for gross deformity of the limb, active bleeding, open wounds, expanding hematomas, and evidence of ischemia. Obvious dislocations or displaced fractures should be reduced as soon as possible. All wounds should be examined for continuity with joint spaces or bone fractures. The limb should be palpated for subcutaneous air, hematomas, and the presence and character of peripheral pulses. A thorough neurologic examination should be undertaken to determine the presence of peripheral nerve deficits. Radiographs of suspected fracture sites should be obtained, and ankle-brachial indices (ABIs) should be measured in the setting of possible vascular injury even if pulses are normal.

J. General. During the secondary survey (and throughout the initial evaluation of the injured patient), any rapid decompensation by the patient should initiate a return to the primary survey in an attempt to identify the cause. Finally, in any penetrating trauma, all entrance and exit wounds must be accounted for during the secondary survey to avoid missing injuries.

V. DEFINITIVE HOSPITAL CARE. With the completion of the primary and secondary surveys, definitive hospital care is undertaken. During this phase of care for the trauma patient, extensive diagnostic evaluations are completed and therapeutic interventions performed. In this section, important therapeutic principles are discussed according to the anatomic location of the injury.

A. Head injuries

   1. Lacerations. Active bleeding from scalp wounds can result in significant blood loss. Initial therapy involves application of direct pressure and inspection of the wound to exclude bone involvement (i.e., depressed skull fracture). If significant bone injury has been excluded, the wound may be irrigated and débrided. A snug mass closure incorporating all the layers of the scalp will effectively control any hemorrhage and should be done as soon as possible (i.e., before CT evaluations).

   2. Intracranial lesions. Traumatic intracranial lesions are diverse. They include extraparenchymal lesions, such as epidural hematomas, subdural hematomas, and subarachnoid hemorrhages, as well as intraparenchymal injuries, such as contusions and hematomas. CT is the diagnostic modality of choice. Acute therapy is focused on controlling ICP and maximizing CPP (see Section II.D.1). There is class 1 evidence against the use of steroids for traumatic brain injury (*J Neurotrauma* 2000;17:457). Induced hypythermia remains controversial, but a recent National Institutes of Health (NIH)–funded randomized trial does not support its use (*N Engl J Med* 2001;344:556). Patients with intracranial hemorrhage should be placed on seizure prophylaxis with phenytoin for 1 week. A neurosurgeon should be consulted early because emergent surgical intervention may be required.

B. Maxillofacial injuries

   1. Lacerations. All lacerations of the face should be meticulously irrigated, débrided, and closed primarily with fine suture. Alignment of anatomic landmarks is essential. Given the highly vascular nature of the face, primary closure can be performed up to 24 hours after an injury (except a bite wound) as long as it is accompanied by adequate irrigation and débridement. Any deep laceration in the region of the parotid or lacrimal ducts should be examined for ductal involvement and consultation with the appropriate specialist undertaken.

2. **Fractures.** Patients with significant craniofacial soft-tissue injury or clinical signs of facial fractures require radiographic evaluation to determine bony integrity. Facial CT has supplanted most facial plain films other than the Panorex view (obtained for mandible fractures) and is often required in complex midface fractures to define fracture fragments in detail. Therapy is predicated on the type of fracture present.

   a. **Frontal sinus fractures.** Nondisplaced anterior table fractures are treated with broad-spectrum antibiotics and observation. Displaced anterior table fractures and posterior table fractures require operative intervention by a specialist.

   b. **Nasal fractures.** Displaced fractures can usually be reduced nonoperatively, with subsequent packing of the nasal cavity for stability. The presence of a septal hematoma requires immediate incision and drainage to prevent avascular necrosis and resultant saddle-nose deformity.

   c. **Maxillary fractures** are classified according to the LeFort system. These fractures often require complex open reduction and fixation by a surgical specialist.

   d. **Mandibular fractures.** Fractures of the mandible typically occur in areas of relative weakness, including the parasymphyseal region, angle, and condyle. These injuries are often treated by maxillomandibular fixation, but such therapy requires a 4- to 6-week interval. Rigid fixation using plates is another option. Patients with open fractures should receive antibiotics covering mouth flora.

C. **Neck injuries**
1. **Penetrating neck wounds.** The diagnostic evaluation of penetrating neck trauma is evolving but has traditionally been determined by both the depth and location of the wound. Lacerations superficial to the platysma should be irrigated, débrided, and closed primarily. Lacerations longer than 7 cm should be evaluated and closed in the operating room to decrease the risk of infection. The traditional approach to wounds deep to the platysma is an evaluation based on the anatomic zone of the injury but is transitioning to a multislice CT angiography–based general approach.

   a. **Zone I injuries.** Thoracic inlet injuries commonly involve the great vessels. Routine four-vessel arteriography had been advocated by many surgeons because of the difficulty of clinical evaluation and operative exposure of this region. In two prospective studies (*Br J Surg* 1993;80:1534, *World J Surg* 1997;21:41), only 5% of zone I injuries required operation for vascular trauma. Furthermore, routine arteriography did not identify any clinically significant vascular injuries that did not already possess "hard" evidence of vascular trauma (severe active hemorrhage, shock unresponsive to volume expansion, absent ipsilateral upper extremity pulse, neurologic deficit) or "soft" evidence (bruit, widened mediastinum, hematoma, decreased upper-extremity pulse, shock responsive to volume expansion). In addition, patients who lacked clinical evidence of vascular trauma and were managed conservatively did not have any morbidity or mortality as a result of missed vascular injuries (*J Trauma* 2000;48:208). Evaluation of the aerodigestive tract can also be approached selectively. Patients with clinical evidence of aerodigestive tract injury (hemoptysis, hoarseness, odynophagia, subcutaneous emphysema, hematemesis) should undergo dual evaluation with bronchoscopy and meglumine diatrizoate (Gastrografin) or thin barium swallow. Esophagoscopy may be substituted for obtunded patients or patients otherwise unable to participate in the swallow study.

   b. **Zone II injuries.** The proper diagnostic algorithm for midneck injuries is somewhat controversial. Little disagreement exists as to the need for immediate operative exploration in the patient with evidence of obvious vascular or aerodigestive tract injury. In stable patients without such signs, multiple approaches have been advocated. These approaches have ranged from routine arteriography with panendoscopy to observation alone (*J Vasc Surg* 2000;32:483). Several studies have suggested that contrast-enhanced CT can be useful by demonstrating the trajectory of the missile to vital structures and thus can aid in decision making regarding further invasive studies or surgical exploration (*Arch Surg* 2001;136:1231, *Trauma* 2001;51:315). Furthermore, studies have shown CT angiography to be useful and comparable to conventional angiography in evaluating for possible vascular injury (*Radiology* 2000;216:356, 2002;224:336, *J Trauma* 2005;58:413). Finally, some authors continue to recommend traditional ipsilateral cervical exploration despite the increased incidence of negative explorations and the associated increased hospital costs. None of these algorithms for management of penetrating zone II injuries has shown superiority over the others, and management is probably best dictated by the manpower and imaging services available to the surgeon.

c. **Zone III injuries.** Upper neck injuries with clinical evidence of vascular involvement require prompt CT angiography owing to the difficulty of gaining exposure and control of vessels in this region. Embolotherapy can be used for temporary or definitive management, except for the internal carotid artery. An injury without clinical evidence of vascular trauma may be managed selectively, with further evaluation by CT. Direct pharyngoscopy suffices to exclude aerodigestive trauma. In neck vascular injuries, endovascular stenting and/or embolization, especially in zones I and III, may be beneficial and should be considered if available.

d. **General approach.** Some authors believe that multislice CT angiography is an appropriate replacement for angiography and advocate an approach that depends on CT findings instead of anatomic of zone (see Fig. 22-1).

e. **Operative therapy.** Regardless of the location of the cervical injury, common operative principles apply once surgical exploration is undertaken. Adequate exposure, including proximal and distal control of vascular structures,

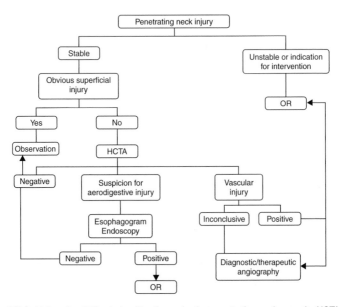

Figure 22-1. University of Miami algorithm for evaluating penetrating neck wounds. HCTA, helical computed tomographic angiography; OR, operating room. (With permission from Munera F, Cohn S, Rivas LA. Penetrating injuries of the neck: use of helical computed tomographic angiography. *J Trauma* 2005;58:413–418.)

is essential. The most common approach is through an incision along the anterior border of the sternocleidomastoid muscle. A collar incision is reserved for repair of isolated aerodigestive injuries or for bilateral explorations (e.g., transcervical injuries). The track of the wound must be followed to its termination. Arterial injuries are repaired primarily if possible. Otherwise, prosthetic vascular grafts can be used. Veins can be ligated, except in the case of bilateral internal jugular injury. Tracheal and esophageal injuries should be repaired primarily using synthetic absorbable sutures. If these injuries occur in tandem, a well-vascularized flap of muscle or fascia should be interposed between the repairs to decrease the incidence of posttraumatic tracheoesophageal fistula. Unexpected laryngeal injuries should be evaluated with endoscopy. A drain may be placed if there is any suspicion of aerodigestive tract violation. This maneuver will allow for controlled cutaneous drainage of any leak, thereby preventing lethal mediastinitis. In the case of combined aerodigestive and vascular injuries, the aerodigestive repair should be drained to the contralateral neck to prevent breakdown of the vascular repair from gastrointestinal (GI) secretions should the aerodigestive repair leak.

   2. Blunt neck trauma. Severe blunt neck trauma can result in significant laryngeal and vascular injuries. In the patient with a stable airway, CT is the best modality for evaluation of a suspected laryngeal injury because it can help to determine the need for operative intervention. Minor laryngeal injuries can be treated expectantly with airway protection, head-of-bed elevation, and possibly antibiotics. Major laryngeal injuries require operative exploration and repair. Blunt vascular trauma usually involves the internal or common carotid artery, but there may also be injury to the vertebral vessels without symptomatology. These injuries can be devastating because they often are not diagnosed until the onset of neurologic deficits. Four-vessel arteriography and CT angiography are the preferred diagnostic modalities. Because the severity of the deficit and the time to diagnosis are strongly associated with outcome, a high index of suspicion is needed. Some authors have even advocated selective arteriography in asymptomatic patients with injury patterns or mechanisms suggestive of a blunt carotid or vertebral artery injury (i.e., severe hyperextension or flexion with rotation of the neck; direct blow to the neck; significant anterior neck soft-tissue injury; cervical spine fracture; displaced midface fractures or mandibular fractures; basilar skull fracture involving the sphenoid, mastoid, petrous, or foramen lacerum) (*Ann Surg* 1998;228:462). The current recommendation is for operative repair of surgically accessible lesions. Systemic anticoagulation (unless contraindicated) with heparin appears to improve neurologic outcome and is therefore recommended for surgically inaccessible lesions. Other anticoagulants are under evaluation for use in this setting.

D. Thoracic injuries. Rapid diagnosis and treatment of thoracic injuries are often necessary to prevent devastating complications.

   1. Chest wall injuries. Lacerations of the chest without pleural space involvement require simple irrigation, débridement, and closure. A chest wound communicating with the pleural space constitutes an open pneumothorax and should be treated accordingly (see Section II.B.4). Significant soft-tissue loss may occasionally be encountered and can be initially repaired with a biologic mesh. Complex myocutaneous flap or prosthetic closure, however, is often required for definitive treatment. Rib fractures are common, especially in blunt trauma. They are readily identified on chest x-ray. Any rib fracture can trigger a progression of pain, splinting, atelectasis, and hypoxemia. Preventing this cascade through the use of adequate analgesia and pulmonary toilet is essential. Parenteral narcotics are often required. In the case of multiple rib fractures, intercostal regional blockade using local anesthetics or epidural analgesia using either narcotics or local anesthetics is often useful. Flail chest often results in significant respiratory embarrassment and must be treated aggressively (see Section II.B.3).

   2. Tracheobronchial injuries often present with massive subcutaneous emphysema. Prompt diagnosis and initial stabilization are essential. The operative approach is dictated by the location of the injury. Upper tracheal injuries require a median sternotomy. Distal tracheal or right bronchial injuries are repaired via a right thoracotomy. Left bronchial injuries mandate a left thoracotomy. Penetrating injuries can be débrided and repaired primarily. Transections resulting from blunt injuries usually require débridement of the tracheobronchial segment with reanastomosis. Tracheal defects involving up to two rings can usually be repaired primarily through adequate mobilization. Complex bronchoplastic procedures or pulmonary resections are rarely required.

3. **Esophageal injuries** are most commonly encountered after penetrating trauma, and they can pose difficult diagnostic and therapeutic challenges. These injuries require prompt recognition because delay in diagnosis is often lethal (mortality can increase threefold when repair is delayed by 24 hours). CT can be helpful in delineating the trajectory of the missile and possible esophageal injury. Esophagoscopy combined with meglumine diatrizoate (Gastrografin) swallow can detect virtually all injuries, but either modality is probably adequate for evaluating the thoracic esophagus. Such evaluations must be performed expeditiously, however, because their use can cause delays that impact the morbidity of an esophageal injury repair (*J Trauma* 2001;50:289). As in the case of tracheobronchial injuries, the operative approach is determined by the location of the injury. A right thoracotomy provides excellent exposure for most thoracic esophageal injuries, particularly those in the midesophagus. A left thoracotomy is recommended for distal esophageal injuries. Primary repair should be undertaken whenever possible and consists of closure using an absorbable synthetic suture. The repair can be buttressed with a vascularized flap (i.e., pleural or pericardial) or fundoplication (for distal injuries). Drain placement near (but not adjacent to) the repair is recommended. Treatment options in late-recognized esophageal injuries include esophageal repair and wide pleural drainage, diversion with injury exclusion, complex flap closure, and esophageal resection (reserved for the esophagus with underlying pathology). Morbidity and mortality are high in this situation.

4. **Pulmonary injuries.** All pulmonary injuries can potentially have an associated pneumothorax (simple or tension). Prompt diagnosis and treatment can be lifesaving (see Section II.B).

   a. **Pulmonary contusion** can be associated with both blunt and penetrating thoracic trauma. These lesions often have adequate perfusion but decreased ventilation. The consequent ventilation–perfusion mismatch results in severe hypoxemia. Diagnosis is often made by chest x-ray. Therapy consists of aggressive pulmonary toilet and respiratory support. Severe contusions often require intubation and mechanical ventilatory support. The management of such patients is extremely challenging because unusual modes of ventilation (e.g., pressure-controlled/inverse-ratio or high-frequency oscillating ventilation) may be needed. Consultation with a critical care specialist is recommended.

   b. **Hemothorax** is typically diagnosed as opacification on chest x-ray, and it commonly arises from penetrating chest injuries. In the majority of cases, tube thoracostomy is sufficient therapy. A chest x-ray obtained after placement of the tube should be inspected for both tube placement and adequacy of drainage of the hemothorax. A persistent hemothorax with a properly placed thoracostomy tube should raise the possibility of persistent hemorrhage within the hemithorax. Operative intervention is often based on the amount of initial sanguinous drainage and ongoing hemorrhage from the tube. Guidelines vary according to institution and should be individualized to the clinical situation. In general, patients who drain *more than 1.5 L of blood at tube insertion or who have an ongoing blood loss greater than 200 mL/hour over 6 hours* should undergo operative thoracotomy for control of hemorrhage. Significant intrathoracic bleeding can result from pulmonary hilar or great-vessel injury (see Section V.D.5). Pulmonary parenchymal hemorrhage can often be controlled with pulmonary tractotomy and oversewing of bleeding intrapulmonary vasculature. Pulmonary resection (lobectomy or pneumonectomy) may be considered for intractable pulmonary hemorrhage (usually from a hilar injury). Morbidity and mortality after pneumonectomy in the trauma setting, however, are significant, and it should therefore be considered a last resort. Air embolism can develop in the setting of significant pulmonary parenchymal injury, especially in the patient on positive-pressure mechanical ventilation. It usually presents as sudden cardiovascular collapse, and therapy consists in placing the patient in steep Trendelenburg, aspirating air from the right ventricle, and providing cardiovascular support. Chest wall intrathoracic hemorrhage usually originates from an intercostal or internal mammary artery and is best treated by ligation.

5. **Great-vessel injury**
   a. **Penetrating trauma.** Thoracic great-vessel injury most commonly occurs secondary to penetrating trauma. These patients often present in profound shock with an associated hemothorax. Occasionally, they present with pericardial tamponade due to a proximal aortic or vena caval injury. Often, diagnostic investigations are not performed because immediate operative intervention is indicated (e.g., massive hemothorax, pericardial tamponade). In certain circumstances, however, diagnostic evaluation is possible and can be rather extensive. For example, the stable patient suffering from a transmediastinal gunshot injury requires evaluation of the thoracic great vessels, esophagus, trachea, and heart unless the trajectory of the missile clearly avoids these structures. Aortography, endoscopy with radiographic swallow study, echocardiography, and CT are all modalities used to evaluate these patients. However, since the late 1990s, advances in technology have allowed spiral CT to take the initial, and the definitive, role in the evaluation of the patient for whom aortic or great-vessel injury is suspected. Aortography was previously used when the results of CT were ambiguous because of technical factors, but additional technical advances now allow for accurate three-dimensional reconstruction and definitive diagnosis. Angiography is now generally limited to patients in whom an endovascular repair is indicated (*Radiol Clin North Am* 2006;44:239).

   The operative approach depends on the vessel involved. Median sternotomy is ideal for access to the proximal aorta, superior vena cava, right subclavian artery, and carotid artery. A left infraclavicular extension ("trapdoor") to the median sternotomy provides exposure to the left subclavian artery, but a high left anterolateral thoracotomy is probably a better approach. Finally, rapid median sternotomy with either right or left infraclavicular extensions is most appropriate in the patient who has undergone resuscitative thoracotomy before arrival in the operating room. Whenever possible, primary repair should be performed for arterial and vena caval injuries. Prosthetic grafting may be necessary for complex reconstructions. Brachiocephalic and innominate venous injuries can be ligated. Endovascular approaches are increasingly used to repair these injuries.

   b. **Blunt trauma** associated with rapid deceleration (e.g., motor vehicle crashes, falls) can result in thoracic great-vessel injury. The descending thoracic aorta just below the origin of the left subclavian artery is particularly prone to rupture from rapid deceleration because it is tethered by the ligamentum arteriosum. Often such a trauma results in complete transection of the aorta and immediate death from exsanguination. In some patients, however, only partial disruption of the aorta occurs, and there is tamponade of the hemorrhage. These patients can arrive at the trauma center alive. If their injury goes unrecognized, however, mortality is near universal. All patients presenting with blunt trauma associated with rapid deceleration therefore must be screened with a chest x-ray, preferably upright. Those patients with positive findings on chest x-ray (widened mediastinum, obscured aortic knob, deviation of the left main-stem bronchus or nasogastric tube, and opacification of the aortopulmonary window) require further evaluation. Helical (spiral) CT is then undertaken, and if it is interpreted as normal, the likelihood of a blunt aortic injury is near zero. If the helical CT is interpreted as indeterminate for aortic injury, immediate four-vessel arteriography is necessary. Arteriographic evidence of an aortic injury mandates prompt operative intervention. In some institutions, direct helical CT evidence of an aortic injury is sufficient to mandate operative repair, whereas in other institutions, it is followed by arteriography. Transesophageal echocardiography is an alternative diagnostic modality in patients who are unable to undergo helical CT or arteriography, but is not preferred because of its limited views of the aortic arch. When a blunt aortic injury is present, operative repair should be undertaken as quickly as possible. A left anterolateral thoracotomy is the preferred approach to this portion of the aorta. Often, a prosthetic interposition graft is inserted at the level of the injury, but primary repair can also be performed. Whether to use partial cardiopulmonary bypass as a circulatory adjunct or the "clamp-and-sew" technique remains controversial. Definitive studies demonstrating the superiority of one method or the other in terms of morbidity and mortality do not exist. Sufficient prospective data do exist, however, to recommend delaying operative repair in patients requiring other emergent interventions (e.g., laparotomy or craniotomy) for more immediately life-threatening injuries or in patients who are poor operative candidates due to age or comorbidities (*J Trauma* 2000;48:1128). These patients require close pharmacologic control of their BP until surgical repair can be accomplished. As in penetrating injury, there is increasing use of endovascular stents in this setting.

6. Cardiac injury

a. Penetrating trauma. Cardiac injury is usually associated with penetrating anterior chest trauma between the midclavicular lines, but it can occur in the setting of penetrating trauma outside these anatomic landmarks. Pericardial tamponade should be suspected in the patient presenting in shock with distended neck veins and diminished heart sounds **(Beck triad).** Tension pneumothorax must be excluded, however, by auscultating the lung fields. In the hemodynamically stable patient with suspicion for an occult penetrating cardiac injury, echocardiography is the diagnostic modality of choice. Transesophageal examination is preferred. The presence of pericardial fluid warrants emergent operative exploration. Another diagnostic modality is immediate subxiphoid pericardial exploration, especially in the setting of multiple injuries requiring emergent interventions. This procedure is performed in the operating room under general anesthesia. The pericardium is exposed via a subxiphoid approach, and a 1-cm longitudinal incision is made along it. The presence of straw-colored fluid within the pericardium constitutes a negative examination. Blood within the pericardium mandates definitive exploration and cardiorrhaphy. In the hemodynamically unstable patient, resuscitative thoracotomy is often the means of diagnosis. The preferred operative approach to the repair of penetrating cardiac injuries is via median sternotomy. Atrial and ventricular cardiac wounds are repaired primarily using interrupted or running monofilament sutures. Skin staples may also be used (especially in the setting of resuscitative thoracotomy). A Foley may also be placed into the cardiac wound and the balloon inflated as a temporary measure until definitive management can be performed in the operating room. Care must be taken to avoid injury to coronary arteries during the repair. Wounds adjacent to major branches of the coronary circulation therefore require horizontal mattress sutures placed beneath the artery. Distal coronary artery branches may be ligated. Early consultation with a cardiothoracic surgeon is essential, especially in cases involving complex repairs or cardiopulmonary bypass.

b. Blunt trauma. Blunt cardiac injury (BCI) should be suspected in all patients presenting with the appropriate mechanism of injury (e.g., motor vehicle crash with chest trauma) or in those manifesting an inappropriate cardiovascular response to the injury sustained (*J Trauma* 1998;44:941). Presentations range from unexplained sinus tachycardia to cardiogenic shock with cardiovascular collapse. Studies suggest that cardiac enzymes have little to no *clinical* value in the diagnosis or treatment of BCI. ECG is the screening modality of choice. A normal ECG excludes significant BCI, whereas the presence of an ECG abnormality (i.e., arrhythmia, ST changes, ischemia, heart block, unexplained sinus tachycardia) in the stable patient warrants admission for 24-hour continuous cardiac monitoring. In the unstable patient, a transthoracic echocardiogram should be performed to identify any dyskinetic/akinetic myocardium or valvular damage. If the transthoracic evaluation is suboptimal, a transesophageal study is mandatory (EAST guidelines, 1998). Patients with frank myocardial or valvular rupture require emergent operative repair. Otherwise, supportive therapy with continuous monitoring and appropriate pharmacologic support (i.e., inotropes and vasopressors) in an ICU setting is warranted. Any arrhythmias are managed according to standard Advanced Cardiac Life Support protocols. Rarely, invasive mechanical cardiac support is necessary. Aneurysmal degeneration can be a long-term complication of blunt cardiac injury.

E. Abdominal injuries. The management of abdominal injuries must often be individualized to meet the needs of each patient, but certain guidelines apply. All patients undergoing laparotomy for trauma should be prepared and draped from the sternal notch to the knees anteriorly and from each posterior axillary line laterally to have access to the thorax if needed and to the saphenous vein for any potential vascular reconstruction.

1. Diaphragmatic injuries occur most commonly as a result of penetrating thoracic or abdominal trauma. Blunt trauma, however, can produce rupture secondary to rapid elevation of intra-abdominal pressure. Frequently, diagnosis is made during celiotomy, but injury can occasionally be recognized on radiographic studies (e.g., chest x-ray or CT). Therapy entails primary repair using monofilament synthetic sutures in a horizontal mattress fashion. Immediate repair prevents the long-term complications associated with diaphragmatic hernias.

2. Abdominal esophageal injuries are managed much like thoracic esophageal wounds (see Section V.D.3). In addition to primary repair and drain placement, the fundus of the stomach can be used to buttress the site via a 360-degree (Nissen) wrap. Exposure of this portion of the esophagus can be difficult. Often, the left lobe of the liver must be mobilized and the crus of the diaphragm partially divided. Finally, placement of a feeding jejunostomy should be considered to allow for enteral nutrition in the postoperative period.

3. Gastric injuries. Injuries to the stomach occur most often in the setting of penetrating trauma. Sanguinous drainage from a nasogastric (or orogastric) tube should raise the possibility of gastric injury. Diagnosis is usually made at laparotomy. Simple lacerations can be repaired in one layer using synthetic absorbable suture. Alternatively, a full-thickness closure can be reinforced with Lembert stitches. Massive devitalization may require formal resection with restoration of GI continuity via gastroenterostomy. In such cases, vagotomy is helpful in reducing the risk of marginal ulcer.

4. Hepatic injuries. The use of CT in blunt trauma has increased the diagnosis of occult liver injuries, making the liver the most commonly injured abdominal solid organ.

    a. Penetrating trauma. The diagnosis of penetrating hepatic injury is usually made at exploratory laparotomy, although CT has been used to identify injuries. Hemorrhage in the setting of hepatic trauma can be massive, and familiarity with maneuvers to gain temporary and definitive control of such bleeding is essential.

        (1) Initial hemostasis. Rapid mobilization of the injured lobe with bimanual compression can often provide initial hemostasis. Perihepatic packing with laparotomy pads placed over the bleeding site and on the anterior and superior aspects of the liver to compress the wound is an extremely effective alternative. Temporary occlusion of the contents of the hepatoduodenal ligament (Pringle maneuver) with a vascular clamp decreases hepatic vascular inflow and is successful in controlling most intraparenchymal bleeding. It is often employed to allow further mobilization of the liver and exposure and repair of injuries. Occlusion times should not exceed 30 to 60 minutes because longer intervals of warm ischemia are poorly tolerated by the liver. Failure of the Pringle maneuver significantly to decrease bleeding suggests major hepatic venous involvement, including juxtahepatic and retrohepatic inferior vena caval injuries. Prompt recognition and temporary vascular control of such injuries via the placement of an atrial-caval shunt (Schrock shunt) can be life-saving. Another option in this setting is total hepatic vascular isolation achieved by placing vascular clamps on the hepatoduodenal ligament (if not already done), the descending aorta at the level of the diaphragm, and the suprahepatic and suprarenal vena cava. Finally, bleeding from deeply penetrating injuries (e.g., transhepatic gunshot wounds) can sometimes be temporarily controlled through placement of an occluding intrahepatic balloon catheter.

(2) Definitive hemostasis is attained via multiple techniques. Raw surface oozing can be controlled by electrocautery, argon beam coagulation, or parenchymal sutures [horizontal mattress stitches placed in a plane parallel to the injury using large absorbable (no. 2 chromic) sutures on a widesweep, blunt-tip needle]. Topical hemostatic agents are also useful (i.e., microcrystalline collagen, thrombin, oxidized cellulose). Deeper wounds are usually managed by hepatotomy and with selective ligation of bleeding vessels. A finger-fracture technique is employed to separate overlying liver parenchyma within a wound until the injured vessel is identified, isolated, and controlled. Major venous injuries should be repaired primarily. Omental packing of open injuries can provide buttressing. Resectional débridement is limited to frankly devitalized tissue. Hepatic artery ligation is reserved for deep lobar arterial injuries where hepatotomy may result in significant blood loss. Formal anatomic resection should be avoided because of its high associated morbidity and mortality. Finally, closed suction drains should be placed near the wound to help to identify and control biliary leaks.

(3) Damage control principles are frequently applied to complex hepatic injuries. Perihepatic packing with ICU admission and resuscitation, followed by return to the operating room in 24 to 48 hours, is common. On occasion, an intrahepatic balloon catheter is used. Liberal use of this algorithm can decrease mortality.

b. Blunt trauma. The management of blunt hepatic trauma has undergone a dramatic change over the last decade, largely due to improvement in CT imaging. CT is the recommended diagnostic modality for evaluation of the stable patient suspected of having blunt hepatic trauma because it can reliably identify and characterize the degree of an injury. Oral and intravenous contrast is necessary to help exclude concomitant hollow viscus injury. In the presence of hepatic trauma, therapy should be predicated on the hemodynamic status of the patient. The unstable patient requires operative exploration and control of hemorrhage as described (see Section V.E.4.a). The stable patient without an alternate indication for celiotomy should be admitted for close hemodynamic monitoring and serial hematocrit determinations. Operative intervention should be promptly undertaken for hemodynamic instability. Evidence of ongoing blood loss in the hemodynamically stable patient warrants angiographic evaluation and embolization of the bleeding source. Transfusions are administered as indicated. The frequency of follow-up CT evaluation of the lesion should be dictated by the clinical status of the patient. Resumption of normal activity should be based on evidence of healing of the injury. Stable patients therefore do not require strict bedrest. Complications of blunt hepatic trauma include biliary leak and abscess formation, both of which are readily amenable to endoscopic and percutaneous therapy. Delayed hemorrhage is rare, but pseudoaneurysm formation can occur with hemorrhage or hemobilia, requiring angiography and embolization.

Nonoperative management is successful in the vast majority of blunt hepatic injuries and has even been reported in certain cases of penetrating hepatic wounds.

5. **Gallbladder injuries.** Injury to the gallbladder frequently coexists with hepatic, portal triad, and pancreaticoduodenal trauma. Treatment consists of cholecystectomy. The gallbladder also provides an effective means of assessing biliary tree integrity via cholangiography.

6. **Common bile duct injuries.** Penetrating trauma is most often responsible for common bile duct injuries. Like gallbladder injuries, they often occur in association with other right–upper-quadrant organ trauma. Most often, diagnosis is apparent at the time of laparotomy, but occult injuries can occur. Intraoperative cholangiography, therefore, is warranted when biliary involvement is suspected. Primary repair of the injured duct over a T tube is the preferred management, but Roux-en-Y choledochojejunostomy is sometimes required (i.e., when significant segmental loss of the duct is present). Choledochoduodenostomy and cholecystojejunostomy are poor options and should be avoided.

7. **Duodenal injuries** frequently coexist with devastating GI and abdominal vascular trauma and, as a result, can represent a diagnostic and therapeutic challenge. The type and severity of duodenal injury determine management.

    a. **Duodenal hematoma.** Intramural duodenal hematomas usually occur after blunt trauma to the upper abdomen. Patients present with abdominal pain, nausea, and vomiting. Diagnosis is made with CT or upper GI fluoroscopy using meglumine diatrizoate (Gastrografin). Therapy consists of long-term nasogastric decompression and nutritional support (parenteral or enteral distal to the level of injury). The majority of duodenal hematomas are effectively treated in this manner, but operative evacuation may be indicated if obstruction persists for more than 14 days and CT reimaging confirms persistent hematoma.

    b. **Duodenal perforation** can be difficult to diagnose. Patients often complain only of vague back or flank pain, and symptoms can evolve slowly. Plane radiographic signs suggestive of perforation include evidence of retroperitoneal gas, blurring of the right psoas muscle, and leftward scoliosis. Upper GI fluoroscopy using water-soluble contrast (meglumine diatrizoate) may also show evidence of a leak. The diagnostic modality of choice, however, is CT using oral and intravenous contrast, with the oral contrast administered in the trauma room. Operative therapy depends on the degree of injury, but complete mobilization of the duodenum (Kocher maneuver) is essential for proper visualization and repair. Most defects (approximately 80%) can be repaired primarily in two layers, with a transverse closure to avoid luminal narrowing. Closed suction drainage placed around the repair is strongly recommended to control any anastomotic leak. Nasoduodenal decompression should be instigated. Alternatively, antegrade or retrograde (preferred) tube duodenostomy can be performed in conjunction with tube gastrostomy and feeding jejunostomy, the so-called triple tube drainage (*J Trauma* 1979;19:334).

    c. **Complex duodenal injuries** are an operative challenge, and management remains controversial, especially in the presence of tissue devitalization. Whenever possible, débridement with primary repair should be performed. The repair should be protected via triple-tube drainage or pyloric exclusion with diverting gastrojejunostomy. For large defects not amenable to primary closure, a retrocolic Roux-en-Y duodenojejunostomy is an option. Finally, pancreaticoduodenectomy (Whipple procedure) should be reserved only for the most complex injuries, including duodenal devascularization or severe combined injuries involving the pancreatic head and bile duct. This procedure has a very high morbidity and mortality in the trauma setting.

8. **Pancreatic injuries.** Injury to the pancreas often occurs as a result of penetrating trauma, although a significant number of cases do involve blunt mechanisms. Associated morbidity and mortality remain significant and increase with the number of associated injuries. However, isolated pancreatic trauma is rare.

Typically, the liver or stomach is also involved, but concomitant duodenal-pancreatic or biliary-pancreatic injuries do happen. CT is the best diagnostic imaging modality available, but occasionally endoscopic retrograde cholangiopancreatography or MR cholangiopancreatography studies should be used to help clarify the presence or absence of pancreatic duct injury. *Pancreatic enzymes are not helpful in the diagnosis.* Treatment focuses on determining the presence and location of major ductal involvement. Commonly, such information is obtained during operative inspection of the gland, but occasionally intraoperative pancreatography (endoscopic or transduodenal) may be necessary. Adequate exploration entails performing a Kocher maneuver (to visualize the head of the pancreas) as well as transecting the gastrohepatic and gastrocolic ligaments (to inspect the body and tail of the pancreas). If necessary, the retroperitoneal attachments along the inferior border are divided (to view the posterior aspect of the pancreas) (*Curr Probl Surg* 1999;36:325). When the pancreatic duct is intact, injuries (e.g., contusions, lacerations) are often treated with débridement and closed drainage. Pancreatorrhaphy is employed when indicated. Transection of the pancreatic duct requires more extensive procedures. For ductal injuries occurring to the right of the superior mesenteric vessels, treatment consists in closing the proximal end of the duct with a stapler or suture and draining the distal end via a Roux-en-Y pancreaticojejunostomy. Distal pancreatectomy (with or without splenectomy) should be used for transections occurring to the left of the superior mesenteric vessels. In addition, it is an option for more-proximal injuries in which resection would preserve greater than 10% of the pancreas. Whatever the procedure, the proximal end of the duct should be closed, and the pancreatic bed should be extensively drained. The liberal use of closed suction drainage helps to decrease morbidity by controlling pancreatic leaks. Finally, severe injury to the head of the pancreas, especially in conjunction with duodenal and biliary trauma, may require pancreaticoduodenectomy but usually not during the initial operation.

9. **Splenic injuries.** The spleen is the second-most-common solid organ injured in abdominal trauma. Like hepatic trauma, the management of splenic injuries has undergone an evolution over the last decade.
   a. **Penetrating trauma.** In general, penetrating splenic injuries are diagnosed at laparotomy, although they are sometimes identified on CT imaging. Management depends on complete mobilization of the spleen. Initial hemostasis is possible through manual compression. Minor injuries contained within the splenic capsule do not require any intervention. Bleeding from small capsular lacerations can be controlled with direct pressure or topical hemostatic agents. More-complex injuries are treated according to the hemodynamic status of the patient. In the stable patient, splenorrhaphy can be employed in an attempt to preserve immune function (requiring salvage of 40% of the splenic mass). Devitalized tissue should be débrided and the wound closed with absorbable horizontal mattress sutures (usually 2-0 chromic). Alternatively, the spleen can be wrapped in absorbable mesh. Partial resection is indicated for isolated superior or inferior pole injuries. In unstable patients or in patients in whom splenic salvage fails, splenectomy should be performed in an expeditious manner. Drainage of the splenic bed is not necessary unless pancreatic injury is suspected. All patients who undergo emergent splenectomy are at risk for overwhelming postsplenectomy sepsis infection. Although this complication is rare (maximum risk is 0.5% in prepubertal children), the mortality is up to 50%. Therefore, all patients undergoing emergent splenectomy require postoperative immunization against *Streptococcus pneumoniae, Haemophilus influenzae,* and *Neisseria meningitidis.* Some authors even recommend penicillin prophylaxis for children because they are at highest risk. Yearly viral influenza vaccines are also recommended for postsplenectomy patients.
   b. **Blunt trauma.** Most blunt splenic injuries are initially treated with nonoperative observation. CT remains the diagnostic modality of choice. All

hemodynamically stable patients without an alternate indication for laparotomy should undergo close observation with continuous monitoring of vital signs, initial bedrest, nasogastric decompression (unless contraindicated), and serial hematocrit determinations. Patients with CT evidence of a contrast "blush" or evidence of continuing blood loss who remain stable should undergo transfusion and selective angiographic embolization. Patients who are hemodynamically unstable or are failing nonoperative management (e.g., require continuing transfusion) should undergo operative exploration and therapy as described (see Section V.E.9.a). Most often, splenectomy is performed. CT reimaging should be performed as clinical status indicates, especially for high-grade injuries.

10. **Small-bowel injuries.** Given its large volume and anatomy (tethering at the duodenojejunal flexure), the small bowel is prone to both penetrating (e.g., gunshot) and blunt (e.g., lap belt) trauma. Diagnosis is made at laparotomy or via radiographic imaging (plane radiograph or CT). Treatment consists of primary repair or segmental resection with anastomosis. Mesenteric defects should be closed.

11. **Large-bowel injuries.** Colonic injuries typically occur secondary to penetrating trauma and are diagnosed at the time of laparotomy. A prospective multicenter study has demonstrated that the surgical management (primary repair vs. diversion) of penetrating colonic injuries did not affect the incidence of abdominal complications regardless of associated risk factors (*J Trauma* 2001;50:765). The only independent risk factors for such complications were severe fecal contamination, large transfusion requirement (>4 units) in the first 24 hours, and single-agent antibiotic prophylaxis. *Primary repair, therefore, should be considered in all penetrating colonic injuries.*

12. **Rectal injuries.** Penetrating trauma is also responsible for most rectal injuries. They often occur in association with genitourinary or pelvic vascular trauma, and they can be diagnosed via proctoscopy, CT, or at laparotomy. Traditional management advocated rectal washout (débridement), diverting sigmoid colostomy creation, and presacral drain placement, although a prospective, randomized trial showed that omission of presacral drains in the management of low-velocity penetrating rectal injuries did not increase infectious complications (*J Trauma* 1998;45:656). Débridement (with primary repair of rectal wounds when possible) and diverting colostomy formation therefore seem sufficient management. The distal stump should be tagged with proline suture to facilitate identification at the time of reversal. Reversal can be undertaken after 6 weeks if barium enema reveals healing of the rectum and the patient is medically stable.

F. **Retroperitoneal vascular injuries.** Injuries to the major retroperitoneal vessels or their abdominal branches can be life-threatening. These wounds usually present with frank intra-abdominal hemorrhage or retroperitoneal hematoma formation. Management is based on both mechanism of trauma and location of injury.

1. **Penetrating trauma.** The majority of retroperitoneal vascular injuries are the result of penetrating trauma. By definition, any hematoma formed by a penetrating mechanism is uncontained and requires prompt exploration.

   a. **Initial access and hemostasis.** At times, vascular injuries present with massive intra-abdominal bleeding, and familiarity with techniques to control such hemorrhage expeditiously and to obtain access to vessels efficiently can be life-saving. Packing the site of injury with laparotomy pads is always a reliable temporizing option. Often, initial control requires occluding the supraceliac aorta at the level of the diaphragmatic hiatus using a vascular clamp, a T bar, or direct pressure. Division of the gastrohepatic ligament and mobilization of the stomach and esophagus can provide access to this section of the aorta. Occasionally, division of the diaphragmatic crus is necessary for more proximal control. Once the proximal aorta has been occluded, definitive identification and repair of vascular injuries require adequate exposure of the involved vessels. A left medial visceral rotation (Mattox maneuver) provides excellent access to the aorta, celiac axis, superior mesenteric artery (SMA), left renal artery, and iliac arteries. A right medial visceral rotation (Catell maneuver) readily exposes the vena cava (with a combined Kocher maneuver), right renal vessels, and iliac veins. The infrarenal aorta may also be approached via a transperitoneal incision at the base of the mesocolon.

b. **Repair of vascular injuries.** Most aortic and iliac arterial injuries can be repaired directly by lateral arteriorrhaphy. On occasion, reconstruction with graft prosthesis or autologous venous graft is necessary for significant circumferential or segmental defects. If enteric contamination is extensive, extra-anatomic bypass with oversewing of the proximal stump is mandatory. Injuries to the celiac root or certain of its branches (left gastric or splenic arteries) can often be ligated without adverse outcome, especially in young patients. Splenectomy must follow splenic artery ligation. Common hepatic artery injuries should be repaired when possible (via lateral arteriorrhaphy, resection and reanastomosis, or graft), but ligation can be tolerated at times. SMA defects must be repaired. Vena caval and iliac venous injuries are repaired by lateral venorrhaphy. Injuries to the superior mesenteric vein (SMV) and portal vein should undergo repair, but cases of successful outcome after ligation have been reported. Because of the risk of postoperative thrombosis leading to portal hypertension or superior mesenteric infarction, SMV and portal venous reconstructions must be closely followed, and anticoagulation is often administered. Finally, major renal arterial and venous injuries require primary repair, whereas partial nephrectomy is recommended for segmental vessel involvement. Endovascular treatment has an expanding role in the treatment of all vascular trauma and may be beneficial.

2. **Blunt trauma** can cause retroperitoneal vascular injury with resultant hematoma formation. Often, these hematomas are discovered at operative exploration, but they are sometimes seen on preoperative imaging. The character and location of the hematoma determine management.

a. **Central abdominal hematomas (zone I).** All central abdominal hematomas caused by blunt trauma require operative exploration. Supramesocolic hematomas are usually due to injuries to the suprarenal aorta, celiac axis, proximal SMA, or proximal renal artery. They should be approached via a left medial visceral rotation. Inframesocolic hematomas are secondary to infrarenal aortic or inferior vena caval injuries and are best exposed by a transperitoneal incision at the base of the mesocolon. As with any vascular repair, proximal and distal control of the involved vessel should be obtained prior to exploration if possible.

b. **Flank hematomas (zone II).** Flank hematomas are suggestive of renal artery, renal vein, or kidney parenchymal injury. Unless they are rapidly expanding, pulsatile, or ruptured, they should not be explored if they are discovered at the time of celiotomy. Radiographic evaluation of the ipsilateral kidney is necessary in this situation to assess its function, usually by means of CT imaging. Evidence of nonfunction should prompt arteriography of the renal artery because blunt abdominal trauma often causes intimal tears, with resulting thrombosis of the artery. If it is discovered within 6 hours of the injury, revascularization is performed, although the success rate is only 20%. Otherwise, nonoperative management is preferred. Nephrectomy is sometimes indicated when laparotomy is performed for associated injuries in a stable patient. In this setting, removal of the nonfunctioning kidney will decrease long-term renal complications (e.g., urinoma, hypertension, delayed bleeding). When operative exploration of a flank hematoma is required, vascular control should be obtained outside of the Gerota fascia. Total or partial (to preserve renal mass) nephrectomy may be necessary for a shattered kidney.

c. **Pelvic hematomas.** Central pelvic hematomas in the setting of blunt trauma are usually due to pelvic fractures. If they are discovered at celiotomy, they should not be explored unless iliac vessel injury is suspected (loss of ipsilateral groin pulse, rapidly expanding hematoma, pulsatile hematoma) or rupture has occurred. Bleeding from pelvic fractures can be massive, and management should focus on nonoperative control. Unstable pelvic fractures in association with hypotension should undergo some form of external stabilization. In extreme circumstances, temporary control of hemorrhage can be achieved by wrapping a pelvic binder tightly around the pelvis. Formal external fixation should follow as soon as possible. It should also be considered in those patients with unstable pelvic fractures who require celiotomy or who are hemodynamically stable but have a need for continued resuscitation. Pelvic angiography with selective embolization is the preferred intervention for patients in whom major pelvic fractures are the suspected source of ongoing bleeding. It should also be considered in patients with major pelvic fractures when CT imaging reveals evidence of arterial extravasation in the pelvis or when bleeding in the pelvis cannot be controlled at laparotomy.

G. Genitourinary injuries. Injuries to the genitourinary tract are discussed in detail in Chapter 35. Three points, however, warrant discussion in the context of trauma. Urethral injuries complicate the placement of an indwelling catheter. Their diagnosis and management have been discussed (Section III.A). In blunt abdominal trauma, **gross hematuria _or_ microscopic hematuria in the setting of hemodynamic instability** mandates urologic evaluation. The absence of hematuria, however, does not always exclude an injury to the urinary tract, especially in the setting of penetrating torso trauma. CT is the best imaging modality for demonstrating urologic injury in the trauma patient who does not require laparotomy for other reasons, and it provides information regarding kidney perfusion. Although once commonly used, excretory urography (IVP) in the trauma patient is often unsatisfactory and is now rarely used. In patients with suspected bladder rupture, especially those with gross _hematuria or pelvic fluid on CT in the presence of pelvic fractures,_ cystography should be performed. **CT cystography** has been demonstrated to be equivalent to conventional cystography in assessing bladder injury (EAST guidelines, 2003).

H. Orthopedic injuries are discussed in detail in Chapter 34, but three important considerations bear mentioning.

1. **Blood loss.** Fractures can produce large blood losses. A broken rib can be associated with a 125-mL blood loss, a forearm fracture with a 250-mL blood loss, a broken humerus with a 500-mL blood loss, a femur fracture with a 1,000-mL blood loss, and a complex pelvic fracture with a blood loss of 2,000 mL or more. Stabilization of fractures can minimize the amount of bleeding. Although the Medical Anti-Shock Trouser (MAST) (pneumatic antishock device) has been largely discredited as a device for raising BP, it may afford transient pneumatic stabilization to lower-extremity and pelvis fractures, thereby attenuating further blood loss while the patient is being prepared for more specific interventions (e.g., traction, fixation, or arteriography and embolization).

2. **Spinal fractures.** Fractures of the spine are multiple in 10% of cases. Complete radiographic evaluation of the spine is necessary, therefore, when a single fracture is discovered.

3. **Joint involvement.** Two joints overlie single-access arteries: the elbow and the knee. Fractures or dislocations of either of these joints increase the risk of ischemic complications of the involved distal limb. The integrity of the underlying artery therefore must be confirmed by duplex ultrasound or arteriography.

I. Extremity injuries. Extremity trauma can result in devastating injuries requiring the coordination of multiple specialists to perform complex reconstructions. The goal of management is limb preservation and restoration of function, and it should focus on ensuring vascular continuity, maintaining skeletal integrity, and providing adequate soft-tissue coverage.

1. **Penetrating trauma.** Penetrating-extremity trauma typically occurs in males younger than 40 years old. Multiple injuries can occur in association with such trauma, and a high index of suspicion is necessary for diagnosing and repairing them expeditiously.

2. **Vascular injuries.** A wounded extremity can tolerate approximately 6 hours of ischemia before the onset of irreversible loss of function. Quickly identifying and

repairing vascular injuries, therefore, is essential in any extremity trauma. Immediate operative exploration is indicated for obvious (hard) signs of vascular involvement (pulse deficit, pulsatile bleeding, bruit, thrill, expanding hematoma) in gunshot or stab wounds without associated skeletal injury. Arteriography should be employed for those patients with hard vascular signs in the setting of associated skeletal injury (fracture, dislocation) or shotgun trauma. Patients with possible (soft) signs of vascular injury (nerve deficit, nonexpanding hematoma, associated fracture, significant soft-tissue injury, history of bleeding or hypotension) require evaluation of vascular integrity. A useful algorithm is to check the ABI initially. If the ABI for the affected limb is greater than 0.9, no further radiographic evaluation is necessary. If it is less than 0.9, noninvasive Doppler ultrasonography, if technically feasible, should follow to exclude vascular injury. If ultrasonography is equivocal, arteriography is indicated; if it is positive, either operative exploration or arteriography can follow. Patients without hard or soft signs do not require arteriography to exclude vascular involvement. Occult vascular injuries can be managed nonoperatively, with subsequent repair as indicated, without an increase in morbidity. Arterial injuries should be repaired within 6 hours to maximize limb salvage rates. The operative approach is similar to elective vascular procedures, and endovascular therapy may be feasible if available. Proximal and distal control of the involved vessel is essential. Primary repair using monofilament suture should be performed for limited arterial lacerations. For complex injuries (large segmental or circumferential defects), resection with reanastomosis, patch angioplasty, or interposition grafting is preferred. Whenever possible, autologous vein should be used instead of polytetrafluoroethylene (PTFE) for patching or grafting because of its higher patency rates. Ligation of single-artery forearm and calf injuries is possible in the presence of normal counterparts. Restoration of blood flow (via temporary shunt or formal repair) should precede any skeletal reconstruction in cases of combined injuries. Completion arteriography should be performed after any arterial repair. Venous injuries should undergo lateral venorrhaphy or resection with end-to-end reanastomosis if the patient is hemodynamically stable. Ligation with postoperative leg elevation and compression stocking placement (to reduce edema) is indicated in all other cases. Multiple compartment fasciotomies should be liberally used, especially after prolonged ischemia or in the presence of associated injuries.

3. **Skeletal injuries** are diagnosed with plane radiography. Restoration of skeletal integrity is attained by means of either internal or external fixation. Temporary vascular shunting should be performed before stabilization of an unstable fracture in the setting of combined injuries. External fixation is preferred in the presence of gross contamination or tissue loss (see Chapter 34 for further details).

4. **Soft-tissue injuries.** Definitive closure of large soft-tissue defects rarely occurs at the initial operation for extremity trauma. Complex wounds are often thoroughly irrigated and débrided, dressed, and reviewed daily in the operating room. Delayed closure is then undertaken and may require advanced soft-tissue flaps (pedicle or free). On rare occasions, a so-called mangled extremity may require primary amputation if there are severe soft-tissue defects, major bone injury, or unreconstructable peripheral nerve injury and loss of limb function.

5. **Blunt trauma.** Blunt extremity trauma can result in debilitating crush or near-avulsion injuries. Diagnosis and management are the same as in penetrating trauma, but limb salvage and preservation of function tend to be worse due to the extent of injury. These wounds often require the coordinated involvement of multiple specialists.

6. **Extremity compartment syndromes.** Compartment syndromes are common in distal extremity trauma. They typically occur in association with prolonged limb ischemia or external pressure, fractures, crush or vascular injuries (especially combined arterial and venous injuries), and burns. **Increased tissue pressure (>30 mm Hg)** within the inelastic fascial compartment leads to occlusion of capillary flow and ischemia. Signs and symptoms of compartment syndrome include **pain (especially on passive motion), pressure, paralysis, paresthesia,**

pulselessness, and pallor (the so-called six Ps). A high index of suspicion is necessary for early diagnosis because signs often occur late in the process, especially the loss of pulses. Serial compartment pressure measurements should therefore be undertaken in any patient with risk factors. Fasciotomy of all involved compartments is necessary when pressures are 30 to 40 mm Hg (or lower if evidence of ischemia exists). In addition, fasciotomy should be performed if pressures cannot be obtained.

J. Damage control surgery. The concept of damage control is well accepted among trauma surgeons as a valuable adjunct in the surgical care of severely injured patients (*Surg Clin North Am* 1997;77:753). Evolving in response to changing patterns of injury in urban American settings, the damage control philosophy centers on coordinating staged operative interventions with periods of aggressive resuscitation to salvage trauma patients sustaining major injuries. These patients are often at the limits of their physiologic reserve when they present to the operating room, and persistent operative effort results in exacerbation of their underlying **hypothermia, coagulopathy, and acidosis,** initiating a vicious cycle that culminates in death. In these situations, abrupt termination of the procedure after control of surgical hemorrhage and contamination, followed by ICU resuscitation and staged reconstruction, can be life-saving. Although often discussed in the context of abdominal trauma, the practice of damage control can be applied to all organ systems. It is divided into three phases: initial exploration, secondary resuscitation, and definitive operation.

1. Phase I (initial exploration). The first phase in the damage control algorithm consists of in performing an initial operative exploration to attain rapid control of active hemorrhage and contamination. The decision to revert to a damage control approach should occur early in the course of such an exploration. In the setting of abdominal trauma, the patient is prepared and draped as previously described (see Section V.E), and the abdomen is entered via a midline incision. Any clot or debris present on entering the abdomen is promptly removed. If exsanguinating hemorrhage is encountered, four-quadrant packing should be performed. The packing is then removed sequentially, and all surgical hemorrhage within a particular quadrant is controlled. Following control of bleeding, attention is directed at containment of any enteric spillage. Any violations of the GI tract should be treated with suture closure or segmental stapled resection. Anastomosis and stoma formation should be deferred until later definitive reconstruction, and any stapled ends of the bowel should be returned to the abdomen. External drains are placed to control any major pancreatic or biliary injuries. Laparotomy packs are then reinserted, especially in the presence of coagulopathic bleeding. Often, primary abdominal fascial closure is not possible secondary to edematous bowel or hemodynamic instability. Alternative methods of closing the abdomen include skin closure via towel clips or running suture, Bogota bag placement, prosthetic mesh insertion, abdominal wall zipper creation, or vacuum closure. Of all these techniques, the vacuum closure is the most commonly used. It is fashioned by placing a nonadherent material (cassette drape) between the bowel and abdominal wall, with gauze and a suction device on top, which is then sealed with an adherent dressing. Closed suction drains covered with a sterile adhesive dressing eases wound care in the ICU. Throughout the initial operative exploration, communication among the surgeons, anesthesia team, and nursing staff is essential for optimal outcome.

2. Phase II (secondary resuscitation). The second phase in the damage control approach focuses on secondary resuscitation to correct hypothermia, coagulopathy, and acidosis. Following completion of the initial exploration, the critically ill patient is rapidly transferred to the ICU. Invasive monitoring and complete ventilatory support are often needed. Rewarming is initiated by elevating the room temperature, placing warming blankets, and heating ventilator circuits. All intravenous fluids, blood, and blood products are prewarmed. As body temperature normalizes, coagulopathy improves, but rapid infusion of clotting factors (fresh-frozen plasma, cryoprecipitate, and platelets) is often still required. Use of recombinant factor VIIa in this setting has been shown to decrease the need for blood transfusion. Circulating blood volume is restored with aggressive fluid and blood product resuscitation, improving end-organ perfusion and correcting acidosis. With these interventions, hemodynamic stability returns, urinary output increases, invasive monitoring parameters improve, and serum lactate levels and blood pH analysis improve. In the setting of abdominal trauma, a potentially lethal complication that can occur during this phase is abdominal compartment syndrome. It is a form of intra-abdominal vascular insufficiency secondary to increased intra-abdominal pressure. Presentation includes abdominal distention, low urinary output, ventilatory insufficiency in association with high peak inspiratory pressures, and low cardiac output secondary to decreased venous return (preload). Diagnosis is made via measurement of urinary bladder pressure (25 to 30 cm H_2O). When present, prompt operative re-exploration is mandated to relieve the increased pressure. Vacuum or Bogota bag closure helps to prevent this complication. If surgical bleeding is found to be the cause of the intra-abdominal hypertension, it should be controlled and the abdomen closed. If severe edema of the intra-abdominal contents is the source of the compartment syndrome, the abdomen should be closed by using a vacuum closure to reduce intra-abdominal pressure. Following correction of the problem, phase II resuscitation is continued.

3. **Phase III (definitive operation).** The third phase of damage control consists of planned re-exploration and definitive repair of injuries. This phase typically occurs 48 to 72 hours following the initial operation and after successful secondary resuscitation. In the setting of abdominal trauma, all complex injuries are repaired, with precedence going to those involving the vasculature. Conservative principles should be applied. Risky GI anastomoses or complex GI reconstructions should be avoided. The abdomen should be closed primarily if possible. Otherwise, biologic mesh or simple skin closure and staged repair of the resulting ventral hernia should be performed. Even though the damage control approach allows for salvage of many severely injured patients, it is still associated with substantial morbidity and mortality. Outcome is often determined by providing excellent supportive care (ventilation, nutrition, appropriate antibiotics, and physical therapy with rehabilitation services).

VI. MISCELLANEOUS ASPECTS OF GENERAL TRAUMA CARE

A. **Resuscitative thoracotomy** is performed in a final attempt to salvage a certain subset of patients presenting in extremis to the emergency department. The goals are to control intrathoracic hemorrhage, relieve cardiac tamponade, cross-clamp the thoracic aorta, and restore cardiac output.

1. **Indications.** The indications for resuscitative thoracotomy have been refined over time. It should be used in the management of penetrating chest trauma associated with significant hemodynamic deterioration (systolic BP of <60 mm Hg) or cardiopulmonary arrest occurring within the emergency department or shortly before arrival. In addition, it can be used in certain cases of penetrating abdominal trauma fulfilling the same criteria.

2. **Technique.** Resuscitative thoracotomy is performed via an anterolateral left thoracotomy in the fifth or sixth intercostal space. The skin, subcutaneous tissues, and intercostal musculature are opened sharply. A Finochietto retractor is placed to spread the ribs and aid in exposure. First, the pericardium is identified and incised vertically anterior to the phrenic nerve. Any clot or debris is removed from around the heart. Specific cardiac injury is then sought, and repair is undertaken as previously described (see Section V.D.6.a). After cardiorrhaphy, air is evacuated from the heart by needle aspiration, and the adequacy of cardiac filling is assessed to determine intravascular volume status. In the absence of associated pulmonary vascular or great-vessel injury, vigorous volume resuscitation is undertaken. If peripheral vascular access is insufficient, direct infusion into the right atrial appendage can be performed. In severely hypovolemic patients, the descending thoracic aorta may be exposed and cross-clamped to maintain coronary and cerebral perfusion. The aorta should also be clamped if any intra-abdominal hemorrhage is suspected. During volume resuscitation, open cardiac massage is employed to provide adequate circulation. After restoration of

adequate circulatory volume, the underlying cardiac rhythm is assessed, and internal cardioversion is used when appropriate. The patient should be transported to the operating room for definitive injury management and wound closure after a successful resuscitation.

3. **Complications of resuscitative thoracotomy** are many. They include lung injury while gaining access to the heart, transection of the phrenic nerve while performing pericardotomy, injury to the coronary vessels during cardiorrhaphy, and esophageal trauma while clamping the descending thoracic aorta. Therefore, care must be taken during each step of the procedure to avoid causing additional injuries.

B. **Diagnostic peritoneal lavage (DPL).** Since the advent of FAST and rapid helical CT imaging, DPL is now rarely used in the evaluation of patients with suspected intra-abdominal injuries. It remains, however, a useful diagnostic modality in certain situations.

1. **Indications.** DPL is useful in excluding the presence of significant intra-abdominal organ injury in the presence of blunt trauma or a stab wound to the abdomen. It should be employed when less invasive techniques (e.g., serial abdominal examinations, CT, or FAST) are unavailable or if the patient develops unexplained hemodynamic instability while in the operating room for another injury. The only absolute contraindication to DPL is a planned celiotomy. Pelvic fracture, pregnancy, and prior abdominal surgery often mandate a change in indication and technique. All patients undergoing DPL require prior evacuation of the stomach via a gastric tube as well as drainage of the bladder by indwelling catheter.

2. **Technique.** Aspiration of 10 mL of gross blood or any enteric contents is considered a positive DPL. In addition, the microscopic presence of 100,000 red blood cells/μL or 500 white blood cells/μL in the setting of blunt abdominal trauma and the presence of 10,000 red blood cells/μL or 50 white blood cells/μL in the setting of penetrating abdominal trauma is considered a positive finding on DPL.

3. **Complications.** DPL can produce false-positive results due to bleeding near the incision or from pelvic fractures hemorrhaging into the anterior preperitoneal space of Retzius. False-negative findings can occur from improper placement of the catheter and infusion of fluid into the space of Retzius. Puncture of viscera is also possible, especially in the setting of pregnancy or adhesions from prior abdominal operations. An open technique is essential in such circumstances. Although it is associated with certain complications, DPL is a safe, simple, and reliable procedure for detecting intra-abdominal injuries with excellent sensitivity (95%).

C. **Deep venous thrombosis** with pulmonary embolus is the leading cause of preventable morbidity and mortality in trauma patients. Some form of prophylaxis is required in all such patients. When neural injuries [i.e., central nervous system (CNS) or spinal cord injuries] are absent, subcutaneous low-molecular-weight heparin should be administered. When lower-extremity injuries do not preclude their use, sequential pneumatic compression devices are beneficial. Therapy combining compression devices with subcutaneous heparin is thought to be synergistic. Therapy should be initiated early because delay in the initiation of prophylaxis is associated with a threefold increase in venous thromboembolism (*J Trauma* 2007;62:557). When the preceding techniques are contraindicated, serious consideration should be given to early placement of a vena caval filter. Although such a filter does not prevent thrombosis, it may decrease the risk of a deadly pulmonary embolus.

D. **Gastroduodenal ulceration.** Injured patients remain at risk for stress gastroduodenal ulceration and concomitant hemorrhage. Prophylaxis is therefore recommended. Enteral feeding remains the most effective method. Parenteral histamine-receptor blockers also prevent posttraumatic GI bleeding in ventilated or coagulopathic patients. Finally, newer intravenous proton-pump inhibitors may find a role in prophylaxis, but their expense may prove prohibitive.

E. **Rehabilitation in trauma care.** Rehabilitation is a crucial aspect of trauma care, and its planning should begin at the time of admission. Contractures and pressure sores can begin within hours of injury, and as a result, standardized prevention must be initiated promptly on the arrival of the patient on the ward. Regular turning of the patient, placement of air mattresses, and elevation of distal extremities (especially the heel) off the bed can decrease the formation of debilitating pressure sores. Specially designed orthotic splints, braces, and stockings prevent joint and scar contractures that can inhibit return of function. Finally, early physical and occupational therapy initiates the recovery process and prepares the patient for the often difficult rehabilitation to daily activity.

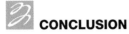 **CONCLUSION**

A chapter of this nature is brief by necessity, but a comprehensive strategy for the care of patients who have been involved with traumatic events will clearly improve outcomes. This care should be coordinated by dedicated general surgeons with an interest or special training in trauma and should ideally use surgical specialty services staffed by individuals with trauma expertise. Although not all institutions will be able to have dedicated trauma-oriented surgeons on staff, the development of statewide trauma systems facilitates the care of patients by directing care of these patients toward those institutions with appropriate resources. For these statewide trauma systems to survive and for the hospitals within the systems to remain financially intact, there needs to be ongoing governmental financial support for the care of trauma victims. Trauma care now costs more than any other disease in the United States and requires comprehensive public health and governmental strategies for managing the complex issues surrounding it.

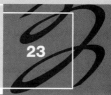

TRANSPLANTATION

Peter O. Simon, Jr., Daniel C. Brennan, and Jeffrey A. Lowell

23

TRANSPLANT ORGAN PROCUREMENT

I. DONOR SELECTION. The greatest obstacle to organ transplantation is the lack of suitable donor organs. Live donation has provided an important source of organs, with annual living kidney donors surpassing deceased donors. Less frequently, live donation is being utilized in liver and lung transplantation. The patients waiting for organs outnumber the available organs, and the waiting list for organ transplants grows each year. In the United States in 2006, more than 94,000 people were awaiting a solid-organ transplant (http://www.unos.org).

II. DECEASED DONORS (formerly known as *brain-dead* or *cadaveric donors*). Strict criteria for establishing brain death include the presence of irreversible coma and the absence of brainstem reflexes (i.e., pupillary, corneal, vestibulo-ocular, or gag reflexes). Other useful diagnostic tests include blood flow scan, arteriography, and an apnea test. **Consent** is required from the family, and inquiries into the donor's medical history are made. Ideally, the donor should have stable hemodynamics, although the use of vasopressors is common. A history of cardiopulmonary resuscitation (CPR) may not preclude donation, particularly in a witnessed arrest with prompt institution of resuscitation and recovery of vital signs. The criteria for donor organ acceptance and use are not absolute; therefore, all patients meeting brain death criteria should be considered as potential donors. Contraindications for organ donation may include a history of intravenous drug abuse or the presence of a malignancy (with the exception of a primary brain tumor). **Exclusion criteria** for specific organs also exist. Potential kidney donors ideally have normal renal function before brain death. Acute tubular necrosis (ATN) in the donor, underlying medical disease (e.g., diabetes, hypertension), or prolonged cold ischemia time may preclude the use of a donor kidney. Selection of a donor liver for a given recipient takes into account donor size, ABO blood type, age, liver function studies, hospital course, hemodynamics, and prior medical and social history. "Expanded-criteria" donors—those not meeting traditional inclusion criteria—have been used with increasing success.

III. DONATION FOLLOWING CARDIAC DEATH (DCD) refers to those who do not meet strict brain death criteria but who are otherwise considered to have nonsurvival neurologic insults. Life support is discontinued in the operating room, and organ procurement is initiated after a specified interval following cardiac asystole.

IV. DECEASED-DONOR ORGAN RECOVERY. The initial dissection identifies hepatic hilar structures, including the common bile duct, portal vein, hepatic artery, and any aberrant arterial blood supply, such as a left hepatic artery branch arising from the left gastric artery or a right hepatic artery from the superior mesenteric artery (SMA). After this dissection, the liver is flushed and cooled with University of Wisconsin (UW) preservation solution (a cold-storage solution containing a high concentration of potassium, lactobionate, hydroxyethyl starch, and other antioxidants) or HTK (histidine-tryptophan-ketoglutarate, a cold-storage solution containing amino acids, potassium, magnesium, calcium, and mannitol) via cannulae placed in the portal vein and the aorta proximal to the iliac artery. A clamp is applied to the supraceliac aorta. The donor liver is removed with its diaphragmatic attachments, a cuff of aorta surrounding the celiac axis and the superior mesenteric artery (SMA), and a portion of the supra- and infrahepatic vena cava. The liver is packaged in UW or HTK solution and surrounded by iced saline during transportation. The remainder of the liver dissection is performed in the recipient's operating room under cold-storage conditions. With the advent of modern preservation solutions, donor livers can be preserved for up to 12 hours before revascularization, with a low incidence of allograft dysfunction. Ideally, cold ischemia time is minimized to less than 8 hours. The donor kidneys are removed *en bloc* and then separated. The ureters are dissected widely to minimize devascularization and are divided near the bladder. This technique minimizes risk of injury to the arteries and allows identification of multiple renal arteries, if present. The pancreas may also be removed for transplantation in a suitable donor. The pancreas, duodenum, and spleen are removed *en bloc.* The blood supply for the pancreas allograft comes from the donor splenic and superior mesenteric arteries, and outflow is via the portal vein. The mesentery below the pancreas is divided with a stapling device.

V. HISTOCOMPATIBILITY. Antibodies to human leukocyte antigen (HLA) do not occur naturally but are produced in response to exposure to foreign histocompatibility antigens that may occur after pregnancy, blood transfusions, or previous transplants. The traditional test used for detecting specific sensitization against donor histocompatibility antigens is termed a **cross-match** or **complement-dependent lymphocytotoxicity assay.** Several methods are available for performing the cross-match, each involving the addition of recipient serum, donor cells (T cells, B cells, or monocytes), and complement. If specific antidonor antibodies are present, antibody binding results in complement fixation and lysis of the donor lymphocytes. Flow cytometry also can be used for cross-matching. This method permits the detection of noncytotoxic antibodies and the definition of cell specificity or antibody binding. Polymerase chain reaction (PCR) and enzyme-linked immunosorbent assay technology are being used increasingly for HLA typing, particularly for the major histocompatibility (MHC) class II HLA antigens. HLA matching is of practical significance only in renal and pancreatic transplantation.

IMMUNOSUPPRESSION

An increasing variety of immunosuppressive medications are available. The protocols outlined in the following section are currently in use at Washington University and are intended only to serve as guidelines. Variations on these protocols are used at other institutions. Most protocols rely on the use of several drugs owing to the different mechanisms and synergies of these medications.

I. IMMUNOSUPPRESSIVE MEDICATIONS

   A. Prednisone or methylprednisolone (Solu-Medrol). Steroids are part of most multiple-drug immunosuppressive regimens and are the first-line drug in the treatment of rejection. Steroids modify antigen processing and presentation, inhibit lymphocyte proliferation, and inhibit cytokine and prostaglandin production. After surgery, patients are placed on a steroid taper and maintained on a low dose of prednisone or eventually withdrawn from the drug altogether. Steroid avoidance and early steroid-withdrawal protocols have had good short-term results. The long-term results are unknown. The acute and chronic side effects of steroid therapy include diabetes mellitus, infections, cataracts, hypertension, weight gain, and bone disease.

   B. Cyclosporine (Sandimmune, Neoral, Gengraf). Cyclosporine is a small fungal cyclic compound, belonging to a class of medications termed calcineurin inhibitors, that blocks T-cell activation, thus inhibiting T-lymphocyte proliferation, interleukin-2 (IL-2) production, IL-2–receptor expression, and interferon-γ release. Two-hour peaks, 12-hour troughs, or both are monitored and adjusted based on time from transplant and HLA matching when known. Side effects include nephrotoxicity, hypertension, tremors, seizures, hyperkalemia, hyperuricemia, hypercholesterolemia, gingival hyperplasia, and hirsutism. Cyclosporine is metabolized by the liver. Common medications that may increase cyclosporine levels include diltiazem, verapamil, erythromycin, fluconazole, ketoconazole, tetracycline, metoclopramide, and cimetidine. Medications that decrease levels include intravenous trimethoprim/sulfamethoxazole, isoniazid, rifampin, phenytoin, phenobarbital, carbamazepine, and omeprazole.

C. **Tacrolimus (FK506, Prograf)** is a macrolide that has a mechanism of action similar to that of cyclosporine but is approximately 100 times more potent. Tacrolimus doses are adjusted to maintain 12-hour trough levels between 5 and 10 ng/mL [fluorescence polarization immunoassay (FPIA)]. The side effect profile is similar to that of cyclosporine but does not include hirsutism and gingival hyperplasia. Alopecia and posttransplant diabetes mellitus (PTDM) are more common with tacrolimus.

D. **Sirolimus (Rapamune)** is an anti–T-cell agent that has a unique inhibitory properties derived from the mammalian target of rapamycin (mTOR) molecule, which blocks T-cell signal transduction. Side effects include thrombocytopenia, hyperlipidemia, mouth ulcers, anemia, proteinuria, and impairment of wound healing.

E. **Mycophenolate mofetil (CellCept, Myfortic)** is a relatively selective inhibitor of T- and B-cell proliferation, cytotoxic T-cell generation, and antibody formation. It is used as an alternative to azathioprine, and is the antimetabolite of choice in most transplant programs. Major toxicities include gastrointestinal disturbances and increased cytomegalovirus infection.

F. **Azathioprine (Imuran)** is an antimetabolite that is a thioguanine derivative of mercaptopurine. This purine analog alters the function or synthesis of DNA and RNA, inhibiting T- and B-lymphocyte proliferation. One of the major side effects of this drug is bone marrow suppression, manifested as leukopenia and thrombocytopenia. An important drug interaction occurs with allopurinol, which blocks the metabolism of azathioprine and increases the degree of bone marrow suppression.

G. **Polyclonal antithymocyte antibodies.** Polyclonal antibodies are immunologic products with antibodies to a wide variety of T-cell antigens, adhesion molecules, costimulatory molecules, cytokines, the T-cell receptor, and class I and II MHC molecules. These agents are used as induction therapy in the perioperative period or as rescue therapy following acute rejection. Two preparations of antithymocyte immunoglobulin are available in the United States: **Thymoglobulin** and **Atgam.** Thymoglobulin, a rabbit-derived product, was recently shown to decrease the incidence of acute rejection in deceased donor renal transplants compared to use of an IL-2–receptor antagonist, basiliximab *(N Engl J Med* 2006;355:1967). Common side effects include fever, leukopenia, and thrombocytopenia.

H. **Monoclonal antibodies. OKT3** is a murine monoclonal antibody that recognizes the T-cell receptor and blocks antigen recognition, hindering T-cell effector functions and potentiating T-cell lysis. OKT3 usually is administered to patients with steroid-resistant, severe rejection. Immediate side effects can include fever, chills, hypotension, respiratory distress, and pulmonary edema, all of which are secondary to the cytokine release syndrome. **Daclizumab (Zenapax)** and **basiliximab (Simulect),** which are IL-2–receptor-specific monoclonal antibodies increasingly being used as induction therapy, are begun immediately prior to transplantation and continued in the immediate postoperative period.

I. **Other immunomodulators** are under investigation and are at varying stages of development.

II. COMPLICATIONS OF IMMUNOSUPPRESSION

A. **Bacterial infections.** Pneumonia and urinary tract infections occur fairly commonly after transplantation. Infectious complications after transplantation from opportunistic organisms are now uncommon because of the use of appropriate prophylactic strategies.

B. **Viral infections.** The most common viral infections after transplantation include **cytomegalovirus (CMV), Epstein-Barr virus (EBV), herpes simplex virus (HSV),** and **BK virus.** See Table 23-1 for a summary of prophylaxis and treatment for common viral and fungal infections.

1. **CMV** infection can occur at any time after transplantation but is most commonly seen 1 to 4 months posttransplant in the absence of prophylaxis. CMV may infrequently infect the recipient's liver, lungs, or gastrointestinal tract. Signs and symptoms of CMV infection include fever, chills, malaise, anorexia, nausea, vomiting, cough, abdominal pain, hypoxia, leukopenia, and elevation in liver transaminases. CMV peripheral blood PCR or antigenemia assays are the most common tools for diagnosing CMV infection. CMV can be associated with significant morbidity

TABLE 23-1	Prophylaxis and Treatment of Infections in Immunosuppressed Patients

Herpes simplex virus (HSV)
  Prophylaxis
    Acyclovir 200 mg PO BID for 3 mo [only D (donor)–/R (recipient)–; otherwise CMV treatment will also cover HSV]
    For liver transplant patients, for 3–6 mo or until prednisone is <10 mg/d
  Treatment
    Decrease immunosuppression
    Acyclovir, 5–10 mg IV for 7–10 d

CMV
  Prophylaxis
    Ganciclovir, 1,000 mg PO TID (1 yr for D+/R–, 6 mo for D+R+, 3 mo for D–/R+, *or*
    Valganciclovir, 900 mg PO QD (reduce dose for renal insufficiency)
  Treatment
    Ganciclovir, 5 mg/kg IV q12h for 3 wk, *or*
    Valganciclovir, 900 mg PO BID for minimum 3 wk and until virus cleared, in the absence of invasive disease
    Consider unselected IgG, 500 mg/kg IV QID for 5 d for pneumonitis or colitis, *or*
    Hyperimmune CMV IgG, 100 mg/kg IV QID for 5 doses for pneumonitis or colitis

Epstein-Barr virus
  Prophylaxis
    Acyclovir, 200 mg PO BID for life (D+/R–)
  Treatment
    Decrease immunosuppression
    Ganciclovir, 5 mg/kg IV q12h for 3 wk
    Chemotherapy for patients with lymphoproliferative disorders

Candida
  Prophylaxis of oral candidiasis
    Nystatin, 5 mL (500,000 units) swish and swallow QID for 3 mo, *or*
    Miconazole, troche suck and swallow QID for 3 mo, *or*
    Fluconazole, 100 mg PO every week for 3 mo
  Treatment of esophageal candidiasis
    Fluconazole, 100 mg PO BID, *or*
    Voriconazole, 200 mg PO BID

Pneumocystis carinii pneumonia
  Prophylaxis (lifetime)
    Trimethoprim/sulfamethoxazole, 1 single-strength tablet PO QD
    Dapsone, 50 mg PO QD for sulfa allergy, *or*
    Pentamidine, 300 mg per nebulizer every month for sulfa allergy and G6PD deficiency

BID, twice daily; CMV, cytomegalovirus; G6PD, glucose-6-phosphate dehydrogenase; IgG, immunoglobulin G; IV, intravenously; PO, orally; q12h, every 12 hr; QD, daily; QID, four times a day.

and even mortality, but it typically responds well to early diagnosis and treatment. There is also evidence that CMV contributes to allograft injury.

Prophylactic administration of ganciclovir (1,000 mg orally three times a day) or valganciclovir (900 mg orally per day) may be useful in any patient who receives a CMV-positive allograft because many of these patients develop a significant CMV infection if left untreated. Treatment consists of decreasing immunosuppression and administering ganciclovir, which inhibits DNA synthesis. Valganciclovir, intravenous ganciclovir, and, to a lesser extent, oral ganciclovir dosing must be adjusted for renal dysfunction. The most common side effects of valganciclovir and ganciclovir are anemia, neutropenia, and thrombocytopenia.

2. **EBV** can infect B cells at any time after transplantation and may be associated with the development of a lymphoproliferative disorder (lymphoma), usually of B-cell origin. Infiltration of the hematopoietic system, central nervous system (CNS), lungs, or other solid organs may occur. The patient usually presents with fever, chills, sweats, enlarged lymph nodes, and elevated uric acid. Diagnosis is made by physical examination; EBV serology; computed tomography (CT) scan of the head, chest, and abdomen (to evaluate lymph nodes or masses); and biopsy of potential sites or lesions. Treatment consists of reducing or withdrawing immunosuppression. Intravenous ganciclovir inhibits EBV-associated DNA polymerase and may be added but is not of proven benefit. Acyclovir prophylaxis for life (200 mg twice a day) may be considered in EBV donor$^+$/recipient$^-$ patients. In addition, standard chemotherapy should be considered for advanced disease or polyclonal tumors that have not responded to other measures.

3. **HSV** causes characteristic ulcers on the oral mucosa, in the genital region, and in the esophagus. Renal transplant patients, if not on ganciclovir, are given prophylactic acyclovir at a dose of 200 mg orally twice a day for 3 months. Active HSV infections are treated by decreasing the patient's immunosuppression and instituting acyclovir therapy (5 to 10 mg/kg intravenously every 8 hours for 7 to 10 days). Side effects of acyclovir are rare but include nephrotoxicity, phlebitis, bone marrow suppression, and CNS toxicity.

4. **BK virus** is a member of the polyoma virus family. Approximately 90% of individuals are seropositive. BK viruria detected by "decoy cell" shedding or PCR develops in 30% of kidney transplant recipients and progresses to viremia in 15% of recipients within the first year. Persistent BK viremia leads to BK nephropathy, which occurs in up to 10% of kidney transplant recipients during the first year. There is no known effective treatment, though low-dose cidofovir (0.25 mg/kg intravenously every 2 weeks) has been tried. Until recently, early graft loss occurred in 50% of patients with BK nephropathy, and the other 50% were left with chronic allograft dysfunction. Recently, prospective monitoring and pre-emptive reduction in immunosuppression has been associated with prevention of nephropathy and better outcomes when nephropathy is diagnosed early.

C. **Fungal infections** can range from mild asymptomatic colonization to lethal invasive infections. Oral **candidiasis** can be prevented and treated with oral nystatin (Mycostatin, 500,000 units orally four times a day for 3 months) or fluconazole. Esophageal candidiasis can be treated with a short course of intravenous amphotericin B or fluconazole (100 mg orally twice a day). Serious fungal infections are treated with intravenous amphotericin B, although use of less nephrotoxic agents such as caspofungin and anidulafungin is increasing.

D. **Other opportunistic infections.** *Pneumocystis jerovecii* (formerly *carinii*) **pneumonia** is a potentially lethal pneumonia that occurs in 5% to 10% of renal transplant patients receiving no prophylactic treatment. Patients typically present with fever, dyspnea, nonproductive cough, hypoxia, and pulmonary infiltrates. The diagnosis is made by bronchoalveolar lavage or a lung biopsy. It can be prevented by low-dose trimethoprim/sulfamethoxazole, dapsone, or inhaled pentamidine. Treatment of pneumonia involves much higher doses of these agents, with a concomitant decrease in immunosuppression.

E. **Malignancies.** Some of the cancers that occur at a higher frequency in transplant recipients than in the general population are squamous cell carcinoma, basal cell carcinoma, Kaposi sarcoma, lymphomas, hepatobiliary carcinoma, and cervical carcinoma. Other common cancers do not have a higher incidence among transplant recipients.

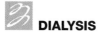 **DIALYSIS**

Acute renal failure (ARF) is defined by a rise in the serum creatinine of more than 0.5 mg/dL (0.04 mmol/L) when the baseline serum creatinine is less than 3 mg/dL (0.27 mmol/L) or by a rise of more than 1 mg/dL (0.09 mmol/L) when the serum creatinine baseline is 3 mg/dL (0.27 mmol/L) or above. **End-stage renal disease (ESRD)** results when the functioning renal mass deteriorates to less than 10% to 20% of normal. ESRD may affect multiple organ systems, resulting in altered fluid and electrolyte homeostasis, accumulation of metabolic waste products, anemia, hypertension, and metabolic bone disease.

I. TREATMENT OF RENAL FAILURE

A. Conservative treatment of renal failure begins with dietary restrictions. Fluid intake is limited to urine output plus insensible losses, usually 1.5 to 2 L/day. Protein is restricted to 0.7 to 1.2 g/kg/day to minimize the rise in blood urea nitrogen (BUN). Sodium chloride is restricted to 2 g/day (sodium, 35 mEq/day), potassium chloride is restricted to 2 g/day (potassium, 25 mEq/day), and phosphorus, magnesium, and aluminum are avoided as much as possible. Control of serum phosphorus can be accomplished through the use of calcium carbonate (500 to 2,500 mg orally within 30 minutes of meals and at bedtime). Sodium bicarbonate (650 mg orally two to three times a day) is used to control acidosis when the serum bicarbonate is less than 20 mg/dL (20 mmol/L). Loop diuretics in combination with thiazide or thiazide-like diuretics are useful adjuncts for maintaining fluid homeostasis. Typically, metolazone (5 mg orally twice a day), followed by furosemide (80 to 200 mg intravenously twice a day or as a continuous infusion of 10 to 20 mg/hour), is given. The thiazide prevents distal tubule adaptation and salt reclamation, which occurs after administration of furosemide. When conservative therapy is inadequate, death ensues without either dialysis or transplantation.

B. Dialysis removes fluids and wastes and adjusts acid-base and electrolyte disturbances by diffusion and osmosis across a semipermeable membrane. This is accomplished in hemodialysis (HD) by the semipermeable membrane of an artificial kidney or in peritoneal dialysis (PD) by the semipermeable peritoneal membrane. Both methods may be used either acutely or chronically.

C. Transplantation is the treatment of choice for many patients with ESRD.

II. INDICATIONS FOR ACUTE DIALYSIS can be remembered by the mnemonic **AEIOU-PP** (**a**cidosis, **e**lectrolyte disturbances, **i**ntoxicants, **o**verload, **u**remia, and **p**ericarditis and **p**olyneuropathy).

A. Acidosis. Dialysis for acidosis should be considered when the serum bicarbonate is less than 10 mEq/L (10 mmol/L).

B. Electrolyte disturbances. A serum potassium acutely greater than 6 mEq/dL (6 mmol/L) is the most common indication for dialysis. Sodium, calcium, and magnesium also can be corrected with dialysis.

C. Intoxicants. Common dialyzable intoxicants include lithium, ethylene glycol, methanol, salicylates, and theophylline.

D. Fluid overload unresponsive to diuretics is another common indication for dialysis.

E. Uremia is a syndrome characterized by vomiting, anorexia, nausea, itching, listlessness, and asterixis associated with renal failure. A patient's symptoms may not correlate directly with the degree of azotemia because many uremic toxins are not yet identified. Furthermore, in ARF, no survival advantage is conferred by early dialysis for patients with azotemic symptoms.

F. Pericarditis and **polyneuropathy** are two absolute indications for dialysis caused by uremia. Pericarditis due to uremia may not necessarily present with elevated ST segments on electrocardiography. Pericardial friction rubs often are ephemeral and may require repeated examinations to detect. Polyneuropathy most commonly manifests as a wrist or foot drop. Without early dialysis, these symptoms may become irreversible.

III. HEMODIALYSIS

A. Types of HD

1. Chronic intermittent maintenance HD usually requires dialysis three times a week for 3 to 4 hours/treatment. Determination of dialysis adequacy uses clearance of BUN as a marker for treatment of uremia. For HD, a urea reduction ratio (predialysis BUN – postdialysis BUN/predialysis BUN) of more than 70% or a **KT/V** of more than 1.3 [where K is the clearance of the dialyzer (in mL per minute),

T is the duration of dialysis in minutes, and V is the volume of distribution of urea (in mL)] confers a survival advantage in chronic renal failure.

2. **Continuous arteriovenous hemofiltration (CAVH), continuous venovenous hemofiltration (CVVH), and continuous venovenous hemodialysis and filtration (CVVHDF).** These modalities, also known as *slow continuous ultrafiltration*, are the methods of HD used most frequently in critically ill patients with hemo-dynamic instability and volume overload. Because the patient's arterial blood pressure (BP) provides the ultrafiltration pressure, a systolic pressure of 80 mm Hg is required to support CAVH. The access for CAVH is obtained by placing a 7-French single-lumen catheter into a femoral artery and a large central vein. CVVH and CVVHDF are accomplished with a double-lumen venous cannula. The ultrafiltrate is essentially plasma, and its rate of collection may exceed 1,000 mL/hour. Clearance in CVVHDF is much higher and depends on the dialysate and replacement fluid rates.

B. **Complications of HD**

1. **Hypotension** commonly occurs with HD and may occur even without ultrafiltration. Measures to prevent it include the use of bicarbonate (rather than acetate) dialysis fluid; low-temperature (35°C) dialysate; infusion of a saline, blood, or albumin prime at the beginning of dialysis or during the dialysis run; high-sodium dialysate; or ultrafiltration without HD during the first hour.

2. **Dyspnea.** The effect of complement and adhesion molecules on circulating leukocytes and endothelium results in leukocyte pooling in the pulmonary circulation and dyspnea. Use of biocompatible cellulose acetate or synthetic membranes helps to prevent dyspnea.

3. **Bleeding** occurs secondary to dysfunctional platelets associated with uremia or the use of heparin. Bleeding can be minimized by performing dialysis with low-dose or no heparin or by preventing clotting with the use of citrate or frequent flushes with saline.

4. **Disequilibrium syndrome** is characterized by mental status deterioration associated with dialysis and is due to the rapid removal of metabolic waste products or fluid and electrolyte shifts. It may be prevented by limiting the percentage reduction in urea to 25% with the first dialysis session.

IV. **PERITONEAL DIALYSIS (PD)**

A. **Technique.** Access is gained through an intraperitoneal soft silicone (Tenckhoff) catheter (*J Am Coll Surg* 2003;196:655). Continuous ambulatory PD requires four to five exchanges of 2 to 3 L of dialysis fluid daily. The dialysis fluid is composed of dextrose at various concentrations (1.5%, 2.5%, or 4%) and electrolytes. Each exchange dwells in the peritoneum for 2 to 4 hours, with the last exchange of the day remaining overnight. A typical exchange takes 20 to 40 minutes. Some patients are able to perform continuous cycler–assisted PD. This form of PD uses a machine to warm, infuse, and drain 10 to 16 L of dialysis fluid overnight while the patient sleeps. For PD, a weekly total KT/V of 2/week and total creatinine clearance of 60 L/week/1.73 m^2 is considered minimally adequate dialysis. Acute PD is used when acute HD cannot be performed, most often owing to hemodynamic instability.

B. **Complications of PD**

1. **Peritonitis.** Despite improvements in equipment and techniques (e.g., Y-system, bagless system, and ultraviolet light box disinfectant bag spiker), one third of patients on PD develop peritonitis each year. The diagnosis is suggested by fever, abdominal pain, cloudy dialysate, more than 100 polymorphonuclear cells per milliliter of PD fluid, bacteremia, or a positive peritoneal fluid Gram stain or culture. The infection is usually caused by Gram-positive organisms. Less frequent causes include Gram-negative bacteria, yeast, and mycobacteria or atypical mycobacteria. Treatment usually is empiric, with antibiotics added to the dialysate or given intravenously. Fungal peritonitis and pseudomonal peritonitis are difficult to eradicate and often require removal of the PD catheter.

2. **Access.** Catheter malposition, obstruction, leakage, and (rarely) bowel perforation are complications associated with PD catheters. Exit-site infections occur

commonly and can often be treated locally. A tunnel infection is more difficult to eradicate and often leads to peritonitis.

3. **Obesity.** Dextrose is the osmotic agent used in PD and provides 200 to 500 calories per exchange. With normal serum glucose, 80% of the dextrose is absorbed. This caloric intake must be considered relative to the patient's needs.

4. **Membrane failure** occurs eventually and more frequently after episodes of peritonitis. After 1 year, only one half of the patients who start PD are able to remain on it.

5. **Other.** Abdominal wall hernias, low back pain, and protein loss are also potential complications of PD.

 KIDNEY TRANSPLANTATION

I. **INDICATIONS** for renal transplantation include the presence of ESRD with an irreversible glomerular filtration rate of less than 20 mL/minute. Excellent short- and long-term results can be achieved regardless of the cause of renal failure (Table 23-2). Renal failure secondary to diabetes mellitus, once thought to be a contraindication to transplantation, is now the most common disease process in the United States requiring renal transplantation, comprising as many as 25% of all cases.

II. **CONTRAINDICATIONS.** Although the indications for transplantation are broad, some conditions must be considered contraindications.

A. **Recent or metastatic malignancy.** In general, most transplantation centers require a significant (2- to 5-year) disease-free interval after the treatment of a malignant tumor. Exceptions include early-stage skin cancers and *in situ* cancers.

B. **Chronic infection.** The presence of any active, life-threatening infection precludes transplantation and the use of immunosuppressive therapy. If the infection can be treated either medically or surgically, the patient should be reconsidered for transplantation after therapy. Infection with the human immunodeficiency virus (HIV) is a contraindication to renal transplantation at most centers.

C. **Severe extrarenal disease** may preclude transplantation in certain circumstances, either because the patient is not an operative candidate or because the transplantation and associated immunosuppression may accelerate disease progression (i.e., chronic liver disease, chronic lung disease, and advanced uncorrectable heart disease). Severe peripheral vascular disease may also be a contraindication.

D. **Noncompliance.** Any patient with a history of repeated noncompliance with medical therapy should be considered high risk. A period of compliance before being placed on the waiting list is generally advised.

E. **Psychiatric illness.** Organic mental syndromes, psychosis, and mental retardation that impairs the patient's capacity to understand the transplantation procedure and its complications are contraindications to transplantation. Patients with alcohol or

TABLE 23-2	Causes of Renal Failure Requiring Transplantation
Type	Characteristics
Congenital	Aplasia, obstructive uropathy
Hereditary	Alport syndrome (hereditary nephritis), polycystic kidney disease, tuberous sclerosis
Neoplastic	Renal cell carcinoma, Wilms tumor
Progressive	Diabetic neuropathy, chronic pyelonephritis, Goodpasture syndrome (anti–glomerular basement membrane disease), hypertension, chronic glomerulonephritis, lupus nephritis, nephrotic syndrome, obstructive uropathy, scleroderma, amyloidosis
Traumatic	Vascular occlusion, parenchymal destruction

TABLE 23-3	Pretransplantation Evaluation of Renal Transplant Recipients

Initial workup
  History and physical examination
  Laboratory analyses: complete blood count; partial thromboplastin time; prothrombin time;
    serum electrolytes; total protein, albumin, cholesterol, glucose, calcium magnesium, and
    phosphorus; liver function tests; intact parathyroid hormone; prostate-specific antigen (men
    >40 yr); viral serologies (herpes simplex virus; Epstein-Barr virus; varicella-zoster virus;
    cytomegalovirus; hepatitis A, B, C; and human immunodeficiency virus); urinalysis and
    culture; purified protein derivative; panel reactive antibody; ABO and human leukocyte
    antigen typing; serum for frozen storage
  Electrocardiography
  Chest x-ray
Routine examinations
  Dental
  Stool guaiac (Hemoccult)
  Pap smear
  Mammogram (women >35 yr)
  Ophthalmologic (diabetic patients)
  Psychosocial
Secondary workup (based on preliminary finding)
  Cardiac: exercise stress electrocardiography, dobutamine stress echocardiography, coronary
    angiography
  Pulmonary: arterial blood gas, pulmonary function tests
  Gastrointestinal tract: upper and lower endoscopy, right upper quadrant ultrasonography
  Genitourinary: voiding cystourethrography, cystoscopy, retrograde ureterography

other drug addiction must enter and successfully complete a rehabilitation program before being offered transplantation.

III. PREOPERATIVE WORKUP AND EVALUATION. Patients referred to a transplantation center are seen by a transplantation surgeon, nephrologist, social worker, and transplantation coordinator. Evaluation of a potential recipient is outlined in Table 23-3. The evaluation identifies coexisting problems or disease entities that must be addressed to improve the outcome of the transplantation. Family history is important because it may provide information about the patient's kidney disease and allows a discussion about potential living donors. When the evaluation is complete, the patient is presented at a multidisciplinary evaluation committee meeting, where a decision is made as to whether to accept the patient as a potential recipient. Allocation of a given organ to a specific patient is done using a computer-generated algorithm run by the United Network for Organ Sharing (UNOS) and is based on specific criteria, which are different for each organ [e.g., blood type, HLA matching, waiting time, prior sensitization (i.e., high panel reactive antibodies [PRA] rating), and medical urgency for kidney allocation]. Once a patient is active on the waiting list, blood is sent monthly to the tissue-typing laboratory for cross-matching and to determine the PRA.

The **PRA (panel reactive antibodies)** helps to predict the likelihood that a patient will have a positive cross-match. It is determined by testing the potential recipient's serum against a panel of cells of various HLA specificities in a manner similar to the cross-match. The percentage of specificities in the panel with which the patient's sera react is the PRA. Most normal individuals do not have preformed anti-HLA antibodies and thus have a low PRA (0% to 5%). Patients who have been exposed to other HLAs through blood transfusions, previous transplantations, or pregnancies or who have autoimmune diseases with antibodies recognizing HLAs may have a high PRA. These patients are more likely to have a positive cross-match.

A. Special considerations. The lower urinary tract should be sterile, continent, and compliant before transplantation. In patients with a history of bladder dysfunction, diabetes mellitus, and recurrent urinary tract infections, a voiding cystourethrogram may be obtained before transplantation. Transplant ureter implantation into the native bladder is preferred and usually can be achieved, even in small bladders and those that have been diverted previously.

B. **Pretransplantation native nephrectomy** has been avoided secondary to the anemia that develops following removal of the kidneys and their endogenous erythropoietin production. It is only performed in patients with chronic renal parenchymal infection, infected renal calculi, heavy proteinuria, intractable hypertension, massive polycystic kidney disease with pain or bleeding, renal cystic disease that is suspicious for carcinoma, and infected reflux nephropathy. Erythropoietin renders pretransplantation nephrectomy more acceptable, especially in patients with intractable hypertension whose posttransplantation management can be difficult without nephrectomy.

C. **Living donors.** Living kidney donation has become an important part of renal transplant practice. Parent–child or sibling combinations are the most common, although biologically unrelated donors are increasingly being used. Advantages of living-donor transplantation include improved short- and long-term graft survival (1-year survival >95%), improved immediate allograft function, planned operative timing to allow for optimization of the recipient's medical condition (and, in many cases, avoidance of dialysis), fewer rejection and infection episodes, and shorter hospital stays. Although expanded-criteria deceased donors (who tend to be older) have increased the donor pool, a living donor, if available, is preferred to a deceased donor.

The primary goal in evaluating a potential living donor is to ensure the donor's well-being and safety. The donor must be in excellent health and must not have any illnesses, such as hypertension or diabetes, that may threaten his or her renal function in the future. The donor anatomy is evaluated preoperatively with arteriography or CT/magnetic resonance (MR) angiography. Donor kidneys are now commonly removed using laparoscopic or mininephrectomy techniques to minimize donor morbidity.

IV. **PREOPERATIVE CONSIDERATIONS.** When a kidney becomes available, the recipient is admitted to the hospital, and the surgeon, nephrologist, and anesthesiologist perform a final preoperative evaluation. Routine laboratory studies and a final cross-match are performed. The need for preoperative dialysis depends on the patient's volume status and serum potassium. Generally, a patient with evidence of volume overload or a serum potassium greater than 5.6 mEq/L (5.6 mmol/L) requires preoperative hemodialysis. Induction therapy with a polyclonal antibody preparation is begun intraoperatively.

V. **OPERATIVE CONSIDERATIONS**

A. **Technique.** In the operating room, a Foley catheter is inserted, and the patient's bladder is irrigated with antibiotic-containing solution. A central venous pressure (CVP) line is inserted, and a first-generation cephalosporin is administered. The renal vein and artery typically are anastomosed to the external iliac vein and artery, respectively. A heparin bolus of 3,000 units is administered before venous clamping. Before reperfusion of the kidney, mannitol (25 g) and furosemide (100 mg) are administered intravenously, and the patient's systolic BP is maintained above 120 mm Hg, with a CVP of at least 10 mm Hg to ensure optimal perfusion of the transplanted kidney. The ureter can be anastomosed to either the recipient bladder or the ipsilateral ureter, although the bladder is the preferred location. Establishing an antireflux mechanism is essential for preventing posttransplantation reflux pyelonephritis. This is accomplished by performing an extravesical ureteroneocystostomy (Litch).

B. **Intraoperative fluid management.** The newly transplanted kidney is sensitive to volume contraction, and adequate perfusion is essential for immediate postoperative diuresis and acute tubular necrosis (ATN) prevention. Volume contraction should not occur, and volume status is constantly monitored by checking the patient's cardiac function, CVP, and BP. The initial posttransplantation urine outputs can vary dramatically based on many factors. It is imperative to know the patient's native urine volume to assess the contribution of the native and the transplanted kidney to posttransplantation urine output. Dopamine may be administered at a level of 2 to 5 μg/kg/minute intravenously to promote renal blood flow and support systemic blood pressure.

VI. POSTOPERATIVE CONSIDERATIONS

A. General care. Many aspects of postoperative care are the same as those for any other general surgical patient. Early ambulation is encouraged, and the need for good pulmonary toilet and wound care is the same. Due to immunosuppression, sutures and skin staples are left in place for 2 to 3 weeks to allow for slower wound healing. The bladder catheter is left in place for 3 to 7 days. Meperidine is avoided because its metabolites are excreted renally and can rise to toxic levels in the patient whose allograft is not functioning immediately after transplantation.

B. Intravenous fluid replacement. In general, the patient should be kept euvolemic or mildly hypervolemic in the early posttransplantation period. Hourly urine output is replaced with one-half normal saline on a milliliter-for-milliliter basis because the sodium concentration of the urine from a newly transplanted kidney is 60 to 80 mEq/L (60 to 80 mmol/L). Insensible fluid losses during this period typically are 30 to 60 mL/hour and essentially are losses of water that can be replaced by a solution of 5% dextrose in 0.45% normal saline at 30 mL/hour. Therefore, during the early posttransplantation period, the patient's intravenous fluid consists of one-half normal saline administered at a rate equal to the previous hour's urine output plus 30 mL of 5% dextrose in 0.45% normal saline. This formula requires the patient's volume status to be assessed repeatedly. If the posttransplantation urine output is low and the patient is thought to be hypovolemic (based on clinical and hemodynamic evaluation), isotonic saline boluses are given. Potassium chloride replacement usually is not required unless the urine output is very high, and even then it should be given with great care. Potassium chloride especially should be avoided in the oliguric posttransplantation patient.

C. Gastrointestinal (GI) tract. Gastritis and peptic ulcer disease occur secondary to steroid therapy in the transplantation patient. Therefore, patients are prophylactically treated with famotidine (20 mg/day orally or intravenously) or lansoprazole (30 mg/day orally).

D. Renal allograft function or nonfunction. If the patient's urine output is low in the early postoperative period (<50 mL/hour), volume status must be addressed first. If the patient is hypovolemic, 250 to 500 mL of isotonic saline should be given in bolus fashion and repeated once, if needed. If the patient is euvolemic, the bladder catheter should be irrigated to ensure patency. If clots are encountered, a larger catheter and/or continuous bladder irrigation may be needed. If the catheter is patent and the patient is euvolemic or hypervolemic, furosemide (100 to 200 mg intravenously for recipients of deceased-donor transplants, 20 to 40 mg intravenously for those with living-donor transplants) should be given. If diuresis follows these maneuvers, urine output is again replaced milliliter for milliliter with one-half normal saline. Early nonfunction of a transplanted kidney is most commonly due to reversible ATN. Ischemia of the kidney is the most frequent cause; it is due to hypotension in the donor, warm ischemia during procurement, prolonged cold ischemia, or excessive warm ischemia during the transplantation procedure. Immunologic injury and reperfusion injury also may play some role in the mechanism of injury leading to ATN. Before the diagnosis of ATN can be made, however, noninvasive studies (renal Doppler ultrasonography or technetium-99m renal scan) demonstrating vascular patency and good renal blood flow in the absence of hydronephrosis (renal ultrasonography) or urinary leak must be obtained. If flow is confirmed, dialysis can be continued until the transplanted kidney recovers.

E. Immunosuppression. A variety of immunosuppressive protocols exist. The protocol in use at Washington University is outlined here. Induction therapy with Thymoglobulin (2 mg/kg intravenously) is given intraoperatively and then daily during the first 2 posttransplantation days. On posttransplantation days 1 to 30, patients receive cyclosporine (4 mg/kg orally twice a day) to maintain a trough level of 250 to 300 ng/mL (FPIA) or tacrolimus (0.05 mg/kg orally twice a day);

azathioprine (2.5 mg/kg orally per day) or mycophenolate mofetil (1,000 mg orally twice a day for 5 days, reduced to 500 mg orally twice a day thereafter); and prednisone (1 mg/kg orally per day for days 1 to 3, 0.5 mg/kg orally per day for days 4 to 14, then 25 mg orally per day, decreasing by 2.5 to 5 mg each week to a goal of 5 mg/day by week 13). Methylprednisolone (7 mg/kg intravenously) is given in the operating room.

VII. REJECTION. There are several different types of rejection; some are preventable, whereas others can be treated with varying degrees of success.

A. Hyperacute rejection occurs when preformed anti-HLA antibodies bind the endothelium of the allograft and initiate a cascade of events culminating in vascular thrombosis and ischemic necrosis of the graft. Hyperacute rejection usually can be prevented by cross-matching donor lymphocytes with recipient serum. Hyperacute rejection usually occurs within minutes of cross-clamp release and is irreversible. Viability of the allograft can be assessed by intraoperative biopsy. The only therapeutic option is to remove the allograft immediately.

B. Accelerated rejection also appears to be antibody-mediated and usually occurs 12 to 72 hours after transplantation. The patient usually is anuric or oliguric and has fever and graft tenderness. Although treatment for this form of rejection is not well defined, administration of an antilymphocyte preparation may salvage the graft. Accelerated rejection can lead to an immunologically mediated ATN from which good renal function recovery can occur.

C. Acute rejection is cell mediated and involves T lymphocytes and soluble mediators called lymphokines. It happens in 10% to 40% of patients and typically occurs 1 to 6 weeks after transplantation. The development of a rising creatinine level should prompt the consideration of rejection. Technetium-99m renal scan demonstrates decreased but persistent perfusion. Diagnosis is confirmed by percutaneous needle biopsy. There are two basic treatment modalities (Table 23-4): high-dose methylprednisolone and an antilymphocyte preparation. The latter generally is reserved for steroid-resistant rejection, although antilymphocyte therapy may be used as first-line therapy for moderate or severe rejections with

TABLE 23-4	Treatment of Rejection

Corticosteroids
  Intravenous pulse, methylprednisolone
    7 mg/kg QD for 3 days
Consider if rejection is early (<3 mo) or mild
  Oral pulse, prednisone
    3 mg/kg QD in 2–4 divided doses for 3–5 d
    After pulse, restart steroids at previous dose
    Use if patient is reliable and rejection is early or mild
Tacrolimus
Target 12-hr trough level 5–15 ng/mL
Antilymphocyte preparations
  Thymoglobulin
  2–3 mg/kg IV for 3–4 d
Mycophenolate mofetil
  1,000 mg PO BID
Rapamycin
  4 mg PO QD, target level 8–20 ng/mL
Plasmapheresis
  Consider for antibody-mediated rejection

BID, twice a day; IV, intravenously; PO, orally; QD, daily.

arteritis. Maintenance immunosuppression may also be switched (i.e., from cyclosporine to tacrolimus). More than 90% of acute rejection episodes can be treated successfully.

D. Chronic rejection is a poorly understood phenomenon that can occur weeks to years after transplantation. Emerging evidence suggests that in addition to calcineurin toxicity, the humoral immune response is an important contributor to chronic rejection. Detection of anti–donor specific antibodies, an elevated posttransplant PRA, or C4d staining on a biopsy are supportive of humoral or antibody-mediated rejection. Plasmapheresis, intravenous immunoglobulin, and rituximab and anti-CD20 antibody have been used to treat antibody-mediated rejection.

VIII. SURGICAL COMPLICATIONS OF RENAL TRANSPLANTATION. Wound seromas, hematomas, and infections are treated according to usual surgical principles. Other complications require special consideration.

A. Lymphoceles are collections of lymph that occur because of lymphatic leaks in the retroperitoneum. They present 1 week to several weeks after transplantation and are best diagnosed by ultrasonography. Most are asymptomatic and are found incidentally. They may produce ureteral obstruction, deep venous thrombosis, leg swelling, or incontinence secondary to bladder compression. Most lymphoceles arise from leakage of lymph from the donor kidney. Treatment of symptomatic lymphoceles consists of percutaneous drainage. Open or laparoscopic internal drainage by marsupialization into the peritoneal cavity may be necessary because repeated percutaneous drainage is not advised and seldom leads to resolution of the lymphocele.

B. Renal artery and vein thrombosis. Arterial and venous thromboses most often occur in the first 1 to 3 days after transplantation. If the kidney had been functioning but a sudden cessation of urine output occurs, graft thrombosis should be suspected. A rapid rise in serum creatinine, graft swelling, and local pain ensue. If the allograft had not been functioning or if the native kidneys make a large amount of urine, there may be no signs of graft thrombosis. The transplanted kidney has no collateral circulation and has minimal tolerance for warm ischemia. The diagnosis is made by technetium-99m renal scan or Doppler ultrasonography. Unless the problem is diagnosed quickly and repair performed immediately, the graft will be lost, and transplantation nephrectomy will be required.

C. Urine leak. The etiology is usually anastomotic leak or ureteral sloughing secondary to ureteral blood supply disruption. Urine leaks present with pain, rising creatinine, and possibly urine draining from the wound. Diagnosis is made by locating the fluid collection with ultrasonography and then aspirating the fluid and comparing its creatinine level to the serum creatinine level. A renal scan demonstrates radioisotope outside the urinary tract. Urine leaks are treated by placing a bladder catheter to reduce intravesical pressure and subsequent surgical exploration. If an anastomotic leak is found, the distal ureter can be resected and reimplanted. If the transplantation ureter is nonviable or of inadequate length, ureteroureterostomy over a double-J stent using the ipsilateral native ureter can be performed. The stent can be removed via cystoscopy several weeks later.

IX. LONG-TERM FOLLOW-UP. Immunosuppression (Table 23-5) and infection prophylaxis (Table 23-1) should be tapered with time. After the initial 3-month period, when acute rejection becomes less of a risk, cyclosporine or tacrolimus and steroid doses are tapered. Chronic long-term immunosuppression can be maintained at lower levels than those required for induction. However, immunosuppression can almost never be discontinued completely. Specific metabolic consequences of cyclosporine administration include hypertension, nephrotoxicity, hypercholesterolemia, and hyperuricemia. Gradual dose reduction can be helpful, but often specific therapy is needed to correct these side effects. Weight gain is the predominant side effect of steroid therapy. Dietary manipulation and gradual dose reduction are important. Long-term complications of steroids include joint deterioration with avascular necrosis, osteoporosis, cataract formation, and diabetes mellitus (10% of patients). The incidence of these problems can be minimized by using as low a dose of prednisone as possible. Antibiotic prophylaxis should be used before any surgical or dental procedure.

TABLE 23-5	Long-Term Maintenance Immunosuppression for Renal Transplantation

Mycophenolate mofetil
  1,000 mg PO BID
  Reduce to 500 mg PO BID when used with tacrolimus and for WBC <5,000/mm^3, diarrhea,
    first week posttransplant

Prednisone
  1 mg/kg QD for days 1–3
  20 mg QD for days 4–14
  15 mg QD for week 3
  10 mg QD for week 4
  5 mg QD for week 5 and onward

Tacrolimus
  5 mg PO BID, target level 5–10 ng/mL (FPIA)
  Levels >15 ng/mL are considered toxic

Cyclosporine
  8 mg/kg QD for first month, 12-hr level 200–300 ng/mL, 2-hr level 800–1,200 ng/mL (FPIA)
  Adjust dose for months 2–3, 12-hour level 100–200 ng/mL, 2-hr level 600–1,000 ng/mL
  >3 mo, 12-hr level 75–150 ng/mL, 2-hr level 400–600 ng/mL
  Trough levels >300 ng/mL are considered toxic; peak (2-hr) levels may be more relevant than
    trough levels

BID, twice daily; FPIA fluorescence polarization immunoassay;
PO, orally; WBC, white blood cell count; QD, daily.

LIVER TRANSPLANTATION

I. INDICATIONS FOR HEPATIC TRANSPLANTATION are complications attributable to end-stage liver disease (ESLD). In the absence of other medical contraindications, virtually any disease resulting in ESLD is amenable to transplantation. The most common diseases for which orthotopic liver transplantation (OLT) is performed are listed in Table 23-6. Common indications for OLT in patients with ESLD include variceal hemorrhage, intractable ascites, encephalopathy, intractable pruritus, and poor synthetic function. Stage I or II hepatocellular carcinoma in a cirrhotic liver is an increasingly common indication for transplantation. Single lesions less than 5 cm or three lesions less than 3 cm may be treated in this way. Experimental protocols for patients with cholangiocarcinoma are also being evaluated (*Surgery* 2006;140:331).

TABLE 23-6	Most Common Indications for Orthotopic Liver Transplantation

Adults
  Chronic hepatitis C
  Alcoholic liver disease
  Chronic hepatitis B
  Primary biliary cirrhosis
  Primary sclerosing cholangitis
  Autoimmune hepatitis

Children
  Extrahepatic biliary atresia
  α-1-Antitrypsin deficiency

II. **CONTRAINDICATIONS.** There are a few absolute contraindications to liver transplantation: multisystem organ failure, extrahepatic malignancy, poor cardiac or pulmonary reserve, refractory pulmonary artery hypertension, severe infection, and ongoing substance abuse. Renal insufficiency, either chronic or acute, increases the morbidity of hepatic transplantation but is not a contraindication. Renal transplantation can be performed at the time of liver transplantation for patients with ESRD. Some degree of preoperative renal insufficiency is often reversible after successful liver transplantation.

III. **PREOPERATIVE EVALUATION.** Referrals to transplantation centers are made on an elective or urgent basis. The evaluation determines the need and urgency for OLT as well as its technical feasibility.

A. **Elective transplantation.** Under elective conditions, the potential candidate is presented to a multidisciplinary committee for evaluation. The patient's evaluation is based on history, physical examination, laboratory evaluation, results of endoscopic procedures, cardiac and pulmonary evaluation, and radiologic examination (Table 23-7). Active infection should be treated promptly, and transplantation should be postponed until the infection resolves. Patients with a recent history of alcohol or other substance abuse should also be evaluated by a specialist prior to transplantation.

B. **Urgent transplantation.** Acceptable results with OLT also can be achieved in selected patients with fulminant liver failure. The pretransplantation evaluation is performed in a manner similar to that outlined for the elective patient; however, timing, neurologic status, and hemodynamic stability may limit the number of tests obtained.

A careful neurologic examination must be done in this setting, and the grade of coma should be determined. Patients in grade IV (unresponsive) coma have been shown in some studies to benefit from continuous perioperative monitoring of intracranial pressure (ICP) because untreated severe elevations in ICP can result in permanent brain injury and death. An attempt is made to keep cerebral perfusion pressure (mean arterial BP minus ICP) above 60 mm Hg. Low mean arterial BP is treated with vasopressors after volume resuscitation. Elevation in ICP is treated with hyperventilation, mannitol, and elevation of the head of the bed more than 45 degrees. ICP monitor placement may be complicated by severe coagulopathy and thrombocytopenia, which is common in these patients.

Patients with acute hepatic failure may develop ARF as well, which can require hemofiltration or HD. Sepsis also is seen in acute hepatic failure and requires broad-spectrum antibiotics and antifungals. Pulmonary insufficiency is a common accompaniment of acute liver failure and may require intubation, high-concentration oxygen, and positive end-expiratory pressure.

IV. **ORGAN ALLOCATION.** Livers are allocated based on the **Model for End-Stage Liver Disease (MELD)** scoring system. The MELD score is derived from the values for bilirubin, serum creatinine, and the international normalized ratio (INR) and ranges from 6 to 40 (http://www.unos.org). Livers are allocated to appropriate patients with the highest MELD scores. Special exception points may be granted, such as in cases of hepatocellular carcinoma. Children are graded based on the Pediatric End-Stage Liver Disease (PELD) score.

V. **DONOR SELECTION.** Selection of an appropriate donor liver takes into account donor size, ABO blood type, age, presence of infection, history of malignancy, liver function studies, hospital course, hemodynamic stability, and prior alcohol or drug use. Absolute contraindications to the use of a donor liver include the presence of extrahepatic malignancy and HIV. The use of expanded donor criteria allows transplantation of organs from older patients, patients with steatotic livers, and patients with positive hepatitis B or C serologies.

VI. **HEPATIC TRANSPLANTATION PROCEDURE**

A. **Whole-organ liver transplantation.** Conceptually, transplantation of the liver can be thought of as comprising three distinct sequential phases. The **first phase** involves the dissection and removal of the recipient's diseased liver. The **second phase,** known as the **anhepatic phase,** refers to the period starting with devascularization of the recipient's liver and ending with revascularization of the newly implanted

TABLE 23-7	Pretransplantation Evaluation of Liver Transplant Recipients

Initial workup

History
   Etiology of liver disease
   Duration of liver disease
   Complications of liver disease
   Previous surgical procedures
   Additional medical problems
   Access to transplant center
   Social support

Physical examination
   Stigmata of chronic liver disease
   Jaundice
   Fluid retention
   Nutritional status
   Abdominal mass
   Asterixis or encephalopathy
   Growth and development (pediatric patients)

Laboratory analysis
   ABO blood type; complete blood count; prothrombin time; partial thromboplastin time; serum electrolytes; urinary electrolytes; total protein, albumin, calcium, magnesium, and phosphorus; total and direct bilirubin; aspartate aminotransferase; alanine aminotransferase; alkaline phosphatase; γ-glutamyl transpeptidase; cholesterol serum ammonia; viral serologies (human immunodeficiency virus; hepatitis A, B, and C; cytomegalovirus; Epstein-Barr virus; and herpes simplex virus); urinalysis and culture; cell count; and culture of ascitic fluid and purified protein derivative

Electrocardiogram

Chest x-ray

Arterial blood gas

Dobutamine stress echocardiography

Pulmonary function tests

Computed tomography or magnetic resonance imaging scan of the abdomen with liver volume

Esophagogastroduodenoscopy

Doppler ultrasonography

Psychosocial evaluation

Optional examinations
   Computed tomography scan of chest and bone scan for patient with malignancy
   Visceral angiogram
   Cardiac catheterization
   Endoscopic retrograde cholangiogram or percutaneous transhepatic cholangiography with brush biopsy for patients with sclerosing cholangitis (10% coincidence of cholangiocarcinoma in these patients)
   Colonoscopy for patients with inflammatory bowel disease, sclerosing cholangitis, Hemoccult-positive stools, family history of colon cancer, previous history of colonic polyps

liver. During the anhepatic phase, venovenous bypass (VVB) may be used. VVB shunts blood from the portal vein and infrahepatic inferior vena cava (IVC) to the axillary, subclavian, or jugular veins. Maintenance of venous return from the kidneys and lower extremities during the anhepatic phase results in a smoother hemodynamic course, allows time for a more deliberate approach to hemostasis, reduces visceral edema and splanchnic venous pooling, and lowers the incidence of postoperative renal dysfunction. The liver allograft is implanted by anastomosing first the suprahepatic vena cava and then the infrahepatic IVC. The portal vein anastomosis is performed, and blood flow to the liver is re-established. Finally, the hepatic arterial anastomosis is performed. If the recipient hepatic artery is not suitable for anastomosis, a donor iliac arterial graft can be used as a conduit from the infra- or suprarenal aorta. The **third phase** includes biliary reconstruction and abdominal closure. Biliary continuity is established via a duct-to-duct anastomosis over a T tube or a choledochojejunostomy. A duct-to-duct anastomosis is preferable, but it may not be possible when there is a donor–recipient bile duct size discrepancy or a diseased recipient bile duct (e.g., with primary sclerosing cholangitis, biliary atresia, and secondary biliary cirrhosis).

In a modification of the foregoing technique, the recipient's retrohepatic IVC is preserved, and the donor suprahepatic IVC is anastomosed to the confluence of the recipient's right, middle, and left hepatic veins. The donor infrahepatic IVC is then oversewn. A temporary end-to-side portacaval shunt is also created at the beginning of the hepatectomy. This technique has all the advantages of VVB without its associated risks and costs.

B. Reduced and split-liver transplantation was developed to support the needs of pediatric patients awaiting appropriately sized transplants. Benefits include the ability to better match the size of the donor liver to the recipient and the option of using a single liver to provide grafts for multiple patients. These benefits have translated to the adult population as well. The liver has a remarkable capacity for regeneration. It can be divided based on the anatomic segments of Couinaud into a left lateral section (segments 2 and 3), a left lobe graft (segments 2 to 4), or a right lobe graft (segments 5 to 8). The left lateral section is most commonly used in children. Comparison of the size of the donor and the recipient is used to determine the appropriate-sized graft. Yersiz and colleagues demonstrated that children receiving a left lateral segment have similar survival outcomes and morbidity to pediatric recipients of similar live donor or whole-organ grafts (*Ann Surg* 2003;238:496).

C. Living-donor liver transplantation has been developed as a result of the success of reduced liver transplantation. The left lateral section or left lobe of the liver is usually used as the donor graft for adult-to-child transplantation. Advantages similar to those observed with living related kidney donors have also been observed, such as reduced ischemic time and the inherent benefits of an elective operation. Adult-to-adult living-donor liver transplantation necessitates the use of the larger right hepatic lobe. An amount of liver approximately equal to 0.1% of patient weight (e.g., 700 g for a 70-kg recipient) is required.

VII. POSTOPERATIVE CARE

A. Hemodynamic. Intravascular volume resuscitation usually is required in the immediate postoperative period secondary to third-space losses, increased body temperature, and vasodilatation. Adequate perfusion is assessed by left and right heart filling pressures, cardiac output, urine output, and the absence of metabolic acidosis. Hypertension is common and should be aggressively treated.

B. Pulmonary. Ventilatory support is required postoperatively until the patient is awake and alert, is able to follow commands and protect the airway, and is able to maintain adequate oxygenation and ventilation.

C. Hepatic allograft function. Monitoring of hepatic allograft function begins intraoperatively after revascularization. Signs of satisfactory graft function include hemodynamic stability and normalization of acid-base status, body temperature, coagulation studies, maintenance of glucose metabolism, and bile production. Reassessment of hepatic allograft function continues postoperatively, initially occurring every 12 hours. Satisfactory hepatic allograft function is indicated by an improving coagulation profile, decreasing transaminase levels, normal blood glucose, hemodynamic stability, adequate urine output, bile production, and clearance of anesthesia. Early elevations of bilirubin and transaminase levels may be indicators of preservation injury. The peak levels of serum glutamic-oxaloacetic transaminase and serum glutamate pyruvate transaminase usually are less than 2,000 units/L and should decrease rapidly over the first 24 to 48 hours postoperatively. After the patient leaves the intensive care unit, liver function tests are obtained daily. Bile is inspected daily; a T-tube cholangiogram may be obtained to ensure adequate biliary drainage and to rule out extravasation. If hepatic dysfunction becomes evident at any time, prompt evaluation must be undertaken and treatment must be initiated. It is important to correctly diagnose the cause of liver dysfunction because each cause has its own unique treatment.

1. **Primary nonfunction and initial poor function.** The use of modern organ preservation solutions for organ preservation has decreased the incidence of primary nonfunction. For poorly understood reasons, however, 1% to 3% of transplanted livers fail immediately after the surgery. Primary nonfunction is characterized by hemodynamic instability, poor quantity and quality of bile, renal dysfunction, failure to regain consciousness, increasing coagulopathy, persistent hypothermia, and lactic acidosis in the face of patent vascular anastomosis (as demonstrated by Doppler ultrasonography). Without retransplantation, death ensues.

2. **Rejection.** Acute rejection is relatively common after liver transplantation, with 60% of recipients experiencing at least one cell-mediated or acute rejection episode. However, rejection is an extremely uncommon cause of graft loss. The most common causes of early graft loss include primary nonfunction and hepatic artery thrombosis.

3. **Technical complications.** A variety of technical problems can lead to liver allograft dysfunction, including hepatic artery stenosis or thrombosis, portal vein stenosis or thrombosis, biliary tract obstruction, bile duct leak, and hepatic vein or vena caval thrombosis. **Hepatic artery thrombosis** that occurs in the early posttransplantation period may lead to fever, hemodynamic instability, and rapid deterioration of the patient, with a marked elevation of the transaminases. An associated bile leak may be noted soon after liver transplantation due to the loss of the bile ducts' main vascular supply. Acute hepatic artery thrombosis may be treated by attempted thrombectomy. If this is unsuccessful, retransplantation is needed. Hepatic artery thrombosis that occurs long after liver transplantation may produce intra- and extrahepatic bile duct strictures and may be an indication for elective retransplantation. Occasionally, hepatic artery thrombosis is completely asymptomatic.

   Portal vein stenosis or thrombosis is rare. When it occurs, the patient's condition may deteriorate rapidly, with profound hepatic dysfunction, massive ascites, renal failure, and hemodynamic instability. Although surgical thrombectomy may be successful, urgent retransplantation is often necessary. Late portal vein thrombosis may allow normal liver function but usually results in variceal bleeding and ascites.

   Bile duct obstruction is diagnosed by cholangiography. A single short bile duct stricture may be treated by either percutaneous or retrograde balloon dilation. A long stricture, ampullary dysfunction, or failed dilation necessitates revision of the biliary tract anastomosis. Fever and abdominal pain in the early posttransplantation period should raise the possibility of biliary anastomotic disruption, which requires urgent surgical revision.

4. **Recurrent infection and neoplasm.** CMV can cause hepatic allograft dysfunction and usually occurs within 8 weeks of transplantation. Diagnosis is made by liver biopsy, with CMV inclusion bodies being found with light microscopy or by PCR in peripheral blood. Treatment consists of decreasing baseline immunosuppression and administering ganciclovir (5 mg/kg every 12 hours via central venous access for 3 weeks).

   Viral hepatitis and malignancy (e.g., hepatoma, cholangiocarcinoma, neuroendocrine tumors) can recur in the hepatic allograft but are uncommon in the early posttransplantation period. The clinical presentation includes elevations on liver function tests. The diagnosis is made by liver biopsy. Imaging studies (e.g., CT scan, liver ultrasonography) are important for following patients transplanted for neoplasms. Patients transplanted for hepatocellular carcinoma also should have surveillance with CT scan and tumor markers at regular intervals.

D. Electrolytes and glucose. The use of diuretics may result in hypokalemia, whereas cyclosporine or tacrolimus toxicity may cause hyperkalemia. Magnesium levels are maintained above 2 mg/dL (0.82 mmol/L) because the seizure threshold is lowered by the combination of hypomagnesemia and cyclosporine or tacrolimus. Calcium should be measured as free ionized calcium and kept above 4.4 mg/dL (1.1 mmol/L). Phosphorus levels should be maintained above 2.5 mg/dL (0.81 mmol/L) to avoid respiratory muscle weakness and altered oxygen hemoglobin dissociation. Glucose homeostasis is necessary because steroid administration may result in hyperglycemia, which is best managed with intravenous insulin because it is short acting and easily absorbed. Cyclosporine and tacrolimus are diabetogenic immunosuppressants and may alter glucose homeostasis. Hypoglycemia is a complication of liver failure, and in the presence of liver dysfunction, glucose administration may be necessary.

E. GI tract. H_2 blockade, proton-pump inhibition, and/or antacids are used to prevent stress ulcers. Endoscopy is performed liberally for any GI bleeding to determine the etiology. Nystatin and GI tract decontamination solution containing gentamicin and polymyxin B are used in the perioperative period to prevent esophageal candidiasis and translocation of bacterial pathogens.

F. Nutrition. Patients who are severely malnourished should be placed on nutritional supplementation as soon as stable fluid and electrolyte status and adequate graft function have been reached. Patients with adequate preoperative nutrition can be maintained on routine intravenous fluids until GI tract function returns (usually 3 to 5 days). Enteral nutrition is used as soon as the postoperative ileus resolves. Total parenteral nutrition (TPN) is indicated when the GI tract is nonfunctional.

G. Infection surveillance. The most common causes of bacterial infection after liver transplantation include line sepsis, urinary tract infection, infected ascites, cholangitis, pneumonia, biliary anastomotic leak, and intra-abdominal abscess. Prophylactic antibiotics covering biliary pathogens are administered for the first 48 hours after liver transplantation. If a fever develops in the liver transplant recipient, a thorough examination should be performed. A chest x-ray and cultures of blood, urine, indwelling lines, and bile also are necessary. A T-tube cholangiogram and Doppler ultrasonography of the liver can be performed to rule out perihepatic fluid collection and to evaluate hepatic vasculature.

Hepatitis B or C recurs in the liver allograft following transplantation. Therefore, protocols are under investigation using different combinations of hepatitis B immune globulin (IG), hepatitis B vaccines, lamivudine, retroviral agents, and monoclonal antibodies. The diagnosis is suspected if the level of liver transaminases increases, and it is confirmed by biopsy. Recurrent disease may be severe enough to lead to life-threatening hepatitis and cirrhosis. Strategies to prevent hepatitis B recurrence include the use of lamivudine before transplant to arrest viral replication and high-dose hepatitis B IG and lamivudine after transplant. Hepatitis C recurrence after transplant, although it is ubiquitous, does not commonly lead to significant problems for many years and is associated with mild transaminitis. Occasionally, hepatitis C recurrence can be early, aggressive, and severe. Antiviral therapy has been used to treat hepatitis C recurrence but with very limited success.

H. Posttransplantation immunosuppression. The immunosuppressive agents used to prevent rejection include corticosteroids and cyclosporine or tacrolimus. Mycophenolate mofetil may be added to reduce cyclosporine or tacrolimus doses in patients, which may be particularly useful in patients with renal disease or autoimmune liver disease.

VIII. REJECTION. Many liver transplant recipients experience at least one acute rejection episode, and it commonly occurs between days 4 and 21 postoperatively. Rejection is characterized by fever, increased ascites, decreased bile quality and quantity, and elevation of total white blood cell and eosinophil count, bilirubin, and transaminase levels. Liver transplant rejection is diagnosed by percutaneous liver biopsy. In the early posttransplantation period, technical causes of hepatic dysfunction are ruled out by Doppler ultrasonography to ensure vascular patency, and T-tube cholangiography is obtained to rule out a bile duct obstruction or leak. Typical biopsy findings consistent with acute rejection include the triad consisting of portal lymphocytes, endothelialitis (subendothelial deposits of mononuclear cells), and bile duct infiltration and damage. The first-line treatment for acute rejection is a bolus of corticosteroids (methylprednisolone, 1 g intravenously). If the rejection responds appropriately, the patient undergoes steroid recycling.

PANCREAS AND ISLET TRANSPLANTATION

I. **INDICATIONS.** Diabetes mellitus (DM) affects 6.3% of Americans and is the sixth-leading cause of death. It is the leading cause of renal failure and blindness in adults. Other long-term complications caused by diabetes include myocardial infarction, stroke, amputation, and neuropathy. Invasive methods for maintaining euglycemia and preventing the long-term complications of DM include the use of autoregulating insulin pumps, pancreatic islet cell transplants, and whole-organ pancreatic transplantation.

Pancreas transplantation is commonly performed in the setting of kidney transplantation (either simultaneously or afterward) for diabetes complicated by end-stage renal disease. Simple pancreas transplants are also performed. Approximately 1,800 pancreas and islet transplants are performed per year in the United States.

II. **CONTRAINDICATIONS** to pancreas transplantation are the same as those for kidney transplantation, including disabilities secondary to DM, such as peripheral gangrene, intractable cardiac decompensation, and incapacitating peripheral neuropathy. Continued tobacco use also is considered a relatively strong contraindication to pancreas transplantation.

III. **PREOPERATIVE WORKUP AND EVALUATION.** Workup of the potential pancreas transplantation patient is similar to that of the kidney recipient and identifies coexisting diseases, as outlined in Table 23-3. To allow identification of beneficial effects of pancreas transplantation on the complications of DM, a careful preoperative evaluation of the patient's neurologic and ophthalmologic status should be performed.

IV. **DONOR PANCREAS PROCUREMENT** occurs as part of a multiorgan retrieval. Contraindications to pancreas donation include the presence of diabetes, pancreatitis, trauma to the pancreas, or significant intra-abdominal contamination. Although the liver and pancreas may share blood supply, combined retrieval can be performed safely without compromising either organ. During the organ retrieval procedure, it is important to identify accessory or replaced hepatic arteries that may arise from the left gastric artery or the SMA. The abdominal viscera are flushed with UW or HTK solution, and the liver, pancreas, duodenum, and spleen are removed *en bloc* and separated under cold-storage conditions. The splenic artery is divided from the celiac, and the SMA is divided at its origin or distal to a replaced right hepatic artery, if present. The mesentery of the small intestine is either oversewn or stapled.

V. **DECEASED-DONOR PANCREAS TRANSPLANTATION OPERATION**

A. **Forms of pancreatic transplantation**

1. **Isolated pancreas transplantation.** The most widely accepted technique of pancreatic transplantation in the United States uses whole-organ pancreas with venous drainage into the systemic circulation and enteric exocrine drainage. Some centers advocate portal venous drainage.

Under cold-storage conditions, the portal vein is isolated. If it is too short to allow for a tension-free anastomosis, an extension autograft is placed using donor iliac vein. The SMA and splenic artery then are reconstructed with a donor iliac artery Y-bifurcation autograft. Only the second portion of the duodenum is retained with the pancreas. Then the portal vein is anastomosed to the iliac vein or the superior mesenteric vein, and the donor common iliac artery graft is anastomosed to the recipient's external iliac artery. The duodenal segment of the transplant is then opened, and a duodenojejunostomy is created. Alternatively, the duodenal segment can be anastomosed to the bladder. The pancreas transplant is left in the right paracolic gutter, and if kidney transplantation is to be performed, it is done on the left side.

2. **Simultaneous kidney-pancreas transplantation** may be considered in insulin-dependent diabetic patients who are dialysis dependent or imminent and have a creatinine clearance of less than 30 mL/minute. Some of the advantages of combined transplantation include the ability to monitor rejection of the pancreas by monitoring renal rejection and the fact that the patient is exposed to only one set of donor antigens.

3. **Pancreatic islet cell transplantation** is still investigational and has not received widespread acceptance. Pancreatic islet cells are isolated and injected into the portal vein for engraftment in the liver. The major problems encountered have been in obtaining enough islet cells to attain glucose homeostasis and failing to achieve long-term insulin independence. A large multicenter trial supported the proof of concept of islet transplantation (*N Engl J Med* 2006;355:1318), Although 58% of patients were able to achieve insulin independence at some time during the trial, only 31% of those achieving insulin independence and 15% of those initially enrolled were insulin independent 1 year after transplantation.

B. **Exocrine drainage**

1. **Enteric drainage.** Most programs now use enteric drainage, which avoids the acidosis, volume depletion, and urologic complications associated with bladder drainage. Enteric drainage can be performed by anastomosing the duodenal segment to small bowel in a side-to-side fashion or via a Roux-en-Y limb. Disadvantages of enteric drainage include the inability to monitor exocrine secretions and a higher rate of technical failure.

2. **Bladder drainage.** Advantages of this technique include the ability to measure urinary amylase, which can facilitate the early diagnosis of rejection. Cystoscopic transduodenal needle biopsy can also be performed in the diagnosis of rejection. The major disadvantages of bladder drainage are fluid and electrolyte disturbances (most commonly a severe metabolic acidosis) and urologic complications (including hematuria, urinary tract infections, urethral strictures, and reflux pancreatitis) caused by the drainage of fluid, bicarbonate, and enzymes into the bladder.

VI. **POSTOPERATIVE MANAGEMENT AND MONITORING**

A. **Immunosuppression** consists of quadruple therapy with antibody induction, tacrolimus, prednisone, and mycophenolate mofetil.

B. **Serum glucose** is followed during and after the transplantation. Intravenous insulin infusions are stopped within the first few hours after pancreas transplantation.

C. **Rejection** of the pancreas transplant is suggested by a rise in serum amylase or a fall in urinary amylase. Rejection of pancreas and kidney transplants usually occurs in parallel but at times may be discordant. The diagnosis of kidney rejection is suggested by a rise in creatinine, which is then confirmed by biopsy. Biopsy of the pancreas transplant is performed percutaneously or via cystoscopy. Rejection is treated with corticosteroids or antilymphocyte preparations.

D. **Graft-related complications.** Besides rejection, complications of pancreas transplantation include metabolic acidosis and dehydration. These are due to the loss of sodium and bicarbonate into the urine from the transplanted duodenum, and they are avoided with enteric drainage. Other common complications include pancreatitis, urinary tract infections, urethritis, and anastomotic leak from the duodenocystostomy. Infections with CMV also may occur.

VII. **EFFECT ON SECONDARY COMPLICATIONS OF DIABETES.** The full effect of pancreatic transplantation on secondary complications of diabetes is unknown. Pancreatic transplantation may prevent the development of diabetic nephropathy in the transplanted kidney. It also may stabilize diabetic retinopathy and improve diabetic neuropathy.

INTESTINAL TRANSPLANTATION

Intestinal failure occurs when the functioning GI tract mucosal surface area has been reduced below the minimal amount necessary for adequate digestion and absorption of food. This

TABLE 23-8	Causes of Intestinal Failure

Superior mesenteric artery thrombosis	Crohn disease
Superior mesenteric artery embolization	Trauma
Necrotizing enterocolitis	Radiation
Volvulus	Malignancy (desmoid, polyposis)
Gastroschisis	Pseudoobstruction
Intestinal atresia	

may be caused by intestinal loss or intestinal disease (Table 23-8). The development of TPN has led to the possibility of long-term survival for infants and adults with intestinal failure. However, TPN has limitations and its own associated morbidity.

I. **INDICATIONS.** Adults and children who have documented intestinal failure without the potential for long-term survival on TPN are candidates for intestinal transplantation. **Intestinal failure** is said to occur when any child younger than 1 year requires more than 50% of his or her caloric needs from TPN after neonatal small-bowel resection or when a child older than 4 years requires more than 30% of calories from TPN. Older children and adults receiving more than 50% of their nutritional requirements from TPN for more than 1 year also should be considered for intestinal transplantation. Other considerations include elevated hepatic enzymes, multiple line infections, thrombosis of two of the central veins, and frequent episodes of dehydration.

II. **DONOR INTESTINAL PROCUREMENT GENERALLY** uses multiorgan recovery techniques. The liver, stomach, duodenum, pancreas, and small intestine are removed *en bloc* and separated under cold-storage conditions. Alternatively, the intestine may be recovered alone or with the liver.

III. **INTESTINAL TRANSPLANTATION OPERATION.** Patients who receive isolated intestinal allografts have vascular anastomoses created between the donor superior mesenteric vein and the recipient portal vein and between the donor SMA and the recipient aorta. Vascular reconstruction for patients who receive combined liver-intestinal grafts parallels that for patients undergoing a standard OLT. Supra- and infrahepatic vena caval anastomoses are completed, and arterial inflow is accomplished after the portal vein anastomosis by using a patch of aorta that contains the SMA and celiac.

IV. **POSTOPERATIVE MANAGEMENT**
   A. **Immunosuppression and infectious prophylaxis.** Posttransplantation immunosuppressive protocols have varied greatly over the last decade, and a universally accepted standard protocol does not exist. Recent studies have demonstrated encouraging results with induction therapy (Thymoglobulin or Campath) followed by maintenance therapy with tacrolimus. Because the allograft ileum is more susceptible to rejection, ileoscopic biopsies through a temporary loop ileostomy are common. Watery diarrhea may be a sign of either rejection or superinfection. With the return of intestinal function, feedings are begun with an elemental diet and then advanced as tolerated. Viral and fungal infection prophylaxis includes ganciclovir, oral antibiotic bowel preparation, low-dose amphotericin B, and early removal of central lines.
   B. **Potential complications.** Inherent risks with intestinal transplantation include up to 50% graft failure (rejection) at 3 years, although recent advances in immunosuppression and perioperative management have promising results (*Lancet* 2003;361:1502). Combined liver–intestine transplantation carries all the additional risks inherent in liver transplantation. Risks that are increased in intestinal transplant recipients include the development of graft-versus-host disease and posttransplantation lymphoproliferative disease. Complications related to tacrolimus-based immunosuppression include diabetes mellitus, headaches, CNS neurotoxicity, peripheral neurotoxicity, and nephrotoxicity. As with any effective immunosuppressant, there is an increased risk of infection and malignancy.

References

Norman DJ, Turka LA, eds. *Primer on Transplantation*, 2nd ed. Thorofare, NJ: American Society of Transplant Physicians; 2001.

Schulak JA. What's new in general surgery: transplantation. *J Am Coll Surg* 2005; 200(3):409–417.

Abu-Elmagd KM. Intestinal transplantation for short bowel syndrome and gastrointestinal failure: current consensus, rewarding outcomes, and practical guidelines. *Gastroenterology* 2006;130:S132–S137.

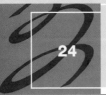

BURNS
Steven J. Schwulst and J. Perren Cobb

*B*urns are tissue injuries resulting from direct contact with flames, hot liquids, gases, or surfaces; caustic chemicals; electricity; or radiation. Most commonly, the skin is injured, which compromises its function as a barrier to injury and infection and as a regulator of body temperature, fluid loss, and sensation. According to a 2002 report of the American Burn Association, more than 1.1 million persons in the United States sustain burns each year, of whom more than 50,000 are hospitalized and 4,500 die. However, the focus on burn care as a subspecialty of surgery in dedicated patient care units has improved overall survival and quality of life.

 ASSESSMENT AND MANAGEMENT OF BURN INJURIES

I. ASSESSMENT

   A. The mechanism of injury identified by the patient or witnesses helps to direct the assessment. Burns sustained in a closed environment, such as a structure fire, often produce inhalation injury in addition to thermal trauma. Explosions can cause barometric injury to the lungs and may cause blunt trauma. Burn source, duration of exposure, time of injury, and environment are documented carefully.

   B. Associated injuries may be present in the burn patient and can result from explosions, falls, or jumping in escape attempts. Fractures, abdominal organ injury, pulmonary contusion, and pneumothorax sometimes occur.

   C. Patient age has a major effect on outcome, with infants and elderly patients being at highest risk. Inpatient, outpatient, or burn unit management decisions also are influenced by patient age. Burns are a common form of child abuse and need to be considered in every child. Important physical exam findings include stocking/glove injury patterns, porcelain-contact sparing, lack of splash marks, and dorsally located contact burns of the hands (*J Burn Care Rehabil* 1993;14:121). Elderly patients often have diminished organ system reserve and comorbid medical problems that place them at increased risk.

   D. State of health. Preexisting medical problems affecting management should be noted, including allergies, medications, hypertension, and diabetes mellitus. A careful review of systems should be obtained, with particular attention paid to cardiac, pulmonary, renal, and gastrointestinal systems.

   E. Prehospital treatment is ascertained and recorded, including care provided by the patient and by the emergency response team. Administered fluids are documented carefully and subtracted from estimated fluid requirements for the first 24 hours of injury. Hypothermia is a significant complication, particularly during transport, and should be addressed both in the field and at the receiving facility. Common effective precautions include preheating patient-receiving areas and minimizing the use of wetted dressings in the prehospital setting.

   F. Primary survey should follow the guidelines established by the American College of Surgeons' Advanced Trauma Life Support Course. Burned patients should be evaluated and treated as victims of polysystem trauma because there is significant morbidity associated with missed injuries secondary to an explosion, fall, and so on.

1. **Airway** assessment and security is the number one priority. Supraglottic tissue edema progresses over the first 12 hours and can obstruct the airway rapidly. The larynx protects subglottic tissue from direct thermal injury but not from injury due to inhaled toxic gases. Inhalation injury should be suspected if the patient was burned in an enclosed structure or explosion. Physical signs include hoarseness, stridor, facial burns, singed facial hair, expectoration of carbonaceous sputum, and presence of carbon in the oropharynx. The decision to intubate the trachea for airway protection should be made early and is preferable to cricothyroidotomy in the edematous and swollen neck. Awake intubation or intubation over a bronchoscope is the safest approach if there is any question about the ease or adequacy of airway exposure (*Curr Opin Anaesthesiol* 2003; 16:183).

2. **Breathing** is evaluated for effort, depth of respiration, and auscultation of breath sounds. Wheezing or rales suggest either inhalation injury or aspiration of gastric contents. Most severely burned patients develop early pulmonary insufficiency and respiratory failure. The etiology of this failure can be direct thermal injury to the upper airways or, more commonly, indirect acute lung injury secondary to activation of systemic inflammation. In addition, the decreased pulmonary compliance and chest wall rigidity of burn patients can lead to iatrogenic ventilator-induced lung injury. The use of lower tidal volumes, permissive hypercapnic, and the "open lung" approach to ventilation can significantly improve outcome (*N Engl J Med* 2000;342:1301).

3. **Circulation.** Circulatory support in the form of aggressive and prompt fluid resuscitation is a cornerstone of early burn management. Burn injury causes a combination of hypovolemic and distributive shock characterized by the release of inflammatory mediators, dynamic fluid shifts from the intravascular compartment to the interstitium, and exudative and evaporative water loss from the burn injury (*World J Surg* 1992;16:30). Full-thickness circumferential extremity or neck burns require escharotomy if circulation distal to the injury is impaired; however, escharotomies are rarely needed within the first 6 hours of injury.

4. **Remove all clothing** to halt continued burn from melted synthetic compounds or chemicals and to assess the full extent of body-surface involvement in the initial examination. Irrigate injuries with water or saline to remove harmful residues. **Remove jewelry** (particularly rings) to prevent injury resulting from increasing tissue edema.

G. **Burn-specific secondary survey**
1. **Depth of burn** (Table 24-1)
   a. **First-degree burns** are limited to the epidermis. The skin is painful and red. There are no blisters. These burns should heal spontaneously in 3 to 4 days.
   b. **Second-degree burns,** which are subdivided into **superficial or deep partial-thickness burns,** are limited to the dermal layers of the skin. **Superficial** partial-thickness burns involve the papillary dermis. They appear red, warm, edematous, and blistered, often with denuded, moist, mottled red or pink epithelium. The injured tissue is very painful, especially when exposed to air. Such burns frequently arise from brief contact with hot surfaces, liquids, flames, or chemicals. **Deep** second-degree burns involve the reticular dermis and thus can damage some dermal appendages (e.g., nerves, sweat glands, or hair follicles). Hence, such burns can be less sensitive, or hairs may be easily plucked out of areas with deep partial-thickness burns. Nonetheless, the only definitive method of differentiating superficial and deep partial-thickness burns is by length of time to heal. Superficial burns heal in less than 2 weeks; deep ones require at least 3 weeks. Furthermore, any partial-thickness burn can convert to full-thickness injury over time, especially if early fluid resuscitation is inadequate.
   c. **Full-thickness** (third- or fourth-degree) burns involve all layers of the skin and some subcutaneous tissue. In **third-degree** burns, all the skin appendages, including hair follicles and sweat and sebaceous glands, and sensory fibers for touch, pain, temperature, and pressure are destroyed. This results in an initially

TABLE 24-1	Treatment Algorithm for the Three Clinically Important Burn Depths[a]

Burn depth[b]	Level of injury	Clinical features	Treatment	Usual result
Superficial partial-thickness	Papillary dermis	Blisters Erythema Capillary refill Intact pain sensation	Tetanus prophylaxis Cleaning (e.g., with chlorhexidine gluconate) Topical agent (e.g., 1% silver sulfadiazine) Sterile gauze dressing[c] Physical therapy Splints as necessary	Epithelialization in 7–21 days Hypertrophic scar rare Return of full function
Deep partial-thickness	Reticular dermis	Blisters Pale white or yellow color Absent pain sensation	As for superficial partial-thickness burns Early surgical excision and skin grafting an option	Epithelialization in 21–60 days in the absence of surgery Hypertrophic scar common Earlier return of function with surgical therapy
Full thickness	Subcutaneous fat, fascia, muscle, or bone	Blisters may be absent Leathery, in classic, wrinkled appearance over bony prominences No capillary refill Thrombosed subcutaneous vessels may be visible Absent pain sensation	As for superficial partial-thickness burns Wound excision and grafting at earliest feasible time	Functional limitation more frequent Hypertrophic scar mainly at graft margins

[a]Epidermal (first-degree) burns present clinically with cutaneous erythema, pain, and tenderness; they resolve rapidly and generally require only symptomatic treatment.
[b]No clinically useful objective method of measuring burn depth exists; classification depends on clinical judgment.
[c]Sterile gauze dressings are frequently omitted on the face and neck.
Reprinted with permission from Monafo WW. Initial management of burns. *N Engl J Med* 1996;335:1581.

painless, insensate dry surface that may appear either white and leathery or charred and cracked, with exposure of underlying fat. **Fourth-degree** burns also involve fascia, muscle, and bone. They often result from prolonged contact with thermal sources or high electrical current. All full-thickness burns are managed surgically, and immediate burn expertise should be sought.

H. Percentage of body surface area (BSA) estimation. The accurate and timely assessment of BSA is a critical aspect of the initial evaluation of burned patients in the emergency department. It will determine whether transfer to a specialized burn

TABLE 24-2	Rule-of-Nines Estimation of Percentage of Body Surface Area					
		Trunk		**Extremity**		
	Head and neck	**Anterior**	**Posterior**	**Upper**	**Lower**	**Genital**
Adult	9	18	18	9	18	1
Infant	18	18	18	9	14	—

center is required as well as the magnitude of initial fluid resuscitation and nutritional requirements (*J Burn Care Res* 2007;28:42).

1. **Small areas: palm of patient's hand equals 1% of BSA** (*Burns* 2001;27:591).
2. **Large areas: "rule of nines":** Regions of the body approximating 9% BSA or multiples thereof are shown in Table 24-2. Note that infants and babies have a proportionally greater percentage of BSA in the head and neck region and less in the lower extremities than adults (*Burns* 2000;26:156).

II. MANAGEMENT

A. Emergency room

1. **Resuscitation.** A surgical consultation is initiated for all patients with major injury (*N Engl J Med* 1996;335:1581).

   a. **Oxygen** should be provided to patients with all but the most minor injuries. A 100% oxygen high-humidity facemask for those with possible inhalation injury assists the patient's expectoration from dry airways and treats carbon monoxide poisoning. Breathing 100% oxygen decreases the half-life of carboxyhemoglobin from 2.5 hours (in room air) to 40 minutes.

   b. **Intravenous access.** All patients with burns of 20% or greater BSA require intravenous fluids. Two 16-gauge or larger peripheral venous catheters should be started immediately to provide circulatory volume support. Peripheral access in the upper extremities is preferred over central venous access because of the risk of catheter-related infection. An intravenous catheter may be placed through the burn if other suitable sites are unavailable. Avoid lower-extremity catheters, if possible, to prevent phlebitic complications.

   c. **Fluid.** Improved survival in the era of modern burn care is largely attributable to early and aggressive volume resuscitation (*Resuscitation* 2000;45:91). Intravenous fluid in excess of maintenance fluids is administered to all patients with burns of 20% or greater BSA and generally follows firmly established guidelines and formulas. Although several formulas have been described, most burn surgeons adhere to crystalloid-based formulations. In particular, fluid resuscitation based on variations of the Parkland formula is widely used and has decreased the occurrence of burn-induced shock (*Ann N Y Acad Sci* 1968;150:874).

   (1) **Modified Parkland formula.** The estimated crystalloid requirement for the first 24 hours after injury is calculated based on patient weight and BSA burn percentage. **Lactated Ringer's solution volume in the first 24 hours = 4 mL × % BSA** (second-, third-, and fourth-degree burns only) × **body weight (kg).** One-half of the calculated volume is given in the first 8 hours after injury, and the remaining volume is infused over the next 16 hours. Fluid resuscitation calculations are based on the time of injury, not the time when the patient is evaluated. Prehospital intravenous hydration is subtracted from the total volume estimate. It should be emphasized that formulas are only estimates, and more or less fluid may be required to maintain adequate tissue perfusion as measured by rate of urine output. Patients with inhalational injury, associated mechanical trauma, electrical injury, escharotomies, or delayed resuscitation require more fluid than that based on the formula alone. Furthermore, for children weighing 30 kg or

less, 5% dextrose in one-quarter normal saline maintenance fluids should supplement the Parkland formula to compensate for ongoing evaporative losses. Patient **body weight** is determined early after the burn as a baseline measurement for fluid calculations and as a daily reference for fluid management.

  (2) Colloid-containing solutions should be held for intravenous therapy until after the first 24 hours postburn. In fact, it has been shown that the use of albumin during the early resuscitative phase increases mortality (*N Engl J Med* 1996;335:1581). If given to patients with inhalation injury early in resuscitation, albumin may move into the interstitium and may increase pulmonary complications. However, by 24 hours postburn, capillary leak diminishes and burn specialists who favor the use of colloids argue that colloid solutions decrease the total volume of fluids infused by half, thereby minimizing the cardiac, electrolyte, and pulmonary complications that arise after large-volume resuscitation (*Am J Physiol* 1995;268:856).

  d. A Foley catheter is used to monitor hourly urine production as an index of adequate tissue perfusion. In the absence of underlying renal disease, a minimum urine production rate of 1 mL/kg/hour in children (weighing ≤ 30 kg) and 0.5 mL/kg/hour in adults is the guideline for adequate intravenous infusion. To minimize edema, consider reducing intravenous hydration if urine output exceeds 1.5 mL/kg/hour in adult patients.

  e. Nasogastric tube insertion with low intermittent suction is performed if patients are intubated or develop nausea, vomiting, and abdominal distention consistent with adynamic ileus. Virtually all patients with burns of greater than 25% BSA have an adynamic ileus.

  f. Escharotomy may be necessary in full-thickness circumferential burns of the neck, torso, or extremities when increasing tissue edema impairs peripheral circulation or when chest involvement restricts respiratory efforts. Full-thickness incisions through (but no deeper than) the insensate burn eschar provide immediate relief (Fig. 24-1). Longitudinal escharotomies are performed on the lateral or medial aspect of the extremities and the anterior axillary lines of the chest (*Arch Surg* 1968;96:502). Usually, they are done at the bedside and require no anesthesia. However, if the digits were burned so severely that desiccation results, midlateral escharotomies have minimal benefit. Escharotomies are rarely required within the first 6 hours after injury. Indications for escharotomy rest on clinical grounds. Traditionally, to aid in assessing peripheral circulation, the documentation of palpable peripheral pulse or the presence of a Doppler signal has been used. However, studies have indicated that correlation of intramuscular pressure with signs and symptoms of extremity compression, including Doppler pulse, is poor (*Am J Surg* 1980;140:825). Infrared photoplethysmography (PPG) (or pulse oximetry) has been a useful adjunct in assessing the need of escharotomies because PPG correlates well with blood flow and direct measurement of compartment pressure (*J Hand Surg* 1984;9:314). More recently, laser Doppler flowmetry has been shown to be predictive of the need for escharotomy and grafting in deep dermal upper extremity burns (*J Trauma* 1997;43:35).

2. Monitors. Continuous pulse oximetry to measure oxygen saturation is useful. One caveat is that falsely elevated levels can be observed in carbon monoxide poisoning.

3. Laboratory examination includes a baseline complete blood cell count, type and cross-match, electrolytes and renal indices, β-human chorionic gonadotropin (in women), arterial carboxyhemoglobin, arterial blood gas evaluation, and urinalysis. A toxicology screen and an alcohol level are obtained when suggested by history or mental status examination. A chest x-ray is obtained with the understanding that it rarely reflects early inhalation injury. Additional chest films are obtained should endotracheal intubation or central line placement become necessary. An electrocardiogram is useful initially, particularly in elderly patients or those with electrical burns. Fluid and electrolyte fluxes during resuscitation and

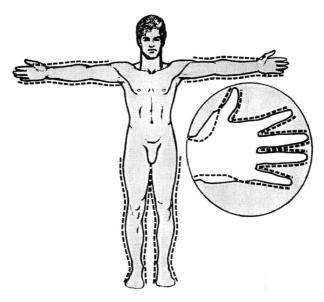

Figure 24-1. Placement of escharotomies. Midaxial escharotomies should be performed if vascular compromise occurs. Incisions should be performed through the dermis and subcutaneous tissue to allow maximal expansion of the underlying fascia. (With permission from Eichelberger M. *Pediatric Trauma*. St. Louis: Mosby; 1993.)

   later mobilization of third-space edema can result in arrhythmias and interval electrocardiographic changes.

4. **Moist dressings** applied to partial-thickness burns provide pain relief from air exposure. Cool water applied to small partial-thickness burns can provide relief but must be avoided in patients with major burns (>25% BSA) and especially in infants, groups that are at high risk for hypothermia. Cold water also can cause vasoconstriction and can extend the depth and surface area of injury.

5. **Analgesia** is given intravenously every 1 to 2 hours to manage pain but in small doses to guard against hypotension, oversedation, and respiratory depression.

6. **Photographs or diagrams** of the BSA involvement and thickness of burns are useful in documenting the injury. They also can facilitate communication between the various members of the team caring for the patient and serve medicolegal purposes in the case of assault or child abuse.

7. **Early irrigation and débridement** are performed using normal saline and sterile instruments to remove all loose epidermal skin layers, followed by the application of topical antimicrobial agents and sterile dressings. In general, it is safe to leave small blisters overlying superficial partial-thickness burns intact because they permit healing in a sterile environment and offer some protection to the underlying dermis. However, in larger and deeper partial-thickness burns, débridement of burn blisters may be protective to the fragile zone of stasis in the early stages of burn injury. The fluid within burn blisters contains numerous inflammatory mediators that have deleterious effects on local microcirculation, including increased capillary permeability and decreased microvascular patency. Furthermore, mechanical pressure from the blister itself on ischemic tissue may contribute to deepening of the wound. These findings support the evacuation of blister fluid to preserve microvascular circulation and to prevent the progression of partial-thickness to full-thickness burns (*J Wound Care* 2001;10:41). Nonviable tissue in the burn wound should be débrided early because it provides a medium on which bacteria can feed and puts the patient at risk for both

local and systemic infection. If the burns resulted from liquid chemical exposure, they are irrigated continuously for 20 to 30 minutes. Dry chemicals are removed from the skin before irrigation to prevent them from dissolving into solution and causing further injury. Corneal burns of the eye require continuous irrigation for several hours and immediate ophthalmologic consultation.

8. **Topical antimicrobial agents** are the mainstay of local burn wound management. Prior to the use of topical antimicrobial agents, the most common organisms causing burn wound infections were *Staphylococcus aureus* and group A streptococci (*J Trauma* 1982; 22:11). Subsequent to the development of topical agents, Gram-negative organisms, particularly *Pseudomonas aeruginosa,* and fungi are the most common causes of invasive burn wound sepsis (*World J Surg* 1992;16:57). Systemic antibiotics are not administered prophylactically but are reserved for documented infection. Bacterial proliferation may occur underneath the eschar at the viable–nonviable interface, resulting in subeschar suppuration and separation of the eschar. Micro-organisms can invade the underlying tissue, producing invasive burn wound sepsis. The risk of invasive infection is higher in patients with multiorgan failure or burns greater than 30% BSA (*World J Surg* 2004;22:135). When the identity of the specific organism is established, antibiotic therapy is targeted to that organism. It may be useful on occasion to diagnose invasive infection. The technique requires a 500-mg biopsy of suspicious eschar and underlying unburned tissue. The presence of micro-organisms in viable tissue confirms the diagnosis. The number of micro-organisms in viable tissue correlates with mortality. Treatment requires infected eschar excision and appropriate topical/systemic antibiotic therapy (*World J Surg* 1998;22:135).

   a. **Silver sulfadiazine** (e.g., Silvadene) is the most commonly used agent because it is not irritating and has the fewest adverse side effects, the worst being a transient leukopenia in the first 1 to 3 days. It is formulated as a cream, which helps to minimize evaporative water and heat loss and thus diminishes caloric requirements. However, silver sulfadiazine has poor Gram-negative and anaerobic bacterial coverage, poor eschar penetration, and is **contraindicated** in patients with glucose 6-phosphatase deficiency.

   b. **Mafenide acetate** (Sulfamylon) is **bacteriostatic** and has better Gram-negative (particularly against *P. aeruginosa*) and anaerobic coverage as well as deeper eschar penetration. Furthermore, burns over avascular cartilage, such as the ear, are ideal for mafenide acetate therapy. However, it is painful and readily absorbed systemically; it can also lead to metabolic **hyperchloremic** acidosis by inhibiting carbonic anhydrase.

   c. **Polymyxin B sulfate** (Polysporin) is tolerated well on facial burns and does not discolor skin, as silver sulfadiazine sometimes can. However, polymyxin B has poor Gram-negative coverage as well as poor eschar penetration.

   d. **Silver nitrate** has lost favor because of the severe electrolyte abnormalities resulting from Na^+, K^+, and Cl^- leaching from the wound and because it readily stains skin and clothing. However, for patients with a sulfa allergy, it is a reasonable choice, provided that electrolytes are closely monitored.

   e. **Acticoat** has recently gained acceptance (*Burns* 2004;30(Suppl 1):S1). This dressing comes as an easy-to-apply sheet, slowly releases silver ions, has good antimicrobial activity, and can be left in place for 3 days. However, its expense may prove prohibitive for some types of injury.

9. **Tetanus prophylaxis** should be administered as tetanus toxoid, 0.5 mL intramuscularly, if the last booster dose was more than 5 years before the injury. If immunization status is unknown, human tetanus immunoglobulin (Hyper-Tet), 250 to 500 units, should be administered intramuscularly using a syringe and injection site different from those used for tetanus toxoid administration.

10. **Critical care issues with burns.** Such issues include burn wound infection, pneumonia, sepsis, ileus, Curling ulcer (gastroduodenal), acalculous cholecystitis, and superior mesenteric artery syndrome.

   a. **Stress ulcer prophylaxis** (e.g., H_2 blockers, antacids, or proton-pump inhibitors) should be provided for patients who have major burns and can receive nothing by mouth, especially those with coagulopathy (*Shock* 1996;5:4).

  b. Deep venous thrombosis (DVT). Burn patients should theoretically be at high risk for DVT secondary to their immobility, repeated operative procedures, and frequent use of indwelling venous catheters. However, the incidence of DVT in burn patients appears to be lower than that of other critically ill patients. Unfortunately, there are no standardized guidelines for DVT prophylaxis in burn patients, and the role of routine prophylaxis has not been clearly defined. Until large-scale prospective trials are completed, most burn surgeons agree that routine heparin prophylaxis is cost-effective, decreasing the incidence of clinically significant thromboembolic episodes without causing significant complications (*Burns* 2004;30:591).

  c. Glucose monitoring is also of paramount importance. In a retrospective study of severely burned pediatric patients, blood glucose levels between 90 to 120 mg/dL were associated with a reduced incidence of infectious complications (*J Trauma* 2005;59:1148). For adult patients, the results of prospective, randomized, placebo-controlled trails of tight glucose control in intensive care unit patients remain the subject of controversy (*Crit Care Med* 2006;34:2843). Thus, the optimal serum glucose level for recovery after burn injury is not known; a goal of less than 140 mg/dL appears prudent based upon available data (*Curr Opin Clin Nutr Metab Care* 2007;10:206).

  d. Sepsis. In patients who survive the first 24 hours after injury, burn sepsis is the leading cause of mortality (*Burns* 2006;32:545). The evidence-based recommendations of the Surviving Sepsis Campaign (*Crit Care Med* 2004;32:858) are under revision based on the results of recent clinical trials, but will likely include antibiotic therapy, source control, crystalloid resuscitation, vasopressor use, a transfusion trigger of hemoglobin of 7 g/dL, an open-lung, low-tidal-volume ventilatory strategy, and maintenance of blood glucose less than 140 mg/dL.

B. Outpatient. Only minor first-degree or partial-thickness injuries should be considered for outpatient management. Whether to use outpatient management depends on many factors, including patient reliability, opportunity for follow-up, and accessibility to health professionals. Surgical consultation is recommended at the time of initial evaluation in all but the most minor injuries.

  1. Dressings are often managed by the patient when the injury is easily accessible. Home health nursing is a useful adjunct when self-application is suboptimal or wounds are in early healing stages, requiring close follow-up. Silver sulfadiazine is often applied as a light coating, followed by sterile dressings once or twice daily.

  2. Antibiotics are not prescribed prophylactically because they allow resistant organisms to multiply. Their use is limited to documented infection of the wounds.

  3. Follow-up usually occurs once or twice a week during the initial healing of partial-thickness burns and split-thickness skin grafts until epithelialization is complete. Thereafter, patients are followed at 1- to 3-month intervals to evaluate and treat scar hypertrophy (application of foam tape or Jobst garments), hyperpigmentation (avoidance of direct sunlight, use of sunscreen), dry skin (unscented lotion massage), pruritus (antihistamines), and rehabilitation potential and therapy (physical, occupational, social, and psychological).

C. Inpatient

  1. Transfer to a burn center should follow the guidelines of the American Burn Association. These criteria reflect multiple studies showing that age and BSA burn percentage remain the two most important prognostic factors.

  a. Patients younger than 10 years or older than 50 years sustaining partial- or full-thickness burns to greater than 10% BSA.

  b. Partial- or full-thickness burns to greater than 20% BSA in other age groups.

  c. Specialized regions, including joints, hands, feet, perineum, genitalia, face, eyes, or ears.

  d. Full-thickness burns to greater than 5% BSA.

  e. **Significant inhalation, chemical, or electrical injury.**
  f. **Burns in combination with significant associated mechanical trauma or preexisting medical problems.**
  g. **Patients requiring specialized rehabilitation, psychological support, or social services (including suspected neglect or child abuse).**
2. **Nutrition.** Early enteral feeding in burn patients helps to attenuate the catabolic response after burn injury and decrease the rate of infectious complications (*Ann Surg* 1984;200:297). The daily estimated metabolic requirement (EMR) in burn patients can be calculated from the Curreri formula: EMR = [25 kcal × body weight (kg)] + (40 kcal ×% BSA). Protein losses in burn patients from both an increased oxidation rate and burn wound extravasation should be replaced by supplying 1.5 to 2 g/kg protein/day (*Lancet* 2004;363:1895). Therapeutic strategies should target prevention of body weight loss of more than 10% of the patient's baseline weight. Losses of more than 10% of lean body mass may lead to impaired immune function and delayed wound healing. Losses of more than 40% lead to imminent death (*Shock* 1998;10:155).
  a. **Enteral** feedings are the preferred route when tolerated and can be administered through an enteral feeding tube positioned in the duodenum. For severe burns, early feeding within the first 24 hours has been shown to improve a number of outcome measures, including overall mortality (*Burns* 1997;23(Suppl 1):519). Increasing feeding beyond the EMR is associated with the development of fatty liver (*Ann Surg* 2002;235:152), hyperglycemia (*J Trauma* 2001;51:540), and impairment of the splanchnic oxygen balance (*Burns* 2002;28:60), all of which have a negative influence on outcome in burned patients. Patients with large burns may remain hypermetabolic for weeks to months after the burn wound is closed; early tapering of nutritional intake in these patients should be avoided.
  b. **Total parenteral nutrition** should be initiated after fluid resuscitation only if the patient is unable to tolerate enteral feeding.
  c. **Daily vitamin** supplementation in adults should include 1.5 g of ascorbic acid, 500 mg of nicotinamide, 50 mg of riboflavin, 50 mg of thiamine, and 220 mg of zinc. Although results from high-dose antioxidant therapy are promising, further clinical trials are needed to define its role in burn patients (*J Burn Care Rehabil* 2005;26:207).
3. **Wound care**
  a. **Analgesia and sedation** for dressing changes are necessary for major burns. Valium (0.1 mg/kg intramuscularly) plus ketamine (0.5 mg/kg intramuscularly) is one sedative regimen that has been used. Alternatively, in patients with a secure airway (typically intubated), intravenous propofol has the desired effects of ease of titration and quick onset and offset of action. Either of these sedative regimens in concert with narcotic analgesia is well tolerated.
  b. **Daily dressing changes.** While the wounds are exposed, the surgeon can properly assess the continued demarcation and healing of the injury. Physical therapy with **active range of motion** is performed at this time, before reapplying splints and dressings.
  c. **Débridement** of all nonviable tissue should take place using sterile technique and instruments when demarcation occurs. Partial-thickness eschar can be abraded lightly, using wet gauze. Enzymatic treatments (i.e., Travase, sutilains ointment) can be useful in dissolving eschar to develop granulation tissue for tissue grafting. All full-thickness eschar should be identified early, excised, and closed or covered before the development of wound colonization and infection.
  d. **Temporary dressings for massive burns with limited donor sites**
   (1) **Biologic.** Fresh or cryopreserved cadaver allografts have been the gold standard (*J Burn Care Rehabil* 1997;18:43). Recently, however, our center has had success using porcine xenografts. This alternative provides the advantages of ease of acquisition and application while providing barrier protection and a biologic bed under which dermis can granulate (*Clin Dermatol* 2005;23:419).

After several days, the allograft can be removed, and a meshed autograft may be replaced for definitive coverage. The use of cultured autologous epithelium, cultured allogeneic epidermis, and allograft dermis has had encouraging results in some burn centers but is largely investigational (*J Cell Mol Med* 2005;9:592).

(2) Using a **synthetic** membrane (e.g., Integra artificial skin, Dermagraft-TC) is an attractive alternative. Integra consists of an epidermal analogue, Silastic film, and a dermal analogue, a collagen matrix with chondroitin 6-sulfate. The patient's dermal fibroblasts can grow into this matrix. Once adequate vascularization is seen through the Silastic film, the film is removed, and an ultrathin autograft is placed onto the artificial dermis. The autograft is thin so that donor sites can be reharvested more quickly. This technique has been reported to give results similar to those obtained using allografts (*J Trauma* 2001;50:358). Dermagraft-TC has had similar success. This bilaminate skin substitute consists of a dermal matrix impregnated with human neonatal fibroblasts and a silicone epidermal analogue. After a few days, the bilaminate artificial skin comes off easily and can be replaced with autograft (*J Burn Care Rehabil* 1997;18:52).

4. Operative management

a. Early tangential excision of burn eschar to the level of bleeding capillaries should follow the resuscitation phase. Debate persists as to the optimal timing of burn wound excision (range is 1 to 10 days). Excision can be performed using a Goulian or Humbly knife for small surfaces and a power- or gas-driven dermatome for larger surfaces. For each trip to the operating theater, consider limiting burn excision to less than 20% BSA or 2 hours of operating time. Even within such limits, aggressive débridement frequently produces profound blood loss and hypothermia (*Crit Care Clin* 1999;15:333).

b. Split-thickness skin grafts are harvested at a thickness of 0.012 to 0.015 in. (*Clin Dermatol* 2005;23:332) with a meshed expansion ratio from 1.5:1 to 3:1 (*Burns* 1995;21:364). The graft is immobilized with absorbable sutures or staples. For very large wounds, 4:1 autograft can be overlaid with meshed allograft skin (Fig. 24-2). However, cosmesis is poor, and graft take may be less; thus, this technique is used on the back, flanks, or other less visible areas. Nonadherent dressings and bolsters are applied to minimize shear forces on the fresh grafts. **Splints or pins** may be required to improve graft survival at joints and to prevent contracture. **Ideal point positions** are extension in the neck, knee, elbow, wrist, and interphalangeal joints, **15-degree flexion** at metacarpophalangeal joints, and **abduction** at the shoulder (*Clin Plast Surg* 1992;19:721).

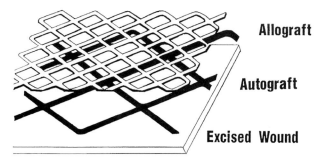

Allograft

Autograft

Excised Wound

Figure 24-2. Combined skin graft to cover burn wounds too extensive for other methods. The widely meshed autograft would allow continued fluid fluxes during the more extended time required for epithelialization. A more narrowly meshed allograft placed superficial to the autograft can accelerate the process by providing temporary coverage while the autograft fills in. (With permission from Eichelberger M. *Pediatric Trauma.* St. Louis: Mosby; 1993.)

D. Follow-up
   1. Wound healing
   a. Infection is minimized by using topical antimicrobial agents.
   b. Granulation tissue that fails to epithelialize at skin graft sites can be cauterized by using an applicator stick tipped with silver nitrate.
   c. Hyperpigmentation is best prevented by avoiding direct sunlight exposure for up to 1 year. When exposure to sunlight is unavoidable, a topical sunblock agent should be used.
   d. Scar hypertrophy is minimized by local tissue compression, inducing the release of prostaglandin E2 (*Burns* 2001;27:215). Tailored Jobst garments, foam sponge, foam tape, silicone gel sheets, and massage regimens are all effective in providing this local tissue compression. Hypertrophic scarring can be described with a rating system such as the Vancouver Scar Scale (VSS). This scale is based on four factors: pigmentation, vascularity, pliability, and height (*J Burn Care Rehabil* 1995;16:535).
   e. Contractures are best prevented by using active range of motion. When present, release (Z-plasty) or excision and skin grafting may be necessary.
   f. Pruritus can be palliated with antihistamines. Recently, doxepin, an antidepressant with strong antihistamine properties, has been approved for topical use.
   g. Rehabilitation with ongoing evaluation is provided by occupational and physical therapists.
III. BURN MECHANISMS: SPECIAL CONSIDERATIONS
   A. Inhalational. Thermal injury to the airway generally is limited to the oropharynx or glottis. The glottis generally protects the subglottic airway from heat, unless the patient has been exposed to superheated steam. Edema formation can compromise the patency of the upper airway, mandating early assessment and constant re-evaluation of the airway (*J Trauma* 1994;36:59). **Gases** containing substances that have undergone incomplete combustion (particularly aldehydes), toxic fumes (hydrogen cyanide), and carbon monoxide can cause tracheobronchitis, pneumonitis, and edema. Mortality may be increased by as much as 20% in these patients. **Carbon monoxide** exposure is suggested by a history of exposure in a confined space with symptoms of nausea, vomiting, headache, mental status changes, and cherry-red lips. Carbon monoxide binds to hemoglobin with an affinity 249 times greater than that of oxygen, resulting in extremely slow dissociation (250-minute half-life with room air) unless the patient is administered supplemental oxygen (40-minute half-life with 100% oxygen via nonrebreathing mask). The arterial **carboxyhemoglobin** level is obtained as a baseline, and if it is elevated (>5% in nonsmokers or >10% in smokers), oxygen therapy should continue until normal levels are achieved. Inhaled chemical products of combustion may include acids, phosgene, and cyanide derived from burning polyvinylchloride and polyurethane. The increased ventilation-perfusion gradient and the reduction in peak airway flow in distal airways and alveoli can be evaluated using a xenon-133 ventilation-perfusion lung scan. **Management** of minor inhalation injury is by delivery of humidified oxygen. Major injuries require endotracheal intubation with a large-bore tube (7.5 to 8 mm) to facilitate pulmonary toilet of viscous secretions and mechanical ventilation with positive pressure. As discussed earlier, decreased pulmonary compliance is often seen after inhalation injury and can lead to iatrogenic ventilator-associated lung injury.
   B. Electrical
   1. Factors influencing severity include the voltage (high is >1,000 V), resistance, type of current, current pathway through the body, and duration of contact with an electrical source (*Annu Rev Biomed Eng* 2000;2:477). Electrical current passes in a straight line between points of body contact with the source and the ground. When current passes through the heart or brain, cardiopulmonary arrest can result. In most cases, these injuries respond to resuscitation and usually do not cause permanent damage (*Ann Intern Med* 2006;145:531). **Severity of injury frequently is underestimated** when only the entrance and exit wounds are considered.

a. **Tissue resistance.** Heat and subsequent injury from thermal necrosis is directly proportional to resistance to current flow. Tissues that have a higher resistance to electricity, such as skin, bone, and fat, tend to increase in temperature and coagulate, causing deep thermal burns. Nerves and blood vessels have low resistance and readily conduct electricity (*Crit Care Clin* 1999;15:319). In addition to direct tissue injury, thrombosis can occur with distal soft-tissue ischemia. Peripheral perfusion should be monitored closely because fasciotomy may become necessary to treat compartment syndrome. Fluid resuscitation requirements often are higher than calculated by published formulas.

b. **Current**

(1) **Alternating** current (household, power lines) can lead to repetitive, tetanic muscle contraction. In fact, when contact is between the palm and an electrical source, alternating current can cause a hand to grip the source of electricity (because of a stronger flexor than extensor tone) and lead to longer electrical exposure (*J Forensic Sci* 1980;25:514). High-voltage injury, which is commonly seen in workers operating near power lines, can present with full-thickness, charred skin at the entrance and exit wounds, with full arrest, and with fractures sustained while current passed through the body or during a fall.

(2) **Direct** current emanates from batteries and lightning and causes a single muscle contraction, often throwing the person receiving the electrical shock away from the source of electricity. With a voltage of at least 100 million volts and a current of 200,000 amperes, lightning kills 150 to 300 people in the United States every year. Injury can result from direct strikes or side flashes. Current can travel on the surface of the body rather than through it, producing a "splashed-on" pattern of skin burn.

2. **Complications** include **cardiopulmonary arrest** (more common with alternating current) (*Br Heart J* 1987;57:279), **thrombosis, associated fractures** related to fall or severe muscle contraction (*Am J Surg* 1977;134:95), **spinal cord injury** (*Neurology* 2003;60:182), and **cataracts** (*J Burn Care Rehabil* 1991;12:458). **Rhabdomyolysis** may occur and result in myoglobin release from injured cells of deep tissues. Precipitation of protein in the renal tubules can cause acute renal failure (*Burns* 2004;30:680). Dark urine is the first clinical indication of myoglobinuria, and intravenous lactated Ringer's solution should be administered to maintain a urine output greater than 100 mL/hour. Concomitant administration of intravenous sodium bicarbonate (three ampules [~150 mEq sodium] in 1 L of 5% dextrose in water) provides an isotonic solution to alkalinize the urine more effectively and potentially minimize nephrotoxicity from myoglobinuria.

C. **Chemical injury** may result from contact with alkali, acid, or petroleum compounds. Removal of the offending agent is the cornerstone of treatment. Dry chemicals should be brushed off or aspirated into a closed suction container before irrigating with copious amounts of water for at least 20 to 30 minutes. Alkali burns, which penetrate more deeply than acid burns, require longer periods of irrigation. Irrigation has a threefold effect: It dilutes the chemicals already in contact with the skin, washes unreacted agent from the skin, and helps to correct the hygroscopic effects that some agents have on tissues (*ANZ J Surg* 2003;73:45). Neutralizing the chemicals is no longer recommended because the resulting reaction has the potential to generate more heat, which can exacerbate the injury. All chemical injuries to the eye are potentially blinding and require copious irrigation with several liters of water and prompt referral to an ophthalmologist (*BMJ* 2004;328:36). **Tar** can cause ongoing burn if not removed. Cool the tar with cold water, and then use an adhesive remover to remove any remaining tar.

D. **Cold injury**

1. **Hypothermia** is defined as a core body temperature less than 35°C. Mild hypothermia is classified as a core body temperature of 32°C to 35°C; moderate hypothermia is 30°C to 32°C; and severe hypothermia is less than 30°C (*CMAJ* 2003;168:305). The elderly, due to their decreased capacity for metabolic heat production, and children, due to their high ratio of body surface area to mass,

are particularly susceptible (*Exp Aging Res* 1997;23:45). Other factors contributing to increased susceptibility include drug or alcohol ingestion, hypothyroidism, immobilization, moisture, sepsis, diabetes mellitus, and cerebral ischemia. Signs of hypothermia include reduced levels of consciousness, dysrhythmias, and skin that appears cold, gray, or cyanotic. Moderate to severe hypothermia is a medical emergency and necessitates maintenance of airway, breathing, and circulation. Core body temperature should be monitored by means of an esophageal or rectal probe. The heart becomes increasingly irritable at core temperatures below 34°C, and cardiac monitoring should be routine in all hypothermic patients (*Ann Emerg Med* 1989;18:72). Asystole may occur below 28°C, and cardiopulmonary resuscitation should be started and maintained until the patient is rewarmed to at least 36°C. Rewarming can be passive or active. Passive rewarming involves using blankets to cover the body and head, and the warming rate ranges between 0.5°C and 2°C per hour. Active rewarming can be external or internal. Active external warming includes the use of heating blankets or a heated forced-air system, which can increase rewarming rates by 1°C per hour as compared to simple cotton blankets (*Ann Emerg Med* 1996;27:479). Active internal rewarming can be started immediately in the case of severe hypothermia and includes the use of warmed intravenous fluids and oxygen, together warming at a rate of 1°C to 2°C per hour (*Resuscitation* 1998;36:101). Although used rarely, active invasive rewarming methods can warm faster, at a rate 1°C to 4°C per hour. Examples of this approach include warmed peritoneal lavage, thoracostomy lavage, and bladder lavage (*Ann Emerg Med* 1990;19:204). Extracorporeal rewarming of blood via a continuous venovenous bypass circuit or heated hemodialysis can rewarm at a rate of 1°C to 2°C every 5 minutes (*N Engl J Med* 1997; 337:1500).

2. Frostbite results from the formation of intracellular ice crystals and microvascular occlusion. Factors affecting severity are temperature, duration of exposure, and environmental conditions promoting rapid heat loss, such as wind velocity, moisture, immobilization, and open wounds. The fingers, toes, and ears are most commonly injured, particularly when reduced tissue perfusion has resulted from other causes, such as shock.

    a. Classification

        (1) First-degree: hyperemia and edema, without skin necrosis.

        (2) Second-degree: superficial vesicle formation containing clear or milky fluid surrounded by hyperemia, edema, and partial-thickness necrosis.

        (3) Third-degree: hemorrhagic bullae and full-thickness necrosis.

        (4) Fourth-degree: gangrene with full-thickness involvement of skin, muscle, and bone.

    b. Treatment consists of rapid rewarming in a warm water bath between 40°C and 42°C until the tissue perfusion returns, which also may help to minimize tissue loss (*Surg Clin North Am* 1991;71:345). Splinting and elevation of the frostbitten extremity may reduce edema and promote tissue perfusion. Because mechanical pressure or friction can injure the tissue further, massage and weightbearing are discouraged. Rewarming can be painful, and therefore intravenous analgesia should be provided. Any ruptured blisters should be débrided and covered with a topical antimicrobial and gauze. Tetanus prophylaxis is administered, and follow-up over several weeks is recommended to allow for demarcation of full-thickness injury. Escharotomy may be required for severe injury. Early amputation is not recommended because improvement in tissue viability can occur weeks after injury.

IV. FUTURE BURN CARE MANAGEMENT. Recently, reported burn mortality rates have improved dramatically. At the U.S. Army Institute of Surgical Research, the LA50, the size of a burn that kills half of patients, is 75.6% SBA in adults and 90% SBA in children younger than 15 years of age (*J Burn Care Rehabil* 1997;18:S2). With aggressive early tangential excision, early coverage, alternative dressings, and better understanding of wound infection pathophysiology, clinicians have an augmented arsenal to combat morbidity and mortality. Earlier detection of bacterial infections of wounds may lead to earlier intervention before serious illness or further wound damage occurs. Molecular diagnostic approaches such as the use of the polymerase chain reaction have been used to identify strains of methicillin-resistant *Staphylococcus aureus* within 2 hours as compared with the days typically required for culture using conventional microbiologic procedures. Ongoing immunologic and clinical studies on burn-induced immunosuppression (*Am J Physiol Lung Cell Mol Physiol* 2003;284:L270), cytokines (*Inflammation* 1999;23:371), and artificial bilaminate skin (*Clin Plast Surg* 2003;30:485) may provide the next advances in burn care. The biggest challenge, however, may still be prevention education.

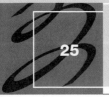

25 SKIN AND SOFT-TISSUE TUMORS
Steven E. Finkelstein and Bruce L. Hall

 **DIAGNOSIS OF SKIN LESIONS
AND SOFT-TISSUE MASSES**

The surgical management of cutaneous oncology has dramatically changed over the last 100 years. As our understanding of tumor cell biology and immunology has improved through dedicated research, so has our ability to apply surgical efforts in a more directed fashion. When a patient presents to a surgeon with a lesion, a focused history and physical examination are crucial to derive the correct diagnosis. Biopsy to obtain a tissue sample followed by histologic examination remains the gold standard for the accurate diagnosis of cutaneous lesions. For large or deep soft-tissue tumors, radiologic evaluation often precedes biopsy.

I. SKIN LESIONS
 A. History. Pigmented lesions with a change in size, borders, and coloration are of concern for malignancy. In addition, the presence of itching, bleeding, or ulceration should be assessed.
 B. Physical examination. The color, size, shape, borders, elevation, location, firmness, and surface characteristics should be noted for each skin lesion. If possible, photographs should be taken. Uniformly colored, small, round, circumscribed lesions are more likely benign. Irregularly colored, larger, asymmetric lesions with indistinct borders and ulceration are worrisome for malignancy.
 C. Biopsy. A tissue diagnosis is needed for lesions that have worrisome features or *change* after a period of observation. Optimally, full-thickness tissue is obtained via punch or excisional biopsy. Punch biopsy uses a cylindrical blade to remove a small core of skin; the sample should be obtained from the thickest portion of the lesion, avoiding areas of crusting, ulceration or necrosis that may underestimate the thickness of the tumor. Excisional biopsy is the same as for soft-tissue masses, discussed in Section II.D. Use of non–full-thickness shave biopsy is generally discouraged because it may lead to inaccurate tumor thickness measurements; however, it does not appear to affect overall patient outcome (*Am J Surg* 2005;190:913). A second consideration is that a shave biopsy site heals by secondary intention, giving an inferior cosmetic outcome.

II. SOFT-TISSUE MASSES
 A. History. Focused history includes location, duration, change in size, and presence of associated symptoms. An enlarging, painless mass is the most common presentation. There is frequently a perceived antecedent trauma. Pain is usually a late symptom. Lesions may be misdiagnosed as hematomas or strained muscle. Any symptom or perception of enlargement is concerning for malignancy.
 B. Physical examination. Key features are size, anatomic relationships with surrounding structures, borders, and mobility. A neurovascular examination of the affected area should be performed.
 C. Radiologic evaluation
  1. Magnetic resonance (MR) scan is the best choice for imaging soft-tissue masses. It can be difficult to distinguish edematous normal tissue from tumor; T2-weighted images and gadolinium enhancement aid with this distinction.
  2. Computed tomography (CT) is used to assess character and extent of larger, deeper tumors. Involvement of adjacent structures and surgical access to the tumor

can be determined. CT-guided core-needle biopsy can be attempted for tumors with difficult surgical access. A CT scan of the chest is useful in patients with soft-tissue sarcomas (STSs) due to its specific pattern of metastasis. CT can also be helpful in evaluating the pelvis and retroperitoneum.

D. Biopsy. Ideally, the surgical oncologist who performs the definitive resection should perform the biopsy.

1. **Incisional biopsy** is the gold standard. A small incision should be made that can be excised at subsequent operation: It should be oriented parallel to the long axis of the extremity. Incisional biopsy rather than excisional biopsy should be performed for a mass greater than 3 cm (or >5 cm if it is consistent with a lipoma). Drains should be avoided; meticulous hemostasis to prevent hemorrhage from spreading tumor is critical. If drains are needed, drain sites should be in line with the incision, to be excised at subsequent operation.

2. **Core-needle biopsy** provides a section of intact tissue for histologic analysis; it can provide the same information as an incisional biopsy if a good core of tissue is obtained. A very small incision allows easy entrance of the needle through the skin. Most indeterminate or negative results should be confirmed by incisional or excisional biopsy.

3. **Excisional biopsy** is performed for tumors that are probably benign or less than 3 cm in diameter. The usual approach is an elliptical incision around the tumor oriented parallel to the long axis of the limb, and when possible along the skin lines of minimal tension. The tumor should be excised completely with a thin margin of normal tissue. Primary closure should be employed whenever possible.

4. **Fine-needle aspiration** (FNA) is the least invasive, but can be the least informative, method of tissue diagnosis. Multiple passes are made through a mass in various directions; the plunger is released before removing the needle from the mass. The specimen is then fixed and sent for cytopathologic evaluation. FNA usually cannot give the grade, but often it can determine the presence of malignancy and the histologic type. Indeterminate results should be followed by further evaluation. FNA is the biopsy method of first choice in the head and neck.

BENIGN LESIONS

I. **SEBORRHEIC KERATOSES** are benign skin growths that originate in the epidermis. These lesions characteristically appear in older people as multiple, raised, irregularly rounded lesions with a verrucous, friable, waxy surface and variable pigmentation from yellowish to brownish black. Common locations include the face, neck, and trunk. If removal is desired, treatment may consist of excision or curettage followed by electrodessication, as well as topical agents, such as trichloroacetic acid, or cryotherapy with liquid nitrogen.

II. **ACTINIC KERATOSES** are caused by sun exposure and are found predominantly in elderly, fair-skinned patients. These lesions are small, usually multiple, flat to slightly elevated lesions with a rough or scaly surface ranging from red to yellowish brown to black and are found in areas of chronic sun exposure. Unlike seborrheic keratoses, these lesions have malignant potential. Indeed, 15% to 20% of lesions become squamous cell carcinoma, although metastases are rare. Benign-appearing actinic keratoses can be observed. When indicated, treatment consists of topical application of 5-fluorouracil twice a day for 2 to 6 weeks.

III. **NEVI.** Junctional nevus cells actually are located in the epidermis and at the dermal-epidermal junction. These nevi are small (<6 mm), well-circumscribed, light brown or black macules found on any area of the body. Nevi rarely develop in people older than 40 years, and any new lesion in someone older than 40 years should be considered a possible early melanoma.

IV. **EPIDERMAL INCLUSION CYSTS** are lined by epidermal cells containing lipid and keratinous material. Asymptomatic cysts may be removed for diagnosis, prevention of infection, or cosmesis. Excision of the cyst should include the entire cyst lining, preferably without interruption of the lining, to prevent recurrence, and should include any skin tract or drainage site.

V. NEUROFIBROMAS are benign tumors that arise from Schwann cells and are seen most frequently in the setting of neurofibromatosis (von Recklinghausen disease). Neurofibromas are soft, pendulous, sometimes lobulated subcutaneous masses that vary widely in size. The overwhelming majority of these tumors do not require excision. These tumors are removed for symptoms of pain, an observed increase in size, or cosmetic reasons.

VI. GANGLION CYSTS are subcutaneous cysts attached to the joint capsule or tendon sheath of the hands and wrists; they are most commonly seen in young and middle-aged women. These lesions present as firm, round masses often seen on the dorsum of the wrist, but can also be found on the radial volar wrist, along the flexor tendon sheaths of the hand, or in the dorsum of the distal interphalangeal joint. After surgical excision, there is an extremely low recurrence rate. To prevent recurrence, the capsular attachment and a small portion of the joint capsule should be removed.

VII. LIPOMAS are benign tumors consisting of fat and are perhaps the most common human neoplasms. There is very little potential for malignancy; sarcomatous elements occur in less than 1% of cases. They are soft, fatty, subcutaneous masses and vary widely in size. Asymptomatic small tumors can be followed clinically, but symptomatic or rapidly growing tumors are of concern and should be removed. Large tumors (>5 cm) should be evaluated by core or incisional biopsy. Every effort should be made to excise lipomas cleanly at the first operation to prevent recurrence.

MALIGNANT LESIONS

I. DERMATOFIBROSARCOMA PROTUBERANS (DFSP) is a locally aggressive tumor that does not metastasize. Margins of 2 to 5 cm should be achieved if possible. Alternatively, Mohs micrographic surgery involves serial excisions of the tumor, with microscopic examination for areas of positive margins that have been mapped and are then re-excised, one section at a time, until a negative margin is reached. Although time consuming and expensive, this surgery has been advocated in the management of dermatofibrosarcoma protuberans for improved tissue conservation, cosmetic advantages, and low recurrence rates (*Curr Opin Oncol* 2006;18:341). DuBay et al. reviewed 62 patients treated for DFSP with wide local excision, Mohs surgery, or a combination approach. At a median follow-up of 4.4 years, there were no local or distant recurrences. Eighty-five percent of the lesions treated initially with Mohs surgery had histologically negative margins. This suggests that Mohs surgery can be effective and that negative margin resection should be achieved (*Cancer* 2004;100:1008).

II. DESMOID TUMORS are nonmetastasizing but locally aggressive tumors that arise from connective tissue. Wide excision with a margin of normal tissue should be performed if possible, but limb function should be spared. Local recurrences are common, and re-excision is often required. Tamoxifen, nonsteroidal anti-inflammatory drugs (e.g., sulindac), or a combination have been used with only anecdotal success and may be attempted as an alternative to surgery. These drugs have been advocated in recurrent or unresectable cases as well. Recommendations as to future pregnancies are conflicting and unclear. Patients with a desmoid tumor should undergo colonoscopy to exclude the diagnosis of familial adenomatous polyposis (*Fam Cancer* 2006;5:275).

III. MELANOMA. The incidence of melanoma continues to rise at an epidemic rate (101.5% increase from 1970s to 1990s). Melanoma represents the fifth-most-common type of cancer (*CA Cancer J Clin* 2006;56:106). The estimated cost of treatment of melanoma by Medicare alone is projected to exceed $5 billion by 2010 (*J Am Acad Dermatol* 2000;42: 820).

   A. Lesions. Most pigmented lesions are benign, but approximately one third of all melanomas arise from pigmented nevi. It is essential to differentiate among benign, premalignant, and malignant lesions.

   1. Premalignant lesions

a. **Dysplastic nevi** have variegated color (tan to brown on a pink base); are large (5 to 12 mm); appear indistinct, with irregular edges; and have macular and papular components. There exists a familial association between dysplastic nevi and a high incidence of melanoma. Melanomas may develop *de novo* or from preexisting dysplastic nevi (*N Engl J Med* 2003;349:2233).

b. **Congenital nevi** are notable by their presence since birth and are commonly referred to as "birthmarks." They can be premalignant; there is an increased risk of melanoma developing from these lesions, particularly for nevi greater than 20 cm.

2. **Malignant lesions**

a. **Superficial spreading melanoma** (SSM) is the most common form of melanoma (80%), with approximately one half arising from a preexisting mole. The lesions usually are slow growing and brown, with small discrete nodules of differing colors. SSM tends to spread laterally but can be slightly elevated. SSM is found most commonly on the back in men and women and on the lower extremities of women.

b. **Nodular melanoma** is the most aggressive form, rapidly becoming a palpable, elevated, firm nodule that may be dense black or reddish blue-black. A distinct convex nodular development indicates deep dermal invasion. Nodular melanomas arise from the epidermal-dermal junction and invade deeply into the dermis and subcutaneous tissue. Approximately 5% are amelanotic.

c. **Lentigo maligna melanoma** usually is found on older patients as a large melanotic freckle on the temple or malar region known as **Hutchinson freckle.** It usually is slow growing but becomes large, often reaching 5 to 6 cm in diameter. Initially, it is flat, but it becomes raised and thicker, with discrete brown to black nodules and irregular edges.

d. **Acral lentiginous melanoma** occurs on the palms, soles, and nail beds, occurs primarily in darker-skinned people, and metastasizes more frequently than do other melanomas, possibly related to later stage at presentation.

e. **In-transit metastases** and **satellites** both signify a poor prognosis with a high risk of local recurrence and distant metastasis. In-transit metastases are lesions in the skin more than 2 cm from the primary lesion; they arise from tumor cells in intradermal lymphatics. Satellites are metastatic lesions in the skin within 2 cm of the primary tumor.

B. **History and risk factors.** A history for melanoma should include an assessment of risk factors and family history.

1. **Risk factors.** Each of the risk factors listed is considered to carry a more-than-threefold increase in risk for melanoma; the presence of three or more risk factors carries approximately 20 times the risk (*Curr Probl Surg* 2006;43:781).

a. **Family or personal history of melanoma.**

b. **Blond or red hair.**

c. **Freckling of the upper back.**

d. **Three or more blistering sunburns before age 20 years.**

e. **Presence of actinic keratosis.**

f. **Blue, green, or gray eyes.**

C. **Clinical features.** Early melanoma and dysplastic lesions can be recognized by the features highlighted in the mnemonic **ABCD: *asymmetry, border** irregularity, **color** variegation, and *diameter* greater than 6 mm. Advanced lesions are more readily apparent and may be nodular or ulcerated.

D. **Staging and prognosis.** Tumor thickness is the most important factor in staging the tumor. Tumors less than 1 mm thick have a cure rate greater than 85%, whereas 10-year survival for lesions more than 4 mm thick is less than 50%. Thickness is also correlated with the risk of regional node and distant metastasis (*J Clin Oncol* 2001;19:3622). The Breslow thickness is a physical depth measurement of the primary tumor and is used to classify the tumor (see "T Classification" in Table 25-1). In contrast, the *Clark's level* describes the *anatomic* level of invasion (Table 25-2). It is also used to classify the primary tumor, but only when the Breslow thickness is less than 1 mm (see "T Classification" in Table 25-1). The revised American Joint

TABLE 25-1	Revised American Joint Committee on Cancer TNM (Tumor, Node, Metastasis) Definitions of Melanoma	
T Classification		
T1	≤1.0 mm	a. without ulceration
		b. with ulceration or level IV or V
T2	1.01–2.0 mm	a. without ulceration
		b. with ulceration
T3	2.01–4.0 mm	a. without ulceration
		b. with ulceration
T4	>4.0 mm	a. without ulceration
		b. with ulceration
Regional lymph nodes (N)		
N1	One lymph node	a. micrometastasis[a]
		b. macrometastasis[b]
N2	2–3 lymph nodes	a. micrometastasis[a]
		b. macrometastasis[b]
		c. in-transit met(s)/satellite(s) without metastatic lymph node(s)
N3	≥4 metastatic lymph nodes, matted lymph nodes, or combinations of in-transit met(s)/satellite(s) and metastatic lymph node(s)	
Distant metastasis (M)		
M1	Distant skin, subcutaneous, or lymph node mets	Normal LDH
M2	Lung mets	Normal LDH
M3	All other visceral or any distant mets	Normal LDH
		Elevated LDH

[a]Micrometastases are diagnosed after sentinel or elective lymphadenectomy.
[b]Macrometastases are defined as clinically detectable lymph node metastases confirmed by therapeutic lymphadenectomy or when any lymph node metastasis exhibits gross extracapsular extension.
LDH, lactic dehydrogenase; mets, metastases.
Modified from Balch CM, Buzaid AC, Soong SJ, et al. New TNM melanoma staging system: linking biology and natural history to clinical outcomes. *Semin Surg Oncol* 2003;21:43–52.

Committee on Cancer (AJCC) system of TNM (tumor, node, metastasis) classification for melanoma (Tables 25-1 and 25-3) is the standard classification system. This system was revised in 2002 to provide more accurate and precise information regarding patient prognosis (*Semin Surg Oncol* 2003;21:43). Older age, male gender, satellitosis, ulceration, and location on the *b*ack, posterolateral *a*rm, *n*eck, or *s*calp (the BANS region) all carry a worse prognosis. The presence of regional node metastasis severely worsens prognosis (10-year survival, 20% to 60%). Distant metastases have a dismal prognosis (median survival, 2 to 11 months).

TABLE 25-2	Clark's Classification (Level of Invasion) of Melanoma
Level I	Lesions involving only the epidermis (*in situ* melanoma); not an invasive lesion
Level II	Invasion of the papillary dermis but does not reach the papillary-reticular dermal interface
Level III	Invasion fills and expands the papillary dermis but does not penetrate the reticular dermis
Level IV	Invasion into the reticular dermis but not into the subcutaneous tissue
Level V	Invasion through the reticular dermis into the subcutaneous tissue

TABLE 25-3	American Joint Committee on Cancer Stage Groupings for Cutaneous Melanoma	
	Clinical staging[a]	Pathologic staging[b]
0	Tis N0 M0	Tis N0 M0
IA	T1a N0 M0	T1a N0 M0
IB	T1b N0 M0	T1b N0 M0
	T2a N0 M0	T2a N0 M0
IIA	T2b N0 M0	T2b N0 M0
	T3a N0 M0	T3a N0 M0
IIB	T3b N0 M0	T3b N0 M0
	T4a N0 M0	T4a N0 M0
IIC	T4b N0 M0	T4b N0 M0
III[c]	Any T N1 M0	
	N2	
	N3	
IIIA		T1–4a N1a M0
		T1–4a N2a M0
IIIB		T1–4b N1a M0
		T1–4b N2a M0
		T1–4a N1b M0
		T1–4a N2b M0
		T1–4a/b N2c M0
IIIC		T1–4b N1b M0
		T1–4b N2b M0
		Any T N3 M0
IV	Any T Any N Any M1	Any T Any N Any M1

[a]Clinical staging includes microstaging of the primary melanoma and clinical/radiologic evaluation for metastases. By convention, it should be used after complete excision of the primary melanoma with clinical assessment for regional and distant metastases.
[b]Pathologic staging includes microstaging of the primary melanoma and pathologic information about the regional lymph nodes after partial or complete lymphadenectomy, except for pathologic stage 0 or stage Ia patients, who do not need pathologic evaluation of their lymph nodes.
[c]There are no stage III subgroups for clinical staging.
Modified from Balch CM, Buzaid AC, Soong SJ, et al. New TNM melanoma staging system: linking biology and natural history to clinical outcomes. *Semin Surg Oncol* 2003;21:43–52.

E. Treatment
1. Surgery
a. Wide local excision is the primary treatment for most melanomas and premalignant lesions. Melanoma *in situ* (MIS) should be excised to clean margins. For all other malignant melanomas, the width of the surgical margin depends on the Breslow tumor thickness: Thin melanomas (Breslow <1 mm) should have a margin of 1 cm; lesions thicker than 1 mm and all scalp lesions should have a margin of at least 2 cm. Several prospective, randomized trials have investigated margin requirements. A seminal trial addressed the efficacy of 2-cm versus 4-cm margins for Breslow's thickness 1 to 4 mm (*Ann Surg* 1993;218(3):262). There was an insignificant difference in the local recurrence rate between the two groups. This trial was recently updated to provide 10 years of follow-up, again revealing no significant differences in the local recurrence rate or disease-free or overall survival (*Ann Surg Oncol* 2001;8:101). These data suggest that a 2-cm margin is both safe and effective for primary melanomas between 1 and 4 mm, with a significant decrease in the need for skin grafting. In general, excisions should be closed primarily, with flaps or

skin grafts reserved for large defects. Mohs micrographic surgery has been advocated for areas where wide and deep excisions are difficult. Trials using this technique for melanoma are ongoing.

b. Elective lymph node dissection (ELND). The term "elective" refers here to lymph node dissection done in the absence of clinically evident, palpable nodes (for palpable nodes, see Section I.E.1.d of this part on therapeutic lymph node dissection). In the past, ELND was at times performed for the staging of patients presenting with localized melanoma. ELND provided an element of local control and reasonably accurate staging for patients with occult lymph node metastases (*Ann Surg* 1991;214:491). Several large trials, such as the World Health Organization trial number 1, World Health Organization trial number 14, the Mayo Clinical Surgical Trial, and the Intergroup Melanoma Surgical Trial, investigated whether ELND provides benefit to patients, particularly regarding survival. The Intergroup Trial showed that elective lymph node dissection in patients with intermediate-thickness tumors (Breslow 1 to 4 mm) improved survival, especially for patients under the age of 60 years. Elective lymph node dissection has not been conclusively shown to benefit other subgroups (*Ann Surg* 1996;224:255). This remains a controversial issue.

c. Sentinel lymph node biopsy (SLNB). SLNB has greatly enhanced accurate staging of melanoma patients. This technique is based on the documented pattern of lymphatic drainage of melanomas to a specific, initial lymph node, termed the *sentinel lymph node*, before further spread. The histology of the SLN is highly (although not perfectly) reflective of the rest of the nodal basin. If the SLN is negative for metastases, a more radical and morbid lymph node dissection can be avoided. This procedure requires expertise and a multidisciplinary approach involving radiology/nuclear medicine and pathology. The SLN can be accurately identified 96% of the time using radiolymphoscintigraphy and intraoperative dye injection and radioprobe guidance. SLNB appears to be most beneficial for intermediate-thickness melanomas (Breslow 1 to 4 mm) (*Ann Surg* 2001;233:250). Data from the Multicenter Sentinel Lymphadenectomy Trial (MSLT)-I, a prospective, randomized, multinational trial, support the role of SLN and immediate (vs. delayed) complete lymphadenectomy if the SLN is positive. In MSLT-I, 1,269 patients with intermediate-thickness melanomas (1.2 to 3.5 mm) were randomized to either wide excision only followed by observation (no SLNB) or to wide excision and SLNB. In the observation-only group, complete lymphadenectomy was performed only when there was clinical evidence of nodal recurrence (delayed), whereas the SLNB group underwent a complete (immediate) lymphadenectomy if nodal micrometastases were detected in any of the SLNs. The results from this landmark trial showed that the mean estimated 5-year disease-free survival rate was significantly higher in the SLNB group than in the observation-only group (78.3% vs. 73.1%, respectively; $p = 0.009$) (*N Engl J Med* 2006;355:1307). Although 5-year melanoma-specific survival rates were similar in the two groups, the presence of metastatic disease within the SLN was found to be the most important prognostic factor predictive of overall survival. The 5-year survival rate was 72.3% in those patients with tumor-positive SLNs and 90.2% in those with tumor-negative SLNs. In summary, SLNB appears to be a better diagnostic procedure than clinical staging or ELND in terms of sensitivity and morbidity, but some controversy remains over its absolute benefit.

d. Therapeutic lymph node dissection should be performed for involved axillary and superficial inguinal lymph nodes unless unresectable distant metastases are present. Ideally, therapeutic LND provides optimal locoregional control of disease and a chance of cure, with 5-year survival rates of 20% to 40% (*Ann Surg Oncol* 1998;5:473). Surgical therapy of the inguinal region includes a superficial inguinal lymphadenectomy with inclusion of the deep pelvic region for either clinical evidence of disease (palpable pelvic nodes) or radiographic or intraoperative evidence of obvious lymph node involvement. Intraoperative pathologic analysis of clinically suspicious lymph nodes may be necessary to determine the presence of metastases and possibly the need for more extensive nodal dissection. The highest superficial inguinal node ("Cloquet's node") can also be analyzed by frozen section to help determine the need for deep dissection. Deep inguinal node dissection should be reserved for patients whose survival is thought to justify the potential morbidity of the procedure. Hughes et al. noted that patients who underwent a superficial and deep nodal dissection ($n = 72$) had a lower regional recurrence rate than those who underwent a superficial dissection only ($n = 60$), although there was no statistical difference in overall survival (*Br J Surg* 2000;87:892). In some cases, nodal dissection will not benefit patients with advanced disease and should therefore be carefully considered.

- **e. Resection of metastases.** The surgical options for patients with metastatic melanoma can be divided into two categories: curative or palliative. Curative interventions for metastatic melanoma should carefully weigh the risks of the surgery against the potential benefits. Recent data on the surgical management of metastatic melanoma note that certain factors are associated with an improved overall survival: (1) ability to achieve a complete resection with negative margins, (2) the initial site of metastasis, (3) extent of metastatic disease (single or multiple sites), (4) disease-free interval after surgical removal of the primary melanoma, and (5) stage of initial disease (*Curr Opin Oncol* 2004;16:155). Favorable sites for resection include the skin, subcutaneous tissue, lymph nodes, lung, and gastrointestinal tract. Skin and subcutaneous metastases demonstrated the best long-term results after resection, with a 20% to 30% 5-year survival and a median survival of 48 months. Unfavorable sites include metastases to the brain, adrenal, and liver (*Arch Surg* 2004;139:961).

2. **Isolated limb perfusion (ILP)** is used for recurrent limb melanoma that is locally advanced and cannot be resected by simple surgical means. ILP delivers high-dose regional chemotherapy and establishes a hyperthermic environment to an extremity while its circulation has been isolated from the rest of the body. Melphalan is commonly used. A large, retrospective meta-analysis reported complete response rates for melphalan with mild hyperthermic ILP range from 40% to 82% (median 54%) (*Eur J Surg Oncol* 2006;32:371). Adding tumor necrosis factor (TNF)-α to melphalan has been suggested to increase the complete response rate to 60% to 85%. Randomized, multicenter data collected through the American College of Surgeons Oncology Group (ACOSOG) comparing hyperthermic ILP with melphalan alone to melphalan plus TNF suggested that addition of TNF did not significantly enhance short-term response rates in locally advanced extremity melanoma; however, addition of TNF was found significantly to increase the overall complication rate (*J Clin Oncol* 2006;24:4196). Patients who are elderly or who have medical comorbidities or systemic metastases are generally not suitable for this therapy.

3. **Immunotherapy.** Endeavors in both animals and humans have established that the immune system can damage or destroy even very large established tumors (*N Engl J Med* 1984;313:1485, *J Exp Med* 2005;202:907). Complete and durable regression of stage IV melanoma has been reported using interleukin-2 (IL-2)–based immunotherapy alone (*J Clin Oncol* 1999;17:2105). Although patients can be cured of metastatic melanoma solely using high-dose IL-2, the response rate is low. This has led to the use of IL-2 in conjunction with other treatments, including vaccines, monoclonal antibodies, and adoptive transfer of T lymphocytes. Recently, a 50% response rate according to Response Evaluation Criteria in Solid Tumors (RECIST) criteria was reported in patients with metastatic melanoma treated with in vitro expanded tumor-infiltrating lymphocytes and IL-2 following a lymphodepleting nonmyeloablative preparative regimen of cyclophosphamide and fludarabine (*Science* 2002;298:850). Intensive studies are ongoing.

F. **Hereditary tumor syndromes: melanoma.** Melanoma is familial in approximately 10% of cases, and in these cases it is often associated with multiple atypical moles. **Familial atypical multiple-mole melanoma syndrome (FAMMM)** has also been called *dysplastic nevus syndrome, B-K syndrome,* and *large atypical nevus syndrome.* A

National Institutes of Health Consensus Conference defined FAMMM using the following criteria: (1) the occurrence of malignant melanoma in one or more first- or second-degree relatives, (2) a large number of melanocytic nevi, usually more than 50, some of which are atypical and variable in size, and (3) melanocytic nevi that have certain histopathologic features, including architectural disorder with asymmetry, subepidermal fibroplasia, and lentiginous melanocytic hyperplasia with spindle or epithelial melanocyte nests. These lesions predominantly occur on the trunk but are also found on the buttocks, scalp, and lower extremities. The relative risk for developing melanoma when multiple atypical moles are present ranges from 5 to 11 based on multiple studies. The median age for melanoma diagnosis is 34. *CDKN2*, a cell cycle protein gene, has been found to contain germline mutations in some kindreds with familial melanoma (*Nat Genet* 1994;8:15). Other malignancies have been related to mutations in the *CDKN2* gene, especially pancreatic cancer. There may be other genes contributing to FAMMM. **Screening** for FAMMM begins at around puberty and consists of yearly physical examinations, including a total-body skin examination. For patients who have a large number of moles, baseline photographs or computerized scanning are helpful. Patients should examine their skin regularly. Suspicious lesions should undergo biopsy. Sun exposure should be avoided. Regular ophthalmologic examinations should be performed due to the increased risk of ocular nevi and ocular melanoma.

OTHER MALIGNANT SKIN TUMORS

I. BASAL CELL CARCINOMA is the most common malignant neoplasm of the skin; it derives from the basal cells of the epidermis and adnexal structures. They are slow growing and very rarely metastasize ($<0.1\%$) but can be locally aggressive. Sun exposure is the most significant epidemiologic factor; consequently, this neoplasm is found most commonly on the skin of the head and neck (85%) in fair-skinned patients older than 40 years.

    A. Lesions. It is particularly important to identify the morpheaform carcinoma because it is more aggressive, with a tendency toward deep infiltration and local recurrence. These carcinomas are flat, indurated lesions with a smooth, whitish, waxy surface and indistinct borders. The noduloulcerative form is the most common and is characterized by shiny, translucent nodules with a central umbilication that often becomes ulcerated, with pearly, rolled, telangiectatic edges.

    B. Treatment

        1. Excisional biopsy is adequate treatment for small tumors, with intraoperative frozen-section analysis (to confirm negative margins) and primary closure. Larger tumors may be diagnosed by incisional or punch biopsy followed by complete removal. A margin of 2 to 4 mm on all sides of visible tumor should be obtained, and positive margins on frozen-section analysis should be re-excised. Margins of dysplasia or actinic changes need not be re-excised because local recurrence generally does not occur in these cases. The patient should be warned about possible pigmentation persistence.

        2. Mohs micrographic surgery may be useful for recurrent tumors or in situations in which tissue conservation is important.

        3. Curettage with electrodessication can be performed for small superficial tumors, with little risk of recurrence.

        4. Liquid nitrogen can be used for tumors less than 1 cm in diameter.

        5. Radiation therapy can be used in certain situations for areas difficult to reconstruct, such as the eyelids. It also can be used for palliation in patients who have large tumors and who might refuse an extensive operation, especially the elderly. Although re-excision is indicated for recurrences or positive margins, radiation therapy can be used in individual circumstances.

II. SQUAMOUS CELL CARCINOMA is the second-most-common skin cancer in fair-skinned people and is the most common cancer in darkly pigmented people. As with the other skin malignancies, sunlight is the major etiology, with the greatest risk in elderly men who have a history of chronic sun exposure. The mean age of presentation is 68 years, and men predominate two to one. Squamous cell carcinoma can be found on any sun-exposed area, including mucous membranes. It also is known to develop from draining sinuses, radiation, chronic ulcers, and scars (particularly burn scars, in which case it is called a **Marjolin ulcer**).

A. **Lesions.** Squamous cell carcinoma presents as small, firm, erythematous plaques with a smooth or verrucous surface and indistinct margins with progression to raised, fixed, and ulcerated lesions. Ulceration tends to occur earlier in aggressive lesions. Most lesions are preceded by actinic keratosis, which results in a slow-growing, locally invasive lesion without metastases. If not preceded by actinic keratosis, the cancer tends to be more aggressive, with more rapid growth, invasion, and metastatic spread. Perineural invasion has a poorer prognosis and higher recurrence rate.

B. **Treatment** is similar to that for basal cell carcinoma. Tumor-free margins of 5 mm for tumors of less than 1 cm and tumor-free margins of 1 to 2 cm for tumors of more than 2 cm in diameter should be obtained. Curettage with electrodessication and laser vaporization have been used for small, superficial squamous carcinomas, but there is no way to assess margins of treatment. Solitary metastases should be resected if possible because there is a relatively high cure rate compared with other cancers.

SOFT-TISSUE SARCOMAS

Soft tissue sarcomas (STSs) represent a heterogeneous group of malignant tumors derived from mesodermal tissues. STS are rare, constituting approximately 1% of adult malignant neoplasms and causing 3,100 deaths annually; many general surgeons will see few of these tumors during their careers. Most of these tumors arise de novo, rarely from premalignant tumors. In a minority of cases, STSs are associated with cancer predisposition syndromes such as von Recklinghausen disease, Werner syndrome, or Li-Fraumeni syndrome. Lymphedema and radiation have been shown to be etiologic factors in certain rare sarcomas (*Am Surg* 2006;72:665).

I. **LESIONS.** Sarcomas are classified by histologic cell type of origin and grade. The most common subtype is malignant fibrous histiocytoma (40%), followed by liposarcoma (25%). Patients typically present with an asymptomatic lump or mass that has grown to be visible or palpable. Retroperitoneal tumor can reach massive proportions before increased abdominal girth and vague symptoms bring it to the physician's attention. Tumors also may grow unnoticed to large sizes in the thigh or trunk.

II. **DIAGNOSIS.** Biopsy (usually core or incisional) is necessary for diagnosis. Care is needed to orient incisions to aid in the definitive operation. Even small, apparently benign lesions should be biopsied or excised. Adequate tissue must be provided to pathology for histologic assessment.

III. **STAGING AND PROGNOSIS** (Table 25-4). The AJCC staging system is based on tumor size, nodal status, histologic grade, and metastasis. Of these, size and grade are the most important.

A. **Grade.** The grade of the tumor is the major prognostic factor. Grade is obtained from histopathologic analysis of biopsy tissue and is generally based on the mitotic index, nuclear morphology, and degree of anaplasia. However, interobserver variability is high, with some centers having different criteria: Rates of discordance even between expert pathologists of up to 40% have been observed.

B. **Staging** for STS includes physical examination and computed tomography (CT) or magnetic resonance (MR) scan to assess the size and extent of tumor. Metastases most commonly are found in the lungs; CT scan of the lungs is a required study for grade II and III lesions. Abdominal CT scan is required for evaluation of retroperitoneal sarcomas. This study can assess for hepatic metastases, which are more common for this primary. Retroperitoneal and truncal STS have worse prognoses than extremity STS.

C. **Prognosis.** Almost 80% of metastases are to the lungs and occur within 2 to 3 years of diagnosis. If the pulmonary disease is resectable, 30% survival at 3 years can be expected. In addition, tumor size, grade, margins after resection, and anatomic location

TABLE 25-4	Soft Tissue Sarcoma Staging

Tumor grade (G)	Stage IA[a]
GX: Grade cannot be assessed	G1, T1a, N0, M0
G1: Well differentiated	G1, T1b, N0, M0
G2: Moderately differentiated	G2, T1a, N0, M0
G3: Poorly differentiated	G2, T1b, N0, M0
G4: Undifferentiated	Stage IB[b]
Primary tumor (T)	G1, T2a, N0, M0
TX: Primary tumor cannot be assessed	G2, T2a, N0, M0
T0: No evidence of primary tumor	Stage IIA[c]
T1: Tumor ≤5 cm in greatest dimension	G1, T2b, N0, M0
T1a: Superficial tumor[d]	G2, T2b, N0, M0
T1b: Deep tumor[d]	Stage IIB[e]
T2: Tumor >5 cm in greatest dimension	G3, T1a, N0, M0
T2a: Superficial tumor[d]	G3, T1b, N0, M0
T2b: Deep tumor[d]	G4, T1a, N0, M0
Regional lymph nodes (N)	G4, T1b, N0, M0
NX: Regional lymph nodes cannot be assessed	Stage IIC[f]
N0: No regional lymph node metastasis	G3, T2a, N0, M0
N1: Regional lymph node metastasis	G4, T2a, N0, M0
Distant metastasis (M)	Stage III[g]
MX: Distant metastasis cannot be assessed	G3, T2b, N0, M0
M0: No distant metastasis	G4, T2b, N0, M0
M1: Distant metastasis	Stage IV[h]
	Any G, any T, N1, M0
	Any G, any T, N0, M1

[a]Stage IA tumor is defined as low grade, small, superficial, and deep.
[b]Stage IB tumor is defined as low grade, large, and superficial.
[c]Stage IIA tumor is defined as low grade, large, and deep.
[d]Superficial tumor is located exclusively above the superficial fascia without invasion of the fascia; deep tumor either is located exclusively beneath the superficial fascia or superficial to the fascia with invasion of or through the fascia or is located superficial and beneath the fascia. Retroperitoneal, mediastinal, and pelvic sarcomas are classified as deep tumors.
[e]Stage IIB tumor is defined as high grade, small, superficial, and deep.
[f]Stage IIC tumor is defined as high grade, large, and superficial.
[g]Stage III tumor is defined as high grade, large, and deep.
[h]Stage IV tumor is defined as any metastasis to lymph nodes or distant sites.
M, metastasis; N, node; T, tumor.

all have an impact on various outcome measures such as local recurrence, overall survival, and tumor-free survival. Local recurrence should be resected aggressively, and long-term follow-up is required because late recurrences may occur.

IV. SURGICAL TREATMENT

- **A. Resection.** Smaller, grade I tumors can be excised with a minimum 1-cm margin, usually without adjuvant radiation. Larger tumors may benefit from a larger margin or radiation to prevent recurrence. Grade II and III tumors, in general, require radiation therapy in addition to excision to avoid more-radical surgery. Depending on the size and grade of tumor, compartment resection may be indicated.

- **B. Limb-sparing resection** combined with radiation therapy offers survival equivalent to that achieved with amputation (*Ann Surg* 1982;196:305). Limb-sparing procedures have a distinct psychological as well as functional advantage and are the procedures of choice for most tumors. The tumor should be removed with an envelope of normal tissue surrounding it, if possible. The resection should include the area of previous incision and biopsy and any drain sites. The resection field should be marked with clips to guide radiation therapy.

C. Gastrointestinal stromal tumors (GISTs) are sarcomatous tumors of the gastrointestinal tract. These tumors are rare and most commonly arise from the stomach. GIST can present with acute or subacute gastrointestinal bleeding, vague abdominal pain, a palpable abdominal mass, or as an incidental mass found on CT scan of the abdomen. These tumors are distinguished from other tumors of the gastrointestinal tract (GI) tract by expression of c-*kit* (CD117). Surgical resection with microscopically negative margins is standard treatment. Gleevec (imatinib mesylate) has been approved to treat patients with unresectable or metastatic GIST.

D. Retroperitoneal sarcomas are considerably more difficult to treat because the tumors often involve vital structures. Operative intervention employs resection of as much tumor as possible with a wide margin. Organs associated with the tumor should be resected *en bloc* to completely remove the tumor. An initial tissue diagnosis is often obtained by core biopsy. Postoperative irradiation may be used in some cases but is associated with relatively high morbidity, often due to irradiation of normal intestines and other organs. Wide margins are often not achievable in the retroperitoneum and limit the effectiveness of surgery. For these reasons, preoperative irradiation therapy, with the tumor in place displacing normal organs, is increasingly favored. Studies are beginning to reveal recurrence and survival benefits. Some surgeons, however, remain concerned about irradiation making surgical dissection more difficult. For tumor recurrences, surgical resection is the therapy of choice. Recently, Gronchi et al. studied 167 consecutive patients who underwent operation for retroperitoneal soft tissue sarcoma; complete resection of all gross disease was achieved in 88% of patients. Overall survival at 10 years was 27% and disease-free survival was 16%. The 10-year disease-free survival rate was 27% for patients who underwent resection for primary sarcomas compared with 5% for patients who underwent resection for recurrent retroperitoneal sarcoma (*Cancer* 2004;100:2448). The data suggest that novel treatment approaches are needed for prevention of local, regional, and distant recurrences.

V. OTHER ADJUVANT THERAPY

A. Interstitial perioperative radiation therapy (brachytherapy) involves the use of catheters or implants placed at the time of surgery to provide radiation directly to the tumor bed. Afterloading involves loading of the radiation source through catheters postoperatively to deliver localized high-dose radiation to the tumor bed. Brachytherapy has at least two advantages: It requires a short course of in-hospital treatment rather than 5 to 6 weeks of outpatient external-beam radiation therapy, and it can provide dose control near sensitive areas, such as joints and blood vessels. There is evidence that it is effective at decreasing local recurrence for high-grade tumors when combined with surgery.

B. Chemotherapy. Several randomized, prospective trials have failed to show any improvement in survival with adjuvant chemotherapy for adult grade II or III sarcomas. The two drugs with the greatest efficacy are doxorubicin and ifosfamide; however, even these have at best a 40% to 60% response rate. Recent data from two institutional prospective sarcoma databases identified patients who underwent resection for high-grade extremity liposarcoma greater than 5 cm in size. Using contemporary cohort analysis, the authors concluded that doxorubicin is not associated with improved disease-specific survival, but that ifosfamide is associated with improved disease-specific survival (*Ann Surg* 2004;240:697).

C. Isolated limb perfusion provides increased delivery of therapy (e.g., hyperthermic therapy and chemotherapy) to an extremity sarcoma while reducing systemic toxicity. There is some suggestion of decreased local recurrence with definite downstaging of the tumor, but there is no improvement in survival (*Ann Surg Oncol* 2007;14:230).

VI. HEREDITARY TUMOR SYNDROMES: SARCOMAS. Soft-tissue sarcomas have been identified in several familial cancer syndromes, including Li-Fraumeni syndrome, hereditary retinoblastoma, and neurofibromatosis types 1 and 2. The prognosis is highly dependent on the tumor grade.

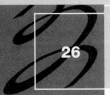

HERNIAS
Ryan C. Fields and Brent D. Matthews

26

I. INGUINAL HERNIAS
A. Incidence. The true incidence and prevalence of inguinal hernia are unknown.
According to the Healthcare Cost and Utilization Project (HCUP), 826,000 inguinal hernia repairs were performed in the United States in 2003, of which 215,000 were bilateral. Laparoscopic studies have reported rates of contralateral defects as high as 22%, with 28% of these going on to become symptomatic during short-term follow-up. The male-to-female ratio is greater than 10:1. Lifetime prevalence is 25% in men and 2% in women. Two thirds of inguinal hernias are indirect. Nearly two thirds of recurrent hernias are direct. Inguinal hernias have an approximate incidence of incarceration of 10%, and a portion of these may become strangulated. Recurrence rates are less than 1% in children and vary in adults according to the method of hernia repair.

B. Terminology and anatomy (Fig. 26-1)
1. **Direct hernias** are those in which viscera protrude through a weakness in the posterior inguinal wall. The base of the hernia sac is medial to the inferior epigastric vessels through the Hesselbach triangle, which is limited by the inferior epigastric artery, the lateral edge of the rectus sheath, and the inguinal ligament.
2. **Indirect hernia sacs** pass through the internal inguinal ring lateral to the inferior epigastric vessels and lie within the spermatic cord. The sac is covered by cremaster muscle fibers.
3. **In combined (pantaloon) hernias,** direct and indirect hernias coexist.
4. A **sliding hernia** (usually indirect inguinal in location) is a hernia in which a part of the wall of the hernia sac is formed by an intra-abdominal viscus (usually colon, sometimes bladder). In a Richter hernia, part (rather than the entire circumference) of the bowel wall is trapped. A Littré hernia is one that contains a Meckel diverticulum. An Amyand hernia is one that contains the appendix.
5. **Incarcerated hernias** cannot be reduced into the abdominal cavity, whereas strangulated hernias have incarcerated contents with vascular compromise. Frequently, intense pain is caused by ischemia of the incarcerated segment.

C. Diagnosis
1. **Clinical presentation**
   a. **Most inguinal hernias** present as an intermittent bulge that appears in the groin, usually related to exertion or long periods of standing. The patient may complain of unilateral discomfort without noting a mass. Often, a purposeful Valsalva maneuver can reproduce the symptoms. In infants and children, a groin bulge often is noted by caregivers during episodes of crying or defecation. Rarely, patients present with bowel obstruction without noting a groin abnormality. All patients with a small-bowel obstruction must be questioned carefully and examined for hernias.
   b. **Physical examination.** The main diagnostic maneuver for inguinal hernias is palpation of the inguinal region. The patient is best examined while standing and straining (cough or Valsalva). Hernias manifest as bulges with smooth, rounded surfaces that become more evident with straining. The hernia sac can also be examined more clearly by invaginating the hemiscrotum to introduce an index finger through the external inguinal ring. This may become uncomfortable for the patient and is unnecessary if an obvious bulge is present.

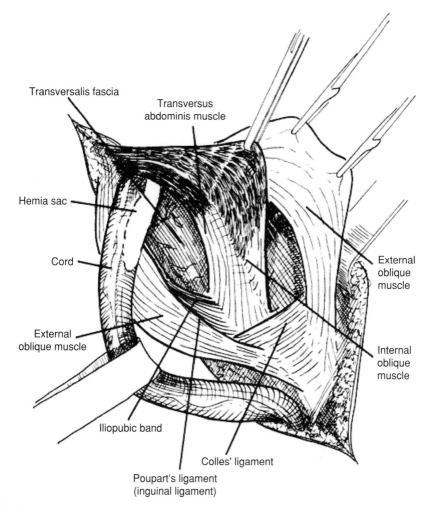

Transversalis fascia

Transversus
abdominis muscle

Hemia sac

Cord

External
oblique muscle

External
oblique
muscle

Internal
oblique
muscle

Iliopubic band

Colles' ligament

Poupart's ligament
(inguinal ligament)

Figure 26-1. Anatomy of the right inguinal region.

Incarcerated inguinal hernias present with abdominal distention, nausea, and vomiting due to intestinal obstruction.

  2. Radiographic evaluation. X-ray studies are rarely indicated. Ultrasonography or CT scanning may occasionally be used to diagnose an occult groin hernia, particularly in the obese patient. Plain abdominal x-rays may verify intestinal obstruction in cases of incarceration.

  D. Differential diagnosis. Inguinal hernias should be distinguished from femoral hernias, which protrude below the inguinal ligament. Inguinal adenopathy, lipomas, dilation of the saphenous vein, epididymitis, testicular torsion, groin abscess, and vascular aneurysms/pseudoaneurysms all should be considered in appropriate situations.

  E. Treatment

  1. Preoperative evaluation and preparation. Most patients with hernias should be treated surgically, although "watchful waiting" may be appropriate for individuals with asymptomatic hernias or elderly patients with minimally symptomatic hernias. Associated abnormalities that can increase intra-abdominal pressure (such as chronic cough, constipation, or bladder outlet obstruction) should be evaluated and remedied to the extent possible before elective herniorrhaphy. In cases of intestinal obstruction and possible strangulation, broad-spectrum antibiotics and nasogastric suction may be indicated. Correction of volume status and electrolyte abnormalities is important when there is an associated small-bowel obstruction.

2. **Reduction.** Temporary management includes manual reduction. In uncomplicated cases, the hernia reduces with palpation over the inguinal canal with the patient supine. If this does not occur, the physician applies gentle pressure over the hernia with the concavity of the palm of his or her hand and fingers. The palm of the physician's hand exerts a steady but gentle pressure and also maintains the direction to be followed: craniad and lateral for direct hernias, craniad and posterior for femoral hernias. If the herniated viscera do not reduce, gentle traction over the mass with compression may allow bowel gas to leave the herniated segment, making the mass reducible. Sedation and the Trendelenburg position may be required for reduction of an incarcerated hernia, but the difficulty of distinguishing between acute incarceration and strangulation should be noted: The inguinal canal can become quite tender with or without ischemic contents. When an incarcerated hernia is reduced nonsurgically, the patient should be observed for the potential development of peritonitis caused by perforation of a loop of strangulated bowel. If there is strong suspicion of strangulation, no attempt should be made to reduce the hernia because of the potential for en masse reduction of a gangrenous segment of bowel with the hernia sac.

3. **Surgical treatment**
   a. **Choice of anesthetic.** Local anesthesia, which has several advantages over general or regional (spinal or epidural) anesthesia, is the preferred anesthetic for elective open repair. Local anesthesia results in better postoperative analgesia, a shorter recovery room stay, and a negligible rate of postoperative urinary retention; it is the lowest-risk anesthetic for patients with underlying cardiopulmonary disorders. Commonly, a mixture of a short-acting agent (lidocaine 1%) and longer-acting agent (bupivacaine 0.25% to 0.50%) is used. The dose limits for local anesthesia are 4.5 mg/kg plain lidocaine or 7 mg/kg lidocaine with epinephrine and 2 mg/kg plain bupivacaine or 3 mg/kg bupivacaine with epinephrine. Use of local anesthesia for herniorrhaphy in our hospital is routinely supplemented by monitored anesthesia care and administration of intravenous midazolam and propofol. Virtually all patients who undergo hernia repair under local anesthesia can be managed as outpatients unless associated medical conditions or extenuating social circumstances necessitate overnight observation in the hospital. Laparoscopic hernia repair has been carried out under local or regional anesthesia but is more commonly done under general anesthesia.
   b. **Treatment of the hernia sac.** The anatomy of the inguinal region is displayed as viewed by the operating surgeon in Figure 26-1. In indirect hernias, the sac is dissected free from the cord structures and cremasteric fibers. The sac should be opened away from any herniated contents. The contents are then reduced, and the sac is ligated deep to the internal ring with an absorbable suture. Alternatively, the hernia sac may be invaginated back into the abdomen without ligation. Large, indirect sacs that extend into the scrotum should not be dissected beyond the pubic tubercle because of an increased risk of ischemic orchitis. Similarly, one should avoid translocating the testicle into the inguinal canal during hernia repair owing to the risk of ischemia. Cord lipomas are frequently encountered during repair and should be excised or reduced into the retroperitoneum to avoid future confusion with a recurrent hernia. Sliding hernia sacs can usually be managed by reducing the sac and attached viscera. Direct sacs are usually too broadly based for ligation and should not be opened, but instead are simply freed from attenuated transversalis fibers and inverted.

In preperitoneal repairs, the sac is usually reduced but not ligated because the repair is situated between the peritoneum and abdominal wall.

c. **Inguinal floor reconstruction.** Some method of reconstruction of the inguinal floor is necessary in all adult hernia repairs to prevent recurrence. Various techniques for inguinal floor repair are available, and factors that influence the choice of repair include the type of hernia as well as the surgeon's preference and expertise. Three broad categories of repairs are available: primary tissue repairs, anterior tension-free mesh repairs, and preperitoneal repairs, including the laparoscopic approach.

(1) **Primary tissue repairs.** Primary repairs without mesh were the mainstay of hernia surgery for decades. The advantages of these repairs are simplicity of the repair and the absence of any foreign body in the groin. Disadvantages include higher recurrence rates (5% to 10% for primary repairs and 15% to 30% for repair of recurrent hernias) due to tension on the repair and a slower return to unrestricted physical activity. Consequently, the vast majority of hernia repairs performed today in the United States use some form of tension-free mesh technique. The principal features of the more commonly performed tissue repairs are the following:

(a) **Bassini repair.** The inferior arch of the transversalis fascia or conjoint tendon is approximated to the shelving portion of the inguinal ligament (iliopubic tract) with interrupted, nonabsorbable sutures. The Bassini repair has been used for simple, indirect hernias, including inguinal hernias in women.

(b) **McVay repair.** The transversalis fascia is sutured to the Cooper ligament medial to the femoral vein and the inguinal ligament at the level of, and lateral to, the femoral vein. This operation usually requires placement of a relaxing incision medially on the aponeuroses of the internal oblique muscle to avoid undue tension on the repair. The McVay repair closes the femoral space and therefore, unlike the Bassini repair, is effective for femoral hernias.

(c) **Shouldice repair.** In this repair, the transversalis fascia is incised (and partially excised if weakened) and reapproximated. The overlying tissues (the conjoint tendon, iliopubic tract, and inguinal ligament) are approximated in multiple, imbricated layers of running nonabsorbable suture. The experience of the Shouldice Clinic with this repair has been excellent, with recurrence rates of less than 1%, but higher recurrence rates have been reported in nonspecialized centers.

(2) **Open tension-free repairs.** The most common mesh inguinal hernia repairs performed today are the tension-free mesh hernioplasty (Lichtenstein repair) and the patch-and-plug technique. In the Lichtenstein repair, a piece of polypropylene mesh approximately 5 × 3 in. is used to reconstruct the inguinal floor (Fig. 26-2). The mesh is sutured to the fascia overlying the pubic tubercle inferiorly, the transversalis fascia and conjoint tendon medially, and the inguinal ligament laterally. The mesh is slit at the level of the internal ring, and the two limbs are crossed around the spermatic cord and then tacked to the inguinal ligament, effectively creating a new internal ring of mesh. This repair avoids the approximation of attenuated tissues under tension, and recurrence rates with this technique have been consistently 1% or less. Moreover, because the repair is without tension, patients are allowed to return to unrestricted physical activity in 2 weeks or less. The mesh plug technique entails placement of a preformed plug of mesh in the hernia defect (e.g., internal ring) that is sutured to the rings of the fascial opening. An onlay piece of mesh is then placed over the inguinal floor, which may or may not be sutured to the fascia. Mesh plugs may be ideally suited for the repair of small, tight defects, such as femoral hernias. Another technique involves the use of a bilayer mesh in which the posterior leaflet is placed in the preperitoneal space and the anterior leaflet is sutured to the same layers as with the Lichtenstein repair.

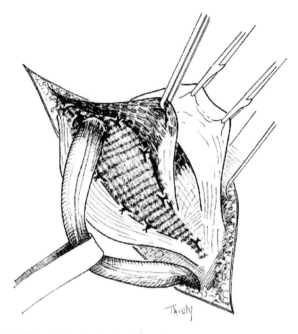

Figure 26-2. Lichtenstein tension-free hernia repair.

(3) Laparoscopic and preperitoneal repairs. Approximately 15% of hernia repairs in the United States are now carried out using a laparoscopic preperitoneal approach. The laparoscopic hernia repair is based on the technique of Stoppa, who used an open preperitoneal approach to reduce the hernia and placed a large piece of mesh to cover the entire inguinal floor and myopectineal orifice. Preperitoneal hernia repairs may also be performed without mesh, an approach that is rarely used today for routine hernia repair but may be a good option in patients with strangulated hernias. Advantages of the preperitoneal approach in this setting are that it may facilitate reduction of the incarcerated or strangulated hernia contents and, if gangrenous bowel is found, resection can be carried out through the preperitoneal incision, whereas this is difficult to accomplish through a standard groin incision.

In **laparoscopic hernia repair,** the preperitoneal space is reached either by a transabdominal [the transabdominal preperitoneal (TAPP) procedure] or a totally extraperitoneal (TEP) repair. With the TAPP repair, the peritoneal cavity is entered by conventional laparoscopy at the umbilicus, and the peritoneum overlying the inguinal floor is dissected away as a flap. With the TEP repair, the preperitoneal space is developed with a balloon inserted between the posterior rectus sheath and the peritoneum (Fig. 26-3). The balloon is then inflated to dissect the peritoneal flap away from the posterior abdominal wall and the direct and indirect spaces, and the other ports are inserted into this preperitoneal space without ever entering the peritoneal cavity. The advantages of the TAPP approach are that there is a large working space, familiar anatomic landmarks are visible, and the contralateral groin can be examined for an occult hernia. The advantages of the TEP repair are that the abdominal cavity is not violated, the peritoneum is not opened, much of the dissection is done by

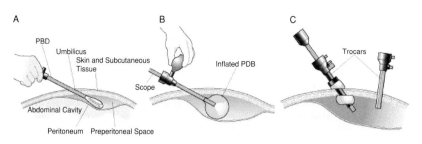

Figure 26-3. Laparoscopic total extraperitoneal (TEP) approach with preperitoneal balloon dilation (PBD) system.

balloon, and the procedure can potentially be performed under regional anesthesia.

After laparoscopic dissection and reduction of the hernia sac, a large piece of mesh (6 × 4 in.) is placed over the inguinal floor. This is stapled superiorly to the posterior abdominal wall fascia on either side of the inferior epigastric vessels, medially to the Cooper ligament and the midline, and superolateral to the fascia above the internal ring. Staples must not be placed in or posterior to the iliopubic tract or lateral to the iliac crest because of the risk of neurovascular injuries to the ilioinguinal, genitofemoral, lateral femoral cutaneous, and femoral nerves as well as the external iliac vessels. Comparative studies of laparoscopic and open hernia repair have shown that laparoscopic repairs are associated with less postoperative pain and faster recovery than open repairs, but hospital costs have been higher for the laparoscopic technique. Operative times, complications, and recurrence rates (<3% for laparoscopic repair) have been similar. A meta-analysis of 29 randomized clinical trials comparing laparoscopic and open inguinal hernia repairs concluded that laparoscopic repair was associated with earlier discharge from hospital, quicker return to normal activity and work, and significantly fewer postoperative complications than open inguinal hernia repair. However, the operating time was significantly longer and there was a nonsignificant trend toward an increase in the relative odds of recurrence after laparoscopic repair (*Br J Surg* 2003;90:1479). Another randomized trial comparing open and laparoscopic mesh inguinal hernia repairs at 14 Veterans Affairs (VA) institutions concluded that the open technique is superior to the laparoscopic technique for mesh repair of primary hernias due to decreased recurrence (4% vs. 10.1%) and complication rates (33.4% vs. 39%) (*N Engl J Med* 2004;350:1819).

Special circumstances in which laparoscopic repair may also be favored include (1) recurrent hernias to avoid the scar tissue in the inguinal canal, (2) bilateral hernias, because both sides of the groin can be repaired with the same three small incisions used for the unilateral repair, (3) individuals with a unilateral hernia for whom a rapid recovery is critical (e.g., athletes and laborers), and (4) obese patients. Laparoscopic hernia repair is contraindicated in patients who have large scrotal hernias or who have undergone prior extensive lower abdominal surgery.

The **Kugel repair** is a preperitoneal repair in which a preformed polypropylene patch with a stiff ring around the edges is placed in the preperitoneal space through an open incision. The preperitoneal space is accessed through an oblique skin incision about 2 to 3 cm above the inguinal ring halfway between the anterior superior iliac spine and the pubic tubercle. After the preperitoneal space is entered, the peritoneum is dissected free by blunt dissection, and the hernia sac is gently reduced. The mesh patch is then placed into the preperitoneal space to cover the hernia defect. The Kugel technique is a preperitoneal alternative to the laparoscopic repair that can be performed under local anesthesia.

d. **Complications.** Surgical complications include wound hematoma, infection, nerve injury (ilioinguinal, iliohypogastric, genital branch of the genitofemoral, lateral femoral cutaneous, femoral), vascular injury (femoral vessels, testicular artery, pampiniform venous plexus), vas deferens injury, ischemic orchitis, and testicular atrophy. Recurrence rates after tension-free mesh repairs for primary hernias are 1% to 2% or less.

e. **Recurrent inguinal hernias** are more difficult to repair because the scar makes dissection difficult and the disease process has continued. Recurrence within 1 year of initial repair suggests an inadequate initial attempt, such as overlooking an indirect hernia sac. Recurrence after 2 or more years suggests progression of the disease process that caused the initial hernia (e.g., increased intra-abdominal pressure, degeneration of tissues). Recurrences should be repaired because the defect usually is small with fixed edges that are prone to complications, such as incarceration or strangulation. Repair can be done by an anterior approach through the old operative field or by a posterior (open preperitoneal or laparoscopic) approach. Prosthetic mesh is almost always used to reinforce attenuated tissues unless the operative field is contaminated.

4. **Watchful waiting.** Another option in patients with minimal symptoms and an easily reducible inguinal hernia is "watchful waiting," consisting of routine follow-up with a health care professional. This strategy was compared to operative repair in a randomized trial, which concluded that this is an acceptable option for men with minimally symptomatic inguinal hernias and that delaying repair until symptoms increase is safe due to a low rate of incarceration. In this study, 23% of patients initially treated with "watchful waiting" crossed over to surgical treatment due to an increase in symptoms, most often hernia-related pain. Only one patient (0.3%) experienced acute hernia incarceration without strangulation within 2 years; a second had acute incarceration with bowel obstruction at 4 years, corresponding to a frequency of acute intervention of 1.8/1,000 patient-years (*JAMA* 2006;295:285).

II. FEMORAL HERNIAS

A. **Incidence.** Femoral hernias constitute up to 2% to 4% of all groin hernias; 70% occur in women. Approximately 25% of femoral hernias become incarcerated or strangulated, and a similar number are missed or diagnosed late.

B. **Anatomy.** The abdominal viscera and peritoneum protrude through the femoral canal into the upper thigh. The boundaries of the femoral canal are the lacunar ligament medially, the femoral vein laterally, the iliopubic tract anteriorly, and the Cooper ligament posteriorly.

C. **Diagnosis**

1. **Clinical presentation**

a. **Symptoms.** Patients may complain of an intermittent groin bulge or a groin mass that may be tender. Because femoral hernias have a high incidence of incarceration, small-bowel obstruction may be the presenting feature in some patients. Elderly patients, in whom femoral hernias occur most commonly, may not complain of groin pain, even in the setting of incarceration. Therefore, an occult femoral hernia should be considered in the differential diagnosis of any patient with small-bowel obstruction, especially if there is no history of previous abdominal surgery.

b. **Physical examination.** The characteristic finding is a small, rounded bulge that appears in the upper thigh just below the inguinal ligament. An incarcerated femoral hernia usually presents as a firm, tender mass. The differential diagnosis is the same as for inguinal hernia.

c. **Radiographic evaluation.** Radiographic studies are rarely indicated. Occasionally, a femoral hernia is found on a CT scan or gastrointestinal contrast study performed to evaluate a small-bowel obstruction.

D. Treatment. The surgical approach can be inguinal, preperitoneal, or femoral.

   1. Inguinal approach. A Cooper ligament repair (McVay) using the inguinal canal approach allows reduction of the hernia sac with visualization from above the inguinal ligament and closure of the femoral space. Occasionally, it may be necessary to divide the inguinal ligament to reduce the hernia. The repair can be performed with or without mesh.

   2. Preperitoneal approach. A transverse suprainguinal incision permits access to the extraperitoneal spaces of Bogros and Retzius. The hernia is reduced from inside the femoral space, and the hernia defect is repaired preperitoneally, usually with mesh, but can be repaired primarily. This approach is especially useful for incarcerated or strangulated femoral hernias. Uncomplicated femoral hernias can also be repaired laparoscopically.

   3. Femoral approach. A horizontal incision is made over the hernia, inferior and parallel to the inguinal ligament. After the hernia sac is dissected free, it can be resected or invaginated. The femoral canal is closed by placing interrupted stitches to approximate the Cooper ligament to the inguinal ligament or by using a plug of prosthetic material.

   4. Complications. Complications are similar to those for inguinal hernia repair. The femoral vein may be especially susceptible to injury because it forms the lateral border of the femoral canal.

III. INTERNAL HERNIAS

A. Incidence. Of patients who present with acute intestinal obstruction, fewer than 5% have an internal hernia. When internal hernias are complicated by intestinal volvulus, there is an 80% incidence of strangulation or gangrene.

B. Etiology. Internal hernias occur within the abdominal cavity owing to congenital or acquired causes. Congenital causes include abnormal intestinal rotation (paraduodenal hernias) and openings in the ileocecal mesentery (transmesenteric hernias). Other, less frequent types are pericecal hernias, hernias through the sigmoid mesocolon, and hernias through defects in the transverse mesocolon, gastrocolic ligament, gastrohepatic ligament, or greater omentum. Acquired causes include hernias through mesenteric defects created by bowel resections or ostomy formation. The small bowel may also herniate beneath an adhesion from previous surgery.

C. Diagnosis

   1. Clinical presentation. These hernias usually are diagnosed because an intestinal segment becomes incarcerated within the internal defect, resulting in small-bowel obstruction. Patients with congenital causes usually have not had prior abdominal surgery. The reported mortality in acute intestinal obstruction secondary to internal hernias is 10% to 16%. **Symptoms** usually are of intestinal obstruction without evidence of an external hernia. When there is intestinal obstruction or intestinal strangulation, the diagnosis is based on clinical rather than on laboratory findings.

   2. Radiographic studies. Plain abdominal films may show small-bowel obstruction. An abdominal CT scan can sometimes establish the diagnosis of an internal hernia preoperatively. Contrast studies may also sometimes be useful.

D. Differential diagnosis includes other causes of intestinal obstruction, such as adhesions, external hernia, malignancy, gallstone ileus, and intussusception.

E. Surgical treatment. The diagnosis of internal hernia is often made at laparotomy for small-bowel obstruction. Intestinal loops proximal to the obstruction are dilated, friable, and edematous above the obstruction and collapsed distal to it. Once the hernia is reduced, intestinal viability is assessed, and nonviable intestine is removed. If a large percentage of bowel is of questionable viability, a limited bowel resection followed by a second-look laparotomy in 24 to 48 hours may preserve small-bowel length. The hernia defect should be closed primarily with nonabsorbable suture.

IV. ABDOMINAL WALL HERNIAS

A. Incidence and etiology

   1. Incisional hernias occur at sites of previous incisions at which there has been dehiscence of the abdominal wall. The causes are multiple and include obesity, wound infections, malnutrition, and technical wound closure factors. Hernias occur in up to 20% of patients undergoing abdominal operations and are most commonly seen with midline incisions. Most incisional hernias are now repaired with a mesh technique either open or laparoscopically.

2. **Umbilical hernias** are congenital defects. They are more frequent in African Americans than in whites. Most newborn umbilical hernias close spontaneously by the second year of life. However, umbilical hernias are also common in adults. Patients with ascites have a high incidence of umbilical hernias. When large, the hernias may cause gastrointestinal tract symptoms. When small, they rarely cause symptoms and may go unnoticed. Umbilical hernias have a fairly high rate of incarceration, usually with preperitoneal fat or omentum.

3. **Epigastric hernias** are hernias of the linea alba above the umbilicus. They occur more frequently in athletically active young men. When small or in obese individuals, epigastric hernias may be hard to palpate, making the diagnosis difficult as well. Usually, they produce epigastric pain that may be falsely attributed to other abdominal diagnoses. The diagnosis is made by palpation of a subcutaneous epigastric mass; most such hernias occur within a few centimeters of the umbilicus and are associated with a small (1 to 2 cm) fascial defect.

4. **Spigelian hernias** protrude through the spigelian fascia, near the termination of the transversus abdominis muscle along the lateral edge of the rectus abdominis near the junction of the linea semilunaris and linea semicircularis. Because the herniated visceral contents are intraparietal (between the abdominal wall muscles), these hernias can be difficult to diagnose and therefore are included in the differential diagnosis of obscure abdominal pain. Ultrasonography, CT scan, or laparoscopy can be useful confirmatory tools in patients with focal symptoms in the appropriate region.

5. The **most common type of lumbar hernia** is an incisional hernia from a previous retroperitoneal or flank incision. Lumbar hernias may also occur in two different triangles: the Petit triangle and the Grynfeltt triangle. Lower lumbar hernias of the Petit triangle are located in a weak area limited posteriorly by the latissimus dorsi, anteriorly by the external oblique muscle, and inferiorly by the iliac crest. Grynfeltt hernias are upper lumbar in location, below the lowest rib.

6. **Obturator hernias** are very rare hernias that occur predominantly in thin, older women and are difficult to diagnose. Patients classically present with bowel obstruction and focal tenderness on rectal examination. Pain along the medial aspect of the thigh with medial thigh rotation, known as the *Howship-Romberg sign*, results from obturator nerve compression and, when present, may aid in the clinical diagnosis of an obturator hernia.

B. **Treatment and operative management.** Small epigastric, umbilical, obturator, and spigelian hernias may be repaired primarily. Most incisional hernias and lumbar and obturator hernias require the use of prosthetic mesh because of their size, the often poor quality of surrounding tissue, and high recurrence rates after primary repair.

1. **Open repairs.** The principles for ventral hernia repair include dissection and identification of all defects and repair with nonabsorbable sutures placed in healthy tissue. Most sizable incisional hernias are now repaired with some type of mesh prosthesis that should be anchored by nonabsorbable sutures placed in healthy fascial tissue several centimeters beyond the margins of the defect. The mesh should be durable and well tolerated by the patient, with a low risk for infection. A variety of mesh products are available for repair, including polypropylene, polytetrafluoroethylene (PTFE, Gore-Tex), and a composite mesh of polypropylene and PTFE. Several newer composite mesh products (Table 26-1) with absorbable barriers coating polypropylene or polyester mesh are available to minimize tissue attachment to intraabdominal structures. Nonsynthetic products available for closure of defects (Table 26-2) in contaminated fields include AlloDerm, which is a decellularized human skin preparation that acts as a matrix for tissue ingrowth, and Surgisis, which is a porcine small intestine submucosa product that also promotes tissue ingrowth. One should try to avoid placing polypropylene mesh in direct contact with the intestine because of the risk of adhesion formation and

| **TABLE 26-1** | Characteristics of Mesh Used for Inguinal Hernia Repair |

	Marlex[a] (heavyweight)	Prolene soft[b] (midweight)	Ultrapro[b] (lightweight)
Material	Polypropylene	Polypropylene	Polypropylene, poliglecaprone
Weight (g/m^2)	95	45	28
Pore size (mm)	0.6	2.4	4
Burst strength (newtons)	1,218	590	576
Stiffness (newtons/cm)	59.1	49.1	43.2

[a]Davol, Inc., Cranston, RI
[b]Ethicon, Inc., Somerville, NJ
Adapted from Cobb WS, Burns JM, Peindl RD, et al. Textile analysis of heavy weight, mid-weight, and light weight polypropylene mesh in a porcine ventral hernia model. *J Surg Res* 2006;136(1):1–7.

fistulization. Rarely, in patients with massive incisional defects and loss of domain of intestinal contents, preoperative pneumoperitoneum can be used to stretch the abdominal wall to provide sufficient autogenous tissue for repair. Peritoneal insufflation of air (500 to 1,000 mL/day for 5 to 10 days) may allow primary closure when not otherwise possible and may obviate the need for a prosthetic graft.

2. **Laparoscopic repairs.** The laparoscopic approach is an increasingly used alternative method for repair of incisional hernias. The repair generally is performed intra-abdominally and involves placement of an intraperitoneal mesh prosthesis to cover the hernia defect. The contents of the hernia should be reduced, but the sac itself is not removed. There should be a 4- to 6-cm margin of mesh lateral to the hernia defect. The mesh should then be anchored in place with sutures and staples. Early results show that the technique is safe, simple, and effective, with results that are equivalent to, if not better than, the results of open repair. Early recurrence rates are reported at 1% to 10% and complication rates at 10% to 25%. Length of hospital stay and pain medication requirements are less than with open repair. A recent meta-analysis of 45 published series comparing open and laparoscopic ventral hernia repairs concluded that laparoscopic repair is associated with fewer wound-related (3.8% vs. 16.8%) and overall complications (22.7% vs. 41.7%) and has a lower rate of recurrence (4.3% vs. 12.1%) when compared to open repairs (Pierce R. et al. *Surg Endosc*, in press). Contraindications to laparoscopic ventral hernia repair include inability to establish pneumoperitoneum safely, an acute abdomen with strangulated or infarcted bowel, loss of abdominal domain, or the presence of peritonitis.

V. **CHOICE OF PROSTHETIC MESH AND BIOMATERIALS FOR USE IN HERNIA REPAIR**

A. **Prosthetic mesh in inguinal hernia repairs**

The choices in mesh for hernia repair differ in their flexibility, weight, burst strength, and inflammatory response. The various mesh options available to surgeons for use in inguinal hernia repairs are summarized in Table 26-1. A recent randomized clinical trial demonstrated that lightweight polypropylene mesh for Lichtenstein hernia repair did not affect recurrence rates but improved aspects of pain and discomfort 3 years after surgery (*Br J Surg* 2006;93:1056). These results support the use of newer, lighter-weight mesh materials in inguinal hernia repair.

B. **Prosthetic mesh in incisional hernia repairs**

The recurrence rate for ventral, incisional hernia repair is 25% to 54% when primarily repaired. The placement of prosthetic biomaterials in the retrorectus, preperitoneal space to repair ventral, incisional hernias as popularized by Rives, Stoppa, and Wantz has reduced the recurrence rate to 14% to 32%. Long-term follow-up of a randomized, controlled trial showed that the use of mesh results in a lower recurrence

TABLE 26-2	Biomaterials for Incisional Hernia Repair

	Product trade name	Manufacturer	Components
Absorbable, barrier composite mesh	Sepramesh	Genzyme Corp., Cambridge, MA	Polypropylene mesh on one side, absorbable sodium hyaluronate/ carboxymethylcellulose on the other side
	Paritex, Parientene	Sofradim Corp., Trevoux, France	Polyester mesh with bovine type I collagen coating covered with absorbable PEG/glycerol layer
	Proceed	Ethicon, Inc., Somerville, NJ	Polypropylene mesh encapsulated with polydioxanone coated on one side with oxidized-regenerated cellulose
Nonabsorbable, barrier composite mesh	Bard Composix	C.R. Bard, Inc., Murray Hill, NJ	Macroporous polypropylene bonded to low-porosity PTFE
	Gore-Tex Dual Mesh	W.L. Gore & Associates, Flagstaff, AZ	PTFE with different architecture on the peritoneal (intra-abdominal) and parietal (abdominal wall) surfaces of the mesh
Bioremodelable materials	Surgisis	Cook Biotech, Inc., West Lafayette, IN	Acellular, extracellular matrix material derived from porcine small intestinal submucosa
	Alloderm	LifeCell Corp., Branchburg, NJ	Acellular dermal matrix harvested from donated human tissue from the American Association of Tissue Banks
	Permacol	Tissue Science Laboratories, Covington, NJ	Acellular, cross-linked porcine dermal collagen implant and its constituent elastin fibers

PEG, polyethylene glycol; PTFE, polytetrafluoroethylene.

rate (32% vs. 63%) and less abdominal pain and does not result in more complications than primary repair (*Ann Surg* 2004;240:578). In clinical studies, the most reliable adhesion-resistant prosthetic biomaterial for intra-abdominal placement during laparoscopic ventral hernia repair has been PTFE (*Ann Surg* 2003;238:391). The microporous architecture and hydrophobicity of ePTFE prevents cellular penetration of intestine or abdominal viscera. Recently, various formulations of absorbable and nonabsorbable biomaterials have been introduced for repair of incisional hernias. Each product has its own characteristics, making it useful in various circumstances. This is summarized in Table 26-2. Currently, there is little outcomes data to support the use of one product over another. However, the use of mesh is superior to primary repair for incisional hernias.

ANATOMY

I. THE BREAST. Breast tissue is located between the subcutaneous fat and the fascia of the **pectoralis major** and **serratus anterior** muscles. Posterior to the breast and anterior to the pectoralis fascia is the *retromammary space*, which contains small lymphatics and vessels. Breast tissue can extend to the clavicle, into the axilla (axillary tail of Spence), to the latissimus dorsi, and to the top of the rectus muscle. Running through the breasts from the deep fascia to the skin are *suspensory ligaments* **(Cooper's ligaments);** involvement of these ligaments by cancer may cause skin dimpling.

  A. Vasculature. The arterial supply is from the **internal thoracic artery,** via perforating branches, and the **axillary artery,** via the long thoracic and thoracoacromial branches. Venous drainage is mainly to the **axillary vein,** as well as the internal thoracic, lateral thoracic, and intercostals veins.

  B. Lymphatic drainage of the breasts occurs via interlobular lymphatic vessels into a subareolar plexus (Sappey's plexus). From this plexus, the majority (75%) of the lymph drains into the axillary lymph nodes. Lymph from the medial breast may drain into the internal mammary nodes or the axillary nodes.

  C. Innervation. Lateral and anterior cutaneous branches of the second to sixth intercostals nerves innervate the breasts.

II. THE AXILLA. The borders of the axilla are defined as the **axillary vein** superiorly, **latissimus dorsi** laterally, and the **serratus anterior** muscle medially.

  A. Axillary lymph nodes are classified according to their anatomic location relative to the **pectoralis minor** muscle.

    1. Level I nodes. *Lateral* to the pectoralis minor muscle

    2. Level II nodes. *Posterior* to the pectoralis minor muscle

    3. Level III nodes. *Medial* to the pectoralis minor muscle and most accessible with division of the muscle

    4. Rotter's nodes. *Between* the pectoralis major and the minor muscles

  B. Axillary nerves. Three motor and several sensory nerves are located in the axilla. Preservation of all is preferred during an axillary lymph node dissection; however, direct tumor invasion may require resection along with the specimen.

    1. Long thoracic nerve: travels from superiorly to inferiorly along the chest wall at the medial aspect of the axilla and innervates the serratus anterior muscle. Injury to this nerve causes a "winged" scapula in which the medial and inferior angle of the scapula abduct away from the chest wall with arm extension.

    2. Thoracodorsal nerve: courses along the posterior border of the axilla from superiorly to inferiorly on the subscapularis muscle and innervates the latissimus dorsi. Injury to this nerve causes weakness in arm abduction and external rotation.

    3. Medial pectoral nerve: travels from the posterior aspect of the pectoralis minor muscle around the lateral border of the pectoralis minor to the posterior aspect of the pectoralis major muscle. It innervates the lateral third of the pectoralis major; injury to this nerve results in atrophy of the lateral pectoralis major muscle.

    4. Intercostal brachial sensory nerves: travel laterally in the axilla from the second intercostal space to the medial upper arm. Transection causes numbness in the posterior and medial surface of the upper arm.

CLINICAL ASSESSMENT

I. HISTORY. Patients seek medical attention most commonly for an abnormal mammogram, a breast mass, breast pain, nipple discharge, or skin changes. History should include the following:

■ Duration of symptoms, change over time, associated pain or skin changes, relationship to pregnancy or the menstrual cycle, previous trauma.

■ Date of last menstrual period and regularity of the menstrual cycle.

■ Age of menarche.

■ Number of pregnancies and age at first full-term pregnancy.

■ Lactational history.

■ Age at menopause or surgical menopause (i.e., oophorectomy).

■ Prior history of breast biopsies or breast cancer.

■ Mammogram history.

■ Oral contraceptive and hormonal replacement therapy.

■ Family history of breast and gynecologic cancer, including the age at diagnosis. This should include at least two generations as well as any associated cancers, such as ovary, colon, prostate, gastric, or pancreatic.

A. Assessment of cancer risks

1. Hormonal, environmental exposure, and **genetics** are correlated to an increased risk for breast cancer. A family history of breast cancer in a first-degree relative is associated with a doubling of risk. If two first-degree relatives (e.g., a mother and a sister) have breast cancer, the risk is further elevated. *These familial effects are enhanced if the relative had either early-onset cancer or bilateral disease.* Breast-feeding may exert a protective effect against the development of breast cancer. Overall, factors that increase a patient's risk by 1.5- to 4-fold include the following:

a. Increased estrogen or progesterone exposure due to early menarche (before age 12 years) or late menopause (age >55 years).

b. Late age at first full-term pregnancy: Women with a first birth after age 30 years have twice the risk of those with a first birth before age 18 years.

c. High body-mass index after menopause.

d. Exposure to ionizing radiation.

2. BRCA1 and BRCA2 are breast cancer susceptibility genes associated with 80% of hereditary breast cancers but account for only 5% of all breast cancers. Women with BRCA1 mutations have an estimated risk of 85% for breast cancer by age 70 years, a 50% chance of developing a second primary breast cancer, and a 20% chance of developing ovarian cancer. BRCA2 mutations carry a lower risk for breast cancer and account for 4% to 6% of all male breast cancers. Screening for BRCA gene mutations should be reserved for women who have a strong family history of breast or ovarian cancer.

3. Prior breast biopsies. Some pathologic features are associated with increased cancer risk.

a. No increased risk is associated with adenosis, cysts, duct ectasia, or apocrine metaplasia.

b. There is a slightly increased risk with moderate or florid hyperplasia, papillomatosis, and complex fibroadenomas.

c. Atypical ductal (ADH) or **lobular hyperplasia (ALH)** carries a 4- to 5-fold increased risk of developing cancer; the risk increases to 10-fold if there is a positive family history. Patients with increased risk should be counseled appropriately and should be followed with semiannual physical examinations and yearly mammograms.

4. Models for breast cancer risk. The original **Gail model** estimates the absolute risk (probability) that a woman in a program of annual screening will develop breast cancer over a defined age interval. The risk factors in this model include current age, age at menarche, age at first full-term pregnancy, previous breast biopsies, presence of ADH on prior biopsy, and number of affected first-degree relatives. The National Surgical Adjuvant Breast and Bowel Project (NSABP) modified this model to project the absolute risk of developing only invasive breast cancer. This **modified Gail model** has been used to define eligibility criteria for entry into chemoprevention trials. The NSABP and the National Cancer Institute offer an interactive online risk assessment tool, which is available at **http://www. cancer.gov/bcrisktool.**

II. PHYSICAL EXAM

A. Inspect the breasts with the patient both in the upright and supine positions. With the patient in the upright position, examine with the patient's arms relaxed and then raised, looking for shape asymmetry, deformity, and skin changes (erythema, edema, dimpling). With the patient in the supine position, examine the entire breast systematically with the patient's ipsilateral arm raised above and behind the head.

1. If a mass is found, determine its size, shape, texture, tenderness, location, fixation to skin or deep tissues, and relationship to the areola. Evaluate the nipples for retraction, discoloration, inversion, ulceration, and eczematous changes.

2. For nipple discharge, note its color and quality, where pressure elicits discharge, and whether it is from a single duct or associated with a mass.

B. The axillary, supraclavicular, and infraclavicular lymph nodes should be palpated with the patient in the upright position, with arms relaxed. The size, number, and fixation of nodes should be noted.

III. BREAST IMAGING

A. Screening for breast cancer. Screening mammogram lowers mortality from breast cancer. It is performed in the **asymptomatic** patient and consists of two standard views, mediolateral oblique (MLO) and craniocaudal (CC). The current recommendation from the National Cancer Institute and American College of Surgeons is **annual screening mammography for women aged 40 years and older.** Breast lesions on mammograms are classified according to the American College of Radiology by **BI-RADS (Breast Imaging Reporting and Database System)** scores:

- **0** = Needs further imaging; assessment incomplete.
- **1** = Normal; continue annual follow-up (risk of malignancy: 1/2,000).
- **2** = Benign lesion; no risk of malignancy; continue annual follow-up (risk of malignancy: 1/2,000).
- **3** = Probably benign lesion; needs 4 to 6 months follow-up (risk of malignancy: 1% to 2%).
- **4** = Suspicious for breast cancer; biopsy recommended (risk of malignancy: 25% to 50%).
- **5** = Highly suspicious for breast cancer; biopsy required (75% to 99% are malignant).
- **6** = Known biopsy-proven malignancy.

1. Malignant mammographic findings
   a. New or spiculated masses.
   b. Clustered microcalcifications in linear or branching array.
   c. Architectural distortion.

2. Benign mammographic findings
   a. Radial scar. Generally due to fibrocystic breast condition (FBC); associated with proliferative epithelium in the center of the fibrotic area in approximately one third of cases. Appearance often mimics malignancy; a biopsy is needed to rule out malignancy.
   b. Fat necrosis. Results from local trauma to the breast. It may resemble carcinoma on palpation and on mammography. The fat may liquefy instead of scarring, which results in a characteristic oil cyst. A biopsy may be needed to rule out malignancy.
   c. Milk of calcium. Associated with FBC; caused by calcified debris in the base of the acini. Characteristic microcalcifications appear discoid on craniocaudal view and sickle-shaped on mediolateral oblique view. These are benign and do not require biopsy.

    d. Cysts cannot be distinguished from solid masses by mammography; ultrasound is needed to make this distinction.

  3. Screening in high-risk patients: For patients with *known BRCA mutations,* annual mammograms and semiannual physical examinations should **begin at age 25 to 30 years.** In patients with a *strong family history of breast cancer but undocumented genetic mutation,* annual mammograms and semiannual physical examinations should begin **10 years earlier than the age of the youngest affected relative and no later than age 40 years.**

  4. Magnetic resonance imaging (MRI) is recommended for screening in *selected high-risk patients* with:

    a. A **lifetime risk of breast cancer greater than 20%** as defined by available risk assessment tools (e.g., BRCAPRO, Gail, Claus, and Tyrer-Cuskick models).

    b. BRCA mutations.

    c. A first-degree relative (parent, sibling, child) with a BRCA1 or BRCA2 mutation.

    d. History of radiation to the chest wall between the ages of 10 to 30 years (e.g., Hodgkin lymphoma patients).

    e. Li-Fraumeni, Cowden, or Bannayan-Riley-Ruvalcaba syndromes.

B. Diagnostic imaging

  1. Diagnostic mammograms are performed in the symptomatic patient or to follow up on an abnormality noted on a screening mammogram. Additional views (spot-compression views or magnification views) may be used to further characterize any lesion. The false-negative and false-positive rates are both approximately 10%. A normal mammogram in the presence of a palpable mass does **not** exclude malignancy and further workup should be performed with an ultrasound, MRI, and/or biopsy.

  2. Ultrasonography is used to further characterize a lesion identified by physical examination or mammography. It can determine whether a lesion is solid or cystic and can define the size, contour, or internal texture of the lesion. Although not a useful screening modality by itself due to significant false-positive rates, when used as an adjunct with mammography, ultrasonography may improve diagnostic sensitivity of benign findings to greater than 90%, especially among younger patients for whom mammographic sensitivity is lower due to denser breast tissue. In those patients with a known cancer, ultrasound is sometimes used to detect additional suspicious lesions and/or to map the extent of disease.

  3. MRI is useful as an adjunct to mammography to determine extent of disease, to detect multicentric disease in the dense breast, to assess the contralateral breast, to evaluate patients with axillary metastases and an unknown primary, and in patients in whom mammogram, ultrasound, and clinical findings are inconclusive. It is also useful for assessing chest wall involvement.

IV. BREAST BIOPSY

  A. Palpable masses

    1. Fine-needle aspiration biopsy (FNAB) is reliable and accurate, with sensitivity greater than 90%. FNAB can determine the presence of malignant cells and estrogen and progesterone receptor status but does not give information on tumor grade or the presence of invasion. Nondiagnostic aspirates require an additional biopsy, either surgical or core needle biopsy (*Am J Surg* 1997;174:372).

    2. Core biopsy is preferred over FNAB. It can distinguish between invasive and noninvasive cancer and provides information on tumor grade as well as receptor status. For indeterminate specimens, a surgical biopsy is necessary.

    3. Excisional biopsy should primarily be used when a core biopsy cannot be done. It is performed in the operating room; incisions should be planned so that they can be incorporated into a mastectomy incision should that subsequently be necessary. Masses should be excised as a single specimen and labeled to preserve three-dimensional orientations.

    4. Incisional biopsy is indicated for the evaluation of a large breast mass suspicious for malignancy but for which a definitive diagnosis cannot be made by FNAB or core biopsy. For inflammatory breast cancer with skin involvement, an incisional biopsy can consist of a skin punch biopsy.

B. Nonpalpable lesions. Minimally invasive breast biopsy is the optimal **initial** tissue acquisition method and procedure of choice for obtaining a pathologic diagnosis of image-detected abnormalities. **Correlation between pathology results and imaging findings is mandatory.** Patients with histologically benign findings on percutaneous biopsy do not require open biopsy if imaging and pathological findings are concordant. Patients with high-risk lesions on image-guided biopsy (ADH, ALH, lobular carcinoma *in situ*, radial scar) may have malignancy at the same site and should undergo a surgical biopsy.

1. **Stereotactic core biopsy** is used for nonpalpable mammographically detected lesions, such as microcalcifications, which cannot be seen with ultrasonography. Tissue can be collected from several foci in disparate quadrants of the breast. Using a computer-driven stereotactic unit, two mammographic images are taken to triangulate the lesion in three-dimensional space. A computer determines the depth of the lesion and the alignment of the needle, which can be positioned within 1 mm of the intended target. Biopsies are taken, and postfire images are obtained of the breast and specimen. **Contraindications** include lesions close to the chest wall or in the axillary tail and thin breasts that may allow needle strikethrough. Superficial lesions and lesions directly beneath the nipple-areola complex are also often not approachable with stereotactic techniques. Nondiagnostic and insufficient specimens should undergo needle-localized excisional biopsy (NLB, see later discussion), as should discordant pathologic findings on core needle stereotactic biopsy.

   a. **Vacuum-assisted biopsy** is generally used during stereotactic core biopsies and ultrasound-guided core biopsies. These devices employ large needles (9 to 14 gauge) to contiguously acquire tissue, which is pulled into the bore of the needle by vacuum suction. Multiple contiguous samples of tissue are collected while the probe remains in the breast. Volumes up to 1 mL can be collected during a single insertion. A metallic marking clip is usually placed through the probe after sampling is complete to allow for identification of the biopsy site should excisional biopsy or partial mastectomy be necessary. This is the preferred approach for lesions presenting with microcalcifications without a visible or palpable mass.

2. **Ultrasound-guided biopsy** is the preferred method if a lesion can be visualized with ultrasound because it is generally easier to perform than a stereotactic core biopsy. Lesions with a cystic component are better visualized with ultrasound, and ultrasound-guided biopsy can be used to aspirate the cyst as well as to provide core biopsy specimens.

3. **Needle localization excisional biopsy** (NLB). A needle and hookwire are placed into the breast adjacent to the concerning lesion under mammographic guidance. The patient is then brought to the operating room for an **excisional biopsy.** Using localization mammograms as a map, the whole hookwire, breast lesion, and a rim of normal breast tissue are removed *en bloc*. The specimen is oriented, and a radiograph is performed to confirm the presence of the lesion within the specimen.

BENIGN BREAST CONDITIONS

I. FIBROCYSTIC BREAST CHANGE (FBC) encompasses several of the following pathologic features: stromal fibrosis, macro- and microcysts, apocrine metaplasia, hyperplasia, and adenosis (which may be sclerosing, blunt-duct, or florid).

A. FBC is common and may present as breast pain, a breast mass, nipple discharge, or abnormalities on mammography.

B. The patient presenting with a breast mass or thickening and suspected FBC should be re-examined in a short interval, preferably on day 10 of the menstrual cycle, when hormonal influence is lowest. Often, the mass will have diminished in size.

C. A persistent dominant mass must undergo further radiographic evaluation, biopsy, or both to exclude cancer.

II. BREAST CYSTS frequently present as tender masses or as smooth, mobile, well-defined masses on palpation. If tense with fluid, its texture may be firm, resembling a solid mass. Aspiration can determine the nature of the mass (solid vs. cystic) but is not routinely necessary. Cyst fluid color varies and can be clear, straw-colored, or even dark green.

A. Cysts discovered by mammography and confirmed as simple cysts by ultrasound are usually observed *if asymptomatic.*

B. *Symptomatic* simple cysts should be aspirated. If no palpable mass is present after drainage, the patient should be evaluated in 3 to 4 weeks. If the cyst recurs, does not resolve completely with aspiration, or yields bloody fluid with aspiration, then mammography or ultrasonography should be performed to exclude intracystic tumor. Nonbloody clear fluid does not need to be sent for cytology.

III. FIBROADENOMA is the most common discrete mass in women younger than 30 years of age. They typically present as smooth, firm, mobile masses.

A. They enlarge during pregnancy and involute after menopause.

B. They have well-circumscribed borders on mammography and ultrasound.

C. They may be managed conservatively if clinical and radiographic appearance is consistent with a fibroadenoma and is less than 2 cm. If the mass is symptomatic, greater than 2 cm, or enlarges, it should be excised.

IV. MASTALGIA. Most women (70%) experience some form of breast pain or discomfort during their lifetime. The pain may be cyclic (worse before a menstrual cycle) or noncyclical, focal or diffuse. Benign disease is the etiology in the majority of cases. However, pain may be associated with cancer in up to 10% of patients. **Features that raise the suspicion of cancer are *noncyclic* pain in a focal area and pain associated with a mass or bloody nipple discharge.** *Once cancer has been excluded,* most patients can be managed successfully with symptomatic therapy and reassurance; a well-fitting supportive bra is an important first step in pain relief. In 15% of patients, the pain may be so disabling that it interferes with activities of daily living.

A. Cyclic breast pain. Often described as a heaviness or tenderness and is usually worse before a menstrual cycle. It may be maximal in the upper outer quadrant and radiate to the inner surface of the upper arm. It resolves spontaneously in 20% to 30% of women but tends to recur in 60%. Many patients experience symptomatic relief by reducing caffeine intake or by taking vitamin E, although there is no scientific evidence supporting this.

B. Noncyclic breast pain. Described as burning or stabbing and frequently occurs in the subareolar area or medial aspect of the breast. It responds poorly to treatment but tends to resolve spontaneously in 50% of women.

C. Treatment of mastalgia

1. **Topical nonsteroidal anti-inflammatory drugs (NSAIDs)** (diclofenac gel) have been proven in a randomized, blinded, placebo-controlled study to have significant efficacy with minimal side effects and should be considered **first-line treatment** (*J Am Coll Surg* 2003;196:525).

2. **Tamoxifen** (an estrogen antagonist) has been shown to provide good pain relief in placebo-controlled trials with tolerable side effects (*Lancet* 1986;1:287), although concerns over increased risks of endometrial cancer limit long-term use.

3. **Danazol** (a derivative of testosterone) has been shown to be efficacious and has been used historically for severe breast pain (*Gynecol Endocrinol* 1997;11:393), but significant side effects (hirsutism, voice changes, acne, amenorrhea, and abnormal liver enzymes levels) limit its use.

4. **Bromocriptine** and **gonadorelin analogs** should be reserved for severe refractory mastalgia due to significant side effects.

5. **Evening primrose oil** is often used but has been shown to have no benefit over placebo in clinical trials (*Am J Obstet Gynecol* 2002;187:1389).

D. Superficial thrombophlebitis of the veins overlying the breast **(Mondor disease)** may present as breast pain. The thrombosed vein or "cord" may be palpated.

NSAIDs and hot compresses can provide symptomatic relief. Antibiotics are not generally indicated.

E. **Breast pain in pregnancy and lactation** can occur from engorgement, clogged ducts, trauma to the areola and nipple from pumping or nursing, or any of the aforementioned sources. Clogged ducts are usually treated with warm compresses, soaks, and massage.

F. **Tietze syndrome or costochondritis** may be confused with breast pain. Patients are locally tender in the parasternal area. Treatment is with NSAIDs.

G. **Cervical radiculopathy** can also cause referred pain to the breast.

V. NIPPLE DISCHARGE

A. **Lactation** is the most common physiologic cause of nipple discharge and may continue for up to 2 years after cessation of breast-feeding. In parous nonlactating women, a small amount of milk may be expressed from multiple ducts. This requires no treatment.

B. **Galactorrhea** is milky discharge unrelated to breast-feeding. Physiologic galactorrhea is the continued production of milk after lactation has ceased and menses resumed and is often caused by continued mechanical stimulation of the nipples.

1. **Drug-related galactorrhea** is caused by medications that affect the hypothalamic-pituitary axis by depleting dopamine (tricyclic antidepressants, reserpine, methyldopa, cimetidine, and benzodiazepines), blocking the dopamine receptor (phenothiazine, metoclopramide, and haloperidol), or having an estrogenic effect (digitalis). Discharge is generally bilateral and nonbloody.

2. **Spontaneous galactorrhea** in a **nonlactating** patient may be due to a pituitary **prolactinoma.** Amenorrhea may be associated. The diagnosis is established by measuring the serum prolactin level and performing a computed tomography (CT) or MRI scan of the pituitary gland. Treatment is bromocriptine or resection of the prolactinoma.

C. **Pathologic nipple discharge** is either (1) bloody or (2) spontaneous, unilateral, and originates from a single duct. *Normal physiologic discharge* is usually nonbloody, from multiple ducts, can be a variety of colors (clear to yellow to green), and requires breast manipulation to produce.

1. **Pathologic discharge** is serous, serosanguineous, bloody, or watery. The presence of blood can be confirmed with a guaiac test.

2. Cytologic evaluation of the discharge is not generally useful.

3. **Malignancy is the underlying cause in 10% of patients.**

4. If physical examination and mammography are negative for an associated mass, the most likely etiologies are **benign intraductal papilloma, duct ectasia,** or **fibrocystic changes.** In lactating women, serosanguinous or bloody discharge can be associated with duct trauma, infection, or epithelial proliferation associated with breast enlargement.

5. A solitary **papilloma** with a fibrovascular core places the patient at marginally increased risk for the development of breast cancer. Patients with persistent spontaneous discharge from a single duct require a surgical microdochectomy, ductoscopy, or major duct excision.

   a. **Microdochectomy:** Excision of the involved duct and associated lobule. Immediately before surgery, the involved duct is cannulated, and radiopaque contrast is injected to obtain a **ductogram,** which identifies lesions as filling defects. The patient is then taken to the operating room, and the pathologic duct is identified and excised, along with the associated lobule.

   b. **Ductoscopy** utilizes a 1-mm rigid videoscope to perform an internal exploration of the major ducts of the breast. Once a ductal lesion is identified, this single associated duct with the lesion is excised.

   c. **Major duct excision** may be used for women with bloody nipple discharge from multiple ducts or in postmenopausal women with bloody nipple discharge. It is performed through a circumareolar incision, and all of the retroareolar ducts are transected and excised, along with a cone of tissue extending up to several centimeters posterior to the nipple.

VI. BREAST INFECTIONS

A. Lactational mastitis may occur either sporadically or in epidemics.

1. The most common causative organism is *Staphylococcus aureus.*

2. It presents as a swollen, erythematous, and tender breast; purulent discharge from the nipple is *uncommon.*

3. In the early cellulitic phase, the treatment is antibiotics. The frequency of nursing or pumping should be *increased.* Approximately 25% progress to abscess formation.

4. **Breast abscesses** occur in the later stages and are often *not* fluctuant. The diagnosis is made by failure to improve on antibiotics, abscess cavity seen on ultrasound, or aspiration of pus. Treatment is cessation of nursing and surgical drainage.

B. Nonpuerperal abscesses result from duct ectasia with periductal mastitis, infected cysts, infected hematoma, or hematogenous spread from another source.

1. They usually are located in the peri/retroareolar area.

2. **Anaerobes** are the most common causative agent, although antibiotics should cover both **anaerobic and aerobic** organisms.

3. Treatment is surgical drainage.

4. **Unresolved or recurring infection requires biopsy to exclude cancer.** These patients often have a chronic relapsing course with multiple infections requiring surgical drainage.

5. Repeated infections can result in a chronically draining periareolar lesion or a mammary fistula lined with squamous epithelium. Treatment is excision of the central duct along with the fistula once the acute infection resolves. The fistula can recur even after surgery.

VII. GYNECOMASTIA: hypertrophy of breast tissue in men.

A. Pubertal hypertrophy occurs in adolescent boys, is usually bilateral, and resolves spontaneously in 6 to 12 months.

B. Senescent gynecomastia is commonly seen after age 70 years, as testosterone levels decrease.

C. Drugs associated with this are similar to those that cause galactorrhea in women, for example, digoxin, spironolactone, methyldopa, cimetidine, tricyclic antidepressants, phenothiazine, reserpine, and marijuana.

D. Tumors can cause gynecomastia secondary to excess secretion of estrogens: testicular teratomas and seminomas, bronchogenic carcinomas, adrenal tumors, and tumors of the pituitary and hypothalamus.

E. Gynecomastia may be a manifestation of **systemic diseases** such as hepatic cirrhosis, renal failure, and malnutrition.

F. During the workup of gynecomastia, cancer should be excluded by mammography and subsequently by biopsy if a mass is found. The cause of gynecomastia should be identified and corrected if possible. If workup fails to reveal a medically treatable cause or if the enlargement fails to regress, excision of breast tissue via a periareolar incision can be performed.

MALIGNANCY OF THE BREAST

I. EPIDEMIOLOGY. Breast cancer is the **most common cancer in women,** with a lifetime risk of **1 in 8 women.** In 2007, approximately 178,000 new cases of invasive breast cancer and 62,000 new cases of noninvasive *in situ* carcinoma of the breast will be diagnosed (*CA Cancer J Clin* 2007;57:43). Approximately 40,000 women will die in 2007 due to breast cancer, making it the second-leading cause of cancer death in women (led by lung cancer).

II. STAGING. The management of breast cancer is guided by the extent of disease and the biologic features of the tumor. Treatment is multidisciplinary, involving surgeons, radiation oncologists, and medical oncologists. The disease is staged by the TNM (tumor, node, and metastasis) system (Tables 27-1 and 27-2). Workup should include the

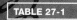

TABLE 27-1 American Joint Committee on Cancer TNM (Tumor, Node, Metastasis) Staging for Breast Cancer

Stage	Description
Tumor	
TX	Primary tumor not assessable
T0	No evidence of primary tumor
Tis	Carcinoma *in situ*
T1	Tumor ≤2 cm in greatest dimension
T1 mic	Microinvasion ≤0.1 cm in greatest dimension
T1a	Tumor >0.1 cm but not >0.5 cm
T1b	Tumor >0.5 cm but not >1 cm
T1c	Tumor >1 cm but not >2 cm
T2	Tumor >2 cm but <5 cm in greatest dimension
T3	Tumor >5 cm in greatest dimension
T4	Tumor of any size with direct extension into the chest wall or skin
T4a	Extension to chest wall (ribs, intercostals, or serratus anterior)
T4b	*Peau d'orange,* ulceration, or satellite skin nodules
T4c	T4a + b
T4d	Inflammatory breast cancer
Regional lymph nodes	
NX	Regional lymph nodes not assessable
N0	No regional lymph node involvement
N1	Metastasis to movable ipsilateral axillary lymph nodes
N2	Metastases to ipsilateral axillary lymph nodes fixed to one anotheror to other structures
N3	Metastases to ipsilateral internal mammary lymph node with or without axillary lymph node involvement, or in clinically apparent clavicular lymph node.
Distant metastases	
MX	Presence of distant metastases not assessable
M0	No distant metastases
M1	Existent distant metastases (including ipsilateral supraclavicular nodes)

With permission from Fleming ID, Cooper JS, Henson DE, et al., eds. *AJCC Cancer Staging Manual,* 5th ed. Philadelphia: Lippincott Williams & Wilkins; 1998.

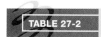

TABLE 27-2 American Joint Committee on Cancer Classification for Breast Cancer Based on TNM (Tumor, Node, Metastasis) Criteria

Stage	Tumor	Nodes	Metastases
0	Tis	N0	M0
I	T1	N0	M0
IIA	T0, 1	N1	M0
	T2	N0	M0
IIB	T2	N1	M0
	T3	N0	M0
IIIA	T0, 1, 2	N2	M0
	T3	N1, 2	M0
IIIB	T4	Any N	M0
	Any T	N3	M0
IV	Any T	Any N	M1

With permission from Fleming ID, Cooper JS, Henson DE, et al., eds. *AJCC Cancer Staging Manual,* 5th ed. Philadelphia: Lippincott Williams & Wilkins; 1998.

following (in addition to breast-specific imaging):

- Complete blood cell count, complete metabolic panel, and chest x-ray.
- A bone scan if the alkaline phosphatase or calcium level is elevated.
- CT scan of the liver if liver function panel is abnormal.
- **Patients with clinical stage III** disease should undergo bone scan and CT scan due to a high probability of distant metastases.

III. **TUMOR BIOMARKERS AND PROGNOSTIC FACTORS** should be evaluated on all tumor specimens.

Tumor size and **grade** are the most reliable pathologic predictors of outcome for patients **without axillary nodal involvement.** The **Nottingham score** combines histologic grade based on *glandular differentiation, mitotic count,* and *nuclear grade.* A higher grade is a *poor* prognostic factor.

A. **Hormone receptors.** Expression of **estrogen receptors (ERs)** and **progesterone receptors (PRs)** should be evaluated by immunohistochemistry. Intense ER and PR staining is a *good* prognostic factor.

B. **Her2/neu (ERB2)** : *Her2/neu* is a member of the epidermal growth factor family and is involved in cell growth regulation. Overexpression due to gene amplification is seen in approximately 30% of patients with breast cancer. *Her2/neu* expression is measured by immunohistochemistry; and if equivocal by fluorescence in situ hybridization overexpression of *Her2/neu* is a *poor* prognostic factor.

C. Other **negative markers** include those tumors that do not express any tumor biomarkers **("triple negative"),** the presence of **lymphovascular invasion,** and other indicators of a high proliferative rate (>5% of cells in the **S phase;** >20% **Ki-67).**

IV. **NONINVASIVE (*in situ*) breast cancer: DCIS** (ductal carcinoma *in situ*) or **LCIS** (lobular carcinoma *in situ*) are lesions with malignant cells that have not penetrated the basement membrane of the mammary ducts or lobules, respectively.

A. **DCIS,** or intraductal carcinoma, is treated as a **malignancy** because DCIS has the potential to develop into invasive cancer.

- It is usually detected by mammography as clustered pleomorphic calcifications.
- Physical examination is normal in the majority of patients.
- It may advance in a segmental manner, with gaps between disease areas.
- It can be **multifocal** (two or more lesions >5 mm apart within the same index quadrant) or **multicentric** (in different quadrants).

1. **Histology**
   a. There are **five architectural subtypes:** papillary, micropapillary, solid, cribriform, and comedo. Specimens are also grouped as *comedo* versus *noncomedo.*
   b. The **high-grade subtype is** often associated with microinvasion, a higher proliferation rate, aneuploidy, gene amplification, and a higher local recurrence rate.
   c. ER and PR expression levels should be obtained if hormone therapy is being considered.

2. **Treatment**
   a. **Surgical excision** alone (via partial mastectomy) with **margins greater than 10 mm** is associated with a local recurrence rate of 14% at 12 years (*Am J Surg* 2006;192:420). The addition of adjuvant radiation reduces the local recurrence rate to 2.5%. Approximately half of the recurrences present as invasive ductal carcinomas. **Surgical options** depend on the extent of disease, grade, margin status, multicentricity of disease, and patient age.
      (1) **Partial mastectomy:** For unicentric lesions. Needle localization is required to identify the area to be excised in most cases. Bracket needle localization (two or more wires to map out the extent of disease to be resected) for more extensive lesions is occasionally used.
      (2) **Mastectomy:** Total (simple) mastectomy with or without immediate reconstruction is recommended for patients with multicentric lesions, extensive involvement of the breast (disease extent relative to breast size), or persistently positive margins with partial mastectomy.
   b. **Assessment of axillary lymph nodes: Axillary dissection** is **not** performed for pure DCIS.

(1) Sentinel lymph node biopsy (SNLB, see later discussion) may be considered when there is a reasonable probability of finding invasive cancer on final pathologic examination (e.g., >4 cm, palpable, or high grade).

(2) Some surgeons perform SLNB in all patients with DCIS undergoing mastectomy because SLNB cannot be performed postmastectomy if an occult invasive cancer is found. This is an area of ongoing controversy and research.

(3) A positive sentinel node indicates invasive breast cancer and changes the stage of the disease; a **completion axillary dissection** is then indicated.

c. Adjuvant therapy

(1) For pure DCIS, there is no added benefit from systemic chemotherapy because the disease is confined to the ducts of the breast. However, in those patients with **ER-positive DCIS,** adjuvant **tamoxifen** can reduce the risk of breast cancer recurrence by 37% over 5 years and the risk of developing a new contralateral breast cancer (NSABP B-24 trial). However, there is no survival benefit. **Aromatase inhibitors** (e.g., **anastrazole, exemestane, letrozole**), which block the peripheral conversion of androgens into estrogens by inhibiting the enzyme aromatase but does not affect estrogen produced by the ovaries, are sometimes used as an alternative in postmenopausal patients.

(2) Adjuvant radiation should be given to patients with DCIS treated with partial mastectomy to **decrease the local recurrence rate** (NSABP B-17 trial). This is especially true for younger women with close margins or large tumors. However, there is no survival benefit. For older patients with smaller, widely excised DCIS of low or intermediate grade, the benefit of radiation therapy is so small that adjuvant radiation is not recommended.

d. The Van Nuys Prognostic Index (Table 27-3) is a numerical algorithm (based on lesion size, margin, tumor grade, presence of necrosis, and age) used to stratify patients with DCIS into three groups to determine which patient is at greatest risk of recurrence and would therefore benefit the most from a more aggressive treatment approach. The low-scoring group may be treated with partial mastectomy alone. The intermediate-scoring group has been shown to benefit from adjuvant radiation therapy, and the high-scoring group should undergo mastectomy because the risk of recurrence with partial mastectomy with or without radiation is high (*Adv Surg* 2000;34:29).

B. LCIS is not considered a preinvasive lesion but rather an indicator for increased breast cancer risk of approximately 1% per year (~20% to 30% at 15 years) (*JNCCN* 2006;4:511) and is not treated as a breast cancer.

TABLE 27-3   Van Nuys Scoring System[a]

	Score		
	1	**2**	**3**
Size (mm)	d15	>15–40	>40
Margins (mm)	S10	<10 but >1	<1
Histology	Non high grade without necrosis	Non high grade with necrosis	High grade with or without necrosis

[a]A score of 13 points is given for each of the prognostic factors described, resulting in a total index score ranging from 3 to 9. Scores of 3 and 4 are considered low index values; scores of 5, 6, or 7 are considered intermediate; and scores of 8 or 9 are considered high.
Modified from Silverstein MJ, Lagios MD, Craig PH, et al. A prognostic index for ductal carcinoma *in situ* of the breast. *Cancer* 1996;77:226–227.

1. It may be multifocal and/or bilateral.
2. The cancer that develops may be invasive ductal or lobular and may occur in either breast.
3. LCIS has loss of **E-cadherin** (involved in cell–cell adhesion), which can be stained for on pathology slides to clarify cases that are borderline DCIS versus LCIS.
4. **Pleomorphic LCIS** is a particularly aggressive subtype of LCIS that is treated more like DCIS; it tends to have less favorable biological markers.
5. **Treatment options** are (1) lifelong close **surveillance,** (2) **bilateral total mastectomies** with immediate reconstruction for selected women with a strong family history after appropriate counseling, or (3) prophylaxis with **tamoxifen.**

V. INVASIVE BREAST CANCER

A. **Histology** consists of five different subtypes: *infiltrating ductal* (75% to 80%), *infiltrating lobular* (5% to 10%), *medullary* (5% to 7%), *mucinous* (3%), and *tubular* (1% to 2%).

B. Surgical options for stage I and II breast cancer:

1. **Mastectomy** with or without reconstruction.

   a. **Modified radical mastectomy** (MRM) involves total (simple) mastectomy **and** axillary lymph node dissection. It is indicated for patients with clinically positive lymph nodes or a positive axillary node based on previous SLNB or FNAB.

   b. **Total (simple) mastectomy with SLNB** is for patients with a clinically negative axilla. A skin-sparing mastectomy (preserves skin envelope and inframammary ridge) may be performed with immediate reconstruction, resulting in improved cosmesis: The nipple-areolar complex, a rim of periareolar breast skin, and any previous excisional biopsy or partial mastectomy scars are excised.

   c. **Immediate reconstruction** at the time of mastectomy should be offered to eligible patients. Options include latissimus dorsi myocutaneous flaps, transverse rectus abdominis myocutaneous flaps, and inflatable tissue expanders followed by exchange for saline or silicone implants. Immediate reconstruction has been shown not to affect patient outcome adversely. The detection of recurrence is not delayed, and the onset of chemotherapy is not changed.

   d. **Follow-up after mastectomy:** physical examination every 3 to 6 months for 3 years, then every 6 to 12 months for the next 2 years, and then annually (*J Clin Oncol* 2006;24:5091). Mammography of the contralateral breast should continue yearly. Regular gynecologic follow-up is recommended for all women (tamoxifen increases risk of endometrial cancer).

2. **Breast conservation therapy (BCT): partial mastectomy** and SLNB (or axillary lymph node dissection; see later discussion) **followed by breast irradiation.**

   a. Several trials have demonstrated that BCT with adjuvant radiation therapy has similar survival and recurrence rates to those for MRM (*J Clin Oncol* 1992;10:976).

   b. Not every patient is a candidate for BCT. **Contraindications for BCT:** A patient who may be unreliable with follow-up or radiation therapy (may involve radiation treatment 5 days a week for 5 to 6 weeks); when the extent of disease prevents adequate negative margins; a high tumor-to-breast size ratio, which prevents adequate resection without major deformity; persistently positive margins on re-excision partial mastectomy; and inability to receive adjuvant radiation (e.g., prior radiation to the chest wall; first- and second-trimester pregnancy in which the delay of radiation to the postpartum state is inappropriate; collagen vascular diseases such as scleroderma).

   c. For patients with large tumors who desire BCT, **neoadjuvant chemotherapy** or **neoadjuvant hormonal therapy** may be offered to attempt to reduce the size of the tumor to make BCT attempt possible.

   d. **Partial mastectomy** incisions should be planned so that they can be incorporated into a mastectomy incision should that prove necessary. Incisions for partial mastectomy and either SLNB or axillary lymph node dissection should be separate.

e. **Adjuvant radiotherapy** decreases the breast cancer recurrence rate from 30% to less than 7% at 5 years and is a required component of BCT.

f. **Follow-up after BCT.** Physical examinations are the same as those for mastectomy (see earlier discussion). A posttreatment mammogram of the treated breast is performed to establish a new baseline, no earlier than 6 months after completion of radiation therapy. Mammograms are then performed every 6 to 12 months after the new baseline mammogram until the surgical changes stabilize and then annually. Contralateral breast mammography remains on an annual basis. Regular gynecologic follow-up is recommended.

3. **Management of the axilla.** Approximately 30% of patients with clinically negative exams will have positive lymph nodes in an **axillary lymph node dissection (ALND)** specimen. The presence and number of lymph nodes involved affect staging and thus prognosis. However, complications are not infrequent (see later discussion). Thus, **sentinel lymph node biopsy** was developed to provide sampling of the lymph nodes without needing an ALND.

a. **SLNB** has been established as a standard of care for predicting axillary involvement in most patients with breast cancer. The procedure requires a multidisciplinary approach, including nuclear medicine, pathology, and radiology.

(1) It involves injection of blue dye (either **Lymphazurin or methylene blue**) in the operating room and/or **technetium-labeled sulfur colloid** (in the nuclear medicine department, radiology suite, or sometimes by the surgeon). The combination of blue dye and radioisotope provides higher node identification rates and increases the sensitivity of the procedure. The goal is to identify the primary draining lymph node(s) in the axillary nodal basin.

(2) A variety of injection techniques are used: **intraparenchymal** versus **intradermal** (intradermal methylene blue will cause skin necrosis at the injection site); **peritumoral** versus **periareolar.**

(3) The SLN is identified by its blue color, and/or by high activity detected by a handheld gamma probe, or by a blue lymphatic seen to enter a nonblue node. Palpable nodes are also sentinel nodes, even if not blue or radioactive.

(4) 20% to 30% of the time more than one SLN is identified.

(5) Experienced surgeons (those who have performed at least 30 SLNBs, with ALND for confirmation) can identify the SLN in greater than 90% of patients, accurately predicting the patients' remaining axillary lymph node status in greater than 97% of cases.

(6) **If the SLN is positive for metastasis** (micrometastasis 0.2 mm or larger, *not isolated tumor cells*), **a standard ALND is performed.** Radiation therapy can be administered to the axilla if the patient refuses ALND.

(7) Serial sectioning and immunohistochemical staining of SLNB specimens may improve accuracy in detecting micrometastatic disease.

(8) Currently, **isolated tumor cells are considered N0** disease, and therapeutic decisions should *not* be based on finding these.

b. **ALND.** Patients with clinically positive lymph nodes, with positive SLN, or with positive should undergo ALND for local control. ALND involves the following:

(1) Removal of **level I** and **level II nodes** and, *if grossly involved,* possibly level III nodes. Motor and sensory nerves are preserved unless there is direct tumor involvement.

(2) An ALND should remove **10 or more nodes.** The number of nodes identified is often pathologist dependent.

(3) Patients with **4 or more positive lymph nodes** should undergo **adjuvant radiation to the axilla.** Selective patients with 1 to 3 positive nodes may also benefit from radiation therapy to the axilla.

(4) **Intraoperative complications:** potential injury to the axillary vessels and neuropathy secondary to injury to the motor nerves of the axilla (the long thoracic, thoracodorsal, and medial pectoral nerves).

(5) Most frequent **postoperative complications**: wound infections and seromas. Persistent seroma may be treated with repeated aspirations or reinsertion of a drain. Other complications include pain and numbness in the axilla and upper arm, impaired shoulder mobility, and **lymphedema.**

Lymphedema occurs in approximately 10% to 40% of women undergoing axillary dissection; radiation to the axilla increases the risk of this complication. The most effective therapy is early intervention with intense physiomassage; graded pneumatic compression devices and a professionally fitted compression sleeve can also provide relief and prevent worsening of lymphedema. Blood draws, blood pressure cuffs, and intravenous lines should be avoided in the affected arm, mainly to avoid infection in it. Infections of the hand or arm should be treated promptly and aggressively with antibiotics and arm elevation because infection can damage lymphatics further and cause irreversible lymphedema. Lymphedema itself increases the risk of developing **angiosarcoma.**

C. Adjuvant chemotherapy is given in appropriate patients after completion of surgery.

1. All **node-positive patients** should receive **adjuvant chemotherapy.**

a. Regimens are guided by the tumor biomarkers. Typical regimens comprise four to eight cycles of a combination of cyclophosphamide and an anthracycline, followed by a taxane administered every 2 to 3 weeks.

b. Patients with **ER-positive tumors** receive **adjuvant hormonal therapy** for 5 years. **Tamoxifen** is given to premenopausal women, and **aromatase inhibitors** are given to postmenopausal women (aromatase inhibitors are not used in premenopausal women).

c. In postmenopausal women older than 70 years, chemotherapy is performed less frequently. In postmenopausal women with tumors with ER or PR positivity, tamoxifen or an aromatase inhibitor is frequently the sole adjuvant medical therapy.

d. In patients with **Her2/neu-positive tumors,** polychemotherapy is combined with biological therapy targeting the *Her2/neu* protein: **Trastuzumab** is a recombinant monoclonal antibody that binds to *Her2/neu* receptor to prevent cell proliferation. The NSABP trial B-31 and the North Central Cancer Treatment Group trial N9831 showed that adding trastuzumab to a chemotherapy regiment of doxorubicin, cyclophosphamide, and paclitaxel was associated with an increase in the disease-free survival by 12% and a 33% reduction in the risk of death at 3 years. It is usually administered intravenously monthly for 12 months. The most serious toxicity with the regiment was cardiac failure (*N Engl J Med* 2005;353:1673).

2. Node-negative patients may have increased disease-free survival from adjuvant chemotherapy and/or hormonal therapy. An individualized approach is crucial and requires thorough discussion with the patient regarding the risks of recurrence without adjuvant therapy, the cost and toxicities treatment, and the expected benefit in risk reduction and survival.

a. Up to 30% of node-negative women die of breast cancer within 10 years if treated with surgery alone.

b. Node-negative patients who are at **high risk** and benefit the most from adjuvant chemotherapy include those with tumors greater than 1 cm, higher tumor grade, *Her2/neu* expression, aneuploidy, Ki-67 expression, increased percentage in S phase, lymphovascular invasion, and ER/PR-negative tumors.

c. The NSABP B-20 trial and the International Breast Cancer Study Group trial IX showed that **polychemotherapy in combination with tamoxifen was superior to tamoxifen alone** in increasing disease-free and overall survival, especially in ER-negative patients, regardless of tumor size.

d. The St. Gallen Consensus Panel in 1998 suggested that patients who have node-negative disease and whose tumors are 1 cm or less and ER-positive may be spared adjuvant chemotherapy but still may benefit from tamoxifen.

    e. The Web site http://www.adjuvantonline.com provides an online tool for physicians to use to calculate the added benefit of hormonal and chemotherapeutic therapies.

D. Adjuvant radiation

    1. Indications for adjuvant radiation to the chest wall and axilla **after mastectomy** include T3 and T4 tumors, attachment to the pectoral fascia, positive surgical margins, skin involvement, involved internal mammary nodes, inadequate or no axillary dissection, four or more positive lymph nodes, and residual tumor on the axillary vein. Presence of one to three positive axillary nodes is a relative indication.

    2. Randomized, prospective trials have shown a significantly decreased recurrence and improved survival in premenopausal women with these indications treated with chemotherapy and radiation therapy (*N Engl J Med* 1997;337:949).

    3. Adjuvant whole-breast radiation **after BCT** decreases the breast cancer recurrence rate from 30% to less than 7% at 5 years.

    4. Complications. Radiation to the chest wall can cause skin changes. Infrequent complications include interstitial pneumonitis, spontaneous rib fracture, breast fibrosis, pericarditis, pleural effusion, and chest wall myositis. Radiation to the axilla can increase the incidence of lymphedema and axillary fibrosis. **Angiosarcoma** can occur as a late complication.

E. Locally advance breast cancer (LABC) comprises T3 or T4, N1 or greater, and M0 cancers **(stages IIIA and IIIB).**

    1. Staging in LABC. Because of the frequency of distant metastasis at the time of presentation, all patients should receive complete blood cell count, complete metabolic panel, bone scan, and CT scan of chest and abdomen before treatment.

    2. Noninflammatory LABC (chest wall or skin involvement, skin satellites, ulceration, fixed axillary nodes)

        a. Patients should receive **neoadjuvant chemotherapy** (often cyclophosphamide combined with an anthracycline and taxane), followed by surgery and radiation. The high response rates seen with this regimen for **stage IIIB** allow **modified radical mastectomy** to be carried out, with primary skin closure. Adjuvant radiation to the chest wall and regional nodes and adjuvant chemotherapy follow surgery. SLNB may be used in selected patients with clinically negative axilla.

        b. Patients with **stage IIIA** disease receiving neoadjuvant chemotherapy who can be converted to **BCT** candidates have no difference in overall survival outcome.

        c. Approximately 20% of patients with stage III disease present with distant metastasis after appropriate staging has been performed.

    3. Inflammatory LABC (T4d)

        a. This is characterized by erythema, warmth, tenderness, and edema (*peau d'orange*).

        b. It represents 1% to 6% of all breast cancers.

        c. An underlying mass is present in 70% of cases. Associated axillary adenopathy occurs in 50% of cases.

        d. It is often misdiagnosed initially as mastitis.

        e. Skin punch biopsy confirms the diagnosis: In two thirds of cases, tumor emboli are seen in dermal lymphatics.

        f. Approximately 30% of patients have distant metastasis at the time of diagnosis.

        g. Inflammatory breast cancer requires **aggressive multimodal therapy** because median survival is approximately 2 years, with a 5-year survival of only 5%.

    4. Follow-up. Due to higher risk for local and distant recurrence, patients should be examined every 3 months by all specialists involved in their care.

F. Locoregional recurrence. Patients with locoregional recurrence should have a **metastatic workup** to exclude visceral or bony disease and should be considered for systemic chemotherapy or hormonal therapy.

1. **Recurrence in the breast after BCT** requires total (simple) mastectomy. Provided margins are negative, survival is similar to that for patients who received mastectomy initially.
2. **Recurrence in the axilla** requires surgical resection followed by radiation to the axilla and systemic therapy.
3. **Recurrence in the chest wall after mastectomy** occurs in 4% to 5% of patients. One third of these patients have distant metastases at the time of recurrence, and greater than 50% will have distant disease within 2 years. Multimodal therapy is essential. For an isolated local recurrence, excision followed by radiotherapy results in excellent local control. Rarely, patients require radical chest resection with myocutaneous flap closure.

VI. CHEMOPREVENTION

A. The NSABP P-1 trial was the first large prospective, randomized chemopreventive trial to evaluate the efficacy of the estrogen antagonist **tamoxifen** to reduce breast cancer incidence in women at risk.

1. Women taking tamoxifen achieved an overall reduction in the risk of developing invasive breast carcinoma of 49% and a reduction in the risk of developing noninvasive breast cancer of 50%.
2. In subgroups of women with a history of **LCIS** and with a history of **ADH**, tamoxifen reduced the risk of developing invasive breast cancer by 65% and 86%, respectively.

B. The NSABP B-24 trial showed that tamoxifen provided a 37% overall risk reduction for all breast cancers (invasive and noninvasive) in women with **DCIS treated with lumpectomy and radiation.**

1. The **toxicities** of the drug include an increased risk of endometrial cancer, thrombotic vascular events, and cataract development. Women on tamoxifen also reported increased vasomotor symptoms (hot flashes) and vaginal discharge.
2. Tamoxifen also provided a significant reduction in hip fractures in women older than 50 years of age. There was no difference noted in the incidence of ischemic heart disease for women taking tamoxifen.
3. Tamoxifen has been approved by the Food and Drug Administration (FDA) for (1) the **treatment of metastatic breast cancer**, (2) **adjuvant treatment of breast cancer**, and (3) **chemoprevention of invasive or contralateral breast cancer in high-risk women.**
4. The **dosage** for chemoprevention is 20 mg/day for 5 years. It is estimated that chemoprevention could prevent as many as 500,000 invasive and 200,000 noninvasive breast cancers over 5 years in the United States alone.
5. The Study of Tamoxifen and Raloxifene (STAR) trial compared tamoxifen to **raloxifene** (a selective estrogen receptor modulator). Raloxifene has not been FDA approved for chemoprevention, but was shown to provide equal risk reduction for the development of invasive breast cancers as tamoxifen. It was not as effective at reducing the risk of developing noninvasive breast cancer. Its side effect profile is somewhat different than that of tamoxifen, so it can be considered in patients with relative contraindications to tamoxifen.

SPECIAL CONSIDERATIONS

I. BREAST CONDITIONS DURING PREGNANCY

A. **Bloody nipple discharge** may occur in the second or third trimester. It results from epithelial proliferation under hormonal influences and usually resolves by 2 months postpartum. If it does not resolve by then, standard evaluation of pathologic nipple discharge should be performed.

B. **Breast masses** occurring during pregnancy include **galactoceles, lactating adenoma, simple cysts, breast infarcts, fibroadenomas,** *and* **carcinoma.** Fibroadenomas may grow during pregnancy due to hormonal stimulation.

1. Masses should be evaluated by ultrasound, and a core needle biopsy should be performed for any suspicious lesion.
2. Mammography can be performed with uterine shielding but is rarely helpful due to increased breast density.
3. If a breast lesion is diagnosed as malignant, the patient should be given the **same surgical treatment** options, stage for stage, as a nonpregnant woman, and the **treatment should not be delayed** because of the pregnancy.

C. **Breast cancer during pregnancy** may be difficult to diagnose due to the low level of suspicion and breast nodularity and density.
1. It occurs in approximately 1 in 5,000 gestations and accounts for almost 3% of all breast cancers.
2. **Workup is the same as in a nonpregnant woman.** The standard preoperative staging workup is performed. Laboratory values such as alkaline phosphatase may be elevated during pregnancy. For advanced-stage disease, MR scan or ultrasound may be used in lieu of CT scan for staging. Excisional biopsy can be safely performed under local anesthesia if there is some contraindication to the preferred core needle biopsy.
3. **Therapeutic decisions** are influenced by the clinical cancer stage and the trimester of pregnancy and must be **individualized.** MRM has been the standard surgical modality for pregnant patients with breast cancer, but BCT can be offered to selected patients. The radiation component of BCT cannot be applied during pregnancy, and delaying radiation therapy is not ideal. For these reasons, BCT is usually not recommended to patients in their first or second trimester. For patients in the third trimester, radiation can begin after delivery. SLNB is starting to be used more frequently; the commonly used radioisotope is approved for use during pregnancy.
4. **Chemotherapy** may be given by the mid-second trimester.

II. **PAGET DISEASE OF THE NIPPLE** is characterized by eczematoid changes of the nipple, which may involve the surrounding areola.
A. Burning, pruritus, and hypersensitivity may be prominent symptoms.
B. Paget disease is almost always accompanied by an underlying malignancy, either invasive ductal carcinoma or DCIS.
C. Palpable masses are present in approximately 60% of patients.
D. Mammography should be performed to identify other areas of involvement. If clinical suspicion is high, a pathologic diagnosis should be obtained by wedge biopsy of the nipple and underlying breast tissue.
E. Treatment is mastectomy or BCT with excision of the nipple-areolar complex (sometimes called a central lumpectomy), followed by radiation therapy. The prognosis is related to tumor stage.

III. **BREAST CANCER IN MEN** accounts for less than 1% of male cancers and less than 1% of all breast cancers. BRCA2 mutations are associated with approximately 4% to 6% of these cancers.
A. Patients generally present with a nontender hard mass. This contrasts with unilateral gynecomastia, which is usually firm, central, and tender.
B. Mammography can be helpful in distinguishing gynecomastia from malignancy. Malignant lesions are more likely to be eccentric, with irregular margins, and are often associated with nipple retraction and microcalcifications. Biopsy of suspicious lesions is essential, and core needle biopsy is preferred.
C. Modified radical mastectomy was traditionally the surgical procedure of choice; however, SLNB has been shown to be effective in men. Thus, total (simple) mastectomy with SLNB is a valid option in men.
D. Eighty-five percent of malignancies are infiltrating ductal carcinoma and are positive for ER.
E. **Adjuvant hormonal, chemotherapy, and radiation treatment criteria are the same as in women.** Overall survival *per stage* is comparable to that observed in women, although men tend to present in later stages.

IV. PHYLLODES TUMORS account for 1% of breast neoplasms.

   A. They present as a large, smooth, lobulated mass and may be difficult to distinguish from fibroadenoma on physical exam.

   B. They can occur in women of any age, but most frequently between ages 35 and 55 years.

   C. Skin ulcerations may occur secondary to pressure of the underlying mass.

   D. FNAB cannot reliably diagnose these tumors; at least a core needle biopsy is needed. Histologically, stromal overgrowth is the essential characteristic for differentiating phyllodes tumors from fibroadenomas.

   E. Ninety percent are benign; 10% are malignant. The biologic behavior of malignant tumors is similar to that of **sarcomas.**

   F. Treatment is **wide local excision to tumor-free margins or total mastectomy.** Axillary assessment with either SLNB or ALND is **not** indicated unless nodes are clinically positive (which is rare).

   G. Currently, there is no role for adjuvant radiation; however, tumors greater than 5 cm in diameter and with evidence of stromal overgrowth may benefit from adjuvant chemotherapy with doxorubicin and ifosfamide (*Cancer* 2000;89:1510).

   H. Patients should be followed with semiannual physical examinations and annual mammograms and chest radiographs.

OTOLARYNGOLOGY: HEAD AND NECK SURGERY

28

Jason T. Rich and Bruce H. Haughey

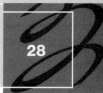

I. INTRODUCTION. Otolaryngology–head and neck surgery (OHNS) is one of a few anatomically defined medical specialties. In addition, there are a significant number of structures concentrated within the head and neck. These factors make OHNS a challenging and exciting field, full of diverse systems and diseases. This chapter provides a brief description of selected diseases thought to be useful to the general surgery practitioner.

II. THE EAR

A. Anatomy and physiology

1. **External ear**

   a. The **auricle (or pinna)** consists of elastic cartilage covered by perichondrium and tightly adherent epithelium. It functions to channel sound waves through the external auditory canal.

   b. The lateral one third of the **external auditory canal** is composed of cartilage and is covered by epithelium containing cerumin glands and hairs. The medial two thirds is composed of bone and is covered by a thin epithelial layer.

2. The **middle ear** is a mucosal-lined sinus within the temporal bone that houses the ossicular chain.

   a. The **tympanic membrane (TM)** converts sound waves into mechanical energy, which is transmitted through the ossicular chain to the cochlea. The TM is adherent to the malleus and is divided into the small **pars flaccida** superiorly and the larger **pars tensa** inferiorly.

   b. The **eustachian tube (ET)** provides communication between the middle ear and nasopharynx. It protects the middle ear from nasopharyngeal pathogens, aerates the middle ear, and drains fluid from the middle ear space. The ET opens during swallowing and yawning, primarily by the action of the tensor veli palatini muscle.

   c. The **mastoid cavity** is a pneumatized bony process within the temporal bone that communicates with the middle ear.

   d. The **ossicular chain** conducts mechanical energy from the tympanic membrane to the oval window of the inner ear. It consists of the **malleus, incus,** and **stapes.** The difference in surface area between the tympanic membrane and the oval window, along with the lever action of the ossicular chain, leads to 22-fold amplification in sound energy.

3. The **inner ear (otic capsule)** encases the sensory end organs of hearing (cochlea) and balance (vestibular system).

   a. The **cochlea** is a snail-shaped structure with two and a half turns that contains the end organ of hearing, the organ of Corti.

   b. The **vestibular system** consists of three semicircular canals oriented at 90 degrees to each other (which sense spatial orientation and angular acceleration) and the utricle and saccule (which sense linear acceleration).

   c. Neuroelectric impulses generated by the cochlea and vestibular system are transmitted centrally via the **vestibulocochlear nerve [cranial nerve (CN) VIII].**

4. The **facial nerve (CN VII)** travels through the temporal bone and middle ear space. In addition to motor innervation of the facial musculature, it innervates

the stapedius muscle and sends off the chorda tympani branch, which supplies taste sensation to the anterior two thirds of the tongue.

B. Hearing loss and tinnitus

1. Hearing loss is classified as sensorineural, conductive, or mixed.

   a. Sensorineural hearing loss (SNHL) is caused by lesions in the cochlea, CN VIII, or the central nervous system. Common causes of SNHL include presbycusis (age-related hearing loss), noise exposure, ototoxicity, viral or bacterial infections, autoimmune diseases, temporal bone trauma, CN VIII tumors, and congenital hearing loss. **Idiopathic sudden SNHL** is treated with systemic or intratympanic corticosteroids. Its etiology is unknown, and the efficacy of current treatments is controversial (*Laryngoscope* 2007;117:3).

   b. Conductive hearing loss is the result of inadequate transmission of sound energy to the inner ear and arises from the external ear canal, tympanic membrane, or middle ear. Common causes include impacted cerumen, tympanic membrane perforation, otitis media, cholesteatoma, ossicular chain fixation (otosclerosis), and ossicular discontinuity.

2. Evaluation of hearing

   a. The **Weber test** entails placing a 512-Hz tuning fork on the patient's forehead or maxillary incisor and asking whether the sound is perceived as louder in one ear or the other. The test is normal if the patient is unable to lateralize the sound to a particular ear. Sound lateralizes to the ear with a conductive hearing loss or contralateralizes to the ear with a SNHL.

   b. The **Rinne test** is performed by placing a tuning fork first lateral to the pinna (air conduction) and then on the mastoid tip (bone conduction). The patient is asked which placement was perceived as louder. Those with normal hearing perceive air conduction louder than bone conduction. Patients with a conductive hearing loss perceive bone conduction as louder than air conduction.

   c. Formal audiometry is able to both qualify and quantify hearing loss. A gap between air and bone thresholds suggests the presence of a conductive hearing loss. Equal drops in both air and bone thresholds suggest sensorineural hearing loss. Decreased word discrimination suggests the presence of retrocochlear pathology (e.g., CN VIII tumors).

   d. Auditory brainstem response (ABR) measures electroencephalogram (EEG) waveforms generated in response to sound and is useful for hearing testing in infants.

   e. Tympanometry, or impedance audiometry, measures tympanic membrane compliance, ear canal volume, and the stapedial reflex (seventh/eighth nerve reflex arc).

3. Surgical treatment of hearing loss

   a. Cochlear implantation (CI) consists of surgically implanting an electrode array into the cochlea. A microphone worn near the ear receives acoustic signals and transmits the stimuli to the implanted cochlear electrode, which then stimulates the cochlear nerve. CI has been shown to be very effective in adults, children, and infants with profound hearing loss (*JAMA* 1995;274: 1955).

   b. Conductive hearing loss can often be successfully treated by restoring the sound conduction pathway through repair of the tympanic membrane (tympanoplasty), ossicular reconstruction, or removal of cholesteatoma. Those who elect not to have surgery may be treated with hearing aids.

4. Tinnitus, or ringing in the ears, is a difficult entity to treat. Life-threatening causes must first be identified and treated, such as CN VIII tumors or arteriovenous malformations. Remaining cases of tinnitus are often referred to comprehensive tinnitus management programs.

C. True vertigo, which originates from the inner ear, must be distinguished from nonotologic causes, such as cardiovascular (orthostatic hypotension, vertibrobasilar insufficiency, cerebellar/brainstem infarction), metabolic (hypoglycemia, hypothyroidism, drug induced), neurogenic (migraines, multiple sclerosis, neoplasm), or psychogenic causes. Nonotologic vertigo is often described as unsteadiness, light-headedness, or syncope, whereas true vertigo is described as a sensation of spinning or being in motion.

1. **Causes of true vertigo** are best organized by the chronology of symptoms.

   a. **Seconds to minutes. Benign paroxysmal positional vertigo (BPPV)** is one of the most common causes of transient vertigo. It is precipitated by changes in head position and is thought to be caused by stimulation of the vestibular system by free-floating calcium carbonate crystals within the semicircular canals. The most common form of BPPV affects the posterior semicircular canal. It is diagnosed by the Dix-Hallpike maneuver, in which torsional nystagmus is induced when the patient is brought rapidly from the upright to the supine position with the head turned 45 degrees toward the affected ear. Canalith repositioning maneuvers (Eppley technique) are immediately effective in 80% of patients with BPPV (*Otolaryngol Head Neck Surg* 2006;135:529).

   b. **Hours. Ménière disease (endolymphatic hydrops)** is classically associated with episodic vertigo, hearing loss, tinnitus, and aural fullness. The pathogenesis is believed to be an increase in endolymph volume within the inner ear. Medical management consists of salt restriction, diuretics, and vestibular suppressants. Refractory cases require transtympanic gentamicin, endolymphatic sac surgery, labyrinthectomy, or vestibular nerve sectioning to control vertigo symptoms.

   c. **Days**

      (1) **Viral labyrinthitis/viral neuronitis** is thought to result from a viral infection of the inner ear. Vertigo can last days or even weeks, and the patient may be left with persistent disequilibrium for months. This is thought to be similar to sudden SNHL (see Section II.B.1.9). Vestibular rehabilitation is helpful.

      (2) **Temporal bone trauma.**

2. **Vestibular testing** includes **electronystagmography (ENG), dynamic posturography, rotational chair analysis, and caloric testing.** The latter entails applying cold and warm water to the external auditory canal in an effort to stimulate **nystagmus.** Nystagmus is defined by its fast phase. The pneumonic COWS (cold opposite, warm same) can be used as a reminder of the direction of nystagmus induced by caloric testing.

D. **Infectious/inflammatory disorders**

   1. **Otitis externa,** or swimmer's ear, is an inflammation of the external auditory canal. A moist ear canal causes changes in the local pH and results in bacterial overgrowth, most commonly by *Pseudomonas aeruginosa*. Symptoms include severe ear pain, drainage, canal swelling, and conductive hearing loss. First-line treatment is aural toilet and antibiotic ear drops (with or without corticosteroids). If the ear canal is extremely swollen, an ear wick may be placed, which both serves as a stent and facilitates contact between the ear drops and the canal wall. **Malignant external otitis (MEO)** is essentially osteomyelitis of the skull base and tends to be a disease of diabetic or immunocompromised patients. MEO can be rapidly fatal and requires aggressive therapy, including intravenous antibiotics and surgical débridement.

   2. **Eustachian tube dysfunction.** The ET provides aeration, clearance, and protection of the middle ear. The ET is nearly horizontal in infants but elongates and assumes a more vertical alignment with facial growth. Failure of the ET to protect the middle ear from nasopharyngeal bacteria is thought to result in acute otitis media, whereas failure to clear middle ear fluid due to an obstructed ET is thought to result in otitis media with effusion.

   3. **Acute otitis media (AOM)** is inflammation of the middle ear space. Symptoms of AOM include fever, otalgia, decreased appetite, and irritability. Examination usually reveals an erythematous, bulging tympanic membrane. Treatment of AOM is controversial. Current guidelines recommend watchful

waiting for uncomplicated cases of AOM in children over 6 months of age to reduce unnecessary antibiotic exposure (*Pediatrics* 2004;113:1451, *Pediatrics* 2005;115:1455). Analgesics should always be prescribed, and if symptoms do not resolve within 48 to 72 hours, antibacterial treatment should be initiated. Common bacterial pathogens associated with AOM include *Streptococcus pneumonia, Haemophilus influenzae,* and *Moraxella catarrhalis.* Complications of AOM are rare and include eardrum perforation, mastoiditis, subperiosteal abscess, labyrinthitis, facial nerve palsy, epidural or subdural abscess, meningitis, brain abscess, sigmoid sinus thrombophlebitis, and otitic hydrocephalus. Four bouts of AOM in 6 months or six episodes in 1 year are indications for tympanostomy tube (TT) placement. TT allows ventilation of the middle ear space and dramatically reduces the incidence of AOM. Chronic tympanic membrane perforation is a rare but real complication of TT.

4. **Otitis media with effusion (OME)** consists of fluid behind the eardrum but without the inflammation associated with acute otitis media. OME predisposes to AOM and can negatively affect hearing and speech development. OME is thought to be a bacterial disease and is treated with antibiotics. If antibacterial therapy fails, OME can be successfully treated with tympanostomy tubes to provide middle ear aeration.

5. **Chronic suppurative otitis media** describes prolonged infection of the middle ear and is often associated with a persistent tympanic membrane perforation. Chronic otorrhea is common. Although some cases may be managed medically, most require surgery.

E. **Cholesteatomas** consist of a keratin matrix surrounded by squamous epithelial cells. Cholesteatomas are slow-growing masses that are usually not symptomatic until later in life. They are classified as **congenital, primary acquired,** or **secondary acquired.** Congenital cholesteatomas are thought to arise from embryonic rests and present as a white cyst medial to an intact eardrum. Primary acquired cholesteatomas result from eustachian tube dysfunction and negative pressure in the middle ear. A retraction pocket develops in the pars flaccida and collects squamous debris. Secondary acquired cholesteatomas arise from tympanic membrane perforations with medial migration of squamous epithelium around the edges of the hole. The cholesteatoma matrix is metabolically active and erodes bone by pressure effect and osteoclast activation. Symptoms include hearing loss, perilymphatic fistula, vertigo, and facial nerve palsy. Treatment requires surgical resection; however, recurrence is not uncommon.

F. **Trauma**
1. Ear trauma is **classified by location.** Trauma to the auricle may result in hematoma that requires incision and drainage. Failure to do so results in cartilage destruction and a deformed "cauliflower" ear. Tympanic membrane perforations usually heal without intervention. Surgical repair is indicated for chronic perforations.

2. **Temporal bone fractures** are classified as longitudinal (80%) or transverse (20%). Although transverse fractures are less common, they are more likely to cause permanent SHNL or facial nerve injury. The decision to pursue surgical intervention is determined by the status of the facial nerve.

G. **Foreign bodies** in the external canal are common. Organic materials expand when moistened and should not be treated with ear drops. Batteries in the ear canal must be removed immediately because they can cause severe scarring and stenosis.

H. **Facial nerve (CN VII) paralysis.** Central paralysis from a supranuclear lesion spares the ipsilateral forehead due to bilateral cortical innervation. Peripheral lesions produce ipsilateral paralysis of the whole face. Facial nerve paralysis can be caused by malignancy, facial neuroma, trauma, or infection. There is a lack of data in the literature regarding treatment of facial nerve paralysis. Delayed-onset facial paralysis is usually treated with corticosteroids (with or without antivirals) and observation. Acute-onset facial paralysis is assessed with nerve stimulation. If the facial nerve loses stimulability, facial nerve exploration is performed for nerve decompression.

1. The diagnosis of **Bell palsy** should be reserved for facial nerve paralysis cases in which no other cause is evident. Bell palsy is thought to be viral in origin. A recent meta-analysis showed a 17% improvement in recovery with corticosteroid treatment (*Laryngoscope* 2000;110:335). The addition of acyclovir and surgical decompression remain controversial.

2. **Ramsay Hunt syndrome** is a facial nerve paralysis caused by herpes zoster reactivation in CN VII. Paralysis is more severe than in Bell palsy and the prognosis is worse. Treatment includes corticosteroids and acyclovir.

III. NOSE AND SINUS DISORDERS

A. Anatomy and physiology

1. The **nose** functions primarily in respiration and olfaction. The **external nose** comprises the nasal bones superiorly and nasal cartilage anteriorly. The **nasal septum** comprises cartilage anteriorly and bone posteriorly. The **inferior, middle, superior, and supreme turbinates** are mucosa-lined bony prominences that project from the lateral nasal walls and serve to filter, warm, and humidify inspired air. The **olfactory nerve** penetrates the **cribriform plate** and is distributed along the superior aspect of the nasal vault. The nose is lined with a mucosa rich in mucous glands, nerves, blood vessels, and inflammatory cells.

2. The **paranasal sinuses** (frontal, maxillary, ethmoid, and sphenoid sinuses) are paired bony cavities of the skull that contribute to voice resonance, decrease the weight of the skull, and cushion cranial contents in the case of head trauma. Mucus produced in the sinuses drains into the nasal cavity through ostia by mucociliary flow.

B. Congenital disorders

1. Congenital midline nasal masses in children can be **encephaloceles, gliomas, or dermoid cysts** and may be present intranasally, extranasally, as a mass or pit. A magnetic resonance image (MRI) should always be obtained to rule out intracranial communication. Treatment is surgical excision.

2. **Choanal atresia** (CA) is persistence of the nasobuccal membrane, which prohibits communication between the nasal cavity and nasopharynx. CA is more common in females, is unilateral in approximately 70% of cases, and is often associated with other anomalies. Because infants are obligate nasal breathers, bilateral CA is often diagnosed shortly after birth. Inability to pass a catheter through the nose into the oropharynx confirms the diagnosis. Bilateral CA requires immediate surgical attention, whereas unilateral CA repair is often delayed to allow the operative site to enlarge.

C. Infectious/inflammatory disorders

1. **Rhinosinusitis** is characterized by nasal congestion, excessive secretions, and postnasal drip. Rhinosinusitis has multiple etiologies that can be grouped into allergic, infectious, or drug induced.

2. **Acute bacterial rhinosinusitis** (ABS) is characterized by facial and dental pain, sinus pressure, fever, and purulent nasal discharge. The most common pathogens are *Streptococcus pneumoniae*, *M. catarrhalis*, and *H. influenzae*. Treatment consists of a 14-day antibacterial regiment (amoxicillin/clavulanate or quinolones), decongestants, mucolytic agents, and humidification, with or without systemic corticosteroids. Surgical intervention is usually not necessary. Clinicians should be vigilant for intraorbital or intracranial complications of ABS.

3. **Chronic bacterial rhinosinusitis (CRS)** is loosely defined as ABS symptoms lasting more than 6 weeks. The pathophysiology of CRS is thought to be multifactorial and includes mechanical obstruction of the paranasal sinus drainage at the **osteomeatal complex,** allergic inflammation, and infection (bacterial or fungal). However, the exact pathogenesis and treatment of CRS are under debate. Coronal computed tomography (CT) scan of the sinuses is the diagnostic study of choice and provides the surgeon with information regarding the bony and soft tissue anatomy, mucosal inflammation, and purulence within the sinus cavities. Patients should first be treated medically for 12 weeks with antibiotics, nasal saline washes, and nasal steroids (*Laryngoscope* 2004;114:923). Patients that have failed medical treatment may be candidates for **functional endoscopic**

sinus surgery (FESS). The objectives of FESS are to re-establish the patency of the sinus ostia, ventilate the sinuses, and remove diseased mucosa or polyps. Studies indicate that patients refractory to medical treatment benefit from FESS (*Curr Opin Otolaryngol Head Neck Surg* 2007;15:6). Immunotherapy might provide another tool in treating CRS; however, data are lacking.

4. **Fungal sinusitis** is most often caused by *Aspergillus* species. Invasive fungal sinusitis is more common in immunocompromised patients and requires intravenous antifungal medications and prompt surgical débridement. Antifungal treatment of chronic rhinosinusitis has not been shown to be successful (*J Allergy Clin Immunol* 2006;118:1149).

D. **Epistaxis** has multiple etiologies, including trauma, tumors, coagulopathies, and granulomatous diseases (Wegener, tuberculosis, sarcoidosis, etc.). Most epistaxis is minor; however, due to the significant vascularity of the nose, hemorrhage can be life-threatening. Always address the ABCs first (airway, breathing, circulation). The patient should be instructed to pinch his or her nose until examined by a clinician. If bleeding persists, pledgets soaked with vasoconstrictors (lidocaine with epinephrine, or cocaine) can be inserted into the nasal cavity. Visualization of the nasal cavity allows for localization of the bleeding (anterior vs. posterior) and allows for cauterization of active bleeding with silver nitrate or electrocautery. The anterior nose can be packed using epistaxis balloons or gauze. Posterior nasal packing can be achieved by passing a Foley catheter through the nares past the choana. The catheter is then inflated and pulled anteriorly until it rests snugly in the posterior choana. Arterial embolization is reserved for refractory cases.

E. **Nasal-sinus trauma**
1. **Nasal fractures** are the result of blunt facial trauma. Epistaxis and airway management are the first priority. Reduction of nasal fractures is recommended between days 3 and 10. This timing allows for resolution of swelling but avoids bony healing. Closed reduction is usually sufficient for most fractures.
2. **Midface fractures** with cosmetic or functional deformities require open reduction and internal fixation. Control of the airway is important in the acute setting. Midface fractures are classified according to the **Le Fort system** (Fig. 28-1). Le Fort I fracture separates the bone containing the maxillary dentition from the rest of the craniofacial skeleton. Le Fort II (pyramidal fracture) extends up through the maxilla, across the orbital floor and nasal bones, and down the other side of the face in similar fashion. Le Fort III fracture represents a true separation of the facial bones from the cranium by involving both zygomas, orbits, and nasal bones.

F. **Nasal septum**
1. **Nasal septal deviation (NSD)** results from nasal trauma or differential growth during postnatal development. The role of NSD in sinus disease is controversial (*Am J Rhinol* 2000;14:175, *Otolaryngol Head Neck Surg* 2005;133:190). Most surgeons correct NSD (septoplasty) in connection with the FESS procedure (see Section III.C.3) if nasal obstruction and sinus disease are present.
2. **Nasal septal hematomas** may occur with any nasal trauma. Blood collects between the mucoperichondrium and cartilage of the nasal septum. Because the cartilage relies on the overlying tissues for its blood supply, the hematoma can cause cartilage necrosis and septal perforation. Treatment is incision and drainage.
3. **Nasal septal perforations (NSPs)** are usually located anteriorly in the cartilaginous portion of the septum. NSPs are most commonly caused by trauma (prior surgery, facial trauma, digital trauma), intranasal cocaine use, or vasculitis. Though NSP is not a life-threatening condition, it can cause substantial morbidity due to continual crusting, bleeding, nasal obstruction, and "whistling" while breathing. Most NSP are not repaired due to the high failure rates of local mucosal flap advancement.

G. **Nasal foreign bodies** are generally found in children or adults with mental retardation. Unilateral, foul-smelling nasal discharge in a child is considered a foreign object until proven otherwise. In adults with similar symptoms, neoplasms must

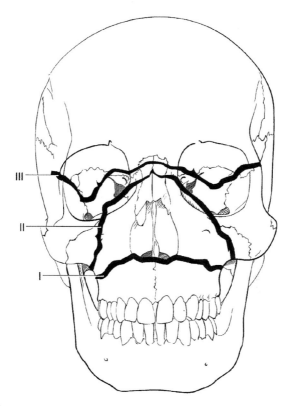

Figure 28-1. Le Fort I, II, and III midface fractures. (With permission from Cummings CW, Haughey BH, Thomas JR, et al., eds. *Cummings Otolaryngology: Head and Neck Surgery,* 4th ed. St. Louis: CV Mosby; 2005.)

be ruled out. Most foreign bodies can be removed in awake patients. However, conscious sedation or general anesthesia with airway protection may be necessary in younger children. Batteries in the nose, ear, trachea, or esophagus constitute a medical emergency requiring urgent removal.

H. The **adenoids** are lymphoid tissue present in the posterior nasopharynx that hypertrophy during childhood and then usually atrophy with age. **Adenoid hypertrophy** can cause recurrent otitis media, snoring, and nasal obstruction, resulting in mouth breathing. Adenoidectomy is often performed in connection with tonsillectomy.

I. **Nasal polyps** are pendulous, edematous, hyperplastic regions of nasal mucosa that often cause sinus drainage obstruction. The etiology of **nasal polyps** is unknown, but they are commonly associated with systemic diseases (cystic fibrosis, allergies, chronic rhinosinusitis, or the clinical triad of aspirin sensitivity, asthma, and nasal polyposis). Nasal polyps are usually treated with nasal steroids and surgical debulking, although the effectiveness of surgical treatment is controversial and requires further investigation (*Health Technol Assess* 2003;7:1).

IV. LARYNX

A. Anatomy and physiology

1. The larynx is divided into the **supraglottis** (which includes the epiglottis, arytenoid cartilages, false vocal folds, and ventricle), the **glottis** (true vocal folds), and **subglottis** (from the true vocal folds to the cricoid cartilage). The **thyroid** and **cricoid cartilages** and the **hyoid bone** provide the rigid support for the larynx.

2. The **superior laryngeal nerve** provides sensory innervation to the supraglottic mucosa and motor innervation to the cricothyroid muscle. The **recurrent laryngeal nerve** provides sensory innervation to the remaining laryngeal mucosa and motor innervation to all the intrinsic laryngeal muscles. Both are derived from the vagus nerve (CN X).

3. The larynx is a critical part of the aerodigestive tract. It contributes to airway protection, deglutition, and phonation. Laryngeal elevation, glottic closure, and retroflexion of the epiglottis help to prevent aspiration during **swallowing.** **Coughing** consists in increasing subglottic pressure by contracting expiratory muscles against a tightly closed glottis. The larynx suddenly opens, resulting in a rapid outflow of air and expulsion of mucus or foreign materials from the airway.

B. Congenital disorders

1. **Laryngomalacia** is the most common congenital laryngeal abnormality. An omega-shaped epiglottis and floppy arytenoid towers prolapse into the airway on inspiration, creating inspiratory stridor. Symptoms generally worsen for the first 18 months of life and then improve. If respiratory or feeding difficulties result in failure to thrive, endoscopic supraglottoplasty is recommended.

2. The second-most-common laryngeal abnormality in the newborn is **vocal cord paralysis.** These are often idiopathic but may be related to central nervous system (CNS) malformations such as the Arnold-Chiari malformation. Most cases resolve spontaneously. Bilateral vocal cord paralysis often requires tracheostomy.

3. Other congenital laryngeal abnormalities include laryngeal atresia, webs, cysts, laryngeal clefts, and **subglottic stenosis.** Subglottic stenosis can be either congenital or acquired. Surgical laryngotracheal reconstruction or cricotracheal resection is often necessary.

C. Trauma

1. **Blunt or penetrating laryngeal trauma** requires rapid airway assessment and control, possibly requiring intubation or tracheostomy. Diagnostic modalities include fiberoptic laryngoscopy, high-resolution CT scan, and operative endoscopy. Laryngeal hematomas and small lacerations are managed conservatively with airway observation and humidified air. Displaced fractures and laryngeal instability require urgent tracheostomy followed by open reduction and internal fixation.

2. **Caustic ingestions** can be classified by the type of material ingested. Alkali ingestions result in liquefactive necrosis of the laryngeal suprastructure, pharynx, and esophagus and put the patient at risk for stenosis. Acidic materials cause coagulative necrosis. Endoscopy is recommended 24 to 48 hours after ingestion. Initial therapy includes nasogastric (NG) tube placement and high-dose systemic steroids. If strictures occur, they are assessed with barium swallow studies and may require periodic esophageal dilation.

D. Infectious/inflammatory disorders

1. **Viral croup,** or viral laryngotracheitis, occurs mostly in children and is an inflammation of the glottis and subglottis caused mainly by parainfluenza viruses 1 and 2. Viral croup is diagnosed clinically, often with a history of a prodromal upper respiratory infection followed by stridor and a barking cough. Treatment of most cases is supportive; however, severe cases respond well to glucocorticoids.

2. **Epiglottitis** is a medical emergency. Children with epiglottitis present acutely (within 2 to 6 hours) with a high fever, drooling, and sitting upright with inspiratory stridor. Airway management is the preeminent concern. In a study, most cases of epiglottitis required intubation (*Laryngoscope* 1994;104:1314). Administration of antibiotics is the main treatment. Widespread vaccination against *H. influenzae* type B has significantly decreased its incidence; however, emerging reports of epiglottitis in fully vaccinated children underscore the importance of clinicians quickly recognizing this disease entity (*Int J Pediatr Otorhinolaryngol* 2003;67:317).

3. **Acute laryngitis** is an inflammation of the laryngeal mucosa and vocal cords resulting in hoarseness. Most cases occur in adults and are of viral origin. Acute laryngitis is usually self-limited and requires strict voice rest.

4. **Laryngopharyngeal reflux** refers to the retrograde movement of gastric contents into the larynx/hypopharynx and is characterized by cervical dysphagia, globus, sore throat, cough, hoarseness, and chronic throat clearing. It is believed to be an esophageal sphincter disorder and is treated with diet, behavior modifications, and high-dose proton-pump inhibitors (*Allergy Asthma Proc* 2006;27:21).

5. Other inflammatory lesions that affect the larynx include sulcus vocalis, contact ulcers, vocal nodules, granulomas, and smoker's laryngitis.

E. **Neuromuscular disorders**

   1. **Chronic aspiration** is caused by a loss of the protective functions of the larynx due to impaired motor activity or sensory loss. Aspiration can result in bronchopulmonary infection and airway obstruction.

      a. **Causes of chronic aspiration** include cerebral damage (stroke, tumor, trauma), degenerative neurologic diseases (Parkinson disease, amyotrophic lateral sclerosis, multiple sclerosis), neuromuscular disorders (myasthenia gravis, muscular dystrophies), and surgical alteration of the larynx (following cancer resection).

      b. **Treatment of chronic aspiration** first requires elucidation of the dysfunction by performing swallowing studies. Focused physical therapy with a speech/swallowing therapist corrects many cases. Refractory cases can be treated with nasogastric, gastric, or parenteral nutrition. Surgical treatments include tracheostomy, vocal cord medialization, and laryngectomy.

   2. **Vocal cord paralysis** occurs when the **recurrent laryngeal nerve (RLN)** is damaged. Due to the lengthy path of the RLN from the vagus nerve down into the thorax and back up to the larynx, the RLN can easily be damaged by surgery, neoplasm, or trauma to the thorax or neck. Recognized iatrogenic injuries should be repaired by primary epineural anastomosis or cable grafting. Patients presenting with a new diagnosis of vocal cord paralysis require a CT scan and/or MRI of the neck and chest to rule out other pathologies. Unilateral vocal cord paralysis puts patients at risk for aspiration and greatly affects phonation. Treatment consists of speech therapy and observation. Partial to full recovery often occurs over many months. Surgical options include injection laryngoplasty (with Gelfoam, fat, or Cymetra), medialization of the vocal cord, and laryngeal reinnervation. Bilateral vocal cord paralysis often results in airway obstruction and is treated with arytenoidectomy, cordectomy, or tracheostomy.

   3. **Spasmodic dysphonia (laryngeal dystonia)** is laryngeal motion disorder. The pathophysiology of spasmodic dysphonia is unknown. It is effectively treated with botulinum toxin injections into the laryngeal musculature.

V. **ORAL CAVITY AND PHARYNX**

A. **Anatomy and physiology**

   1. The oral cavity plays a crucial role in articulation and deglutition. The oral cavity includes the lips, oral mucosa, tongue, base of the tongue, floor of the mouth, alveolar ridges, and hard and soft palates. The pharynx is divided into the nasopharynx, oropharynx, and hypopharynx. Swallowing is a complex task involving soft palate elevation, elevation and retrusion of the tongue, laryngeal elevation, glottic closure, epiglottic retroflexion, and pharyngeal/esophageal peristalsis.

   2. **Waldeyer's ring** is a ring of lymphoid tissue in the superior pharynx. It is composed of the lingual tonsils, palatine tonsils, and adenoids.

B. **Congenital disorders**

   1. A variety of congenital abnormalities can affect the oral cavity and pharynx and are often associated with genetic syndromes. The **Pierre-Robin sequence** includes micrognathia, glossoptosis, and a U-shaped cleft. A variety of syndromes such as Apert craniosynostosis, Crouzon craniosynostosis, Treacher Collins syndrome, and velocardiofacial syndrome may also create breathing and swallowing problems through midface abnormalities. Airway obstruction and feeding difficulties can be treated with prone positioning, glossopexy, mandibular advancement, closure of the cleft palate, or tracheostomy.

2. **Cleft lip and palate.** Clefts form as a result of failed fusion of the midface processes during embryogenesis. Clefts may be complete or incomplete, unilateral or bilateral, and can involve the primary and/or secondary palates. Patients with cleft lip and palate deformities should be managed by a multidisciplinary cleft team that can address feeding, hearing, respiratory, cosmetic, speech, and psychosocial issues. Cleft lips are usually closed during the first year of life, and cleft palate surgery is undertaken between 6 months and 2 years of life. These procedures are staged and may require multiple surgeries as the child ages.

C. **Trauma**

1. **Mandible fractures** (MFs) occur most commonly at the angle and parasymphyseal regions of the mandibular body and at the condylar neck (*Plast Reconstr Surg* 2006;117:48e). Panorex radiographs are usually sufficient to diagnose MF and visualize postreduction. However, cervical spine radiographs and/or CT scan of the face and spine should be performed if maxillofacial and spinal injuries are also suspected. MFs are not surgical emergencies and should be addressed after stabilization of life-threatening conditions in the multiply injured patient. Fixation within 3 days has been shown to result in more favorable outcomes (*Laryngoscope* 2005;115:769). Minimally displaced fractures can be treated by closed reduction and external fixation [mandibulomaxillary fixation (MMF), or "wiring the jaw shut"]. MMF is less involved and less expensive (*J Oral Maxillofac Surg* 2000;58:1206; discussion, 1210) but requires fixation for 4 to 8 weeks. Open reduction and internal fixation with lag screws and/or plates allows for more precise reduction and is useful in treating complex or comminuted fractures. Although MF is considered a contaminated fracture due to oral flora, a recent study demonstrated no increased benefit from postoperative antibiotics when administered in uncomplicated MF (*J Oral Maxillofac Surg* 2001;59:1415). Complications of MF include wound infection, malocclusion, nonunion, tooth loss, temporomandibular joint ankylosis, and paresthesias.

D. **Infectious/inflammatory disorders**

1. **Ulcers** in the oral cavity are common and are usually related to viral infections, nutritional deficiencies, or glandular changes. Treatment is generally supportive, although a variety of oral rinses are available that contain antifungals, antihistamines, antibiotics, steroids, and coating agents.

2. **Tonsillopharyngitis** is caused by bacteria in approximately 40% and 10% of children and adults seeking medical care, respectively. Of those, group A β-hemolytic streptococci are by far the most common pathogens (*Ann Emerg Med* 1995;25:390). Due to the high incidence of nonbacterial tonsillopharyngitis and to minimize unnecessary antibiotic therapy, new validated guidelines have emerged that recommend antibiotic treatment for *only* rapid test–positive or throat culture–positive cases (*JAMA* 2004;291:1587, *Ann Intern Med* 2001;134:509). Because β-hemolytic streptococci have never shown resistance to penicillin, the recommended antibiotic is still penicillin (oral or intramuscular), with erythromycin reserved for penicillin-allergic patients. Current guidelines recommend tonsillectomy with or without adenoidectomy in children with six or more episodes of tonsillopharyngitis per year or three episodes per year for 2 years.

3. **Peritonsillar abscess** (PTA) refers to purulence between the tonsil bed and capsule. It is characterized by severe throat pain, unilateral swelling of the soft palate, trismus, drooling, and a muffled "hot potato voice." The physical exam reveals a bulging erythematous tonsil and soft palate with uvular deviation. Needle aspiration or incision and drainage is the recommended treatment of PTA. In young patients who will not tolerate an awake incision and drainage or in whom recurrence of PTA is suspected, an immediate (Quinsy) tonsillectomy is indicated.

4. **Retropharyngeal abscesses** occur primarily in children under the age of 2 years. The retropharyngeal space extends from the cranial base to the mediastinum and becomes infected from suppurated retropharyngeal lymph nodes.

Children usually present with irritability, fever, stiff neck, muffled speech, and cervical lymphadenopathy. Examination reveals unilateral posterior pharyngeal swelling. A CT scan with contrast can help to delineate the extent of infection. Oral intubation followed by transoral incision and drainage is the treatment of choice.

5. **Parapharyngeal space abscess** occurs when purulence collects posterolateral to the pharynx and may track down the carotid sheath into the mediastinum. Patients present with fever, leukocytosis, and pain. Treatment consists of aggressive antibiotic therapy. Often, an external surgical approach is necessary for treatment.

E. **Obstructive sleep apnea (OSA)** refers to dysfunctional respiration during sleep due to airway obstruction. OSA is thought to be an underdiagnosed and undertreated entity in both adults and children. Symptoms of OSA in children often include behavioral, learning, and growth problems, whereas OSA in adults is usually manifest by excessive daytime sleepiness. Untreated OSA can lead to pulmonary hypertension and cor pulmonale in both age groups. The most common cause of OSA in children is adenotonsillar hypertrophy, whereas in adults the most common cause is obesity. Overnight polysomnography is the gold standard for diagnosing OSA. Treatment of OSA in children is mainly surgical (adenotonsillectomy), whereas in adults OSA is successfully treated with continuous positive airway pressure (CPAP). Surgery (uvulopalatopharyngoplasty, tongue base reduction, maxillomandibular advancement, or tracheostomy) is reserved for refractory cases.

VI. THE NECK

A. **Anatomy and physiology**

1. The **anterior triangle** is bounded by the sternocleidomastoid, the body of the mandible, and the midline of the neck. It can be further subdivided into the submandibular, carotid, and muscular triangles. The anterior triangle contains the common carotid artery with both its external and internal branches, the internal jugular vein, the ansa cervicalis nerve, and cranial nerves IX, X, XI, and XII.

2. The **posterior triangle** is posterior to the sternocleidomastoid, anterior to the trapezius, and superior to the clavicle. It contains the accessory nerve (CN XI).

3. The neck is also divided by multiple fascial layers. The **superficial cervical fascia** lies directly under the skin. The **deep cervical fascia** is divided into three layers. The **external layer of the deep fascia** is deep to the platysma and invests the strap muscles, sternocleidomastoid, and trapezius. The **middle layer of the deep fascia** (or visceral fascia) encloses the trachea, esophagus, and thyroid gland. The **deep layer of the deep fascia** (or prevertebral fascia) encloses the vertebral column and deep musculature of the neck.

4. **Lymphatic drainage** of the neck is extensive and can be divided into six lymphatic levels. Level I contains the submental and submandibular nodes, levels II to IV parallel the jugular vein, level V is in the posterior triangle, and level VI is the central compartment medial to the carotid artery. The retropharyngeal nodes also form a distinct nodal group.

B. **Congenital disorders**

1. **Thyroglossal duct cysts.** The thyroid gland descends from the foramen cecum at the tongue to its position anterior to the first three tracheal rings by week 7 of gestation. As the gland descends, the residual thyroglossal duct is obliterated. Persistence of the duct may give rise to cystic, midline masses at any point along the tract. These sometimes enlarge during upper respiratory tract infections or can get infected. Prior to resection, the surgeon must make sure that the cyst is not the patient's only functioning thyroid tissue. The cyst is excised surgically using the Sistrunk procedure, which involves resecting the mass, a central portion of the hyoid bone, and a small block of the tongue base.

2. **Branchial anomalies.** Persistence of any portion of the embryologic branchial apparatus results in a cyst (most common), a sinus, or a fistula. A cyst is an epithelium-lined structure with no external or visceral connection (no opening), a sinus is a tract that has an internal or external opening (one opening), and a

fistula is a connection from the upper digestive tract to the skin (two openings). **First branchial anomalies** usually present as painless swellings in the region of the parotid gland, ear, or high sternocleidomastoid muscle. **Second branchial anomalies** are the most common and course from the tonsillar fossa to the skin anterior of the sternocleidomastoid muscle. **Third branchial fistulas** connect the pyriform sinus to the skin. Infected branchial anomalies require antibiotics and/or incision and drainage. Definitive management of these lesions requires complete excision once the inflammation has subsided.

3. **Cystic hygroma** is an older term for macrocystic lymphatic malformations of the head and neck. These masses are soft, compressible, and usually nontender. MRI is the imaging modality of choice, and surgical resection is the preferred therapy. Care is taken to preserve all vital neural and vascular structures during resection.

4. **Teratomas and dermoid cysts.** Teratomas are composed of ectoderm, mesoderm, and endoderm, whereas dermoids contain ectoderm and mesoderm. Tissues within these masses can have varying degrees of differentiation. Treatment entails surgical excision.

C. **Infectious/inflammatory disorders**

1. Fascial compartments in the head and neck can develop **deep neck space infections.** Although a dental source is most common, these can also result from trauma, tonsillitis, or suppuration of lymph nodes. **Ludwig's angina** is inflammation in the sublingual and submandibular spaces. These patients appear septic, presenting with a firm floor of mouth and retrusion of the tongue. Treatment is intravenous antibiotics. Surgery is reserved for débridement of necrotic tissue. Swelling can easily compromise the airway, and a recent study cited that 75% of patients with Ludwig angina required tracheotomies (*Ann Otol Rhinol Laryngol* 2001;110:1051).

VII. **SALIVARY GLANDS**

A. **Anatomy and physiology.** The **major salivary glands** include the parotid, submandibular, and sublingual glands. Hundreds of minor salivary glands exist in the palate, oral mucosa, and tongue. Salivary glands supply 1 to 1.5 L of saliva per day. Saliva provides lubrication during mastication, inhibits bacterial growth, helps to maintain dental health, and contains some digestive enzymes.

1. The **parotid gland** is the largest of the salivary glands. Its secretions are primarily serous, and it is the dominant producer of saliva during mastication. It lies anterior to the ear on the surface of the masseter muscle. The parotid duct (Stensen's duct) empties into the oral cavity adjacent to the second maxillary molar. The facial nerve (CN VII) travels through the parotid gland.

2. The **submandibular gland** lies inferomedial to the mandible. It produces a mixture of mucinous and serous saliva. The submandibular duct (Wharton's duct) empties into the floor of the mouth just lateral to the lingual frenulum.

3. The **sublingual gland** lies below the floor of the mouth mucosa. Its multiple ducts empty directly into the floor of the mouth and secrete primarily mucinous saliva.

B. **Inflammatory diseases of the salivary glands**

1. **Acute sialadenitis** is a bacterial inflammation of the salivary glands, usually involving the parotid gland. It occurs from retrograde bacterial contamination from the oral cavity due to salivary stasis. It is more common in elderly, diabetic, immunocompromised, or dehydrated individuals. Treatment includes hydration, antibiotics, and sialogogues (agents that increase the flow of saliva, such as lemon drops). Surgical drainage is rarely needed.

2. **Chronic sialadenitis** is caused by recurrent episodes of salivary gland inflammation. The gland becomes fibrotic and firm, and treatment is surgical resection of the gland.

3. **Mumps** is caused by *paramyxovirus* and results in acute parotitis. Treatment of parotitis involves supportive measures. Due to widespread vaccinations, the incidence of mumps is low in the United States.

4. **Sialolithiasis** most frequently affects the submandibular gland. Calculi consist of organic and crystalline components, which cause glandular swelling and pain

prior to eating. Calculi can be diagnosed by palpation or radiography. Ductal calculus may be removed transorally using probing instruments, whereas parenchymal calculi require surgical removal of the gland.

C. Trauma. Facial lacerations can involve the parotid parenchyma, Stensen's duct, and branches of the facial nerve. Loss of facial function mandates exploration and epineural repair of the nerve. Injury to the parotid duct requires repair of the duct over a stent.

VIII. NEOPLASMS OF THE HEAD AND NECK. An in-depth review of the diverse neoplasms affecting the head and neck is beyond the scope of this chapter. Squamous cell carcinoma and other selected neoplasms are addressed.

A. Squamous cell carcinoma (SCC) arising from the aerodigestive tract is the most common neoplasm of the head and neck. SCC is strongly associated with tobacco and alcohol use. Despite advances in tumor resection, reconstruction techniques (which allow for larger surgical margins), and adjuvant treatments, the 5-year rate of disease-free survival is still approximately 50% (*N Engl J Med* 2004;350:1937). This is thought to be due to the extensive lymphatic system of the head and neck (which increases the incidence of metastasis), anatomic constraints on achieving adequate surgical margins, the invasive nature of SCC, the multiplicity of primary tumors, and the concurrence of other alcohol- and tobacco-related illnesses present in this patient population.

1. **Workup** of malignancies includes a thorough head and neck physical examination and history, CT or MRI scan, positron emission tomography (PET) scan, and intraoperative endoscopic biopsies (to assess extent of the tumor, metastasis, presence of multiple primaries, and to obtain tissue for pathologic analysis). **Treatment** of SCC involves a multidisciplinary team consisting of head and neck surgeons, radiation oncologists, medical oncologists, pathologists, and speech/swallowing therapists.

2. **Treatment of SCC** is complex and based on location, nodal involvement, local invasion, and metastasis. Most tumors are treated by surgical resection and neck dissection, followed by postoperative radiotherapy. Recent studies suggest that surgical resection followed by *concurrent* radiotherapy and chemotherapy improve local/regional control and disease-free survival (*N Engl J Med* 2004;350:1937, *N Engl J Med* 2004;350:1945). However, this intense combined treatment results in significant adverse effects. Due to the complex anatomy and physiology of the head and neck and the variable presentation of SCC, surgical approach and resection must be individualized on a case-by-case basis.

3. Molecular targeting of **epidermal growth factor-receptor** and **tyrosine kinase** has shown promising results with less toxicity than chemotherapy and may prove to be a mainstay treatment of SCC (*Br J Cancer* 2007;96:408).

4. **Anatomic distribution of SCC**
   a. **Laryngeal SCC** often presents with sore throat (supraglottic), hoarseness, stridor, dysphagia, and persistent cough. Small lesions are successfully treated with local laser resection or radiotherapy alone. Moderate-sized lesions are also managed with laser resection; however, increasing evidence has shown these cancers to be highly responsive to primary concurrent chemoradiotherapy (*N Engl J Med* 2003;349:2091). Advanced SCC of the larynx requires partial or total laryngectomy with creation of a tracheoesophageal speech fistula.
   b. **Nasopharyngeal SCC** is most common in Asia and Africa, where it is associated with the Epstein-Barr virus. Current treatment consists of combined chemotherapy, with surgical resection reserved for residual disease (*Lancet* 2005;365:2041). Metastasis is very common.
   c. **Oral cavity SCC** usually presents as nonhealing ulcers. Treatment is primarily surgical followed by postoperative radiotherapy. At times, the mandible is involved, necessitating mandibulectomy followed by reconstruction.
   d. **Tongue base SCC** is often detected at advanced stages and is among the most difficult malignancies to treat. Emerging transoral laser resection has

decreased the complications of surgical resection, but aspiration remains a significant concern following treatment.

    e. A **neck mass** in an adult must be considered malignant until proven otherwise. These neck masses are generally metastatic SCC from the upper aerodigestive tract, especially the base of the tongue and tonsil. Primary tumors arising in the neck are less common but include lymphoma, soft-tissue sarcomas, thyroid carcinoma, salivary gland carcinoma, and neuroendocrine malignancies.

  5. Other malignancies of the head and neck

    a. Mucoepidermoid carcinoma, adenoid cystic carcinoma, and **adenocarcinoma** can arise from the major or minor salivary glands or aerodigestive tract. Treatment includes resection followed by radiotherapy. Injury to the facial nerve (CN VII) is the most common complication of surgery when the parotid gland is involved. Five-year survival is approximately 50%.

    b. Melanoma of the head and neck can be cutaneous, mucosal, or metastatic from an unknown primary. Head and neck melanoma represents 25% of all cutaneous melanomas. Melanoma is treated by complete surgical resection with wide excision. Melanoma is highly metastatic and notoriously chemo- and radioresistant, with 5-year survival rates of 6% to 30% for advanced disease (*J Clin Oncol* 2001;19:3635).

B. Benign neoplasms of the head and neck

  1. Nasopharyngeal neoplasms

    a. Papillomas are benign, wartlike growths on the septum or lateral nasal wall and are associated with a 10% incidence of squamous cell carcinoma. Wide local excision is necessary to prevent recurrence.

    b. Juvenile nasopharyngeal angiofibromas occur in adolescent boys and usually present with nasal obstruction and recurrent epistaxis. Treatment is complete surgical excision. Angiography and embolization of the vascular supply 24 hours prior to resection helps to minimize blood loss.

  2. Oral cavity benign lesions include papillomas, hemangiomas, lymphatic malformations, mucous cysts, and granular cell tumors. Premalignant changes include leukoplakia (white hyperkeratotic patches) and erythroplakia (velvet red patches).

    a. Ameloblastoma is a locally invasive tumor that occurs most frequently in the mandible. It often requires partial resection and reconstruction of the mandible.

  3. Neck

    a. Paragangliomas arise from the paraganglionic cells of the autonomic nervous system. These are classified as jugulotympanic, vagal, sinonasal, laryngeal, and carotid body tumors. Approximately 3% of paragangliomas produce catecholamines. Angiography allows for embolization prior to surgical excision (within 24 to 48 hours).

    b. Schwannomas are tumors derived from the Schwann cells of peripheral nerves and have a predilection for the head and neck. Treatment is excisional.

    c. Neurofibromas also arise from peripheral nerves and are usually associated with neurofibromatosis type I. These may form massive plexiform accumulations in the neck. Treatment is excisional.

  4. Salivary gland. Pleomorphic adenoma is the most common of all salivary gland tumors, followed by **Warthin tumor** (cystadenoma lymphomatosum). Pleomorphic adenomas grow slowly over many years, are painless, and commonly occur in the parotid gland. Facial nerve palsy is rare. Diagnosis can be made with fine-needle aspiration, and treatment consists of surgical resection.

  5. Acoustic neuromas (ANs) are benign schwannomas of CN VIII that arise at the skull base. ANs can be nonhereditary or associated with neurofibromatosis type 2. Early signs of AN are hearing loss, vertigo, or facial paralysis due to compression of cranial nerves. AN requires surgical resection.

IX. FACIAL PLASTICS AND RECONSTRUCTION

A. Fellowship-trained otolaryngologists perform facial cosmetic procedures including face-lift, blepharoplasty, rhinoplasty, and so on. As with any cosmetic procedure, careful patient selection is critical.

B. Reconstruction of the head and neck is often required following tumor resection or trauma or to treat congenital disorders. **Microvascular free tissue transfers** can provide skin, muscle, mucosal, and/or bone tissue. They represent a powerful tool for reconstruction of the tongue, oropharynx, mandible, esophagus, and hypopharynx. Most commonly used microvascular free flaps include the radial forearm, scapular, and fibular. The pedicled pectoralis major flap is also commonly used to reconstruct pharyngeal defects.

29 PLASTIC AND HAND SURGERY

Marissa J. Tenenbaum, Jason M. Rovak, and Susan E. Mackinnon

$\mathcal{P}$lastic surgeons are charged with the broad task of maximizing form and function in the setting of trauma, burn, congenital defects, postoncologic defects, general reconstruction, and elective cosmetic improvements. Operative sites may be from head to toe, with subspecialties including pediatrics, hand surgery, craniofacial surgery, peripheral nerve surgery, microsurgery, and aesthetic surgery. Although the entirety of plastic surgery is too broad to cover in one chapter, we discuss topics germane to the general surgeon, with special emphasis on trauma.

BASIC TECHNIQUES AND PRINCIPLES

I. **THE RECONSTRUCTIVE LADDER.** When considering a reconstructive challenge, the simplest approach is often the best. The reconstructive ladder of soft-tissue coverage begins with consideration of the simplest approach (healing by secondary intention) and culminates with the most complex (free tissue transfer), maximizing opportunities for success.

A. Healing by **secondary intention** is the simplest approach but is not always feasible. Absolute contraindications include exposed vessels, nerves, tendons, viscera, or bone. Relative contraindications include a large or poorly vascularized wound with a prolonged (>3 weeks) anticipated period of healing and undesirable aesthetic consequences.

B. **Primary closure** may provide the most aesthetically pleasing result, but excessive tension on the skin may cause displacement of neighboring structures (e.g., lower eyelid) or necrosis of the skin flaps.

C. **Skin grafting** is the most common method of large-wound closure. Skin grafts require a healthy, uninfected bed, protected from shear forces, to survive. Wound surfaces such as bare tendon, dessicated bone or cartilage, or infected tissue beds will not support skin graft survival. In addition, exposed vessels, nerves, or viscera are relative contraindications for skin grafting.

D. **Local tissue transfers** of skin, fascia, and muscle may be used in regions with healthy adjacent tissue. If the adjacent tissue cannot be adequately mobilized or the wound requires more bulk than is locally available, the sole use of local flaps may not be adequate.

E. **Distant tissue transfers** were the mainstay of difficult wound closure until the advent of free tissue transfer in the 1970s. This involves transferring healthy tissue into the wound bed while leaving it attached to its native blood supply. The pedicle is divided in a subsequent procedure. Inherent disadvantages of this technique include multiple operations, prolonged wound healing, immobilization for at least 3 weeks, and a limited choice of donor sites.

F. **Free tissue transfer** is the most technically demanding approach to wound closure but has several potential advantages, including single-stage wound closure, a relatively wide variety of flaps to ensure closure specifically tailored to coverage needs, and, in many cases, an aesthetically pleasing outcome.

G. **Vacuum-assisted closure** has altered wound management by decreasing bacterial load and accelerating granulation. Wounds may be treated adequately with vacuum-assisted closure that would not traditionally be candidates for healing by secondary intention. Furthermore, it may convert a wound that would otherwise need adjacent or free tissue transfer into a wound that needs only split-thickness skin grafting.

II. TYPES OF GRAFTS

A. Skin grafts

1. **Split-thickness grafts** consist of epidermis and a variable thickness of dermis. Thinner grafts (<0.016 in.) have a higher rate of engraftment, whereas thicker grafts, with a greater amount of dermis, are more durable and aesthetically acceptable. Common donor sites are the thigh, buttock, and scalp.

2. **Full-thickness grafts** include epidermis and a full layer of dermis. Common donor sites include groin and postauricular and supraclavicular sites, but the hypothenar eminence and instep of the foot can also be used. The donor site is usually closed primarily. These grafts are generally used in areas for which a high priority is placed on the aesthetic result (e.g., face and hand). Thinner grafts have greater secondary contraction and do not grow commensurate with the individual. They have fewer adnexal cells and therefore have variable pigment, less hair, and less sebum, with a proclivity toward dryness and contractures. Full-thickness grafts, with more dermis and the requisite adnexal structures, exhibit less contraction and better cosmesis.

3. Grafts can be meshed in **expansion ratios** from 1.5:1 to 6:1. Meshing a graft allows coverage for a wider area using the same-size donor site and decreases the risk of serous fluid accumulating under the graft without a method of egress. The interstices are covered within 1 week by advancing keratinocytes. However, because the entire area is not covered by dermis, meshed grafts are less durable, and the meshing pattern remains after healing, making them inappropriate for aesthetically important areas, such as the face.

4. **Graft healing.** Initial metabolism is supported by **imbibition** or diffusion of nutrients from the wound bed. Revascularization occurs between days 3 and 5 by ingrowth of recipient vessels into the graft **(inosculation).** Therefore, for a graft to take, the bed must be well vascularized and free of infection, and the site must be immobilized for a minimum of 3 to 5 days. Prevention of shear forces is particularly important during this period of inosculation. Although bare bone and tendon do not engraft, periosteum and peritenon can support skin grafts, especially if they are first left to form a layer of granulation tissue. Graft failures are most often the result of hematoma, seroma, or shear force prohibiting diffusion and vascular ingrowth.

B. Tendon grafts are used to replace or augment tendons. Preferred donor sites are palmaris longus and plantaris tendons.

C. Bone grafts are used for repair of bony defects. Iliac bone is commonly used for donor cancellous bone, and ribs or outer table of cranium are commonly used for donor cortical bone.

D. Cartilage grafts are used to restore the contour of the ear, nose, and eyelid. Preferred donor sites include costal cartilage, concha of ear, and nasal septum.

E. Nerve grafts are used to repair damaged nerves when primary repair is not feasible. Preferred donor sites include the sural nerve and lateral or medial antebrachial cutaneous nerves. Allogeneic nerve grafting has been described using a short course of immunosuppression (*Plast Reconstr Surg* 1992;90:695).

F. Dermal or dermal-fat grafts are used for contour restoration. Preferred donor sites include back, buttock, and groin. The long-term survival of grafted fat is variable but is generally unreliable.

III. TYPES OF FLAPS. A flap is any tissue that is transferred to another site with an intact blood supply.

A. Classification based on blood supply

1. **Random cutaneous flaps** have a blood supply from the dermal and subdermal plexus without a single dominant artery. They generally have a limited length-to-width ratio (usually 3:1), although this varies by anatomic region (e.g., the face has a ratio of up to 5:1). These flaps are usually used locally to cover adjacent tissue defects but can be transferred to a distant site by use of a staged procedure.

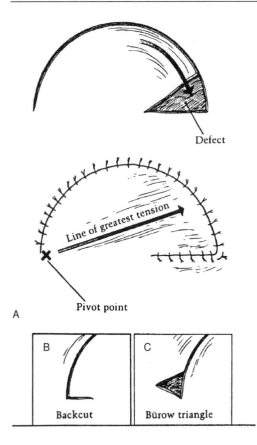

Figure 29-1. Rotation flap. **A:** The edge of the flap is four to five times the length of the base of the defect triangle. **B, C:** A backcut or Burow triangle can be useful if the flap is under tension.

Depending on the size of the defect to be covered, moving a local tissue flap can create a donor defect, which may require skin grafting. All local flaps are comparatively easier to use with the loose skin of the elderly.

a. Flaps that rotate around a pivot point include rotation flaps (Fig. 29-1) and transposition flaps (Fig. 29-2). Planning for shortening of the effective length through the arc of rotation is important when designing these flaps. More complex rotation flaps include bilobed flaps (Fig. 29-3) and rhomboid flaps (Fig. 29-4).

b. Advancement of skin directly into a defect without rotation can be accomplished with a simple advancement, a V-Y advancement (Fig. 29-5), or a bipedicle advancement flap.

2. **Axial cutaneous flaps** contain a single dominant arteriovenous system. This results in a potentially greater length-to-width ratio.

a. Peninsular flaps are those in which the skin and vessels are moved together as a unit.

b. Island flaps are those in which the skin is divided from all surrounding tissue but maintained on an isolated, intact vascular pedicle.

c. Free flaps are those in which the vascular pedicle is isolated and divided. The flap and its pedicle are then moved to a new location and microsurgically anastomosed to vessels at the recipient site, allowing for long-distance transfer of tissue.

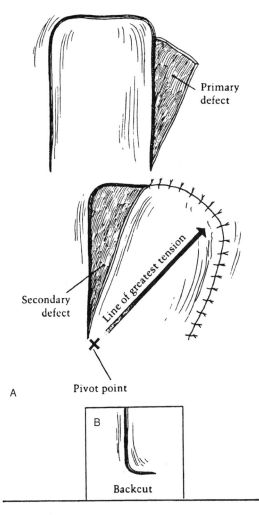

Figure 29-2. A: Transposition flap. The secondary defect is typically covered with a skin graft. **B:** A backcut may be added to reduce tension at the pivot point.

B. Classification based on tissue type
1. **Cutaneous flaps** include the skin and subcutaneous fat. These are generally random flaps because the axial blood supply is deep to the fat.
2. **Fasciocutaneous flaps** are axial flaps with a single dominant blood supply contained in the deep fascia along with the overlying fat and skin. A wide variety of fasciocutaneous flaps have been described, but those commonly used include radial forearm, parascapular, lateral arm, and groin flaps. These flaps are often utilized for coverage of mobile structures such as tendons.
3. **Muscle flaps** use the specific axial blood supply of a muscle to provide well-vascularized soft-tissue bulk. These flaps can often be transferred with the overlying skin as a myocutaneous flap. Alternatively, they may be transferred without the overlying skin to fill a cavity or may be covered with a skin graft.

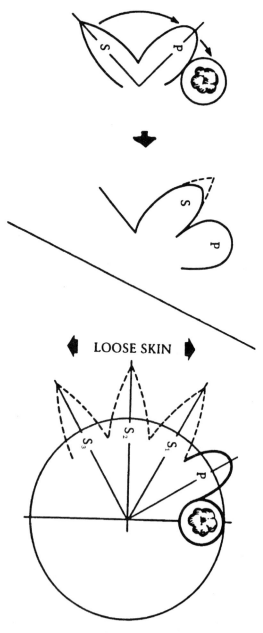

LOOSE SKIN

Figure 29-3. Bilobed flap. After the lesion is excised, the primary flap (P) is transposed into the initial defect, and the secondary flap (S) is moved to the site vacated by the primary flap. The bed of the secondary flap is then closed primarily. The primary flap is slightly narrower than the initial defect, whereas the secondary flap is half the width of the primary flap. To be effective, this must be planned in an area where loose skin surrounds the secondary flap site. Three choices for the secondary flap are shown (S_1, S_2, S_3).

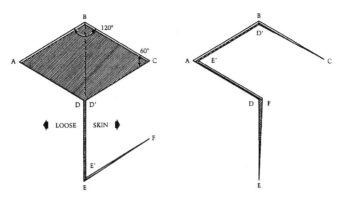

Figure 29-4. Rhomboid or Limberg flap. The rhomboid defect must have 60- and 120-degree angles so that the length of the short diagonal is the same as the length of the sides. The short diagonal is extended by its own length to point *E*. The line *EF* is parallel to *CD,* and they are equal in length. There are four possible Limberg flaps for any rhomboid defect; the flap should be planned in an area where loose skin is available to close the donor defect primarily.

Considerations in the transfer of vascularized muscle include the pattern of circulation, arc of rotation, donor-site contour, and donor-site functional defects. Commonly used muscle flaps include the latissimus dorsi, pectoralis major, rectus abdominis, gastrocnemius, soleus, gracilis, tensor fascia lata, trapezius, and gluteus maximus, but any muscle can potentially be transferred as a flap.

 4. **A musculocutaneous flap** involves transfer of a muscle with the overlying skin and subcutaneous tissue. The skin is vascularized via myocutaneous or septocutaneous perforating vessels.

C. Specialized flaps

 1. **Fascial flaps** are used when thin, well-vascularized coverage is needed (e.g., for coverage of ear cartilage or the dorsum of the hand or foot). The temporoparietal fascia flap is a classic example, but other fasciocutaneous flaps (see Basic Techniques and Principles, Section III.B.2) can be transferred without the overlying skin.

 2. **Vascularized bone flaps** are designed to meet specific reconstructive needs, as dictated by loss of bony structure. Because they must be transferred to a specific location, they are generally transferred as free flaps. They may or may not include muscle and/or overlying skin. Commonly used bone flaps include free fibula, scapular spine, iliac (with overlying internal oblique muscle), and rib (with pectoralis major or intercostal muscle).

 3. **Functional muscle** may be transferred with its accompanying dominant nerve. Common functional muscle transfers include transfer of gracilis for restoration of facial movement or latissimus for replacement of biceps function.

 4. **Segmental muscle flaps** can be used when multiple sources provide blood supply to the muscle. A portion of the muscle is used as a flap, leaving behind a vascularized, innervated, functional muscle. This technique minimizes donor-site

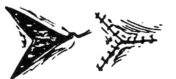

Figure 29-5. V-Y advancement. The skin to the sides of the V is advanced.

functional loss. Portions of the serratus anterior and gluteus maximus can be transferred as segmental flaps.

IV. TISSUE EXPANSION is a reconstructive technique that uses an inflatable silicone balloon to serially expand surrounding skin. This expansion adjacent to the wound provides donor tissue of similar color, texture, thickness, and sensation, with minimal scar formation and donor-site morbidity. The technique takes advantage of the skin's ability to accommodate a slowly enlarging mass beneath it by increasing its surface area. The idea is to create and develop donor tissue, harvest it, and leave the original donor site preserved.

A. The advantages include lower donor-site morbidity and the provision of donor tissue of similar quality to the recipient tissue. Tissue expansion is a simple and versatile technique that provides robust tissue.

B. The disadvantages are that it is a staged technique, there is a visible deformity during the period of expansion, it requires frequent visits for expansion, and there is a relatively high rate of complications, including infection and extrusion.

C. Technique

1. **Preoperative planning** involves assessing the defect size, locating matching tissue to be expanded, and deciding where final scars will be.

2. **Expander placement** is usually performed through an incision at the junction of the lesion and the area of proposed expansion. The length of the incision is controversial. Some authors propose one third the length of the expander (it should be big enough to ensure full pocket creation). The filling port can be incorporated into the expander or placed in a separate pocket. In addition, the port may be externalized to minimize anxiety and pain during filling, especially in the pediatric population. Partially filling the expander on initial placement may reduce the duration of the expansion phase and reduce mechanical implant failure due to folding.

3. **The expansion phase** begins 2 to 3 weeks after expander placement. The expander is inflated weekly with saline, using sterile technique. The amount infused with each fill depends on patient comfort, skin tension, and blanching of overlying skin. A rough guide is 10% of expander volume per injection. The duration of the expansion phase can vary from 6 weeks to 3 months. Waiting 2 to 3 weeks after the desired volume is achieved allows the expanded skin to soften, decreasing the contraction at the time of flap transposition.

4. **Removal of expander** is straightforward. However, infection, exposure, or rupture may necessitate early explant.

5. **The expanded tissue** is usually in the form of a random flap (rotation, advancement, or transposition). If more than one flap is necessary using expanded tissue, one must ensure that all flaps have adequate blood supply.

D. The **origin of the new tissue** is not completely understood. One potential source is new tissue created in response to the expansion process. Alternatively, tissue may derive from recruitment of adjacent tissues by stretching or creep and by stress relaxation. These possibilities are not mutually exclusive. Studies have shown that expansion gives rise to an increase in the thickness of the epidermis, a decrease in the thickness of the dermis, and atrophy of the underlying muscle and fat (*Clin Plast Surg* 1987;14:435).

E. Tissue expanders are indicated for patients who cannot, or choose not to, tolerate the longer operative procedures or rehabilitation associated with more distant flaps. In areas where little suitable tissue is available (e.g., scalp), tissue expansion can be the aesthetically superior option. The patient must be motivated and understand the process. Common indications include burn alopecia, congenital nevi, male pattern baldness, and postmastectomy breast reconstruction.

F. Relative contraindications include malignancy or an open wound, active infection, and unwillingness to comply with multiple procedures. Similarly, tissue expanders cannot be placed under burned tissue, scar, skin graft, or a prior incision. In addition, tissue expanders are less effective in areas that will be irradiated because the skin in those areas thickens, scars, and contracts, minimizing the degree of expansion possible.

G. **Complications** include pain, seroma, hematoma (rates widely variable), infection (1% to 5%), exposure or extrusion (5% to 10%), and skin necrosis. Less common complications include striae, resorption of underlying bone, and neurapraxia.

 ACUTE INJURIES

I. **FACIAL TRAUMA**

A. **Examination.** A facial trauma exam should assess soft-tissue, nerve, and underlying bony injuries, with special attention to periorbital injuries. Note the location of lacerations and abrasions that may indicate underlying facial nerve injuries or fractures. Gingival lacerations and step-offs between the teeth may be a sign of a mandibular fractures. The examiner should query the five branches of the facial nerve (temporal, zygomatic, buccal, marginal mandibular, cervical) by having the patient raise the eyebrows, squeeze the eyelids shut, smile, and frown, noting any paresis or asymmetry. The facial skeleton should be palpated for bony step-offs indicating fractures. A brief ocular exam should include an assessment of gross vision, pupil reactivity, and intact extraocular movements. Examine the ears for lacerations as well as intact tympanic membranes. One should note gross deviations in the nose externally, and examine the nasal septum with an otoscope to assess for septal hematoma.

B. **Imaging.** A computed tomography (CT) scan with fine cuts through the facial bones is a fast, sensitive, and specific means of determining the location and orientation of facial fractures. A Panorex may be useful in the setting of isolated mandible fractures; however, many facial reconstructive surgeons want a more complete picture of the anatomy with a CT scan as a guide for the reconstructive plan, regardless of the diagnosis of a fracture on plain film.

C. **Other workup.** Any patient with a mandible fracture should be examined for C-spine injuries. Mandible fractures are associated with a 10% incidence of C-spine fractures. Patients with bony orbital fractures should have an ophthalmology evaluation to rule out associated ocular injuries.

D. **Soft-tissue repair.** Facial lacerations should be copiously irrigated, and obviously devitalized tissue should be débrided. The wound edges may be reapproximated using a few interrupted deep dermal 4-0 Vicryl or Monocryl sutures. A running superficial layer of 6-0 fast gut suture may be used to close the epidermis. If nonabsorbable sutures are used on the face, they should be removed within 5 days to prevent permanent suture marks.

Eyelid lacerations should be referred to a facial reconstructive surgeon or ophthalmologist. Full-thickness lacerations of the ear and nose should be copiously irrigated, cartilage reapproximated with an absorbable monofilament suture [polydioxanone (PDS)], and skin closed in the usual manner. Full-thickness lip lacerations may be repaired using a three-layer closure. The orbicularis muscle should be reapproximated with 5-0 PDS, the mucosa repaired with 5-0 chromic, and the vermillion carefully aligned with 6-0 fast gut suture. Lacerations overlying fractures should be copiously irrigated and closed until definitive fracture fixation can be achieved.

E. **Fractures.** In the absence of airway compromise or ocular muscle entrapment, most facial and mandible fractures may be fixed electively within 1 to 2 weeks with good results and low incidence of infection. Patients with mandible fractures may be temporized until definitive fixation with a liquid diet, pain control, antibiotics covering intraoral flora (clindamycin), and good oral hygiene including Peridex (chlorhexidine) swish and spit three times per day. Indications for fracture reduction and fixation include dental alteration in dental occlusion with mandible and midface fractures, ocular muscle entrapment and inadequate eye support associated with orbital fractures, midface instability, and displaced fractures with obvious cosmetic implications. In light of these indications, not all facial fractures require operative intervention.

F. **Special situations**

1. Facial nerve injuries may be managed expectantly if they are medial to the lateral canthus because facial nerve branches, such as the buccal branch, are extensively

arborized in these locations. Function will usually return without operative intervention, and it is exceedingly difficult to localize and repair nerve branches in this area. Facial nerve injuries should be referred to a facial plastic surgeon as soon as possible.

2. Eyelid lacerations situated in the medial aspect of the lid may be associated with injury to the lacrimal drainage system. These injuries should be evaluated by a facial plastic surgeon or ophthalmologist.

II. HAND TRAUMA

A. **Assessment** must be done using a systematic, efficient, and reproducible approach. Underestimating the extent of a hand injury or infection can lead to extended recovery or permanent loss of function.

1. **History.** The mechanism and timing of the injury, hand position at the time of injury, hand dominance, and patient occupation are all important to diagnosis and treatment.

2. **Examination**

a. **Inspect the position of the patient's hand,** paying attention to the resting position of the digits and any swelling or asymmetry as compared with the contralateral hand.

b. **Vascular assessment** requires observation of color, temperature, capillary refill, and the presence of pulses (palpable or Doppler) and an Allen test to verify the integrity of the palmar arches. Bleeding is controlled by application of direct pressure, not by blindly clamping tissue, because this often results in serious injury to surrounding structures. The use of tourniquets should be reserved for life-threatening exsanguinations because serious and irreversible damage may result.

c. **Motor examination,** both active and passive, involves testing for integrity of the tendons.

(1) **Flexor digitorum profundus (FDP)** is tested by stabilizing the proximal interphalangeal (PIP) joint in extension and having the patient flex the distal interphalangeal (DIP) joint.

(2) **Flexor digitorum superficialis (FDS)** is tested by blocking all other fingers in full extension before asking the patient to flex at the PIP joint.

(3) **Extensor tendons** are tested by having the patient extend each finger individually. It should be noted that connections between neighboring tendons (juncturae tendinum) can mask a proximal laceration.

d. **Sensory testing** includes gross examination of the ulnar, radial, and median nerves, which innervate the muscles in the hand and forearm (Table 29-1). It also involves careful examination of two-point discrimination on the palmar aspect of both the radial and ulnar sides of the digits and comparison with the uninjured hand. Normal two-point discrimination is 3 to 6 mm at the distal tip of the digit. The Strauch 10-10 test is also extremely useful in determining degrees of sensory loss. For this test, the patient rates his or her level of light touch sensation in an injured area on a scale of 1 to 10 as compared to the

TABLE 29-1	Unambiguous Tests of Hand Nerve Function		
Test	**Radial nerve**	**Median nerve**	**Ulnar nerve**
Sensory	Dorsum first web	Index fingertip	Little fingertip
Extrinsic motor	Extend wrist	FDP index	FDP small
Intrinsic motor	None	Abduct thumb perpendicular to palm	Cross long finger over index (interossei)

FDP, flexor digitorum profundus.

contralateral normal region, which is by definition a 10. This test should be used over multiple visits to chart the patient's subjective improvement with operative intervention or spontaneous reinnervation.

   e. **Skeletal examination** involves palpating for any tenderness, soft-tissue swelling, or deformity of the bones. Joint integrity is assessed by gently stressing the ligaments and noting any instability, crepitus, or pain. Any suspicion of fracture or dislocation requires radiographic examination.

3. **Diagnostic radiology.** Plain radiographs of the injured area, including the joint above and below if the physical examination warrants it, are indicated for almost all hand trauma and should be considered in cases of hand infections, particularly in penetrating trauma. Images should include true posteroanterior, lateral, and oblique views. If the injury involves the digits, separate laterals of the involved digits are indicated. The description of the fracture pattern should include the following: the bone(s) involved, simple versus comminuted, displaced versus nondisplaced, transverse versus oblique versus spiral, angulation or rotation of the distal fragment, and intra-articular versus extra-articular. Fractures in children involving the growth plate use the Salter-Harris classification.

B. **Fractures**
1. **Principles of management**
   a. **Reduction of displaced fractures** can be attempted in the emergency room using local or regional anesthesia. However, early referral to a hand surgeon is essential for all hand fractures.
   b. **Postreduction radiographs** should be done for all fractures after splinting or casting.
   c. **Splinting the fracture** in a position that does not impair function during the healing phase is imperative. A splint made of plaster or fiberglass, appropriately padded and with the hand in the "intrinsic-plus" position, may be used for almost all hand injuries. The intrinsic-plus position places ligamentous structures in their longest position and minimizes stiffness should immobilization be required to treat the fracture. The interphalangeal (IP) joints are in full extension, the metacarpophalangeal (MCP) joints are at 60 to 90 degrees of flexion, and the wrist is at 20 to 30 degrees of extension. Individual digits can be splinted without involving the remainder of the patient's hand and wrist. A thumb spica splint is used for fractures that involve the thumb proximal to the IP joint. The MCP joint is placed in extension, the thumb abducted, and the wrist placed in 20 to 30 degrees of extension. Even if operative management of the fracture is planned, a reduction with splinting in the emergency room is still appropriate for patient comfort and to prevent stiffness.
   d. **Early motion** is used whenever possible to minimize joint stiffness.
   e. **Operative intervention** is considered if closed treatment does not obtain or maintain reduction of the fracture. Contaminated open fractures, associated soft-tissue injuries, malalignment (uncorrected rotated, angulated, or shortened deformities of the digit), and articular incongruity of greater than 1 mm are also indications for operative management.

2. **Specific fractures**
   a. **Phalangeal fractures** require closed reduction and protective splinting for 4 to 6 weeks. Fractures of the distal phalanx may involve the nail bed apparatus or insertion of either the flexor or extensor mechanisms. Disruption of the extensor mechanism at the distal phalanx results in a mallet finger deformity (see Hand Surgery, Section IV.B.1) and can be treated by splinting the DIP joint in extension. Other fractures of the distal phalanx can generally be treated with a protective splint. Stable middle and proximal phalanx fractures can be adequately treated by taping the injured finger to its neighbor. Certain fracture patterns are considered unstable and require operative fixation. As always, the goal of early motion is desirable.
   b. **Boxer's fracture** is a common transverse fracture at the distal portion of the ring or small finger metacarpal, with volar angulation of the distal fragment. Volar angulation of the distal fragment of up to 45 degrees is acceptable in the

fifth metacarpal because of its mobility, although this may cause prominence of the metacarpal head in the palm. Less angulation is accepted in the fourth metacarpal, and angulation greater than 15 degrees is unacceptable in the second and third metacarpals. Any rotation or scissoring of the finger must be corrected by reduction as well. It is unnecessary to immobilize the MCP joint, and protection with a volar splint brought to the middle palmar crease is used until the patient sees a hand surgeon. Buddy taping of the ring and small fingers may also be helpful.

- c. **Transverse metacarpal shaft fractures** are caused by axial loading and follow the same guidelines as neck fractures in terms of angulation. Oblique and spiral fractures result from torsional forces and are often best treated with operative fixation, protective splinting, and early range-of-motion exercises.
- d. **Bennett fracture** is an intra-articular fracture at the base of the first metacarpal resulting from an axial load to the thumb. The distal fragment subluxes radially through the pull of the abductor pollicis longus and angulates volarly through the force of the adductor pollicis. The ulnar fragment of the base is held fixed by the volar beak ligament. Closed reduction and splinting often yield a reduction that is anatomic; however, the deforming forces usually move the fragments out of reduction, and these fractures are best treated with open reduction and fixation. Less common is the "baby Bennett," or "reverse Bennett," fracture of the fifth metacarpal base; it is similar to the Bennett fracture, with the extensor carpi ulnaris representing the deforming force on the distal fragment.
- e. **Epiphyseal fractures in children** can lead to alterations in the growth of the involved bone. Treatment is similar to that for adults, although healing is often faster and immobilization is more acceptable because joint stiffness is less of a problem in children. Although reduction of the fracture is important, bone remodeling allows for angulation deformities of up to 20 or 30 degrees in the phalanges and metacarpals, provided it is in the anteroposterior plane. Rotatory deformity or deviation in the coronal plane should not be accepted because remodeling does not correct these deformities (*Clin Orthop* 1984;188:12).
- f. **Open fractures** require adequate irrigation, reduction, and fixation as necessary, with prophylactic antibiotic coverage.

C. **Dislocations and ligament injuries**
  1. **Principles of management**
     a. **Pre- and postreduction films** to confirm joint alignment and look for associated fractures.
     b. **Joint stability assessment** by stressing the periarticular structures and putting the joint through its range of motion. If instability is demonstrated, operative management should be considered. A stable joint is managed with protective splinting and early range-of-motion exercise.
     c. **Distal neurovascular assessment** before and after manipulation.
  2. **Specific dislocations**
     a. **DIP joint and thumb IP joint dislocations** are uncommon injuries treated with closed reduction followed by splinting for 3 weeks, along with early protective range-of-motion exercise, provided tendon function is normal.
     b. **PIP joint injuries** are commonly known as "jammed fingers" and require careful assessment and follow-up to prevent long-term stiffness.
        (1) **Dislocations may be dorsal or volar.** Volar dislocations may be difficult to reduce owing to interposition of the extensor apparatus. Volar dislocations may also result in disruption of the extensor tendon central slip and need close observation to watch for boutonniere deformity. Postreduction care consists of early hand therapy, or operative management if unstable or irreducible.
        (2) **Volar plate injuries** are common and result from hyperextension of the PIP joint. The ligament can be strained, ruptured, or avulsed from the base of the middle phalanx with or without a bone fragment. If the injury is to soft tissue only or the avulsion represents less than 20% of the articular surface with

a stable joint, treatment involves buddy taping or extension block splinting with the joint in 30 degrees of extension and immediate range of motion. If the bone fragment represents 20% or more of the articular surface and there is associated instability, open reduction and internal fixation or volar plate arthroplasty are required.

c. **Finger MCP joint dislocations** are usually caused by forced hyperextension and are most often seen in the index and small fingers. The dislocation is usually dorsal and is usually reducible in the emergency room. If the volar plate is interposed in the joint, however, open reduction may be required. If the joint is stable after reduction, it should be splinted for protection and early motion started. Occasionally, the metacarpal head can be held volarly by the flexor tendons on one side and the intrinsic muscles on the other side such that longitudinal traction tightens the "noose" around the head and prevents reduction. Open reduction is required in these situations.

d. **Thumb MCP joint dislocations** are uncommon. The dislocation is usually dorsal and results from forced abduction. Closed reduction with a thumb spica splint and early range of motion is the usual treatment. The ulnar collateral ligament can be partially or completely torn and may avulse with a bone fragment from the proximal phalanx. If there is joint stability and congruity, the MCP joint is splinted for 4 weeks, leaving the IP joint free. If the joint is unstable or the proximal portion of the torn ulnar collateral ligament is displaced superficial to the adductor pollicis (Stener lesion), open reduction and internal fixation are required. **Of note, a stable lesion may be converted into an unstable (Stener) lesion by inexperienced examiners aggressively stressing the joint.**

e. **Carpometacarpal injuries** are usually dislocations with or without fractures. Ligamentous injuries are less common because the carpometacarpal articulation has less movement than do other joints. Dorsal dislocations with and without fractures result from a direct blow and are more common on the ulnar part of the hand. Closed reduction is frequently possible, but maintaining the reduction often requires percutaneous pinning of the joint.

D. Tendon injuries

1. **Flexor tendons** are frequently lacerated during everyday activities. Assessment and management of these injuries by a hand surgeon are critical to a satisfactory outcome.

a. **The assessment** involves a careful history and examination; the examiner should look for a change in the resting tone of the digits (cascade) and assess the profundus and superficialis tendons independently. If flexion against resistance elicits pain, a partial laceration must be suspected. A careful neurovascular examination, including evaluation of two-point discrimination, should be performed to evaluate for concomitant nerve or vessel injury.

b. **Emergency room management** involves a thorough examination, then irrigation and closure of the wound, dorsal splinting with the patient's wrist in 20 to 30 degrees of flexion, the MCP joint at 90 degrees of flexion, and the IP joints in extension. Operative exploration and repair are appropriate for all lacerations through the tendon sheath because wrist and digit position at the time of injury can result in significant retraction with respect to skin laceration.

c. **Anatomy: flexor tendon zones**

(1) **Zone I:** distal to the superficialis (FDS) insertion.

(2) **Zone II:** from proximal A1 pulley (distal palmer crease) to FDS insertion.

(3) **Zone III:** from distal transverse carpal ligament (carpal tunnel) to A1 pulley.

(4) **Zone IV:** within the carpal tunnel.

(5) **Zone V:** proximal to the carpal tunnel.

d. **Technique of repair** involves a core, locking suture and an epitendinous repair. For tendon ruptures and lacerations within 1 cm of the FDP insertion, advancement and reinsertion of the tendon are used. A dorsal splint is applied, and a strict protected motion protocol directed by a hand therapist is started within 24 to 72 hours after repair and continues for 6 to 8 weeks.

2. **Extensor tendon injuries** result from lacerations and closed axial loading of the digits.

   a. **Zone I: over the DIP joint.** Mallet finger is a very common injury that results from forced flexion of the tip of the finger, with rupture of the terminal tendon from the distal phalanx. This leads to inability to extend the DIP. Mallet finger may be associated with an avulsion fracture or joint subluxation. These injuries are treated with splinting of the DIP joint in extension for 6 weeks. Operative management with reduction of the fracture and joint is only occasionally indicated. For open injuries, the tendon should be repaired and the joint pinned or splinted in extension for 6 weeks.

   b. **Zone II: over the middle phalanx.** Lacerations in this zone should be repaired using a figure-of-eight or mattress technique. The DIP joint may be transfixed with a pin or splinted for 4 to 6 weeks.

   c. **Zone III: over the PIP joint.** A complicated injury because injury can occur to the central slip or lateral bands. A clue to central slip injury is the inability of the patient to initiate PIP extension from 90 degrees. If the patient is able to fully extend the PIP and DIP, at least one lateral band is intact. If untreated, these injuries can result in a boutonnière deformity (PIP flexion and DIP hyperextension) of the digit. For open injuries, the tendon should be repaired and the joint transfixed with an oblique pin for 3 to 5 weeks. For tendon injuries associated with a fracture that is displaced, reduction and fixation of the fracture are advised. Protective splinting of the joint should be maintained for 6 weeks.

   d. **Zone IV: over the proximal phalanx.** The lacerations are often partial because of the width of the tendon at this level. Splinting of the PIP joint in extension for 3 to 4 weeks is often sufficient for these injuries. Repair of the tendon is required if there is any extension lag of the IP joints.

   e. **Zone V: over the MCP joint.** These injuries often occur as a result of a punching incident, particularly with a blow to the mouth. Contamination of the wound with oral flora can produce serious infection (see Hand Surgery, Section VI.B.5). Aggressive wound exploration must be undertaken to rule out joint space involvement because intra-articular infection can rapidly destroy the delicate cartilaginous surfaces. This often requires elongation of the laceration for adequate visualization and irrigation of the full extent of the wound. Only after the full extent of the wound has been evaluated and the wound aggressively cleansed can the tendon or tendons be repaired and the joint splinted in 20 to 30 degrees of flexion. The wrist is splinted in 30 degrees of extension. Dynamic splinting is useful to avoid adhesions and improve early motion.

   f. **Zone VI: over the dorsum of the metacarpals and carpus.** Repair and splint as for zone V injuries.

   g. **Zone VII: at the level of the extensor retinaculum.** Repair and splint as for zone V.

   h. **Zone VIII: proximal to the extensor retinaculum.** Injury is often at the musculotendinous junction. Repair and splinting for 4 to 6 weeks are required.

E. **Amputation**

   1. **Replantation or revascularization**

      a. **Indications** for replantation include amputation of the thumb, amputation of multiple digits, amputation at the metacarpal, wrist, or forearm level, and amputation at any level in a child. More-controversial indications include amputation of the proximal arm and amputation of a single digit distal to the FDS insertion.

      b. **Contraindications** for replantation include coexisting serious injuries or diseases that preclude a prolonged operative time, multiple levels of amputation, severe crush or degloving injury to the part, and prolonged ischemia time (12 hours for fingers and 6 hours for proximal limb amputations). Avulsion injury is a relative contraindication to replantation because of the extensive vascular and soft-tissue trauma.

      c. **Preparation for transfer** involves a moist dressing on the stump and splinting for comfort. The amputated part should be wrapped in saline-moistened gauze and placed in a clear plastic bag on a mixture of ice and water. The part should never be placed directly on ice or immersed in saline. Radiographs of the stump and the amputated part are essential and can be done at the transferring facility, provided that this does not significantly delay transfer to the microsurgery center. Intravenous fluids, prophylactic antibiotics, and tetanus toxoid, when indicated, should be begun immediately to facilitate prompt transfer to the appropriate facility for replantation. The sequence of repair involves identification of neurovascular structures and tendons and preparation of the bone for fixation. After providing bony stability, the arteries are repaired, followed by repair of the tendons and then veins, nerves, and skin. The postoperative care involves careful monitoring of the splinted part (temperature, color, and turgor) and adequate intravenous hydration in a warm environment.

   2. Revision amputation (nonreplantable amputation) management
   - **a. Principles**
     - **(1) Complete assessment,** including radiographs.
     - **(2) Antibiotics** when bone is involved or soft tissues are crushed or contaminated.
     - **(3) Preservation of length.**
     - **(4) Maintenance of sensation and motion.**
     - **(5) Aesthetics.**
     - **(6) Early motion.**
   - **b. Fingertip injuries** are optimally managed using primary closure without shortening. If this is not possible, lateral V-Y advancement or volar advancement flaps or skin grafts can be used to obtain closure. An alternative for small wounds (with no vital structures exposed) is closure by secondary intention.
   - **c. More proximal amputations** involve shortening and contouring the bone, shortening the tendons, and identifying digital nerves and allowing them to be transposed away from the skin closure.
   - **d. A protective dressing** that allows joint motion is recommended, with early referral to a hand therapist for range-of-motion exercises and later desensitization of the tip of the stump.

F. Infections
   1. Management. Infections in the hand can progress rapidly via potential spaces and may risk the viability of tendons, bones, joints, and neurovascular structures by creating increased pressure from pus and edema in closed spaces.
   - **a. Surgical drainage** is required in most hand infections.
   - **b. Antibiotic coverage** should be directed against common skin flora such as *Staphylococcus aureus, Staphylococcus epidermidis,* and *Streptococcus* species.
   - **c. Gram stain and culture of wound.**
   - **d. Splinting and elevation of the hand.**
   - **e. Tetanus prophylaxis when appropriate.**
   2. Local infections
   - **a. Paronychia** is a soft-tissue infection of the skin and soft tissue of the lateral nail fold; an **eponychial infection** may extend from this and involves the proximal nail fold. These localized infections often arise from self-inflicted trauma by nail biting or foreign-body penetration, such as a needle-stick. Treatment requires incision and drainage, with removal of the nail when the infection extends deep to the nail plate. Oral antibiotics are used if a cellulitis is present. **Chronic paronychia** is sometimes associated with underlying osteomyelitis or fungal organisms.
   - **b. Felon** is a localized infection involving the pulp of the volar digit and usually originates with a puncture wound, although a paronychial infection may spread volarly. Purulent fluid is usually under pressure in the fibrous septa of the tip of the digit. Management involves incision and drainage of the abscess (which can be between septa) and systemic antibiotics if there is an associated cellulitis. In general, the incision is located where the felon is "pointing"; however, it should be carefully planned to avoid sensitive scars and destabilization of the pulp of the finger. As with a paronychia, aggressive cleansing with soap and water after

incision and drainage promotes drainage and avoids premature closing of the wound.

c. **Cellulitis** in the hand usually occurs secondary to a laceration, abrasion, or other soft-tissue injury. Management involves draining an abscess if present. The fluid should be sent for culture and sensitivity, and oral or intravenous antibiotics should be administered, depending on the severity. When associated with swelling of the digits and hand, splinting in the intrinsic-plus position and elevation prevent stiffness.

d. **After an animal bite,** the wound must be thoroughly irrigated to decrease the bacterial load and to remove any foreign body, such as a tooth. Bite wounds should be treated with oral antibiotics prophylactically and with intravenous antibiotics when an established infection is present. Although a greater percentage of cat bites become infected than do dog bites, the jaws of a dog are significantly more powerful and can inflict other injuries. The organisms most often involved from dog or cat bites include *Pasteurella multocida, S. aureus, Bacteroides* species, and *Streptococcus viridans.* Recommended oral antibiotics are amoxicillin-clavulanate or clindamycin with either ciprofloxacin or trimethoprim/sulfamethoxazole.

e. **Human bites** can involve particularly virulent organisms and frequently present in association with extensor tendon injuries or fractures sustained during physical altercations. An open wound, particularly if it overlies the dorsum of the hand with signs of infection or underlying soft-tissue or bony injuries, should prompt patient questioning about the source of the laceration. Typical organisms cultured from human bite wounds are *S. viridans, S. epidermidis,* and *S. aureus,* as well as anaerobic bacteria, such as *Eikenella corrodens* and *Bacteroides* species. Amoxicillin-clavulanate should be used prophylactically, and when signs of infection are present, treatment with ampicillin-sulbactam, cefoxitin, or clindamycin plus either ciprofloxacin or trimethoprim/sulfamethoxazole is recommended. Wound exploration should be carried out.

G. Surgical emergencies

1. **Compartment syndrome** is seen in the hand and forearm and results from increased pressure within an osseofascial space, leading to decreased perfusion pressure. If it is left untreated, muscle and nerve ischemia may progress to necrosis and fibrosis, causing Volkmann ischemic contracture.

   a. **Etiology.** Fractures that cause bleeding, crush and vascular injuries, circumferential burns, bleeding dyscrasias, reperfusion after ischemia, or tight dressings can lead to the syndrome.

   b. **Diagnosis** is based on a high index of suspicion, clinical examination, and symptoms of pain that are exacerbated with passive stretch of the compartment musculature, paresthesias, paralysis, or paresis of ischemic muscles. Pulselessness may occur and indicates a late finding (and is usually also a sign of irreversible damage) or the presence of major arterial occlusion rather than compartment syndrome. Measurement with a pressure monitor of a compartment pressure of greater than 30 mm Hg confirms diagnosis.

   c. **Treatment** for incipient compartment syndrome involves close observation and frequent examinations and should include removal of tight casts and dressings. Elevation of the extremity to, or slightly above, the level of the heart is recommended. Acute or suspected compartment syndrome requires urgent fasciotomies of the involved areas. Decompression within 6 hours of established compartment pressures is necessary to prevent irreversible muscle ischemia. Forearm fasciotomies involve volar, carpal tunnel, and dorsal compartments. Hand fasciotomies include dorsal incisions for interossei and adductor pollicis, thenar, and hypothenar compartments, as well as midaxial incisions of the digits (ulnar for the index, long, and ring fingers and radial for the thumb and small finger).

2. **Suppurative tenosynovitis** involves infection of the flexor tendon sheath, which is usually caused by a puncture wound to the volar aspect of the digit or palm.

    a. Diagnosis: cardinal signs of Kanavel
      (1) Finger held in flexion.
      (2) Fusiform swelling of the finger.
      (3) Tenderness along the tendon sheath.
      (4) Pain on passive extension.
    b. Management involves urgent incision and drainage in the operating room, with placement of an irrigating catheter, such as a pediatric feeding tube, in the sheath for continuous irrigation with saline. Irrigation is maintained for 24 to 48 hours. Intravenous antibiotics are administered. Frequent reassessment to verify resolution is critical to avoiding ischemic injury to the tendon secondary to the contained infection.

  3. Palmar abscess is usually associated with a puncture wound. The fascia divides the palm into thenar, midpalmar, and hypothenar spaces; each involved space must be incised and drained. As with other infections, splinting, elevation, and intravenous antibiotics are required.

  4. Necrotizing infections threaten both limb and life. The incidence of invasive group A streptococcal infection is on the rise (*N Engl J Med* 1996;335:547) and can occur after surgery or trauma. Aggressive surgical débridement, high-dose penicillin, and supportive management are the mainstays of treatment. Additional therapy with gentamicin or clindamicin provides antibacterial synergy and blocks production of bacterial toxins. Immune globulin and hyperbaric oxygen are adjuvant therapies.

  5. High-pressure injection injuries result from grease or paint injected at up to 10,000 lb/in.^{2}. Although the external wounds are often small and unassuming, deep-tissue injury can be severe. Injury to the tissue is the result of both direct physical damage and chemical toxicity, and it leads to edema, thrombosis, and subsequent infection. Management involves urgent, thorough débridement, irrigation, decompression, systemic antibiotics, and splinting, with frequent reassessments and repeat débridement in 24 hours as required. When a digit has sustained significant injection, amputation may be required.

SPECIFIC PROBLEMS IN RECONSTRUCTIVE PLASTIC SURGERY

I. PERIPHERAL NERVE
  A. Clinical assessment of neuropathy requires evaluation of both motor and sensory function as well as electrodiagnostic evaluation of nerve conduction and muscle innervation.
    1. Standard classification schemes are available for classification of motor nerve function (Table 29-2). In addition, specific testing of moving or static two-point

TABLE 29-2	Classification of Motor Function

Grade	Motor function
M0	No contraction
M1	Perceptible contraction in proximal muscles
M2	Perceptible contraction in proximal and distal muscles
M3	All important muscles powerful enough to act against gravity
M4	Muscles act against strong resistance; some independent movement possible
M5	Normal strength and function

Adapted from SE Mackinnon, AL Dellon. *Surgery of the Peripheral Nerve.* New York: Thieme; 1988:118.

discrimination, vibration and pressure thresholds, or grip strength may be appropriate.

2. **Diagnostic studies** for quantification of nerve dysfunction include nerve conduction studies (NCSs) and electromyography (EMG). A nerve conduction study characterizes the conduction of large-diameter, myelinated nerves, and normal values may be present despite partial nerve injury. NCSs are useful in determining the degree of nerve dysfunction, the presence of segmental demyelination or axonal degeneration, the site of injury, and whether the injury is unifocal, multifocal, or diffuse. EMG samples the action potentials from muscle fibers and can detect individual motor unit potentials, which may indicate early reinnervation, and fibrillations, which represent denervation owing to axonal degeneration.

B. **Acute nerve injury** results from transection, crush, or compression and represents the loss of nerve function distal to the area of injury. Axons are myelinated by Schwann cells and organized into fascicles surrounded by the perineurium. The fascicles are bundled into nerves by the epineurium. The prognosis of injury to a peripheral nerve is dictated by which structures are disrupted. It is important to recognize in the acute setting that an injured nerve may be responsive to stimuli distally for 48 to 72 hours after transection. The severity of nerve injury has been organized into a grading scheme (Table 29-3). Operative repair is indicated for fourth- through sixth-degree injury.

1. **The technique of nerve repair** affects the eventual degree of recovery. Several basic concepts are used to optimize outcome.

   a. **Microsurgical technique** should be used, including magnification and microsurgical instruments and sutures. When conditions allow, a **primary repair** should be performed. The repair should be tension free.

   b. Positioning a limb or digit in extreme flexion or extension to facilitate an end-to-end repair is discouraged because of the joint and ligamentous problems that result. If a tension-free repair cannot be achieved in **neutral position**, transposing the nerve or placing an interposition nerve graft should be used.

   c. An **epineural repair** is typically performed, but a grouped fascicular repair should be performed whenever the internal topography of the nerve is segregated into motor, sensory, or regional components.

   d. **Postoperative motor and sensory reeducation** will help to optimize outcome.

2. **Indications** for peripheral nerve repair include partial or complete transection or in-continuity conduction block. These represent fourth- to sixth-degree nerve injuries and can be difficult to distinguish from lesser grades of injury based on clinical examination alone. This is true because all grades of injury can lead to

TABLE 29-3 **Classification of Nerve Injuries**

Sunderland[a]	Seddon[b]	Structure injured	Prognosis
First degree	Neurapraxia	Schwann cell (demyelination)	Complete recovery within 12 wk
Second degree	Axonotmesis	Axon (wallerian degeneration)	Complete recovery regeneration 1 mm/d
Third degree		Endoneurium	Incomplete recovery
Fourth degree		Perineurium	No recovery
Fifth degree	Neurotmesis	Epineurium	No recovery
Sixth degree		Mixed injury, neuroma incontinuity[c]	Unpredictable recovery

[a]Sunderland S. A classification of peripheral nerve injuries producing loss of function. *Brain* 1951;74:491.
[b]Seddon HJ. Three types of nerve injury. *Brain* 1943;66:237.
[c]Mackinnon SE. New direction in peripheral nerve surgery. *Ann Plast Surg* 1989;22(3):257–273.

complete loss of function. Some guidelines for surgical intervention are listed in the following sections.

  a. **Nerves inadvertently divided** during operation are fifth-degree injuries and should be repaired immediately.

  b. **Closed-nerve injuries that localize near an anatomically restrictive site** (e.g., the ulnar nerve at the elbow or the common peroneal nerve at the knee) can result in neurologic deficit secondary to conduction block from edema and compression. If no recovery occurs within 3 weeks, management includes surgical decompression at that site. Iatrogenic nerve deficit from positioning during long operative procedures is managed similarly.

  c. **Closed-nerve injury from blunt trauma or traction** is usually a first-, second-, or third-degree injury, and full recovery can be expected in most cases. Patients are closely followed for signs of recovery, including an advancing Tinel sign, indicating regenerating axons. Baseline NCS and EMG are obtained at 6 weeks. If there is no evidence of return of function at 3 months, repeat studies are obtained. If there is no improvement, the nerve is explored and repaired.

  d. **Nerve deficit after sharp trauma** (e.g., a stab wound) usually is the result of partial or complete transection, and the nerve should be explored and repaired urgently.

  e. **Loss of nerve function after gunshot or open blunt trauma** is usually the result of first- or second-degree injury, and recovery can be expected in most cases. These cases are usually treated as for closed injuries. If the nerve is visible or the wound is explored for other reasons (e.g., vascular repair), the nerve is explored. If the nerve is in continuity, it is managed as for a closed injury. If the nerve is not in continuity, it is usually best to tag the ends of the nerve for ease of identification and delay definitive repair until the zone of injury to the nerve is clearer (generally by 3 weeks).

  f. **Nerve deficit from compartment syndrome** is treated by emergent fasciotomy. If decompressed early (within 6 hours), there is usually a rapid return of function.

  g. **Decompression of injured nerves** (e.g., ulnar nerve transposition or carpal tunnel release) at sites distal to trauma can be useful to avoid retardation of nerve regeneration across these areas. Multiple sites of injury or compression can have additive effects, and for first- through third-degree injuries, decompression can improve outcome.

  h. **Division of a sensory nerve** can lead to a painful neuroma as the regenerating axons grow into the surrounding soft tissue. If the resulting neural deficit results in loss of function or protective sensation, these nerves can be repaired. If not, the neuroma is excised and the cut end of the nerve is transposed proximally well away from the wound, preferably into a nearby muscular environment.

C. **Compression neuropathy** due to compression or repetitive trauma is a common clinical problem. Typically involved nerves include the median nerve at the wrist (carpal tunnel syndrome), the ulnar nerve at the elbow or wrist (cubital tunnel syndrome), the anterior or posterior interosseous nerves in the forearm, the brachial plexus at the thoracic outlet, the common peroneal nerve at the knee, and the posterior tibial nerve at the ankle (tarsal tunnel syndrome).

  1. **Clinical assessment** of these conditions involves assessment of motor and sensory function, as well as provocative testing (reproducibility of symptoms with extrinsic nerve compression) and determination of whether the Tinel sign is present. EMG and NCS are appropriate if the clinical picture is unclear.

  2. **Initial management** is usually physical therapy, behavior modification, and splinting to avoid repetitive compression. A period of at least 6 weeks of nonsurgical management without improvement is usually recommended before operation, although nerve compression at the cubital tunnel or thoracic outlet typically requires prolonged nonsurgical management. Operations generally involve **decompression** of the affected nerve or transposition to an unrestricted site.

II. SCALP, CALVARIAL, AND FOREHEAD RECONSTRUCTION

A. Anatomy

1. The **scalp** consists of five layers: skin, subcutaneous tissue, galea aponeurotica, loose areolar tissue, and pericranium.

2. **Five major paired vessels** provide the scalp with an ample collateral blood supply: the supraorbital, supratrochlear, superficial temporal, posterior auricular, and occipital arteries.

3. The **scalp receives sensory innervation** from the supraorbital and supratrochlear, branches of cranial nerve V1, the lesser occipital branch of C2 or C3, the greater auricular nerve, and the auriculotemporal branch of cranial nerve V3. The motor innervation to the frontalis derives from the frontal branch of the facial nerve.

B. Scalp lacerations are common concomitant sequelae of blunt trauma to the head.

As such, there may be associated skull, cervical spine, or intracranial injuries. The rich blood supply to the scalp can produce significant blood loss, and hemostasis is important to prevent subgaleal hematoma. Radical débridement is seldom indicated, and primary repair is usually feasible. Repair of the galea generally helps to prevent hematoma formation.

C. Partial-thickness scalp loss from avulsion usually occurs at the subaponeurotic

layer. Large avulsions may be skin grafted. One can expect 20% to 40% contraction of the skin graft over the first 6 to 8 months. After this has leveled off, the grafted area can be removed by serial excisions.

D. Full-thickness scalp loss can occur from trauma or tumor extirpation. The optimal

treatment varies depending on the size of the defect.

1. **Small defects** (<3 cm) can often be closed primarily after undermining of flaps. Local flaps, either random or based on blood supply, can be raised. Scoring the galea in a grid pattern of perpendicular lines spaced 1 cm apart can allow for expansion of the flap. Rotation flaps should involve a margin of at least five times the length of the defect. Bipedicled flaps are well suited for coverage of the poles of the head (forehead, temporal areas, and nape of neck).

2. **Medium-sized defects** (3 to 10 cm) are usually covered with a scalp flap combined with skin grafting of the donor pericranium. Several specific flaps have been described for medium-sized defects, including the pinwheel flap, three-flap, and four-flap techniques described by Orticochea. All have been used with variable success.

3. **Large defects** (>10 cm) often require free tissue transfer. If the deficit is due to trauma, replant may be attempted. Because most of these injuries are from industrial accidents involving avulsion, however, the injury to the arterial intima can extend far into the scalp. Latissimus dorsi or omental free flaps with split-thickness skin grafts are described for complete scalp loss.

E. Calvarial defects in the parietal or occipital regions require cranioplasty for protec-

tion. Temporal defects are somewhat protected by the temporalis muscle.

1. **Alloplastic material** can be used to cover these defects, including calcium hydroxyapatite and methylmethacrylate. Polymethylmethacrylate (PMMA) is the most commonly employed because it is both durable and easy to use. However, it is exothermic on initial application, it has reported infection rates of approximately 5%, and the rates can be as high as 30% with infection nearby. Newer alloplastic materials are being developed to promote bony ingrowth and decrease the risk of infection. Some can be custom made, based on three-dimensional reconstructions of computed tomographic scans.

2. **Autogenous tissue for cranioplasty** includes split-rib grafts, split-table calvarial bone grafts, and bone paste. These are somewhat more difficult to use but have the advantage of a lower complication rate.

III. TRUNK

A. Breast

1. **Postmastectomy breast reconstruction** offers restoration of an important symbol of femininity and sexual intimacy. Reconstruction of breast symmetry can lead to a significant improvement in body image and is an important part of cancer rehabilitation for many women (*Scand J Plast Reconstr Surg* 1984;18:221).

a. **The aims of reconstruction** are to create symmetric breast mounds and, if desired, a new nipple-areola complex. The aesthetic goal is defined by the patient and includes a symmetric appearance both clothed and unclothed. Extensive preoperative consultation is required to allow women to explore their options. It should be emphasized that each approach to breast reconstruction usually requires at least two procedures and that the reconstructed breast will never completely replicate the original. Reconstruction can be accomplished with or without the use of an implant, and most procedures can be performed either immediately at the time of the mastectomy or in a delayed fashion.

b. **Reconstruction of the breast mound** is accomplished with an implant in approximately two thirds of cases (*Probl Gen Surg* 1996;13:75). In most cases, enough skin is removed with the mastectomy that the desired size of the breast precludes closure of the wound without tension. When this is the case, a tissue expander is placed and serial expansions performed until the desired size is reached (usually after 6 weeks of expansion). At this time, the expander is replaced with a permanent implant filled with silicone gel or saline. The advantages of this approach to reconstruction are that minimal operative time is required, additional scars are minimized, and the recovery period is shorter. The disadvantages include the risks of permanent implants (rupture, infection) and the inability to reproduce certain natural contours.

c. **Autologous tissue** can be used to recreate a breast mound in the form of pedicled (rectus abdominis, latissimus dorsi) or free (rectus abdominis, gluteus maximus) myocutaneous flaps. The advantages include a more natural appearance for some patients, permanent reconstruction without the potential for future procedures to replace a ruptured implant, and fewer complications with subsequent radiation therapy. Disadvantages include a relatively long procedure, additional scars, and potential donor-site morbidity.

d. **Reconstruction of the nipple-areola complex** is chosen by approximately 50% of patients undergoing breast reconstruction. A variety of methods are used and include local flaps or nipple-sharing grafts to reconstruct a nipple-like prominence. Split-thickness skin grafting or tattooing can be used to recreate an areola.

e. **Procedures on the contralateral breast to improve symmetry** may be performed concomitantly or subsequently and include modification of an inframammary fold, removal of dog ears, liposuction of flaps, or reduction mammoplasty or mastopexy of the contralateral side. Symmetry procedures are almost always covered by insurance.

2. **Reduction mammoplasty** is performed for women with a variety of physical complaints and aberrations in body image.

a. **Common symptoms** are listed as follows and are considered indications for reduction mammoplasty:

(1) **Personal embarrassment and psychosocial problems.**

(2) **Shoulder and back pain.**

(3) **Grooving of the soft tissue of the shoulders by bra straps.**

(4) **Chronic inframammary skin breakdown, rash, or infection (intertrigo).**

(5) **Inability to engage in vigorous exercise.**

(6) **Symptoms of brachial plexus compression (rare).**

b. A variety of procedures are designed to **reduce breast size.** All of them move the nipple-areola complex superiorly on the chest wall. The nipple-areola complex is maintained on a pedicled blood supply when possible, but in certain instances (e.g., pedicle length >15 cm or a patient who smokes), tenuous blood supply to the nipple-areola complex may require a full-thickness graft. There are always scars resulting from the movement of the nipple and resection of excess skin, and the configuration of these scars varies by the procedure chosen.

B. **Chest wall reconstruction**

1. **Before beginning chest wall reconstruction,** one must ensure complete resection of tumor and radiation-damaged or infected tissue.

2. **Dead space** in the chest allows for potential empyema and must be obliterated. This space is best filled with pedicled muscle (latissimus dorsi, pectoralis major, serratus anterior, or rectus abdominis) or omental flaps.

3. **Skeletal stabilization** is required if more than four rib segments or 5 cm of chest wall are missing. This can be achieved using autologous (rib, dermis, or fascial grafts or bulky muscle flaps) or prosthetic (Prolene mesh, Gore-Tex, Marlex-methylmethacrylate sandwich) material.

4. **Optimal soft-tissue coverage** usually requires pedicled myocutaneous flaps but can be achieved with pedicled muscle or omentum covered with split-thickness skin graft. Rarely, free tissue transfer is required.

5. **Median sternotomy dehiscence** owing to infection occurs in 1% to 2% of cardiac procedures. Predisposing factors include bilateral internal mammary artery harvest, diabetes mellitus, obesity, and multiple operations. Closure requires removal of wires and débridement of all infected tissue, including bone and cartilage. Closure of the resultant dead space is usually accomplished by advancing or rotating the pectoralis major and/or rectus abdominis muscles. The rectus abdominis muscle cannot be used as a rotational flap if the ipsilateral internal mammary artery has been harvested. Pedicled omental flaps are reserved as alternatives in case of initial failure.

C. Abdominal wall reconstruction

1. **Reconstruction of full-thickness abdominal wall defects** includes re-creation of a fascial barrier and skin coverage. Restoration of a functional muscle layer is also helpful in maintaining abdominal wall functionality.

2. **Complete absence of all layers of the anterior abdominal wall** is usually the result of direct trauma or infection, with or without intra-abdominal catastrophe. The open abdomen can be temporized by skin grafts placed directly on bowel serosa, omentum, or absorbable mesh through which granulation tissue has formed. This allows for resolution of intra-abdominal edema and maturation of adhesions but usually results in a large ventral hernia.

3. **Primary closure of fascial defects** represents the best approach and can be assisted by sliding myofascial advancement flaps. Lateral release of the external oblique fascia, or "component separation," is ideal for midline musculofascial defects greater than 3 cm in size. Using bilateral relaxing incisions and release, a total of 10, 18, and 6 to 10 cm of advancement may be obtained in the upper, middle, and lower thirds of the abdomen, respectively (*Plast Recon Surg* 1990;86:519). The anterior sheath of one or both rectus muscles can be divided and turned over to provide additional fascia for closure. Synthetic mesh may be used when fascial defects cannot be primarily closed. AlloDerm, freeze-dried cadaveric dermis devoid of antigenic cells, also may be utilized for large fascial defects. **Muscle flaps** are required when the existing fascia is insufficient for closure after advancement. The most frequently used flaps are the tensor fascia lata, rectus femoris, and vastus lateralis. These flaps are usually not useful for closing defects of the upper abdomen.

4. **Skin coverage** is accomplished with split-thickness skin grafts, the cutaneous portion of a myocutaneous flap, or local tissue rearrangement (e.g., bipedicled flap, V-Y advancement flap). Because skin grafts cannot survive directly on synthetic mesh, a muscle flap may be required to provide an adequate bed for skin grafting.

D. Pressure sores

1. The **etiology and staging criteria** are described in Chapter 6.

2. **Principles of nonoperative management** of pressure sores include (1) relief of pressure by positioning changes and appropriate cushioning; (2) bedside débridement of devitalized tissue; (3) optimization of the wound environment with aggressive wound care; (4) avoidance of maceration, trauma, friction, or shearing forces; and (5) reversal of underlying conditions that may predispose to ulcer development as well as optimizing nutritional status. This type of aggressive nonoperative management is often optimally coordinated by specially trained wound care nurses.

3. **Operative management** with soft-tissue flap closure is only indicated for large, deep, or complicated ulcers and then only in patients who are able to care for their wounds. A high degree of cooperation from the patient and caregivers is essential because the recurrence of pressure sores at the same site or new sores at other sites after operation is high. This is especially true for individuals who have spinal cord transection from firearm injuries, whose rate of recurrence is 91%, with a mean time to recurrence of 18 months (*Adv Wound Care* 1994;7:40). This is most likely the result of breakdown in the postoperative support and care systems in this population. Most surgeons, therefore, require demonstration of the patient's ability to care for wounds before embarking on operative closure. Flaps commonly used for closure of pressure ulcers around the pelvic girdle include gluteus maximus, tensor fascia lata, hamstring, or gracilis-based rotation or advancement flaps.

IV. **LOWER EXTREMITY.** Soft-tissue defects from trauma to the lower extremity are common. A multidisciplinary approach involving orthopedic, vascular, and plastic surgeons provides optimal care.

A. Lower-extremity injuries are first assessed according to **advanced trauma life support guidelines.** The general sequence of priorities is as follows:

1. The first priority is assessment for **concomitant life-threatening injuries and control of active bleeding.** Blood loss from open wounds is often underestimated, and patients must be adequately resuscitated.

2. The **neurovascular status** is determined. If a nerve deficit is progressive during observation in the emergency room, it is likely the result of ischemia from arterial injury or compartment syndrome.

3. **Bony continuity** is assessed by radiographs of all areas of suspected injury.

4. **Operative management** addresses bone stabilization followed by venous and arterial repair. Fasciotomies are indicated for compartment pressures greater than 30 mm Hg and by clinical suspicion from preoperative neurovascular examination. Fasciotomy must be performed within 6 hours to avoid ischemic contracture. Nonviable tissue is débrided, and an assessment is made about delayed or immediate soft-tissue coverage.

B. **Soft-tissue defects of the thigh** are usually closed by primary closure, skin grafts, or local flaps. The thick muscular layers ensure adequate local tissue for coverage of bone and vessels and adequate vascular supply to any fracture sites.

C. **Open tibial fractures** frequently involve degloving of the thin layer of soft tissue covering the anterior tibial surface. The distal tibia is a watershed zone, and fracture with loss of periosteum or soft tissue leads to increased rates of infection and nonunion.

TABLE 29-4   **Gustilo Open Fracture Classification**

Classification	Characteristics
I	Clean wound <1 cm long
II	Laceration >1 cm long; no extensive soft-tissue damage, flaps, or avulsions
III	Extensive soft-tissue laceration, damage, or loss; open segmental fracture; or traumatic amputation
IIIa	Adequate periosteal cover of the bone despite extensive soft-tissue damage; high-energy trauma with small wound
IIIb	Extensive soft-tissue loss with periosteal stripping and bone exposure; usually associated with massive contamination
IIIc	Arterial injury requiring repair

Adapted from RB Gustilo, JT Anderson. Prevention of infection in the treatment of one thousand and twenty-five open fractures of long bones: retrospective and prospective analysis. *J Bone Joint Surg Am* 1976;58A:453.

1. Open tibial fractures are classified according to the scheme of **Gustilo** (Table 29-4).
2. **Gustilo types IIIb and c** frequently require flap coverage of exposed bone.
   a. The **proximal third** of the tibia or knee can often be covered by a pedicled hemigastrocnemius flap.
   b. The **middle third** of the tibia is often covered by a pedicled hemisoleus flap.
   c. **Large defects of the distal third** of the tibia generally require coverage by free muscle transfer.

D. **Limb salvage reconstruction for neoplasm** differs from that for trauma, in that large segments of bone, nerve, or vessels may require replacement. **Skeletal replacement** can be accomplished using an endoprosthesis, allogeneic bone transplant, or vascularized free bone (fibula) transfer.

E. **The foot** is divided into regions for purposes of soft-tissue defects caused by trauma or ischemic, diabetic, or infectious ulceration. Optimal coverage of the plantar surface provides a durable, sensate platform.
   1. **Small defects of the heel** can be covered using the non–weight-bearing skin of the midsole. Larger defects require free muscle transfer and split-thickness skin grafting.
   2. **The metatarsal heads** are often successfully covered using plantar V-Y advancement and fillet of toe flaps. Multiple fillet of toe flaps or free muscle transfer may be required for large defects.
   3. **For fitting of proper footwear,** coverage of the dorsum of the foot must be thin. If paratenon is present, the dorsum can usually be covered with a skin graft. Small areas of exposed tendon may granulate, but larger areas require thin fascial free flaps (temporoparietal, parascapular, or radial forearm) covered by skin grafts.

CARDIAC SURGERY

Spencer J. Melby, Nader Moazami,
and Ralph J. Damiano, Jr.

30

$\mathscr{T}$his chapter focuses on the adult patient undergoing common cardiac operations, particularly coronary artery bypass grafting (CABG) and valve replacement. It also discusses the surgical treatment of heart failure and arrhythmia.

I. ANATOMY

A. Coronary arteries. The left and right coronary arteries arise from within the sinuses of Valsalva just distal to the right and left coronary cusps of the aortic valve.

1. The **left main coronary artery** travels posterior toward the pulmonary artery, then divides into its main branches, the **left anterior descending artery (LAD)** and the **left circumflex artery (LCx).** The LAD runs in the interventricular groove and arborizes into **septal** and **diagonal** branches. The LCx runs in the posterior atrioventricular groove and gives off **obtuse marginal** branches. In 10% to 15% of patients, the LCx gives off the **posterior descending artery (PDA),** termed a **left dominant coronary circulation.**

2. The **right coronary artery (RCA)** descends in the anterior atrioventricular groove, where, in **right dominant coronary circulation** (80% to 85% of cases), it gives off the PDA. In addition, the RCA gives off **acute marginal** branches.

B. Coronary veins. There are three principal venous channels for coronary venous drainage.

1. The **coronary sinus** is located in the posterior atrioventricular groove and receives venous drainage mainly from the left ventricular system. Its main tributaries are the great, middle, and small cardiac veins.

2. **Thesbian veins** are small venous channels that drain directly into the cardiac chambers.

3. The **anterior cardiac veins** drain the right coronary system, ultimately into the right atrium.

C. Valves. The valves of the heart are critical to the pump function of the heart. Their proper functioning is essential for the maintenance of pressure gradients and ante-grade flow through the heart chambers.

1. **Atrioventricular (AV) valves.** The function of the AV valves is to prevent atrial regurgitation during ventricular contraction. These valves are fibrous and continuous with the **annuli fibrosi** at the base of the heart. Furthermore, the leaflets are joined at their commissures and are further secured by **chordae tendineae,** which attach the free leaflets to the interventricular papillary muscles.

   a. The **tricuspid valve** separates the right chambers and consists of a large anterior leaflet, a posterior leaflet on the right, and a septal leaflet attached to the interventricular septum.

   b. The **mitral (bicuspid) valve** separates the left chambers and consists of a large anterior (aortic) leaflet and a posterior (mural) leaflet.

2. **Semilunar valves.** The **pulmonary** and **aortic** valves are essentially identical, except that the coronary arteries arise just distal to the aortic valve. The valves consist of three cusps, and each cusp comprises two lunulae. The lunulae extend from the commissure and meet at the midpoint, a thickening known as the **nodulus of Arantius.** During diastole, the three nodules coapt, forming a seal. Just distal to the valves are gentle dilations of the ascending aorta, known as **sinuses of**

Valsalva. These structures play an important role in the maintenance of sustained laminar blood flow.

II. PHYSIOLOGY

A. Electrophysiology. Like all neuromuscular tissue, the myocardium depends on efficient and predictable electrical activation. The myocardium has specialized tissue responsible for the rapid and orderly dispersal of myocardial electrical activation. The myocardial cells communicate through **gap junctions.**

1. The **sinoatrial (SA) node** is located at the junction of the anteromedial aspect of the superior vena cava and the right atrial appendage. The **cardiac pacemaker** is determined by the cells that have the most frequent rate of spontaneous depolarization. In most instances, the pacemaker is at the SA node **(sinus rhythm),** which represents an area in the right atrium with the fastest **automaticity.** In general, all myocardium demonstrates automaticity.

2. The **atrioventricular (AV) node** is located in the interatrial septum, on the ventricular side of the orifice of the coronary sinus. It is designed to protect the ventricle from high atrial rates. In the event of SA node dysfunction, the AV node can assume a pacemaker role because this specialized tissue has one of the next-highest rates of spontaneous depolarization.

3. The **bundle of His** originates in the AV node and descends through the membranous interventricular septum, just inferior to the septal cusp of the tricuspid valve. Also referred to as **Purkinje fibers,** it separates into the right and left branches at the junction of the membranous and muscular portions of the interventricular septum. In normal anatomy, this is the only electrical connection between the atria and the ventricles. The bundle of His functions to rapidly distribute the depolarization to ventricular myocardium, starting with the ventricular septum; to the apex; then throughout the ventricle via gap junctions.

B. Mechanics. The heart functions to convert electrical stimuli to chemical energy and eventually to mechanical energy. The mechanical forces are governed by the pressure, volume, and contractile state of the cardiac chambers. The determination of **rate, rhythm, preload, afterload,** and **contractility** are critical to understanding effective cardiac mechanical function.

1. The **cardiac cycle** describes the relationship between the electrical status of myocardial membranes and the mechanical condition of the cardiac chambers. As the mitral valve opens, diastolic filling commences. Following atrial depolarization and contraction, the ventricle depolarizes and isovolumetric contraction begins [at **end-diastolic volume** (EDV)]. Once intraventricular pressure exceeds aortic pressure, the aortic valve opens and **ventricular ejection** occurs. As the aortic pressure overcomes ventricular pressure (at EDV), the aortic valve closes. Isovolumetric relaxation commences until intraventricular pressure is lower than left atrial pressure, and the mitral valve opens.

2. **Preload** is defined as the end-diastolic volume of the ventricle. It is practically measured by central venous or **pulmonary capillary wedge pressure.**

3. **Afterload** is most widely defined as "resistance to ejection." It is more practically described as the **aortic pressure gradient.**

4. **Starling's law** describes the relationship between EDV and contractility. As EDV is increased, ventricular contraction is increased as the optimal sarcomere length is reached. However, once the optimal length is exceeded, contractility can decrease, as can be seen in pathologic states.

III. PREOPERATIVE EVALUATION.

The preoperative evaluation of patients undergoing cardiac surgery is similar to the evaluation of patients undergoing any major operation. All patients should have a complete history and physical examination. Laboratory studies usually include a complete blood cell count; determination of serum electrolyte, creatinine, and glucose levels; determination of prothrombin (PT) and partial thromboplastin times (PTT); and urinalysis. An arterial blood gas measurement is indicated in patients with chronic obstructive pulmonary disease, heavy tobacco abuse, or other pulmonary pathology. In general, 2 to 4 units of packed red blood cells should be available for use during operation. For elective operations, this may be pre-donated autologous blood. A chest radiograph (posteroanterior and lateral) should be obtained to evaluate calcification of the aortic arch and assess the proximity of the cardiac silhouette to the sternum in patients undergoing repeat sternotomy. The chest radiograph is also examined for the presence of other intrathoracic pathology. The height and weight of the patient should be measured, and the body-surface area (in square meters) should be calculated.

A. Organ-specific evaluation

1. **Neurologic complications** after cardiac surgery can be devastating. Perioperative cerebrovascular accidents (CVA) occur in 1% to 2% of low-risk patients but in up to 10% of the elderly (*Ann Thorac Surg* 1995;59:1296). CVA may result from aortic atherosclerotic or air emboli that are loosened by cannulation, cross-clamping, or construction of proximal anastomoses. Postoperative arrhythmias such as atrial fibrillation are also a common cause of CVA following cardiac surgery. Underlying cerebrovascular disease in conjunction with alterations in cerebral blood flow patterns during cardiopulmonary bypass (CPB) may play a role in some patients. Patients with a history of transient ischemic attack, amaurosis fugax, or CVA should undergo noninvasive evaluation of the carotid arteries with Doppler ultrasonography before operation. Because of the strong association between carotid artery and left main coronary artery stenoses, patients with left main disease should undergo carotid Doppler examination preoperatively. Evaluation of asymptomatic carotid bruits is more controversial. In general, **carotid stenoses** greater than or equal to 80% are addressed by carotid endarterectomy or stenting before or in combination with the planned cardiac surgical procedure.

2. **Pulmonary disease,** particularly the obstructive form, occurs commonly in patients with cardiac disease because cigarette smoking is a risk factor for both disease processes. A preoperative chest x-ray may demonstrate suspicious pulmonary pathology and can be used in combination with a preoperative arterial blood gas evaluation to identify patients who are at high risk for difficulty in being weaned from the ventilator postoperatively. Pulmonary function tests are indicated in high-risk patients. Smoking should be discontinued before operation, when possible.

3. **Peripheral vascular examination.** The presence and quality of arterial pulses in the radial, brachial, femoral, popliteal, dorsalis pedis, and posterior tibial arteries should be documented preoperatively as a baseline for comparison if postoperative arterial complications arise. Blood pressure should be measured in both arms to evaluate for subclavian artery stenosis. Significant subclavian artery stenosis may preclude the use of an internal thoracic (mammary) artery (ITA) as a conduit. A preoperative Allen test should also be performed to assess the palmar arch and the feasibility of using the radial artery for bypass conduit. For patients with varicosities of the saphenous veins or a history of vein stripping, preoperative vein mapping with ultrasonography can be done to assess the availability and quality of saphenous vein for conduit.

4. **Infection.** Operation should be delayed, if possible, in patients with systemic infection or sepsis and in those with cellulitis or soft-tissue infection at the site of planned incisions. Specific infections should be identified preoperatively, if possible, and treated with appropriate antibiotic therapy. In patients who have fever or leukocytosis but require an immediate operation, cultures should be obtained from all potential sources (including central venous catheters), and broad-spectrum intravenous antibiotics should be administered preoperatively.

5. **Medications.** The cardiac surgery patient may be taking a variety of medications before operation. In general, nitrates and β-adrenergic blocking agents should be continued throughout the entire perioperative period (*Circulation* 1991; 84(5 Suppl):III236). Unless a specific contraindication exists, statins should be given to all patients because a reduction of recurrent coronary artery disease (CAD) and postoperative stroke rates has been established (*Eur J Cardiothorac Surg* 2006;30:300). If possible, antiplatelet agents (e.g., aspirin or Plavix) are stopped before surgery to prevent hemorrhagic complications. Digoxin and calcium channel blockers generally are discontinued at the time of operation and

restarted only as needed in the postoperative period. For patients receiving heparin preoperatively for unstable angina, the heparin should not be discontinued before operation because this may precipitate an acute coronary syndrome. For patients receiving warfarin preoperatively (including patients with mechanical valves), the warfarin should be discontinued several days before operation. Once the prothrombin time [International Normalized Ratio (INR)] has normalized, anticoagulation can be accomplished using intravenous heparin.

B. Cardiac testing

1. The **electrocardiogram (ECG)** is an important tool for the evaluation of the heart. It demonstrates the electrical activity of the cardiac cycle. **Stress testing** is used to detect CAD or to assess the functional significance of coronary lesions. The exercise ECG is used to evaluate patients who have symptoms suggestive of angina but no symptoms at rest. A positive test is the development of typical signs or symptoms of angina pectoris and/or ECG changes (ST-segment changes or T-wave inversion).

2. A **pulmonary artery catheter (Swan-Ganz)** is often used in the perioperative setting; it is placed prior to the start of a cardiac procedure. The PA catheter allows for measurement of intravascular and intracardiac pressures, cardiac output, and mixed-venous oxygen saturation (see Table 30-1).

3. The use of **echocardiography** is essential in modern practice. The real-time assessment of chamber size, wall thickness, ventricular function, and valve appearance and motion are possible. It also is an invaluable aid in assessing the presence of intracardiac air prior to weaning from cardiopulmonary bypass. With the addition of Doppler imaging, blood flow characteristics can be easily determined. Both **transthoracic** and **transesophageal** echocardiography are widely available. Transesophageal imaging is particularly helpful intraoperatively.

4. **Thallium imaging** is used to identify ischemic myocardium. The thallium in the blood is taken up by the normal myocytes in proportion to the regional blood flow. Decreased perfusion to a region of the myocardium during exertion with subsequent reperfusion suggests reversible myocardial ischemia, whereas the lack of reperfusion suggests irreversibly scarred, infarcted myocardium. In patients who cannot exercise, thallium imaging can be performed after administration of the coronary vasodilator dipyridamole or **adenosine.**

5. **Coronary arteriography** is used to document the presence and location of coronary artery stenoses. Separate injections are made of the right and left main coronary arteries. In general, the atherosclerotic process involves the proximal portions of the major coronary arteries, particularly at or just beyond branch points. A 75% decrease in cross-sectional area (50% decrease in luminal diameter)

TABLE 30-1   **Normal Hemodynamic Parameters**

Parameter	Normal value	Unit
Central venous pressure	2–8	mm Hg
Right ventricular pressure (syst/diast)	15–30/2–8	mm Hg
Pulmonary artery pressure (syst/diast)	15–30/4–12	mm Hg
Pulmonary capillary wedge pressure	2–15	mm Hg
Left ventricular pressure (syst/diast)	100–140/3–12	mm Hg
Cardiac output	3.5–5.5	L/min
Cardiac index	2–4	L/min/m^2 BSA
Stroke volume index	1	mL/kg
Pulmonary vascular resistance	20–130	dynes · sec/cm^5
Systemic vascular resistance	700–1600	dynes · sec/cm^5
Mixed-venous oxygen saturation	65–75	percent

BSA, body-surface area; diast, diastolic; syst, systolic.

is considered a significant stenosis. Indications for coronary arteriography include suspected CAD (e.g., positive stress test), preparation for coronary revascularization, typical or atypical clinical presentations with normal or borderline stress testing when a definitive diagnosis of CAD is needed, and planned cardiac surgery (e.g., valve surgery) in patients with risk factors for CAD. Concomitant **ventriculography** can be used for assessing left ventricular function.

IV. MECHANICAL CARDIOPULMONARY SUPPORT AND OFF-PUMP CABG

  A. **Cardiopulmonary bypass (CPB),** first introduced in 1954 by Gibbon, allowed for the development of modern cardiac surgery. It is intended as a support system during surgery and requires systemic anticoagulation.

   1. A **venous reservoir** stores blood volume and allows for escape of bubbles prior to infusion. There are several varieties of **oxygenators,** but all perform the same gas exchange function. A **heat exchanger** is necessary to maintain hypothermia when needed and to assist with patient rewarming. The **arterial pump** is usually a roller pump and requires frequent calibration to ensure accurate flows. The **cannulae** and pump tubing are constructed of Silastic or latex, which remain supple when cold. A **left atrial vent** can be used to remove any blood that enters the left-side circulation.

   2. **Myocardial protection** strategies are critical to good outcome. Hyperkalemic perfusate (warm or cold) based on blood or crystalloid may be infused into the aortic root and coronary ostia (antegrade) or via the coronary sinus (retrograde).

   3. During CPB, the perfusionist, working with the surgeon, can effectively control perfusion rate, temperature, hematocrit, pulmonary venous pressure, and glucose and arterial oxygen levels.

   4. CPB is generally considered safe, but side effects do exist. Most notably, **postperfusion syndrome** is characterized by a diffuse, whole-body inflammatory reaction that can lead to multisystem organ dysfunction. It is believed that most patients experience some form of inflammatory reaction following CPB, but only a fraction develop this syndrome. Other factors contributing to poor CPB tolerance are length of support (e.g., >4 hours) and patient age.

  B. **Extracorporeal membrane oxygenation (ECMO)** is primarily used in infants with severe cardiopulmonary failure but can be used in adults. It is not a treatment modality but rather an intermediate-term (days to weeks) artificial heart and lung support system. Most commonly, it is used to allow patients to recover from reversible severe adult respiratory distress syndrome or pulmonary insufficiency of various etiologies.

  C. **Off-pump coronary bypass** is an alternative method of doing CABG. In recent years, this method has been promoted by some as a way to decrease morbidity associated with the use of cardiopulmonary bypass. This technique of doing bypass grafting on the beating heart while supporting the myocardium with stabilizers has shown a decrease in morbidity by some groups (*J Thorac Cardiovasc Surg* 2003;125:797, *BMJ* 2006;332:1365). However, it is more technically challenging than on-pump techniques, and long-term outcomes were similar in a multicenter, randomized trial comparing on- and off-pump CABG in low-risk patients (*JAMA* 2007;297:701). Patients at high risk (e.g., those with severe atheromatous aortic plaque or renal failure or the elderly) may benefit, especially when done by surgeons experienced with this technique.

V. DISEASE STATES AND THEIR TREATMENT

  A. **Coronary artery disease** is the leading cause of death in adults in North America. Risk factors for CAD include cigarette smoking, hypertension, diabetes mellitus, hyperlipidemia, male gender, obesity, advanced age, rheumatoid arthritis, and a family history of CAD. The clinical presentation of CAD is determined by the distribution of the atherosclerotic lesions, the severity of stenosis, the level of myocardial oxygen demand, and the relative acuity or chronicity of the oxygen supply–demand mismatch. The three most common presentations for patients with CAD are angina pectoris, myocardial infarction (MI), and chronic ischemic cardiomyopathy.

   1. **Angina pectoris** is a symptom complex resulting from reversible myocardial ischemia without cellular necrosis. Patients typically complain of retrosternal chest pain or pressure that often radiates to the left shoulder and down the left arm

or into the neck. Stable angina occurs with reproducible increases in myocardial oxygen demand (e.g., exercise) and resolves with rest or the administration of nitrates. Unstable angina refers to chest pain that occurs at rest or episodes of pain that are increasing in frequency, duration, or severity. Silent myocardial ischemia occurs when there is ECG evidence of myocardial ischemia in the absence of any angina or angina-equivalent symptoms.

2. **Acute MI** results from interruption of myocardial oxygen supply with irreversible muscle injury and cell death. The patient typically presents with protracted and severe chest pain, possibly associated with nausea, diaphoresis, or shortness of breath. There are increases in the troponin isozyme, creatine kinase-MB isozyme, or serum lactate dehydrogenase. ECG changes include ST-segment elevation, T-wave inversions, and the development of new Q waves. Early and late sequelae of acute MI can include atrial or ventricular arrhythmias, heart failure, rupture of the interventricular septum or ventricular free wall, dysfunction or rupture of the papillary muscle(s) and new mitral regurgitation (MR), and the development of a ventricular aneurysm.

a. **Arrhythmias** are common during the first 24 hours after acute MI. In addition to potentially fatal ventricular arrhythmias, patients can develop supraventricular tachycardia, atrial fibrillation, atrial flutter, heart block of any degree, or junctional rhythms.

b. **Congestive heart failure** (CHF) may result when a large portion (usually >25%) of the left ventricular myocardium is infarcted. Cardiogenic shock and death often occur with loss of more than 40% of the left ventricular myocardium. The extent to which the patient's activity is limited can be graded according to the **New York Heart Association (NYHA) classification:** class I, no symptoms; class II, symptoms with heavy exertion; class III, symptoms with mild exertion; class IV, symptoms at rest. There is additional discussion of CHF in Section D.

c. **Rupture of the interventricular septum** occurs in approximately 2% of patients after MI (anterior wall in 60%, inferior wall in 40%) and leads to a **ventricular septal defect (VSD).** Septal perforation typically occurs when the myocardium is at its weakest, approximately 3 to 5 days after an acute MI, but it may develop 2 or more weeks later. An acute VSD is suggested by a new holosystolic murmur and an oxygen step-up from the right atrium to the pulmonary artery, as evaluated with a pulmonary artery catheter. This is determined by comparing the oxygen saturation of samples drawn simultaneously from the central venous port and the distal pulmonary artery port. A step-up of greater than 9% is generally held to be diagnostic of a left-to-right shunt. The diagnosis can be confirmed with echocardiography. More than 75% of patients survive the initial event and are candidates for urgent surgical repair of the VSD before they develop the sequelae of low-output syndrome (i.e., multiorgan system failure), which greatly increases the operative risk. An intra-aortic balloon pump (IABP) is indicated to support the failing circulation until surgical correction is possible. Ventricular free-wall rupture results in hemopericardium and cardiac tamponade, which usually is fatal. For those patients who survive, emergent surgical repair is indicated.

d. **Acute mitral regurgitation** is caused by papillary muscle dysfunction or rupture after an infarction that has extended into the region of the papillary muscles (usually the posteroinferior wall). The failing circulation should be supported with an IABP or percutaneous cardiopulmonary bypass (CPB), if necessary, until emergent operation can be performed.

e. **Ventricular aneurysm,** a well-defined fibrous scar that replaces the normal myocardium, develops in 5% to 10% of individuals after acute MI. The majority of aneurysms develop at the anteroseptal aspect of the left ventricle after infarction in the distribution of the LAD coronary artery. Large dyskinetic left ventricular aneurysms can reduce the left ventricular ejection fraction substantially, resulting in signs and symptoms of congestive heart failure. These scars can also serve as the substrate for ischemic reentrant ventricular arrhythmias.

In addition, the pooled blood that collects in the aneurysm can clot and shower emboli into the peripheral circulation.

3. **Chronic ischemic cardiomyopathy** can develop after several MIs. Diffuse myocardial injury results in diminishing ventricular function and, eventually, signs and symptoms of heart failure. This presentation is most common in patients with diffuse small-vessel disease (e.g., in patients with diabetes mellitus).

4. **Coronary revascularization** may be accomplished via percutaneous transluminal coronary angioplasty (PTCA) or CABG. Indications depend on the patient but generally include intractable symptoms and proximal coronary stenoses that place a significant portion of myocardium at risk.

   a. **PTCA** is often used for focal symmetric stenoses in proximal coronary vessels. It is generally contraindicated if there is significant left main coronary disease, three-vessel disease, or complex obstructive lesions (N Engl J Med 2005;352:2174). PTCA is associated with restenosis, which may be reduced with the concomitant placement of an endoluminal stent. The newer **drug-eluting stents,** which prevent neointimal hyperplasia, have improved outcomes but have not eliminated the problem of need for reintervention (J Am Coll Cardiol 2007;49:616).

   b. **CABG** is indicated for patients with documented atherosclerotic CAD in several settings: (1) patients with unstable angina for whom maximal medical therapy has failed; (2) patients with severe chronic stable angina who have multivessel disease or left main or proximal LAD stenoses; (3) patients with severe, reversible left ventricular dysfunction (documented by stress thallium scan or dobutamine echocardiography); (4) patients who develop coronary occlusive complications during PTCA or other endovascular interventions; (5) patients who develop life-threatening complications after acute MI, including VSD, ventricular free-wall rupture, and acute MR; and (6) patients with diabetes mellitus and multivessel disease (J Am Coll Cardiol 2004;44:1146).

   c. Compared with balloon angioplasty alone, the need for repeat revascularization has dramatically decreased for patients in whom a stent was placed, from 50% of angioplasty patients to approximately 20% of stented patients at 1 year (Lancet 2002;360:965). More recent studies have shown the reintervention rate to be lower, from 5% to 7% depending on the type of stent used (J Am Coll Cardiol 2007;49:616). This decrease has been due to improved delivery systems and the development of drug-eluting stents. For patients with hemodynamic instability or refractory angina after failed angioplasty, IABP support or percutaneous CPB may be helpful before an emergent operation can be performed.

   d. **CABG** results in initial elimination of angina in more than 90% of patients. Perioperative mortality ranges from 1% to 2% in low-risk patients to more than 10% to 15% in high-risk patients. Graft patency after CABG is related to the bypass conduit used and the outflow vessel. In one study, the left internal thoracic artery patency at 5 years was 98%, at 10 years it was 95%, and at 15 years it was 88%. The right internal thoracic artery patency at 5 years was 96%, at 10 years it was 81%, and at 15 years it was 65%. The radial artery patency at 1 year was 96%, and at 4 years it was 89% (Ann Thor Surg 2004;77:93). Reverse saphenous vein grafts have 10-year patency rates of approximately 80% to the LAD and 50% to the circumflex or right coronary artery. Antiplatelet therapy using aspirin (81 to 325 mg/day) beginning immediately after operation and continued indefinitely is recommended to increase the graft patency rate.

B. **Valvular heart disease**

   1. **Aortic valve**

      a. **Aortic stenosis (AS).** Left ventricular outflow obstruction can occur at the subvalvular, the supravalvular, or (most commonly) the valvular level. Aortic valvular stenosis is usually the result of senile degeneration and calcification of a normal or a congenitally bicuspid aortic valve. Less frequently, AS develops many years after an episode of acute rheumatic fever. AS places a pressure overload on the left ventricle. Adequate cardiac output is usually maintained until late in the course of AS, but at the expense of **left ventricular hypertrophy.** Physical signs include a systolic ejection murmur, diminished carotid pulses, and a sustained, forceful, nondisplaced apical impulse. Symptoms often develop when the valve area decreases to 1 cm^2 or less. **Angina pectoris** develops in approximately 65% of patients with severe AS and results from ventricular hypertrophy (e.g., increased myocardial oxygen demand and reduced coronary perfusion) and the high incidence of concomitant CAD. **Syncope** (25% incidence) probably results from fixed cardiac output and decreased cerebral perfusion during systemic vasodilatation. Congestive heart failure is the presenting symptom in approximately one third of patients and usually manifests as dyspnea on exertion. The effect of aortic valve replacement on patients with aortic valve stenosis is dramatic and well documented by several studies. For example, survival was 87% at 3 years in operated and 21% in unoperated patients in one study (*Circulation* 1982;66:1105).

    b. Aortic insufficiency (AI) is usually the result of valve leaflet pathology from rheumatic heart disease (often associated with mitral valve disease) or myxomatous degeneration. AI also may result from other causes of leaflet dysfunction or aortic root dilation, including endocarditis, syphilis, connective tissue diseases (e.g., Marfan syndrome), inflammatory disease (e.g., ankylosing spondylitis), hypertension, and aortic dissection. Chronic AI results in volume overload of the left ventricle, causing chamber enlargement and wall thickening (although a relatively normal ratio of wall thickness to volume is usually maintained). Gradual myocardial decompensation often progresses either without symptoms or with subtle symptoms (e.g., weakness, fatigue, or dyspnea on exertion). Physical signs include a hyperdynamic circulation with markedly increased systemic arterial pulse pressure, known as **Corrigan's water-hammer pulse;** forceful and laterally displaced apical impulse; and a decrescendo diastolic murmur. Acute AI is not well tolerated because of the lack of compensatory chamber enlargement and thus often results in fulminant pulmonary edema, myocardial ischemia, and cardiovascular collapse.

    c. Aortic valve replacement (AVR) is indicated for symptomatic patients with severe AS (defined as valve area <1 cm^2, or mean gradient >40 mm Hg or jet velocity >4 m/second). Surgery is also indicated in asymptomatic patients with severe AS undergoing CABG or other cardiac surgery and in patients with severe AS and left ventricular systolic dysfunction (i.e., ejection fraction <0.50). AVR may also be considered for (1) asymptomatic patients with severe AS and hypotension or symptoms with exercise, (2) patients who have a high likelihood of rapid progression (age, calcification, and coronary artery disease), (3) patients undergoing CABG who have mild to moderate AS with moderate to severe calcification of the valve, and (4) low-risk patients with extremely severe AS (valve area <0.6 cm^2 or gradient >60 mm Hg or jet velocity >5 m/second). Elderly patients (>80 years old) have had acceptable morbidity and mortality rates undergoing AVR, with greater than 50% 5-year survival (*Ann Thorac Surgery* 2007;83(5):1651).

    For symptomatic patients with AI, indications for surgery include (1) severe AI, (2) chronic moderate to severe AI and left ventricular dysfunction (ejection fraction <0.5), and (3) patients with chronic severe AI who are undergoing other cardiac surgery. Patients without symptoms and normal left ventricular function but who have severe left ventricular dilatation (end diastolic dimension >75 mm) are also reasonable candidates.

2. Mitral valve

    a. Mitral stenosis (MS) is caused by rheumatic fever in most cases. Other, less common causes include collagen vascular diseases, amyloidosis, and congenital stenosis. MS places a pressure overload on the left atrium, with relative sparing of ventricular function. Left atrial dilation to more than 45 mm is associated with a high incidence of atrial fibrillation and subsequent thromboembolism. A transvalvular pressure gradient is present when the valve area is greater than 2 cm², and critical MS occurs when the valve area is 1 cm² or less. Physical signs include an apical diastolic murmur, an opening snap, and a loud S_1. Symptoms usually develop late and reflect pulmonary congestion (e.g., dyspnea), reduced left ventricular preload (e.g., low–cardiac-output syndrome), or atrial fibrillation (e.g., thromboembolism).

b. Mitral regurgitation results from abnormalities of the leaflets (e.g., rheumatic disease, myxomatous degeneration, endocarditis), annulus (e.g., calcification, dilation, or destruction), chordae tendineae (e.g., rupture from endocarditis or MI, fusion, or elongation), or ischemic papillary muscle dysfunction or rupture. The most common cause of MR in the United States is myxomatous degeneration. MR places a volume overload on the left ventricle and atrium, causing chamber enlargement and wall thickening, although a relatively normal ratio of wall thickness to volume is usually maintained. Systolic unloading into the compliant left atrium allows enhanced emptying of the left ventricle during systole, with only slight increases in oxygen consumption. Atrial fibrillation often develops because of left atrial dilation. Physical signs include a hyperdynamic circulation and a brisk, laterally displaced apical impulse; a holosystolic murmur; and a widely split S_2. Gradual myocardial decompensation often progresses in the absence of symptoms (e.g., dyspnea on exertion, fatigue). In acute MR, adaptation is not possible, and fulminant cardiac decompensation often ensues.

c. Repair of the mitral valve is preferred over replacement whenever possible. Anticoagulation after surgery for 3 months after repair is reasonable. Surgery is indicated in patients with moderate to severe MS and symptoms or asymptomatic patients with severe pulmonary hypertension if percutaneous mitral balloon valvotomy is unavailable. Repair may be considered for patients with recurrent embolic events in spite of adequate anticoagulation. Surgery is indicated in symptomatic patients with acute severe MR, or chronic severe MR with NYHA class II, III, or IV heart failure. Asymptomatic patients with chronic severe MR and mild to moderate left ventricular dysfunction (ejection fraction 0.3 to 0.6) are also candidates for surgery. MV repair is indicated for asymptomatic patients with chronic severe MR when (1) the likelihood of successful repair is greater than 90% or (2) there is new onset of atrial fibrillation or (3) pulmonary hypertension. Patients with atrial fibrillation and indications for MR repair/replacement should be considered for a Cox-Maze procedure at the time of surgery.

Mitral valve repair or replacement is indicated for patients with symptomatic MR, new-onset atrial fibrillation, or objective evidence of left ventricular dysfunction (same as for AI). Operation is indicated in symptomatic MS or asymptomatic patients with critical MS (valve orifice <1 cm²). With the advent of mitral valve repair, operation is often undertaken earlier if the valvular anatomy suggests that the valve can be repaired rather than replaced.

3. Tricuspid valve

a. Tricuspid insufficiency (TI) most often results from a functional dilation of the valve annulus caused by pulmonary hypertension, which, in turn, may be caused by intrinsic mitral or aortic valve disease. Causes of primary TI include rheumatic heart disease, bacterial endocarditis (usually in intravenous drug users), carcinoid tumors, Ebstein anomaly, and blunt trauma. Patients have a systolic murmur, a prominent jugular venous pulse, and a pulsatile liver. Mild to moderate TI usually is well tolerated.

b. Significant **tricuspid regurgitation** may be repaired at the time of surgery for other cardiac anomalies. Intervention for isolated TI is uncommon. The majority of tricuspid valves can be repaired with simple annuloplasty techniques rather than replacement.

4. Selection of a prosthetic valve must be individualized for each patient. Despite many years of research, there still is no ideal prosthetic valve. The general considerations for selecting an appropriate prosthetic valve are summarized in Table 30-2.

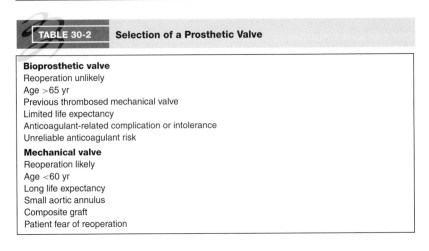

TABLE 30-2 Selection of a Prosthetic Valve

Bioprosthetic valve
Reoperation unlikely
Age >65 yr
Previous thrombosed mechanical valve
Limited life expectancy
Anticoagulant-related complication or intolerance
Unreliable anticoagulant risk

Mechanical valve
Reoperation likely
Age <60 yr
Long life expectancy
Small aortic annulus
Composite graft
Patient fear of reoperation

a. **Bioprostheses** are made from animal tissues, usually the porcine aortic valve or bovine pericardium. Examples include the Carpentier-Edwards, Hancock, St. Jude Biocor, and Edwards Perimount stented valves and the St. Jude Toronto SPV, Sorin, and Medtronic Freestyle stentless valves. These prostheses are associated with a low rate of thromboembolism, even without long-term anticoagulation. However, they are less durable than mechanical valves. Their rate of deterioration depends on the patient's age and is relatively faster in younger patients and slower in the elderly. Overall, the mean time to failure is approximately 10 to 15 years. However, the bioprosthetic material life may be prolonged in newer valves due to modern preservation methods. In general, bioprostheses are the preferred valves for older patients (>65 years) or patients with a contraindication to anticoagulation (e.g., young women who desire future pregnancies).

b. **Mechanical valves** have excellent long-term durability, but the high rate of thromboembolic complications (0.5% to 3% per year) necessitates lifelong anticoagulation. All of these valves are manufactured from **pyrolytic carbon,** which was first discovered in 1966 and has the unique quality of thromboresistance. Examples include the St. Jude, Medtronic Hall, CarboMedics, Starr-Edwards, and Björk-Shiley valves. These valves typically are used in young patients who have a long life expectancy and can tolerate lifelong anticoagulation.

c. **Allograft and autograft valves** are useful for replacement of the aortic valve, particularly in the setting of endocarditis (*J Heart Valve Dis* 1994;3:377). These prostheses have excellent durability and a low incidence of thromboembolism, but experience with them is limited by the supply of allografts and the relative difficulty of the autograft (Ross) procedure, in which a patient's pulmonic valve is used to replace the diseased aortic valve.

5. **Endocarditis.** The main indications for operation include hemodynamic instability, congestive heart failure, recurrent septic emboli, and persistent evidence of infection despite appropriate antibiotic therapy. Relative indications include severe acute mitral or aortic valvular insufficiency, heart block, and intracardiac fistulas. The risk for reoperation for recurrent infective endocarditis is about 17% for intravenous (IV) drug users and 5% for non–IV drug users (*Ann Thorac Surg* 2007;83:30). Antibiotic therapy alone may be sufficient for some late infections, but expeditious valve replacement usually is required.

6. **Perivalvular leak** occurs when the implanted valve separates from the valve annulus. This may lead to clinically significant valvular regurgitation, which can be documented by echocardiography. Hemolytic anemia may be documented by an

increased reticulocyte count, increased serum lactate dehydrogenase level, and increased urinary iron excretion. Replacement of the valve is indicated for perivalvular leak associated with symptoms, moderate to severe valvular regurgitation, or severe hemolysis.

7. **Thrombosis and thromboembolism.** Thrombus formation may occur on the surface of the artificial valve and lead to valve thrombosis or embolism. Embolic complications may include transient ischemic attack, stroke, or embolism to the kidneys or extremities. The use of appropriate anticoagulation with mechanical valves may reduce the risk of thromboembolism to the level (approximately 0.5% per year) associated with bioprosthetic valves (*Chest* 2004;126:457S). The target INR for aortic valves is 2 to 3 and for mitral valves is 3 to 4.

8. **Hypertrophic obstructive cardiomyopathy (HOCM)** is characterized by asymmetric hypertrophy and fibrosis of the myocardium, causing obstruction of the outflow tract. The overall annual death rate of patients with HOCM is about 2% per year. In hypertrophic cardiomyopathy without obstruction of the outflow tract, the annual death rate is about 1% per year. Hypertrophic cardiomyopathy (with or without obstruction) is the most common cause of sudden cardiac death in young people. Medical therapy of β-blockade or calcium channel blockade is preferred. Nifedipine, nitroglycerin, angiotensin-converting enzyme inhibitors, and angiotensin II blockers are all generally contraindicated due to vasodilation properties. Surgical treatment for HOCM is myectomy, with a postoperative mortality of 1% to 3%. By convention, surgery is recommended for patients who are symptomatic with a documented at-rest outflow tract gradient of at least 30 mL/mm Hg. Although long-term follow-up data are lacking, short-term results with success rates greater than 90% have been reported for catheter-based septal alcohol ablation (*Circulation* 2005;112:293).

C. **Atrial fibrillation** affects more than 2.2 million people in the United States, with approximately 160,000 new cases per year. It affects nearly 10% of individuals older than the age of 80 years. Morbidity includes patient discomfort, hemodynamic compromise, and thromboembolism.

1. Nonsurgical management of atrial fibrillation includes antiarrhythmic drugs, cardioversion, and percutaneous transcatheter ablation. Although drugs can induce **chemical cardioversion,** the failure rate is high (60% at 2 years in some series) (*Cardiology* 2001;95:1). When cardioversion fails, the use of chronic anticoagulation for stroke prevention has significant associated morbidity. Because the pulmonary veins have been shown to be the source of ectopic foci in many patients with paroxysmal atrial fibrillation (*Circulation* 1999;100:1879), the use of catheter-based ablation and isolation of the pulmonary veins has gained popularity. Success rates have been improving, with the best centers achieving success rates of greater than 70% in patients with paroxysmal atrial fibrillation (*Circulation* 2005;111:1100). In patients with continuous or permanent atrial fibrillation, results have been worse.

2. Surgical indications for atrial fibrillation include patients who have failed medical therapy and one or more of the following: drug or arrhythmia intolerance, cerebrovascular accident, contraindication to chronic anticoagulation, and concomitant coronary artery or valve disease requiring operation. The **Cox-Maze procedure,** first performed in the late 1980s, was designed to eliminate multiple macroreentrant circuits in the atria that were felt to be responsible for fibrillation. Through a median sternotomy, a series of incisions on both atria, excision of the atrial appendages, and isolation of the pulmonary veins was performed. Long-term results have been outstanding, with a freedom from atrial fibrillation of 97% at a median of 5.4 years and an operative mortality of less than 2% (*J Thorac Cardiovasc Surg* 2003;126:1822). This "cut and sew" procedure is difficult to perform, and consequently only a few groups routinely did the surgery. Recently, less invasive surgical procedures have been developed that have replaced the surgical incisions with linear lines of ablation. These techniques include the use of cryosurgery, radiofrequency or microwave energy, and ultrasound. These new approaches have made the adoption of the procedure feasible for more surgeons

and have had promising early success (*Ann Surg* 2006;244:583). If the entire Cox-Maze lesion set is performed, ablation-assisted procedures with appropriate ablation technology have had identical success rates (*J Thorac Cardiovasc Surg* 2007;133:389).

D. Heart failure. It is estimated that approximately 300,000 people suffer from advanced heart failure in the United States. The management of heart failure involves medical and surgical care and both acute and chronic interventions. The surgical management of heart failure is discussed here.

    1. The **intraaortic balloon pump** is used as the first-line device to provide circulatory support in acute heart failure (*Ann Thorac Surg* 1992;54:11).

        a. Physiology. The principal effect of the IABP is a reduction in left ventricular afterload. This occurs due to deflation of the balloon at the time of the opening of the aortic valve. The resulting effects include improved ventricular ejection and reduction in myocardial oxygen consumption. The IABP inflates during early diastole, increasing diastolic blood pressure (BP) and thus also diastolic coronary artery blood flow.

        b. Indications for the IABP vary in relation to the timing of operation. In the preoperative period, the IABP is indicated for low–cardiac-output states and for unstable angina refractory to medical therapy (e.g., nitrates, heparin, and β-adrenergic blocking agents). Intraoperatively, the IABP is used to permit weaning from CPB when inotropic agents alone are not sufficient. In the postoperative period, the IABP is used primarily for low–cardiac-output states. The IABP can be used to support the circulation during periods of refractory arrhythmias and can also be used to provide support to the patient awaiting cardiac transplantation.

        c. Insertion of the IABP generally is accomplished percutaneously via the common femoral artery. Sheathless devices, because of their narrower diameter, may have decreased the incidence of lower-extremity ischemic complications. Correct placement should be confirmed by chest x-ray. The radiopaque tip of the balloon is positioned just below the aortic knob and just distal to the left subclavian artery. At operation, the IABP may be placed directly into the transverse aortic arch, with the balloon positioned down into the descending aorta. Before **removal of the IABP,** the platelet count, PT, and PTT should be normal. Manual pressure should be applied for 20 to 30 minutes after removal to achieve hemostasis and avoid the formation of a femoral artery pseudoaneurysm or arteriovenous fistula.

        d. Management of the device after placement focuses on ensuring proper diastolic inflation and deflation. The ECG and the femoral (or aortic) pressure waveform are monitored continuously on a bedside console. The device may be triggered using either the ECG or the pressure tracing for every heartbeat (1:1) or less frequently (1:2, 1:3). Anticoagulation during IABP support is optional. If the balloon must be repositioned or removed, the device should be turned off first. IABP support is withdrawn gradually by decreasing the augmentation frequency from 1:1 to 1:3 in steps of several hours each.

        e. Complications of IABP therapy include incorrect placement of the device, resulting in perforation of the aorta; injury to the femoral artery; and reduction in blood flow to the visceral or renal arteries. Ischemia of the lower extremity, evidenced by diminished peripheral pulses or other sequelae, may necessitate removal of the IABP or performance of an inflow arterial bypass procedure (e.g., femoral-to-femoral artery). Rupture of the balloon is an indication for immediate removal because blood may clot within the ruptured balloon, necessitating operative removal.

    2. Ventricular remodeling. The progression of heart failure leads to dilation and structural changes in the ventricle by a process known as remodeling. Initially, these changes are compensatory, but eventually they result in pathologic states—including high wall stress, increased neurohormonal levels, and increased inflammatory mediators—that lead to congestive heart failure.

a. **Partial left ventriculectomy.** There are several techniques described to reduce the diameter of the left ventricle. In most series, after an initial improvement, heart failure parameters returned to their preoperative state. For the most part, these procedures have been abandoned in favor of assist devices and transplantation.

b. **Ischemic cardiomyopathy.** The repair of ischemic left ventricular aneurysms or akinetic infarctions, either by direct excision or patch repair (**Dor proce-dure**), may play a role in end-stage heart failure. Based on the concept that ventricular contraction begins in the apex, the direct exclusion or patch ven-triculoplasty removes both the stagnant blood as well as the low-resistance chamber within the ventricle. The Dor procedure remodels the ventricle from the pathologic spherical shape toward the normal and mechanically more fa-vorable elliptical shape.

3. **Mitral valve surgery** has gained recent popularity for the therapy of congestive heart failure. Mitral regurgitation secondary to ventricular dilatation depends on ventricular geometry and results from mitral annular dilatation and leaflet length-ening, leading to poor leaflet coaptation. The use of a mitral ring annuloplasty has been shown to be safe and effective for improving NYHA class, left ventric-ular ejection fraction, cardiac output, and left ventricular end-diastolic volume (*Eur J Heart Fail* 2000;35:365). In fact, it has been estimated that up to 10% of patients undergoing heart transplant evaluation may benefit from mitral valve repair (*J Heart Valve Dis* 2002;11:S26). However, the long-term results of mi-tral valve repair remain controversial (*J Heart Valve Dis* 2000;9:364). In cases in which papillary muscle dysfunction due to ischemia has changed valvular ge-ometry considerably, mitral valve replacement rather than repair may be more appropriate.

4. **Ventricular assist devices (VADs)** may be used to support the left side of the circulation (LVAD) or the right side of the circulation (RVAD). When both an LVAD and an RVAD are used, the combination is termed a **biventricular assist device (BiVAD).**

a. The **physiologic effect** of a VAD is decompression of the left or right ventricle (or both) and restoration of cardiac output, resulting in decreased myocardial oxygen consumption. The goal is either to permit recovery of myocardium that is not irreversibly injured (e.g., "stunned" myocardium) or to support the circulation in patients with a failing heart until a heart transplantation is possible.

b. **Indications for a VAD** include (1) inability to separate from CPB despite in-otropic and IABP support ("bridge to recovery"), (2) intermediate-term car-diac support ("bridge to transplant"), and (3) permanent replacement therapy ("destination therapy").

c. **VAD subtypes**

(1) **Nonpulsatile devices**

(a) **Centrifugal pumps** (BioMedicus Bio-pump and 3M Sarns Delphin) have been used most frequently as bridges to recovery in patients with postcardiotomy cardiogenic shock. Technologies are available for per-cutaneous support using the femoral vessels (Tandem Heart device) for high-risk interventions or achieving hemodynamic stability in pa-tients with cardiogenic shock (e.g., after myocardial infarction). In the subgroup of patients in whom recovery does not occur, if patients are eligible, they become transplant candidates. Advantages include widespread availability, low cost, and simplicity. Disadvantages include the need for systemic anticoagulation, limited duration of support, and the need for continuous supervision by specially trained personnel.

(b) **ECMO.** See Section IV.B.

(c) **Axial flow pumps** (Jarvik 2000 Flowmaker, MicroMed DeBakey VAD, Thoratec HeartMate II) are small pumps, consume less power, and are completely implantable. These devices are designed for longer-term support (months to years). The devices have an impeller suspended by bearings and provide continuous flow. The speed of the pump and the adequacy of left ventricular preload determine output. All of these pumps have a cable that is externalized from the right lower quadrant of the abdomen that connects to the controller system. These devices are undergoing clinical trials in the United States.

   (2) Pulsatile devices

     (a) External devices (Abiomed BVS 5000, AB Ventricle, and Thoratec Ventricular Assist Device) generally have the same indications as centrifugal pumps, although the duration of support may be somewhat longer. These devices can be used as a bridge to recovery in patients with acute fulminant myocarditis or myocardial infarction. Advantages are that the devices are designed to allow sternal closure (centrifugal pumps require an open chest) and that they may have a lower incidence of thromboembolism and generally support higher flow. A disadvantage is that systemic anticoagulation is still required. Typically these devices are implanted in a preperitoneal pocket.

     (b) Long-term implantable devices (WorldHeart Novacor and Thoratec HeartMate) are used primarily as bridges to transplantation in patients with chronic heart failure. See destination therapy in Section V.D.4.g below.

  d. Insertion of VADs. In general, RVADs receive inflow from the right atrium and return outflow to the pulmonary artery using flexible cannulae or grafts. LVADs receive inflow from the left atrium or ventricle and return outflow to the ascending aorta.

  e. Management of the VAD after placement focuses on maintaining proper function and adequate anticoagulation. The activated clotting time should be monitored frequently and maintained at approximately 200 seconds. Patients should receive medications to ensure adequate sedation, analgesia, and muscle paralysis. Factors that affect **a low-flow-state status post-LVAD** include right ventricular dysfunction, pulmonary hypertension, hypovolemia, and tamponade. It is therefore critical that adequate ventilatory support be provided to correct hypoxemia and acidosis. Pulmonary vasodilators such as NO or inhaled prostacyclin are frequently used to lower pulmonary vascular resistance.

  f. Complications of VAD therapy include excessive bleeding, thrombus formation, embolization, and hemolysis, which are most common with temporary support devices. Associated complications not related to the device specifically include respiratory failure (due to infection or fluid overload) and renal failure. For chronic devices, long-term complications include infections at the drive-line site, thromboembolism, and device failure.

  g. Destination therapy. The recent Randomized Evaluation of Mechanical Assistance for the Treatment of Congestive Heart Failure (REMATCH) trial compared assist devices with best medical therapy and demonstrated a decrease in mortality of 48% at 2 years in 129 patients. The most dramatic increase in survival occurred in those who required inotropic support at randomization (104% at 1 year). In addition, there was a significant quality-of-life improvement (*N Engl J Med* 2001;345:1435). The Thoratec HeartMate XVE Left Ventricular Assist System (LVAS) has been approved for destination therapy by the Food and Drug Administration.

5. Cardiac transplantation can provide relief from symptoms in patients with end-stage cardiomyopathy who are functionally incapacitated despite medical therapy and who are not candidates for any other cardiac operation. The first successful heart transplant occurred in 1967 in South Africa. There were 2,029 heart transplants performed in the United States in 2006, making this intervention an infrequently used but important modality in the management of heart failure. The 1-year survival following heart transplant exceeds 87% (United Network for Organ Sharing database, 2004).

a. **Accepted indications for heart transplant** include cardiomyopathy that is ischemic, idiopathic, postpartum, or chemotherapy induced. These patients are in class III or IV NYHA CHF, have a Heart Failure Survival Score of high risk, and have a peak oxygen consumption of less than 14 mL/kg/minute after reaching an anaerobic threshold. Relative indications include instability in fluid balance or renal function despite best medical therapy, recurrent unstable angina not amenable to revascularization, and intractable ventricular arrhythmias.

b. **Relative contraindications to transplantation** include age older than 65 years, irreversible pulmonary hypertension (>4 Wood units), active infection, recent pulmonary embolus, renal dysfunction (serum creatinine >2.5 mg/dL or creatinine clearance <25 mL/min), hepatic dysfunction (bilirubin >2.5 or alanine aminotransferase/aspartate aminotransferase >2× normal), active or recent malignancy, systemic disease such as amyloidosis, significant carotid or peripheral vascular disease, active or recent peptic ulcer disease, brittle diabetes mellitus, morbid obesity, mental illness, substance abuse, or psychosocial instability.

c. **Donor pool expansion.** Due to the shortage of acceptable donors, the use of an expanded donor pool has been advocated. Some centers have tolerated size mismatch, increased age (>55 years), malignancy, infection, or even donor bypass grafting for carefully selected high-risk recipients.

d. **Immunosuppressive therapy** generally includes a calcineurin inhibitor (cyclosporine or tacrolimus), steroids, and an antimetabolite (mycofenolate or mofetil). Cyclosporine usually is started preoperatively. The dosage is adjusted to achieve circulating plasma levels of 250 to 350 ng/mL. Levels significantly above this range may cause nephrotoxicity. Steroid therapy is initiated in the operating room. When rejection episodes occur, the majority can be reversed with bolus doses of intravenous steroids. When rejection episodes are resistant to increased steroid doses, the monoclonal antibody OKT3 or rabbit antithymocyte serum can be added to the treatment regimen. Immunosuppression is covered in more detail in Chapter 23.

e. **Acute allograft rejection** is diagnosed by **endomyocardial biopsy.** Biopsy forceps are passed into the right ventricle percutaneously, using fluoroscopic or echocardiographic guidance, usually via the right internal jugular or femoral vein, and several biopsies are taken to document the presence and degree of rejection histologically. During the early postoperative period, biopsies are performed several times each month. After the first 6 months, the frequency of biopsies is decreased to one or two times per year. Whenever a patient develops evidence of a rejection episode, a biopsy is performed. Complications of endomyocardial biopsy are rare but include ventricular perforation, pneumothorax, transient ventricular or supraventricular arrhythmias, hematoma, and infection. **Coronary artery vasculopathy (CAV),** thought to represent **chronic vascular rejection,** occurs in a significant percentage of cardiac transplant recipients and is a major limitation on the long-term success of cardiac transplantation. CAV is usually not amenable to conventional revascularization owing to small-vessel, nonfocal disease and often requires retransplantation. Routine echocardiography is also performed frequently to evaluate allograft function.

6. **Future therapy for heart failure**
   a. **Device therapy.** There has been a substantial improvement in devices over the last two decades. They have become smaller, more durable, and less prone to thrombotic complications. Continued advances in this area will likely improve the acceptability of these devices for long-term support (destination therapy).
   b. **Myocyte regeneration.** Several approaches, including those using embryonic stem cells, cardiomyocytes, cryopreserved fetal cardiomyocytes, skeletal myoblasts, bone marrow–derived mesenchymal cells, and dermal fibroblasts, are under investigation.

     c. **Xenotransplantation.** The primary difficulty in xenotransplantation is the management of rejection and cross-species infection, and to date such management has been unsuccessful. The data do not yet justify clinical trials.

VI. POSTOPERATIVE MANAGEMENT. Postoperative care of the cardiac surgery patient is provided in three phases: in the intensive care unit (ICU), in the step-down unit, and after discharge from the hospital.

  A. Intensive care. ICU care resources generally are required for 1 to 3 days after an operation requiring CPB.

    1. Initial assessment. Information on the patient's history, indications for operation, and technical details of the operation (e.g., coronary arteries bypassed, conduits used, CPB time, and aortic cross-clamp time) should be related to the ICU staff by the surgeon. The anesthesiologist should relate information about the intraoperative course, including preoperative and intraoperative hemodynamic parameters (especially cardiac filling pressures) and current medications. A thorough physical examination should be performed, with attention to the cardiovascular system. A chest x-ray and ECG are usually obtained.

    2. Monitoring in the immediate postoperative period is usually extensive. Continuous recordings are made of arterial, central venous, and pulmonary artery pressures; the ECG; and arterial oxygen saturation using pulse oximetry. The pulmonary artery wedge pressure is measured as indicated by the patient's status, and calculations are made of the cardiac output, cardiac index (cardiac output per unit of body-surface area), stroke volume, pulmonary vascular resistance, and systemic vascular resistance (by thermodilution technique). Normal values for these parameters are listed in Table 30-1. Immediate attention is necessary to determine the etiology and to correct deviations from normal values of any of these parameters. **Body temperature** is monitored continuously using a pulmonary artery thermistor. Because early postoperative hypothermia may increase afterload (systemic vascular resistance) and adversely affect blood clotting, hypothermia is treated aggressively (e.g., air-warming blankets). Warming is discontinued when the core temperature reaches 36°C. For patients with persistent fever, a search should be made for active infection.

    3. Cardiovascular. Cardiac pump function is assessed as described earlier. A cardiac index of 2 L/minute/m^2 is generally a minimum acceptable value for an average body habitus. A mixed-venous oxygen saturation of less than 60% suggests inadequate peripheral tissue perfusion and increased peripheral oxygen extraction. Etiologies include reduced oxygen-carrying capacity (e.g., low hematocrit), reduced cardiac output, and increased oxygen consumption (e.g., shivering). Common causes of low cardiac output in the early postoperative period are hypovolemia, increased systemic vascular resistance due to persistent hypothermia or increased circulating catecholamines, and decreased contractility secondary to myocardial stunning.

     a. Preload is increased by administering crystalloid solution (e.g., lactated Ringer's solution) or colloid solution (e.g., 6% hetastarch, 5% albumin) as needed to maintain the pulmonary arterial wedge pressure in the target range, as determined by the patient's diastolic compliance and systolic performance. Using blood products in a judicious manner is mandatory.

     b. Afterload reduction in the volume-restored patient increases ejection fraction and cardiac output and decreases myocardial oxygen consumption. The body temperature should be returned to the normal range, and hypertension should be controlled. In general, the mean arterial BP should be maintained near the preoperative level. For patients with valve replacement or aortic replacement, the systolic BP should be carefully controlled to prevent postoperative bleeding. Afterload is often initially titrated with parenteral infusions of sodium nitroprusside, nitroglycerin, or nicardipine, followed by a change to longer-acting parenteral or enteral agents.

     c. Contractility. Inotropic agents are used only after ensuring an adequate preload and an appropriate afterload. Selection of a particular inotropic agent must be individualized based on the agent's specific effects on the heart rate,

BP, cardiac output, systemic vascular resistance, and renal blood flow. All of these agents increase the work of the heart and increase myocardial oxygen consumption and thus should be used judiciously. **Mechanical support** in the form of an IABP or a VAD can be considered if other measures are ineffective in restoring adequate ventricular ejection.

d. **Rate control.** The heart can be paced using temporary epicardial pacing electrodes (placed at the time of operation) at 80 to 100 beats/minute to increase the cardiac output. Pacing can be performed using only the atrial leads (atrial pacing, or AAI mode), only the ventricular leads (ventricular pacing, or VVI mode), or with both sets of leads (atrioventricular sequential pacing or atrial tracking with ventricular pacing). Optimal pacing always involves maintaining atrioventricular synchrony. VVI pacing should only be used in patients with atrial tachyarrhythmias. If epicardial pacing is not necessary, the epicardial pacemaker generator is set in a backup mode to provide ventricular pacing only in the event of marked bradycardia. The pacemaker output threshold (in milliamperes) should be set to approximately twice the minimum threshold required to capture.

e. **Arrhythmias,** including bradycardia from resolving hypothermia, heart block secondary to persistent cardioplegia effect, and supraventricular tachyarrhythmias (e.g., atrial fibrillation or flutter) can be associated with reduced cardiac output and should be corrected. **Arrhythmias** occur in 40% to 60% of patients after cardiac surgical procedures and are more common in patients who receive inotropic support. Advanced cardiovascular life support guidelines should be followed.

(1) **Supraventricular arrhythmias** (atrial fibrillation, atrial flutter, paroxysmal atrial tachycardia) are most common and are associated with an increased risk of transient or permanent neurologic deficit (*J Card Surg* 2005;20:425). To reduce the incidence of postoperative arrhythmias, patients receiving β-adrenergic blocking agents and/or statins preoperatively should continue to be given these medications postoperatively. Patients with supraventricular arrhythmias and hemodynamic compromise should undergo immediate electrical cardioversion (with 50 to 100 J). Because the most frequent etiology is hypoxia or hypokalemia, the new onset of a supraventricular arrhythmia should be evaluated by measurement of the arterial oxygen saturation and the serum potassium. In many patients with hemodynamically stable arrhythmias, prompt correction of the partial pressure of oxygen (to >70 mm Hg) and the serum potassium level (to >4.5 mg/dL) may terminate the arrhythmia. For patients with **atrial flutter,** overdrive pacing may be used to terminate the arrhythmia. The patient's atrial temporary epicardial pacing wires are connected to a pacemaker generator, and either burst pacing (700 to 800 beats/minute for 3 to 4 seconds) or decremental pacing (stepwise decrease from 10% above the flutter rate to 180 beats/minute) is used.

(2) **Ventricular arrhythmias** in the postoperative period are treated as they are in other patients. Ventricular arrhythmias other than premature ventricular contractions suggest significant underlying ischemic pathology.

f. **Cardiac tamponade** is a potentially lethal cause of low cardiac output early after operation. Clinical features include narrowed pulse pressure, increased jugular venous distention, rising cardiac filling pressures, pulsus paradoxus, widened mediastinal silhouette on chest radiograph, and decreased urine output. Definitive diagnosis is usually made by equalization of diastolic heart pressures or transthoracic or transesophageal echocardiography.

g. **Perioperative MI** occurs in approximately 1% to 2% of patients and can be diagnosed by ECG changes, biochemical criteria (e.g., elevated troponin-I or creatine kinase-MB), or echocardiography. Survival may be adversely affected if complications such as cardiogenic shock or ventricular arrhythmias develop.

h. **Postoperative hemorrhage** is common after cardiac surgery and necessitates reexploration in up to 5% of patients. Hematologic parameters (complete blood count, PT, PTT) are measured on admission to the ICU and as needed. CPB requires heparinization, causes platelet dysfunction and destruction, and activates the fibrinolytic system. Aprotinin, but not aminocaproic or tranexamic acid, has been shown to increase renal dysfunction and has also been associated with increased long-term mortality; therefore its use is discouraged except in very high risk patients (*JAMA* 2007;297:471). Initial focus is on adequate BP control, metabolic stability, maintenance of normothermia, and adequate reversal of heparin with protamine. For patients with significant postoperative bleeding (>200 mL/hour), consideration should be given to platelet transfusion to maintain the platelet count at greater than 100,000/μL and transfusion of fresh-frozen plasma if the INR is abnormal. Although definitive randomized studies have not been conducted, the use of recombinant factor VIIa in patients experiencing life-threatening, unresponsive bleeding has been effective in rare cases and should be considered in this situation (*Ann Thorac Surg* 2007;83:707). Some surgeons advocate stripping the chest tubes every hour to prevent clotting. If clotting becomes apparent, sterile suction tubing can be used to evacuate blood clot. The formation of undrained clot in the mediastinum may result in cardiac tamponade. Indications for operative reexploration for bleeding include (1) prolonged bleeding (>200 mL/hour for 4 to 6 hours), (2) excessive bleeding (>1,000 mL), (3) a sudden increase in bleeding, and (4) cardiac tamponade. Pleural and mediastinal chest tubes generally are removed when the drainage is less than 200 mL in 8 hours.

4. **Pulmonary. Mechanical ventilation** is used in the initial postoperative period with typical settings: intermittent mandatory ventilation, 10 to 16 breaths/minute; inspired oxygen concentration, 1; tidal volume, 10 to 15 mL/kg; and positive end-expiratory pressure, 5 cm H_2O. The patient can be extubated when (1) he or she is fully awake and has had a normal neurologic examination; (2) weaning parameters are satisfactory (e.g., respiratory rate <20 breaths/minute; minute ventilation <12 L/minute; negative inspiratory pressure >20 mm H_2O); (3) the arterial blood gas, with only continuous positive airway pressure, is satisfactory (pH approximately 7.40; CO_2 tension <45 mm Hg; oxygen tension >70 mm Hg); (4) there is little mediastinal bleeding (<100 mL/8 hours); and (5) there is hemodynamic stability. Most patients can be extubated shortly after operation. After extubation, oxygen is administered by high-humidity facemask with an initial inspired oxygen concentration of 0.4. The oxygen can be weaned, as tolerated, to keep the arterial oxygen saturation above 94%.

5. **Renal. Renal dysfunction** in the postoperative period can be due to decreased perfusion pressure during CPB or to inadequate perfusion of the kidneys in the postoperative period. Treatment of acute renal insufficiency in the postoperative period includes ensuring adequate hydration and avoiding nephrotoxic medications. Fluid and electrolyte balance is evaluated immediately after operation and then as needed. Early after operation, intravenous fluids are administered slowly (<30 mL/hour). A useful measure of a patient's intravascular volume status is the body weight, which is measured daily and compared to the preoperative weight. Serum potassium levels are maintained at greater than 4.5 mg/dL to prevent atrial and ventricular arrhythmias, and concomitant repletion of magnesium is warranted (to >2 mg/dL). Metabolic acidosis can reflect a low–cardiac-output state.

6. **Neurologic. Neurological examination** of the patient is performed on admission to the ICU and periodically as needed. Changes in the neurologic examination warrant immediate investigation. Shivering increases oxygen consumption and should be treated in the early postoperative period by warming the patient or by the administration of meperidine (50 to 100 mg intramuscularly or intravenously every 3 hours) or, for the ventilated patient, pancuronium (0.04 to 0.10 mg/kg intravenously) or vecuronium (0.08 to 0.10 mg/kg slow intravenous bolus, then 1 to 5 mg/hour intravenous continuous infusion). **Pain control** is accomplished using parenteral narcotics or nonsteroidal anti-inflammatory agents, or both, during the early postoperative period.

7. **Nutrition.** The patient is given nothing by mouth until after extubation. A clear liquid diet then is begun and is advanced to a regular diet as tolerated. Patients with prolonged ventilation should receive either enteral feedings or parenteral nutrition.

8. **Infection.** Infectious complications are uncommon after cardiac surgical procedures but may lead to substantial morbidity and mortality. Perioperative antibiotics should be started prior to surgery and administered for 24 hours because use of second-generation cephalosporins has been associated with a fivefold decrease in wound infection rates (*J Thorac Cardiovasc Surg* 1992;104:590). **Wound infection** occurs in 1% to 2% of sternotomy incisions and a higher proportion of saphenous vein harvest sites. Risk factors for deep sternal wound infection include diabetes mellitus, male gender, and, possibly, the use of bilateral internal thoracic arteries during CABG procedures in patients older than 74 years (*Ann Thorac Surg* 1998;65:1050). Serous drainage from the skin incision is worrisome and should be treated by application of a sterile dressing twice daily and the administration of intravenous antibiotics. Purulent wound drainage, a sternal click, gross movement of the sternal edges, or substernal air on the chest x-ray may indicate a deep sternal infection. A computed tomography scan of the chest can confirm this diagnosis. In general, deep sternal infections require operative débridement of devitalized sternal and substernal tissues, with cultures of the tissue; administration of broad-spectrum intravenous antibiotics; and vascularized muscle flap closure of the soft-tissue defect.

9. **Gastrointestinal. Gastrointestinal (GI) complications** are uncommon after cardiac surgical procedures. Stress gastritis can occur after CPB and is thought to be secondary to subclinical ischemia of the gut mucosa. Although overt GI hemorrhage is uncommon, when it does occur, it is associated with a high mortality. Patients should receive proton-pump inhibitor or H_2-receptor–antagonist therapy until a regular diet is begun. GI bleeding may arise from throughout the GI tract. Acute cholecystitis, usually acalculous, is associated with high mortality.

B. **Step-down unit.** Step-down unit care focuses on convalescence, management of fluid balance, activity level, and diet.

1. **Fluid status.** The patient is weighed daily. Patients receiving diuretics preoperatively resume the same regimen postoperatively. For patients who were not receiving diuretics preoperatively, oral diuretics are administered until the patient's weight falls to the preoperative value. For most patients, no restrictions are placed on the daily oral fluid intake.

2. **Activity.** The patient is encouraged to be out of bed to a chair and to ambulate as early as possible after operation. Patients are instructed not to perform any heavy lifting (>10 lb) for a period of 6 weeks postoperatively.

3. **Diet.** A mild postoperative ileus may be present for several days after operation. A regular diet is begun as early as possible after operation. Some patients require a stool softener. Attention should be paid to maintaining a prudent diet that is low in salt and cholesterol.

C. **Postdischarge care.** Care after hospital discharge focuses on continued risk factor modification and surveillance for late complications. Common difficulties during the first 6 to 8 weeks after operation include decreased motivation, decreased appetite, depression, and insomnia. In general, these conditions are temporary, and the physician can provide reassurance.

1. **Physical rehabilitation** with a daily exercise program begins early after operation and continues after discharge from the hospital. Vigorous walking, with increasing distances and longer periods of activity, is the most useful form of exercise for most patients. Bicycling and swimming are acceptable alternatives after 6 to 8 weeks. Patients who were working before operation should return to work within 2 months after operation.

2. **Risk factor modification** may slow or possibly reverse the progression of atherosclerosis in bypass grafts after CABG.

   a. **Smoking** should be discontinued. Referral to organizations with smoking cessation programs should be made before operation, if possible.

   b. Obesity. Patients should reach an ideal body weight through planned exercise
   and dieting.
   c. Hyperlipidemia is a major risk factor for the development of graft atherosclerosis and should be treated aggressively, with diet modification and treatment
   with statins.
   d. Hypertension must be controlled.
   e. Postpericardiotomy (Dressler) syndrome is a delayed pericardial inflammatory reaction characterized by fever, anterior chest pain, and pericardial
   friction rub, and it may lead to mediastinal fibrosis and premature graft occlusion. Treatment includes nonsteroidal anti-inflammatory drugs for 2 to
   4 weeks or corticosteroids for refractory cases.

31

GENERAL THORACIC SURGERY
Felix G. Fernandez and Richard J. Battafarano

$\mathcal{T}$horacic surgery encompasses the management of both benign and malignant conditions of the esophagus, lung, pleura, and mediastinum. In this chapter, we focus on the systematic evaluation and treatment of the most common conditions. Disease processes of the esophagus are discussed in Chapter 8.

I. LUNG CANCER. Cancer of the lung remains the leading cause of cancer death in the United States. Approximately 173,000 cases of lung cancer were diagnosed in 2005, and more than 164,000 people died from this disease. Most newly diagnosed cases are not amenable to surgical resection and have poor prognosis. Lung cancer carries an overall 15% 5-year survival. **Cigarette smoking** remains the leading risk factor and influences risk stratification in the evaluation of a suspicious lesion. Increasing **age** also increases the probability of malignancy. Although trials conducted more than two decades ago to screen for lung cancer by either sputum cytology or chest x-ray imaging failed to show benefit, annual spiral computed tomography (CT) scanning can detect lung cancers that are curable (*N Engl J Med* 2006;355:1822). However, questions remain as to whether the test is sufficiently effective to justify screening people at high risk for lung cancer.

A. Radiographic presentation

1. **Solitary pulmonary nodule (SPN).** Due to the widespread application of CT technology, an estimated 150,000 SPNs are diagnosed each year. By definition, these are circumscribed lung lesions in an asymptomatic individual. Lesions greater than 3 cm are called **masses**.

2. **Radiographic imaging by CT** is used to both follow these lesions and predict outcome. The first step in the evaluation of an SPN is to evaluate any prior films. **Factors favoring a benign lesion** include absence of growth over a 2-year period, size of the lesion, and pattern of calcification. Calcifications that are diffuse, centrally located, "onion skinned" (laminar), or popcornlike are generally benign. Eccentric or stippled calcifications may indicate malignancy. Lesion greater than 2 cm, intravenous contrast enhancement, or irregular borders **predict malignancy.**

3. **Positron emission tomography (PET) scanning** has demonstrated 95% sensitivity and 80% specificity in characterizing solitary pulmonary nodules. PET imaging has a high negative predictive value for most lung cancers; however, bronchoalveolar carcinoma and carcinoid tumor can be negative by PET scan, and inflammatory and infectious processes can be falsely positive. The patient's overall risk factor profile must be considered. In the setting of low risk (e.g., young age, nonsmoker, favorable features on CT), a negative PET scan has a high negative predictive value, but the same result in an elderly smoker is less reassuring, and further evaluation is warranted.

4. **Tissue biopsy** remains the gold standard for diagnosis. Tissue may be obtained by bronchoscopy in patients with central lung lesions or by CT-guided biopsy. This latter technique has an 80% sensitivity for a malignant process and requires technical expertise. Surgical biopsy of SPN by either minimally invasive techniques or open technique can provide a definitive diagnosis and definitive treatment.

B. Pathology

The **two main classes** of lung tumors are small-cell (oat cell) carcinoma and non–small-cell carcinoma.

1. **Small-cell carcinoma** accounts for approximately 20% of all lung cancers. It is highly malignant, usually occurs centrally near the hilum, occurs almost exclusively in smokers, and rarely is amenable to surgery because of wide dissemination by the time of diagnosis. These cancers initially respond to chemotherapy, but overall 5-year survival remains 10%.

2. **Non–small-cell carcinomas** account for 80% of all lung cancers and make up the vast majority of those treated by surgery. The three subtypes are **adenocarcinoma** (30% to 50% of cases), **squamous cell** (20% to 35%), and **large cell** (4% to 15%). Most tumors are histologically heterogeneous, possibly indicating common origin. **Bronchioloalveolar carcinoma** is a variant of adenocarcinoma and is known for its ability to produce mucin and its multifocal nature. Over the last decade, it has been appreciated that carcinoid tumors (grade I), atypical carcinoid tumors (grade II), large-cell carcinoma, and small-cell tumors represent important subgroups of bronchogenic neuroendocrine carcinoma. This may explain the more aggressive behavior of large-cell carcinoma relative to other non–small-cell cancers.

C. Symptomatic presentation of lung cancer implies a worsening stage and is associated with an overall lower rate of survival.

1. **Bronchopulmonary features** include cough or a change in a previously stable smoker's cough, increased sputum production, dyspnea, and new wheezing. Minor hemoptysis causing blood-tinged sputum, even as an isolated episode, should be investigated with flexible bronchoscopy, especially in patients with a history of smoking who are 40 years of age or older. Lung cancer may also present with postobstructive pneumonia.

2. **Extrapulmonary thoracic symptoms** include chest wall pain secondary to local tumor invasion, hoarseness from invasion of the left recurrent laryngeal nerve near the aorta and left main pulmonary artery, shortness of breath secondary to malignant pleural effusion, and superior vena cava syndrome causing facial, neck, and upper-extremity swelling. Pancoast tumor (superior sulcus tumor) can lead to brachial plexus invasion, as well as invasion of the cervical sympathetic ganglia, which causes an ipsilateral Horner syndrome (ptosis, miosis, and anhidrosis). Rarely, lung cancer can present as dysphagia secondary to compression or invasion of the esophagus by mediastinal nodes or by the primary tumor.

   The most frequent **sites of distant metastases** include the liver, bone, brain, adrenal glands, and the contralateral lung. Symptoms may include pathologic fractures and arthritis from bony involvement. Brain metastasis may cause headache, vision changes, or changes in mental status. Adrenal involvement infrequently presents with Addison disease. Lung cancer is the most common tumor causing adrenal dysfunction.

3. **Paraneoplastic syndromes** are frequent and occur secondary to the release of hormonelike substances by tumor cells. They include Cushing syndrome (adrenocorticotropic hormone secretion in small-cell carcinoma), syndrome of inappropriate antidiuretic hormone (SIADH), hypercalcemia (parathyroid hormone–related protein secreted by squamous cell carcinomas), hypertrophic pulmonary osteoarthropathy (clubbing of the fingers, stiffness of joints, and periosteal thickening on x-ray), and various myopathies.

D. Accurate clinical and pathologic staging is critical in the management of patients with non–small-cell carcinoma because surgery is the primary mode of therapy for all stage I and II patients and selected stage IIIa patients who have enough physiologic reserve to tolerate resection. It is critical to exclude metastatic disease prior to resection. The essential elements of staging include evaluation for lymph node involvement and evaluation for adrenal, brain, and bone metastasis. An anatomic staging system using the classification for tumor, nodal, and metastatic status was most recently modified in 1997 (Table 31-1).

TABLE 31-1	American Joint Committee on Cancer Staging System of Lung Cancer

Tumor status (T)

T1	<3 cm without invasion of visceral pleura proximal to lobar bronchus
T2	>3 cm or any size with associated atelectasis or obstructive pneumonitis that does not involve the entire lung; may invade visceral pleura; proximal extent must be >2 cm from carina
T3	Any size with direct extension into chest wall, diaphragm, mediastinal pleura, or pericardium without involvement of great vessels or vital mediastinal structures; cannot involve carina; atelectasis or obstructive pneumonitis of the entire lung
T4	Any size with invasion of heart or mediastinal vital structures or carina, malignant pleural effusion, satellite lesions

Nodal involvement (N)

N0	None
N1	Peribronchial or ipsilateral hilar lymph nodes
N2	Ipsilateral mediastinal lymph nodes, including subcarinal
N3	Contralateral mediastinal or hilar lymph nodes, ipsilateral or contralateral scalene or supraclavicular lymph nodes

Distant metastases (M)

M0	None
M1	Distant metastases present

STAGE	
Ia	T1 N0 M0
Ib	T2 N0 M0
IIa	T1 N1 M0
IIb	T2 N1 M0; T3 N0 M0
IIIa	T3 N1 M0; T1,2,3 N2 M0
IIIb	Any T N3 M0; T4, any N, M0
IV	Any T, any N, M1

Reprinted with permission from Fleming ID, Cooper JS, Henson DE, et al., eds. *AJCC Cancer Staging Manual,* 5th ed. Philadelphia: Lippincott Williams & Wilkins; 1998.

1. **Chest CT to include the upper abdomen** provides useful information on location, size, and local involvement of tumor and also allows evaluation for liver and adrenal metastasis. CT scanning alone does not accurately determine the resectability of tumor adherent to vital structures. Patients with localized disease may require intraoperative staging to determine resectability. CT also can identify mediastinal lymphadenopathy. However, the sensitivity for identifying metastatic lymph nodes by CT is only 65% to 80% and the specificity is only 65%. With nodes larger than 1 cm, the sensitivity decreases but the specificity increases.

2. **PET imaging** is often used in the staging of patients with non–small-cell carcinoma, but its accuracy for detecting primary tumors and metastatic disease may be limited by the presence of inflammation and ongoing infection. In regions endemic for inflammatory processes such as histoplasmosis, the usefulness of PET imaging for investigating mediastinal lymph nodes is limited. However, it can be useful for identifying occult distant metastatic disease to the liver, adrenals, and bone.

3. **Mediastinoscopy** is the most accurate method for staging mediastinal lymph nodes, and it provides access to the pretracheal, subcarinal, and paratracheal node stations. Although invasive, it is safe, with less than a 1% complication rate. We favor the routine use of this technique in the staging of patients with non–small-cell carcinoma, with the exception of patients with clinical stage I lung cancer staged by CT and PET, who benefit little from mediastinoscopy (*J Thorac*

Cardiovasc Surg 2006;131:822). The timing of mediastinoscopy, whether at the time of thoracotomy or before a planned resection, is controversial and depends on the surgeon's preference and the availability of expert pathologic evaluation of mediastinal lymph node frozen sections.

4. **CT or magnetic resonance (MR) imaging of the brain** to identify brain metastases is mandatory in the patient with neurologic symptoms but is controversial as a routine part of the workup of symptomatic patients. Given the reported, albeit low, incidence of CNS metastasis in the setting of even small primary tumors, we advocate the routine use of brain imaging.

5. **Bone scan** is obtained in all patients with specific symptoms of skeletal pain and selectively as part of the preoperative metastatic workup. The routine use of PET imaging in many centers has eliminated the need for this modality.

6. **Fiberoptic bronchoscopy** is important in diagnosing and assessing the extent of the endobronchial lesion. Although peripheral cancers rarely can be seen with bronchoscopy, preoperative bronchoscopy is important for excluding synchronous lung cancers (found in approximately 1% of patients) prior to resection. Bronchial washings with culture can be taken at the time of bronchoscopy in patients with significant secretions.

E. **Preoperative assessment of pulmonary** function and estimation of postoperative pulmonary assessment is the most critical factor in planning lung resection for cancer.

1. **Pulmonary function tests** and **arterial blood gas analysis** are the standard by which the risk of developing postoperative pulmonary failure is determined. In general, pulmonary resection can be tolerated if the preoperative FEV_1 (forced expiratory volume in 1 second) is greater than 60% of predicted. If the FEV_1 is less than 60% of predicted, measurement of **diffusion capacity, quantitative ventilation-perfusion scan, and exercise testing** are indicated. These tests allow the surgeon to determine how much of the area of resection contributes to the overall pulmonary function. In general, an **estimated postresection FEV_1** of 800 cc or greater suggests that the patient will tolerate a pneumonectomy. Preoperative hypercapnia (arterial carbon dioxide tension >45 mm Hg) precludes resection.

2. **Evaluation of cardiac disease** is critical for minimizing perioperative complications. Patients with lung cancer are often at high risk for coronary disease because of extensive smoking histories. A detailed history and physical examination to elicit signs and symptoms of ischemia and a baseline electrocardiogram (ECG) are the initial steps. Any abnormal findings should be aggressively pursued with stress tests or coronary catheterization.

3. **Smoking cessation** preoperatively for as little as 2 weeks can aid in the regeneration of the mucociliary function and pulmonary toilet and has been associated with fewer postoperative respiratory complications.

F. In summary, all patients should have a posteroanterior and lateral chest x-ray and a chest CT scan to evaluate the primary tumor and the mediastinum and to check for metastatic disease to the brain and adrenals. PET imaging or bone scan is required to exclude bone metastasis. Cervical mediastinoscopy with biopsy of the lymph nodes in the paratracheal and subcarinal space should be performed to exclude mediastinal lymph node metastasis prior to resection, except possibly in patients with clinical stage I disease. All patients should undergo a fiberoptic bronchoscopy by the surgeon before thoracotomy; this is usually done at the same setting as mediastinoscopy.

G. **Operative principles.** In the patient able to tolerate resection, the minimal extent of resection should be an anatomic lobectomy. Even in stage I disease, a more limited resection, such as a wedge resection, results in a threefold higher incidence of local recurrence and a decreased overall and disease-free survival. Patients with limited pulmonary reserve may be treated by segmental or wedge resection. Most centers report operative mortality of 2% to 3% with lobectomy and of 6% to 8% with pneumonectomy. Minimally invasive techniques for anatomic resection are in clinical trial.

H. Five-year survival rates are 67% for stage Ia (T1N0) disease and 57% for stage Ib (T2N0) disease. Stage I disease is generally treated with surgical resection alone. The presence of ipsilateral intrapulmonary lymph nodes decreases the overall survival to 55% for stage IIa (T1N1) disease and 39% for stage IIb (T2N1) disease. Stage II cancers are also treated with surgical resection. However, adjuvant chemotherapy has been associated with improved 5-year survival and is now routinely recommended in patients with stage II or stage III disease. Adjuvant radiation therapy is considered in patients with close surgical margins or central N1 lymph node metastasis.

Certain patients with stage IIIa disease appear to benefit form surgical resection alone (T3N1M0). However, selected patients with mediastinal lymph node metastasis (N2 disease) may be candidates for surgical resection after neoadjuvant chemoradiation therapy. Patients with bulky, diffuse mediastinal lymphadenopathy are often treated using definitive chemoradiation. The optimal regimen of chemotherapy, radiation, or a combination of both is being investigated in clinical trials. Stage IIIb tumors involve the contralateral mediastinal or hilar lymph nodes, the ipsilateral scalene or supraclavicular lymph nodes, extensive mediastinal invasion, intrapulmonary metastasis, or malignant pleural effusions. These tumors are considered unresectable. Stage IV tumors have distant metastases and are also considered unresectable. However, selected patients with node-negative lung cancer and a solitary brain metastasis have achieved long-term survival with combined resection.

II. TUMORS OF THE PLEURA. The most common tumor of the pleura is the rare but deadly **mesothelioma.** Less common tumors include lipomas, angiomas, soft-tissue sarcomas, and fibrous histiocytomas.

A. Asbestos exposure is associated with mesothelioma 70% of the time. Mesotheliomas arise from mesothelial cells but differentiate into a variety of histologic patterns. It is often difficult to differentiate mesothelioma from other tumors without the benefit of special stains or immunohistochemistry.

B. Epidemiologically, mesothelioma is primarily a disease of men in the fifth through seventh decades of life. Patients may have been exposed to asbestos decades before (latency >30 years). Patient presentation may be variable. Although benign mesothelioma variants are not associated with asbestos exposure and are asymptomatic, patients with the more common malignant form often report chest pain, malaise, cough, weakness, weight loss, and shortness of breath with pleural effusion. One third of patients report paraneoplastic symptoms of osteoarthropathy, hypoglycemia, and fever.

C. CT scan is useful in differentiating pleural from parenchymal disease. Malignant mesothelioma usually appears as a markedly thickened, irregular, pleural-based mass or nodular pleura with a pleural effusion. Occasionally, only a pleural effusion is seen. Routine use of MR imaging has not been shown to have significant advantages over use of CT. However, it has been useful for identifying transdiaphragmatic extension of tumor into the abdomen.

D. Diagnosis based purely on cytology of thoracentesis sample is difficult. Thoracoscopic or open pleural biopsy is usually necessary to confirm the diagnosis.

E. Classification is based on histologic evaluation: Epithelial, sarcomatous, and mixed forms have been identified.

F. Median survival in untreated patients with malignant mesothelioma is 4 to 12 months. Patients with mixed or sarcomatous mesothelioma have a poor prognosis and do not appear to benefit from surgical resection. Current aggressive multimodality therapy consists of pleurectomy and decortication or extrapleural pneumonectomy to decrease tumor mass, followed by chemotherapy and radiotherapy. Adjuvant therapy is not beneficial in the setting of incomplete resection. However, patients with epithelial histology, no evidence of lymph node metastasis, and complete resection appear to benefit from an aggressive combined modality approach. The most encouraging studies report a 5-year survival of 39%.

III. TUMORS OF THE MEDIASTINUM. The location of a mass in relation to the heart helps the surgeon to form a differential diagnosis (Table 31-2). On the lateral chest x-ray, the mediastinum is divided into thirds, with the heart comprising the middle segment.

TABLE 31-2	Differential Diagnosis of Tumors Located in the Mediastinum	
Anterior	**Middle**	**Posterior**
Thymoma	Congenital cyst	Neurogenic
Germ cell	Lymphoma	Lymphoma
Teratoma	Primary cardiac	Mesenchymal
Seminoma	Neural crest	
Nonseminoma		
Lymphoma		
Parathyroid		
Lipoma		
Fibroma		
Lymphangioma		
Aberrant thyroid		

Modified from Young RM, Kernstine KH, Corson JD. Miscellaneous cardiopulmonary conditions. In: Corson JD, Williamson RCN, eds. *Surgery.* Philadelphia: Mosby; 2001.

A. **Epidemiology.** In the totality of all age groups, lymphoma is the most common mediastinal tumor. Neurogenic tumors are more likely in children. The likelihood of malignancy is greatest in the second to fourth decades of life. The presence of symptoms is more suggestive of a malignant lesion. Symptoms are often nonspecific and include dyspnea, cough, hoarseness, vague chest pain, and fever.

B. **Evaluation.** Chest x-ray is often used as a screening tool and can lead to the diagnosis of a mass. This should be followed by a CT scan to further delineate the anatomy.

C. **Tumors.** Due to the prevalence of germ cell tumors, all anterior mediastinal masses should be evaluated with biochemical markers β-human chorionic gonadotropin (β-HCG) and α-fetoprotein (AFP).

  1. Teratomas are usually benign and often contain ectodermal components such as hair, teeth, and bone. Elevation of both β-HCG and AFP suggests a malignant teratoma. Treatment is surgical resection.

  2. Seminomas do not present with an elevation in AFP, and fewer than 10% present with an elevation in β-HCG. Their treatment is primarily nonsurgical (radiation and chemotherapy), except in the case of localized disease.

  3. Nonseminomatous germ cell tumors present with an elevation of both tumor markers. Again, the treatment is primarily nonsurgical, with the exception of obtaining tissue for diagnosis.

  4. Tissue diagnosis is often crucial for the diagnosis and treatment of **lymphoma.** Treatment is primarily nonsurgical. Cervical lymph node biopsy, CT-guided biopsy, or mediastinoscopy with biopsy may be required. These lesions often present as irregular masses on CT scan.

  5. Patients with paravertebral or posterior mediastinal masses should have their catecholamine levels measured to rule out **pheochromocytomas.**

IV. THYMECTOMY/THYMOMA

A. The role of the **thymus gland in myasthenia gravis** is poorly understood. However, it appears to be important in the generation of autoreactive antibodies directed against the acetylcholine receptor. Anti–acetylcholine-receptor antibodies may be used to evaluate for myasthenia gravis. Greater than 80% of cases demonstrate complete or partial response to thymectomy. Chances of improvement are increased if thymectomy is performed early in the course of disease (first signs of muscle weakness) and if the myasthenia is not associated with a thymoma.

B. A **thymoma** is a focal mass in the thymus gland composed primarily of thymic epithelial cells. Most are benign, but the presence of invasion of its fibrous capsule defines malignancy. Whereas 15% of myasthenia gravis patients have a thymoma, approximately 50% of patients with a thymoma have paraneoplastic syndromes, including myasthenia gravis, hypogammaglobulinemia, and red cell aplasia.

C. Preoperative preparation of the patient with myasthenia gravis involves reduction of corticosteroid dose, if appropriate, and the weaning of anticholinesterases. Plasmapheresis can be performed preoperatively to aid in discontinuation of anticholinesterase agents. Muscle relaxants and atropine should be avoided during anesthetic induction.

D. The **operative approach** for thymectomy for myasthenia in cases in which noninvasive imaging **does not indicate the presence of a thymoma** or a mass lesion is controversial. The options range from median sternotomy to a transcervical thymectomy. The **transcervical approach** involves a low collar incision and is facilitated by using a table-mounted retractor to elevate the manubrium and expose the thymic tissue for resection. The transcervical approach has lower morbidity, but there are questions as to whether it is as efficacious as the transsternal approach.

E. In instances of bulky thymic disease, a median sternotomy approach is preferred to **provide maximal exposure for complete resection.**

V. PNEUMOTHORAX

A. Pneumothorax is the presence of air in the pleural cavity, leading to separation of the visceral and parietal pleura. This disruption of the potential space disrupts pulmonary mechanics, and, if left untreated, it may progress to tension physiology. In tension pneumothorax, cardiac compromise occurs and presents a true emergency. The etiology may be spontaneous, iatrogenic, or due to trauma. The etiology will determine the most appropriate short- and long-term management strategies.

B. Physical examination may demonstrate decreased breath sounds on the involved side if the lung is more than 25% collapsed. Hyperresonance on the affected side is possible. Common symptoms include dyspnea and chest pain. Careful examination for signs of tension pneumothorax (including deviation of the trachea to the opposite side, respiratory distress, and hypotension) must be performed. If there is no clinical evidence of tension pneumothorax, an upright chest x-ray will be required to establish the diagnosis. Smaller pneumothoraces may only be evident on expiration chest x-rays or CT scan. The clinical setting will influence their management.

C. Management options include observation, aspiration, chest tube placement with or without pleurodesis, and surgery. The etiology of the pneumothorax influences management strategy.

1. Observation is an option in a healthy, asymptomatic patient. This should be reserved for small pneumothoraces, unlikely to recur, because failure to fully resolve may lead to fibrous entrapment of the lung. Supplemental oxygen may help to reabsorb the pneumothorax by affecting the gradient of nitrogen in the body and in the pneumothorax.

2. Aspiration of the pneumothorax may be done using a small catheter attached to a three-way stopcock. This should be reserved for situations with low suspicion of an ongoing air leak.

3. Percutaneous catheters may be placed using Seldinger technique. Multiple commercial kits exist and allow for the catheter to be placed to a Heimlich valve or to suction. The catheters in these kits are generally of small caliber, and their use is limited to situations of simple pneumothorax.

4. Tube thoracostomy remains the gold standard, especially for larger pneumothoraces, for persistent air leaks, when there is an expected need for pleurodesis, or for associated effusion.

a. Chest tubes may be connected either to a **Heimlich flutter valve,** to a **simple underwater-seal system,** or to **vacuum suction.** The two most commonly used systems are the Pleurovac and Emerson systems. Both systems may be placed to a water seal (providing –3-cm to –5-cm H_2O suction) or to vacuum suction (typically –20 cm).

b. If the water-seal chamber bubbles with expiration or with coughing, this is evidence that an air leak persists. Newer Pleurovac systems allow as much as –40-cm H_2O suction to be applied to the pleural space.

5. **Bedside pleurodesis.** Sclerosing agents may be administered through the chest tube to induce fusion of the parietal and visceral pleural surfaces. Doxycycline, bleomycin, and talc have all been described.

   a. Bedside pleurodesis **can be associated with an inflammatory pneumonitis** in the lung on the treated side. In patients with limited pulmonary reserve, this may present as clinically significant hypoxia. Pleurodesis can be quite uncomfortable for the patient, and adequate analgesia is mandatory. Patient-controlled analgesic pump and bolus administration of ketorolac (if tolerated) are effective.

   b. **Doxycycline** is used as the sclerosing agent for benign processes.

      (1) It is administered as 500 mg in 100 mL of normal saline. Doxycycline is extremely irritating to the pleural surfaces; therefore, 30 mL of 1% lidocaine can be administered via the chest tube before the doxycycline is given and used to flush the drug again. The total dose of lidocaine should not exceed the toxic dose, which is usually 5 mg/kg.

      (2) In patients with large air leaks, the chest tube should not be clamped, to prevent the development of a tension pneumothorax. Instead, the drainage bottle or suction device should be elevated to maintain the effective water-seal pressure at –20 cm H_2O.

      (3) The patient (with assistance) is instructed to roll from supine to right lateral decubitus to left lateral decubitus every 15 minutes for 2 hours. Prone, Trendelenburg, and reverse Trendelenburg positions should also be part of the sequence if the patient is able to tolerate it.

      (4) The chest tube may be unclamped (if done for the procedure) and returned to suction after the procedure.

   c. **Talc** is a less painful sclerosing agent. Due to concern about introducing a potentially carcinogenic agent and permanent foreign body, it is generally limited to patients with underlying malignant conditions (see Effusions, Section VII.A.4.a).

      (1) Talc, 5 g in 180 mL of sterile saline split into 360-mL catheter syringes, is administered via the chest tube and then flushed with an additional 60 mL of saline.

      (2) The patient is instructed to change positions as described previously.

6. **Surgery** is performed using a video-assisted approach or by thoracotomy. Patients who have a persistent air leak secondary to a ruptured bleb but are otherwise well should be considered for surgery. By this point, patients have already undergone stabilization by chest tube placement (see Section V.D.3 for specific indications for surgery).

D. **Etiology**

1. **Iatrogenic** pneumothoraces usually are the result of pleural injury during central venous access attempts, pacemaker placement, or transthoracic or transbronchial lung biopsy. A postprocedure chest x-ray is mandatory. Often the injury to the lung is small and self-limited. The extent of pneumothorax and associated injury should determine the need for invasive procedures. Observation or percutaneous placement of a chest tube may be appropriate in a patient who is not mechanically ventilated.

2. **Spontaneous** pneumothorax is nearly always caused by rupture of an apical bleb. Up to 80% of patients are tall, young adults, and men outnumber women by 6 to 1; it is more common in smokers than in nonsmokers. The typical patient presents with acute onset of shortness of breath and chest pain on the side of the collapsed lung. Patients older than 40 years usually have significant parenchymal disease, such as emphysema. These patients present with a ruptured bulla and often have a more dramatic presentation, including tachypnea, cyanosis, and hypoxia. There is a significant risk of recurrence, and pleurodesis or surgical intervention may be indicated even after the first occurrence. Other etiologies of spontaneous pneumothorax include cystic fibrosis and, rarely, lung cancer.

3. **Indications for operation** for spontaneous pneumothorax include (1) recurrent ipsilateral pneumothoraces, (2) bilateral pneumothoraces, (3) persistent air leaks

on chest tube suction (usually >5 days), and (4) first episodes occurring in patients with high-risk occupations (e.g., pilots, divers) or those who live a great distance from medical care facilities. The risk of ipsilateral recurrence of a spontaneous pneumothorax is 50%, 62%, and 80% after the first, second, and third episodes, respectively. Some authors recommend chemical pleurodesis as the minimal therapy for the first occurrence.

Operative management consists of stapled wedge resection of blebs or bullae, usually found in the apex of the upper lobe or superior segment of the lower lobe. Pleural abrasion (pleurodesis) should be done to promote formation of adhesions between visceral and parietal pleurae. Video-assisted thoracoscopic techniques have allowed procedures to be less morbid in most cases. Using three small port incisions on the affected side, thoracoscopic stapling of the involved apical bulla and pleurodesis can be done. Alternatively, a transaxillary thoracotomy incision gives excellent exposure of the upper lung through a limited incision.

4. **Traumatic** pneumothoraces may be caused by either blunt or penetrating thoracic trauma and often result in lung contusion and multiple rib injury.
   a. **Evaluation and treatment** begin with the initial stabilization of airway and circulation. A chest x-ray should be obtained.
   b. **Prompt chest tube insertion** is performed to evacuate air and blood. In 80% of patients with penetrating trauma to the hemithorax, exploratory thoracotomy is unnecessary, and chest tube decompression with observation is sufficient. Indications for operation include immediate drainage of greater than 1,500 mL of blood after tube insertion or persistent bleeding of greater than 200 mL/hour. Patients who have with multiple injuries and proven pneumothoraces or significant chest injuries should have prophylactic chest tubes placed before general anesthesia because of the risk of tension pneumothorax with positive-pressure ventilation.
   c. **Pulmonary contusion** is associated with traumatic pneumothorax. The contusion usually is evident on the initial chest x-ray (as opposed to aspiration, in which several hours may elapse before an infiltrative pattern appears on serial radiographs), and it appears as a fluffy infiltrate that progresses in extent and density over 24 to 48 hours.
   d. The contusion may be associated with multiple rib fractures, leading to a **flail chest.** This occurs when several ribs are broken segmentally, allowing for a portion of the chest wall to be "floating" and to move paradoxically with breathing (inward on inspiration). The paradoxical movement and splinting secondary to pain and the associated pain lead to a reduction in vital capacity and to ineffective ventilation.
   e. All patients with suspected contusions and rib fractures should have **aggressive pain** control measures, including patient-controlled analgesia pumps, epidural catheters, and/or intercostal nerve blocks.
   f. **Intravenous fluid should be minimized** to the extent allowed by the patient's clinical status because of associated increased capillary endothelial permeability. Serial arterial blood gas measurements are important for close monitoring of respiratory status. Close monitoring and a high index of suspicion for respiratory decompensation are necessary. Intubation, positive-pressure ventilation, and even tracheostomy are often necessary.
   g. **A traumatic bronchopleural fistula** can occur after penetrating or blunt chest trauma. If mechanical ventilation is ineffective secondary to the large air leak, emergent thoracotomy and repair are usually necessary. On occasion, selective intubation of the uninvolved bronchus can provide short-term stability in the minutes before definitive operative treatment.
   h. The unusual circumstance known as a **sucking chest wound** consists of a full-thickness hole in the chest wall greater than two thirds the diameter of the trachea. With inspiration, air preferentially flows through the wound because of the low resistance to flow. This requires immediate coverage of the hole with an occlusive dressing and chest tube insertion to reexpand the

lung. If tube thoracostomy cannot be immediately performed, coverage with an occlusive dressing taped on three sides functions as a one-way valve to prevent the accumulation of air within the chest, although tube thoracostomy should be performed as soon as possible.

VI. HEMOPTYSIS can originate from a number of causes, including infectious, malignant, and cardiac disorders (e.g., bronchitis or tuberculosis, bronchogenic carcinoma, and mitral stenosis, respectively).

A. Massive hemoptysis requires emergent thoracic surgical intervention, often with little time for formal studies before entering the operating room. The surgeon is called primarily for significant hemoptysis, which is defined as more than 600 mL of blood expelled over 48 hours or, more often, a volume of blood that is impairing gas exchange. Because the volume of the main airways is approximately 200 mL, even smaller amounts of blood can cause severe respiratory compromise. Prompt treatment is required to ensure survival. As baseline lung function decreases, a lower volume and rate of hemoptysis is capable of severely compromising gas exchange.

1. A **brief focused history** can often elucidate the etiology of the bleed, such as a history of tuberculosis or aspergillosis. A recent chest x-ray may reveal the diagnosis in up to half of cases. Chest CT is rarely helpful in the acute setting and is contraindicated in patients who are unstable. Trace amounts of hemoptysis can be evaluated by radiologic examinations in conjunction with bronchoscopy.

2. **Bronchoscopy** is the mainstay of diagnosis and initial treatment. Although it may not eliminate later episodes of bleeding, it can allow for temporizing measures, such as placement of balloon-tipped catheters and topical or injected vasoconstrictors. In a setting of massive hemoptysis, the patient should be prepared for a rigid bronchoscopy, which is best performed in the operating room under general anesthesia. Asphyxiation is the primary cause of death in patients with massive hemoptysis. Rigid bronchoscopy allows for rapid and effective clearance of blood and clot from the airway, rapid identification of the bleeding side, and prompt protection of the remaining lung parenchyma (with cautery, by packing with epinephrine-soaked gauze, or by placement of a balloon-tipped catheter in the lobar orifice).

3. In cases in which the **etiology** and the precise bleeding source are not identified by bronchoscopy, ongoing bleeding requires protection of the contralateral lung. Selective ventilation, either with a double-lumen tube or by direct intubation of the contralateral main-stem bronchus, may be critical to avoid asphyxiation.

4. **After isolation of the bleeding site, angiographic embolization** of a bronchial arterial source may allow for lung salvage without the need for resection. The bronchial circulation is almost always the source of hemoptysis. Bleeding from the pulmonary circulation is seen only in patients with pulmonary hypertension.

5. **Definitive therapy** may require thoracotomy with lobar resection or, rarely, pneumonectomy. Infrequently, emergent surgical resection is necessary to control the hemoptysis. The etiology of the bleeding and the pulmonary reserve of the patient are important because many patients are not candidates for surgical resection.

VII. PLEURAL EFFUSION

A. Pleural effusion may result from a wide spectrum of benign, malignant, and inflammatory conditions. By history, it is often possible to deduce the etiology, but diagnosis often depends on the analysis of the pleural fluid. The presentation of symptoms depends on the underlying etiology, and **treatment is based on the underlying disease process.**

1. **Chest x-ray** is often the first diagnostic test. Depending on radiographic technique, an effusion may remain hidden. Although decubitus films are the most sensitive for detecting small, free-flowing effusions, the same volume may remain hidden in a standard anteroposterior film. A concave meniscus in the costophrenic angle on an upright chest x-ray suggests at least 250 mL of pleural fluid. **CT scan** and **ultrasound** can be particularly helpful if the fluid is not

free flowing or if history suggests a more chronic organizing process such as empyema.

2. **Thoracentesis**
   a. **The technique** of thoracentesis is described in Chapter 37.
   b. **The fluid should be sent for culture and Gram stain, biochemical analyses [pH, glucose, amylase, lactate dehydrogenase (LDH), and protein levels], and a differential cell count and cytology to rule out malignancy.**
   c. In general, thin, yellowish, clear fluid is common with transudative effusions; cloudy and foul-smelling fluid usually signals infection or early empyema; bloody effusions often denote malignancy; milky white fluid suggests chylothorax; and pH less than 7.2 suggests bacterial infection or connective tissue disease.
   d. Larger volumes (several hundred milliliters) can often aid the cytopathologists in making a diagnosis. White blood cell count greater than $10,000/mm^3$ suggests pyogenic etiology. A predominance of lymphocytes is noted with tuberculosis. Glucose is decreased in infectious processes as well as in malignancy.
   e. Pleural effusions are broadly categorized as either **transudative** (protein-poor fluid not involving primary pulmonary pathology) or **exudative** (resulting from increased vascular permeability as a result of diseased pleura or pleural lymphatics). Protein and LDH levels measured simultaneously in the pleural fluid and serum provide the diagnosis in nearly all settings.
   f. Exudative pleural effusions satisfy at least one of the following criteria: (1) ratio of pleural fluid protein to serum protein greater than 0.5, (2) ratio of pleural fluid LDH to serum LDH greater than 0.6, or (3) pleural fluid LDH greater than two thirds the upper normal limit for serum.

3. **Transudative pleural effusion** can usually be considered a secondary diagnosis; therefore, therapy should be directed at the underlying problem (e.g., congestive heart failure, cirrhosis, or nephrotic syndrome). Therapeutic drainage is rarely indicated because fluid rapidly reaccumulates unless the underlying cause improves.

4. **Exudative pleural effusion** may be broadly classified based on whether its cause is benign or malignant.
   a. **Malignant** effusions are most often associated with cancers of the breast, lung, and ovary and with lymphoma. Diagnosis is often made by cytology, but in the event that this process is not diagnostic, pleural biopsy may be indicated. Given the overall poor prognosis in these patients, **therapy offered by the thoracic surgeon is generally palliative.**
      (1) **Drainage** of effusion to alleviate dyspnea and improve pulmonary mechanics by reexpanding the lung may be done with chest tube placement.
      (2) **Pleurodesis** with talc or doxycycline may prevent reaccumulation of the effusion.
   b. **Benign exudative effusions** are most often a result of pneumonia **(parapneumonic).** The process begins with a sterile parapneumonic exudative effusion and leads to a suppurative infection of the pleural space, **empyema,** if the effusion becomes infected. The initially free-flowing fluid becomes infected and begins to deposit fibrin and cellular debris (5 to 7 days). Eventually, this fluid becomes organized, and a thick, fibrous peel entraps the lung (10 to 14 days).
      (1) **Empyema.** Fifty percent of empyemas are complications of pneumonia; 25% are complications of esophageal, pulmonary, or mediastinal surgery; and 10% are extensions from subphrenic abscesses. Thoracentesis is diagnostic but is sufficient treatment in only the earliest cases.
      (2) The **clinical presentation** of empyema ranges from systemic sepsis requiring emergent care to chronic loculated effusion in a patient who complains of fatigue. Other symptoms include pleuritic chest pain, fever, cough, and dyspnea.

(3) The **most common offending organisms** are Gram-positive cocci (*Staphylococcus aureus* and streptococci) and Gram-negative organisms (*Escherichia coli* and *Pseudomonas* and *Klebsiella* species). *Bacteroides* species are also common.

(4) Management includes control of the infection by appropriate antibiotics, drainage of the pleural space, and obliteration of the empyema space. Once the diagnosis is made, treatment should not be delayed. Specific management depends on the phase of the empyema, which depends on the character of the fluid. **If the fluid does not layer on posteroanterior and lateral and decubitus chest x-ray, a CT scan should be done.**

(a) Early or **exudative empyema** is usually adequately treated with simple tube drainage.

(b) Fibropurulent empyema may be amenable to tube drainage alone, but the fluid may be loculated. The loculations of empyema cavities are composed of fibrin.

(c) In advanced or **organizing empyema,** the fluid is thicker and a fibrous peel encases the lung. Thoracotomy may be necessary to free the entrapped lung.

(d) If a patient has a **persistent fluid collection with an adequately placed tube** as evidenced by chest CT, intrapleural fibrinolytic therapy may be indicated. Intrapleural streptokinase, 250,000 units, is divided into three doses, each in 60 mL of normal saline. A dose is administered and flushed with 30 mL of normal saline. The tube is clamped and the patient rolled as described for pleurodesis; then the tube is returned to suction. The procedure is repeated every 8 hours. Alternatively, 250,000 units can be administered daily for 3 days. The adequacy of treatment is determined by resolution of the fluid collection and complete reexpansion of the lung.

(e) A **postpneumonectomy empyema** is one of the most difficult complications to manage in thoracic surgery. Typically, there is a dehiscence of the bronchial stump and contamination of the pneumonectomy space with bronchial flora. The finding of air in the pneumonectomy space on chest x-ray is often diagnostic. The incidence of major bronchopleural fistula after pulmonary resection varies from 2% to 10% and has a high mortality (16% to 70%). Initial management includes thorough drainage (either open or closed) of the infected pleural space, antibiotics, and pulmonary toilet.

(f) Definitive surgical repair of the fistula may include primary closure of a long bronchial stump or closure of the fistula using vascularized muscle or omental flaps. The residual pleural cavity can be obliterated by a muscle transposition, thoracoplasty, or delayed Clagett procedure.

(i) Initially, a chest tube is inserted to evacuate the empyema. Great caution should be taken in inserting chest tubes into postpneumonectomy empyemas. A communicating bronchial stump–pleural fistula can contaminate the contralateral lung rapidly when decompression of the empyema is attempted. The patient should be positioned with the affected side down so that the remaining lung is not contaminated with empyema fluid. This procedure might best be handled in the operating room.

(ii) After the patient is stabilized, the next step usually is the creation of a **Clagett window** to provide a venue for daily packing and to maintain external drainage of the infected pleural space. This typically involves reopening the thoracotomy incision at its anterolateral end and resecting a short segment of two or three ribs to create generous access to the pleural space. The pleura is then treated with irrigation and débridement. After a suitable interval (weeks to months), the wound edges can be excised, and the pneumonectomy space is closed either primarily or with a muscle flap after it has been filled with 0.25% neomycin solution. Alternatively, the space can be filled with vascularized muscle flap.

VIII. CHRONIC OBSTRUCTIVE PULMONARY DISEASE (COPD), LUNG VOLUME REDUCTION, AND TRANSPLANTATION

A. The long-term consequences of smoking lead not only to lung cancer but also to **COPD**.

1. **Destruction of lung parenchyma** occurs in a nonuniform manner. As lung tissue loses its elastic recoil, the areas of destruction expand. This expansion of diseased areas, in combination with inflammation, leads to poor ventilation of relatively normal lung.

2. This leads to the **typical findings of hyperexpanded lungs** on chest x-ray: flattened diaphragms, widened intercostal spaces, and horizontal ribs. On pulmonary function testing, patients present with increased residual volumes and decreased FEV_1.

3. Despite maximal medical and surgical treatment, the **disease is progressive.** Surgical treatment is generally reserved for the symptomatic (dyspnea) patient who has failed maximal medical treatment, with the goal of improving symptoms.

4. The **goals of surgery** are to remove diseased areas of lung and allow improved function of the remaining lung tissue.

B. The mainstays of surgical treatment have been bullectomy, lung volume reduction, and transplantation. Prior to any surgical intervention, **patients must be carefully selected. Smoking cessation for at least 6 months is mandatory, as is enrollment in a supervised pulmonary rehabilitation program.**

1. **Bullectomy.** Patients with emphysema may have large bullous disease. Emphysematous bullae are giant air sacs and may become secondarily infected.

2. **Lung volume reduction** may be indicated in patients who have predominantly apical disease, with FEV_1 greater than 20% of predicted, and patients who may be too old for transplantation. Through a sternotomy incision, one or both lungs have areas of heavily diseased lung resected. Patients with diffuse emphysema are not candidates for this procedure.

3. Emphysema and α_1-antitrypsin deficiency have become the leading indications for lung transplantation. Other common indications include cystic fibrosis, pulmonary fibrosis, and pulmonary hypertension.

   a. Patients selected for lung transplantation generally are younger, have diffuse involvement of emphysema, and have FEV_1 less than 20%.

   b. Both single-lung and bilateral-lung transplantation have been performed for emphysema, although bilateral transplant patients have improved long-term survival.

   c. The only absolute indication for bilateral lung transplantation is cystic fibrosis because single-lung transplantation would leave a chronically infected native lung in an immunocompromised patient.

   d. Long-term, chronic allograft dysfunction in the form of bronchiolitis obliterans occurs in 50% of patients.

IX. ISSUES IN THE CARE OF THE THORACIC PATIENT

A. Postoperative care of the thoracic surgery patient focuses on three factors: **control of incisional pain, maintenance of pulmonary function, and monitoring of cardiovascular status.**

1. The **thoracotomy incision is one of the most painful and debilitating** in surgery. Inadequate pain control contributes heavily to nearly all postoperative complications. Chest wall splinting contributes to atelectasis and poor pulmonary toilet. Pain increases sympathetic tone and myocardial oxygen demand, provoking arrhythmias and cardiac ischemic episodes. The routine use of epidural catheter anesthesia perioperatively and during the early recovery period has improved pain management significantly. Other effective analgesic maneuvers include intercostal blocks with long-acting local anesthetic before closure of the chest and

intrapleural administration or local anesthetic via catheters placed at the time of thoracotomy.

2. **Maintenance of good bronchial hygiene** is often the most difficult challenge facing the postthoracotomy patient. A lengthy smoking history, decreased ciliary function, chronic bronchitis, and significant postoperative pain all contribute to the ineffective clearance of pulmonary secretions. Even aggressive pulmonary toilet with incentive spirometry and chest physiotherapy delivered by the respiratory therapist, along with adequate analgesia, are insufficient on occasion. **Diligent attention must be paid,** including frequent physical examination and daily chest x-ray and arterial blood gas evaluation to detect any changes in gas exchange. **Atelectasis** and **mucus plugging** can lead to ventilation-perfusion mismatch and ensuing respiratory failure. The clinician should make liberal use of nasotracheal suctioning, bedside flexible bronchoscopy, and mechanical ventilatory support if needed.

3. All physicians caring for the postthoracotomy patient should be familiar with **chest tube placement, maintenance, and removal.** The purpose of chest tube placement after thoracotomy and lung resection is to allow drainage of air and fluid from the pleural space and to ensure reexpansion of the remaining lung parenchyma.

   a. **Chest-tube drainage** is not used routinely with pneumonectomy unless bleeding or infection is present. Some surgeons place a chest tube on the operative side and remove it on postoperative day 1. Balanced pneumonectomy Pleurovacs have been advocated to balance the mediastinum during the first 24 to 48 hours. A chest tube in the patient with a pneumonectomy space should not be placed to conventional suction because of the risk of cardiac herniation.

   b. **Chest tubes are removed after the air leak has resolved and fluid drainage decreased** (usually <100 mL over 8 hours). Chest tubes usually are removed one at a time. The patient is instructed to take a large inspiratory breath and hold it while the tube is removed swiftly and the site is simultaneously covered with an occlusive dressing. The technique of chest tube removal is critical to preventing air entry through the removal site.

4. **Cardiovascular complications** in the postoperative period are second in frequency only to pulmonary complications because the population that develops lung cancer is at high risk for heart disease. The three most common sources of cardiac morbidity are **arrhythmias, myocardial infarctions, and congestive heart failure.** A negative preoperative cardiac evaluation does not preclude the development of postoperative complications.

   a. **Cardiac arrhythmias** occur in up to 30% of patients undergoing pulmonary surgery. The highest incidence occurs in elderly patients undergoing pneumonectomy or intrapericardial pulmonary artery ligation. All patients should have cardiac rhythm monitoring after thoracotomy for at least 72 hours.

   b. A number of trials have failed to reach consensus on optimal regimen for prophylaxis.

   c. **Treatment** of any rhythm disturbance begins with an assessment of the patient's hemodynamic status. Manifestations of these arrhythmias vary in acuity from hemodynamic collapse to palpitations. If the patient is hemodynamically unstable, the advanced cardiac life support protocol should be followed. After the patient has been examined and hemodynamic stability confirmed, an electrocardiogram, arterial blood gas sample, and serum electrolyte panel should be obtained. Frequently, supplementary oxygen and aggressive potassium and magnesium replenishment are the only treatment necessary. Premature ventricular contractions often are signs of myocardial ischemia. They should be treated expediently with electrolyte correction, optimization of oxygenation, and evaluation for ischemia.

   d. **Chest pain associated with myocardial infarction** often goes unnoticed by caretakers and patients due to thoracotomy incisional pain and narcotic administration.

e. **Perioperative fluid management** of thoracic surgery patients differs from that of patients after abdominal surgery. **Pulmonary surgery does not induce large fluid shifts.** In addition, collapse and reexpansion of lungs during surgery can lead to pulmonary edema. Pulmonary edema should be treated with aggressive diuresis. This is largely due to the limited pulmonary reserve, most graphically demonstrated in the pneumonectomy patient in whom 100% of the cardiac output perfuses the remaining lung. Judicious fluid management, including avoiding fluid overload and pulmonary edema, is critical in patients with limited pulmonary reserve. Discussions regarding intraoperative fluid management should be held with the anesthesiologist before surgery. Physicians may need to accept transiently decreased urine output and increased serum creatinine. Mild hypotension may be treated with intravenous α-agonists such as phenylephrine. Cardiac dysfunction may also be the source of postoperative oliguria, pulmonary edema, and hypotension and should always be considered in patients who are not responding normally. Echocardiography or placement of a Swan-Ganz catheter may guide treatment.

X. THORACOSCOPY

A. **Diagnostic thoracoscopy** (*Surg Gynecol Obstet* 1922;34:289)

  1. **Video-assisted thoracoscopic surgery (VATS)** is performed in patients after thoracentesis and percutaneous pleural biopsy have failed to provide a diagnosis of suspected pleural disease. VATS frequently is used to diagnose malignancy in a solitary peripheral nodule. It is contraindicated in patients with extensive intrapleural adhesions or those who are unable to tolerate single-lung ventilation.

  2. **VATS is approximately 95% accurate** for diagnosis of pleural disease.

B. **Therapeutic thoracoscopy**

  1. **VATS has been performed** for peripheral lung biopsy, closure of leaking blebs, parietal pleurodesis, pericardiectomy, and excision of mediastinal cysts. Fewer lobectomies, pneumonectomies, and esophagectomies have been performed owing to concern about adequacy of complete tumor resection, and therefore they should be considered investigational procedures at this time.

      a. **Absolute contraindications** include extensive intrapleural adhesions or the inability to tolerate single-lung anesthesia.

      b. **Relative contraindications** include previous thoracotomy, tumor involvement of the hilar vessels, and previous chemotherapy or radiotherapy for lung or esophageal tumors.

  2. The **patient is placed** in the lateral decubitus or semioblique position. Thoracoscopy requires selective intubation to allow collapse of the ipsilateral lung and to create a working space within the thorax (thus, insufflation gases are not needed). For most procedures, three incisions are required. The thoracoscope is placed through a port in the seventh or eighth intercostal space in the midaxillary line. Working ports for instruments generally are at the fourth or fifth intercostal space in the anterior axillary line and posteriorly near the border of the scapula. The endoscopic stapler, electrocautery, or laser can be used for resection. A chest tube is generally placed through one of the port sites.

  3. **Complications** include hemorrhage, perforation of the diaphragm, air emboli, prolonged air leak, and tension pneumothorax.

  4. **Postoperative thoracoscopy management**

      a. **A chest x-ray** is taken and checked for residual air or fluid.

      b. **Chest tubes,** if any, are usually removed in 1 to 2 days.

      c. **Analgesia** is provided by patient-controlled anesthesia or orally administered medication as needed.

      d. **Diet** is usually advanced by postoperative day 1.

      e. **Physical activity** is as tolerated with a chest tube. Depending on the procedure and diagnosis, patients can return to work in approximately 1 week.

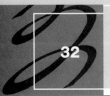

PEDIATRIC SURGERY

Trudie A. Goers and Patrick A. Dillon

$\mathcal{S}$ urgery involving children is predicated on the fundamental facts that infants and children differ from adults in anatomy, physiology, and particularly their reaction to operative trauma and that the necessary adjustments of surgical procedures are not merely matters of scale. Although some disease processes are managed similar to those in adults, this chapter addresses the more pediatric-specific surgical issues.

I. FLUID, ELECTROLYTES, AND NUTRITION

A. Fluid requirements

1. Children's **normal daily fluid requirements** are higher than those of adults due to higher insensible losses as a result of the high ratio of body-surface area to volume and the limited ability of immature kidneys to concentrate urine (Table 32-1).

2. **Postoperative fluid replacement:** daily requirements plus losses (measurable and insensible).

   a. **Total body water** is a higher percentage of body weight (75%) than in adults (60%).

   b. **Total blood volume in the newborn** is approximately 8% of body weight, which decreases to 5% in older infants.

   c. The **total fluid administered** should be adjusted to support urine output between 1 and 2 mL/kg/hour.

   d. **Output from tubes and drains** should be matched by replacement fluid with similar electrolyte composition.

B. Electrolytes

1. **Children younger than 6 months old** should be given 10% dextrose in 0.25% saline with potassium chloride, 20 mEq/L.

2. **Children older than 6 months old** should be given 5% dextrose in 0.45% saline with potassium chloride, 20 mEq/L.

3. Daily **sodium** requirements are 2 to 3 mEq/kg.

4. Daily **potassium** requirements are 1 to 2 mEq/kg.

C. Nutrition

1. Calories (Table 32-2):

   Total daily caloric need (kcal/kg/day) = Resting energy expenditure (REE) + (REE × additional factor),

   where the additional factors are as follows:

   > Normal maintenance: 0.2
   > Activity: 0.1 to 0.25
   > Fever: $0.13/(°C >38°C)$
   > Simple trauma: 0.2
   > Multiple trauma: 0.4
   > Burns: 0.5 to 1

2. A **newborn weight gain** of 15 to 30 g/day is expected.

3. **Carbohydrates** should supply 40% to 45%, **lipids** 35%, and **protein** 15% of total calories in the diet.

TABLE 32-1	Normal Fluid Requirements in Children

Weight (kg)	24-hr fluid requirements
<2 (premature)	150 mL/kg
1–10	100 mL/kg
11–20	1,000 mL + 50 mL/kg for each kg >10
>20	1,500 mL + 20 mL/kg for each kg >20

Weight (kg)	Hourly fluid requirements
0–10	4 mL/kg
10–20	2 mL/kg
>20	1 mL/kg

4. Most **infant formulas** contain 20 kcal/oz; therefore, caloric needs can be calculated by the following formula:

Weight (kg) × 6 oz = Volume of formula necessary to deliver 120 kcal/kg.

5. **Enteral nutrition** is the preferred method of delivering calories to a patient. However, for patients for whom enteral nutrition in contraindicated, parenteral nutrition should be initiated early.
   a. Glucose

Glucose infusion rate (mg/kg/minute) = % dextrose × infusion rate (mL/hour)/weight (kg) × 6,

where dextrose 3.4 kcal/g = % dextrose × 10.
Goal is 13 to 15 mg/kg/minute.
   b. Protein
      (1) <1 year of age: TrophAmine.
      (2) >1 year of age: Travasol.
      (3) Goal:

         ○ Preterm infant: 3.5 to 4 g/kg/day.
         ○ Term infant: 2 to 3 g/kg/day.
         ○ Child: 1.5 to 2.5 g/kg/day.

TABLE 32-2	Normal Daily Calorie Needs in Children

Age (yr)	REE (kcal/kg/d)	Average (kcal/kg/d)
<36 wk		120
0–0.5	53	108
0.5–1	56	98
1–3	57	102
4–6	48	90
7–10	40	70
11–14	32	55
15–18	27	45
11–14	28	47
15–18	25	40

REE, resting energy expenditure.

TABLE 32-3	Nothing-by-Mouth Requirements in Children	
Age	Clear liquids	Solids/formula/breast milk
<6 mo	3 hr	4 hr
>6 mo	4 hr	6 hr
>12 yr	6 hr	6 hr

   c. **Lipids**
      (1) 20% intralipid = 2 kcal/mL.
      (2) Goal: 2 to 3 g/kg/day or 30% to 40% of total calories.
II. **PREOPERATIVE PREPARATION**
   A. **History and physical**
   B. **Laboratory tests.** Without major comorbidities, usually a hematocrit is sufficient.
   C. **Nothing-by-mouth (NPO status) (Table 32-3).** Studies have indicated that clear liquids ingested 2 to 3 hours before induction of anesthesia do not increase the risk of aspiration (*Anesthesiology* 1990;72:593). **Aspiration risks** can also be reduced by administering H_2-receptor antagonists, metoclopramide, and buffering agents such as sodium citrate.
   D. **Preoperative antibiotic prophylaxis** indications
      1. Patients with cardiac anomalies.
      2. Patients with ventriculoperitoneal shunts.
      3. Patients with implanted prosthetic material.
      4. Most common regimen: **ampicillin** (50 mg/kg) and gentamicin (1.5 mg/kg) given usually 1 hour before and 6 hours after the procedure.
III. **VASCULAR ACCESS**
   A. **Peripheral venous access.** Usual candidates for access: dorsal vein of the hand, antecubital vein of the arm, saphenous vein at the ankle, dorsal vein in the foot, median tributary at the wrist, external jugular vein, and scalp veins.
   B. **Percutaneous central venous catheter insertion.** Central venous access may be needed if peripheral access is exhausted or if drugs or nutrition need to be given centrally or for a prolonged period of time. Access to central veins can be accomplished directly or via peripheral veins [i.e., peripherally inserted central catheter (PICC) placement]. Sites most often chosen are the subclavian vein, internal jugular vein, and femoral vein.
   C. **Intraosseous (IO) access** should be used in an emergency setting when other attempts at obtaining vascular access have failed. A location 1 to 3 cm distal to the tibial tuberosity is the recommended site. The needle should be directed inferiorly during insertion. Alternatively, the femur may be reached by inserting the needle in a cephalad direction 3 cm proximal to the condyles. Either a bone marrow aspiration needle or a 16- to 19-gauge butterfly needle is adequate. Contraindications to IO access include a fracture of the bone or previous IO catheter.
   D. **Arterial catheters** are needed in some neonates and infants. The potential sites for placement of an arterial catheter include the umbilical, radial, femoral, posterior tibial, and temporal arteries; however, the radial artery is used most frequently. The typical catheters are 22 to 24 gauge and can be placed percutaneously or by cutdown. In a neonate who is within the first 2 to 4 days of life, the umbilical artery can often be cannulated through the umbilical stump.
IV. **COMMON NEONATAL SURGICAL PROBLEMS**
   It must be remembered that congenital anomalies rarely occur independently. When a defect is identified, laboratory and radiologic investigations must be employed to uncover associated developmental abnormalities (e.g., **VACTERL syndromes** involving *v*ertebral defects, imperforate *a*nus, *c*ardiac defects, *t*racheo*e*sophageal malformations, *r*enal dysplasia, and *l*imb anomalies).

A. Congenital diaphragmatic hernia (CDH)

- **Incomplete diaphragm development** at 8 weeks' gestation results in herniation of abdominal organs into the chest, preventing normal lung development.
- **Left leaflet occurs in 90% of cases,** and right leaflet in 10%.
- **Bochdalek** (posterolateral defect; 85% of cases); **Morgagni** (anterior, parasternal; fewer pulmonary and systemic complications).
- A 1:1 male-to-female ratio.

1. Diagnosis

   a. Antenatal **ultrasound and maternal-fetal magnetic resonance imaging (MRI).** Polyhydramnios is detected in up to 80% of cases.

   b. Physical exam

   (1) Cardiorespiratory distress.

   (2) Asymmetric "funnel" chest.

   (3) Reduced breath sounds on the affected side.

   (4) Scaphoid abdomen.

   c. Chest x-ray

   (1) Herniated abdominal viscera within the chest.

   (2) Mediastinal shift.

2. Mortality

   a. Approximately 35%.

   b. May be higher in patients with severe pulmonary hypoplasia and hypertension or in the presence of associated congenital anomalies.

3. Management

   a. Immediate postnatal care

   (1) Supplemental oxygen.

   (2) Endotracheal intubation is indicated if significant respiratory distress is present. Avoid bag-mask ventilation, which exacerbates gastrointestinal (GI) distention and further impedes lung ventilation.

   (3) Intravenous access is necessary for the administration of fluids to maintain organ perfusion.

   (4) GI decompression by orogastric or nasogastric intubation reduces distention of the stomach and within the thoracic cavity.

   b. Intensive care

   (1) Conventional ventilation utilizing permissive hypercapnia to minimize barotrauma.

   (a) Once stabilized, wean fraction of inspired oxygen (FiO_2) for preductal oxygen saturation greater than 90%.

   (b) Arterial carbon dioxide tension of 60 to 70 mm Hg is acceptable.

   (c) Maintain pH greater than 7.20.

   (d) Peak airway pressures less than 25 cm H_2O.

   (e) Mean airway pressures less than 12 cm H_2O.

   (2) High-frequency oscillating ventilator (HFOV)

   (a) May be used if conventional ventilation failed.

   (b) Possibly limit barotrauma.

   (3) Inhaled **nitric oxide may decrease severity of pulmonary hypertension.**

   (4) Extracorporeal membrane oxygenation (ECMO) is considered for patients with severe preductal hypoxemia or right-to-left shunting due to high pulmonary hypertension. Patients with overwhelming pulmonary hypoplasia may not be not candidates for ECMO.

   c. Operative intervention

   (1) Usually deferred until the patient's pulmonary status is stable.

   (2) A subcostal incision on the affected side allows the herniated abdominal contents to be replaced in the peritoneal cavity.

   (3) Repaired primarily or with a synthetic patch, depending on the size of the defect.

   d. Complications: long-term respiratory insufficiency, GI reflux, neurologic sequelae from prolonged hypoxia, recurrence of hernia.

B. Tracheoesophageal malformations
- This is a spectrum of anomalies, including esophageal atresia (EA) and tracheoesophageal fistula (TEF), separately or in combination (Fig. 32-1).
- Interruption in the normal budding of the trachea from the foregut during embryonic development.
- A 1:1 male-to-female ratio.

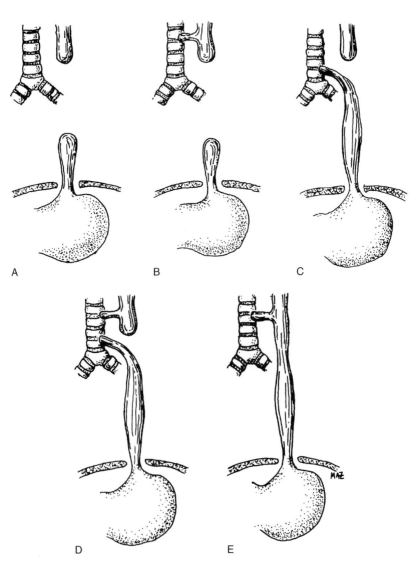

Figure 32-1. Variants of tracheoesophageal fistula. **A:** Atresia without fistula (5% to 7% of cases). **B:** Proximal fistula and distal pouch (<1% occurrence). **C:** Proximal pouch with distal fistula (85% to 90% of cases). **D:** Atresia with proximal and distal fistulas (<1% of cases). **E:** Fistula without atresia (H type) (2% to 6% occurrence).

1. **Diagnosis**
   a. **Physical exam**
      (1) **Excessive drooling.**
      (2) **Regurgitation** of feedings.
      (3) **Choking, coughing, or cyanosis** during feeding.
   b. **Radiology**
      (1) **Coiled orogastric tube** in the esophageal pouch.
      (2) **Gas in the GI tract** implies the presence of a distal TEF.
2. **Management**
   a. Prevent aspiration and pneumonia.
      (1) **Supine position** with the **head elevated 30 to 45 degrees.**
      (2) Insert an **orogastric or nasogastric tube** into the proximal esophageal pouch for decompression and to prevent aspiration.
      (3) Administer **ampicillin (50 mg/kg) and gentamicin (2.5 mg/kg)** intravenously.
   b. **Operative intervention**
      (1) Right extrapleural thoracotomy.
      (2) **Ligation of the fistula** and **repair of the EA** with esophagoesophagostomy.
   c. **Complications**
      (1) Stricture of esophagus, leak of esophageal anastomosis, recurrence of fistula.
      (2) Gastrointestinal reflux disorder (GERD), esophageal dysmotility.
C. **Gastroschisis**
   - This abdominal wall defect is believed to arise from an **isolated vascular insult** in the developing mesenchyme.
   - It usually **occurs to the right of a normal umbilical cord** with any combination of abdominal organs herniating through the defect.
   - **In contrast to omphalocele,** there is **no membranous sac** covering the eviscerated abdominal organs. The **incidence of associated anomalies** in gastroschisis is low, but approximately 10% may have intestinal atresia.
1. **Diagnosis**
   a. **Ultrasound examination**
      (1) Evident after 13 weeks' gestation.
      (2) Intestine free within the amniotic fluid apart from the umbilical cord.
   b. **Physical exam**
      (1) Abdominal defect to the right of the umbilical cord.
      (2) No encompassing sac.
      (3) Exposed bowel may develop a **serositis.**
2. **Management**
   a. **Prenatal management**
      (1) Serial ultrasound: If bowel dilation and mural thickening of the eviscerated bowel are detected, delivery at the time of lung maturity may be indicated (*Surg Obstet Gynecol* 1993;81:53).
      (2) Delivery should be planned at a tertiary care center with both high-risk obstetrics service and pediatric surgical expertise.
   b. **Postnatal management**
      (1) **Intravenous fluids**
         (a) Normal saline, 20-mL/kg bolus.
         (b) Maintenance intravenous fluid (IVF) to achieve a urine output of 1.5 to 2 mL/kg/hour.
      (2) **Heat and fluid losses** can be decreased by covering the exposed bowel with moistened gauze and then wrapping the bowel with Saran/plastic wrap.
      (3) **Position** the neonate in a lateral position to prevent kinking of the bowel and vascular compromise.
      (4) **Extension of the fascial defect** in the midline for 1 to 2 cm can be done if the bowel mesentery appears to be compressed by a narrow opening.

(5) Operative intervention

(a) Viscera may be reduced primarily, but if this is not possible, viscera are placed in a spring-loaded or self-made silo, which is secured beneath the fascial edge.

(b) Silo and viscera are reduced gradually over time.

(c) The abdominal wall defect is then repaired in a primary fashion on an elective basis. Fewer complications may arise with this method of management compared with immediate reduction of viscera and early primary closure (*J Pediatr Surg* 2000;35:843).

(6) Complications: bowel ischemia, short gut, bowel nonrotation, feeding intolerance.

D. Omphalocele

■ This is an abdominal wall defect of the umbilical ring in which the intestines protrude through the base of the umbilical cord and herniate into a sac.

■ High incidence (50%) of related anomalies (cardiac, chromosomal).

1. Diagnosis

a. Antenatal ultrasound

(1) Evident after 13 weeks' gestation.

(2) Bowel can be seen herniating through the base of the umbilical cord into an echogenic sac.

(3) Because of the high incidence of related anomalies, the presence of an omphalocele should direct a thorough search for other birth defects by ultrasonography and amniocentesis.

b. Amniotic fluid *α*-**fetoprotein** (AFP) levels are elevated.

c. Physical examination

(1) Abdominal wall defect at the base **of the umbilical cord.** The size of the defect varies from a few centimeters to absence of most of the abdominal wall.

(2) The presence of a sac covering the herniated viscera.

(3) Rupture of the sac is infrequent, but it is distinguished from gastroschisis by the presence of residual sac in continuity with the umbilical cord.

2. Management. The care of a patient with an omphalocele should be conducted according to the same principles as for gastroschisis (see Section IV.C.2). Rupture of the sac requires that the defect be treated as a gastroschisis.

3. Due to the presence of other anomalies associated with omphalocele, **the overall prognosis** for infants with omphalocele is significantly worse than that for gastroschisis.

E. Necrotizing enterocolitis (NEC)

■ This **acute fulminating, inflammatory disease of the intestine** is associated with focal or diffuse ulceration and necrosis of the small bowel, colon, and, rarely, the stomach.

■ Cause is unknown; however, the pathogenesis is thought to be multifactorial, involving an **immature gut barrier defense and virulent bacteria.**

■ The incidence of NEC is 1 to 3/1,000 live births.

■ It primarily affects **premature infants,** and occurs in 10% of all babies born weighing less than 1,500 g.

1. Diagnosis

a. High index of suspicion.

b. History and physical exam

(1) Lethargy.

(2) Skin pallor or mottling.

(3) Temperature instability.

(4) Apnea.

(5) High gastric residuals.

(6) Vomiting or bilious nasogastric tube drainage.

(7) Hematochezia.

(8) Diarrhea.

(9) Abdominal distention.

(10) Intra-abdominal mass.

(11) Edema or erythema of the abdominal wall may indicate peritonitis, local response to inflamed bowel, or perforation of bowel.

c. Laboratory tests

(1) Metabolic acidosis.

(2) Thrombocytopenia.

(3) Leukocytosis or leukopenia.

d. Radiologic studies

(1) Dilated bowel loops.

(2) Pneumatosis intestinalis.

(3) Ascites.

(4) Intrahepatic portal vein gas.

(5) Pneumoperitoneum.

(6) Ultrasonography may reveal portal venous gas, pneumatosis, and the presence of free peritoneal fluid.

(7) Contrast imaging is often avoided due to the risk of perforation.

2. Management

a. Nonoperative treatment

(1) Bowel rest.

(2) Nasogastric decompression.

(3) Removal of umbilical catheters.

(4) Maintenance of proper fluid balance.

(5) Parenteral nutrition.

(6) Broad-spectrum antibiotics.

(7) Serial abdominal examinations.

(8) Serial radiographs.

(9) Laboratory studies.

b. Indications for operative treatment

(1) Pneumoperitoneum.

(2) Portal vein gas.

(3) Enteric organisms present in paracentesis fluid.

(4) Intestinal obstruction.

(5) Intra-abdominal abscess.

(6) Sepsis unresponsive to treatment.

c. Choice of procedure

(1) Bowel resection of involved bowel with the creation of stomas. When intestinal viability is questionable, reexploration within 24 hours is essential.

(2) Open peritoneal drainage.

(a) Temporizing measures in critically ill infants until they can tolerate a laparotomy.

(b) Primary therapy for extremely low birth weight infants (<1,000 g) (*J Pediatr Surg* 1990;25:1034).

V. ALIMENTARY TRACT OBSTRUCTION

A. Congenital causes

1. Intestinal malrotation

a. Intestine fails to undergo its normal rotation and fixation during embryologic development.

b. Incidence 1/500 to 1/6,000 live births.

c. Associated anomalies are present in 30% to 59% of patients.

d. Symptoms most often present in the neonatal period but may present in adulthood.

(1) Diagnosis

(a) History and physical

(i) Bilious emesis

(ii) Hematemesis

(iii) Abdominal distention

         (iv) Abdominal tenderness

         (v) Hematochezia

      (b) Radiologic studies

         (i) Plain radiographs. "Double-bubble" is indicative of duodenal obstruction but not diagnostic of volvulus.

         (ii) Contrast imaging

- Necessary to establish diagnosis.
- **Failure of the duodenum to cross to the right of the midline** with right-sided jejunum characterizes intestinal malrotation.
- Hallmark signs for volvulus include the "**bird's beak**" sign and a **corkscrew appearance of the proximal small intestine.**

    (2) Management

      (a) Observation for signs of obstruction.

      (b) Operative intervention. Ladd procedure:

         (i) Correct volvulus by counterclockwise rotation of bowel and division of peritoneal (Ladd's) bands.

         (ii) Position colon on the left side of the abdomen and the small bowel on the right.

         (iii) Perform appendectomy.

B. Intestinal atresia or stenosis

- This results from intrauterine **vascular insult.**

1. Location. Distal ileum > proximal jejunum > duodenum > colon.

2. Diagnosis

  a. Antenatal **ultrasound**

    (1) Polyhydramnios.

    (2) Dilated intestinal loops.

  b. Neonatal history and physical

    (1) Symptoms appear shortly after birth for atresia but may take weeks to months for stenosis.

    (2) Bilious vomiting.

    (3) Abdominal distention.

    (4) Failure to pass meconium.

    (5) Failure to thrive.

    (6) Poor feeding.

  c. Radiology

    (1) A **"double-bubble" sign** is diagnostic of duodenal obstruction.

    (2) Contrast enema may be used to identify a distal intestinal atresia and can also identify obstruction secondary to meconium ileus or meconium plug syndrome.

3. Management

  a. Nasogastric decompression.

  b. Intravenous fluid.

  c. Ampicillin (50 mg/kg) and gentamicin (2.5 mg/kg) should be given preoperatively.

  d. Operative intervention

    (1) Primary anastomosis, which may require resection or tapering of the dilated proximal segment.

    (2) For **duodenal** atresia, a duodenoduodenostomy or duodenojejunostomy is created to bypass the obstruction.

    (3) Saline should be infused into the distal bowel to rule out synchronous intestinal atresias.

C. Hirschsprung disease

- Variable length of intestinal aganglionosis of the hindgut.
- Rectosigmoid is the aganglionosis transition point for 80% of patients.
- Familial or sporadic.
- Up to 7.8% of cases occur in patients for whom more than one family member is affected.

- Mutations in the *RET* protooncogene have been found in both familial and sporadic cases.
1. **Diagnosis**
   a. **History**
      (1) **Neonates:** abdominal distention, infrequent defecation, failure to pass meconium within the first 48 hours of life, or enterocolitis with sepsis.
      (2) **Older infants** and **children** present with chronic constipation or failure to thrive.
   b. **Radiology**
      (1) **Plain abdominal radiographs** commonly show a pattern of distal obstruction.
      (2) **Barium enema**
         (a) Usually demonstrates a **transition zone** between distal nondilated bowel and proximal dilated bowel.
         (b) Most common in the rectosigmoid, but may be seen anywhere in the colon.
         (c) Total colonic aganglionosis: no transition zone.
   c. **Pathology**
      (1) **Rectal biopsy** is essential for making the diagnosis.
      (2) **Full-thickness** specimens are the ideal tissue samples to allow identification of the absence of ganglion cells.
      (3) In neonates, **rectal suction biopsy** often is sufficient for diagnosis.
2. **Preoperative management**
   a. **Colonic decompression** to prevent enterocolitis. Saline enemas may be used to evacuate impacted stool.
   b. **Nasogastric tube** should be placed if the child is vomiting.
3. **Operative treatment**
   a. Goals of surgical management are removal of aganglionic bowel and reconstruction of the intestinal tract by bringing the innervated bowel down to the anus while maintaining normal sphincter function.
   b. **Primary pull-through**
      (1) Swenson.
      (2) Duhamel.
      (3) Soave.
      (4) Laparoscopic endorectal pull-through (Georgeson).
      (5) Transanal endorectal pull-through (Langer).
          Each of these operations has been modified to improve functional results and may be performed in the newborn period, although surgery may delayed to allow for increased weight gain or resolution of enterocolitis. Advocates of the last two approaches cite decreased recovery time, decreased hospital stay, decreased complications, a potential for decreased adhesions, and decreased cost as some of the advantages of minimal-access approaches in comparison with open transabdominal procedures (*Ann Surg* 1999;229:678, *J Pediatr Surg* 2000;35:820).
   c. **Diverting colostomy**
      (1) Performed proximal to aganglionic segment in patients who are unstable or who have massively dilated bowel.
      (2) Daily rectal irrigations may obviate the need for a colostomy.
D. **Anorectal anomalies**
   Classification system (*Am J Surg* 2000;180:370):
   - **Males:** perineal fistula, rectourethral bulbar fistula, rectourethral prostatic fistula, rectovesical (bladder neck) fistula, imperforate anus without fistula, rectal atresia and stenosis.
   - **Females:** perineal fistula, vestibular fistula, imperforate anus with no fistula, rectal atresia and stenosis, persistent cloaca.
   - The lesions may also be classified as low, intermediate, or high depending on whether the atresia is below, at the level of, or above the puborectalis sling, respectively.

1. **Diagnosis**
   a. Physical examination.
   b. Plain radiographs: obstructive series, invertogram, sacral abnormalities.
   c. Contrast studies: mucous fistulogram.
   d. Magnetic resonance.
2. **Management**
   a. Define associated defects.
      (1) VACTERL syndromes.
      (2) Cardiovascular anomalies occur in conjunction with anorectal malformations 12% to 22% of the time.
   b. Inspection of the perineum is required to help distinguish the type of defect. The presence of meconium on the perineum within 24 hours of birth may signify a perineal fistula (low defect), which may be safely repaired without a colostomy.
   c. A high defect with probable rectourethral or rectovaginal fistula requires a colostomy and mucous fistula for initial management.
   d. If the anatomy is unclear, lateral radiographs of the pelvis with the infant in a prone position can be obtained.
3. **Definitive operative repair**
   The main goal of caring for a baby with an anorectal malformation is bowel and urinary continence. For perineal fistulas, primary repair may be performed without a protective colostomy. For the more complex anorectal anomalies, a three-step methodology is advocated with a diverting colostomy after birth, posterior sagittal anorectoplasty (PSARP), and colostomy closure. Of note, laparoscopic management of anorectal anomalies has been performed.

E. **Omphalomesenteric duct abnormalities**
   ■ These represent failure of complete involution of the vitelline duct.
   ■ They occur in the ileum 60 cm or less from the ileocecal valve.
   ■ Common presentations:

   > **Meckel diverticulum.** A true diverticulum on the antimesenteric border.
   > **Patent duct** between the ileum and the umbilicus.
   > **Umbilical cyst** lined by intestinal mucosa.
   > **Fibrous cord** between an ileal diverticulum and the umbilicus or mesentery.

1. **Diagnosis**
   a. **Meckel diverticulum**
      (1) More than 50% **present before 2 years of age.**
      (2) Painless hemorrhage. Ectopic gastric mucosa that is frequently present results in peptic ulceration and hemorrhage in 22% of cases.
      (3) Bowel obstruction
         (a) Internal hernia around a vitelline duct band (13%).
         (b) Diverticulitis with abdominal pain (2%.)
      (4) Intussusception (*Arch Surg* 1987;122:542).
      (5) Technetium-99m pertechnetate scintiscan. Isotope is taken up by the ectopic gastric mucosa within the diverticulum.
   b. **Patent duct.** Leakage of ileal contents through the child's umbilicus.
   c. **Umbilical cysts.** Secretion of mucoid fluid via the child's umbilicus.
   d. **Fibrous band.** Usually presents as an internal hernia or intestinal volvulus around this cord of tissue, with the accompanying signs of intestinal obstruction.
2. **Management**
   a. **Operative intervention**
      (1) Diverticulectomy
         (a) Open or laparoscopic resection of the diverticulum.
         (b) Stapling of diverticulum or resection with anastomosis.
         (c) Dissection with ligation of feeding mesenteric vessel.
            When radiographic reduction of an **intussusception** is unsuccessful:

  (d) Surgical reduction of invaginated intestine.
  (e) Diverticulectomy.
  (f) If gangrenous bowel is present, bowel resection with primary anastomosis should be done.
  (2) Infants or young children who have a Meckel diverticulum discovered **incidentally** at laparotomy should usually undergo diverticulectomy.
F. Meconium ileus
  ■ This is a neonatal intestinal obstruction caused by inspissated meconium that may occur in the setting of cystic fibrosis.
  1. Diagnosis
    a. Prenatal ultrasound. Polyhydramnios.
    b. History and physical exam
      (1) Abdominal distention.
      (2) Bilious vomiting.
      (3) Failure to pass meconium within 24 to 48 hours of life.
      (4) Pneumoperitoneum.
      (5) Peritonitis.
      (6) Abdominal wall inflammation.
      (7) Hypovolemia.
      (8) Sepsis.
    c. Radiology. Plain film.
      (1) Dilated loops of small bowel.
      (2) Ground-glass appearance of air and meconium mixture.
      (3) Intra-abdominal calcifications suggest prenatal perforation and subsequent meconium peritonitis.
      (4) Ascites or **pneumoperitoneum** suggests perforation.
      (5) Up to 35% of infants with complicated meconium ileus show no radiographic abnormalities.
      (6) Water-soluble contrast enema. Confirms diagnosis by demonstrating a **microcolon** and inspissated meconium in the ileum.
  2. Management
    a. Nonsurgical treatment
      (1) Intravenous fluid.
      (2) Broad-spectrum antibiotics.
      (3) Hyperosmolar, water-soluble contrast enema, which is both diagnostic and therapeutic. This solution draws fluid into the bowel lumen and causes an osmotic diarrhea.
    b. Operative intervention
      (1) Indicated for complicated meconium ileus or when enema therapy fails.
      (2) Enterotomy followed by irrigation with 1% to 2% acetylcysteine solution. If gentle irrigation does not flush out the meconium, a 14-French ileostomy tube may be placed, and routine irrigations are done beginning on postoperative day 1.
      (3) If intestinal volvulus, atresia, perforation, or gangrene complicates the illness:
        (a) Resect nonviable bowel.
        (b) Create end ileostomy with mucous fistula.
        (c) Institute routine irrigation.
        (d) Perform primary anastomosis 2 to 3 weeks later.
        (e) Advance oral feeds.
        (f) Institute pancreatic enzyme supplementation.
G. Meconium plug syndrome
  ■ This refers to altered colonic motility or viscous meconium believed to cause impaired stool transit and obstruction of the colonic lumen.
  ■ Patients **do not** have cystic fibrosis.
  1. Diagnosis (see meconium ileus, Section V.F).
  2. Management (see meconium ileus, Section V.F).
    a. Operative intervention is **rarely** needed to relieve the obstruction.

    b. Suction biopsy to rule out Hirschsprung disease.

    c. Sweat chloride test to ensure that cystic fibrosis is not the etiology of the disease.

H. Intestinal duplications
- These are cystic or tubular structures lined by various types of normal GI mucosa.
- They are located dorsal to the true alimentary tract.
- They frequently share a common muscular wall and blood supply with the normal GI tract.
- In 20% of cases, enteric duplications communicate with the true GI tract.
- They are most commonly located in the ileum but may occur anywhere from the mouth to the anus.

  1. Diagnosis
    a. Prenatal ultrasound.
    b. History and physical exam.
      (1) Emesis.
      (2) Abdominal pain.
      (3) Abdominal distention may occur if the duplication compresses the lumen of the adjacent hollow viscus.
      (4) Abdominal mass.
    c. Abdominal ultrasound.
    d. GI contrast studies. External compression or displacement of the normal alimentary tract.
    e. Technetium radioisotope scans. Aid in diagnosis if the cyst contains gastric mucosa.

  2. Operative intervention
    a. Resection.
    b. Internal drainage.
      (1) Minimizes the risk of damage to the biliary system in the case of duodenal duplication.
      (2) May be indicated if duplication would require extensive bowel resection.
      (3) When gastric mucosa is found in a cyst, it is stripped, and the cyst lumen is joined to the adjacent intestine.

I. Acquired causes of alimentary tract obstruction
  1. Pyloric stenosis
- This is the most common surgical cause of nonbilious vomiting in infants.
- It occurs in 1 of 400 live births.
- The male-to-female ratio is 4:1.

    a. Diagnosis
      (1) History and physical
        (a) Occurs generally in neonates who are **2 to 5 weeks of age.**
        (b) Vomiting
          (i) Characteristically forceful or projectile and occurs 30 to 60 minutes after feeding.
          (ii) Formula intolerance initially suspected but does not resolve with change of feeds.
        (c) Dehydration
          (i) Lethargy.
          (ii) Absence of tears.
          (iii) Sunken anterior fontanelle.
          (iv) Dry mucous membranes.
          (v) Decreased urine output.
        (d) The "olive" mass
          (i) Mass palpated to the right and above the umbilicus.
          (ii) Approximately 2 cm in diameter, firm, and mobile.
        (e) Abdominal ultrasonography
          (i) Pyloric **diameter greater than 14 mm,** muscular **thickness greater than 4 mm,** and **pyloric length greater than 16 mm** are diagnostic

of pyloric stenosis with 91% to 100% sensitivity and 100% specificity (*J Pediatr Surg* 1987; 22:950).

(f) Upper GI contrast study
  (i) Enlarged stomach.
  (ii) Poor gastric emptying.
  (iii) Elongated, **narrow pyloric channel or "string sign."**

b. Management
  (1) Preoperative fluid resuscitation
    (a) 20-mL/kg bolus.
    (b) 5% dextrose in normal saline to achieve urine output of 2 mL/kg/hour.
    (c) Addition of potassium and changing to 5% dextrose in 0.45% normal saline occurs when urine output is adequate.
  (2) Correction of the hypochloremic hypokalemic metabolic alkalosis.
  (3) Operative intervention
    (a) Indicated only after adequate resuscitation and correction of metabolic alkalosis.
    (b) Pyloromyotomy
      (i) Division of the hypertrophied pyloric muscle, leaving the mucosa intact.
      (ii) Open or **laparoscopic technique.**
    (c) Postoperative feeding
      (i) Begin electrolyte solution by mouth 6 hours after pyloromyotomy.
      (ii) Over the next 12 hours, formula or pumped breast milk can be started and should reach goal within 24 hours.
      (iii) Parents should be advised that vomiting may occur postoperatively as a result of swelling at the pyloromyotomy, but this problem is self-limited.
      (iv) If the pyloric mucosa is perforated and repaired during surgery, nasogastric drainage is recommended for 24 hours.

2. Intussusception
  • This refers to an invagination of proximal intestine into adjacent distal bowel, with resultant obstruction of the lumen (most common: ileocolic intussusception). A lead point of the intussusception is identified in only 5% of patients and is most commonly a Meckel diverticulum (see Section V.E.1).
  • This obstruction may compromise the arterial inflow and venous return.
  • Highest incidence is at 5 to 10 months of age.

a. Diagnosis
  (1) History and physical exam
    (a) A previously healthy infant who presents with periods of abrupt **crying and retraction of the legs** up to the abdomen.
    (b) Attacks usually subside over a few minutes but recur every 10 to 15 minutes.
    (c) In 30% of cases, a recent viral gastroenteritis or upper respiratory infection may precede onset of symptomatology.
    (d) "Currant jelly" stool. Dark-red mucoid material, which is sloughed mucosa.
    (e) Emesis.
    (f) Hyperperistaltic rushes may be heard during an episode.
    (g) A **sausage-shaped abdominal mass** may be palpated, or the tip of the intussusception may be felt on rectal examination.
  (2) Ultrasound can be used for screening in suspected cases of intussusception.
  (3) Barium or air-contrast enema confirms the diagnosis by demonstrating a **"coiled spring" sign.**

b. Management
  (1) Early surgical consultation.

(2) Nasogastric drainage.

(3) Intravenous fluid resuscitation.

(4) Broad-spectrum antibiotics.

(5) Pneumatic or hydrostatic reduction.

  (a) Air insufflation under radiographic guidance should be attempted if no evidence of peritonitis exists and the patient is stable.

  (b) This technique has a 90% success rate.

  (c) The maximum safe intraluminal air pressure for young infants is 80 mm Hg, and that for older children is 110 to 120 mm Hg.

  (d) Recurrent intussusception in children less than 1 year old can be treated with repeated enema therapy.

  (e) Postreduction course

    (i) Observation for 24 hours.

    (ii) Liquid diet with advancement can be started once the child is alert.

    (iii) Recurrent intussusception occurs in **8% to 12%** of patients.

(6) Operative intervention

  (a) Indications:

    (i) Failure of nonoperative reduction.

    (ii) Child presents with peritonitis, sepsis, or shock.

    (iii) Recurrence after enema reduction in an older child is indicated due to small-bowel tumors, which can serve as the lead point more frequently in this age group.

  (b) A transverse incision can be made to deliver the bowel. Gentle retrograde pressure is applied to the telescoped portion of the intestine in an attempt at manual reduction. Proximal and distal segments should not be pulled apart because of the risk of injury to the bowel.

  (c) If manual reduction is not possible, **resection** of the involved segment and primary anastomosis should be done.

  (d) An incidental appendectomy should also be performed.

  (e) Recurrence of intussusception after operative treatment is approximately **1%.**

3. Distal intestinal obstruction syndrome (DIOS), formerly known as *meconium ileus equivalent*

  • This intestinal obstruction is caused by impaction of inspissated intestinal contents in older patients with cystic fibrosis.

  • This problem occurs in 10% to 40% of patients with cystic fibrosis who are followed long term.

  a. Diagnosis

    (1) High index of suspicion in a child with cystic fibrosis who presents with chronic or recurrent abdominal pain and distention, vomiting, and constipation.

    (2) Inciting cause

      (a) Abrupt cessation of pancreatic enzyme supplementation.

      (b) Dehydration.

      (c) Dietary change.

      (d) Exacerbation of respiratory symptoms.

    (3) Plain abdominal radiographs

      (a) Ground-glass appearance of the intestine.

      (b) Dilated small-bowel.

      (c) Air-fluid levels.

    (4) Water-soluble contrast enemas demonstrate the inspissated intestinal contents.

  b. Management

    (1) Water-soluble contrast enemas induce an osmotic diarrhea to flush the intestine and relieve the obstruction.

(2) GoLytely solution may be used in selective cases to relieve the obstruction from above.

c. **Surgical intervention**

(1) Indicated when enemas or conservative therapy is unsuccessful.

(2) Indicated when intussusception or volvulus complicates DIOS.

VI. JAUNDICE

- This is a yellowing of the skin that reflects the presence of hyperbilirubinemia.
- In jaundiced infants, the total serum bilirubin usually exceeds 7 mg/dL.
- This elevated bilirubin may reflect a rise in either the **conjugated (direct)** or **unconjugated (indirect)** bilirubin, or both. This distinction is integral for establishing a differential diagnosis for jaundice.

A. **Unconjugated hyperbilirubinemia**

1. This occurs when bilirubin that has not been metabolized in the liver rises above normal serum values.

2. Most common causes:

a. Hemolytic disorders.

b. Breast-feeding.

c. Physiologic jaundice of the newborn.

d. Indirect causes of increased enterohepatic circulation of bilirubin (rare)

(1) Meconium ileus.

(2) Hirschsprung disease.

(3) Pyloric stenosis.

3. Treatment

a. Phototherapy.

b. Exchange transfusion.

c. Correction of primary diseases.

B. **Conjugated hyperbilirubinemia**

- This occurs when excess monoglucuronides and diglucuronides in the liver result in elevated levels of bilirubin in the serum. Most common causes:
  - Biliary obstruction
  - Hepatitis (infectious, toxic, or metabolic etiology)
  - TORCH (*t*oxoplasmosis, *r*ubella, *c*ytomegalovirus, and *h*erpes simplex virus) infections
- Treatment
  - Identify and treat etiologies of hepatitis.
  - Surgical interventions are only possible with the obstructive causes of direct hyperbilirubinemia discussed here.

1. **Biliary atresia**

a. Most common cause of infantile jaundice that requires surgical correction.

b. Etiology is unknown.

c. Disease characteristics

(1) Progressive obliteration and sclerosis of the biliary tree.

(2) With age, obliteration of the extrahepatic bile ducts, proliferation of the intrahepatic bile ducts, and liver fibrosis progress at an unpredictable rate.

d. **Diagnosis**

(1) Clinical and laboratory information is often nonspecific.

(2) Jaundice.

(3) Alcoholic stools.

(4) Dark urine.

(5) Hepatomegaly.

(6) Percutaneous liver biopsy. Biopsy results range from classic biliary tree fibrosis to those unable to be differentiated from α1-antitrypsin deficiency or neonatal hepatitis.

(7) Technetium-99m iminodiacetic acid hepatobiliary imaging

(a) Aids in differentiation between liver parenchymal disease and biliary obstructive disease.

(b) In biliary atresia, the liver readily takes up this tracer molecule, but no excretion into the extrahepatic biliary system or duodenum is seen.

(8) Ultrasonography. Shrunken extrahepatic ducts and a noncontractile or absent gallbladder.

e. Management

(1) Open **liver biopsy** and **cholangiogram**

(a) The common bile duct is visualized by cholangiography in only 25% of patients with biliary atresia.

(b) Cholangiography in the remaining 75% of patients demonstrates an atretic biliary tree.

(2) Operative intervention

(a) Kasai procedure

(i) "Hepatoportoenterostomy."

(ii) Excision of obliterated extrahepatic ducts with hepaticojejunostomy.

(iii) When the distal common bile duct is patent, a choledochojejunostomy is constructed.

(iv) The overall results have shown that in children treated with a Kasai procedure, one third show long-term improvement, one third obtain temporary benefit, and one third experience treatment failure. Five-year survival for infants treated with a Kasai procedure before 2.5 months of age was 50% (*Ann Surg* 1989;210:289).

(b) Liver transplantation. Recommended option when liver failure occurs or the Kasai procedure fails.

2. Choledochal cysts

- This spectrum of diseases is characterized by cystic dilation of the extrahepatic and intrahepatic biliary tree.
- They are believed to be an embryologic malformation of the pancreaticobiliary system.
- **Type I:** fusiform cystic dilation of the common bile duct (most common form).
- **Type II: diverticulum of the extrahepatic bile duct.**
- **Type III: choledoochocele.**
- **Type IV:** cystic disease of the intra- or extrahepatic bile ducts.
- **Type V:** single or multiple intrahepatic ducts.

a. Diagnosis

(1) Approximately 50% of children present within the first 10 years of life.

(2) History and physical exam.

(a) Asymptomatic jaundice.

(b) Abdominal pain.

(c) Jaundice.

(d) Abdominal mass.

(e) Cholangitis.

(f) Pancreatitis.

(g) Portal hypertension.

(h) Hepatic abscess.

(i) Cyst rupture.

(3) Ultrasonography.

(4) Hepatobiliary scintigraphy.

(5) Transhepatic cholangiography.

(6) Magnetic resonance cholangiopancreatography (MRCP).

(7) Endoscopic retrograde cholangiopancreatography. Superior definition of intrahepatic and extrahepatic ductal disease.

b. Management

(1) Cyst excision

(a) Entire cyst excision when possible.

(b) Shelling out the inner wall and cyst contents.

(c) It is important to identify the entrance of the pancreatic duct into the biliary tree before the excision is complete.

    (2) Choledochojejunostomy.

    (3) Hepatic resection. Disease is intrahepatic and limited to a lobe or segment of the liver.

    (4) Liver transplantation. For diffuse intrahepatic disease.

VII. GROIN MASSES

A. Indirect inguinal hernias

- Approximately 1% to 5% of children are affected.
- Boys are affected more than girls, with an 8:1 ratio.
- Prematurity increases the incidence of inguinal hernia to between 7% and 30%.
- Incidence of bilateral hernias ranges from 10% to 40%.
- Bilateral hernias occur more frequently in premature infants and in girls.

1. Diagnosis. History and physical examination:

    a. Groin bulge extending toward the scrotum or vulva either by history or observation.

    b. Sometimes reproduced only when child laughs, cries, or stands.

    c. Thickened spermatic cord.

2. Management

    a. Reducible hernias

        (1) Elective repair with high ligation of sac through a low abdominal incision.

        (2) Hernia sac is anterior and medial to the spermatic cord in boys and more difficult to locate among the muscle fibers running through the external ring in girls.

        (3) Sac can contain small bowel, omentum, or ovary.

    b. Incarcerated hernias

        (1) Most can be reduced with gentle direct pressure on the hernia.

        (2) Simultaneously applying caudal traction on the testicle in addition to direct pressure on the hernia may be necessary in some cases.

    c. Strangulated hernias

        (1) Emergent operative repair is indicated.

        (2) Even if a severely incarcerated/strangulated hernia is reduced, the child should be admitted and scheduled for urgent herniorrhaphy.

        (3) If viability of sac contents is in question, the bowel must be examined before abdominal closure.

B. Hydroceles

- Fluid collections within the processus vaginalis that envelop the testicle.
- Occur in approximately 6% of full-term male newborns.

1. Communicating

    a. Free flow of peritoneal cavity fluid down to scrotum.

    b. Processus vaginalis is patent.

    c. Must be regarded as a hernia, with elective repair encouraged to prevent subsequent incarceration.

2. Noncommunicating

    a. A portion of the processus vaginalis obliterates normally.

    b. Fluid remains confined to the scrotum.

    c. Usually self-limiting and resolve in 6 to 12 months.

VIII. ABDOMINAL PAIN

A. Common complaint in the pediatric age group (see Table 32-4)

B. Differential diagnosis must take the following into consideration:

    1. Age.

    2. Gender.

    3. Duration of symptoms.

    4. Circumstances at onset.

    5. Modifying factors.

C. History of the present illness

    1. This is often difficult to obtain from a child; therefore, parents should be present to corroborate accurate information.

TABLE 32-4	Etiologies of Pediatric Abdominal Pain	
Very common causes	**Less common causes**	**Rare causes**
Acute appendicitis	Intussusception	Henoch-Schönlein purpura
Viral infection	Lower lobe pneumonia	Nephrotic syndromes
Gastroenteritis	Intestinal obstruction	Pancreatitis
Constipation	Urinary tract obstruction	Hepatitis
Genitourinary tract infection	Inguinal hernia	Diabetic ketoacidosis
Trauma	Meckel diverticulum	Lead poisoning
	Cholecystitis	Acute porphyria
	Intra-abdominal mass	Herpes zoster
		Sickle cell anemia

   2. Characteristics of pain:
      a. Quality (sharp/dull, episodic/constant).
      b. Onset.
      c. Location.
      d. Duration.
      e. Presence of exacerbating or relieving factors.
   3. Associated symptoms:
      a. Emesis (bilious/nonbilious, bloody/foul).
      b. Diarrhea/constipation.
      c. Melena/hematochezia.
      d. Fever.
D. Physical examination
   1. General toxic appearance.
   2. Patient's ease and comfort are integral to a thorough and accurate physical exam.
   3. Elicit presence of **peritonitis**
      a. Palpation.
      b. Percussion.
      c. Manipulation of the hip.
      d. Deep respiratory movements.
      e. Rectal examination.
   4. Palpate **masses.**
   5. Localize pain.
   6. Bimanual pelvic exam in age appropriate patient.
IX. TUMORS AND NEOPLASMS
   A. Neuroblastoma
      ■ Neoplasm of the sympathochromaffin system.
      ■ Incidence of approximately 8 new cases per million children per year.
      ■ Most common extracranial tumor of childhood.
      ■ Accounts for 10% of all pediatric malignancies.
      ■ Median age at diagnosis is 2 years, with 85% of the tumors being diagnosed before age 5 years.
      1. Diagnosis
         a. Incidental finding on radiographic studies performed for other reasons.
         b. Detection of abdominal mass by the parents or pediatrician.
         c. Rarely, children present with symptoms of fever, malaise, or abdominal pain.
         d. At the time of discovery, up to 75% of neuroblastomas are metastatic.
         e. Regional lymph nodes.
         f. Liver.
         g. Skin.
         h. Bone.
         i. Orbits.

TABLE 32-5	International Neuroblastoma Staging System

Stage	Characteristics
1	Localized tumor confined to the area of origin; complete gross excision with or without microscopic residual disease; identifiable ipsilateral and contralateral lymph nodes negative microscopically
2A	Unilateral tumor with incomplete gross excision; identifiable ipsilateral and contralateral lymph nodes negative microscopically
2B	Unilateral tumor with complete or incomplete gross excision; with positive ipsilateral regional lymph nodes; identifiable contralateral lymph nodes negative microscopically
3	Tumor infiltrating across the midline with or without regional lymph node involvement; or unilateral tumor with contralateral regional lymph node involvement; or midline tumor with bilateral tumor involvement
4	Dissemination of tumor to distant lymph nodes, bone, bone marrow, liver, or other organs (except as defined in stage 4S)
4S	Localized primary tumor as defined for stage 1 or 2 with dissemination limited to liver, skin, or bone marrow

    2. International Neuroblastoma Staging System

      a. This system places patients in low-, intermediate-, or high-risk groups based on age, surgical staging, and status of **N-*myc* oncogene** because these factors significantly predict outcome.

      b. Children younger than 12 months at the time of diagnosis have a better prognosis for cure, whereas in older patients with disseminated disease, the prognosis remains poor.

      c. Incorporates **clinical, radiographic,** and **surgical** information to define the tumor stage (Table 32-5).

        (1) Plain radiographs of the chest and skull.

        (2) Bone scan.

        (3) CT scan.

        (4) Bone marrow aspirate.

        (5) ^{131}I-meta-iodobenzylguanidine (MIBG) scan.

        (6) Operative evaluation may also be necessary for accurate staging.

    3. Surgical treatment

      a. Local disease

        (1) Complete excision of the tumor.

        (2) Lymph node sampling.

      b. Bulky or **metastatic** disease

        (1) Tumor biopsy.

        (2) Chemotherapy.

        (3) Radiotherapy.

        (4) If tumor shrinkage occurs with chemo and radiotherapy, delayed resection can take place.

B. Wilms tumor

    ■ This tumor accounts for 6% of all malignancies in children.

    ■ It is the most common renal malignancy in children.

    ■ Most children are diagnosed between 1 and 3 years of age.

    ■ Annual incidence is approximately 5 to 7.8 per 1 million children younger than 15 years.

    ■ Bilateral in 5% of cases.

    ■ Gender distribution is equal.

    1. Diagnosis

      a. History

    (1) Abdominal pain.

    (2) Fever.

    (3) Hematuria.

    (4) Urinary tract infection.

  b. Physical examination

    (1) 85% of these children have a palpable flank or abdominal mass.

    (2) Associated anomalies:

      (a) Hemihypertrophy (2%).

      (b) Aniridia (1%).

      (c) Genitourinary anomalies (5%).

  c. Abdominal ultrasonography

    (1) Distinguish an intrarenal mass (Wilms tumor) from an extrarenal mass (neuroblastoma).

    (2) Rule out tumor extension into the renal vein or vena cava.

  d. Abdominal and chest CT scans

    (1) Necessary for staging.

    (2) Evaluate contralateral kidney.

    (3) Screen for pulmonary metastases.

  e. Histologic examination confirms the diagnosis.

2. Management

  a. Surgery and **chemotherapy** together result in a better than 90% chance of cure.

  b. Surgical intervention.

    (1) Radical nephrectomy.

    (2) Sample para-aortic lymph nodes.

    (3) Isolation of the hilar vessels and examination of the contralateral kidney also are required.

    (4) If the Wilms tumor is found initially to be unresectable because of size or bilaterality, a second-look operation can be done after chemotherapy.

  c. Chemotherapy. Vincristine, doxorubicin, and dactinomycin are used, depending on the stage of the Wilms tumor.

  d. Radiotherapy is used for advanced stages of Wilms tumor.

C. Hepatic tumors

  ■ These make up fewer than 5% of all intra-abdominal malignancies.

  ■ They are malignant in 70% of cases.

  ■ **Hepatoblastoma**

    • 39% of liver tumors.

    • 90% occur before 3 years of age.

    • 60% are diagnosed by 1 year of age.

  ■ **Hepatocellular carcinoma**

    • Presents in older children.

    • Approximately one third of these patients have cirrhosis secondary to an inherited metabolic abnormality.

1. Diagnosis

  a. History and physical exam

    (1) Abdominal pain.

    (2) Enlarging abdominal mass.

  b. Elevated serum **AFP**

  c. Radiology

    (1) CT or **MR scan.**

    (2) Angiography.

2. Management

  a. Surgical intervention

    (1) Primary tumor resection and lymph node sampling. Intraoperative histologic analysis of the liver margins is necessary to confirm complete removal of the tumor.

    (2) Hepatoblastoma that is not initially resectable undergoes chemotherapy and reexploration for curative resection.

D. Teratomas

- These are composed of tissues from all germ layers (endoderm, ectoderm, and mesoderm).
- In neonates, sacrococcygeal teratomas are the most common.
- They are more common in girls (4:1).

1. Diagnosis
   a. Prenatal/antenatal ultrasound.
   b. CT scan.
   c. Rectal exam.

2. Management
   a. Antenatal diagnosis may necessitate delivery by cesarean section.
   b. Surgical intervention:
      (1) Resection through a chevron-shaped buttocks incision during the first week of life.
      (2) Principles important in resection of the tumor include preservation of the rectal sphincter muscles, resection of the coccyx with the tumor, and early control of the midsacral vessels that supply the tumor.
      (3) May require combined abdominal and perineal approach for large intra-abdominal teratomas.
   c. Chemotherapy for malignant teratomas. May shrink the tumor and allow for resection.

3. Complications
   a. Hemorrhage.
   b. Recurrence. High rate of recurrence if the coccyx incompletely resected.
   c. Malignancy
      (1) Rarely seen in neonates but increases with the age of the child.
      (2) If the tumor is malignant, a thorough search for metastases is needed.

E. Soft-tissue sarcomas

- These account for 6% of childhood malignancies.
- Greater than one half are rhabdomyosarcomas.

1. Diagnosis
   a. CT scan.
   b. MR scan.
   c. Incisional biopsy usually is required to determine the histologic type preoperatively.

2. Management
   a. Consultation with a radiotherapist and oncologist before initiating therapy is advised.
   b. Nonrhabdomyosarcomas. Wide surgical excision.
   c. Rhabdomyosarcoma
      (1) Treatment is determined by the location of the tumor.
      (2) Complete resection of **head and neck tumors** is rarely possible, and they usually are treated with biopsy followed by chemotherapy.
      (3) Trunk and retroperitoneal tumors are treated with wide excision.
      (4) Extremity tumors also are treated with wide excision, but resection of muscle groups and the use of radiotherapy or brachytherapy should also be considered (*Surg Clin North Am* 1992;72:1417).
      (5) A biopsy of the regional lymph nodes should be included in all procedures.

X. FETAL SURGERY

Most disorders diagnosed in the antenatal period are best managed after birth. However, a few disorders with devastating developmental consequences may benefit from fetal treatment. The fundamental conflict in fetal surgery is balancing the risks to both mother and fetus against the potential benefit to only the fetus. Over two decades of rigorous groundwork has resulted in safe surgical intervention for several anomalies.

A. Congenital diaphragmatic hernia
   1. To promote growth of the lungs and reverse the effects of potentially lethal pulmonary hypoplasia.

    2. Method of repair.
      a. Tracheal balloon occlusion with lung distension
        (1) Eligibility criteria: CDH with liver in chest and a ratio of lung to head of less than 1.4.
        (2) Pilot study survival: 75% versus 45% to 50% controls repaired after birth.

B. Obstructive uropathy
    1. Posterior urethral valves lead to oligohydramnios, pulmonary hypoplasia, and death.
    2. Percutaneous vesicoamniotic shunt placement.

C. Congenital cystic adenomatoid malformation
    1. Most fetuses diagnosed with a cystic pulmonary lesion either undergo surveillance with spontaneous resolution or require neonatal treatment.
    2. A small subset with large lung lesions who become hydropic and deteriorate may benefit from maternal hysterotomy, fetal thoracotomy, and resection of the mass.

D. Sacrococcygeal teratoma
    1. High blood flow into the tumor can result in cardiac failure and fetal hydrops.
    2. Maternal hysterotomy and resection can be lifesaving.
    3. Recently, radiofrequency ablation of tumor's arterial flow has shown promise, but it carries a high risk to the fetus (*Am J Obstet Gynecol* 2001;184:503).

E. Twin–twin transfusion syndrome
    1. Placental vascular connections result in one twin "stealing" the blood supply from the other twin, resulting in death of both twins.
    2. Randomized, controlled trials are under way in both Europe and the United States comparing fetoscopic laser ablation of abnormal placental vessels with amnioreduction (*Am J Obstet Gynecol* 2001;185:708).

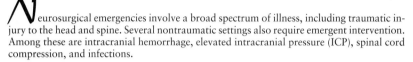

NEUROSURGICAL EMERGENCIES

Daniel Refai, James Johnston, and Michael R. Chicoine

33

*N*eurosurgical emergencies involve a broad spectrum of illness, including traumatic injury to the head and spine. Several nontraumatic settings also require emergent intervention. Among these are intracranial hemorrhage, elevated intracranial pressure (ICP), spinal cord compression, and infections.

NEUROSURGICAL TRAUMA

I. INTRACRANIAL TRAUMA

A. Evaluation. Initial management of head injury focuses on hemodynamic stabilization through establishment of an adequate airway, ventilation, and support of circulation, followed by the rapid diagnosis and treatment of intracranial injuries.

1. **Airway and ventilation.** Severe head injury frequently leads to failure of oxygenation, ventilation, or airway protection; therefore, intubation in these cases is essential. A rapid neurologic assessment performed before sedation and paralysis are induced is critical. A low threshold for intubation must be present for agitated patients requiring sedation. When possible, cervical spine films should be assessed before intubation. In situations of acute compromise, intubation should proceed even before complete evaluation of the cervical spine. Two-person in-line intubation is performed, with the second individual securing the patient's neck with axial traction to avoid extension of the neck during intubation. Nasal intubation can be performed if craniofacial injuries do not otherwise contraindicate this procedure. Associated cervical spine injuries should be assumed in the patient with a head injury until they are ruled out.

2. **Circulatory support** requires aggressive fluid resuscitation for treatment of arterial hypotension, followed by blood products, if necessary, and identification of the etiology of the hypotension. Head injury with intracranial hemorrhage is almost never the sole cause of systemic hypotension (in the absence of profuse scalp bleeding). Impairment in mental status cannot be adequately assessed until mean arterial pressure (MAP) and thus cerebral perfusion pressure (cerebral perfusion pressure = MAP – intracranial pressure) are corrected. In addition, the use of hypotonic fluids should be avoided in patients with head injuries because this could exacerbate cerebral edema.

B. Neurologic evaluation

1. **A rapid but systematic** neurologic examination is performed on the scene and is repeated frequently during transport and on initial presentation to the emergency room. Examination focuses on the three components of the **Glasgow Coma Scale** (GCS) (Table 33-1): eye opening, verbal response, and motor response (*Lancet* 1974;2:81). This score indicates injury severity and measures changes in the impairment of consciousness. Pupillary response, extraocular movements, and facial movements should be examined, and the remainder of the cranial nerve examination should be performed. The pupils of a head-injured patient should never be pharmacologically dilated in the acute setting because changes in pupillary reaction can be early signs of herniation. Strength and symmetry of the extremities should be noted as part of the search for evidence of cerebral or spinal cord damage. The sensory examination should be performed as thoroughly as the level

TABLE 33-1	Glasgow Coma Scale[a]
Component	**Points**
Eye opening	
Spontaneous	4
To voice	3
To stimulation	2
None	1
Motor response	
To command	6
Localizes	5
Withdraws	4
Abnormal flexion	3
Extension	2
None	1
Verbal response	
Oriented	5
Confused but comprehensible	4
Inappropriate or incoherent	3
Incomprehensible (no words)	2
None	1

[a]Glasgow Coma Score = best eye opening + best motor response + best verbal response. If patient is intubated, the verbal score is omitted and an addendum of "T" is given to the best eye opening + best motor response score.

of consciousness permits. Useful landmarks for sensory dermatomes include the nipple (T4 level) and the umbilicus (T10 level). Reflexes and sphincter tone should also be assessed. Finally, the head-injured patient has a high incidence of associated injuries. Cervical spine evaluation is obligatory (see Sections IV.A.3 and IV.A.4). Thorough examination is essential, even in patients believed to have an isolated closed-head injury. Unnecessary sedation and prolonged pharmacologic paralysis in head-injured patients can make neurologic assessment difficult and should be avoided.

2. **Systemic causes** of mental status impairment must be ruled out. Metabolic (electrolyte or acid-base abnormalities, hypo- and hyperglycemia), toxic (drugs, uremia), hypothermic, or respiratory (hypoxia, hypercapnia) derangements can underlie mental status changes, even if closed-head injury is present. Recent seizures or cardiac arrest can also impair neurologic function severely.

C. **Radiographic evaluation** begins with cervical spine plain x-rays, including anteroposterior, lateral, open-mouth (odontoid) views, and a lateral swimmer's view if needed (see Section IV.A.4.a). The initial emergency room evaluation should proceed rapidly to head computed tomographic (CT) scanning. Delay caused by evaluation of non–life-threatening injuries should be avoided until the patient's head is imaged. Centers without this capability should stabilize the vital signs, secure the airway, and arrange for rapid transfer of the patient to a facility with head CT scanning and neurosurgical facilities.

D. **Initial therapies**

1. **If elevated intracranial pressure** is suspected, such as with signs of herniation or acute neurologic deterioration, therapy should be initiated until the ICP can be measured. If the patient is hemodynamically stable, high-dose **mannitol** (0.25- to 1-g/kg intravenous bolus) is effective in controlling raised ICP acutely. A Foley catheter should be placed to follow the osmotic diuresis closely after mannitol administration. Fluid replacement may be necessary to avoid hypotension because a euvolemic, hyperosmolar situation is desirable. Ventilatory support to maintain

a mildly hypocapnic partial pressure of carbon dioxide (PCO_2) ($\sim$35 mm Hg) should be instituted. For refractory elevated ICP, **hyperventilation** (PCO_2 $\sim$30 mm Hg) may be used only in the acute setting for brief periods. Prolonged use of hyperventilation should not be used to control elevated ICP and may worsen ischemia by compromising cerebral blood flow. There is no proven role for steroids in the management of acute head injury.

2. **Seizures** should be controlled rapidly in patients with head injury. Intravenous lorazepam can be administered in 1-mg boluses and repeated until seizures are controlled. Airway protection must be available if significant doses of benzo-diazepines are to be given. Phenytoin (Dilantin) should also be administered for seizures and is indicated for seizure prophylaxis in patients at high risk for early posttraumatic seizures (GCS = 10 or less, intracranial hematoma, depressed skull fracture, cortical contusion visible on CT, penetrating or open injuries) for a duration of no more than 7 days if the patient remains seizure free (*N Engl J Med* 1990;323:497). A loading dose of phenytoin or fosphenytoin (Cerebyx) in patients with poor intravenous access or status epilepticus may be given. Maintenance doses of phenytoin should then be started and drug levels followed to guide dosing. In patients with hepatic disease, an alternative to Dilantin use is levetiracetam (Keppra). Keppra can be loaded orally at 1,000 mg and then continued at 500 to 1,000 mg orally twice a day. However, there are no class I data on the use of Keppra and the prevention of early posttraumatic seizures.

II. TYPES OF HEAD INJURY

A. **Focal (mass) lesions** are best diagnosed by emergent CT scan of the head without contrast. Hemiparesis, unilateral pupillary dysfunction (the fixed and dilated pupil), or both can herald brainstem herniation from mass lesions, but these are imperfect localizing signs (*Neurosurgery* 1994;34:840); therefore, CT scan is imperative. Relative indications for surgical evacuation include neurologic symptoms referable to the mass lesion, midline shift greater than 5 mm, and elevated ICP that is refractory to medical management. Posterior fossa mass lesions can be particularly dangerous because brainstem herniation may have very few specific warning signs before death occurs (see Section V.A.2.b).

1. **Epidural and subdural hematomas (SDHs)** can cause rapid deterioration and usually require surgical evacuation. Classically, epidural hematomas present with a "lucid interval" after injury, which precedes rapid deterioration. This sign is inconsistent and nonspecific and may also be seen with SDHs. Epidural hematomas appear on head CT scan as biconvex hyperdensities that typically respect the suture lines, and they are operated on emergently if they are causing significant mass effect, symptoms, or both.

2. **Acute SDHs** typically appear on head CT scan as hyperdense crescents as the blood spreads around the surface of the brain. Often, SDHs are associated with severe intracranial injury. If surgical evacuation is indicated and delayed for more than 4 hours, these lesions have a high mortality (*J Neurosurg* 1991;74:212, *N Engl J Med* 1981;304:1511).

3. **SDHs** also can present, especially in the elderly, days to weeks after head injury. These **chronic SDHs** can cause focal neurologic deficit, mental status changes, metabolic abnormalities, and seizures. If necessary, a symptomatic chronic SDH can be treated with burr-hole drainage with subdural drain placement (*J Neurosurg* 1986;65:183). Prophylactic anticonvulsants should be considered, and steroids may be beneficial. Diagnosis is best made with CT scan.

B. **Nonfocal** sequelae of head injury include **cerebral edema** and **diffuse axonal injury (DAI).** Hallmarks of cerebral edema on head CT scan include obliteration of the basal cisterns and coronal sulci and loss of differentiation of the gray and white matter. In DAI, severe head injury can be associated with minimal changes on head CT scan (*J Neurosurg* 1982;56:26). DAI represents the pathologic result of shearing forces on the brain. Often, small hemorrhages are seen in corpus callosum, midbrain, or deep white matter. Microscopic injury to axons may result in severe neurologic dysfunction.

C. **Open injuries and fractures. Open skull fractures** require operative irrigation, débridement of nonviable tissues, and dural closure. Evaluation of scalp lacerations should include attention to the presence of underlying skull fractures. Prophylactic antibiotics may reduce the risk of infection. Surgical treatment of **depressed skull fractures** usually is required for depressions greater than the thickness of the skull table. Open, depressed skull fractures require elevation and débridement of depressed skull fragments as well as devitalized tissue, followed by a course of antibiotics. Fractures through the paranasal air **sinuses,** especially with associated pneumocephalus and dural tears, may require repair. Often, repair is performed in combination with repair of associated facial fractures. The prophylactic use of broad-spectrum antibiotics to prevent meningitis in these cases is controversial.

D. **Basilar skull fractures** can be complicated by **cerebrospinal fluid (CSF)** leaks, and are managed nonoperatively. The use of prophylactic antibiotics is controversial. If drainage continues or recurs, a lumbar drain or surgical repair may be required because persistent leakage can lead to meningitis. Temporal bone fractures can be associated with damage to the seventh and eighth cranial nerves, the middle ear apparatus, or both.

E. **Missile injuries** require débridement, closure, and prophylactic antibiotics similar to those used for other open-head injuries. However, injuries from gunshot wounds present several associated problems. Shock waves can result in widespread destruction of brain tissue and vasculature. Operative management must address removal of accessible foreign bodies and bone fragments, evacuation of intracranial hematomas, débridement of entrance and exit wounds, and closure of dura and scalp. Overaggressive débridement near large vessels should be avoided to prevent further damage to vascular structures.

III. MANAGEMENT OF ELEVATED ICP

A. Monitoring

1. **Indications.** ICP monitoring generally is recommended in head injury if serial neurologic examinations cannot be used as a reliable indicator of progressive intracranial pathology. The current standard for ICP monitoring is in patients with abnormal head CT scans and GCS scores less than 8, or in individuals with normal head CT scans but GCS scores greater than 8, if two of the following three criteria are met: (1) age greater than 40 years, (2) unilateral or bilateral motor posturing, and (3) systemic blood pressure less than 90 mm Hg on admission (*J Neurosurg* 1982;56:650).

2. **ICP pressure monitors** are of several types. The **parenchymal bolt** consists of a fiberoptic or strain gauge catheter tip that measures ICP at the brain surface. **Intraventricular catheters** (ventriculostomy) are placed in the lateral ventricle with the tip at the foramen of Monro. In addition, intraventricular catheters allow for the drainage of CSF in the treatment of elevated ICP (see Section I.D.1). Newer monitors include devices that measure intracranial pressure, cerebral temperature, and brain tissue oxygenation, and the utility of such devices is under investigation.

B. Treatment

1. In addition to initial treatment of elevated ICP (e.g., mannitol, mechanical ventilation), **simple measures** are taken, such as head elevation to 30 degrees, a neutral head position to enhance venous drainage, avoidance of circumferential taping around the patient's neck when securing the endotracheal tube, appropriate fitting of cervical spine collars if indicated, and adequate sedation before any stimulation, such as intubation. Elevated intrathoracic pressures (as with coughing, straining, or high positive end-expiratory pressure) can elevate ICP. Fever can also exacerbate ICP, and aggressive treatment with antipyretics, cooling blankets, and intravascular cooling devices should be instituted to prevent hyperthermia.

2. Further treatment is aimed at keeping ICP less than 20 mm Hg (*J Neurosurg* 1991;75:S59), usually with **high-dose mannitol** (25- to 50-g intravenous boluses every 6 hours). High-dose mannitol may have a beneficial effect on mortality when compared with phenobarbital (*Cochrane Database Syst Rev* 2005;4:CD003983). Hypertonic saline has recently emerged as a useful adjunct to mannitol in the control of elevated intracranial pressure (*Crit Care Med* 2003;31:1683). Fluid

balance, serum electrolytes, and serum osmolarity should be carefully monitored; euvolemia must be maintained. Diuretics generally are held if serum osmolarity exceeds 320 mOsm/L. In addition, hypotension should be avoided in these patients, and there are some data that suggest that better outcomes occur with maintenance of cerebral perfusion pressure (MAP – ICP) of 60 mm Hg or greater (see Section III.C.1).

3. **Sedation** can also be used to control ICP. Benzodiazepine or narcotic (e.g., fentanyl) infusions can be given and titrated to effect, with a goal of 3 on the Ramsay sedation scale (*Br Med J* 1974;11:659). Intubation and mechanical ventilation usually are needed. Refractory elevation of ICP may require neuromuscular paralysis or even barbiturate coma with invasive hemodynamic monitoring.

4. **Surgical interventions** are directed primarily at removal of **mass lesions,** if present. In the absence of a mass lesion, uncontrollable ICP and a deteriorating neurologic examination may require **craniectomy,** with removal of a large bone flap to relieve pressure on the intracranial contents. Retrospective studies suggest that decompressive hemicraniectomy for uncontrolled intracranial hypertension may decrease mortality and improve outcomes in certain patients (*J Neurosurg* 2006;104:469). Multicenter, prospective studies are underway to better evaluate the indications for surgical intervention in this difficult patient population (*Acta Neurochir Suppl* 2006;96:17). Removal of CSF by **ventriculostomy** can reduce ICP; however, the small intracranial volume occupied by the CSF limits this effect.

C. **Frequently associated complications**
1. **Cardiac considerations.** Adequate blood pressure should be maintained in the setting of elevated ICP, with care taken to avoid hypotension (systolic blood pressure <90 mm Hg), which has been associated with worse outcome in severely head injured patients (*Br J Neurosurg* 1993;7:267). Maintenance of cerebral perfusion pressure greater than 60 mm Hg (or MAP >80 to 90 mm Hg) can be used as a treatment guideline (*Crit Care* 2000;9(6):R670).

2. **Respiratory considerations.** Early airway control is essential in the head-injured patient. Severe head injury is also associated with ventilation-perfusion mismatch and development of pulmonary edema or adult respiratory distress syndrome.

3. **Gastrointestinal (GI) considerations.** Patients with severe head injury and increased ICP are at risk of developing Cushing (stress) ulcers and GI bleeding. These patients should undergo prophylaxis with H_2 antagonists, proton-pump inhibitors, or sucralfate.

4. **Fluid and electrolytes.** Head-injured patients are at risk for development of either diabetes insipidus or the syndrome of inappropriate antidiuretic hormone. Initially, the use of isotonic saline (with glucose and, if necessary, potassium) avoids exacerbating cerebral edema. Close monitoring of electrolytes is essential because alterations in sodium and water balance are common. **Diabetes insipidus** can develop rapidly and must be treated aggressively. Fluid hydration should match output. Often, the process is self-limiting, but persistent output of large amounts (>300 mL/hour) of urine with a low specific gravity (<1.005) may necessitate vasopressin treatment [desmopressin (DDAVP), 1 μg intravenously every 12 hours]. If the syndrome of inappropriate antidiuretic hormone with hyponatremia develops, treatment with restriction of free water intake usually is sufficient, although infusion of hypertonic (1.5% NaCl) saline may be necessary.

5. **Hematologic considerations.** Disseminated intravascular coagulopathy can occur with severe head injury, such as missile injuries, often developing several hours after the disruption of brain tissue. Coagulopathies should be aggressively treated with fresh-frozen plasma and vitamin K (10 mg/day intramuscularly), especially if intracranial hemorrhage is present.

6. **Nutrition.** Nutritional demands are increased in head injury (*Neurosurg Clin North Am* 1991;2:301). High-osmolarity tube feedings can reduce the risk of cerebral edema and provide adequate caloric intake. If tube feedings are not tolerated, parenteral nutrition may be necessary.

7. **Associated injuries.** A thorough assessment for other systemic and orthopedic injuries is essential. The unconscious patient should always be assumed to have

a cervical spine injury until this is ruled out with appropriate radiographic tests. A growing body of evidence demonstrates increased sensitivity of computed tomography in detecting spine fractures in blunt trauma patients compared with plain radiography (*J Trauma* 2006;61:382).

8. **Deep venous thrombosis prophylaxis.** Patients with severe head injury are at high risk for deep venous thrombosis and subsequent pulmonary embolism. Early use of intermittent pneumatic compression devices is highly recommended. Although efficacy remains controversial, recent studies suggest no increased risk of intracranial hemorrhage in head-injured patients who receive subcutaneous heparin (*J Trauma* 2002;53:38) or enoxaparin (*Arch Surg* 2002;137:701) within 72 hours of admission.

9. **Mild head injury.** Management of the patient with a mild head injury (presenting GCS score of 13 to 15) focuses on detecting and rapidly treating those at risk for subsequent deterioration (*J Neurosurg* 1986;65:203). Selection of those at higher risk for delayed mass lesion, associated fracture, elevated ICP, and CSF leaks is needed. A normal CT scan without altered level of consciousness, neurologic deficit, or open injuries may allow the patient to be discharged to home with reliable supervision. Any exceptions may indicate a more severe injury with a higher risk of associated or delayed lesions and may require the patient to be admitted for observation.

IV. **SPINAL TRAUMA. Evaluation** for spinal injury is indicated if focal pain, neurologic examination, or mechanism of injury warrants. Neurologic deficit involving the lower extremities after trauma may require evaluation of the entire spine to find an injury.

A. **Initial support**
1. **Airway and breathing.** Intubation should be performed early in patients demonstrating respiratory fatigue or otherwise requiring airway protection or ventilatory support. In the presence of cervical spine injury, fiberoptic intubation requires less manipulation and reduces the risk of further neurologic injury.

2. **Circulation.** Nonneurologic sources of hypotension must be pursued thoroughly. In patients with obvious external hemorrhage or suspected hypovolemic shock, standard fluid resuscitation should be initiated. In the paraplegic or quadriplegic patient, if no blood loss is suspected and fluid challenges do not improve perfusion, diagnosis of **spinal shock** should be considered. Hypotension associated with the loss of sympathetic tone seen in some high thoracic and cervical spine injuries does not respond to fluids alone. Pressors (e.g., dopamine) reduce peripheral vasodilatation and improve cardiac output. Excessive fluid administration can worsen respiratory difficulty and spinal cord edema.

3. **Neurologic examination.** This includes a careful assessment of motor and sensory function and deep tendon reflexes. Multiple sensory modalities (light touch, pinprick, temperature sensation, and joint position sense) should be assessed, especially in the patient with an incomplete lesion. Deep tendon reflexes, sphincter tone, and cremasteric and bulbocavernosus reflexes should be documented. Incomplete lesions are common and, as with sacral sparing of sensory function, carry prognostic significance (*Neurosurgery* 1987;20:742).

4. **Radiographic evaluation**
   a. Standard radiographic evaluation of the cervical spine includes **anteroposterior, lateral, and open-mouth (odontoid)** views. A **swimmer's** view may be necessary to visualize C7 and the C7–T1 interspace, which is essential in complete evaluation of the cervical spine. CT scanning with coronal and sagittal reconstructions is necessary if adequate plain films cannot be obtained and is replacing radiography as the standard of care in patients with blunt trauma (*J Trauma* 2006;61:382). Of note, flexion extension films remain the best means of surveying for fractures or subluxations that may suggest occult ligamentous instability that may not be visualized on computed tomography. Anteroposterior and lateral views of the thoracic and lumbar spine are obtained as indicated or may be reconstructed from chest, abdominal, and pelvic CT if available. If a spinal fracture is found, the entire spine should be imaged because of the high rate of coincident injuries (*J Spinal Disord* 1992;5:320).

b. Other imaging modalities include **CT scans** to further evaluate known or suspected fractures. **Magnetic resonance imaging** is sensitive for ligamentous injuries, intraspinal hemorrhage, and protruded intervertebral discs (*J Neurosurg* 1993;79:341), which can cause deficit with or without bony abnormalities seen on plain films. Damage to the vertebral artery can occur with cervical injuries, especially if fracture of the foramen transversarium occurs. CT angiography, conventional digital subtraction angiography, or magnetic resonance angiography are pursued if neurologic damage is referable to vertebral artery injury.

B. Instability. Spinal instability must be suspected until ruled out. Ligamentous injury can occur in the absence of fracture, and instability can occur with normal plain films. Point tenderness, severe midline pain, or apprehension of neck movement also warrants careful assessment. In the minimally symptomatic, alert patient, cervical flexion/extension films can aid in the assessment of spinal stability. Flexion and extension must be done under the patient's own power, and motion should be stopped if pain or other symptoms arise. Limited flexion and extension motion on physical exam may significantly decrease the utility of flexion/extension radiography in detecting ligamentous instability (*J Trauma* 2002;53:426). These patients should be left in a cervical collar and may require additional cross-sectional imaging to exclude occult injury.

C. Treatment

1. Methylprednisolone may improve outcome from spinal cord injury if given within 8 hours (*N Engl J Med* 1990;322:1405). Patients seen between 3 to 8 hours after injury should be treated emergently with **methylprednisolone, 30-mg/kg intravenous bolus** over 15 minutes, followed 45 minutes later by a **5.4-mg/kg/hour intravenous infusion** continued over the next 48 hours (*JAMA* 1997;277:1597). If steroids are administered within 3 hours of injury, intravenous infusion is given for only 24 hours. If patients are seen more than 8 hours after injury, this protocol is not of proven benefit and is contraindicated. Steroids are also contraindicated in cases of penetrating spinal injury (*Neurosurgery* 1997;41:576). Because of the significantly increased risks of medical complications associated with its use, methylprednisolone is recommended only as an option in the treatment of spinal cord injury, given that evidence suggesting harmful side effects is more consistent than that of clinical benefits (*Neurosurgery* 2002;50:S63).

2. Immobilization and reduction. Suspected or known spine injuries require immobilization, initially with a rigid cervical collar and long backboard. Cervical spine subluxations and dislocations must be reduced under neurosurgical supervision. Fractures may be treated by external immobilization (e.g., halo external fixation) or by operative fusion, depending on the nature of the fracture and degree of instability.

Thoracic and lumbar spine fractures are managed with operative stabilization or immobilization with an orthosis. Injuries with associated neurologic deficit, with excessive displacement or angulation of the spinal column, or with loss of vertebral body height are more likely to require operative stabilization. Before stabilization, patients are managed with bedrest with frequent log-rolling. Although early surgical decompression and stabilization promote mobilization of the patient, the timing of surgery and the role of emergency surgery in the patient with acute neurologic deficit remain somewhat controversial (*Neurosurgery* 1994;35:240).

3. Cervical spine injuries are associated with the development of adult respiratory distress syndrome, hyponatremia, hypotension, bradyarrhythmias, ileus, and urinary retention. Patients with cervical spine injuries may require cardiorespiratory monitoring, isotonic fluid support, nasogastric decompression, urinary catheter placement, laxatives, and stool softeners to address these issues. Bladder and bowel dysfunctions also are seen with lower spine injuries, although autonomic problems are rare in injuries below the upper thoracic spine.

4. Penetrating injuries to the neck and torso may result in fractures of the spine or penetration of the spinal canal, along with other injuries.

5. **Venous thromboembolism risk** is significantly elevated in patients with spinal cord injury. Intermittent pneumatic compression devices with subcutaneous heparin or enoxaparin have been demonstrated to be equally safe in the acute management of spinal cord injury (*J Trauma* 2003;54:1116).

V. OTHER EMERGENCIES

A. Nontraumatic intracranial hypertension and herniation syndromes

1. **Etiology.** Elevation of the ICP may lead to compression of neurologic structures and irreversible neurologic damage. Nontraumatic causes include hemorrhagic and nonhemorrhagic mass lesions.

   a. Spontaneous **intraparenchymal hemorrhages** may occur owing to hypertension, vascular malformations (arteriovenous malformations or aneurysms), tumor, angiopathy, vasculitis, or secondary hemorrhage into a large infarction.

   b. **Nonhemorrhagic lesions** include tumor, infection, and mass effect from edema after cerebral infarction.

2. Clinical **herniation syndromes** exist with presentations referable to the location of the lesion.

   a. **Supratentorial** sites of herniation include uncal, central transtentorial, and subfalcine herniation. Progressive lethargy, unilateral pupillary dysfunction, and/or hemiparesis suggest uncal herniation. Compression of vascular and brain structures requires immediate intervention. **Uncal** herniation often is the result of temporal lobe lesions. **Central transtentorial** herniation results from downward compression of brainstem structures. Unresponsiveness, deep coma, and cranial nerve dysfunction are observed. Central transtentorial herniation suggests a bilateral process or an interhemispheric lesion. **Subfalcine** herniation results from lesions causing a shift across the inferior aspect of the falx and can present with only lethargy or lower-extremity weakness. Both falcine and uncal herniation can progress to a central transtentorial picture as further structures are compressed.

   b. **Infratentorial** herniation results from posterior fossa masses compressing the brainstem or from herniation of the cerebellar tonsils through the foramen magnum. Signs of infratentorial herniation include lower cranial nerve dysfunction and the rapid onset of respiratory or cardiac arrest with little warning.

3. **Treatment** of herniation requires control of the ICP. The obtunded patient must have his or her airway controlled. Mannitol can be used, often with ICP monitoring (see Section III.A) to guide medical treatment. Mass lesions may need to be evacuated.

B. Nonhemorrhagic lesions.
Diffuse cerebral edema also can produce ICP elevations that require treatment. **Metabolic derangements,** such as those seen in hepatic encephalopathy, can elevate the ICP. Edema can also develop secondary to large **infarctions** in the cerebral hemispheres, leading to delayed deterioration. Management of elevated ICP may be indicated in large cerebral infarctions, whether hemorrhagic or nonhemorrhagic.

1. **Brain tumors** rarely are surgical emergencies. Presenting symptoms include progressive headache, seizures, and localizing neurologic deficit. Uncommonly, acute neurologic deterioration is seen, usually suggestive of hemorrhage into the tumor. Evaluation and treatment are similar to those for any other acute intracranial mass lesion. High-dose **steroids** may have a potent effect on the brain edema associated with tumors. Urgent **surgical resection** of the mass lesion occasionally is required.

2. **Hydrocephalus** may result from a variety of causes and can lead to rapid neurologic deterioration.

   a. **Cerebellar tumors** or other mass lesions may cause fourth ventricle obstruction without preceding symptoms. Tuberculosis and bacterial meningitis also can cause hydrocephalus. Patients classically present with lethargy, headache, papilledema, sixth nerve palsy, or abnormalities of upward gaze ("setting-sun" sign). **Treatment** involves urgent placement of a catheter for external **ventricular drainage** (see Section III.A.2) to relieve the buildup of CSF.

    b. Shunt malfunction. Internal ventricular drainage systems (shunts) require special attention. Malfunction can present with warning symptoms, such as headache or nausea, or with rapid deterioration of mental status, such as somnolence. Imaging, such as an emergency CT scan, can help in the diagnosis, but emergent operative revision may be indicated if mental status deterioration is present and shunt malfunction is suspected. A shunt series (plain films of the head, neck, chest, and abdomen) can visualize the entire course of the shunt and its connections, possibly leading to identification of a shunt tube fracture or stricture.

C. Intracranial hemorrhage. Spontaneous intracranial hemorrhage requires emergent intervention, and the sequelae of the associated mass effect also need to be addressed.

    1. Subarachnoid hemorrhage (SAH) secondary to aneurysmal hemorrhage is a common neurosurgical emergency. The clinical **presentation** usually includes a history of severe sudden headache, nuchal rigidity, photophobia, lethargy, agitation, or a comatose state. Acute blood from an SAH appears bright on CT scan. Blood usually is seen in the cisterns or sylvian fissure. Lumbar puncture can make the diagnosis if the history is suggestive, even with a normal CT scan, but is not required when the scan is diagnostic. The principal goal of treatment is the prevention of rebleeding by surgical clipping or endovascular techniques. Without treatment, rebleeding occurs in 50% of patients with a ruptured aneurysm in the first 6 months (*J Neurosurg* 1985;62:321).

    2. Spontaneous intraventricular hemorrhage may result from vascular malformations, hypertensive hemorrhage, or extension of intraparenchymal hemorrhage. Angiography can be used in determining the etiology. Patients are observed for the development of hydrocephalus, which requires external CSF drainage (ventriculostomy).

    3. Pituitary apoplexy occurs after hemorrhage into the pituitary gland, usually related to an underlying pituitary adenoma. Patients typically present with acute headache and visual symptoms, such as decreased acuity, visual field cut, ptosis, or diplopia, which result from compression of nearby cranial nerves. Life-threatening panhypopituitarism can occur. Treatment involves hormonal replacement, correction of any electrolyte abnormalities, and emergent CT or MR scan to evaluate for hemorrhagic pituitary lesions. Emergent evacuation of hematoma may preserve vision.

D. Infections

    1. Cerebral abscesses can result from hematogenous or local traumatic spread of a septic process. Infections may also involve the epidural or subdural spaces. Underlying abnormalities are common, such as an immunocompromised state or systemic arteriovenous shunting. Presenting symptoms include those of increased ICP, focal deficits, and seizures. A head CT scan with intravenous contrast shows an enhancing lesion. Early-stage cerebral abscess may respond to medical management alone. Abscesses larger than 3 cm, failure of medical management, and the need for tissue diagnosis are common indications for surgical drainage by open craniotomy or stereotactic drainage. Prolonged intravenous antibiotics are indicated.

    2. Spinal epidural abscesses can become a surgical emergency. Severe neck or back pain in the setting of fever should raise concern. Although neurologic deficit may not occur initially, often progressive evidence of cord compression exists. MR scan or myelography demonstrates the lesion. Surgical evacuation is most often necessary, although antibiotics alone can be attempted if neither neurologic compromise nor a large collection is present. Even with surgical drainage, an extended course of antibiotics is required. Disc space infection and spinal osteomyelitis can occur in association with or separately from spinal epidural abscesses. Antibiotic therapy usually is effective. An elevated erythrocyte sedimentation rate generally is present and falls with effective treatment.

E. Spinal cord compression

    1. Diagnosis. Nontraumatic spinal cord compression can result from metastatic tumor or another adjacent mass lesion. Patients present initially with pain, followed by progressive or sudden neurologic symptoms. Lung, breast, and prostate are the most common sources of metastases (*Neurosurgery* 1987;21:676). Examination usually reveals weakness, long-tract signs (spasticity, hyperactive reflexes, upgoing toes), or sphincter dysfunction. It is important to distinguish myelopathy from radiculopathy. The latter presents with pain, sensory changes, and weakness in a dermatomal pattern. Emergent MR scan or myelography to demonstrate the presence and level of the lesion confirms diagnosis of cord compression. Imaging should extend to higher spinal levels if no lesion is found because, for example, a cervical lesion can present with only lower-extremity symptoms; alternatively, multilevel involvement can be present.

2. **Treatment** begins with **steroids** (dexamethasone, 10 mg intravenously, followed by 4 to 10 mg orally or intravenously every 6 hours; higher doses frequently are given for severe deficits); these are administered immediately if spinal cord compression is suspected. The neurosurgical priorities include **decompression** if a deficit is present and spinal **stabilization and fusion** if bony destruction is prominent (*Neurosurgery* 1985;17:424). Vertebral corpectomy and reconstruction with internal fixation is often required because a simple laminectomy may not be helpful (*Lancet* 2005;366(9486):643). Emergent **radiation therapy** to the area of compression may be preferable to surgical intervention in some cases.

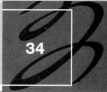

ORTHOPEDIC INJURIES

34

Jason Robison and William M. Ricci

TREATMENT OF ORTHOPEDIC INJURIES

I. INITIAL ASSESSMENT

A. Priorities of management. Assessment and management of ABCs (*a*irway, *b*reathing, and *c*irculation) take precedence over extremity injuries. Multisystem-injured patients benefit from early aggressive treatment of extremity and pelvic trauma.

B. History. In addition to standard medical history, the mechanism of injury, especially the relative energy associated with the injury (e.g., low energy fall vs. high-energy motor vehicle crash), is important to elucidate and helps to direct assessment, management, and prognosis of patients with musculoskeletal injuries. An orthopaedic history should also include preinjury functional level.

C. Examination

1. An orthopedic examination includes inspection, palpation, range-of-motion, strength, stability, and body region–specific tests. A systematic approach includes comparison to the unaffected side in isolated injuries and a complete skeletal evaluation in the multiply injured patient. **Inspect** the extremities for bruising, swelling, lacerations, abrasions, deformity, and asymmetry. Systematically **palpate** all extremities, noting tenderness, crepitus, and deformity of the underlying bone. Assess joint **range of motion,** stressing the joint in nonmotion planes to determine **stability. Special tests** are indicated for the further evaluation of specific injuries and can be found in comprehensive texts. In suspected cervical spine injury, maintain immobilization in a cervical collar until cervical spine injury is ruled out radiographically and/or clinically. Logroll the patient to examine and palpate the spine.

2. **Assess extremity vascular status** by checking pulses, capillary refill, temperature, and color and comparing to the opposite side.

3. **Sensorimotor evaluation.** Muscle strength evaluation in the setting of acute spinal cord injury or peripheral nerve injury is critical, and serial exams are often required. A sensory examination includes light touch in dermatomal and peripheral nerve distributions. In upper-extremity or cervical spine trauma, two-point discrimination of the fingers should be assessed.

4. **Associated injuries.** Severe or multiple injuries can mask other injuries. Especially important in this setting is a complete primary evaluation and then a secondary survey.

II. RADIOLOGIC EXAMINATION.
All trauma and unconscious patients should have screening chest, pelvis, and cervical spine radiographs. Lateral cervical spine radiographs must visualize all cervical vertebrae to the C7-T1 junction. Assessment of extremity fractures and dislocations should include a minimum of two views 90 degrees to each other [usually anteroposterior (AP) and lateral views] of the affected area and should include both the joint above and the joint below the injury. Dislocations should be reduced as soon as possible, without the benefit of radiographs if necessary, because they are often associated with neurovascular and soft-tissue compromise.

III. FRACTURES AND DISLOCATIONS
A. Terminology and classification

1. Accurate descriptions of fractures and dislocations begin with the bone or joint involved. For fractures, the **anatomic region** refers usually to the proximal, middle, or distal portion of the bone. *Epiphyseal, metaphyseal,* and *diaphyseal* (also *head, base,* and *shaft*) are acceptable descriptive terms of the fracture location. The **quality** of the fracture is described based on its **orientation** and the **number of fracture fragments.** A fracture is **transverse** if it runs relatively perpendicular to the long axis of the bone and **oblique** if it is angled. **Spiral** fractures propagate around and along a long bone and are caused by a twisting injury. **Comminuted** fractures have, by definition, more than two fragments. **Intra-articular** fractures involve the joint surface.

2. **Alignment** always references the distal fragment relative to the proximal fragment. Key components are **angulation, translation, rotation,** and **shortening.** **Angulation** is angular deformity in the coronal or sagittal plane, **rotation** is deformity about the long axis of the bone, **translation** is nonangular coronal or sagittal displacement with decreased bony **apposition,** and **shortening** is loss of bone length though the fracture.

3. **Stable** fractures and dislocations are not likely to displace after reduction (the "setting" of a fracture or dislocation) and appropriate immobilization, whereas **unstable** fractures are either unable to be reduced or are likely to lose reduction despite adequate immobilization.

4. **Soft-tissue injury. Open** or "compound" (an outdated term) fractures are those with a disruption of the overlying skin and tissue such that the fracture communicates with the external environment. **Closed** fractures are those that do not communicate with the external environment. Abrasions or lacerations that do not communicate with the fracture site are considered closed. Fractures complicated by associated neurovascular, ligamentous, or muscular injury require prompt recognition and injury-specific treatment.

5. Joint **subluxation** refers to joint disruption and instability with decreased contact between joint surfaces. **Dislocation** refers to complete loss of contact between joint surfaces. Both are described by the position of the distal bone in relation to its proximal articulation.

B. General management principles

1. **Dislocation.** All dislocated joints, especially in the setting of **neurovascular compromise,** should be reduced emergently. This can generally be accomplished via gentle longitudinal traction. Successful reduction reduces the risk and degree of soft-tissue injury (e.g., pressure necrosis) and neurovascular compromise. Postreduction radiographs are essential to confirm adequate reduction and to re-evaluate for associated fractures previously not visualized because of deformity associated with the dislocation. Persistently diminished or absent pulses may require arteriography and further evaluation. See specific injury sections for joint-specific issues.

2. **Fracture.** A diagnosis of fracture is suspected by **history** of injury, symptoms of pain, loss of motion, and swelling. **Physical examination** findings include crepitus, tenderness, swelling, and/or deformity. Confirmation of fracture is obtained via appropriate **radiographs.**

   a. **General treatment principles.** Treatment of fractures first includes reduction, if indicated, and then appropriate immobilization. Appropriate immobilization helps to prevent further injury to the surrounding soft tissues and is usually required for fracture healing. Nondisplaced fractures and those that can be adequately reduced (with regard to fracture alignment) in a closed manner can often be treated without surgery. However, this requires sufficient stability to predictably maintain reduction through healing. Fractures that cannot be reduced closed, are too unstable to maintain adequate reduction, or have significant joint involvement are generally treated surgically with open reduction and either internal fixation (plates, screws, and wires), intramedulary nailing, external fixation, or, in some cases, primary joint arthroplasty (joint replacement). Certain stable fractures, such as hip fractures, are usually treated surgically because of the increased morbidity associated with prolonged immobilization associated with nonoperative management. Open fractures have specific considerations and treatments that are discussed later (see Section VI.C).

b. Pediatric musculoskeletal fractures

(1) Children, especially those with open growth plates, have a greater potential for bony remodeling than adults, and therefore a greater amount of malalignment is acceptable. Despite this, however, at least limited reduction of deformity is often necessary to decrease the risk of permanent deformity. As in the adult, inability to achieve and obtain an acceptable reduction is a relative indication for surgical treatment. Fracture evaluation principles of history, physical exam, and radiographs are the same as in the adult.

(2) Physeal plate injuries ("growth plate") are common because this is the weakest part of the bone. The Salter-Harris classification categorizes these fractures into five types of increasing severity and likelihood of future growth disturbance. Type I injuries involve a fracture through the growth plate without any metaphyseal or epiphyseal involvement. Type II injury occurs when disruption of the growth plate is associated with a metaphyseal fracture, and type III when it is associated with an epiphyseal fracture. Fracture through the metaphysis, across the growth plate, and exiting the epiphysis constitute a type IV injury. A type V injury is a severe crush injury to the growth plate.

c. Hazards in fracture management. Patients must be observed closely for possible compartment syndrome (see Section VI.B), especially those with leg and forearm injuries. Neurovascular compromise after plaster immobilization usually is secondary to swelling, and splints and bandages should be loosened to accommodate anticipated swelling. Circumferential casting in the acute setting should generally be avoided, but in a low-energy, nondisplaced fracture in a child, casting may be appropriate. If the patient is to return home, he or she should be instructed on the warning signs of early compartment syndrome and told to return to the hospital immediately if these symptoms develop.

IV. SOFT-TISSUE INJURY

A. Principles of management. In general, isolated soft-tissue injuries, such as ligament sprains and muscle strains, are treated with *r*est, *i*ce, *c*ompression bandage, and *e*levation (**RICE therapy**) with or without immobilization.

1. Skin lacerations/defects. All devitalized tissue should be débrided. If the wound cannot be closed due to excessive tension, it should be covered with a moist saline dressing, and a delayed primary closure or skin grafting should be planned.

2. Muscle

a. Mechanism. Strains of the **musculotendinous unit** are usually secondary to violent contraction or excessive stretch. Injury spans the range from stretch of the fibers to a complete tear with loss of function.

b. Physical examination. Swelling, tenderness, and pain with movement occur. A defect may be palpable. RICE-type treatment of the muscle involved is adequate for most such injuries.

3. Tendon. Lacerated, ruptured, or avulsed tendons, especially those of the upper extremity, should be surgically repaired because such injuries result in loss of function. Examination reveals loss of motion or weakness. Open wounds with a tendon laceration are irrigated thoroughly, débrided, and closed primarily with early planned repair of the tendon in the operating room. In grossly contaminated wounds, incision and débridement in the operating room are needed. Splints are applied with the extremity in a functional position.

4. Ligament. Ligament **sprains** range from mild stretch to complete tear and are commonly sports related. Pain, localized tenderness, and joint instability may be present on examination. Radiographs may reveal joint incongruence. If the joint is clinically or radiographically unstable, treatment involves immobilization in a reduced position. If no evidence of instability is present, treatment based on the RICE principle is used, and early range of motion is encouraged.

V. SPECIFIC INJURIES BY ANATOMIC LOCATION

A. Shoulder

1. **Fractures: clavicle, scapula, and proximal humerus**

   a. **Typical mechanism:** a fall onto an outstretched hand or onto a shoulder. Proximal humerus fractures are commonly caused by a low-energy fall in the elderly. Scapula fractures are a marker of very high energy chest trauma, usually involving a motor vehicle.

   b. **Typical physical signs.** A clavicle fracture is often palpable under the skin. Deformity is common with displaced fractures. Proximal humerus fractures can present with decreased range of motion, swelling, ecchymosis, and pain. The neurovascular exam is critical. Test for **isometric** (contraction without joint motion, usually against resistance) deltoid muscle function and lateral shoulder sensation to determine axillary nerve function. Median, radial, and ulnar nerve function is tested in the distal extremity. Observe for signs of pneumothorax or other chest trauma with scapula fractures.

   c. **Usual radiographic evaluation.** Oblique radiographs of the clavicle are obtained to provide orthogonal views. Radiographic evaluation of the shoulder and proximal humerus should include three orthogonal views: an AP of the glenohumeral joint, scapular Y, and axillary. A dislocation can be missed if one relies solely on an AP and scapular Y-view, and an axillary view is mandatory. A scapula fracture is often first noted on chest computed tomography (CT) in the evaluation of coexisting chest injuries and is the best way to evaluate for joint involvement.

   d. **Typical management**

      (1) Most **clavicle fractures** heal with nonoperative treatment and can be managed with a sling. Figure-of-eight splints offer no benefit over a sling, are usually poorly tolerated by patients, and therefore are usually not indicated.

      (2) **Proximal humerus fractures,** if nondisplaced and stable, can be treated with a sling and early, controlled mobilization. Significant comminution, especially of the greater and lesser tuberosities, and displacement place the humeral head at risk of avascular necrosis and are indications for surgical reduction and fixation, especially in the young. For such a fracture in the elderly, a primary shoulder arthroplasty (replacement) may be considered if stabile internal fixation cannot be achieved.

      (3) **Scapula fractures** are treated in a sling unless intra-articular glenoid displacement necessitates surgical fixation.

   e. **Pitfalls and pearls.** A fracture-dislocation of the shoulder is difficult to reduce closed and may have associated neurovascular compromise. Often, a pneumothorax or other chest injuries are associated with high-energy chest trauma. The subcutaneous location of the clavicle places it at risk of an open fracture, and careful observation is necessary to avoid overlooking this component of the injury.

2. **Dislocations (sternoclavicular, acromioclavicular, and glenohumeral)**

   a. **Common mechanism.** Same as with fractures (fall onto an outstretched hand or onto a shoulder). Anterior shoulder dislocations (most common, ~85%) occur with forced shoulder abduction or external rotation (or both). Less common posterior shoulder dislocations are associated with seizure and electrical shock. Most shoulder dislocations do not spontaneously reduce, which helps to distinguish between subluxation and dislocation.

   b. **Typical physical signs.** Variable deformity and instability can be seen with acromioclavicular (AC) and sternoclavicular dislocations; side-to-side asymmetry must be evaluated. Pain with motion and tenderness to palpation are seen with sprains of the AC and sternoclavicular joints. **Hoarseness, dyspnea,**

dysphagia, or engorged neck veins are red flags for posterior sternoclavicular joint dislocations with neurovascular compromise and should prompt emergent evaluation and treatment. Shoulder dislocation presents with decreased and painful range of motion, and the humeral head may be palpable anteriorly or posteriorly. A "sulcus sign," or indentation between the acromion and humeral head, is suggestive of dislocation. As with fractures, a thorough neurovascular examination is critical and should be documented prior to and following any reductions.

c. **Usual radiographic evaluation.** See fracture section. Stress views of the AC joint are taken holding 5- to 10-lb weights, comparing side to side for displacement; however, this can be quite uncomfortable and is not generally necessary. A CT scan may be indicated to evaluate the sternoclavicular joint to determine anterior or posterior displacement and to visualize adjacent neurovascular structures. If shoulder dislocation is suspected, radiographs must include an axillary view. Evidence of glenoid rim fractures or humeral head impaction fractures (Hill-Sach lesion) associated with shoulder dislocations should be sought.

d. **Typical management**
   (1) **Anterior sternoclavicular dislocation** can be treated with a sling or shoulder immobilizer, whereas **posterior dislocations** commonly require reduction because of potential neurovascular and airway compromise. This should be done in the operating room under general anesthesia with general or thoracic surgery backup in case of injury to the lung or great vessels.
   (2) **AC joint sprains/dislocations** (e.g., shoulder separation) can be treated with a sling and early motion in most cases. Significant displacement and deformity may require reduction and fixation, especially if the skin or soft tissue is tented or otherwise at risk.
   (3) **Shoulder dislocations** should be reduced and immobilized in the position of greatest stability: internal rotation for anterior dislocations and external rotation for posterior dislocations. Radiographs should be repeated to demonstrate reduction, and a postreduction neurovascular exam should be done. Reduction is performed under sedation with axial traction and bringing the arm up in to full abduction above the head. **Fracture-dislocations** frequently require open reduction and internal fixation. Closed reduction, if performed, should be done cautiously to avoid neurovascular injury and to avoid displacement of an otherwise nondisplaced fracture. The redislocation rate is inversely proportional to patient age and correlated with activity level and demand.

e. **Pitfalls and pearls.** Neurovascular and airway compromise often coexist with sternoclavicular joint dislocations. Posterior shoulder dislocations can be missed with traditional films if there is not an adequate axillary view. Care should be taken with the elderly with any reduction because it is possible to fracture osteoporotic bone with minimal force.

3. **Soft-tissue injury**
   a. **Rotator cuff tears.** In the young, rotator cuff tears are caused by repetitive overuse (throwing in athletes) or by acute trauma. In the elderly, tears are commonly degenerative and chronic, but they can be acute. They are often associated with shoulder dislocation. History reveals shoulder pain and weakness, especially with overhead activities, and decreased range of motion. This is confirmed on examination with pain and weakness with shoulder abduction, forward elevation, and external rotation with decreased active as compared to passive shoulder motion. In the young, treatment consists of open or arthroscopic tendon repair. In the elderly, function may not be as severely affected, and physical therapy for improved strength and motion may suffice. Failure of nonoperative care is an indication for surgery.
   b. **Pectoralis major rupture.** This is most often caused by heavy lifting or other injury. In addition to weakness and pain, there is often significant bruising, a

palpable defect, and a visibly changed muscle contour. Initial treatment consists of sling immobilization. An open repair gives best results when performed early.

B. Arm and elbow

1. Fractures (humeral shaft, distal humerus [supracondylar] and elbow)

a. **Typical mechanism.** Commonly caused by a fall onto an outstretched arm or directly onto the elbow. Supraconylar humerus fractures are the most common elbow fracture in both children and the elderly and are commonly caused by falls onto outstretched arms.

b. **Typical physical signs. Humerus shaft fractures** are often rotationally unstable and can demonstrate shortening. **Olecranon fractures** may have a palpable defect if displaced. **Radial head fractures** present with tenderness to palpation and pain with forearm rotation. Swelling and ecchymosis are often seen with supracondylar and other elbow fractures. The amount of swelling about the joint and of the muscle compartments should be carefully noted, as well as other signs of possible developing compartment syndrome (see Section VI.B). All displaced elbow fractures and dislocations place the neurovascular structures at risk, and a complete neurovascular exam should be performed testing both motor and sensory function of the radial, median, and ulnar nerves. In mid-diaphyseal fractures, the radial nerve is especially vulnerable to injury because it is directly adjacent to the posterior humeral shaft in this region.

c. **Usual radiographic evaluation.** Orthogonal views of the fracture should be obtained, as well as imaging of the joint above and below the site of injury. For supracondylar fractures in adults, stress views taken with gentle longitudinal traction can help to delineate the fracture pattern, especially in cases with significant comminution or deformity. A CT scan may be indicated for additional fracture characterization to aid in surgical planning. A CT can similarly be useful to evaluate the extent and nature of fractures involving the radial head. Nondisplaced elbow fractures in children may present only with a "sail sign" caused by the superior displacement of the anterior and posterior elbow fat pads by a joint effusion.

d. **Typical management**

(1) Following reduction, **humeral shaft fractures** are initially immobilized with a coaptation splint for approximately 1 to 2 weeks with subsequent placement into a fracture brace. Operative fixation is indicated in cases of polytrauma (to afford use of the upper extremity to expedite and ease mobilization), open fracture, segmental fractures, ipsilateral forearm fracture, radial nerve palsy development after fracture reduction, and inadequate closed reduction or failed closed treatment.

(2) **Supracondylar fractures in children** can be treated in a splint acutely if they are nondisplaced but require percutaneous pinning and casting if they are displaced. Significant swelling and neurovascular embarrassment are indications for urgent reduction followed by close observation. In adults, displaced fracture is an indication for open reduction with internal fixation.

(3) Nondisplaced **olecranon fractures** are treated with a posterior splint followed by early range of motion, but when they are displaced, surgical fixation is indicated.

(4) **Radial head fractures** with minimal involvement of the articular surface (<30%) can be treated nonoperatively in a splint followed by early range-of-motion exercises. Increasing head involvement is an indication for surgical management. Open reduction and internal fixation are performed when stable fixation is achievable (usually three or fewer fragments), or, in adults, excision or replacement is performed if comminution precludes adequate repair.

e. **Pitfalls and pearls.** Neurologic complications are possible and must be carefully looked for. Secondary (following closed reduction) radial nerve palsy is considered an indication for surgical management to rule out incarceration of the nerve within the fracture. However, primary radial nerve dysfunction usually resolves spontaneously (over a period of months) and can be treated nonoperatively. A compartment syndrome may occur with a supracondylar fracture, and a high index of suspicion must be maintained both before and after any reduction or surgical treatment. Care should be exercised when placing splints because tight, circumferential dressings can contribute to a developing compartment syndrome or prevent adequate serial examinations.

2. **Dislocations (elbow [ulnohumeral] and radial head)**
    a. **Typical mechanism:** fall onto an outstretched hand.
    b. **Typical physical signs.** Examination reveals pain, swelling, bruising, and deformity with loss of elbow flexion and extension and forearm supination and pronation. Posterior dislocations are most common but can also occur anteriorly, medially, or laterally. The dislocated segment can often be palpated. As with other elbow injuries, signs of neurovascular complications must be sought. Ulnar shaft fractures associated with radial head dislocation are termed Monteggia injuries.
    c. **Usual radiographic evaluation.** AP and lateral radiographs of the elbow confirm the diagnosis and reveal the direction of dislocation and major associated fractures. Postreduction radiographs are essential to demonstrate concentric joint reduction and more reliably identify any associated fractures. Coronoid process and radial head fractures can be seen with elbow dislocations, and ulna fractures can be seen with radial head dislocations. A CT scan may aid in complex fracture-dislocations.
    d. **Typical management.** Initial treatment consists of prompt reduction (typically accomplished with axial traction and flexion) and assessment of stability. The joint should be splinted in a stable position. Postreduction radiographs are taken and neurovascular status documented. Associated fractures must be addressed for stability. Stable dislocations benefit from early, controlled motion, whereas unstable fractures may require surgical stabilization of fractures or ligament reconstruction. Most Monteggia fractures in children can be treated with closed reduction and splinting, but in adults and in unstable fractures in children, surgery is indicated.
    e. **Pitfalls and pearls.** Beware of neurovascular compromise. Identify associated fractures, and ensure adequate reduction with adequate radiographs. After reduction, examine and document stable positions and range of motion to aid in treatment planning. Frequent follow-up evaluations are required to assure maintained stability.

3. **Soft-tissue injury**
    a. **Bicep tendon rupture/avulsion** is usually secondary to violent contracture or excessive stretch. Loss of power, pain with resisted elbow flexion, local swelling, and ecchymosis are seen, along with an abnormal muscle contour, proximal retraction. Examine for side-to-side differences. Initial treatment is sling immobilization followed by early surgical repair.

C. **Forearm and wrist**
    1. **Fractures (radius and ulna fractures)**
        a. **Typical mechanism.** These are commonly caused by falls onto the elbow or outstretched arm and are common in both children and the elderly. A direct blow can cause fracture such as in the "night-stick fracture," a typically midshaft fracture of the ulna caused by a forceful blow to the arm positioned to protect the face, often with a bat or club during an assault.
        b. **Typical physical signs.** Examination reveals deformity, pain, and focal tenderness. Fractures involving the wrist joint result in painful and limited range of motion. Variable amounts of swelling can be seen, and diaphyseal fractures can cause a compartment syndrome, so careful, serial examination may be needed (see Section VI.B). A Galeazzi fracture is a fracture of the distal half of the radius associated with disruption of the distal radioulnar joint (DRUJ); this joint must be tested for stability. A distal fracture with spread of

the hematoma into the carpal tunnel may present as an **acute carpal tunnel syndrome** with associated median nerve sensory and motor dysfunction. Note wrist swelling and ecchymosis, and test two-point discrimination of the fingers (normally <5 to 7 mm) and test motor strength of the thumb abductors.

c. **Usual radiographic evaluation.** AP and lateral radiographs that include the entire forearm including the elbow and wrist are the minimum required. Splinted postreduction films are obtained to confirm reduction, and inspection of the DRUJ for involvement should be repeated. Rarely, a CT scan to evaluate a complex, comminuted intra-articular fracture is necessary.

d. **Typical management.** In children, most diaphyseal and wrist fractures can be managed with closed reduction and long-arm posterior splinting. Unstable growth-plate fractures or midshaft fractures may require operative reduction and fixation. In adults, shaft fractures that involve both bones are almost always surgically treated after initial closed reduction and splinting. Isolated radius and ulna fractures can be treated nonoperatively if they are minimally displaced. Wrist fractures require additional fixation if they are unstable, are inadequately reduced, or have displaced intra-articular fragments.

e. **Pitfalls and pearls.** An acute carpal tunnel syndrome requires urgent surgical release and will often be missed if not looked for specifically. Closed reduction of wrist factures can be greatly aided by hematoma blocks (see Section VII.B) and the use of finger traps. Watch for development of compartment syndrome in shaft fractures. Be vigilant to detect radial head dislocations associated with ulna fractures (Monteggia injury) and DRUJ disruption with radius fractures (Galeazzi injury).

D. Wrist and hand

1. Fractures

a. **Typical presentation:** a fall onto an outstretched hand or a crushing injury.

b. **Typical physical signs.** A **scaphoid fracture** is the most common of the carpal fractures and presents with local swelling, pain with wrist motion, and focal tenderness in the "anatomic snuffbox." **Metacarpal fractures** present with swelling and bruising, often with flexion of the distal fragment causing the knuckle to be less prominent; the most common is the distal fifth metacarpal or so-called **"boxer's" fracture.** Check for rotational deformity by observing for finger divergence with flexion of the metacarpal phalangeal joints and comparing to the contralateral side. Distal phalanx fractures are often seen in the setting of nail-bed injuries.

c. **Usual radiographic evaluation.** Obtain AP and lateral radiographs of involved areas. Oblique views can be useful in evaluating the carpal bones.

d. **Typical management.** Nondisplaced **scaphoid fractures** are treated in a thumb spica splint. Fractures with greater than 1 mm of displacement are at risk of nonunion and avascular necrosis and benefit from internal fixation. **Metacarpal fractures** are reduced and splinted in a thumb spica or ulnar gutter splint, reexamining for rotational malalignment. Prefabricated aluminum splints are generally adequate for **phalanx fractures. Intra-articular fractures** and unstable or inadequately reduced fractures often require pinning or internal fixation.

e. **Pitfalls and pearls.** Scaphoid fractures are at risk of nonunion and/or avascular necrosis, especially with fractures of the proximal pole. It is critical to adequately immobilize even suspected fractures to minimize this risk. Metacarpal fractures generally heal reliably, but rotational malalignment is poorly tolerated.

2. Dislocations

a. **Typical mechanism.** Lunate and perilunate dislocations usually occur after forced wrist hyperextension. Fracture dislocations can occur at any metacarpal or interphalangeal joint but are most common at the base of the first and fifth metacarpals, occurring with forced hyperabduction.

b. **Typical physical signs. Perilunate dislocations** present with pain, limited wrist motion, tenderness, and possibly signs of median neuropathy caused by compression of the median nerve in the carpal tunnel by the displaced lunate. **Carpometacarpal dislocations** are rare and difficult to diagnose clinically because of considerable swelling. **Interphalangeal dislocations** result in an obvious deformity.

  c. Usual radiographic evaluation. AP and lateral views of involved joints are the minimum required. Oblique views aid in evaluating the position of displaced carpal bones. Scaphoid, capitate, and radial styloid fractures should be ruled out as associated injuries with lunate dislocations. Close examination of the carpal bones and their articulations will reveal an otherwise difficult-to-make diagnosis.

  d. Typical management. Perilunate dislocations are reduced using axial traction and hyperextension of the wrist while pressure is applied to the lunate. These usually require surgical treatment with stabilization of associated fractures and disrupted intercarpal ligaments. Most other hand dislocations are reduced with longitudinal traction and splinted in a "safe" position (see Section VII.A.2.d). Irreducible and unstable dislocations may require open reduction to remove interposed soft tissue or to treat associated bony or ligamentous injury.

  e. Pitfalls and pearls. Perilunate dislocations can be difficult to diagnose, and care is required to avoid missing such injuries. Any derangement in the position and orientation of the carpal bones should prompt further evaluation. Observe closely for signs of acute carpal tunnel syndrome. Avoid splinting the wrist in a flexed position because this increases risk of median nerve compression. Metacarpal-phalangeal joints should be splinted in flexion to avoid joint contractures.

3. Soft-tissue injury

  a. Subungual hematomas are decompressed by burning a hole in the nail with electrocautery or with a large-bore needle after a digital block.

  b. Nail-bed injuries require removal of the overlying nail with repair of the nail bed using absorbable suture and splinting open of the nail fold with sterile Vaseline-impregnated gauze or with the Betadine-soaked nail.

  c. Tip amputations involving only soft tissue can often be allowed to heal by secondary intent or, if the area is greater than 1 cm^2, treated with local flaps. Exposed bone is resected back to a level that allows soft tissue coverage.

E. Pelvic fractures

1. Typical mechanism. Pelvic fractures in the young are typically of very high energy, as from a motor vehicle collision or a fall from a height. In the elderly, low-energy falls from a standing height often cause pubic ramii fractures.

2. Typical physical signs. Crepitus, pelvic instability, or pain with iliac wing compression or distraction should alert the examiner to possible pelvic ring injury. Inspect for soft-tissue injury including a degloving injury. Rectal and vaginal examinations are performed to check for blood, open communication with a fracture, or a high-riding prostate. Blood at the urethral meatus at time of catheterization is a sign of lower urogenital injury. Pelvic bleeding may result in a loss of 2 to 3 L of blood or more, and signs of hypovolemic shock must be monitored along with aggressive fluid replacement. High-energy pelvic fractures rarely occur in isolation, and significant associated injuries are likely. Palpate for spinal tenderness or step-offs, and treat all patients initially with spinal precautions. A thorough primary and secondary survey must be undertaken and documented.

3. Usual radiographic evaluation. An AP pelvis view is part of the standard trauma panel. The use of an abdominal-pelvic CT scan is becoming standard part of the trauma workup and is extremely useful in evaluating pelvic, sacral, and lumbar spine fractures. An L5 transverse process fracture suggests posterior pelvic ligamentous disruption. Once stabilized, pelvic ring fractures are further evaluated with pelvic inlet and outlet views. If genitourinary injury is suspected, a retrograde urethrogram and cystogram should be obtained. Other standard radiographs such as chest and c-spine films should be reviewed.

4. **Typical management**

   a. The initial treatment consists of adherence to standard **trauma ABCs.** Maintenance of adequate intravascular volume and systolic blood pressure is essential in the hemodynamically unstable patient. In the persistently unstable patient, sources of bleeding other than the pelvis should be ruled out followed by emergent fixation of the pelvic ring in the emergency department, usually with a linen sheet tied around the pelvis or with a specialized pelvic binder to reduce pelvic volume until an anterior pelvic external fixation can be applied. Angiogram and embolization of bleeding pelvic vessels may precede or follow operative placement of provisional external fixation. If the patient is hemodynamically and otherwise stable, surgical intervention can be delayed to allow complete assessment of associated injuries and resuscitation of the patient.

   b. Fractures involving non–weight-bearing regions (e.g., pelvic rami) or those without pelvic ring disruptions are treated symptomatically with graduated weight bearing. Fractures in weight-bearing areas require protection from weight-bearing and possible surgical fixation. Sacral fractures and sacroiliac joint disruptions can often be treated with percutaneous screws. Unstable fractures may require external fixation while awaiting definitive surgical stabilization.

5. **Pitfalls and pearls.** Associated injuries (abdominal, pelvic, spinal, head, etc.) occur commonly with high-energy pelvic injuries and are the source of significant morbidity and mortality and should not be missed. An open pelvic fracture has a very high morbidity, and a diverting colostomy should be considered. Pelvic binders that remain in place for more than several hours must be often re-evaluated to rule out associated pressure necrosis of the skin. Because binders can cause increased patient discomfort and skin breakdown, they should be removed if patients remain hemodynamically stable or the fracture pattern does not allow decreased pelvic volume with lateral compression. Patients are at high risk of developing a deep venous thrombosis (DVT) in association with these injuries, and appropriate prophylaxis should be initiated.

F. **Hip and femur**

1. **Fractures of the hip and femur** (acetabular fractures, femoral neck fractures, peritrochanteric hip fractures)

   a. **Typical mechanism.** Acetabular and femoral shaft fractures, like pelvic fractures, are generally the result of high-energy trauma. "Hip" fractures (femoral neck and peritrochanteric fractures) are commonly the result of low-energy falls or direct blows in the elderly, but in the young they are generally a result of more significant trauma. A stress fracture of the femoral neck typically presents as groin or medial thigh pain associated temporally with a recent increase in activity level or training.

   b. **Typical physical signs.** Shortening of the limb may be seen in addition to pain with motion and the inability to bear weight. Rotational stability is typically lost with shaft and displaced hip fractures, with the leg falling into a shortened, externally rotated posture. A sciatic palsy is possible with a posterior acetabular dislocation that can occur with a fracture. A high index of suspicion must be maintained in the elderly after a low-energy fall presenting with complaints of groin or medial thigh pain (site of referred pain from the hip joint) because these may be the only signs of a nondisplaced hip fracture.

   c. **Usual radiographic evaluation.** With regard to the hip, an AP pelvis view and hip films (AP and lateral views) are usually diagnostic. For acetabular fractures, oblique views of the pelvis (Judet views) are obtained in addition to a fine-sliced spiral CT scan. These are very useful in evaluating the fracture. Shaft fractures of the femur are evaluated with orthogonal views showing both the hip and knee. **An ipsilateral femoral neck fracture must be excluded in patients with femoral shaft fracture.** The femoral neck can easily be evaluated on a trauma pelvic CT if available. If history suggests a hip fracture in the elderly or a stress fracture in the young but no fracture is seen, magnetic resonance imaging (MRI) or bone scan is indicated to rule out the occult fracture.

d. Typical management

(1) Skeletal traction may be indicated for **fractures of the acetabulum,** depending on the size and location of the fracture and presence of an associated dislocation (see also Section V.F.2). Fractures involving the weight-bearing portion of the acetabulum are usually treated with surgical reduction and fixation.

(2) Displaced femoral neck fractures in the young require urgent anatomic reduction and internal fixation to reduce the **risk of avascular necrosis,** whereas stress fractures are treated with protected weight bearing. In the elderly, surgical treatment is generally the rule for hip fractures. Stable femoral neck fractures are usually treated with internal fixation (most commonly, percutaneous screws) and unstable femoral neck fractures with hip arthroplasty (hemi- or total hip arthroplasty). Peritrochanteric fractures are treated with a variety of internal fixation methods, including the use of compression screw and plate or intramedulary nail. The utility of skin traction to increase patient comfort prior to surgery is controversial.

(3) Femoral shaft fractures need initial long-leg splinting and occasionally skeletal traction to increase comfort and stability while maintaining length and protecting the soft tissues (traction splints placed by emergency personnel should be promptly removed at time of initial evaluation). Even closed femur fractures can be a source of significant blood loss, and appropriate blood replacement, especially in the multiply injured patient, is important. Serial exams for compartment syndrome should be performed. Most shaft fractures are treated with intramedullary nailing soon after the injury to allow early mobilization and decrease the risk of additional complications. In the unstable, multiply injured patient, external fixation may be the initial treatment of choice to minimize adverse systemic effects caused by the additional trauma of surgery.

e. Pitfalls and pearls. Any fracture can be sufficiently distracting to preclude the identification of additional injuries, and so secondary surveys and adequate radiographic examinations are critical. Pulmonary and other complications are decreased with early femoral shaft fracture treatment. Fat embolism can occur after any long-bone fracture and may be exacerbated with intramedullary nailing of such fractures; increased O_2 requirements, dyspnea, and tachycardia are early signs. Arterial blood gas examination may show decreased O_2 tension, whereas chest x-ray will show patchy infiltrates and an electrocardiogram may show inverted T waves, right-bundle-branch block, and depressed ST segments. Treat fat embolism with supportive measures including fluid resuscitation, appropriate respiratory support and close observation. Serial exams will prevent missing a developing compartment syndrome. DVTs are common after pelvic and leg bone fractures, so prophylaxis (mechanical with or without chemical) is essential. In the elderly with a hip fracture, no more than 10 lb of skin traction (Buck's) should be used, and skin breakdown or sloughing can occur. If traction causes discomfort, then it should be discontinued.

2. Dislocation (hip)

a. Typical mechanism: high-energy motor vehicle crash, often associated with acetabular fracture. In patients with previous hip replacement, dislocation is typically atraumatic, caused primarily by exceeding positioning precautions given after hip replacement.

b. Typical physical signs. Anterior dislocations typically leave the extremity abducted and externally rotated. Posterior dislocations cause greater shortening with an adducted and internally rotated posture. Sciatic nerve function should be assessed for palsy with posterior dislocations (the peroneal division is most commonly affected).

c. **Usual radiographic evaluation.** Obtain appropriate pelvic films to evaluate for acetabular, femoral head, or hip fracture (see previous section) and to determine the direction of dislocation (requires adequate lateral view). In hip replacement, check for component positioning, loosening, or periprosthetic fractures.

d. **Typical management.** Immediate closed reduction, operatively if unsuccessful, to reduce **risk of avascular necrosis** should be done. Stable range of motion and postreduction neurologic exam are necessary. Skeletal traction is indicated when the hip remains unstable. Postreduction radiographs, including AP, lateral, and Judet views, are needed to confirm reduction and assess for associated fractures. Associated fractures are stabilized surgically. Patients with dislocated hip arthroplasties can usually be reduced closed and benefit from abduction bracing.

e. **Pitfalls and pearls.** Time to reduction is critical. Closed reduction prior to obtaining additional imaging of the pelvis should be done. After reduction of posterior dislocations (most common), keep legs abducted with an abduction pillow, brace, or equivalent. Traumatic dislocations of native hips (without arthroplasty) typically reduce with longitudinal traction. The typical reduction maneuver for dislocated total hip arthroplasties includes in-line traction with hip flexion, internal rotation, and adduction. Most failed attempts at closed reduction are due to inadequate sedation and muscle relaxation, which are essential. Persistent failure of closed reduction can be caused by buttonholing of a prosthetic head through the capsule or fractured or displaced acetabular liners. In the case of fracture dislocations, incarcerated fracture fragments can commonly prevent concentric reduction.

G. **Knee and tibia**

1. **Fractures (supracondylar femur, patellar, tibial plateau and shaft)**

   a. **Typical mechanism:** can be low energy in the elderly, generally higher energy in younger patients. Motor vehicle collision, fall from a height, direct blow, and pedestrian versus car are all common. Patella fractures are commonly caused by falling onto the knee or striking a dashboard. Spiral fractures of the tibia are caused by twisting injury.

   b. **Typical physical signs:** deformity and swelling about the knee with loss of rotational stability. Patella fractures often have a palpable defect and have an associated inability to perform a straight-leg raise. The subcutaneous location of the tibia predisposes to open fractures. Observation and probing lacerations and skin defects for communication to underlying bone or fracture are necessary. Check nerve function and the presence of pulses and foot perfusion compared to the contralateral side. Plateau and tibial shaft fracture are particularly at risk for compartment syndrome and should be monitored appropriately (see Section VI.B).

   c. **Usual radiographic evaluation.** Four views of the knee (AP, lateral, and two obliques) help to identify fractures involving the knee. Traction views taken with gentle longitudinal traction for comminuted and displaced periarticular fractures may be necessary to understand the fracture pattern. A CT scan may be helpful for preoperative planning for complex tibial plateau fractures. Tibial shaft fractures require an AP and lateral of the tibia and views of the knee and ankle. Diminished perfusion persistent after reduction should prompt an arteriogram.

   d. **Typical management**

      (1) Displaced **supracondylar femur fractures** are treated operatively with open reduction internal fixation or with retrograde intramedullary nailing.

      (2) **Patella fractures** with displacement, joint incongruity, or loss of knee extension require reduction and surgical fixation. Nondisplaced fractures can be treated with a knee immobilizer and weight bearing as tolerated.

      (3) **Tibial plateau fractures** are treated with splinting and early motion if they are nondisplaced and stable but require reduction and internal fixation for articular incongruity, significant displacement, deformity, or

instability. Most plateau fractures associated with significant soft tissue swelling or compartment syndrome are treated with a temporary, spanning external fixator across the knee followed by open reduction internal fixation (ORIF) or circular external fixation as definitive management. Stable **tibial shaft fractures** can be treated with casting; however, most are treated with intramedulary nailing to allow early weight bearing and motion. Open tibial shaft fractures often require multiple surgical débridements and soft-tissue coverage.

  e. **Pitfalls and pearls.** Be vigilant to detect a developing compartment syndrome. Strict elevation above the level of the heart is invaluable in managing such swelling.

2. **Dislocations (patella and knee)**

  a. **Typical mechanism.** Patella dislocations are usually lateral and occur with a twisting force while in extension, often during sports. Most spontaneously reduce. Knee dislocations are very high energy injuries and require multiple ligamentous disruption to occur.

  b. **Typical physical exam.** Patella dislocations cause a hemarthrosis, increased lateral translation of the patella while in extension, and tenderness to palpation about the patella and the femoral medial epicondyle. Knee dislocations present with deformity, shortening, ligamentous instability, and often signs of significant neurovascular compromise. Check side-to-side differences in pulse examination serially.

  c. **Usual radiographic evaluation.** For suspected patellar fracture, AP, lateral, and merchant views should suffice. Look for associated fractures with knee dislocations with four views of the knee *after* reduction. Angiography is often performed with knee dislocations (see later comments). Obtain an MRI of the knee in the subacute setting to evaluate the associated ligamentous injuries.

  d. **Typical management.** Most patella dislocations are treated nonoperatively unless recurrent instability ensues. A patella-centralizing brace may be used. Knee dislocations require immediate, emergent reduction. The incidence of concomitant vascular injury is approximately 30%, and pedal pulse examination has a low sensitivity (79%) for detecting significant vascular injury and a very low threshold for arteriography; a vascular surgery consultation is mandatory. If vascular repair is necessary, a spanning external fixator can be placed to stabilize the knee. After any vascular repair, prophylactic fasciotomy should be considered. Often, delayed ligamentous reconstruction is necessary to restore knee stability.

  e. **Pitfalls and pearls.** Knee dislocations that spontaneously reduce are easier to miss. An exam demonstrating multiligamentous instability in the setting of significant trauma should be treated as a knee dislocation. As with other high-energy traumas, do not miss a developing compartment syndrome.

3. **Soft-tissue injuries**

  a. **Quadriceps and patellar tendon ruptures** are caused by violent contraction or excessive stretch. Palpable defects and a high-riding (with patella tendon rupture) or low-riding (with quadriceps rupture) patella on physical exam or lateral radiographs are hallmarks. Partial tears that do not affect the integrity of the extensor mechanism can be managed without surgery with protected motion. Injuries affecting the extensor mechanism require surgical repair.

  b. **Knee ligament disruption** is commonly seen with sports injuries involving a pivoting injury or a bending moment. A hemarthrosis is common. Physical exam demonstrates joint instability with testing. Common ligamentous injuries include anterior cruciate (ACL) and medial collateral ligaments.

  c. **Meniscal tears** are more common than ligamentous injury and often occur in association with them. They present with a joint effusion, pain with deep flexion, and joint line tenderness. Rarely, a displaced segment can cause locking of the knee joint. Meniscal tears can be treated nonoperatively or, if symptoms persist, with arthroscopic débridement or repair.

H. Distal tibia and ankle
 1. **Fractures**
   a. **Typical mechanism.** Distal tibial intraarticular fractures **(pilon fractures)** are associated with an axial loading mechanism such as falls from a height or floor board injury from a motor vehicle accident. Ankle fractures are commonly caused by a twisting mechanism.
   b. **Typical physical exam.** Note deformity and instability of the lower leg and ankle joint. Perform and document a neurovascular exam. Note soft-tissue injury, which is often significant with pilon injuries, including location of fracture blisters and whether blood filled (marker of deeper injury). With ankle fractures, note the precise location of tenderness and swelling.
   c. **Usual radiographic exam.** Obtain three views of the ankle (AP, lateral, and mortise) for both pilon and ankle fractures. Foot films are used to evaluate for concomitant talus, calcaneous, or other foot fractures associated with high-energy pilon fractures. With ankle fractures of questionable joint stability, obtain a stress mortise view by stabilizing the distal tibia and externally rotating the patient's foot and look for widening of greater than 2 mm of the medial joint space. Comparison views to the uninjured ankle can be helpful. Traction views and a postreduction CT of pilon fractures help with fracture characterization and surgical planning.
   d. **Typical management**
     (1) Pilon fractures with significant shortening, comminution, or soft-tissue injury are best managed initially with closed reduction and placement of a spanning external fixator. External fixation is then maintained until the soft tissues can tolerate a formal open procedure.
     (2) Stable, nondisplaced **fractures of the ankle** can be treated with immobilization and protected weight bearing. Unstable fractures (one with both medial and lateral injuries) and fractures with joint subluxation benefit from open reduction and internal fixation. All fractures should be reduced at presentation under adequate anesthesia (see Section VII.B) with postreduction radiographs demonstrating adequate joint and fracture reduction.
   e. **Pitfalls and pearls.** Soft-tissue management is critical in the presence of these injuries, especially pilon fractures. If adequate joint reduction cannot be achieved or maintained, early surgical treatment is indicated to prevent further joint damage.
 2. **Dislocations (ankle)**
   a. **Typical mechanism. Simple** (not associated with fracture) ankle dislocations are uncommon. Fracture dislocations are caused by similar, but higher-energy, mechanisms as those in other ankle fractures.
   b. **Typical physical exam.** Look for deformity and pain with inability to bear weight. Dislocations are often associated with open fractures about the ankle. Document a neurovascular exam because significant soft-tissue injury and deformity place neurovascular structures at risk.
   c. **Usual radiographic examination:** same as for ankle fractures.
   d. **Typical management:** urgent closed reduction under adequate anesthesia. Open injuries should be treated appropriately (see Section VI.C). Dislocations represent unstable injuries, and associated fractures are treated surgically. As with pilon fractures, spanning external fixation may be an appropriate initial treatment.
   e. **Pitfalls and pearls:** similar to fractures.
 3. **Soft-tissue injuries**
   a. **Ankle sprains** are commonly caused by inversion or eversion of the foot. Patients present with swelling, ecchymosis, and maximal tenderness along the injured ligaments medially or laterally. Radiographs are normal or reveal insignificant cortical avulsions. Initial treatment based on the RICE principle (see Section IV.A) is usually adequate, followed by physical therapy for proprioceptive training to reduce the risk of reinjury.

b. A **ruptured Achilles tendon** usually occurs during running, jumping, or vigorous activity, with sudden pain and difficulty in walking. Examination can reveal a palpable defect, weak plantar flexion, and (if a complete rupture) no passive ankle plantar flexion on squeezing the patient's calf (positive Thompson sign). Nonoperative treatment in a splint with the ankle plantar flexed is associated with higher rerupture rates than surgical management.

I. Foot

1. Fractures (talus, calcaneous, metatarsal, and toe)

a. Typical mechanism. Calcaneous fractures are the most common tarsal fracture and are usually the result of an axillary load such as a fall from height, often in a young laborer. Talus fractures (the second most common) are also generally higher energy (motor vehicle collision or falls) and are usually caused by forced dorsiflexion (e.g., slamming on the brake at the time of impact). **Metatarsal fractures** can be seen with lower-energy trauma. **Stress fractures** can occur in runners or others who have recently increased their distance or activity.

b. Typical physical exam. Calcaneal fractures are associated with considerable swelling and blister formation, heel widening, and significant tenderness and ecchymosis extending to the arch. Associated fractures are common and include those seen with an axial loading mechanism. Talus fractures can also present with significant swelling, and when they are associated with a dislocation of the tibiotalar joint and/or the subtalar joint, a significant deformity can be present. A careful neurologic exam should be performed and followed. Stress fractures may present only with tenderness to palpation at the level of the injury.

c. Usual radiographic examination. Obtain three views each of the ankle and the foot. A Harris view evaluates the calcaneal width and profiles the subtalar joint. A CT scan is usually obtained with displaced calcaneal fractures and often with talus fractures to evaluate the myriad of articular surfaces of the tibiotalar and subtalar joints, which are difficult properly to evaluate with plain radiographs. Obtain lumbar spine films to evaluate for associated fracture. Metatarsal stress fractures, if suspected and not apparent on initial radiographs, may be seen on MRI or bone scan.

d. Typical management

(1) Calcaneal fractures should be placed in a well-padded splint and observed for compartment syndrome. Significant subtalar joint depression and comminution may require open reduction with internal fixation once soft-tissue swelling allows. Regardless of treatment, outcomes are often disappointing and result in significant disability.

(2) Talus fractures can be treated with cast immobilization if they are absolutely nondisplaced, but most talar neck fractures are treated with ORIF to decrease the risk of nonunion and avascular necrosis.

(3) Metatarsal fractures can generally be treated nonoperatively with splinting. First metatarsal fractures may be treated operatively if displaced. Transverse fractures of the proximal fifth metatarsal diaphysis (**Jones fracture**), due to being in a vascular watershed region, are prone to healing complications and require more aggressive treatment than other metatarsal fractures, including either strict non-weight bearing with cast immobilization or surgery. An avulsion of the base of the fifth metatarsal, the so-called "pseudo-Jones fracture," can be treated with early weight bearing.

(4) Toe injuries are best treated by "buddy taping" to the adjacent digit and giving the patient a hard-soled shoe for more comfortable ambulation.

e. Pitfalls and pearls. The **diabetic foot** requires special attention and care. Because of neuropathic changes, casts and splints must be well padded and adapted to any deformity of the foot. Typically, foot and ankle fractures in the diabetic require twice the normal period of immobilization. A hot, swollen foot in a diabetic patient should be examined radiographically for neuropathic fractures (the Charcot foot) and immobilized. This should be differentiated from cellulitis and infection with laboratory tests, although they can occur simultaneously.

2. Dislocations (talar, LisFranc)

a. Typical mechanism. The level of energy is similar to that for calcaneal and talar fractures. Talar dislocation occurs with forced foot inversion. **LisFranc** injuries are disruptions of the tarsal-metatarsal joints by either dislocation or fracture dislocation and are caused by a bending or twisting force through the midfoot.

b. Typical physical exam. With **talar dislocations,** there is often significant deformity. Dislocation of the talar body can commonly impinge on adjacent neurovascular structures and can be entrapped by tendons. Neurovascular compromise is possible and must be identified and treated emergently. Fracture-dislocations of the tarsometatarsal joint **(LisFranc)** are associated with significant swelling and midfoot tenderness. Both injuries can have associated compartment syndrome of the foot.

c. Usual radiographic evaluation. With a talus dislocation, obtain views of both the ankle and the foot. If it is associated with a fracture, perform imaging as noted previously. LisFranc fractures are diagnosed radiographically by incongruity of the tarsometatarsal joints, most commonly between the medial base of the second metatarsal and the medial edge of the middle cuneiform, which normally are collinear. A CT scan may be useful if a significant fracture component is present.

d. Typical management

(1) Talar dislocations are treated with emergent reduction to decrease the risk of avascular necrosis, neurovascular injury, and skin compromise. Soft-tissue interposition can prevent closed reduction, in which case open reduction is required. Associated fractures must be anatomically reduced and stabilized as described previously.

(2) LisFranc injuries are splinted, iced, and elevated in preparation for eventual operative reduction and fixation. An attempt at closed reduction should be made to help decrease soft-tissue swelling.

e. Pitfalls and pearls: Concerns are similar to those for fractures.

VI. OTHER ORTHOPEDIC CONDITIONS

A. Infection must be considered in any patient with localized findings (pain, redness, swelling, warmth) or systemic findings (fever, malaise, and tachycardia). **Acute infections** often respond to medical treatment with appropriate antibiotic therapy (cellulitis) and surgical decompression (abscess, septic bursitis).

1. Septic arthritis usually occurs in association with immunosuppression, systemic infection, preexisting joint disease, previous joint surgery, or intravenous drug abuse. It is of special concern in patients with joint replacements.

a. Examination reveals tenderness, effusion, increased warmth, and **pain with motion.** Laboratory tests may demonstrate an elevated erythrocyte sedimentation rate (ESR), C-reactive protein (CRP), and/or white blood cell (WBC) count. Diagnosis is confirmed by needle aspiration and laboratory analysis of synovial fluid for cell count and differential, Gram stain, routine aerobic and anaerobic cultures, and crystal analysis. **Baseline radiographs** are obtained at the time of presentation (note that significant changes occur late, after 7 to 10 days).

b. Treatment with broad-spectrum intravenous antibiotics (usually vancomycin, with or without gentamicin) should be initiated **after** adequate joint fluid specimens are obtained. If septic arthritis is diagnosed, some means of joint lavage should be performed (serial aspirations, arthroscopic or open débridement) to prevent progressive cartilage degradation and further systemic illness.

2. Osteomyelitis. Childhood osteomyelitis most commonly results from hematogenous spread of bacteria to the metaphysis. Adult osteomyelitis typically occurs from direct inoculation via surgery, an open fracture, or chronic soft-tissue ulceration. Hematogenous spread may occur in cases of intravenous drug abuse, sickle cell disease, and immunosuppression.

    a. Physical examination findings are similar to those in septic arthritis, if located about a joint, but may also reveal bony tenderness and drainage. Assess the soft tissues about the region. Examine for infective sources.

    b. Appropriate **imaging studies** start with plain radiographs of the area. Bone scan, MRI, or tagged WBC scan may be useful to confirm the diagnosis. Laboratory examination includes ESR, CRP, peripheral WBC count, and blood cultures.

    c. Treatment typically involves an extended course of empiric intravenous antibiotics (guided by cultures if available). Response to treatment is gauged clinically and with ESR and CRP. If response is inadequate, bone biopsy can be done to obtain further cultures for sensitivities. Débridement of the infected bone is sometimes required. Associated septic arthritis is treated as outlined previously.

  3. Suppurative flexor tenosynovitis. Patients present with tenderness along the flexor sheath, the finger held in a semiflexed position, pain with finger extension, and fusiform swelling of the entire finger (**Kanavel signs**). Look for associated skin wounds (may appear quite innocuous). The patient's entire hand must also be examined because infection can extend into other spaces. Immediate surgical decompression, irrigation, and débridement are indicated in addition to initiation of intravenous antibiotics.

  4. Abscess

    a. Hand. Numerous potential spaces exist that can become infected. All present with pain, erythema, tense swelling, induration, and tenderness to palpation. Systemic signs of infection may or may not be present. Immediate surgical drainage is required.

    b. Olecranon and prepatellar bursa can become infected and present with pain, redness, heat and fluctuance, often with a zone of cellulitis. Treatment is decompression and packing in addition to a course of oral antibiotics. A significant cellulitis may necessitate a brief course of intravenous antibiotics.

    c. Others. Infection in the soft tissue may occur anywhere and presents with pain, tenderness, swelling, fluctuation, and induration. Fluid collections are often readily localized with large-bore needle aspiration. Surgical decompression can often be performed in the emergency department at presentation or nonurgently (unless clinically septic) in the operating room under anesthesia.

B. Compartment syndrome is characterized by an increase in tissue pressure within a closed osteofascial space sufficient to compromise microcirculation, leading to irreversible damage to tissues within that compartment, including muscle and nerves. This can cause nerve dysfunction and muscle loss, which in turn can progress to rhabdomyolysis and acute renal failure. The end result can be a chronically wasted, contracted, paralytic extremity.

  1. Location. Although it occurs most frequently in the anterior, lateral, or posterior compartments of the leg or the volar or dorsal compartments of the forearm, it can also occur about the elbow or in the thigh, hand, or foot.

  2. Causes. Long-bone fracture, crush, or vascular injuries are common risk factors. Increased capillary permeability secondary to postischemic swelling, trauma, or burns may also contribute to compartment syndrome. Muscle hypertrophy, tight dressings, and pneumatic antishock garments (e.g., military antishock trousers) are less common causes.

  3. Examination

    a. Based on injury and physical findings, patients at risk for compartment syndrome should be identified early and examined frequently. The **five "P's"** are classically used to aide in diagnosis: **Pain** out of proportion to the injury, particularly an increasing and disproportionate narcotic demand and unexpectedly poor response to appropriate pain medication, and **pain** with passive motion of involved muscles or tendons traversing the involved compartment are relatively early signs. **Paresthesias** in the distribution of the peripheral nerves traversing the involved compartment occur at an intermediate time. **Paralysis, pallor, and pulselessness** are late signs and likely indicate irreversible soft-tissue injury. If pulses are altered or absent, major arterial occlusion rather than compartment syndrome should be considered in the diagnosis.

b. In the awake patient, compartment syndrome is a clinical diagnosis. However, when the clinical picture and physical examination are sufficiently uncertain or in the unresponsive patient, **compartment pressures** should be measured. Multiple measurements should be taken in different locations. Comparison to uninvolved compartments may be helpful.

4. Treatment. Circumferential bandages, splints, or casts should be removed. Extremities should be elevated to above the level of the heart. Excessive elevation can be counterproductive. If the clinical picture deteriorates or physical examination worsens, then fasciotomy should be performed. Generally, if clinical suspicion warrants the measurement of compartment pressure, a fasciotomy is likely indicated. For pressures within 30 mm Hg of the diastolic blood pressure with equivocal clinical examination, fasciotomy is in order.

C. Open fractures and joints. Lacerations or wounds near fractures or joints can communicate and should be carefully evaluated. If exposed bone is not evident, wounds should be probed to determine whether communication to fracture is present. Joints may be distended with sterile saline to check for extravasation from adjacent wounds, but this method is associated with poor sensitivity. Air in the joint on x-ray and fat droplets in blood from the wound also confirm communication with a joint or fracture, respectively.

1. Treatment. Assess wounds, irrigate grossly contaminated wounds with normal saline, apply moist saline-soaked dressing, reduce the fracture or joint, and splint the extremity. Administer tetanus prophylaxis and intravenous antibiotics based on fracture severity. Type I open fractures, defined as having a skin opening less than 1 cm, require a first-generation cephalosporin. With type II and III injuries (skin opening >1 cm and significant soft-tissue stripping from bone), an aminoglycoside should be added. Farm injuries require administration of penicillin to cover for *Clostridium perfringens*.

2. Gunshot injuries

a. It is helpful to identify the **weapon caliber and type.** High-energy injuries (shotgun, rifle, or high-caliber (.357 or.44) handguns may require operative débridement secondary to severe soft-tissue or bony damage. With lower-energy injuries (most handguns, .22 rifles), débridement is generally not needed because less damage occurs.

b. Neurovascular status should be checked closely and followed in high-energy injuries. Deficits are usually due to concussive injury and not laceration, but developing deficits are a sign of compartment syndrome. Obtain radiographs to assess for bony involvement. If the wound is near a joint with concern for intra-articular involvement, aspirate to check for hemarthrosis and sterilely distend the joint capsule with saline, looking for extravasation from the wound. If the injury is not fresh, the track may have sealed and give a false-negative exam.

c. Treatment. Clean the skin, débride the wound edges, and irrigate thoroughly. Apply a dressing and splint the extremity if a fracture is found. If no neurovascular compromise or compartment syndrome exists, isolated soft-tissue injury is treated with local wound care with or without oral antibiotics.

3. Traumatic amputation. A team approach is needed to evaluate for possible reimplantation, and all necessary consultants should be contacted early.

a. Management. The proximal stump is cleaned, and a compressive dressing is applied. Tourniquets are not used. Amputated parts are wrapped in moist gauze, placed in a bag, and cooled by placing on ice (must avoid freezing damage). The amputated part can be sent to the operating room before the patient for preparation. Reimplantation is most likely to be successful with a sharp amputation and not likely possible with crush injuries or other injuries with a wide zone of injury. Timing is of the essence, and a rapid and efficient evaluation is critical.

VII. PRACTICAL PROCEDURES

A. Common splints and casts. Splints and casts stabilize bones and joints and limit further soft-tissue injury and swelling and help to minimize pain. They also facilitate further clinical and radiographic evaluation. Splints are not circumferential as cast are, and so splints allow for swelling better than casts but are less durable. Air splints are used only in the emergency setting because they increase pressure in the extremity and can compromise blood flow.

1. Preparation and application. Prefabricated splints and immobilizers can be used if available. Plaster splints consist of plaster and cast padding. The required length to include a joint above and below the injury is measured from the uninjured side. Two layers of soft roll are applied against the skin, and extra padding is placed over bony prominences. A ten-layer-thick stack of plaster splint material is wetted in cold to lukewarm water and squeezed until damp. Hot water should be avoided because increased water temperature leads to a decreased setting time and an increased setting temperature that can lead to burns. The splint is applied over the soft-roll padding and wrapped lightly with an elastic bandage. The extremity is held in the appropriate position (without making indentations that can lead to skin breakdown) until the plaster is firm.

2. Upper-extremity splints. Removal of all of the patient's jewelry is mandatory.

  a. Commercial shoulder immobilizers, Velpeau dressing, and sling and swathe are used for shoulder dislocations, humerus fractures, and some elbow fractures. A pad is placed in the axilla to prevent skin maceration.

  b. Figure-of-eight slings can be used for clavicle fracture stabilization but are often poorly tolerated by adults and offer little advantage over slings for these injuries.

  c. Posterior and sugar tong splints are used in elbow, forearm, and wrist injuries. They are applied with the patient's elbow flexed to not greater than 90 degrees, the wrist in neutral to slight extension, and forearm in neutral rotation.

  d. Thumb spica, ulnar/radial gutter, and volar/dorsal forearm splints are used for forearm, hand, and wrist injuries. Finger injuries may be treated with prefabricated aluminum splint material. For wrist and hand injuries, immobilization is performed with the patient's hand and wrist in a so-called **safe position:** the wrist in 20 to 30 degrees of extension, the metacarpophalangeal joints in 70 to 80 degrees of flexion, and the interphalangeal joints extended.

3. Lower-extremity splints

  a. Thomas/Hare traction splints are used by primary responders for femur fractures. Traction is applied by an ankle hitch, with counter traction across the ischial tuberosity. The splint should not be left in place for longer than 2 hours because sloughing of the skin can occur around the ankle and groin.

  b. A Jones dressing with or without plaster reinforcements is used in acute knee, ankle, calcaneous, and tibial pilon fractures or any other foot or lower leg injury where considerable swelling is expected. The injured extremity is wrapped with cotton, followed by a lightly wrapped elastic bandage. Plaster splints can be applied to the posterior, medial, and lateral aspects for added stability. Circumferential plaster should be avoided.

  c. Short leg splints are used in acute leg or foot trauma. They extend from below the knee to the toes and include posterior, medial, and lateral plaster slabs. Posterior slabs alone are inadequate. The ankle should be immobilized in the neutral position.

4. Precautions. Bony prominences should be padded. Casts or circumferential splints are avoided in acute trauma when swelling is anticipated.

B. Anesthesia for fracture and joint reduction

1. Local anesthesia. Appropriate sterile technique must be used.

    a. Digital nerve block: The digital nerves of the fingers or toes can be blocked by infiltrating 2 to 5 mL of lidocaine with or without the addition of a longer-acting agent (such as bupivacaine) into the web spaces adjacent to the injured digit ensuring infiltration to the palmar or plantar skin. Ring blocks are needed for the thumb and great toes and involve circumferential subcutaneous infiltration about the digit. **Epinephrine-containing products are contraindicated in digits.**

    b. Hematoma block involves direct injection of lidocaine into a fracture site and is especially effective with fractures of the distal radius. A 21-gauge needle is inserted into the fracture site through the dorsal forearm. Aspiration of blood confirms the appropriate position of the needle in the fracture site. Approximately 8 to 10 mL of 1% of lidocaine without epinephrine is then infiltrated. A hematoma block in conjunction with light sedation often provides excellent analgesia and relaxation for reduction.

    c. Intra-articular injection is used to provide analgesia for reduction of intraarticular fractures and dislocations. Under **sterile conditions**, the joint is entered with a needle with verification of placement by aspiration of blood (in the case of fracture) and the easy flow of the anesthetic from the syringe. The **ankle** may be entered anteriorly adjacent to either malleolus, and the **elbow** laterally in the triangle formed by the lateral epicondyle, radial head, and olecranon. Finally, the shoulder is entered either anteriorly 1 cm lateral to the coracoid process or posteriorly 2 cm distal and 2 cm medial to the posterolateral edge of the acromion aiming toward the corocoid.

  2. Sedation. For safety reasons, the person performing a reduction cannot be in charge of the sedation and its monitoring. Midazolam (Versed) and fentanyl are administered intravenously slowly over 2 to 5 minutes to achieve easily arousable sedation and pain control (usually a total of 2 to 5 mg midazolam is needed). Close observation of respiratory status and monitoring with a pulse oximeter are required. Midazolam sedation is readily reversed with flumazenil (Romazicon) and fentanyl with naloxone hydrochloride (Narcan). Patients are generally monitored for 60 minutes after manipulation.

C. Technique for reduction of fracture or dislocation (see also specific injury sections)

  1. Dislocation. After adequate analgesia and sedation as noted, longitudinal traction of the affected extremity (avoiding sudden, forceful movements) is applied. Start gently and progress with increasing force until reduction is achieved. The dislocated fragment is manipulated by applying pressure in the direction of reduction. Gentle rotation, flexion, or extension may help but is performed cautiously because long-bone fracture may occur. **Great care should be taken in the elderly to avoid fracture.**

  2. Fracture. Traction is applied first in the direction of the angulation (recreating the injury to release the impaction of the bony ends) and then in-line with the long axis of the limb to correct the alignment, rotation, and length. Pressure is applied to the distal fragment in the direction of the reduced position. Postreduction x-rays are obtained in all cases, and the joint or extremity is immobilized in the reduced position.

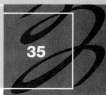
 EVALUATION OF HEMATURIA

I. HEMATURIA is the hallmark of disease in the genitourinary tract and warrants a thorough investigation. Pain associated with hematuria may suggest a benign etiology such as cystitis or urinary calculi. However, painless hematuria should be regarded as secondary to a tumor until proven otherwise.

A. All of the following warrant a hematuria workup:

1. Any episode of gross hematuria.

2. At least three red blood cells (RBCs) per high-power field on two of three urine specimens.

B. Evaluation of hematuria

1. Freshly voided urine is evaluated with a dipstick and microscopic analysis for the following:

   a. Specific gravity is noted because RBC rupture occurs in hypotonic urine (specific gravity <1.008).

   b. Urinary pH can aid in the diagnosis of disease.

   c. Microscopic analysis evaluates RBC morphology, casts, crystals, white blood cell (WBC) count, and bacteria.

   d. The presence and character of **clots** can be revealing; upper tract bleeding may cause vermiform (wormlike) clots, whereas bladder clots may be amorphous.

2. Complete blood cell (CBC) count and coagulation parameters should be studied with gross hematuria. Serum creatinine is essential before performing a contrast study of upper tracts.

3. Radiologic evaluation of the upper urinary tract is mandatory. Computed tomography (CT) urogram is the preferred imaging modality because it provides greater detail of the renal parenchyma and collecting system in comparison to the older routine of an intravenous pyelogram (IVP) and renal ultrasound. In addition, there is the obvious benefit of viewing the remainder of the abdomen.

4. The lower urinary tract is visualized with **cystoscopy.**

5. Urine is sent for culture and cytology.

6. If the etiology of the hematuria is not revealed with the foregoing, the patient should have a repeat urinalysis (UA), urine cytology, and a blood pressure measurement at 6, 12, 24, and 36 months (*Urology* 2001;57:604).

C. Treatment. Gross hematuria requires urgent evaluation.

1. Patients passing blood clots may require irrigation and initiation of continuous bladder irrigation with normal saline via a three-way Foley catheter (22 to 24 French). Prostatic bleeding may be controlled with gentle catheter traction.

2. Bladder irrigation with 1% alum or 1% silver nitrate can alleviate persistent bleeding. It is imperative that the bladder be free of clots before initiating alum or silver nitrate irrigation. Silver nitrate and alum are astringents that act by protein precipitation over the bleeding surfaces. Initiation of intravenous ε-aminocaproic acid [Amicar; 5 g in 250 mL of dextrose 5% in water (D5W) infused over 1 hour, then 1-g/hour continuous infusion] can also be used to help control bleeding. ε-Aminocaproic acid is an inhibitor of fibrinolysis and can be associated with thromboembolic complications. It should be used judiciously and should not be used in any patient suspected of disseminated intravascular coagulopathy. It may also be given orally or administered intravesically.

3. **Persistent bleeding** on continuous bladder irrigation or significant gross hematuria in the unstable patient requires immediate cystoscopic evaluation to localize and control bleeding.

 DISEASES OF THE KIDNEY

I. EVALUATION OF RENAL MASSES

A. Increased use of abdominal CT scanning and ultrasonography has resulted in detection of more asymptomatic **renal masses.** These masses must be characterized as benign or malignant.

B. The vast majority of masses are benign cysts (*Radiology* 1991;179:307).

C. Renal cysts occur in one half of persons older than 50 years. Other **benign lesions** include infarction, abscess, hemangioma, angiomyolipoma, and adenoma. **Most solid renal masses** (85% to 90%) are renal cell carcinomas (RCCa). Up to 33% of these malignancies are diagnosed incidentally by imaging obtained for other reasons (*Abdom Imaging* 2002;27:629). Over the last 20 years, the incidence of RCCa has been increasing. Improved imaging and early diagnosis have dramatically increased the number of patients who present with curable disease. **Other malignant lesions** that present as renal masses include transitional cell carcinoma, oncocytoma (benign in the vast majority of cases), sarcoma, lymphoma, leukemia, and metastatic tumor (lung, breast, gastrointestinal, prostate, pancreatic tumors, and melanoma).

D. Presentation. The historical triad of flank pain, hematuria, and flank mass occurs less than 10% of the time.

E. From 10% to 40% of renal cell carcinomas are associated with **paraneoplastic syndromes.**

1. Hypertension from **renin overproduction** is common.
2. **Stauffer syndrome** (nonmetastatic hepatic dysfunction) is seen in some patients and resolves after tumor removal.
3. **Hypercalcemia** from parathyroid hormone–like protein produced by the tumor also may occur.
4. **Erythrocytosis** can occur as a result of production of erythropoietin by the tumor.

F. Staging. The most common sites of renal cell carcinoma metastasis are bone, liver, and lungs. In addition to a complete history and physical examination, it is imperative to stage RCCa prior to initiating any therapy. Blood testing should include a complete blood count, electrolytes, calcium, creatinine, and liver function tests. All patients need a chest radiograph and cross-sectional abdominal imaging [CT or magnetic resonance imaging (MRI) scan with contrast]. Radionuclide bone scan is not necessary in patients without skeletal symptoms who have normal alkaline phosphatase and serum calcium levels. The TNM (tumor, node, metastasis) staging system for RCCa is outlined in Table 35-1.

G. Imaging modalities

1. **CT scan** with and without intravenous contrast is the preferred diagnostic study for evaluating a renal mass. Precontrast images may be hypodense, isodense, or hyperdense compared with normal renal parenchyma; renal cell carcinomas generally enhance, but to a lesser degree than surrounding parenchyma. CT also provides staging information, including local extent of the tumor, presence of regional lymphadenopathy, and presence of distant metastatic lesions (lung, liver, or adrenal gland).

2. **Ultrasonography** is the modality of choice in determining whether a lesion is solid or cystic. **Doppler ultrasonography** is useful for evaluating vena caval involvement.

   a. The **Bosniak** classification of renal cysts (*Radiology* 1991;179:307) is as follows:

   (1) Category I: simple cyst.

   (2) Category II: high-density cyst; thin, smooth septa; or linear calcification.

TABLE 35-1	American Joint Committee on Cancer Staging of Kidney Cancer		
Stage	Tumor (T)[a]	Node (N)[b]	Metastasis (M)[c]
I	T1	N0	M0
II	T2	N0	M0
III	T1	N1	M0
	T2	N1	M0
	T3	N0, N1	M0
IV	T4	N0, N1	M0
	Any T	N2, N3	M0
	Any T	Any N	M1

[a]T1, tumor ≤7 cm in greatest dimension, limited to the kidney; T2, tumor >7 cm in greatest dimension, limited to the kidney; T3, tumor extends into major veins or invades adrenal gland or perinephric tissues, but not beyond Gerota's fascia; T3a, tumor invades adrenal gland or perinephric tissues, but not beyond Gerota's fascia; T3b, tumor grossly extends into renal vein or vena cava below diaphragm; T3c, tumor grossly extends into vena cava above the diaphragm; T4, tumor grossly extends beyond Gerota's fascia.
[b]N0, no regional lymph node metastasis; N1, metastasis in a single regional lymph node, 2 cm in greatest dimension; N2, metastasis in a single regional lymph node, >2 cm but not >5 cm in greatest dimension, or multiple lymph nodes, none >5 cm in greatest dimension; N3, metastasis in a lymph node >5 cm in greatest dimension.
[c]M0, no distant metastasis; M1, distant metastasis.

> (3) **Category IIF (requires follow-up):** multiple smooth, thin septae or thickened, nonenhancing septa; high-density cyst greater than 3 cm.
> (4) **Category III:** indeterminate lesions; numerous or thick septa, or both; thick calcification. These lesions require surgical management.
> (5) **Category IV:** high probability of malignancy with cystic component, irregular margins, and solid vascular elements. These lesions require surgical management.
> **3. MR scan** is useful for staging renal tumors (especially in patients with renal insufficiency or allergy to contrast dye) and for detecting tumor thrombus in the renal vein and inferior vena cava.

II. MANAGEMENT OF RENAL MASSES

A. Radical nephrectomy remains the most effective treatment modality for stage T1 and T2 disease. Radical nephrectomy involves removing the kidney outside of Gerota's fascia. Ten-year survival after nephrectomy for Robson stage I and II lesions was greater than 78% in one modern series (*J Urol* 1998;159:192). Laparoscopic radical nephrectomy has been shown to provide equivalent oncologic results in several single institutional reports (*J Urol* 2005;174:1222, *J Endourol* 2005;19:803, *Urology* 2003;62:1018). Nephron-sparing surgery (partial nephrectomy) has become the standard of care for small T1 (<4 cm) lesions (*J Urol* 2004;171:2181). For smaller tumors, laparoscopic partial nephrectomy, cryoablation, and radiofrequency ablation remain experimental.

B. Renal cell carcinoma is resistant to radiation and chemotherapy. Immunotherapy protocols using interferon and interleukin-2 have demonstrated increased survival after nephrectomy for metastatic renal cell carcinoma in patients with excellent functional status (*J Urol* 2000;163:154S).

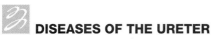

DISEASES OF THE URETER

I. URETEROPELVIC JUNCTION OBSTRUCTION (UPJO)

A. UPJO is often a **congenital anomaly** that results from a stenotic segment of ureter. Acquired lesions may include tortuous or kinked ureters as a result of vesicoureteral reflux, benign tumors such as fibroepithelial polyps, or scarring as a result of stone disease, ischemia, or previous surgical manipulation of the urinary system. The role of crossing vessels (present in one third of cases) has not been firmly established, although their presence may be associated with treatment failures.

B. Presentation. Although UPJO can be a congenital problem, patients may present at any age. Common symptoms are flank pain (which may be intermittent), hematuria, infection, and, rarely, hypertension.

C. Radiographic studies help to determine the site and functional significance of the obstruction. Useful studies include IVP, diuretic renal scintigraphy, and retrograde pyelography. Ultrasound may demonstrate hydronephrosis, but this is not diagnostic of functional obstruction.

D. Open pyeloplasty is the gold standard treatment, with success rates greater than 90%. Recently, a variety of minimally invasive procedures have been developed to avoid the morbidity of open surgery. Options include laparoscopic pyeloplasty, percutaneous endopyelotomy, and ureteroscopic or retrograde endopyelotomy with a balloon-cutting device.

II. UROLITHIASIS

A. Epidemiology. The peak incidence of urinary calculi is in the third to fifth decades. Stones are more prevalent in men than in women. Stone incidence is increased during the late summer months. Dietary factors leading to stone formation include low water intake and high protein or oxalate (leafy green vegetable) consumption. Calcium restriction is not recommended as a means of preventing stone formation; however, a low-sodium diet may decrease calciuria. Citrus juices, particularly lemonade, may increase urinary levels of citrate, an inhibitor of stone formation (*J Urol* 1996;156:907). Various drugs, including high-dose vitamins C and D, acetazolamide, triamterene, and some protease inhibitors (indinavir) (*Lancet* 1997;349:1294), have been associated with stone formation. Disease states, such as inflammatory bowel disease, and metabolic disorders, such as type I renal tubular acidosis or cystinuria, can also contribute to stone formation.

B. Clinical features. Acute onset of severe flank pain or renal colic, often associated with nausea and vomiting, results from urinary obstruction by the stone. Common locations for stones to become impacted include the renal infundibulum, the ureteropelvic junction, the crossing of the iliac vessels, and the ureterovesical junction, which is the most constricted area through which the stone must pass. Patients may present with microscopic or gross hematuria, but 15% of patients may have no hematuria.

C. Types of calculi

1. Calcium stones make up approximately 70% of all stones. Disorders of calcium metabolism, such as increased intestinal absorption or increased renal excretion of calcium or oxalate, can cause calcium stones. Systemic disorders, such as hyperparathyroidism, sarcoidosis, immobilization (causing calcium resorption from bone), and type I renal tubular acidosis, can lead to these derangements of calcium metabolism.

2. Uric acid stones make up approximately 10% of all stones. They occur as a result of hyperuricosuria, persistently acidic pH, and low urine volumes.

3. Cysteine stones account for 4% of stones. They are caused by a defect in tubular reabsorption of cysteine that is inherited in an autosomal recessive manner. Hexagonal crystals in the urine are highly suggestive of cysteine stones.

4. Magnesium ammonium phosphate or struvite stones account for 15% of stones and are associated with urinary tract infection, commonly with urea-splitting organisms, and a chronically alkaline urinary pH (>7.2). Urinalysis may demonstrate rectangular "coffin lid" crystals.

D. Evaluation of urinary calculi

1. Urinalysis, including microscopic examination and urine culture, should be performed on all patients suspected of having calculi.

2. Serum electrolytes, including calcium, and creatinine levels are also part of the standard workup. In addition, uric acid levels and parathyroid hormone levels may be helpful. A CBC with differential can be obtained in patients with signs of concurrent infection.

3. **Noncontrast spiral CT** has replaced IVP as the diagnostic study of choice in the acute setting (*J Urol* 1998;160:679). For patients with suspected nephrolithiasis but atypical symptoms, CT may elucidate other causes of abdominal pain. Signs of obstruction include hydroureteronephrosis and perinephric fat stranding.

4. **KUB (kidneys, ureters, bladder)** should be used to monitor stone passage in patients with already documented nephrolithiasis and to evaluate whether the stone is amenable to extracorporeal shock-wave lithotripsy (ESWL).

E. **Management of urinary calculi**

1. **Hydration.** Intravenous fluids are required if the patient is nauseated and cannot take oral fluids. Normal saline usually is initiated at 150 mL/hour in appropriate patients.

2. **Pain management.** Patients whose pain is not adequately managed with oral analgesics require hospitalization for administration of parenteral narcotics. Parenteral nonsteroidal compounds, such as ketorolac, can be effective in reducing the pain of renal colic but should not be used in patients who may undergo lithotripsy. ESWL is contraindicated within 72 hours of administration of nonsteroidal analgesics to minimize the risk of renal hematoma.

3. **Urine should be collected and strained** to retrieve the stone. The stone should be analyzed for composition.

4. **Any patient found to have an obstructing stone in the presence of infection or fever needs emergent decompression** with percutaneous nephrostomy tube or stent placement. This situation can deteriorate quickly into a life-threatening crisis, particularly in the diabetic or immunosuppressed patient.

5. **Ninety-five percent of stones 4 mm or smaller in size pass spontaneously** (*J Urol* 1997;158:1915). Patients may be given up to 4 weeks to pass a partially obstructing stone without permanent renal damage. Patients with stones larger than 4 mm or with intractable symptoms of pain, nausea, or vomiting may need early surgical treatment to relieve obstruction with a ureteral stent, shock-wave lithotripsy, or ureteroscopy with stone ablation or retrieval.

6. Patients who have had one episode of nephrolithiasis do not require further workup. Those who have recurrent episodes require a 24-hour urine collection for volume, creatinine, pH, sodium, calcium, magnesium, phosphorous, oxalate, citrate, uric acid, and protein measurement.

7. Potassium citrate may help to prevent stone recurrence by increasing urinary citrate levels and alkalizing the urine. Uric acid stones may dissolve by increasing urinary pH, and calcium stones may be prevented with thiazide diuretics.

 DISEASES OF THE URINARY BLADDER

I. **BLADDER CANCER.** Bladder cancer is found in up to 10% of patients with microscopic hematuria.

A. **Transitional cell carcinoma** accounts for up to 90% of bladder tumors in the United States; squamous cell carcinoma and adenocarcinoma are less common. Transitional cell carcinoma has been linked directly to cigarette smoking, aniline dye and aromatic amine exposure, and chronic phenacetin use. Patients who have received cyclophosphamide are at increased risk for developing transitional cell carcinoma; use of the uroprotectant mesna (2-mercaptoethane sodium sulfonate) may reduce this risk as well as reduce the risk of hemorrhagic cystitis.

B. **Transitional cell cancer is categorized as superficial or invasive.** Staging is outlined in Table 35-2.

C. **Superficial tumors** are exophytic papillary lesions that do not invade the muscular bladder wall. These tumors can be treated with transurethral resection. Between 65% and 85% of superficial tumors recur; therefore, diligent follow-up is necessary. Recurrent tumors are treated with transurethral resection and intravesical therapy (bacillus Calmette-Guérin or mitomycin C). In 10% to 15% of patients with superficial

TABLE 35-2	American Joint Committee on Cancer Staging for Bladder Cancer		
Stage	**Tumor (T)**[a]	**Node (N)**[b]	**Metastasis (M)**[c]
0_a	Ta	N0	M0
0_{is}	Tis	N0	M0
I	T1	N0	M0
II	T2a	N0	M0
	T2b	N0	M0
III	T3a	N0	M0
	T3b	N0	M0
IV	T4a	N0	M0
	T4b	N0	M0
	Any T	N1–3	M0
	Any T	Any N	M1

[a]Ta, noninvasive papillary carcinoma; Tis, carcinoma *in situ*; T1, tumor invades subepithelial connective tissue; T2, tumor invades muscle; T2a, tumor invades superficial muscle (inner half); T2b, tumor invades deep muscle (outer half); T3, tumor invades perivesical tissue; T3a, microscopically; T3b, macroscopically (extravesical mass); T4, tumor invades any of the following prostate, uterus, vagina, pelvic wall, or abdominal wall; T4a, tumor invades prostate, uterus, or vagina; T4b, tumor invades pelvic wall or abdominal wall.
[b]N0, no regional lymph node metastasis; N1, metastasis in a single lymph node ≤2 cm in largest dimension; N2, metastasis in a single lymph node >2 cm but not >5 cm in greatest dimension, or multiple lymph nodes, none >5 cm in greatest dimension; N3, metastasis in a lymph node >5 cm in greatest dimension
[c]M0, no distant metastasis; M1, distant metastasis.

bladder tumors, the tumors progress to muscle-invasive disease; their tendency to progress depends on stage and grade.

D. Muscle-invasive transitional cell carcinoma is treated with radical cystectomy and urinary diversion. Radical cystectomy involves radical cystoprostatectomy (removal of bladder, prostate, and possibly urethra) in the male and anterior exenteration (removal of bladder, urethra, uterus, cervix, and anterior wall of vagina) in the female. Appropriate metastatic evaluation for patients with invasive bladder cancer includes chest radiograph, CT urogram, bone scan, and liver function tests. Despite this aggressive management, only 50% of patients with invasive bladder cancer are rendered completely free of tumor because many have occult metastases at the time of surgery.

E. Chemotherapy is the treatment of choice for locally advanced or metastatic bladder cancer. MVAC [methotrexate, vinblastine, doxorubicin (Adriamycin), and *cis*-platinum] has been the traditional regimen, but recent studies have shown the combination of gemcitabine and *cis*-platinum to have equivalent oncologic efficacy with an improved side effect profile (*J Clin Oncol* 2005;23:4602).

DISEASES OF THE PROSTATE

I. PROSTATE CANCER
A. Prostate examination. Digital rectal examination (DRE) of the prostate is an important part of the physical examination. The **normal prostate** is chestnut sized and measures 3.5 cm wide at the base, 2.5 cm long, and 2.5 cm deep; it weighs approximately 20 g. The prostate should feel smooth and have the consistency of the contracted thenar eminence of the thumb. The prostate is best examined when the patient is standing with the knees slightly flexed and elbows resting on a table or in the lateral decubitus position with the hips flexed.

B. Prostate nodules usually are small (pea sized) or larger firm areas within the peripheral zone of the prostate. Fifty percent of prostate nodules represent prostate cancer and must be evaluated with transrectal ultrasonography (TRUS) and prostate biopsy. Serum prostate-specific antigen (PSA) is a more sensitive test than DRE for detection of prostate cancer, but the tests should be used together to maximize cancer detection (*J Urol* 1994;151:1283).

C. Prostate cancer is the most common noncutaneous malignancy in American men and the second leading cause of cancer death. Twenty percent of men with prostate cancer die of the disease. Prostate cancer rarely causes symptoms until it becomes locally advanced or metastatic.

D. Current American Urological Association and American Cancer Society guidelines recommend that men age 50 years and older begin prostate cancer screening with a yearly DRE and PSA measurement. African American men and men with a family history should begin screening at age 45 years (*Oncology* 2000;14:267). Abnormalities in either the DRE (manifest as indurated nodules) or the PSA greater than 2.5 ng/mL should be evaluated by TRUS and needle biopsy of the prostate (*National Comprehensive Cancer Network Clinical Practice Guidelines in Oncology* 2006, http://www.nccn.org).

E. Appropriate staging workup includes DRE and PSA. Table 35-3 outlines current staging for prostate cancer. Bone scan is not necessary for patients with well-differentiated or moderately differentiated tumors and a PSA less than 10. CT is of limited value for patients with well-differentiated or moderately differentiated tumors and a PSA less than 20.

F. Prostate cancer is graded by the **Gleason scoring system,** which is based on the histologic architectural pattern of the prostate gland. The two most predominant architectural patterns are assigned a grade 1 through 5 (1 being the most differentiated and 5 being the least differentiated). The two patterns are added together to give the overall Gleason score. The Gleason score is reported as the most prevalent grade plus the second most prevalent grade, followed by the sum (e.g., $4 + 3 = 7$). Well-differentiated tumors have a Gleason sum of 2 to 4, moderately differentiated tumors have a sum of 5 or 6, and poorly differentiated tumors have a sum of 8 to 10. For Gleason sum 7, patients with $3 + 4$ are considered moderately differentiated, and those with a $4 + 3$ are considered poorly differentiated.

TABLE 35-3	American Joint Committee on Cancer Staging of Prostate Cancer		
Stage	**Tumor (T)**[a]	**Node (N)**[b]	**Metastasis (M)**[c]
I	T1a	N0	M0[d]
II	T1a	N0	M0
	T1b	N0	M0
	T1c	N0	M0
	T2a,T2b	N0	M0
III	T3	N0	M0
IV	T4	N0	M0
	Any T	N1	M0
	Any T	Any N	M1

[a]T1, clinically inapparent tumor neither palpable nor visible by imaging; T1a, tumor incidental histologic finding in ≤5% of tissue resected; T1b, tumor incidental histologic finding in >5% of tissue resected; T1c, tumor identified by needle biopsy (e.g., because of elevated prostate-specific antigen levels); T2, tumor confined within the prostate; T2a, tumor involves one lobe; T2b, tumor involves both lobes; T3, tumor extends through the prostatic capsule; T3a, extracapsular extension (unilateral or bilateral); T3b, tumor invades seminal vesicles; T4, tumor is fixed or invades adjacent structures other than the seminal vesicle(s) structures, bladder neck, external sphincter, rectum, levator muscles, and/or pelvic wall.
[b]N0, no regional lymph node metastasis; N1, metastasis in regional lymph node(s).
[c]M0, no distant metastasis; M1, distant metastasis; M1a, nonregional lymph node(s); M1b, bone(s); M1c, other site(s).
[d]Includes only well-differentiated (Gleason grade 2–4) tumors.

G. Treatment options for men with organ-confined prostate cancer include radical prostatectomy, external-beam radiation therapy, and interstitial radiotherapy (brachytherapy).

1. **Radical prostatectomy** compared to active surveillance offers a **44%** relative reduction in 10-year prostate cancer related mortality, a **26%** relative reduction in 10-year overall mortality, a **40%** reduction in the risk of distant metastasis, and a **67%** relative reduction in local progression in men with early prostate cancer (*N Engl J Med* 2005;352:19).

2. **External-beam radiotherapy** with delivery of 6,500 to 7,500 cGy achieves disease-free rates of 45% to 85% for localized disease (*N Engl J Med* 1994;331: 996). High-risk patients benefit from adjuvant hormonal therapy in addition to radiotherapy (*Lancet* 2002;360:103, *JAMA* 2004;292:821).

3. **Technical improvements in dosimetry and implantation** combined with reports of low morbidity have led to a renewed interest in brachytherapy. Some authors have suggested that brachytherapy alone may have a higher rate of PSA progression than other treatment modalities (*Urology* 1998;51:884).

4. **Hormonal therapy** with either bilateral orchiectomy or luteinizing hormone–releasing hormone agonists usually is reserved for men with locally advanced or metastatic disease.

5. **Active surveillance** may be appropriate for men with low-grade prostate cancer (*J Urol* 2004;172:S48). The optimal form of treatment for clinically localized prostate cancer has not been conclusively determined.

II. PROSTATITIS is a diagnosis that spans a spectrum of disease entities. The classification and diagnostic criteria for the different forms of prostatitis recently have been changed in an effort to standardize diagnosis to improve research and clinical treatment.

A. Signs and symptoms of urinary tract infection mark acute bacterial prostatitis; many patients have significant voiding complaints, fevers, and malaise. DRE reveals a tender, boggy prostate. Repeat exams should be minimized to avoid spread of infection. Fluoroquinolones are the mainstays of treatment and should be continued for 4 to 6 weeks. Patients with high fevers may require admission for intravenous antibiotics. Drainage of the urinary bladder via a suprapubic tube or a small urethral catheter may be required for patients in urinary retention.

B. Chronic bacterial prostatitis is differentiated from other categories by the presence of documented recurrent bacterial infection of expressed prostatic secretions, postprostatic massage urine, or semen. Treatment is with antibiotics; fluoroquinolones have excellent prostatic penetration.

III. BENIGN PROSTATIC HYPERPLASIA (BPH) is a histologic diagnosis and represents an increase in the number of epithelial and stromal elements of the prostate. Men with BPH and benign prostatic enlargement (BPE) on examination do not necessarily have lower urinary tract symptoms (LUTS).

A. Evaluation. Common signs and symptoms of BPH include hesitancy, decreased force of stream, frequency, urgency, postvoid dribbling, double voiding, incomplete bladder emptying, and nocturia. LUTS is a symptom complex of obstructive and irritative voiding problems. Bladder outlet obstruction (BOO) is objective evidence of obstructive voiding problems and can include a demonstrated decrease in maximum urinary flow rate, increase postvoid residual urine (PVR), and cystoscopic findings of obstruction.

B. Treatment

1. **Medical Therapy. BPH** is most commonly treated medically with α-blockers, such as doxazosin, terazosin, tamsulosin, and alfuzosin. Another class of medications, 5-α-reductase inhibitors, such as finasteride or dutasteride, are also used to treat BPH. The Medical Therapy of Prostatic Symptoms Trial (MTOPS) showed that combination therapy with an α-blocker and a 5-α-reductase inhibitor reduced the risk of overall clinical progression of BPH significantly more than did treatment with either drug alone (*N Engl J Med* 2003;349:2387).

2. **Surgical Therapy.** If medications are ineffective, intervention with some form of prostatectomy is warranted. Microwave thermotherapy is an office-based, transurethral procedure that uses heat energy to cause tissue necrosis, decreased

prostate volume, and improved voiding. The gold standard is the transurethral prostatectomy (TURP), but transurethral resection using various forms of laser energy is being more commonly performed.

IV. **URINARY RETENTION** may result from BPH, prostate cancer, or urethral stricture disease. Retention also can be associated with pelvic trauma, neurologic conditions, or various medications or the postoperative setting.

A. **Evaluation.** A history usually elicits the cause of retention. Patients with BPH who are treated with decongestants containing an α-agonist may develop urinary retention from increased smooth-muscle tone at the bladder neck and the prostate.

B. **Physical examination** reveals a distended lower abdomen. Prostatic enlargement is common on DRE. Serum electrolytes including creatinine level, urinalysis, and urine culture should be obtained. Serum PSA concentration obtained during acute urinary retention often is spuriously elevated and is best measured at least 4 to 6 weeks after the acute event.

C. **Treatment**
   1. **Bladder decompression with a Foley catheter is the mainstay of treatment.** The proper technique of urethral catheter placement involves passing the catheter to the hub and inflating the balloon *only* after the return of urine.
   2. **When a standard Foley catheter cannot be passed easily,** sterile 2% viscous lidocaine can be injected through the urethra. This anesthetizes and relaxes the sphincter, allowing gentle passage of a 16- to 22-French Coudé tip catheter. The catheter is passed gently with the tip directed upward. If the Coudé tip catheter does not pass easily, a urology consultation is required.
   3. **Catheterization should not be attempted when a urethral injury is suspected.** Urethral stricture requires calibration and dilation or placement of a suprapubic tube by a urologist. Urinary clot retention usually requires bladder irrigation.
   4. **Patients should be monitored for postobstructive diuresis, especially if the patient is azotemic.** This is a physiologic response to a hypervolemic state. Occasionally, it can become a pathologic diuresis and may warrant hospital observation, with fluid and electrolyte replacement. Five-percent dextrose in 0.45% saline should be used for hydration. Urine output greater than 200 mL/hour for more than 2 hours should be replaced with 0.5 mL of intravenous 0.45% saline for each 1 mL of urine. Electrolytes should be checked every 6 hours initially and replaced as needed.

 DISEASES OF THE PENIS

I. **PRIAPISM** is a persistent erection that is not associated with sexual stimulation or that continues after orgasm. The corpora cavernosa are affected, but the corpus spongiosum usually is spared. Priapism can be classified as low flow or high flow.

A. **Ischemic priapism** is characterized by little or no blood flow to the corpora and is considered a urologic emergency. Symptoms include pain and tenderness. History should elicit various etiologies of priapism including: (1) hematologic abnormalities, such as **sickle cell disease;** (2) **drugs,** including antihypertensives (hydralazine, guanethidine, prazosin), anticoagulants, antidepressants and psychotropic agents (especially Trazodone), alcohol, marijuana, cocaine, and intracavernous injection of vasoactive substances (prostaglandin E_1, phentolamine, papaverine) used to treat erectile dysfunction; and (3) **neoplasm (especially leukemia),** with venous occlusion, stasis, and emboli. Physical examination reveals firm corpora and a flaccid glans. Stasis, thrombosis, fibrosis, and scarring of the corpora cavernosa eventually can result in erectile dysfunction if priapism is not treated promptly. Of note, phosphodiesterase type 5 (PDE5) inhibitors, which are used for the treatment of erectile dysfunction (see Section II.E.2), are rarely associated with ischemic priapism.

B. **Treatment** (*American Urological Association Clinical Guidelines* 2003)

1. **First-line treatment** involves corporal irrigation and aspiration of old blood from the corpora via a 21-gauge needle.
2. An α-**adrenergic agent** (phenylephrine, 250 to 500 μg) can then be injected. The solution is prepared by mixing 1 mL of phenylephrine (10 mg/mL) in 19 mL of sterile normal saline. Each milliliter contains 500 μg of phenylephrine. Doses can be repeated every 5 to 10 minutes. Patients should be monitored for the possible hemodynamic effects of phenylephrine. Topical or subcutaneous injection of lidocaine before therapeutic injection or irrigation can be helpful for patient comfort. Injections and aspiration should be performed laterally at the 3 o'clock and 9 o'clock positions to avoid the dorsal blood supply of the penis.
3. For patients with sickle cell disease, treatment involves aggressive hydration, supplemental oxygen, and blood transfusion if the hematocrit is low.
4. If evacuation of old blood and injection of a-adrenergic agents fails, **surgical shunting** should be considered. Distal corpus cavernosum-to-glans penis (corpus spongiosum) shunting (**Winter or Al-Ghorab shunt**) is the initial surgical treatment. If distal shunting fails, then a more proximal **side-to-side cavernosospongiosal shunt (Quackel shunt) or cavernosaphenous shunt** may be necessary.

C. **High-flow priapism** is a nonischemic state usually brought about by perineal or genital trauma. A traumatic pudendal arterial fistula or cavernosal artery laceration may give rise to a high-flow state. Diagnosis is confirmed by aspiration of bright-red, well-oxygenated blood. Blood gas analysis can be helpful in differentiating low-flow priapism from high-flow priapism. Treatment is accomplished by embolization of the ipsilateral branch of the pudendal artery.

II. **ERECTILE DYSFUNCTION (ED)** recently has received increasing attention from the public and lay media as a result of new treatment modalities. ED affects 52% of men aged 40 to 70 years of age according to the Massachusetts Male Aging Study; incidence increases with age, but the degree of mild ED remains fairly constant from age 40 to 70 years. Unfortunately, only 20% of men with ED discuss this condition with a health care provider. The overwhelming majority of men have an organic etiology of their ED.

A. **Initial evaluation** entails a frank discussion of the complaint to define the true sexual disorder; one must differentiate ED from premature ejaculation, inability to climax, infertility, and loss of libido. Unlike men with organic ED, those with psychogenic ED have sudden onset and continue to have nocturnal erections. Loss of libido may signal hormonal disturbances. A complete history and physical examination are done to elicit possible underlying causes of ED, including heart disease, hypertension, diabetes, dislipidemia, renal insufficiency, and endocrine disease (hypogonadism). Smokers have a twofold higher incidence of ED. Previous pelvic or penile surgery may be associated with ED.

B. **Attention should be paid to medications,** such as antihypertensives [central-acting agents (clonidine), α-adrenergic blocking agents (prazosin), β-blocking agents], antipsychotics, tricyclic antidepressants, and histamine (H_2) blockers, that may be associated with ED. Heavy use of alcohol and social drugs can also lead to ED.

C. **Physical examination** should focus on genital development and signs of endocrinologic or neurologic abnormalities.

D. **Appropriate laboratory testing** includes serum chemistries, creatinine, CBC, urinalysis, and, when indicated, a limited hormonal evaluation (testosterone and prolactin). In addition, screening for diabetes and hypercholesterolemia should be done. For the majority of patients, ED is multifactorial, and no single cause is identified.

E. **Treatment.** The initial recommendation should be for lifestyle modification and management of the underlying disease. Smoking cessation, diet modification, and exercise have all been shown to improve erectile function and overall health. It is appropriate to counsel patients about available nonsurgical and surgical options for treatment and to encourage treatment until a satisfactory solution is found.

1. **Hormone replacement.** Exogenous testosterone is available in a variety of delivery methods, including parenteral preparations and transdermal therapy. Liver function tests should be monitored. This treatment is best suited for patients with a low libido and documented hypogonadism. The effect of testosterone on erectile function is variable.

2. **Oral therapies.** PDE5 inhibitors should be offered as first-line therapy. Medications include sildenafil (Viagra), tadalafil (Cialis), and vardenafil (Levitra). PDE5 inhibitors inhibit the breakdown of cyclic guanosine monophosphate, allowing smooth-muscle relaxation in the corpus cavernosum. Side effects include headache, facial flushing, and dyspepsia. PDE5 inhibitors are contraindicated in patients who are taking nitrates because of a synergistic effect that results in hypotension.

3. **Intracavernosal therapy.** Injection of vasoactive medications, such as alprostadil (prostaglandin E_1), directly into the corpus cavernosum is effective in 70% to 80% of patients. Side effects are pain with injection, hematoma or ecchymosis, and priapism. An intraurethral alprostadil suppository is also available and is effective in some men.

4. **Vacuum erection device (VED).** For men who fail or are not candidates for medical therapy, a vacuum pump is efficacious, but many couples find it cumbersome and uncomfortable. Patients with difficulty in maintaining an erection due to cavernosal venous insufficiency may benefit from a constriction band.

5. **Surgical options.** For patients who are refractory to noninvasive therapy, consideration may be given to a surgically placed penile implant. These devices have a high degree of success, and they are placed via small genital incisions. There are potential complications, such as infection (2%) and mechanical malfunction (2%).

DISEASES OF THE SCROTUM AND TESTICLES

I. **MANAGEMENT OF SCROTAL EMERGENCIES.** Acute scrotal pathology can result in significant morbidity, testicular loss, and infertility. The diagnosis can be difficult to make and may require scrotal exploration.

A. **Testicular torsion** develops most often in the peripubertal (12 to 18 years old) age group, although it can occur at any age.

1. The **clinical picture** is one of acute onset of testicular pain and swelling, commonly associated with nausea and vomiting. Some patients give a history of a prior episode that spontaneously resolved (intermittent torsion). There usually is no history of voiding complaints, dysuria, fever, or exposure to sexually transmitted diseases.

2. **Physical examination** reveals an extremely tender, swollen testicle high riding in the scrotum with a transverse lie. The cremasteric reflex (elicited by stroking the inner thigh) is absent on the affected side. In contrast to epididymitis, elevation of the scrotum does not provide relief of pain (Prehn sign) in torsion. Normal urinalysis and the absence of leukocytosis help to rule out epididymitis. Testicular torsion is a clinical diagnosis, and if enough suspicions exist, the patient needs to be explored without delay.

3. When the **clinical diagnosis** is equivocal or suspicion is low, color Doppler ultrasound can help to confirm or exclude the diagnosis. Doppler ultrasound has a low false-positive rate and a high sensitivity and specificity (*Pediatrics* 2000;105:604).

4. **Treatment** should not be delayed to obtain imaging. If testicular torsion is suspected, urgent scrotal exploration is indicated. Manual detorsion of the testicle may be attempted in the emergency room, but bilateral orchiopexy is still indicated. Typically, the testicle is detorsed by rotating from a medial to lateral direction. Testicular viability is a function of the reestablishment of perfusion (Table 35-4). Contralateral testicular fixation should be performed at the time of surgery.

B. **Torsion of testicular appendage (appendix testis)** can present with symptoms similar to those of torsion of the testicle, usually in a prepubertal boy. The onset commonly is over 12 to 24 hours.

1. **Extreme tenderness over the appendage** exists, usually on the superior aspect of the testicle. The "blue dot" sign may be present when the ischemic appendage can be seen through the scrotal skin. The testicle has a normal position and lie.

TABLE 35-4	Rate of Salvage in Testicular Torsion

Duration of ischemia (hr)	Salvage rate (%)
0–6	85–97
6–12	55–85
12–24	20–80
>24	<10

Adapted from American Urological Association. *Torsion of the Testis: Changing Concepts* (AUA Update Series IX). Linthicum, MD: American Urological Association; 1990.

Careful examination reveals that the testicle and the epididymis are not diffusely tender or swollen. The cremasteric reflex usually is present. Imaging studies may be necessary if the clinical diagnosis is unclear.

2. **Torsion of the testicular appendage** usually is managed expectantly. Pain is best controlled with anti-inflammatory agents and gradually resolves over 7 to 14 days.

C. **Mild epididymitis** usually presents with a 1- to 2-day onset of unilateral testicular pain and swelling associated with dysuria or urethral discharge.

1. Typically, the **findings** include a painful, indurated epididymis and pyuria. Urinalysis, urine culture, and CBC count are obtained. When clinically indicated, urethral swabs for gonococci and chlamydiae are sent for culture.

2. With **appropriate antibiotic coverage,** these patients can be managed as outpatients. For patients in whom the etiology is gonococcal or chlamydial, ceftriaxone (125 to 250 mg intramuscularly) is given in the emergency room, followed by doxycycline (100 mg orally two times a day for 7 days). Azithromycin, 1 g orally as a one-time dose, is as effective as doxycycline in the treatment of chlamydial infections (*MMWR* 1998;47:51). In older men (>35 years of age), enterobacteria are more common, and a fluoroquinolone, such as ciprofloxacin (500 mg orally two times a day), provides broad coverage until culture sensitivities can be obtained. Nonsteroidal analgesics and scrotal elevation can reduce inflammation and provide symptomatic relief.

3. Moderate to severe cases of epididymitis may require hospital admission. Symptoms usually have been present for several days. Fever and leukocytosis are present. Broad-spectrum antibiotics and supportive measures of bedrest with scrotal elevation should be instituted. Ultrasonography can be useful to rule out abscess formation and assess testicular perfusion.

D. **Fournier gangrene** is a severe polymicrobial soft-tissue infection involving the genitals and perineum. Although the term *Fournier gangrene* usually is applied to men, necrotizing fasciitis of this area can occur in women. Prompt diagnosis and institution of treatment may be lifesaving. Roughly 25% of the patients have a genitourinary source, 25% have an anorectal source, up to 10% have an intra-abdominal source, and nearly 40% have an unidentified source. Diabetic, alcoholic, and other immunocompromised patients appear to be more susceptible. The clinical course is one of abrupt onset with pruritus, rapidly progressing to edema, erythema, and necrosis, often within a few hours. Fever, chills, and malaise are accompanying signs.

1. **Physical examination** reveals edema and erythema of the skin of the scrotum, phallus, and perineal area. This may progress rapidly to frank necrosis of the skin and subcutaneous tissues, with extension to the skin of the abdomen and back, reaching as high as the clavicles and down the thighs. Crepitus in the tissues suggests the presence of gas-forming organisms.

2. **Laboratory evaluation** should include a CBC, serum electrolytes, creatinine, arterial blood gas, coagulation parameters, urinalysis, urine, and blood cultures. A KUB plain film may reveal subcutaneous gas.

3. **The patient should be stabilized and prepared emergently for the operating room.** Broad-spectrum antibiotics that are active against both aerobic and anaerobic organisms should be started immediately. Aerobic and anaerobic wound cultures are usually polymicrobial.

4. **Wide débridement** is required, with aggressive postoperative support. The testicles are often spared because they have a blood supply discrete from the scrotum; orchiectomy is rarely indicated. Wound closure and dermal coverage often is an extensive process, and recovery requires intense physical therapy and wound care. Despite improvements in critical care, antibiotics, and surgical technology, **mortality** ranges from 3% to 45% (*Br J Surg* 2000;87:718).

II. NONACUTE SCROTAL MASSES

A. **Hydroceles** generally are asymptomatic fluid collections around the testicle that **transilluminate.** Ultrasound evaluation is recommended to rule out serious underlying causes such as testicular malignancies. If hydroceles do enlarge and become symptomatic, they can be repaired by a variety of transscrotal techniques. Hydroceles in infants may be associated with a patent processus vaginalis; parents give a history of intermittent scrotal swelling. These hydroceles usually resolve by 1 year of age. Those that persist can be repaired by an inguinal approach.

B. **Spermatoceles** are benign cystic dilations involving the tail of the epididymis or proximal vas deferens.

C. **Varicoceles** are abnormal tortuosities and dilations of the testicular veins within the spermatic cord. On physical examination, they feel like a "bag of worms." A varicocele may diminish in size when the patient is supine. Because the left gonadal vein drains directly into the renal vein, varicoceles are much more common on the left side. Right-sided varicoceles may be associated with obstruction of the inferior vena cava. Varicoceles are the most common surgically correctable cause of male infertility; however, most men with varicoceles remain fertile. Varicocele repair results in improved semen quality in approximately 70% of patients. Surgical treatment of varicoceles is indicated for diminished testicular growth in adolescents, infertility, or significant symptoms. Any patient who presents with a new-onset varicocele later in life warrants retroperitoneal imaging to rule out a malignancy causing venous obstruction.

III. TESTICULAR TUMORS are the most common solid tumors in 15- to 35-year-old men.

The estimated lifetime risk for testicular malignancy is 1 in 500. Owing to improved multimodality therapy, overall 5-year survival for testis cancer is now 95%.

A. **The typical clinical finding is a painless testicular mass,** although one third of patients may present with pain. Pulmonary or gastrointestinal complaints or the presence of an abdominal mass may reflect advanced disease. Scrotal sonography is mandatory; seminomas appear as a hypoechoic lesion, and nonseminomatous tumors appear inhomogeneous. α-Fetoprotein, β-human chorionic gonadotropin, and lactic acid dehydrogenase are serum tumor markers that help to identify the tumor type and completely stage the tumor. The markers are used to monitor the effectiveness of therapy and to screen for recurrence.

B. **Staging of testicular tumors** is outlined in Table 35-5. Serum tumor markers have recently been added to the staging system.

C. **Initial therapy** for all testicular tumors is radical inguinal orchiectomy. The type of tumor and the stage of the disease determine further therapy.

1. **Seminomas** constitute 60% to 65% of germ-cell tumors. Low-stage seminomas are treated with adjuvant radiation therapy to the retroperitoneum. Advanced disease is usually treated with a platinum-based chemotherapy regimen.

2. **Nonseminomatous tumors** include the histologic types of embryonal carcinoma, teratoma, choriocarcinoma, and yolk sac elements, alone or in combination. Nonseminomatous tumors are more likely to present with advanced disease. Patients with clinically negative retroperitoneal nodes with normal tumor markers are treated with retroperitoneal lymph node dissection, prophylactic chemotherapy, or close observation. Patients with high-stage disease with elevated markers receive platinum-based chemotherapy followed by retroperitoneal node dissection if there is residual disease.

| TABLE 35-5 | American Joint Committee on Cancer Staging of Testicular Cancer |

Stage	Tumor(T)[a]	Node (N)[b]	Metastasis (M)[c]	Serum tumor markers (S)
0	Tis	N0	M0	S0
IA	T1	N0	M0	S0
IB	T2–4	N0	M0	S0
IS	Any T	N0	M0	S1–3
IIA	Any T	N1	M0	S0
	Any T	N1	M0	S1
IIB	Any T	N2	M0	S0
	Any T	N2	M0	S1
IIC	Any T	N3	M0	S0
	Any T	N3	M0	S1
IIIA	Any T	Any N	M1a	S0
	Any T	Any N	M1a	S1
IIIB	Any T	Any N	M0	S2
	Any T	Any N	M1a	S2
IIIC	Any T	Any N	M0	S3
	Any T	Any N	M1a	S3
	Any T	Any N	M1b	Any S

	Serum tumor markers		
	Lactate dehydrogenase	Human chorionic gonadotropin (mIU/mL)	α-Fetoprotein (ng/mL)
S0	≤Normal	≤Normal	≤Normal
S1	<1.5 × N	<5,000	<1,000
S3	1.5–10 × N	5,000–50,000	1,000–10,000
S3	>10 × N	>50,000	>10,000

[a]Tis, intratubular germ-cell neoplasia; T1, limited to testis; T2, beyond tunica albuginea or into epididymis; T3, invades spermatic cord; T4, invades scrotum.
[b]N0, no node metastasis; N1, one node metastasis, <2 cm; N2, one node metastasis, 2–5 cm, or multiple nodal metastasis, each <5 cm; N3, node metastasis >5 cm.
[c]M0, no metastasis; M1, nonregional nodal or pulmonary metastasis; M2, nonpulmonary visceral metastasis.

GENITOURINARY TRAUMA

Genitourinary injuries should be identified during the secondary survey after life-threatening injuries have been addressed and initial resuscitation has been undertaken.

- **I. RENAL INJURY** is a component of approximately 10% of abdominal traumas. Blunt trauma accounts for 80% to 90% of renal injuries. Penetrating trauma occurs as a result of gunshot wounds or stab wounds and accounts for 10% to 20% of renal injuries. The grading system for renal injuries is shown in Table 35-6.
  - **A. Blunt renal trauma** should be suspected in patients with abdominal tenderness, lower rib fractures, vertebral fractures, or flank contusions.
  - **B. Microscopic hematuria** (>3 RBCs per high-power field) or gross hematuria is present in more than 95% of patients with a renal injury. A voided specimen is

TABLE 35-6	Renal injury scale of the American Association for the Surgery of Trauma

Renal injury scale	Injury	Description
I	Contusion	Microscopic or gross hematuria; urologic studies normal
	Hematoma	Nonexpanding perirenal hematoma confined to the renal retroperitoneum
II	Hematoma	Subcapsular, nonexpanding without parenchymal laceration
	Laceration	<1 cm parenchymal depth of renal cortex without urinary extravasation
III	Laceration	>1 cm parenchymal depth of renal cortex without collecting system rupture or urinary extravasation
IV	Laceration	Parenchymal laceration extending through the renal cortex, medulla, and collecting system
	Vascular	Main renal artery or vein injury with contained hemorrhage
V	Laceration	Completely shattered kidney
	Vascular	Avulsion of renal hilum that devascularizes the kidney

best for urinalysis, but if the patient cannot void or is unconscious and no blood is at the meatus, a well-lubricated urethral catheter should gently be passed.

C. All patients with **gross hematuria and blunt trauma** should be evaluated with a CT scan using intravenous contrast. If the patient is stable, 10-minute-delayed imaging is helpful to evaluate for collecting system injuries. Patients with microscopic hematuria and shock (systolic blood pressure <90 mm Hg) should be imaged with a CT scan after they are stabilized. Patients with microscopic hematuria, no shock, and no evidence of significant deceleration or renal injury do not need radiographic evaluation of their urinary system (*J Urol* 1989;141:1095).

D. The **degree of hematuria** does not correlate with the severity of the injury (*J Urol* 1978;120:455), and any patient with a suspected renal injury due to rapid deceleration requires radiographic evaluation. Disruption of the ureteropelvic junction should be considered in children with deceleration or hyperextension injuries.

E. The majority of **blunt renal injuries** can be managed conservatively; fewer than 10% of blunt renal injuries require surgery (*World J Urol* 1999;17:71).

F. **Penetrating renal trauma** with microscopic hematuria (>3 RBCs per high-power field) or gross hematuria requires radiographic assessment with CT scan or an IVP. Preferably, this is done before exploration to evaluate the injured kidney and to confirm function of the contralateral kidney. The presence of a normal contralateral kidney may influence the surgeon's decision (repair vs. nephrectomy) on management of the injured kidney. Intraoperative palpation of a contralateral kidney may be misleading.

G. A **high-dose, single-shot IVP** with a 2-mL/kg bolus injection of contrast followed by a single film at 10 minutes can be performed in the trauma suite or in the operating room without interfering with other critical elements of the trauma evaluation and resuscitation.

H. **Absolute indications for intraoperative renal exploration** include hemodynamic instability, expanding or pulsatile perirenal mass, or injury to the renal pelvis or ureter (*J Trauma* 2005;59:491).

II. **URETERAL INJURIES** account for approximately 3% of all urologic traumas. A high index of suspicion often is necessary to make the diagnosis, and many ureteral injuries have a delayed presentation.

A. The most common scenario is **penetrating trauma with multiple associated injuries.** The absence of gross or microscopic hematuria has been documented in 30% of patients.

B. Radiographic findings include extravasation and, more commonly, delayed function; proximal dilation; and deviation of the ureter. A CT may demonstrate medial extravasation; delayed images are necessary to assess ureteral patency. Retrograde pyelography is the most sensitive diagnostic tool but may be difficult to obtain in the setting of acute trauma.

C. Adequately visualizing the ureter during laparotomy is important for diagnosing ureteral injury; intravenous or intraureteral injection of indigo carmine or methylene blue may help to assess the integrity of the urothelium.

D. For purposes of determining the **type of repair,** the ureter is divided into thirds.

1. Injuries to the distal one third of the ureter are best managed by **ureteral reimplantation.** Additional length to provide a tension-free anastomosis may be gained by using a Psoas hitch and, if necessary, a Boari bladder flap.

2. Injuries of the middle or upper third of the ureter are best managed by **ureteroureterostomy.** An omental wrap may be used to protect the repair. Stents and drains are recommended for all ureteral repairs (*World J Urol* 1999;17:78).

III. BLADDER INJURIES result from blunt trauma, penetrating trauma, and iatrogenic injury during surgical procedures.

A. Ninety-five percent of bladder injuries present with **gross hematuria** (*Urol Clin North Am* 2006;33:676). Anyone with a history of blunt or penetrating trauma, gross hematuria, and difficulty in urinating should be evaluated with a cystogram.

B. Cystogram. A **Foley catheter** is placed if a urethral injury is not suspected (see Section IV). A scout film is obtained. Standard radiographic contrast is diluted to a 50:50 mix with saline and is **infused under gravity.** When 100 mL have been instilled, an anteroposterior radiograph is taken. If no extravasation is seen, the bladder is filled to 350 mL or until the patient experiences a strong urge to void under gravity, and an anteroposterior and oblique radiograph is obtained. A postdrainage film is mandatory.

C. Upper tract imaging can then be done. If a CT scan is obtained, a CT cystogram may be substituted for a plain radiographic or fluoroscopic cystogram. The bladder should be filled retrograde by gravity via an indwelling Foley catheter with 350 mL of dilute (3% to 5%) contrast. Postdrainage films are not necessary; merely clamping the Foley to allow bladder filling with excreted contrast does not constitute an adequate study. An IVP or CT scan alone is not adequate to evaluate bladder trauma.

D. Management

1. All patients with penetrating trauma to the bladder and intraperitoneal extravasation of contrast require **surgical exploration and repair** of the bladder (*Urol Clin North Am* 2006;33:67).

2. Often, patients with blunt trauma and extraperitoneal extravasation of contrast can be managed nonoperatively with **catheter drainage** for 10 days. A cystogram should be performed prior to catheter removal.

IV. GENITAL AND URETHRAL INJURIES

A. Urethral injuries occur in 5% of patients with pelvic fractures. Posterior urethral injuries involve the prostatic and membranous urethra to the level of the urogenital diaphragm. These injuries are caused mainly by blunt trauma.

B. Urethral injury should be suspected when blood is at the meatus or the mechanism of injury is such that urethral injury might have occurred. Physical examination in patients with urethral injury may reveal penile and scrotal edema and ecchymosis. Rectal examination can reveal a high-riding prostate or boggy hematoma in the expected position of the prostate.

C. If a urethral injury is suspected, a **retrograde urethrogram** must be performed prior to Foley catheter placement. It is performed by placing a 14- or 16-French Foley catheter into the urethra **without lubrication** so that the balloon is 2 to 3 cm beyond the meatus. The balloon is inflated with 1 to 2 cc to seat it in the fossa navicularis. With the patient in a 30-degree oblique position, 25 to 30 mL of half-strength contrast medium is injected through the catheter. The radiograph is exposed when the contrast is nearly completely injected. If the urethra is normal, the balloon can be deflated, the catheter advanced into the bladder, and a cystogram performed.

D. Anterior urethral injuries include injuries to the bulbous and penile urethra distal to the urogenital diaphragm. Straddle injuries and penetrating trauma are the most common causes of these types of injuries. Injuries contained by Buck's fascia often have a characteristic "sleeve of penis" pattern, whereas urethral or penile injuries in which Buck's fascia is disrupted are contained by the Colles fascia and have a "butterfly" appearance on the perineum.

E. Posterior ureteral injuries can be managed by primary endoscopic realignment and delayed repair. Unstable patients require suprapubic tube placement and realignment when stable. These injuries are often associated with formation of urethral strictures and with impotence (*Urol Clin North Am* 2006;33:87).

F. Minor penile lacerations and contusions can be managed in the emergency room. **Serious blunt or penetrating trauma** with injury to the corpus cavernosum require surgical exploration, débridement, and repair of the corporal injury. A retrograde urethrogram or flexible cytoscopy is necessary to rule out urethral injury. Broad-spectrum antibiotics should be given, particularly in human bite injuries.

G. Testicular injury may occur as a result of blunt or penetrating trauma. History and physical examination are the keys to diagnosis of testicular rupture. The presentation is marked by acute and severe pain, often with associated nausea and vomiting. Physical examination may reveal a hematoma or ecchymosis of overlying skin. All penetrating scrotal gunshot wounds deep to the dartos fascia require surgical exploration. **Ultrasonography** can help to diagnose testicular injury associated with blunt trauma with a 100% sensitivity and a specificity of 93.5% (*J Urol* 2006;175:175). The orchiectomy rate is less than 10% for ruptured testicles explored within 72 hours after injury. Repair consists of hematoma evacuation, débridement of the necrotic tubules, and closure of the tunica albuginea (*World J Urol* 1999;17:101).

H. Scrotal avulsion and skin loss are most often a result of motor vehicle accidents. Because of the redundancy and vascularity of scrotal skin, a variety of options are available for local flaps and coverage of the testicles. Wounds should be copiously irrigated and débrided; clean wounds may be closed in layers, whereas grossly contaminated wounds should be cleaned and packed with sterile gauze dressings.

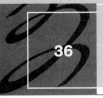

OBSTETRIC AND GYNECOLOGIC SURGERY

36

Rebecca A. Brooks and Premal H. Thaker

 OBSTETRIC AND GYNECOLOGIC DISORDERS

I. **VAGINAL BLEEDING** to an abnormal degree may result from a variety of causes. A thorough history including pattern and intensity of bleeding and physical examination is sufficient to determine the etiology. A pregnancy test must be performed in all women of reproductive age. Hemoglobin (Hgb) and hematocrit (Hct) should be drawn to determine whether the abnormal bleeding is chronic or heavy. An endometrial biopsy should be performed in all postmenopausal women with bleeding to rule out endometrial carcinoma. The evaluation and treatment of vaginal bleeding depend on the presentation and etiology.

A. **Obstetric etiologies.** Approximately 30% to 40% of all pregnancies are associated with some vaginal bleeding, and approximately half of these are spontaneously aborted.

1. **Terminology**

a. **Threatened abortion:** any vaginal bleeding during the first half of pregnancy, cervix closed.

b. **Missed abortion:** fetal death with retention of products of conception (POC), cervix closed.

c. **Inevitable abortion:** cervical dilation with or without ruptured membranes.

d. **Incomplete abortion:** partial passage of POC, cervix open.

e. **Complete abortion:** expulsion of all POC from the uterine cavity, cervix closed.

2. **Presentation and clinical features.** Classically, patients present with vaginal bleeding and crampy midline lower abdominal pain. Bleeding from the urethra or rectum or from lacerations of the cervix or vagina should be excluded. Passage of tissue may represent a complete or incomplete abortion.

3. **Physical examination.** Vital signs are within normal ranges unless extensive vaginal bleeding or septic abortion occurs with resultant tachycardia and hypotension. Septic abortions can cause elevated temperatures, marked suprapubic tenderness, or purulent discharge through the cervical os.

4. **Laboratory investigation**

a. **Hgb and Hct.** Plasma volume expansion in pregnancy may result in a lower mean Hgb during the second trimester. With acute blood loss, the Hgb and Hct can be normal until compensatory mechanisms restore normal plasma volume.

b. **White blood cell (WBC) count with differential** is useful to evaluate febrile morbidity. Septic abortion is associated with a left shift and an elevated WBC count.

c. **Blood type and screen** are essential to identify Rh-negative patients at risk for isoimmunization. Any woman with pregnancy-related vaginal bleeding who is Rh-negative should be given Rho immune globulin (RhoGAM) if she has not received it within the last 12 weeks (see Section I.A.6.g).

d. **Quantitative β subunit of human chorionic gonadotropin (hCG).** The sensitivity of a pregnancy test (urine or serum) can vary depending on the type of test performed (i.e., latex agglutination, enzyme-linked immunosorbent assays, radioimmunoassay). A urine pregnancy test gives a rapid qualitative result, although the sensitivity is variable. Serum pregnancy tests are more sensitive and yield a quantitative level of hCG that assists in evaluating the status of a pregnancy. Serial serum hCG values may be used along with ultrasonography to distinguish an early viable pregnancy from an abnormal pregnancy. In most normal intrauterine pregnancies (IUPs) near 6 weeks' gestation, hCG increases by at least 66% every 48 hours (ACOG Practice Bulletin 3. In: *Compendium of Selected Publications.* Washington, DC: American College of Obstetrics and Gynecology; 2007:883). Patients with stable clinical examinations can be followed with serial hCG values until they reach the sonographic threshold values at which ultrasound visualization of an IUP is possible (see Section I.A.5).

   e. Progesterone levels in excess of 15 ng/mL usually are associated with a normal IUP. Below this range, pregnancy is likely abnormal.

5. **Imaging studies.** Ultrasonography may be useful in demonstrating a viable pregnancy. Vaginal probe ultrasonography should demonstrate an intrauterine gestational sac (if it exists) at hCG levels greater than 1,500 to 2,000 mIU/mL. For abdominal ultrasonography, the threshold is greater than 6,000 mIU/mL. Cardiac activity can be seen at 10,000 mIU/mL.

6. **Treatment**

   a. **Threatened abortion.** Patients with a pregnancy that is viable or of indeterminate viability, vaginal bleeding, and a closed internal cervical os are followed expectantly with either a repeat ultrasound in 7 days, repeat hCG in 48 hours, or both. A normal IUP should show at least a 66% increase in hCG level every 48 hours.

   b. **Missed abortion.** Patients may be followed expectantly or undergo evacuation. If they are followed expectantly, weekly coagulation studies [i.e., complete blood cell (CBC) count, prothrombin time, partial thromboplastin time, fibrinogen, and fibrin degradation products] should be monitored because of the risk of disseminated intravascular coagulopathy (DIC). Patients should be counseled to bring any tissue passed back to the hospital for pathologic verification. If the patient has not passed the tissue within 3 weeks, evacuation should be scheduled.

   c. **For inevitable abortion,** the uterus usually begins to contract, resulting in expulsion of products. Patients occasionally are followed expectantly with monitoring for infection but typically undergo uterine evacuation. If fever develops, intravenous antibiotics with polymicrobial coverage are administered, followed by evacuation of the uterus. These patients require admission and careful monitoring of coagulation factors because they are at risk of DIC.

   d. **For incomplete abortion,** bleeding, cramping, and an open internal os usually are found. Uterine evacuation is indicated. If POC are not recovered, ectopic pregnancy should be considered.

   e. **For complete abortion,** all POC have been expelled, and the cervix is closed. Bleeding and cramping are minimal. Only short-term observation is necessary.

   f. **Evacuation of the uterus.** Suction curettage is done safely in the first trimester and can be performed in the emergency room if significant cervical dilation exists. A stable patient with a first-trimester missed abortion can undergo dilation and curettage (D & C) as an outpatient. In the second trimester, a dilation and evacuation or medical induction of labor under gynecologic consultation is performed. After curettage, prophylactic antibiotics (doxycycline, 100 mg orally two times a day for 7 days), ergot alkaloids (methylergonovine maleate, 0.2 mg orally three times a day for 2 to 3 days) for uterine contraction, and antiprostaglandins (ibuprofen, 800 mg orally every 8 hours as needed for pain) commonly are prescribed. If heavy vaginal bleeding, abdominal pain, or fever occurs after evacuation, investigation for retained POC, uterine perforation, and endometritis is warranted.

   g. **Rho immune globulin** is given to any pregnant patient with vaginal bleeding who is Rh negative and has a negative antibody screen. The recommended dose of RhoGAM is 300 μg intramuscularly after the first trimester. For

TABLE 36-1	Nonobstetric Causes of Vaginal Bleeding		
Differential diagnosis	**Laboratory data**	**Signs and symptoms**	**Treatment**
Menses	CBC count, urine hCG	Cyclic bleeding every 21–35 d	Iron therapy if indicated
Dysfunctional uterine bleeding	CBC count, urine hCG, endometrial biopsy if >35 yr, duration >6 mo	Noncyclic bleeding; may have associated dysmenorrhea, fatigue, or dizziness	Hormonal therapy if patient is hemodynamically stable; if hemodynamically unstable, transfuse as needed, IV estrogen or high-dose oral contraceptive pills
Infection: gonorrhea/chlamydia cervicitis	Cervical culture, wet prep	Purulent vaginal discharge, possible spotting	Ceftriaxone, 125 mg IM × 1; azithromycin, 1 g PO × 1
Trichomonas vaginitis	Wet prep	Yellow-green frothy vaginal discharge, possible spotting	Metronidazole, 500 mg PO BID × 7 days or 2 g PO × 1 (if pregnant, defer treatment to second trimester)
Sexual trauma	Rape kit	Vaginal bleeding and/or discharge	Emergency contraception, prophylactic treatment for sexually transmitted diseases; if laceration, pack vagina, possible surgical repair
Malignancy	Endometrial biopsy, Pap smear, cervical biopsy	Postmenopausal bleeding, postcoital bleeding, intermenstrual bleeding	Refer to gynecologic oncologist

BID, twice daily; CBC, complete blood cell; hCG, human chorionic gonadotropin; IM, intramuscular; IV, intravenous; PO, oral.

first-trimester events, 50 μg intramuscularly is sufficient (ACOG Practice Bulletin 4. In: *Compendium of Selected Publications*. Washington, DC: American College of Obstetrics and Gynecology; 2007:475).
- **h. Pathology.** Any tissue passed or obtained on uterine evacuation must be evaluated for chorionic villi. If villi are not identified, further investigation is necessary to exclude ectopic pregnancy or incomplete abortion.
- **B. Nonobstetric etiologies of vaginal bleeding** (Table 36-1).
II. ABDOMINAL PAIN. The differential diagnosis for nongynecologic etiologies includes appendicitis, gastroenteritis, irritable bowel, ischemic bowel, ureteral colic, urinary tract infection, and cholecystitis. Pregnancy should be excluded in all women of reproductive age.
- **A. Ectopic pregnancy** occurs when the blastocyst implants outside the uterine cavity; 97% of cases occur in a fallopian tube (tubal pregnancy).
  - **1. Presentation and clinical features.** Although more than 90% of patients with tubal pregnancies have abdominal or pelvic pain, some may be asymptomatic. Early (unruptured) ectopic pregnancies often present with amenorrhea, vaginal spotting, and colicky, vague lower abdominal pain, whereas patients with ruptured ectopic pregnancies often present with severe pain, syncope, and dizziness. Pleuritic chest pain and shoulder pain from diaphragmatic irritation by blood can also occur.

2. **Physical examination.** Vital signs vary greatly, from normal blood pressure and pulse to hypotension and tachycardia due to cardiovascular collapse secondary to hemorrhage. Whereas patients with unruptured ectopic pregnancy may demonstrate only mild tenderness, peritoneal signs including marked tenderness, rigidity, guarding, and rebound may also be found. Pelvic masses sometimes are palpable, but lack of a mass does not exclude ectopic pregnancy. The uterus may appear small for presumed gestational date.

3. **Laboratory investigation**
   a. **CBC.** Hgb and Hct may indicate the degree of hemorrhage, except in acute loss. The WBC count typically is normal or slightly elevated and does not demonstrate increased percentage of immature neutrophils.
   b. **Blood type and screen** should be obtained to identify Rh-negative patients and to cross-match blood for possible transfusion (see Section I.A.6.g).
   c. **hCG.** Although ectopic pregnancy can occur with any quantitative serum hCG value, these data can be useful for ultrasound interpretation. Serial hCG values that do not increase appropriately are suspicious for an ectopic pregnancy (see Section I.A.4.d).
   d. **Progesterone** values rarely aid in the diagnosis of ectopic pregnancy (see Section I.A.4.e).

4. **Imaging studies.** Ultrasonography is most useful in excluding a tubal pregnancy by demonstrating an intrauterine gestational sac or fetus. With a quantitative hCG less than 1,500 mIU/mL, this may not be possible, and stable patients should be followed with serial hCG titers. However, an hCG greater than 2,500 mIU/mL and absence of a gestational sac in the uterus indicate either a nonviable intrauterine or an ectopic pregnancy. Ultrasound findings consistent with ectopic pregnancy include a uterus without a well-formed gestational sac—although a pseudosac (intrauterine fluid collection) may be present—free intraperitoneal fluid, and sometimes an adnexal mass representing the tubal pregnancy.

5. **Diagnostic studies**
   a. **Culdocentesis** is useful for detecting hemoperitoneum, although it is used infrequently because sonographic evaluation for free intraperitoneal fluid often is sufficient. A culdocentesis is performed by passing a needle aseptically into the posterior vaginal fornix. Aspiration of clear yellow fluid is normal. If no fluid is obtained, the test is nondiagnostic. Aspiration of clotting blood is likely from an intravascular source and nondiagnostic, whereas nonclotting blood with an Hct above 15% is consistent with hemoperitoneum.
   b. **D & C** can be performed to differentiate between ectopic pregnancy and incomplete abortion after excluding a normal early intrauterine pregnancy. Curettage products that float in saline are suggestive of chorionic villi. If villi are not identified, laparoscopy to exclude ectopic pregnancy is indicated.

6. **Treatment**
   a. **Surgical therapy.** The majority of ectopic pregnancies are treated surgically.
      (1) **Laparoscopy** is preferred for diagnosis and treatment of tubal pregnancy; however, laparotomy is indicated if the patient is hemodynamically unstable.
      (2) **Conservative surgical therapy** is recommended in patients who wish to preserve reproductive potential. **Linear salpingostomy** in the antimesosalpinx portion of the tube performed with fine-tip electrocautery is preferable when the ectopic pregnancy is unruptured and is located in the ampulla of the tube, although this may increase the risk of future ectopic pregnancies. After removal of the pregnancy from the tube, the base is irrigated, and hemostasis is achieved with cautery. The tube is left to heal by secondary intention. **Segmental resection** often is performed when the tube is ruptured, and the ectopic pregnancy is in the isthmic portion of the tube.
      (3) **Nonconservative surgical therapy** includes **salpingectomy** (removal of tube) for tubal rupture or severe hemorrhage and **cornual resection** for interstitial pregnancies. Pregnancy rates after salpingectomy have been

shown to be equivalent to those following linear salpingostomy, although the incidence of recurrent ectopic pregnancy may be slightly higher with salpingostomy.

(4) Follow-up. Patients treated with conservative surgical management or after rupture or spillage of trophoblastic tissue have a 5% incidence of persistent viable trophoblastic tissue. Weekly quantitative hCG values should be followed until negative. If the levels plateau or increase, reevaluation is indicated.

b. Medical therapy with methotrexate, a folic acid antagonist, can be used in compliant outpatients who are hemodynamically stable. Indications for ectopic pregnancy treatable with methotrexate include size of ectopic pregnancy equal to or less than 3.5 cm in diameter, an intact tube, no fetal heart motion, no evidence of hemoperitoneum, and an hCG less than 10,000 mIU/mL. Baseline laboratory tests including hCG, Rh factor, CBC, and hepatic enzymes should be obtained. The most common side effects of therapy are bloating and flatulence. Transient rise in hepatic enzymes may be observed. Less frequent side effects include stomatitis, hair loss, and anemia. Repeat quantitative hCG levels should be drawn on days 4 and 7. If hCG levels fail to decline less than 15% between days 4 and 7, a second dose of methotrexate should be administered and a new day 1 assigned. Quantitative hCG values are followed until negative. Approximately 20% of patients have an inappropriate fall in hCG levels and require surgical intervention. *Separation pain* refers to the increase in abdominopelvic discomfort that is commonly experienced by patients undergoing treatment and is thought to be caused by tubal stretching during resolution of the pregnancy. Patients are counseled to rest and take oral analgesics but warned to seek immediate reevaluation to rule out rupture if pain does not resolve within 1 hour. They should also avoid alcohol and folic acid because these may interfere with methotrexate and avoid intercourse because this may increase the risk of rupture (Copeland LJ. *Textbook of Gynecology,* 2nd ed. Philadelphia: WB Saunders; 2000).

B. Pelvic inflammatory disease (PID) is a polymicrobial infection of the upper genital tract. The majority of cases occur in sexually active 15- to 30-year-old women. It rarely occurs in nonmenstruating women and during pregnancy. Factors promoting progression of infection from the lower to upper genital tract include events that cause breakdown of the cervical mucus barrier, such as douching, intrauterine device (IUD) insertion, hysteroscopy, D & C, endometrial biopsy, and hysterosalpingography. Risk factors include a history of sexually transmitted diseases or PID, multiple sexual partners, and age less than 25 years. Causative pathogens are primarily *Neisseria gonorrhoeae* and *Chlamydia trachomatis,* although other vaginal flora microorganisms, such as anaerobes, *Gardnerella vaginalis, Haemophilus influenzae,* enteric Gram-negative rods, *Streptococcus agalactiae,* as well as cytomegalovirus, *Mycoplasma hominis, Ureaplasma urealyticum,* and *Mycoplasma genitalium,* have been associated with PID.

1. Presentation and clinical features. Patients with PID typically have lower abdominal and pelvic pain, which may be constant, dull, sharp, or crampy. PID is aggravated by movement and often occurs around or during menses. Approximately 75% of patients have purulent vaginal discharge; fewer than 50% have abnormal vaginal bleeding; only 33% manifest fever. Nausea and vomiting with associated ileus may occur but are usually late symptoms.

2. Physical examination reveals lower abdominal tenderness, including peritoneal signs of guarding and rebound, adnexal tenderness, and cervical motion tenderness; adnexal fullness or a mass may be found. PID is often accompanied by a mucopurulent vaginal discharge. Cervical motion tenderness is a nonspecific sign of peritoneal irritation that can be elicited in any female patient with peritonitis from any cause; therefore, it is not pathognomonic of PID.

3. Laboratory investigation. Pregnancy must be excluded. Elevated WBC count and elevated erythrocyte sedimentation rate (ESR) suggest a severe infection. A wet-smear examination of a drop of vaginal discharge in a few drops of isotonic saline under high magnification usually reveals numerous WBCs. If no WBCs are demonstrated on wet prep and the discharge appears normal, PID is unlikely. A cervical swab for DNA probe analysis of *N. gonorrhoeae* and *C. trachomatis* should be obtained. Bloody samples may give false-negative results. Alternatively, cultures for *N. gonorrhoeae* and *C. trachomatis* can be obtained by using a voided urine assay (URIprobe). Women diagnosed with PID should also be screened for HIV.

4. **Imaging studies.** Ultrasonography is used to detect tubo-ovarian abscess (TOAs) if a mass is palpated on examination or if no improvement is noted after 48 hours of antibiotic treatment. Abdominal plain films, ultrasonography, or computed tomographic (CT) scan also may be used to investigate other etiologies of a patient's pain if the diagnosis is uncertain.

5. **Diagnostic studies**

   a. The Centers for Disease Control and Prevention (CDC) issued guidelines for diagnosis of acute PID that are intended to serve as clinical criteria for initiating treatment. **Minimum criteria** include lower abdominal tenderness, adnexal tenderness, and cervical motion tenderness. **Additional criteria** include temperature greater than 101°F (38.3°C), abnormal cervical/vaginal discharge, elevated ESR, elevated C-reactive protein, and documented infection with *N. gonorrhoeae* or *C. trachomatis*. **Definitive criteria** include histopathologic evidence of endometritis on endometrial biopsy, transvaginal ultrasound showing fluid-filled tubes or TOAs, and laparoscopic abnormalities consistent with PID.

   b. **Culdocentesis** seldom is necessary to make the diagnosis of PID. However, aspiration of purulent material confirms an infectious process (see Section II.A.5.a).

   c. **Laparoscopy** revealing erythema and edema of the fallopian tubes and purulent material confirms the diagnosis and provides the opportunity to collect direct cultures of infected organs, although laparoscopy should not be considered a routine means of establishing a diagnosis.

6. **Treatment** of PID depends on the severity of the infection.

   a. **Inpatient therapy** is indicated for patients with nausea and vomiting, possible surgical emergencies, pregnancy, suspicion for TOA, immunodeficiency, or failed outpatient therapy or for patients in whom preservation of reproductive potential is very important. According to 2006 CDC guidelines, inpatient treatment is provided by cefotetan 2 g intravenously every 12 hours or cefoxitin 2 g intravenously every 6 hours and doxycycline 100 mg orally or intravenously every 12 hours (alternatively, clindamycin 900 mg intravenously every 8 hours and gentamicin 2-mg/kg intravenous load followed by 1.5 mg/kg intravenously every 8 hours can be used). Oral doxycycline is preferred due to pain with intravenous administration. Other alternative regimens include ofloxacillin 400 mg intravenously every 12 hours and metronidazole 500 mg intravenously every 8 hours; ampicillin/sulbactam 3 g intravenously every 6 hours and doxycycline 100 mg intravenously or orally every 12 hours; and ciprofloxacin 200 mg intravenously every 12 hours, doxycycline 100 mg intravenously or orally every 12 hours, and metronidazole 500 mg every 8 hours. Inpatient treatment is continued until the patient is afebrile for 48 hours and has decreased pain on pelvic examination. Patients then are treated with oral doxycycline for a total of 14 days. Patients with discrete pelvic fluid collections and TOAs may be candidates for drainage by interventional radiologists; concurrent antibiotics should be administered.

   b. **Outpatient therapy** includes one dose of ceftriaxone 250 mg intramuscularly, followed by doxycycline 100 mg orally twice daily for 14 days (alternatively, ofloxacin 400 mg orally twice daily, and metronidazole 500 mg orally twice daily for 14 days can be used) (*MMWR Recomm Rep* 2002;51(RR-6):1). Patients should be followed up within 48 to 72 hours to ensure adequate improvement.

   c. In patients with TOAs who are not responding to intravenous antibiotics after 48 hours, **surgery** should be considered. Generally, surgery should be reserved for patients with symptomatic pelvic masses or for ruptured TOAs in patients failing intravenous antibiotics. Ultrasound-guided transvaginal aspiration of TOAs and pelvic drain placement by interventional radiology are additional options that may benefit patients who do not respond to intravenous antibiotics.

C. **Corpus luteal cysts** develop from mature follicles in the ovary. Intrafollicular bleeding can occur 2 to 4 days after ovulation creating a hemorrhagic cyst. Corpus luteal cysts usually are less than or equal to 4 cm in diameter but can be greater than 12 cm. Diagnosis can be difficult in pregnancy because a cyst may be confused with ectopic pregnancy.

1. **Presentation and clinical features.** Patients can be asymptomatic or may present with unilateral, dull lower abdominal and pelvic pain. If the cyst has ruptured, the patient may complain of sudden, severe lower abdominal pain.

2. **Physical examination** reveals adnexal enlargement, tenderness, or both; if the cyst has ruptured, signs of peritoneal irritation can be present. Hemodynamic stability must be ensured because some patients can bleed significantly from a hemorrhagic cyst.

3. **Laboratory investigation.** A CBC and an hCG should always be obtained. Ultrasound can aid in visualizing a cyst or free fluid in the pelvis, indicative of recent cyst rupture. Culdocentesis may be performed to search for blood in the cul-de-sac in cases of suspected cyst rupture.

4. **Treatment** usually is conservative, allowing for spontaneous resolution. Oral contraceptive pills (OCPs) to suppress ovulation and future cyst formation and nonsteroidal antiinflammatory drugs (NSAIDs) or short courses of narcotics for pain can be prescribed. Surgical treatment with laparoscopic cystectomy is rarely indicated unless significant ongoing intraperitoneal hemorrhage is present.

D. **Adnexal torsion** accounts for an estimated 3% of gynecologic emergencies requiring immediate operative intervention. Torsion occurs when the ovary, tube, or both structures twist on the infundibulopelvic ligament. Incomplete torsion results in occlusion of the venous and lymphatic channels, causing cyanotic and edematous adnexa. With complete torsion, the arterial supply is interrupted, with subsequent ischemia and necrosis of the adnexa. Adnexal torsion occurs most commonly in the reproductive age group, more frequently on the right side, and typically with large ovaries or ovarian masses. In 20% of cases, concurrent pregnancy is present; in 50% to 60% of cases, a benign ovarian tumor may be present (Copeland LJ. *Textbook of Gynecology*, 2nd ed. Philadelphia: WB Saunders; 2000).

1. **Presentation and clinical features.** Patients with torsion present with acute, severe, sharp, intermittent, unilateral lower abdominal or pelvic pain and nausea. Intermittent torsion may present with periodic pain for days to weeks from twisting and untwisting of the adnexa. The pain often is related to a sudden change in position.

2. **Physical examination** can reveal tachycardia or bradycardia (from vagal stimulation) and fever if there is necrosis. Unilateral abdominal tenderness or a tender adnexal mass often is found on pelvic examination. Peritoneal signs may be present as the ovary undergoes necrosis.

3. **Diagnostic studies.** Ultrasonography may visualize an adnexal mass. Doppler ultrasound has moderate sensitivity and specificity in diagnosing torsion. Blood flow around the adnexa is reassuring but does not exclude torsion, which is mainly a clinical diagnosis. Visualization by laparoscopy confirms the diagnosis.

4. **Treatment** involves immediate surgical intervention. If only partial torsion or no evidence of tissue necrosis exists and the patient desires future fertility, preservation of adnexa with untwisting and transfixation of the ovarian pedicle is possible. Cyst resection and exclusion of underlying malignancy (rare) should be performed. If necrosis of the adnexa is present or the ovary is felt to be nonviable, salpingo-oophorectomy should be performed.

E. **Fibroids or leiomyomas** are benign tumors of uterine smooth muscle that vary in size from less than 1 to greater than 20 cm.

1. **Presentation and clinical features.** Although most fibroids are asymptomatic, one third of patients have dysmenorrhea or abnormal menstrual bleeding, including menorrhagia (heavy menses) or metrorrhagia (intermenstrual bleeding). Symptoms also can result from pressure on the bladder or rectum. Fever and acute pain responsive to high-dose NSAID therapy may be associated with fibroid degeneration, which occurs more commonly in pregnancy.
2. **Physical examination** may reveal an enlarged, irregular uterus.
3. **Diagnostic studies.** Ultrasonography confirms uterine size and the presence of myomas. In patients older than 35 years with abnormal bleeding, an endometrial biopsy should be performed to rule out endometrial pathology, including hyperplasia and carcinoma.
4. **Treatment** is determined by symptoms and the patient's desire for future fertility. Prostaglandin synthetase inhibitors, including ibuprofen (200 to 800 mg every 6 to 8 hours) or naproxen sodium (220 to 550 mg every 6 hours), can be used for pain. Hormonal therapy, including OCPs and medroxyprogesterone acetate, can be used to regulate bleeding, and gonadotropin-releasing hormone agonist (Lupron) can also be used to shrink fibroids. Surgery (myomectomy or hysterectomy) is reserved for patients who failed medical management.

F. **Dysmenorrhea** is painful lower abdominal cramping that occurs just before and during menses. It affects 40% of women of reproductive age and often is accompanied by other symptoms, including diaphoresis, tachycardia, headache, nausea, vomiting, and diarrhea.
1. The **etiology** of dysmenorrhea is thought to be related to increased prostaglandin levels.
2. **Treatment** includes prostaglandin synthetase inhibitors, such as ibuprofen or naproxen sodium beginning before the onset of menses, or OCPs to suppress ovulation.

G. **Adnexal masses** are often found incidentally either on pelvic examination or intraoperatively. To guide the surgeon in their management, criteria have been developed that aid in assessing the malignant potential of adnexal masses.
1. **Presentation and clinical features.** Most adnexal masses are asymptomatic unless they are associated with torsion or are large enough to compress surrounding structures. Less than 2% of adnexal masses are malignant, although up to 34% may be malignant in postmenopausal women.
2. **Physical examination** may reveal adnexal fullness or a discrete mass. Attention should be paid to the mobility of the mass and to the texture of the mass (solid vs. cystic).
3. **Diagnostic studies.** Ultrasound can reveal the size and characteristics (i.e., complex, simple, nodular, etc.) of adnexal masses. CT is less useful for visualizing the pelvis.
4. **Treatment.** A large (>10 cm) adnexal mass warrants surgical exploration. Smaller masses in premenopausal women may be observed for 6 to 8 weeks unless certain factors make it likely to be malignant, and these patients should be counseled on the warning signs of torsion. If the mass grows or persists on repeat ultrasound, surgery is indicated. Controversy exists regarding the management of small, asymptomatic adnexal masses in postmenopausal women. Small, unilocular cysts may be observed for some time, although most practitioners have a lower threshold for surgery in these patients because the risk of malignancy increases with increasing age. Laparoscopy has been shown to be as effective and safe as laparotomy for the removal of masses less than 10 cm, with decreased morbidity and shorter hospital stays. Fixed and solid masses or those associated with ascites require laparotomy and a gynecologic oncologist on standby. Benign adnexal masses frequently encountered include cystic teratomas (dermoid cysts), endometriomas, and serous and mucinous cystadenomas. Dermoids and serous cystadenomas are frequently bilateral and warrant close inspection of the contralateral ovary. Mucinous cystadenomas can be associated with pseudomyxoma peritonei. In those cases, inspection of the appendix is important because appendiceal mucoceles and carcinomas can also result in pseudomyxoma.

Other benign, solid ovarian tumors include Brenner tumors, fibromas, and thecomas.

III. NONOBSTETRIC SURGERY IN THE PREGNANT PATIENT. Common indications for surgery in the pregnant patient are appendicitis, adnexal mass, and cholecystitis. It is preferable to treat pregnant patients conservatively and if possible defer surgery to the postpartum period; however, delay of an indicated surgical procedure can be devastating. If nonemergent surgery is required, it is safest to proceed in the second trimester. Surgery in the first trimester carries a risk of fetal loss and malformation because organogenesis occurs. Surgery in the third trimester carries a risk of inducing preterm labor.

  A. Preoperative considerations. Patients are at increased risk for aspiration because of upward displacement of the stomach and the inhibitory effects of progesterone on gastrointestinal motility. A nonparticulate antacid should be given shortly before induction of anesthesia. In the second half of pregnancy, the left lateral position should be used to decrease vena caval and aortic compression. Fetal heart tones should always be documented pre- and postoperatively.

  B. Laparoscopic trocar placement in pregnancy is best accomplished by an open technique with the additional trocars inserted under direct visualization. Laparoscopy in pregnancy has primarily been used for cholecystectomy. The second trimester is the maximum gestational age for safe laparoscopy in pregnancy because the uterus is not large enough to obstruct visualization and room for manipulation exists. Intra-abdominal carbon dioxide insufflation appears safe up to 14 mm Hg and is unlikely to alter the acid-base balance in the fetus. Preliminary data suggest that laparoscopic surgical procedures may result in decreased morbidity and mortality, a reduced cost with shorter hospitalizations, and a decreased risk of thromboembolic disease compared with laparotomy.

  C. Anesthetic selection is based on the maternal condition and the planned surgical procedure. For general anesthesia, all patients should be intubated using cricoid pressure to minimize the risk of aspiration. Anesthetic inhalation agents and narcotic analgesia commonly are used. Regional anesthesia may be complicated by hypotension, which is potentially poorly tolerated by patient and fetus.

  D. Postoperatively, fetal-uterine monitoring and tocolytic agents are used, depending on gestational age and degree of maternal symptoms.

IV. TRAUMA IN PREGNANCY

  A. Presentation and clinical features. Trauma is the leading cause of morbidity and mortality in the United States in women less than 40 years of age and is a frequent event in pregnancy. After initial interventions are aimed at stabilization of the mother according to advanced cardiac trauma life support protocols and extent of injury, then establishment of fetal age and monitoring of fetal heart tone (if feasible) are performed.

  B. Types of abdominal trauma

    1. Penetrating trauma places the uterus and fetus at great risk during the later stages of pregnancy. Evaluation and treatment are similar to those in the nonpregnant patient; surgical exploration is usually necessary. Amniocentesis to establish fetal lung maturity or to detect bacteria or blood may be helpful if time permits.

    2. Blunt trauma in pregnancy is associated most often with motor vehicle accidents. Despite the concern for abdominal seat-belt injuries, restrained pregnant patients fare better than those who are unrestrained. Intrauterine or retroplacental hemorrhage must be considered because 20% of the cardiac output in pregnancy is delivered to the uteroplacental unit.

    3. Abruptio placentae occurs in 1% to 5% of minor and 40% to 50% of major blunt traumas. Focal uterine tenderness, vaginal bleeding, hypertonic contractions, and fetal compromise frequently occur. DIC may occur in almost one third of abruptions, and a disseminated intravascular coagulation panel including fibrinogen and a Kleihauer-Betke screen to assess for fetal-maternal hemorrhage in Rh-negative patients should be obtained.

      a. Management of abruptio placentae depends on fetal age, degree of placental separation, and blood loss as estimated on ultrasonography. At viability, continuous fetal heart monitoring is done, and the route of delivery is dictated by both fetal and maternal cardiovascular stability. However, immediate cesarean section is undertaken if evidence of severe compromise exists after the threshold of viability (usually 24 weeks). The immediate maternal and fetal threat must be weighed against the morbidity associated with prematurity, with the threshold for delivery decreasing with increasing gestational age.

C. **Special considerations of trauma in pregnancy**

1. **Fetal-uterine monitoring** is effective in determining fetal distress, abruptio placentae, and preterm labor caused by trauma for gestations greater than 20 weeks. Doppler auscultation of fetal heart tones is sufficient for previable pregnancies after 12 weeks of gestation.

2. **Ultrasonography** is an effective tool for establishing gestational age, fetal viability, placental characteristics, and placental location.

3. In **positioning** the pregnant patient, avoid placing her supine to optimize venous return. During cardiopulmonary resuscitation, a 15-degree wedge into the left lateral decubitus position should be used if possible.

4. **Tetanus prophylaxis** should be administered in the same manner and for the same indications as in the nonpregnant patient.

5. **Peritoneal lavage,** usually by the open, above-the-fundus technique, can be used to detect intraperitoneal hemorrhage while avoiding the uterus, which is localized by examination and ultrasonography (ACOG Practice Bulletin 251. In: *Compendium of Selected Publications.* Washington, DC: American College of Obstetrics and Gynecology; 2007:873).

6. **Radiation** in the form of diagnostic studies places the fetus at potential risk for spontaneous abortion (first several weeks of pregnancy), teratogenesis (weeks 3 to 12), and growth retardation (>12 weeks of gestation). These effects and secondary childhood cancers are unlikely at doses of <10 rads (chest film, <1 rad; CT scan of abdomen and pelvis, 5 to 8 rads). Uterine shielding should be used when possible. Studies should be ordered judiciously, but imaging deemed important for evaluation should not be omitted (ACOG Education Bulletin 236. In: *Compendium of Selected Publications.* Washington, DC: American College of Obstetrics and Gynecology; 2007:859).

7. **Perimortem or postmortem cesarean section** should be accomplished within 10 minutes of maternal cardiopulmonary arrest to optimize neonatal prognosis and maternal response to resuscitation.

8. **Isoimmunization** must be considered in the Rh-negative patient, and RhoGAM is administered when fetal maternal hemorrhage is suspected (see Section I.A.6.g).

9. All **blood product transfusions** should be screened and negative for cytomegalovirus.

10. **Prophylactic cephalosporins** are safe in all trimesters of pregnancy.

V. **GYNECOLOGIC MALIGNANCIES.** The female genital tract accounts for more than 78,290 new cases of invasive carcinoma annually in the United States, resulting in approximately 28,020 deaths in 2007 (*CA Cancer J Clin* 2007;57:43). Mortality can be reduced by earlier detection. Five-year survival rates after proper treatment of cancers diagnosed at stage I (confined to primary organ) approach 90% but fall to 30% to 50% when diagnosed at advanced stages. A brief overview of vulvar, cervical, endometrial, and ovarian cancers is presented with emphasis on diagnosis and initial management. A complete discussion of gynecologic malignancies including less common cancers (vaginal, fallopian tube, and gestational trophoblastic disease) is beyond the scope of this manual. Patients should be referred to a gynecologic oncologist for comprehensive management.

A. **Vulvar carcinoma.** Vulvar cancer is primarily a disease of postmenopausal women, and the average age at diagnosis is 68 years. The etiology has been linked to human papillomavirus infection in younger patients, and vulvar cancer is associated with chronic vulvar conditions including dystrophies, lichen sclerosis, and condylomata. Squamous cell histology predominates (90%), followed by melanoma and adenocarcinoma.

1. **Presentation and clinical features.** Vulvar cancer often presents as a hyper- or hypopigmented lesion. It may be ulcerated, pruritic, painful, or asymptomatic

and may have been treated with a variety of antibiotics and ointments before diagnosis.

2. **Diagnosis.** Accurate diagnosis requires biopsy and histopathologic evaluation of suspicious areas.

3. **Treatment** of vulvar cancer depends on the stage. Surgery ranging from local excision to radical vulvectomy with bilateral inguinal lymph node dissection generally is the primary treatment. Local, groin, and pelvic adjuvant radiation is administered, depending on the pathologic findings. Basal cell carcinoma requires only a wide local excision.

4. **Prognosis** depends on stage. Patients with stage I tumors have a 5-year survival of 90% or better, whereas those with positive lymph nodes have a 5-year survival of approximately 50% to 60%, depending on the number and location of positive lymph nodes (*Am J Obstet Gynecol* 1991;164:997).

B. **Cervical carcinoma.** Although detection of preinvasive disease has increased, the incidence of invasive cervical cancer has dramatically decreased in the United States due to widespread screening by cervical cytology (Papanicolaou smears). However, cervical cancer remains the leading cause of cancer related deaths among women in developing countries (National Cervical Cancer Coalition Web site, http://www.nccc-online.org/). In the United States, approximately 14,000 new cases and 3,900 deaths occur annually. The goal of evaluating abnormal Papanicolaou smears with colposcopy-guided biopsies for appropriate patients is to diagnose and treat disease of the cervix in the preinvasive state [Stoler MH, Schiffman M; Atypical squamous cells of undetermined significance-low-grade squamous introepithelial lesion triage study (ALTS) group. Interobserver reproducibility of cervical cytologic and histologic interpretations: realistic estimates from the ASCUS-LSIL Triage Study. *JAMA.* 2001;285:1500–1505]. Risk factors for cervical cancer include a history of sexually transmitted diseases, HIV infection, multiple sexual partners, early age of first intercourse, lower socioeconomic status, smoking, and human papilloma virus (HPV) infection. Because the majority of squamous cell cancers of the cervix contain high-risk HPV DNA, an HPV vaccine (Gardasil) has been developed and should be administered to females between the ages of 9 and 26 years, although the impact in eradicating cancer will take several decades.

1. **Presentation and clinical features.** Patients may be asymptomatic or present with irregular or postcoital vaginal bleeding or a foul-smelling or watery discharge. Advanced stages may present with leg pain (sciatic nerve involvement), flank pain (ureteral obstruction), renal failure, or rectal bleeding.

2. **Diagnosis** is by biopsy via speculum examination of a visible or palpable lesion. Staging remains clinical and is based on a thorough bimanual and rectovaginal examination, cystoscopy, and proctoscopy. Appropriate adjuvant radiographs include chest x-ray, intravenous pyelogram, and barium enema. Positron emission tomography (PET) scan is a useful diagnostic modality for assessing distant disease activity. Stage, which is never changed by intraoperative findings, remains the most important prognostic factor, with an 88% 5-year survival for stage I disease and a 38% 5-year survival for stage III disease (Table 36-2).

3. **Treatment** depends on stage and lymph node status.

   a. **Microinvasive disease** (stage IA1, depth of invasion <3 mm, diameter <7 mm, negative lymph vascular space invasion) can be treated with cervical conization alone or with extrafascial hysterectomy. Reproductive age patients desiring fertility (preferably with a cervical lesion <2 cm) may be offered a radical vaginal or abdominal trachelectomy with a lymph node dissection and cerclage placement. Lesions with greater depth of invasion, multifocal disease, or upper-vaginal involvement (stages IA2 to IIA) require a radical hysterectomy (removing the parametria and upper vagina) and a complete pelvic and sometimes para-aortic lymphadenectomy. Although radical hysterectomy is only appropriate for a subset of patients, radiotherapy is applicable to any patient with early-stage cervical cancer. The most common complication after radical hysterectomy is bladder dysfunction. Ureteral fistulas, infection, hemorrhage, and lymphocyst formation are less common.

TABLE 36-2		Cervical Cancer Staging

TNM	FIGO	Definition
T1	I	Cervical carcinoma confined to the uterus (extension to the corpus should be disregarded)
T1a	IA	Preclinical invasive carcinoma, diagnosed by microscopy only
T1a1	IA1	Microscopic stromal invasion no greater than 3 mm in depth and no wider than 7 mm
T1a2	IA2	Tumor with stromal invasion between 3 and 5 mm in depth and no wider than 7 mm
T1b	IB	Tumor confined to the cervix but larger than IA2
T1b1	IB1	Clinical lesions no greater than 4 cm in size
T1b2	IB2	Clinical lesions greater than 4 cm in size
T2	II	Tumor invades beyond the cervix but not to the pelvic side wall or the lower third of the vagina
T2a	IIA	Tumor without parametrial involvement
T2b	IIB	Tumor with parametrial involvement
T3	III	Tumor extends to the pelvic side wall and/or involves the lower one third of the vagina and/or causes hydronephrosis or nonfunctioning kidney
T3a	IIIA	Tumor invades lower third of the vagina with no extension to the pelvic side wall
T3b	IIIB	Tumor extends to the pelvic side wall and/or causes hydronephrosis or a nonfunctioning kidney
T4	IVA	Tumor invades mucosa of the bladder or rectum and/or extends beyond the true pelvis
M1	IVB	Distant metastasis

FIGO, International Federation of Gynecology and Obstetrics; TNM, tumor, node, metastasis.

    b. Radiotherapy is the appropriate treatment for advanced-stage disease. Combined surgery and radiotherapy for advanced-staged disease does not improve survival but dramatically increases the rate of treatment-related complications such as ureteral and bowel obstruction, strictures, and fistula formation. The nature of radiation is based on stage, lesion size, and lymph node status. Both external-beam (teletherapy) and intracavitary (brachytherapy) radiation are used in various combinations. Complications from radiotherapy depend on dose, volume, and tissue tolerance. Acute complications include transient nausea and diarrhea. Early complications including skin ulceration, cystitis, and proctitis occur within the first 6 months after treatment and. Late complications (>6 months after treatment) may include bowel obstruction secondary to strictures, fistulas, hemorrhagic cystitis, and chronic proctosigmoiditis. Recent studies indicate that adding cisplatin to radiation decreases the risk of dying from cervical cancer by 30% to 50% over radiation alone (*Lancet* 2001;358:781).

    c. Patients with **pelvic recurrence** after radical hysterectomy are often treated with radiation. Patients with isolated central recurrence may be candidates for pelvic exenteration. Five-year survival ranges from 20% to 62% after exenteration, with an operative mortality of 10%. Response to chemotherapy alone in recurrent cervical cancer is poor.

4. Uncontrolled vaginal bleeding from cervical cancer occasionally is encountered in the emergency department. In most cases, bleeding can be stabilized with tight vaginal packing, after which a transurethral Foley catheter should be placed. Acetone-soaked gauze is the most effective packing for vessel sclerosis and control of hemorrhage from necrotic tumor. Emergent radiotherapy or embolization may be necessary.

C. Endometrial carcinoma. Endometrial carcinoma is the most common gynecologic malignancy in the United States. Approximately 39,080 new cases will be diagnosed in 2007. Most (approximately 90%) of these tumors are adenocarcinomas arising from the lining of the uterus. Risk factors for endometrial cancer include white race, obesity, early menarche and late menopause, nulliparity, tamoxifen therapy, estrogen replacement therapy, infertility, hereditary nonpolyposis colon cancer (HNPCC), and factors leading to unopposed estrogen exposure. Pregnancy and oral contraceptive use appear to be protective. Complex atypical endometrial hyperplasia, a precursor lesion, progresses to carcinoma in 29% of cases if left untreated. Only 1% to 3% of cases of hyperplasia without atypia progress to carcinoma. Hyperplasia can be treated conservatively with progestins and close observation with follow-up endometrial biopsy. Extrafascial hysterectomy is suggested for persistent hyperplasia in patients who have completed their childbearing.

1. **Presentation and clinical features.** The most common symptom is abnormal vaginal bleeding, often in a postmenopausal patient. Approximately three fourths of patients present with stage I disease. Endometrial sampling should be considered mandatory in all postmenopausal women. Although endometrial carcinoma is rare in women younger than 35 years, patients in this age group who have persistent noncyclic vaginal bleeding, are nonresponsive to medical management, or are morbidly obese should undergo endometrial assessment (ACOG Practice Bulletin 65. In: *Compendium of Selected Publications.* Washington, DC: American College of Obstetrics and Gynecology; 2007:1128).

2. **Physical examination** should include an assessment for obesity, hirsutism, and other signs of hyperestrogenism. The uterus may be enlarged or of normal size.

3. **Diagnosis** is by transcervical aspiration (e.g., Pipelle), which usually is performed as an office procedure, or by hysteroscopy/D & C, which is performed in the operating room. Ultrasound can help to suggest an intrauterine abnormality.

4. **Treatment** generally consists of a laparoscopic or open staging procedure including pelvic washings, extrafascial total hysterectomy, bilateral salpingo-oophorectomy, and sometimes omentectomy. Pelvic and para-aortic lymphadenectomy is considered both diagnostic and therapeutic and should be performed in all patients. Intraoperative evaluation of the uterus should be performed by bivalving the uterus and obtaining a frozen section as needed. Adjuvant radiotherapy and/or chemotherapy is used postoperatively in patients with poor prognostic factors who are at high risk for recurrence. Hormonal therapy or chemotherapy is used for advanced disease, but response to chemotherapy has been poor.

5. **Prognosis** generally is favorable, with 5-year survival greater than 90% for patients with surgical stage I tumors (Table 36-3). Prognosis depends on the grade of tumor as well as the depth of myometrial invasion, adnexal involvement, pelvic cytology, lymph vascular space invasion, and lymph node spread. Rarer histologies, such as clear-cell or papillary serous cancers and the sarcomas arising from the wall of the uterus, do not share the overall good prognosis of early-stage adenocarcinomas. African American women have mortality rates nearly twice that of white women.

D. Ovarian carcinoma. Ovarian cancer is the deadliest of all the gynecologic malignancies. There will be approximately 22,430 new cases diagnosed in 2007. More than two thirds of patients in whom epithelial ovarian cancer is diagnosed eventually die from this disease (15,280/year in the United States) (*Cancer J Clin* 2007;57:43). Besides tumors arising from the ovarian coelomic surface, which are the most common, germ cell (often in younger patients) and stromal primary tumors can occur. Two thirds of epithelial ovarian cancers are diagnosed at advanced stages with extraovarian metastasis. Incidence increases steadily with advancing age to a total lifetime incidence of 1 in 68. Risk factors include nulliparity, late menopause, early menarche, use of infertility drugs, and personal or family history of breast or ovarian cancer. Genetic cancer syndromes including the presence of *BRCA1* or *BRCA2* mutations and hereditary nonpolyposis colon cancer also have been associated with an increased risk of ovarian cancer, and prophylactic removal of ovaries and fallopian tubes

TABLE 36-3		Endometrial Cancer Staging
TNM	**FIGO**	**Definition**
T1	I	Tumor confined to the corpus uteri
T1a	IA	Tumor limited to the endometrium
T1b	IB	Tumor invades less than or up to half of the myometrium
T1c	IC	Tumor invades more than half of the myometrium
T2	II	Tumor invades the cervix but does not extend beyond the uterus
T2a	IIA	Endocervical glandular involvement only
T2b	IIB	Cervical stromal invasion
T3	III	Local and/or regional spread as specified
T3a	IIIA	Tumor involves the serosa and/or adnexa and/or positive washings
T3b	IIIB	Vaginal involvement
N1	IIIC	Metastasis to the pelvic and/or para-aortic lymph nodes
T4	IVA	Tumor invades the bladder mucosa or the rectum and/or bowel mucosa
M1	IVB	Distant metastasis including intra-abdominal and/or inguinal lymph nodes

FIGO, International Federation of Gynecology and Obstetrics; TNM, tumor, node, metastasis.

decreases the risk of gynecologic cancer in these patients. Use of oral contraceptives, pregnancy, and tubal ligation appear to be protective.

1. **Presentation and clinical features.** Women with early-stage disease are generally asymptomatic. In advanced stages, patients may present with vague abdominal pain or pressure, nausea, early satiety, weight loss, or swelling.

TABLE 36-4		Ovarian Cancer Staging
TNM	**FIGO**	**Definition**
T1	I	Tumor limited to one or both ovaries
T1a	IA	Tumor limited to one ovary; capsule intact, no tumor on ovarian surface, no malignant cells in ascites or peritoneal washings
T1b	IB	Tumor limited to both ovaries; capsule intact, no tumor on ovarian surface, no malignant cells in ascites or peritoneal washings
T1c	IC	Tumor limited to one or both ovaries with any of the following: capsule ruptured, tumor on ovarian surface, malignant cells in ascites or peritoneal washings
T2	II	Tumor involves one or both ovaries with pelvic extension
T2a	IIA	Extension and/or implants on uterus and/or tubes; no malignant cells in ascites or peritoneal washings
T2b	IIB	Extension to other pelvic tissues; no malignant cells in ascites or peritoneal washings
T2c	IIC	Pelvic extension with malignant cells in ascites or peritoneal washings
T3	III	Tumor involves one or both ovaries with microscopically confirmed peritoneal metastasis outside the pelvis and/or regional lymph node metastasis
T3a	IIIA	Microscopic peritoneal metastasis beyond the pelvis
T3b	IIIB	Macroscopic peritoneal metastasis beyond the pelvis ≤2 cm in greatest dimension
T3c	IIIC	Peritoneal metastasis beyond the pelvis >2 cm in greatest dimension and/or regional lymph node involvement
M1	IV	Distant metastasis (excludes peritoneal metastasis)

FIGO, International Federation of Gynecology and Obstetrics; TNM, tumor, node, metastasis.

2. **Diagnosis** of ovarian cancer at early stages has proved to be clinically difficult (Table 36-4). No cost-effective screening test has proven to be reliable in detecting stage I disease (confined to the ovaries). Bimanual examination remains the most effective means of screening, followed by surgery for histologic diagnosis. Ultrasonography of the pelvis (preferably transvaginal) and CT scan are effective adjuncts. CA 125 antigen is not effective for mass screening but serves as an effective tumor marker in patients with initial elevations once diagnosis has been established and treatment is initiated.

3. **Treatment** is primarily aggressive surgical debulking for all patients. Complete staging includes pelvic washings on entering the peritoneum, total abdominal hysterectomy, bilateral salpingo-oophorectomy, omentectomy, pelvic and para-aortic lymph node dissection, and peritoneal biopsies. Optimal cytoreduction (residual disease <1 cm) improves response to adjuvant chemotherapy and overall survival. In young women with early-stage disease, fertility-sparing surgery can often be performed with removal of the uterus and contralateral ovary after childbearing is completed. However, complete staging at initial surgery is still necessary. Patients with disease outside the ovary are treated with six cycles of paclitaxel and platinum–based chemotherapy either intravenously or intraperitoneally.

4. **Prognosis** correlates directly with stage and with the residual disease after debulking. Median survival depends on optimal cytoreduction at initial laparotomy. Median survival for optimally debulked advanced-stage tumors is nearly 80% at 1 year; the 5-year relative survival rate for all stages is 45% (*Cancer J Clin* 2007; 57:43).

COMMON SURGICAL PROCEDURES

Li Ern Chen and Bradley D. Freeman

37

INTRODUCTION

This chapter reviews concepts, indications, and technical aspects of procedures commonly performed in hospitalized surgical patients, focusing on central venous catheterization, thoracic and peritoneal drainage procedures, airway access, and laparoscopy.

Basic rules govern the successful performance of surgical procedures: (1) Necessary equipment, supplies, lighting, and assistance should be available prior to starting the procedure; (2) the patient should be positioned to optimize exposure; (3) patient comfort must be ensured, and appropriate analgesia and sedation must be provided so that the patient can cooperate with and tolerate the procedure; and (4) sterile technique should be practiced when appropriate

I. CENTRAL VENOUS CATHETERIZATION. Central venous catheterization is commonly used in surgical patients both for diagnosis [central venous pressure (CVP) determination] and treatment (fluid infusion, mechanical device, (e.g., pacemaker or inferior vena cava filter insertion). Several approaches to the central venous system exist, each with advantages and disadvantages. Before placement of a central venous access device (CVAD), the patient should be evaluated for the presence of an indwelling central venous device, such as a transvenous pacemaker, and signs of central venous obstruction, such as distended collateral veins about the shoulder and neck. **Contraindication:** Venous thrombosis is an absolute contraindication to catheter placement at the affected site. Relative contraindications include coagulopathy [International Normalized Ratio (INR) >2 or partial prothrombin time (PTT) >2 times control] refractory to correction and thrombocytopenia (platelet count <50,000/μL). For an elective procedure, the INR should be corrected to less than 1.5, PTT to less than 1.5 times control, and platelet count to greater than 50,000/μL.

A. Types of catheters. Catheters are classified on the basis of number of lumens, location (artery, vein), lifespan (short, intermediate, long term), site of insertion (subclavian, internal jugular, femoral, peripheral), subcutaneous tunneling, anti-infective features (Dacron and/or antibiotic cuff, heparin, or antibiotic impregnation), and tip structure (valved, nonvalved).

    1. Short-term (nontunneled) CVADs. The advantages of single-lumen and multilumen nontunneled catheters include low cost, bedside placement and removal, and ease of exchange of damaged catheters. Examples include the **triple-lumen catheter,** the **Mahurkar catheter,** and the **Hemo-Cath pheresis catheter.**

    2. Intermediate-term, peripherally inserted CVADs. Peripherally inserted central catheters (PICCs) are composed of Silastic or polyurethane and can be kept in place for up to 6 months. These are commonly used for home total parenteral nutrition (TPN) or intravenous antibiotic administration (4 to 12 weeks). PICCs can be inserted using local anesthetic at the bedside via cephalic, basilic, or median cubital veins. Proper position should be radiographically documented. These catheters have low risk of insertion-related complications, such as pneumothorax, and infection. Disadvantages of PICCs result from their small diameter and length (40 to 60 cm), including problems with withdrawal occlusion and risk for thrombophlebitis (*JVIR* 2000;11:1309).

3. **Intermediate-term, nontunneled CVADS.** These catheters contain a silver-impregnated gelatin cuff (Vitacuff), which is designed to be positioned subcutaneously and to serve as a barrier to migration of bacteria from the skin. The gelatin dissolves within a short time, facilitating removal. The **Hohn catheter** is the prototypical CVAD of this type, and it may remain in place for as long as 6 months.

4. **Long-term, tunneled CVADS.** Tunneled catheters enable indefinite venous access for prolonged nutritional support, chemotherapy, antibiotics, hemodialysis, or blood draws. The subcutaneous portion of the catheter contains a double cuff that functions to induce scar formation, anchoring the catheter in place and preventing bacterial migration from skin. Most tunneled catheters are manufactured using silicone, which is more flexible and durable than other materials. Examples include the **Hickman** and **Broviac catheters.** The **Groshong catheter** differs by the presence of a slit valve at the tip, which seals it from the bloodstream. Unlike other catheters, which require daily or weekly heparinized saline injections, Groshong catheters are flushed with normal saline, and thus they are well suited for patients with history of heparin allergy or heparin-induced thrombocytopenia.

5. **Implanted venous ports.** Ports are used primarily for chronic therapy (>6 months) and for which only intermittent access is needed. Common indications include chemotherapy and frequent hospitalization (e.g., patients with sickle cell disease or cystic fibrosis). Access is preferably obtained via the internal jugular vein and a reservoir placed in a subcutaneous pocket created in the infraclavicular fossa. Smaller port devices (e.g., **PASport**) are designed for upper-extremity implantation. Most models contain a silicone or polyurethane catheter connected to a metal or plastic reservoir with a dense silicone septum for percutaneous needle access. Advantages of ports over other CVADs include a lower incidence of infection and less maintenance (monthly heparin flushes when not in use). Plastic ports are magnetic resonance scan compatible (e.g., **MRI port**) and are as durable as ports with reservoirs constructed of metal. Port access requires skin puncture using a special noncoring (Huber) needle to prevent deterioration of the septum.

B. **Internal jugular approach**

1. **Indications.** The internal jugular vein is easily and rapidly accessible in most patients. Advantages of this site include decreased risk of pneumothorax compared with the subclavian approach and ready compressibility of the vessels in case of bleeding. For the unsedated or ambulatory patient, this may be an uncomfortable site and may hinder his or her neck movement. Maintaining a sterile dressing on the insertion site can be difficult. This is a commonly used site of central venous access for placement of tunneled catheters and ports where the catheter's exit site is on the chest.

2. **Technique.** Imaging devices (such as ultrasound) are being increasingly used to delineate the vascular anatomy and enhance the safety of vascular access procedures. If available, such devices should be used, particularly in patients in whom anatomic landmarks are obscure. The pulse of the common carotid artery is palpated at the medial border of the sternocleidomastoid (SCM) muscle at midneck. The internal jugular vein is located lateral to the common carotid artery and courses slightly anterior to the artery as it joins the subclavian vein (Fig. 37-1). Two equally effective approaches to the internal jugular vein are described: the central and posterior approaches. The physician stands at the head of the bed. The patient is placed in the Trendelenburg position at an angle of 10 to 15 degrees with his or her head flat on the bed and turned away from the side of the procedure. The skin is prepared with 70% propanal/0.5% chlorhexidine followed by 10% povidone-iodine, which has been shown in a prospective randomized trial (*J Intens Care Med* 2004;30:1081) to be superior in prevention of catheter colonization. One percent (1%) lidocaine is infiltrated subcutaneously over the belly and lateral border of the SCM. For the central approach, a 21-gauge "seeker" needle is introduced approximately 1 cm lateral to the carotid pulse into the belly of the SCM. At a 45-degree angle, the needle is slowly advanced toward the ipsilateral nipple. For the posterior approach, the seeker needle is introduced at

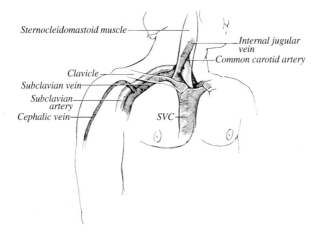

Figure 37-1. Anatomy of the upper chest and neck, including the vasculature and important landmarks. SVC, superior vena cava.

the lateral edge of the SCM and directed toward the sternal notch at a 45-degree angle. The vein should be entered within 5 to 7 cm with both approaches. If the vein is not entered, the needle should be withdrawn and redirected for another attempt. Redirection of the needle should be done just below the surface of the skin because of the potential of the needle tip to lacerate adjacent vessels. Constant negative pressure is exerted on the syringe, and entry into the vein is confirmed by the return of venous blood. A 14-gauge needle is then introduced just inferior to the seeker needle and is advanced along the same path until venous blood is aspirated. The **Seldinger technique** is carried out, whereby a flexible guidewire is passed into the vein through the 14-gauge needle, the needle is removed over the wire, and a nick is made in the skin at the puncture site to allow passage of the dilator. It is important to maintain control of the guidewire at all times. The dilator creates a tract for the passage of the less rigid central venous catheter. The catheter is introduced over the wire and advanced to 15 to 20 cm so that its tip is at the junction of the superior vena cava (SVC) and the right atrium. In patients with difficult anatomy or indwelling devices (vena cava filters, pacemakers), fluoroscopy may be used to guide placement. Aspiration of blood from all ports and subsequent flushing with saline confirm that the catheter is positioned in the vein and that all of its ports are functional. The catheter is then secured to the patient's neck at a minimum of two sites, and a sterile dressing is applied. A chest x-ray is obtained to confirm the location of the catheter tip and to rule out the presence of a pneumothorax.

3. **Complications**
    a. **Pneumothorax.** All percutaneously placed neck lines carry a risk of pneumothorax. Every attempt at placement of a central venous catheter, successful or unsuccessful, should be followed by an erect chest x-ray before the catheter is used or line placement is attempted at another site.
    b. **Carotid artery injury.** Carotid artery puncture complicates internal jugular cannulation in as many as 10% of cases, representing 80% to 90% of all insertion-related complications. Inadvertent carotid artery puncture is usually tolerated in the noncoagulopathic patient and treated by direct pressure over the carotid artery. If the carotid artery is punctured, no further attempts at central venous access should be made on either side of the patient's neck and the patient must be observed for the development of a neck hematoma and resultant airway compromise. Although carotid artery puncture is usually benign, it can be life threatening when it results in inadvertent intra-arterial cannulation,

stroke, hemothorax, or carotid artery–internal jugular vein fistula. In the hemodynamically unstable or poorly oxygenating patient, it is not always possible to distinguish venous blood from arterial blood by appearance. This can lead to inadvertent cannulation of the carotid artery. If the dilator or catheter is 7 French or smaller, it can usually be removed and direct pressure held over the carotid puncture site without further detrimental sequelae. Catheters larger than 7 French should be removed in a setting in which operative repair of the arteriotomy can be performed.

   c. **Guidewire-related complications.** Advancement of the guidewire into the right atrium or ventricle can cause arrhythmia, which usually resolves once the wire is withdrawn. Central venous catheter insertion in patients with indwelling devices (such as vena cava filters or pacemakers) must be performed under fluoroscopic guidance to minimize the possibility of entanglement of the guidewire with these structures.

   d. **Venous stenosis.** Venous stenosis can occur at the site where the catheter enters the vein, which can lead to thrombosis of the vessel. Because the upper extremities and neck have extensive collateralization, stenosis or thrombosis is usually well tolerated.

   e. **Other.** Air embolus, perforation of the right atrium or ventricle with resultant hemopericardium and cardiac tamponade, and injury to the trachea, esophagus, thoracic duct, vagus nerve, phrenic nerve, or brachial plexus can all complicate the placement of central venous catheters.

4. **Catheter-related bloodstream infection (CRBSI)** occurs with a prevalence ranging from 3% to 7% and has a mortality rate of up to 15% (*Infect Control Hosp Epidemiol* 2000;21:375). Catheter colonization—or bacterial growth from the catheter tip—occurs in 20% of central venous catheters.

   a. **Epidemiology.** CRBSIs are generally caused by coagulase-negative staphylococci (37%), followed by enterococci (13.5%), coagulase-positive *Staphylococcus aureus* (12.6%), and *Candida albicans* (8%). Treatment of these organisms has become increasingly difficult now that 60% of *S. aureus* isolates and 90% of coagulase-negative *Staphylococcus* isolates are resistant to oxacillin. The percentage of enterococcal isolates resistant to vancomycin has also increased, from 0.5% in 1989 to 28.5% in 2003 (*Am J Infect Control* 2004;32:470). For lower-extremity CVAD, Gram-negative rods represent the most frequent organisms of infection, along with enterococci. The majority of catheter infections are monomicrobial.

   b. **Pathogenesis.** Infection occurs by two routes. First, endogenous skin flora at the insertion site migrate along the external surface of the catheter and colonize the intravascular tip. Second, pathogens from contamination at the hub colonize the internal surface of the catheter and are washed into the bloodstream when the catheter is infused. Occasionally, catheters may become hematogenously seeded from another focus of infection. Rarely, infusate contamination or break in sterile technique leads to CRBSI.

   c. **Definitions and diagnosis.** Catheter colonization is defined as greater than 15 colony-forming units of microorganisms on semiquantitative culture. The definition of CRBSI requires bacteremia or fungemia in a patient with CVAD and meeting of the following criteria: (1) clinical signs of infection (fever, chills, tachycardia, hypotension, leukocytosis), (2) no identifiable source for bloodstream infection other than the CVAD, and (3) isolation of the same organism from semiquantitative culture of the catheter and from the blood (drawn from a peripheral vein taken within 48 hours of each other) (*Clin Infect Dis* 2001;32:1249). Diagnosis of CRBSI with coagulase-negative staphylococci requires two positive blood cultures or a positive catheter culture.

   d. **Presentation.** Catheter infections may manifest with local, regional, or systemic signs.

      (1) **Local catheter-related infections.** Exit-site infections may present with erythema and drainage. In the absence of systemic signs and negative blood cultures, treatment consists of routine antibiotics for skin flora and more

frequent dressing changes and care. Catheter removal is required in only about 10% of cases.

(2) Regional catheter infections. Tunnel infections or pocket infections present with erythema, induration, and tenderness along the catheter tract or over the pocket, often with a clear demarcation of the affected area. Often there are systemic manifestations (e.g., leukocytosis, positive blood culture). If regional infection is diagnosed, the CVAD is usually removed, and in some cases, the tunnel or pocket is débrided. Antibiotic treatment alone is rarely successful.

(3) Bacteremia. Bacteremia is the most severe manifestation of a catheter-related infection. In the setting of bacteremia, indwelling catheters generally should be removed. However, in patients with limited access and other potential sources for infection, broad-spectrum antibiotics can be initiated and continued for 10 to 14 days. Persistent bacteremia requires catheter removal. One exception is the presence of fungemia, which requires the catheter to be removed, with immediate initiation of antifungal treatment.

e. Risk factors. Several factors increase the risk of CVAD-related infections, including neutropenia, malignancy, parenteral feeding, intensive care unit (ICU) admission, mechanical ventilation, hyperalimentation, increasing number of catheter lumens, and thrombus. The risk for infection varies with the catheter insertion site, with the femoral vein associated with a much higher infection rate than subclavian vein access (19.8% vs. 4.5%) (*JAMA* 2001;286:700). Jugular venous catheterization carries an intermediate risk of infection. The likelihood of infection directly correlates with length of time a catheter has been in position.

f. Antimicrobial-impregnated catheters. Antimicrobial-coated catheters, ionic silver cuffs, antibiotic-impregnated hubs, and intraluminal antibiotic locks have all been shown to reduce the incidence of CRBSI in critically ill patients and should be used in this patient population. In a multicenter, randomized, double-blind, controlled trial, second-generation chlorhexidine-silver sulfadiazine (CHSS)–impregnated CVADs reduced microbial colonization compared to uncoated catheters (*Ann Intern Med* 2005;143:570). In addition, a recent meta-analysis found that rifampin/minocycline–impregnated CVADs reduced the rate of microbial colonization and CRBSI (*J Antimicrob Chemother* 2007;59:359). Comparison of second-generation CHSS-coated catheters to rifampin/minocycline–impregnated catheters has not been made. The emergence of resistant organisms resulting from the use of antimicrobial-impregnated catheters remains a potentially important concern.

g. Routine (elective) catheter replacement. Routine catheter replacement (either changing position to a new site or rewiring an existing catheter after an arbitrary length of time) has not been demonstrated to decrease the incidence of catheter-related infections. Thus, CVADs should be left in place until discontinuation is clinically indicated.

C. Subclavian vein approach

1. Indications. The subclavian approach to the central venous system is generally most comfortable for the patient and easiest to maintain. The Centers for Disease Control and Prevention (CDC) published guidelines in 2002 that recommend subclavian access as the preferred site in patients at risk for CVAD infection (*MMWR Recomm Rep* 2002;51:1). A prospective observational study found that CRBSI incidence was lowest in subclavian access, higher in jugular access, and highest in femoral access, and recommended that sites for CVAD placement be considered in that order (*Crit Care* 2005;9:R631). In the presence of an open wound, tracheostomy, and tumors of the head and neck, CVAD should be placed in the subclavian position to minimize infectious risk.

2. Technique. The subclavian vein courses posterior to the clavicle, where it joins the internal jugular vein and the contralateral veins to form the SVC (Fig. 37-1). The subclavian artery and the apical pleura lie just posterior to the subclavian vein. The patient is placed in the Trendelenburg position with a rolled towel between the scapulas, which allows the shoulders to fall posteriorly. The skin is prepared with 70% propanal/0.5% chlorhexidine followed by 10% povidone-iodine, and 1% lidocaine is infiltrated subcutaneously in the infraclavicular space near the middle and lateral third of the clavicle. The infusion is carried into the deep soft tissue and to the periosteum of the clavicle. A 14-gauge needle is introduced at the middle third of the clavicle in the deltopectoral groove. The needle is kept deep to the clavicle and parallel to the plane of the floor and is slowly advanced toward the sternal notch. Constant negative pressure is applied to the syringe. Once the needle enters the subclavian vein, the guidewire, dilator, and catheter are introduced using the **Seldinger technique.** As with the other approaches, all catheter ports are aspirated and flushed to ensure that they are functional. A chest x-ray is obtained to confirm the location of the catheter tip and to evaluate for pneumothorax.

   3. **Complications.** The complications of subclavian venous catheterization include those described in the previous section. Puncture of the subclavian artery can be troublesome because the clavicle prevents the application of direct pressure to achieve homeostasis. Therefore, this approach should be avoided in the patient with uncorrectable coagulopathy. If the artery is punctured, the patient should be placed on hemodynamic monitoring for the next 30 to 45 minutes to ensure that bleeding is not ongoing. Inadvertent cannulation of the subclavian artery with the dilator or catheter is a potentially fatal complication. The dilator or catheter should be left in place and an angiogram performed. Removal of the catheter should be done in the operating room so that open arteriotomy repair may be performed if necessary. Particular attention must be paid to the placement of left subclavian catheters to avoid injuring the thoracic duct, brachiocephalic vein, and SVC with the needle or dilator. Attention must be paid to the final position of the catheter tip when placed on the left side to avoid abutting the SVC wall, which poses the immediate or delayed risk of SVC perforation.

D. Femoral vein approach

   1. **Indications.** The femoral vein is the easiest site for obtaining central access and is therefore the preferred approach for central venous access during trauma or cardiopulmonary resuscitation. This approach does not interfere with the other procedures of cardiopulmonary resuscitation. It should be remembered that a femoral vein catheter does not actually reach the central circulation and may not be ideal for the administration of vasoactive drugs. This may be the only site available in patients with upper-body burns. The femoral approach is also favored during trauma resuscitation except when there is an injury to the inferior vena cava. The femoral vein catheter inhibits patient mobility, and the groin is a difficult area in which to maintain sterility. Therefore, it should not be used in elective situations, except when upper-extremity and neck sites are not available.

   2. **Technique.** The femoral artery crosses the inguinal ligament approximately midway between the anterosuperior iliac spine and the pubic tubercle. The femoral vein runs medial to the artery as they cross the inguinal ligament (Fig. 37-2). The skin is prepared with 70% propanal/0.5% chlorhexidine followed by 10% povidone-iodine, and 1% lidocaine is infiltrated in the subcutaneous tissue medial to the femoral artery and inferior to the inguinal ligament. The pulse of the femoral artery is palpated below the inguinal ligament, and a 14-gauge needle is introduced medial to the pulse at a 30-degree angle. It is directed cephalad with constant negative pressure until the vein is entered. The catheter is placed using the **Seldinger technique.** When a femoral pulse cannot be palpated, as in cardiopulmonary arrest, the position of the femoral artery can be estimated to be at the midpoint between the anterosuperior iliac spine and the pubic tubercle, with the vein lying 1 to 2 cm medial to this point. Once the catheter is successfully placed, all three ports are aspirated and flushed to ensure that they are functional.

   3. **Complications.** Injury to the common femoral artery or its branches during cannulation of the femoral vein can result in an inguinal or retroperitoneal hematoma,

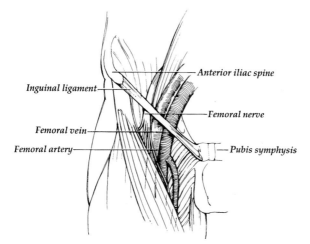

Figure 37-2. Anatomy of the femoral vessels.

a pseudoaneurysm, or an arteriovenous fistula. The femoral nerve can also be damaged. Injury to the inguinal lymphatic system can result in a lymphocele. The possibility of injuring peritoneal structures also exists, particularly if an inguinal hernia is present. Errant passages of the guidewire and the rigid dilator run the risk of perforating the pelvic venous complex and causing retroperitoneal hemorrhage. Late complications include infection and femoral vein thrombosis.

E. Catheter maintenance. Proper care of access sites and devices is crucial to their long-term function. Short-term and tunneled CVADs require sterile, occlusive, transparent dressings that are changed weekly by trained personnel using meticulous technique. More frequent dressing changes may be needed for those patients who are immune compromised. Application of topical antibiotic beneath an occlusive dressing may provide a moist culture medium for bacterial growth. Catheter lumens should be flushed on a regular basis to prevent thrombosis.

F. Thrombosis (*J Natl Compr Cancer Netw* 2006;4:889). Difficulty in aspirating blood or infusing fluid may be indicative of partial or complete catheter blockage. Blockage may be due to kinking of the catheter, occlusion of the catheter tip on a vessel wall, or luminal thrombosis. The spectrum of thrombotic complications ranges from fibrin sleeve formation around the catheter to mural or occlusive thrombus. Although only 3% to 5% of central venous catheters develop clinically significant thromboses, ultrasonography with color Doppler imaging has been found to detect venous thrombosis in 33% to 67% of patients when the indwelling time of the CVAD was greater than 1 week. A negative Doppler ultrasound in a symptomatic patient should be followed by venographic assessment because thrombi in the central upper venous system (superior vena cava, brachiocephalic, and subclavian veins) are better detected by venography.

1. Patient-related risk factors include prothrombotic states associated with underlying coagulation disorders, malignancy, chronic disease, hydration state, nutritional status, and prior history of CVAD placement

2. Catheter-related risk factors include size, position, infection, and duration of placement. Risk of catheter-related thrombosis varies according to site of insertion, with reported rates of 21.5% in femoral catheters compared to only 1.9% with subclavian access (*p* <0.001) (*JAMA* 2001;286:700). Catheters in the subclavian or innominate veins are at higher risk for producing symptomatic central venous stenosis than are those that are placed in the right internal jugular vein.

More-pliable and smoother catheter material, such as silicone, is less thrombogenic than stiffer materials, such as polyurethane. Risk of infection is strongly correlated to the presence of thrombus. Regular flushing protocols may reduce the incidence of thrombotic complications.

3. **Intervention.** Thrombolytic intervention with urokinase or alteplase is generally an effective and safe means of restoring CVAD function and blood flow without resorting to catheter replacement. If this procedure fails or if the patient is symptomatic, the catheter should be removed and systemic anticoagulation should be initiated.

II. THORACIC DRAINAGE PROCEDURES

A. Thoracentesis

1. **Indications.** Diagnostic thoracentesis is indicated for pleural effusion of unknown etiology. Pleural effusions are categorized as transudative or exudative. This differentiation is based on its gross, microscopic, and biochemical characteristics. Several laboratory studies are available for studying pleural fluid. A pleural fluid–serum lactate dehydrogenase (LDH) ratio greater than 0.6 and a fluid–serum protein ratio greater than 0.5 indicate an exudative effusion, whereas a fluid–serum LDH ratio less than 0.6 and a fluid–serum protein ratio less than 0.5 indicate a transudative effusion. Fluid pH, glucose level, amylase level, and lipid level may be measured when analyzing pleural fluid to aid in diagnosis. Cytologic examination for malignant cells should be obtained when a malignant effusion is considered. If an infectious etiology is suspected, Gram stain and culture for bacteria and fungi are necessary. Therapeutic thoracentesis is indicated to relieve shortness of breath or discomfort from large pleural effusions. When repeated therapeutic thoracentesis is needed to treat recurrent pleural effusions, chest tube drainage and pleurosclerosis should be considered.

2. **Technique.** Erect and lateral decubiti chest radiographs or equivalent imaging studies [such as computed tomography (CT) scanning] should be obtained to assess the size and location of the effusion as well as whether the effusion is free flowing or loculated. For free-flowing effusions, the patient is seated upright and slightly forward. The thorax should be entered posteriorly, 4 to 6 cm lateral to the spinal column and one to two interspaces below the cessation of tactile fremitus and where percussion is dull. Loculated effusions can be localized by ultrasonography, and the site for thoracentesis is marked on the skin. The site is prepared with povidone-iodine and draped with sterile towels. Lidocaine 1% is infiltrated into the subcutaneous tissue covering the rib below the interspace to be entered. The infiltration is carried deep to the periosteum of the rib. Next, with negative pressure placed on the syringe, the needle is advanced slowly over the top of the rib to avoid injury to the neurovascular bundle. The needle is advanced until pleural fluid is returned; then it is withdrawn a fraction, and lidocaine is injected to anesthetize the pleura. Lidocaine is then infiltrated into the intercostal muscles as the needle is withdrawn.

Most thoracentesis kits contain a long, 14-gauge needle inserted into a plastic catheter with an attached syringe and stopcock. The needle-catheter apparatus is introduced at the level of the rib below the interspace to be entered. With negative pressure applied to the syringe, the needle is slowly advanced over the top of the rib and into the pleural cavity until fluid is returned. Aspiration of air bubbles indicates puncture of the lung parenchyma; the needle should be promptly removed under negative pressure. Once the needle is in the pleural space, the catheter is advanced over the needle toward the diaphragm. Special attention is taken not to advance the needle as the catheter is being directed into the pleural space. A drainage bag is attached to the stopcock to remove the pleural fluid. The amount of fluid removed depends on the indication for the thoracentesis. A diagnostic thoracentesis requires 20 to 30 mL of fluid for the appropriate tests, and a therapeutic thoracentesis can drain 1 to 2 L of fluid. A chest x-ray should be obtained after the procedure to evaluate for pneumothorax and resolution of the effusion.

3. **Complications.** Pneumothorax is the most common complication of thoracentesis. It must be treated with a tube thoracostomy and negative suction until the air leak seals. An exception is that if the pneumothorax is small and the patient is stable with regard to hemodynamics and respiratory status, one may check another chest radiograph in 6 hours. Re-expansion pulmonary edema can occur in rare situations when a large amount of fluid is removed. Hemothorax, infection, injury to the neurovascular bundle, and subcutaneous hematoma are other potential complications.

B. Tube thoracostomy

1. **Indications and contraindications.** Tube thoracostomy is indicated for a pneumothorax, hemothorax, recurrent pleural effusion, chylothorax, and empyema. Profound coagulopathy is a relative contraindication to the placement of a chest tube, and efforts should be made to correct the coagulopathy before the tube is placed.

2. **Tubes.** The size of the thoracostomy tube needed depends on the material to be drained. Generally, a 32- to 36-French tube is used for the evacuation of a hemothorax or pleural effusion. In a pneumothorax, a 24- to 28-French tube is used. Alternatively, a percutaneous small-bore (18-French) chest tube (Thal-Quik) can be placed by Seldinger technique.

3. **Anatomy.** A good understanding of thoracic anatomy is needed to prevent injuries to the lung parenchyma, diaphragm, intercostal neurovascular bundles, and mediastinum during chest tube placement. The lung may have adhesions to the chest wall that make insertion and advancement of the thoracostomy tube difficult. The intercostal neurovascular bundle runs in a groove on the inferior aspect of each rib; therefore, the tube should be passed over the top of the rib to avoid injury. Because during normal respiration, the diaphragm can rise to the level of the fourth intercostal space, insertion of the chest tube lower than the sixth interspace is discouraged.

4. **Technique.** The patient is placed in the lateral position with the unaffected side down, and the head of the bed is inclined 10 to 15 degrees. The patient's arm on the affected side is extended forward or above the head. With the skin prepared, 1% lidocaine is infiltrated over the fifth or sixth rib in the middle or anterior axillary line by the technique described in the previous section. A 2- to 3-cm transverse incision is made through the skin and subcutaneous tissue. A curved clamp is used bluntly to dissect an oblique tract to the rib (Fig. 37-3A). With careful spreading, the clamp is advanced over the top of the rib. The parietal pleura is punctured with the clamp, and an efflux of air or fluid is usually encountered. A finger is introduced into the tract to ensure passage into the pleural space and to lyse any adhesions at the point of entry (Fig. 37-3B), ensuring that there is no lung adherent to the thoracic wall. With the clamp as a guide, the chest tube is introduced into the pleural space (Fig. 37-3C); the tube is directed posteriorly or basally for a dependent effusion and apically for a pneumothorax. A clamp placed at the free end of the chest tube prevents drainage from the chest until the tube can be connected to a closed suction or water-seal system. The chest tube is advanced until the last hole of the tube is clearly inside the thoracic cavity. When the tube is positioned properly and functioning adequately, it is secured to the skin with two heavy silk sutures and covered with an occlusive dressing to prevent air leaks. A U-stitch around the chest tube is commonly placed to be used as a purse-string suture to close the tract once the tube is removed. A chest x-ray is obtained after the procedure to assess re-expansion of the lung and the tube position. Under certain circumstances, radiographic guidance is required for tube placement (e.g., loculated pleural effusion, prior thoracic surgery).

5. **Complications.** Low placement of a chest tube can result in injury to the diaphragm and adjacent viscera. Failure to guide the tube into the pleural space can result in dissection of the extrapleural plane. This can be a difficult diagnosis, but anteroposterior and lateral chest radiographs should reveal a lung that

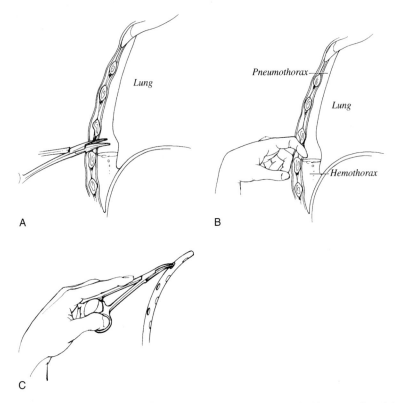

Figure 37-3. Tube thoracostomy placement. **A:** Pleural space entered by blunt spreading of the clamp over the top of the adjacent rib. **B:** A finger is introduced to ensure position within the pleural space and to lyse adhesions. **C:** The chest tube is placed into the tunnel and directed with the help of a Kelly clamp. The tube is directed posterior and caudal for an effusion or hemothorax and cephalad for a pneumothorax.

has failed to re-expand and suggest a chest tube placed outside the thorax. The tube should be removed and placed within the thoracic cavity to re-expand the lung. Parenchymal or hilar injuries or cardiac injuries can occur with overzealous advancement of the tube or dissection of pleural adhesions. Other complications include subcutaneous emphysema, re-expansion pulmonary edema, phrenic nerve injury, esophageal perforation, contralateral pneumothorax, and neurovascular bundle injury. Late complications include empyema, infection along the chest tube tract, and abscess. Infectious complications may be minimized by following strict sterile technique during thoracostomy tube placement.

III. PERITONEAL DRAINAGE PROCEDURE

A. Paracentesis

1. **Indications.** Paracentesis is a useful diagnostic and therapeutic tool. The most common indication for diagnostic paracentesis in the surgical patient is to determine whether ascites is infected. Accordingly, ascites should submitted for cell count, Gram stain, microscopy, and culture. A therapeutic paracentesis is indicated for patients with respiratory compromise or discomfort caused by tense ascites and in patients with ascites refractory to medical management. Relative contraindications include previous abdominal surgery, pregnancy, coagulopathy, and progressive liver failure with encephalopathy or hepatorenal syndrome.

2. **Technique.** Patients should be in a supine position. The bladder should be empty. Level of the ascites can be determined by locating the transition from dullness to tympany with percussion. Depending on the height of the ascites, a midline or lateral approach can be used. Care must be taken with the midline approach because the air-filled bowel tends to float on top of the ascites. The skin at the site of entry should be prepared and draped. Lidocaine 1% is infiltrated subcutaneously and is carried to the level of the peritoneum. For the midline approach, a needle is introduced at a point midway between the umbilicus and the pubis symphysis. For the lateral approach, the point of entry can be in the right or left lower quadrant in the area bounded by the lateral border of the rectus abdominis muscle, the line between the umbilicus and the anterior iliac spine, and the line between the anterior iliac spine and the pubis symphysis. A simple diagnostic tap can be achieved by inserting a 22-gauge needle into the peritoneal cavity and aspirating 20 to 30 mL of fluid. Constant negative pressure should be applied to the syringe, and care should be taken not to advance the needle beyond the point where ascites is encountered. For a therapeutic paracentesis, a 14-gauge needle fit with a catheter allows for efficient drainage of larger volumes of ascites. With either the midline or the lateral approach, once ascites is returned, the catheter is advanced over the needle and directed toward the pelvis. A drainage bag is attached to the catheter to collect and measure the fluid removed.

3. **Complications.** Injuries to the bowel or bladder can occur with paracentesis. Emptying the bladder prior to the procedure, avoiding the insertion of the needle near surgical scars, and maintaining control of the needle once inside the peritoneum will help to minimize these injuries. Intraperitoneal hemorrhage from injury to a mesenteric vessel can occur. Laceration of the inferior epigastric vessels can lead to a hematoma of the rectus sheath or the abdominal wall. In patients with large, recurrent ascites, a persistent leakage of ascites from the site of entry can result. Peritonitis and abdominal wall abscess can also result.

IV. EMERGENCY AIRWAY ACCESS

A. Endotracheal (ET) intubation

1. **Indications.** Establishment of a secure airway is the first priority in the management of an acutely ill patient. The airway can be secured either mechanically, with an ET tube, or surgically, with a tracheostomy or cricothyroidotomy. The oral approach under direct vision is the most common method of intubating the trachea. Other approaches include nasotracheal and endoscopic intubation; however, only orotracheal intubation is described here. Relative contraindications to orotracheal intubation include maxillofacial trauma, laryngeal injury, and cervical spine injury. A thorough description of this topic is beyond the scope of this text. A brief overview of the salient aspects of this technique is provided.

2. **Technique.** Preoxygenation with a bag-valve-mask apparatus and 100% oxygen, suction, adequate sedation, and muscle relaxation; an appropriately sized ET tube; and a functional laryngoscope are required. Two types of laryngeal scope blades are available: a straight blade (Miller) and a curved blade (Macintosh). The straight blade may provide better visualization in children, and the curved blade may be better for patients with short, thick necks. The physician should be comfortable using either blade. With the physician at the patient's head, the head is positioned so that the pharyngeal and laryngeal axes are in alignment (Fig. 37-4A). The patient's head and neck are fully extended into the "sniffing" position. With the nondominant hand, the physician opens the patient's mouth with the thumb and index finger on the patient's lower and upper teeth, respectively. Using the middle finger, the physician sweeps the patient's tongue to the side. The oropharynx is inspected, and foreign bodies or secretions are removed. The blade of the laryngoscope is introduced and advanced with gentle traction upward and toward the patient's feet. Once the epiglottis is visualized, the tip of the blade is positioned in the vallecula. Great care must be taken not to use the handle as a lever against the patient's teeth and lips. The glottic opening and vocal cords should come into view (Fig. 37-4B). If not, gently increasing the upward and caudal traction or having an assistant place external pressure on the cricoid and

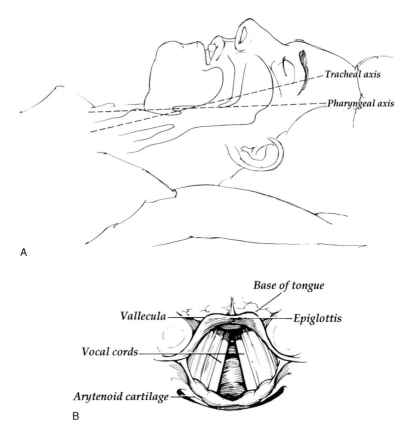

Figure 37-4. Orotracheal intubation. **A:** Fully extending the patient's head into the "sniffing" position aligns the pharyngeal and laryngeal axes. This allows for the best visualization of the airway. **B:** View of the larynx and airway during oral intubation of the trachea.

thyroid cartilage can be helpful. If the glottic opening still cannot be visualized, the blade should be removed and the patient oxygenated and repositioned prior to additional attempts. Once the glottic opening is adequately visualized, the ET tube is advanced under direct vision until the cuff passes through the vocal cords. The cuff is inserted roughly 2 cm past the vocal cords, and the patient's incisors should rest between the 19- and 23-cm markings on the tube. The stylet and laryngoscope are carefully removed while maintaining control and the position of the ET tube. The cuff is inflated, and proper position is confirmed by osculating bilateral breath sounds and determining end-tidal carbon dioxide. Once position is confirmed, the ET tube is secured to the patient. An anteroposterior chest x-ray is obtained to confirm position. Ideally, the tip of the ET tube should be 2 to 4 cm above the carina.

3. **Complications.** If attempts to establish a translaryngeal airway are unsuccessful and the patient cannot be manually ventilated, an emergent surgical airway must be secured (see later discussion). Intubation of the esophagus or right-main-stem bronchus can readily be diagnosed by absent breath sounds associated with epigastric gargling on manual ventilation and right-sided breath sounds with absent left-sided breath sounds, respectively. Chipped teeth, emesis and aspiration, vocal

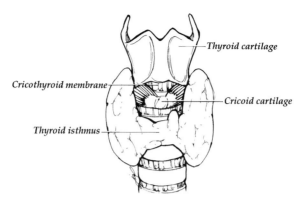

Figure 37-5. Anatomy of the larynx.

cord injury, laryngospasm, and soft-tissue injury to the oropharynx can all complicate ET intubation.

B. Cricothyroidotomy

   1. **Indications.** Cricothyroidotomy is indicated when attempts at oral or nasal intubation fail or maxillofacial injury prohibits oral or nasal intubation. In cases of trauma, blood or maxillofacial injuries may prevent direct visualization of the larynx; cricothyroidotomy is the procedure of choice. Other indications for a surgical airway include cervical spine injuries that preclude optimal positioning for translaryngeal intubation. Laryngeal tracheal separation and laryngeal trauma are contraindications to this procedure. Percutaneous dilational cricothyroidotomy is a safe and effective method of emergently obtaining an airway, and it is gaining widespread use.

   2. **Technique.** Because the vast majority of cricothyroidotomies are done in emergent situations, an excellent understanding of the anatomy in the region of the trachea is necessary to minimize complications. The thyroid cartilage is easily identified in the midline of the neck (Fig. 37-5). The cricoid, the only complete cartilaginous ring, is the first ring inferior to the thyroid cartilage. The cricothyroid membrane joins these two cartilages and is an avascular membrane. Inferior to the cricoid and straddling the trachea is the isthmus of the thyroid gland. The thyroid lobes lie lateral to the trachea, and the superior poles can extend to the level of the thyroid cartilage. If time permits, the area is prepared, draped, and anesthetized with 1% lidocaine. A vertical skin incision is made. The cricoid cartilage is identified and held firmly and circumferentially in the physician's nondominant hand until the end of the procedure. With a no. 11 or 15 blade, a small, 3- to 5-cm transverse incision is made over the cricothyroid membrane. The incision is carried deep until the airway is entered through the cricothyroid membrane. The index finger of the physician's nondominant hand can be used to identify landmarks as the dissection proceeds. The tract is widened using a clamp, a tracheal dilator, or the end of the scalpel handle. The tracheostomy tube is inserted along its curve into the trachea, the cuff is inflated, and bilateral breath sounds are confirmed. If breath sounds are present, the tracheostomy is secured to the skin by suturing the tabs to the skin with heavy, nonabsorbable, monofilament suture. A chest x-ray is obtained to document the location of the tracheostomy tube and to rule out a pneumothorax. Traditionally, cricothyroidotomy was converted to a formal tracheostomy. However, it has been suggested that a cricothyroidotomy may be used long term without an increase in acute complications (*South Med J* 2003; 96:465).

   3. **Complications.** Creation of a false passage when inserting the tracheostomy tube is the most common complication. This should become evident by the absence of

breath sounds and the development of subcutaneous emphysema. Pneumothorax can also occur. Injury to surrounding structures, such as the thyroid, parathyroids, esophagus, anterior jugular veins, and recurrent laryngeal nerves, can occur in situations of urgency. Subglottic stenosis and granuloma formation are potential long-term complications.

C. Percutaneous tracheostomy

1. **Indications.** The advantages of percutaneous tracheostomy (PT) over surgical tracheostomy (ST) are primarily related to reduced tissue trauma and ease of performance at the bedside, which avoids transportation of critically ill patients to the operating room. Several studies support the cost-effectiveness of this approach (*Crit Care Med* 2001;29:926). Contraindications include unstable cervical spine, inability to identify anatomic landmarks, refractory coagulopathy, and difficult oropharyngeal anatomy such that re-establishing a translaryngeal airway would be difficult in the event of airway loss. Percutaneous tracheostomy should only be performed electively.

2. **Technique.** This procedure should be performed under bronchoscopic guidance. The patient should be adequately sedated and positioned in a moderate degree of neck extension. The aim of the fiberoptic scope is to ensure correct initial placement of the introducer needle (midline through the second or third tracheal rings). Subsequent to this, it is used to monitor dilation of the trachea and ensure the introducer does not remain in the trachea. After an initial 1.5-cm skin incision over the first tracheal ring, blunt dissection is performed down to the level of the pretracheal fascia using a mosquito hemostat, and the existing endotracheal tube is withdrawn into the subglottic position, permitting a needle to be introduced between the first and second or second and third tracheal rings. Placement of a guidewire is followed by progressive dilation of the tracheal stoma using beveled plastic dilators **(Seldinger technique).** Once the stoma has been adequately dilated, the tracheostomy tube is introduced into the trachea over the same guidewire, using a dilator as an obturator. An anteroposterior chest x-ray is obtained to confirm position.

3. **Complications.** In many studies, there was no significant difference in the rate of intraprocedural complication between PT and ST (*Chest* 2000;118:1421). Postoperative complications include accidental decannulation, bleeding, and stoma infection. The complications associated with cricothyroidotomy can also occur with PT.

V. LAPAROSCOPY.
An overview of general laparoscopic principles is provided. Readers are referred elsewhere in this manual for information pertaining to specific disease processes.

A. Advantages.
Laparoscopic procedures, when compared with open techniques, may result in less patient discomfort, shorter hospitalizations, and more rapid convalescence.

B. Contraindications

1. **Absolute contraindications** include the inability to tolerate general anesthesia and uncorrectable coagulopathy.

2. **Relative contraindications**
   a. **Prior abdominal surgery** may require alternative port locations to avoid intra-abdominal adhesions and laparoscopic adhesiolysis to improve exposure.
   b. **Peritonitis** may limit access secondary to adhesions.
   c. **First- and third-trimester pregnancy.** Laparoscopy is more safely undertaken in the second trimester for conditions that require urgent surgical management (i.e., cannot be safely delayed until after delivery).
   d. **Severe cardiopulmonary disease** may be exacerbated by hypercarbia that occurs secondary to insufflation of carbon dioxide and changes in pulmonary and cardiovascular mechanics during periods of increased intra-abdominal pressure. These effects can be minimized by using lower intra-abdominal pressures (8 mm Hg) in conjunction with abdominal wall lift devices.

    e. Massive abdominal distention may result in an increased risk of iatrogenic bowel injury.

C. Access and pneumoperitoneum. A working space is created in the patient's abdomen by insufflating carbon dioxide after access is obtained either by a closed or open technique. Both techniques have been shown to be safe, although a recent study showed a lower complication rate with open direct insertion (*Surg Laparosc Endosc Percutan Tech* 2005;15:80). Optical access trocars have been advocated in the morbidly obese population (*Surg Endosc* 2006;20;1238).

   1. Closed technique. A Veress needle is placed most commonly at the umbilicus through a small skin-stab incision. Two serial clicks are heard as the needle penetrates the fascia and peritoneum, respectively. The surgeon aspirates the needle with a 10-mL syringe partially filled with saline to look for blood or enteric contents. The surgeon injects 3 to 5 mL of saline through the needle. If any resistance is met, the syringe is most likely in the abdominal muscle or omentum and should be repositioned. If no resistance is met, the surgeon aspirates the syringe again and removes the plunger. Observing the saline pass freely into the abdomen with gravity (drop test) confirms proper intra-abdominal placement. The abdominal cavity is insufflated via an automatic pressure-limited insufflator to 10 to 15 mm Hg. The initial intra-abdominal pressure should be less than 10 mm Hg. As the abdomen expands, pneumoperitoneum is confirmed with percussion. After insufflation, the abdominal wall is stabilized manually, the Veress needle is removed, and the initial trocar and port are inserted blindly in a direction away from critical abdominal structures.

    a. Elevated pressure with low flow (1 L/minute) on insufflation usually indicates placement of the Veress needle into a closed space (e.g., pre- or retroperitoneal, within the omentum).

      (1) First, the port's insufflation valve should be confirmed to be open.

      (2) If so, the Veress needle is removed and reinserted with a subsequent drop test.

      (3) If the **needle position is in doubt,** an open insertion technique should be used.

    b. Return of blood, cloudy or bilious fluid, or enteric contents after Veress needle placement mandates needle repositioning and inspection of the violated abdominal organ.

   2. Open insertion of the initial port uses a direct cutdown through the abdominal fascia. A Hasson (wedge-shaped) port is placed under direct vision and secured to the abdominal fascia with stay sutures.

   3. Complications

    a. Gas embolism is life threatening. With right ventricular outflow obstruction, expired end-tidal carbon dioxide falls, with concomitant hypotension and a "mill-wheel" heart murmur.

      (1) Insufflation is stopped and the pneumoperitoneum released.

      (2) The patient should be placed in a steep Trendelenburg position with the right side up to float the gas bubble up toward the right ventricular apex and away from the right ventricular outflow tract.

      (3) Air from the right ventricle is aspirated through a central venous catheter.

    b. Brisk bleeding after trocar insertion warrants emergent conversion to open laparotomy. The trocar should not be removed until proximal and distal control of the injured vessel is achieved.

   4. Alternatives to carbon dioxide pneumoperitoneum have been advocated because of the potentially deleterious effects of hypercapnia. Alternative pneumoperitoneum gases such as nitrous oxide, helium, and argon have been evaluated experimentally. Increased intra-abdominal pressure can occur with any insufflation gas (e.g., compression of the vena cava with decreased venous return to the heart, resultant hypotension, decreased renal blood flow, and diminished urinary output). External abdominal wall lift devices are available to create a working space without pneumoperitoneum.

D. Port placement. The location of ports has been standardized for most procedures, and several general rules for port placement have been established. All additional ports should be placed under direct video visualization. Prior to inserting the port, the surgeon indents the abdominal wall manually and identifies the location with the video camera. Transilluminating the abdominal wall identifies significant vessels to avoid. The skin and peritoneum are anesthetized locally. The surgeon makes a small stab incision with a no. 11 blade. The trocar is introduced in a direct line with the planned surgical target to minimize torque intraoperatively. The tip of the trocar should be visualized as it passes through the peritoneum.

1. The **camera port** should be behind and between the surgeon's two operative ports to maintain proper orientation.
2. **Working ports** are placed lateral to the viewing port, with the operative field ahead. All ports should be at least 8 cm apart to avoid the interference of instruments with one another. Ports should be approximately 15 cm from the operative field for the site to be reached comfortably by standard 30-cm instruments and to maintain a 1:1 ratio of hand-instrument tip movement.

E. Suturing and knot tying are essential skills for the surgeon to master before attempting advanced laparoscopic procedures. It is important to remember and anticipate suturing when considering port placement.

1. **Extracorporeal knotting techniques** are generally simpler to perform and are recommended for more durable tissues that can tolerate the pulling through of the excess suture material (e.g., the gastric wall or diaphragmatic crura). Extracorporeal techniques usually require more than 32 cm of suture and use a "knot pusher" to advance the throw down the port and make the knot snug. To avoid disruption, the knot pusher should be envisioned as an extension of the surgeon's finger while pushing the knot down to the tissue. Tension should be maintained on the other arm of the suture without pulling up on the tissue. An air leak occurs whenever suture is introduced or withdrawn through the introducer sheath. This can be reduced by having an assistant occlude the reducer orifice with a fingertip.
2. **Loop ligatures** provide preformed sliding knots on a thin stylet to allow rapid ligation of structures. A grasping instrument is placed through the loop and grasps the tissue or vessel. The loop is then closed and tightened around the pedicle.
3. **Intracorporeal suturing** is preferred for delicate tissues, such as the intestine, bile duct, or esophagus. Sutures should be 8 to 12 cm long. Laparoscopic instrument tying is similar to that of open surgery. A variety of specific techniques have been developed to accomplish knot tying. The surgeon should be facile with at least one technique and be able to tie a square knot without undue tissue trauma or time. The square knot is performed similarly to an instrument tie performed in open surgery.

F. Exiting the abdomen. The surgeon should survey the abdomen at the conclusion of the procedure to detect any visceral injury or hemorrhage. The operative site is irrigated, and hemostasis is obtained. Inspection of the peritoneal side of all port sites as the trocars are removed allows verification of hemostasis. Port-site fascial incisions that are larger than 5 mm should be closed with permanent or long-term absorbable suture to avoid the risk of incisional herniation. This can be done through the port-site incision or under video guidance with a fascial closure device (also known as a "suture passer"), which is particularly helpful in obese patients.

G. Converting to open surgery. A laparoscopic case may need to be converted to an open case for a number of reasons.

1. **Elective conversion**
   a. **Surgeon experience** is critical. The surgeon's threshold for conversion should be low while gaining experience.
   b. **Failure to progress** is the most common reason to convert. This can be secondary to adhesions, inflammatory changes, poor exposure, or altered or aberrant anatomy. In cases of unclear anatomy, avoiding injuries should take precedence over avoiding laparotomy.
   c. The surgeon may discover **a disease not appropriate for minimally invasive methods** (e.g., gallbladder cancer or colon cancer invading adjacent organs).

    d. Technical problems or instrument malfunction may occasionally require conversion. The surgeon must check that all equipment is in working order prior to starting the operation.

  2. Emergent conversion should be performed in the event of severe bleeding or complex bowel injuries if repair is beyond the skill level of the surgeon.

H. Postoperative management for most laparoscopic procedures is similar to that for open procedures, although laparoscopic surgery is associated with less postoperative pain and shorter hospital length of stay and recuperation time.

Note: Page numbers followed by "*f*" indicate figure and followed by "*t*" indicate table.

Schecter 2012 ed   d...
2/14/14